10 0578300 9

KV-370-017

Goat Medicine

Second Edition

Goat Medicine

Second Edition

Mary C. Smith, DVM

Diplomate, American College of Theriogenologists
Professor, Department of Population Medicine and Diagnostic Sciences
New York State College of Veterinary Medicine
Cornell University
Ithaca, New York

David M. Sherman, DVM, MS

Diplomate, American College of Veterinary Internal Medicine
Clinical Associate Professor
Department of Environmental and Population Health
Cummings School of Veterinary Medicine at Tufts University
North Grafton, Massachusetts

WILEY-BLACKWELL
A John Wiley & Sons, Inc., Publication

First Edition first published 1994, Lea & Febiger
Second Edition first published 2009

Blackwell Publishing was acquired by John Wiley & Sons in February 2007. Blackwell's publishing program has been merged with Wiley's global Scientific, Technical, and Medical business to form Wiley-Blackwell.

Editorial Office
2121 State Avenue, Ames, Iowa 50014-8300, USA

For details of our global editorial offices, for customer services, and for information about how to apply for permission to reuse the copyright material in this book, please see our Website at www.wiley.com/wiley-blackwell.

Library of Congress Cataloguing-in-Publication Data

Smith, Mary C.
Goat medicine / Mary Smith, David Sherman. – 2nd ed.
p. cm.
Includes bibliographical references and index.
ISBN-13: 978-0-7817-9643-9 (alk. paper)
ISBN-10: 0-7817-9643-1 (alk. paper)
1. Goats–Diseases. 2. Goats–Diseases–Tropics. I. Sherman, David M. II. Title.

SF968.S63 2009
636.3'9089–dc22

2008049843

A catalog record for this book is available from the U.S. Library of Congress.

Set in 10/12 pt Palatino by SNP Best-set Typesetter Ltd., Hong Kong
Printed in Singapore by Markono Print Media Pte Ltd

1 2009

Middle and lower cover photos courtesy of Christine and Vincent Maefsky, Poplar Hill Dairy Goat Farm, Scandia, Minnesota. Top cover photo courtesy of Russ and Rita Kellogg, Side Hill Acres, Candor, New York.

Dedication

From D.M.S.

For my wife, Laurie, with abiding love and great appreciation for her support during the preparation of this work.

From M.C.S.

For my parents, Randall and Lelah Cole, who have always encouraged me to "do it myself," and my husband, Eric Smith, and our children, Kalmia and Ross, who have patiently awaited completion of this manuscript.

Contents

Preface to the First Edition

The writing of this book was undertaken in recognition of the need for a comprehensive veterinary text addressing health and disease issues of goats raised under varying conditions around the world. The authors' primary experiences are with intensively managed dairy and fiber goats in temperate zones. However, because most of the world's goats live in tropical and subtropical regions, serious effort has been made to fully cover disease entities and production constraints in those areas. Much of the material presented on tropical diseases is derived from the published literature. The authors invite readers whose personal and clinical experience with these diseases in goats varies from our presentation to share their knowledge with us for the purpose of improving later editions.

We intend this book for veterinary practitioners dealing with diagnosis and treatment of individual goats as well as for those striving to improve the health and productivity of commercial herds and flocks throughout the world. Veterinarians involved in formulation of animal health policy, regulatory medicine, and livestock development should also find this information valuable.

We expect this book to be useful also for academic clinicians, researchers, and veterinary students with a special interest in goats. Others who might find this book a useful reference are animal scientists, extension agents, herd managers, and hobbyists.

David M. Sherman
Mary C. Smith

Preface to the Second Edition

The first edition of Goat Medicine was well received and we are pleased to have the opportunity to produce a second edition. Since the first edition appeared in 1994, the global landscape for veterinary medicine has changed dramatically. In 1996, bovine spongiform encephalopathy was recognized to be a zoonotic disease, causing variant Creutzfeldt-Jakob disease (vCJD) in humans. In 1999, West Nile virus infection reached the United States and in a short time was endemic throughout the country. In 2001, there was a major outbreak of foot and mouth disease in northern Europe, with devastating effects in the United Kingdom. That same year, the specter of bioterrorism emerged with the use of anthrax as a weapon against citizens in the United States.

These events underscored the continued importance of infectious diseases in what has become an intimately interconnected, global society. These events also emphasized the need for veterinary practitioners everywhere to have knowledge of and be able to recognize diseases which traditionally have been considered exotic to their own countries. International issues influencing contemporary veterinary medicine are discussed further in David Sherman's other textbook "Tending Animals in the Global Village", also available from Wiley-Blackwell.

Global infectious disease trends also have affected goat medicine. In 2005, the first case of bovine spongiform encephalopathy was confirmed in a goat in France. Peste des petits ruminants, a serious viral disease of goats and sheep, has extended its range from Africa through the Middle East and well into Asia, causing widespread hardship for subsistence farmers and herders who depend on goats for their livelihoods. Repeated outbreaks of Rift Valley fever in Kenya have also taken a toll on goat populations and the people who rely on them. As such, the second edition of Goat Medicine continues to maintain a global perspective and provide information on goat diseases as they occur throughout the world.

Another significant development since the publication of the first edition has been the advent of the Internet and the increased availability of information on all subjects, including the diseases of goats. Some of this information is very good and some is not so good. As in the first edition, we have strived to provide the most accurate information available on the diseases of goats, their diagnosis, treatment, and control. We have avoided whenever possible extrapolating information from other species and we continue to strive, as in the first edition, to provide definitive information that is specific to goats and supported by citations from the world's veterinary literature as well as our own expanded experience in dealing with goat diseases in various locations around the world.

As with the first edition, we intend this book primarily for veterinary practitioners but believe that academic clinicians, veterinary students, regulatory veterinarians, researchers working with goats, animal scientists, extension agents, livestock development workers, and goat owners will also find it useful.

David M. Sherman, Kabul, Afghanistan
Mary C. Smith, Ithaca, New York

Acknowledgments

I would like to acknowledge with great appreciation and sincere thanks, the substantial contributions of the following colleagues: Dr. Gerrit Uilenberg, retired, for his extensive inputs on anaplasmosis, babesiosis, cowdriosis, eperythrozoonosis, theileriosis, and trypanosomosis; Dr. Peter Roeder, Taurus Animal Health, for his careful review and valuable inputs on peste des petits ruminants, rinderpest and Rift Valley fever; Dr. William G. Gavin, GTC Biotherapeutics, Framingham, Massachusetts, for his major contributions in Chapters 1 and 20 on the content related to transgenic goats; Dr. Linda Detwiler, Virginia-Maryland Regional College of Veterinary Medicine, for her detailed review and comments on bovine spongiform encephalopathy; Dr. Wilfred Goldmann, Roslin Institute and the University of Edinburgh, for his detailed review and comments on scrapie; Dr. Christophe Chartier, Agence Française de Sécurité Sanitaire des Aliments, Laboratoire d'études et de Recherches Caprines, Niort, for his comprehensive review of nematode gastroenteritis; Dr. Robin A.J. Nicholas, Veterinary Laboratories Agency (Weybridge) for his valuable inputs on mycoplasma arthritis; Dr. Etienne Thiry, University of Liege, for his most helpful review of caprine herpesvirus vulvovaginitis and balanoposthitis; and, Dr. Valgerdur Andrésdóttir, University of Iceland, for his comments on maedi-visna.

I would also like to acknowledge the cooperation and inputs of Dr. Daan Dercksen of GD Animal Health Service Deventer in the Netherlands on clinical aspects of foot and mouth disease in goats; Dr. Felix Ehrensperger, University of Zürich, on Borna disease; Dr. Truske Gerdes, Onderstepoort Veterinary Institute, on diagnostic tests for Wesselsbron disease and Rift Valley fever; Dr. D.T.J. Littlewood, the Natural History Museum, London, on schistosomiasis; Dr. John C. Reagor, Texas Veterinary Medical Diagnostic Laboratory on hard yellow liver disease; and, Dr. Ann Wells, Springpond Holistic Animal Health, on organic livestock production. Any errors which might occur in the chapters for which these colleagues have provided inputs are solely the responsibility of the author.

I would especially like to thank Ms. Suzanne Duncan, Ms. Jane Cormier and Ms. Carolyn Ziering from the Webster Veterinary Library, Cummings School of Veterinary Medicine at Tufts University for their wonderful assistance in gathering goat literature from around the world to make the completion of my chapters possible. Most of all, I owe a debt of gratitude and heartfelt thanks to my wife, Laurie Miller, without whose patience, support and encouragement, I would never have completed this task.

David M. Sherman

I would like to thank my colleagues at the New York State College of Veterinary Medicine, Cornell University, Ithaca, New York who have graciously reviewed manuscripts during revision of various chapters in preparation for this edition: Dr. Danny W. Scott (skin), Dr. Nita L. Irby (ocular system), Dr. Robert O. Gilbert (reproductive system), Dr. Linda Tikofsky (mammary gland and milk production), and Dr. Andrea L. Looney (anesthesia). I am also indebted to Dr. Marie S. Bulgin of the Caine Veterinary Teaching Center, University of Idaho, Caldwell, Idaho for her helpful critique of the chapter on subcutaneous swellings and Dr. Dan L. Brown of the Department of Animal Science, Cornell University, Ithaca New York and Dr. Pierre Morand-Fehr from the INRA Laboratoire de Nutrition et Alimentation, Institut National Agronomique Paris-Grignon, Paris, France for their assistance with the chapter on nutrition. Dr. Gareth F. Bath of the Faculty of Veterinary Science, University of Pretoria,

Onderstepoort, South Africa and Dr. Ray M. Kaplan from the College of Veterinary Medicine of the University of Georgia, Athens, Georgia were also very gracious about answering specific questions.

The many members of the American Association of Small Ruminant Practitioners were instrumental in the creation of this text because of the questions asked and answers provided through the association's on-line discussion list. Likewise, many goat owners and their animals contributed to my education and photo collection. I would also like to thank Susanne K. Whitaker and Michael A. Friedman of the Flower-Sprecher Veterinary Library, New York State College of Veterinary Medicine, Ithaca, New York for assistance in obtaining reference material. Finally, my husband Eric Smith deserves the greatest thanks for encouraging the writing of this manuscript and tolerating the time and attention that it has required of me.

Mary C. Smith

Goat Medicine

Second Edition

1

Fundamentals of Goat Practice

OVERVIEW

Distribution of Goats

According to the Food and Agriculture Organization (FAO) of the United Nations, in 2006 there were an estimated 837.2 million goats in the world, approximately 64.2% of which were in Asia, 28.8% in Africa, 4.3% in South and Central America, 2.2% in Europe, 0.3% in North America, and 0.1% in Oceania. Approximately 4.2% of the world's goats are found in developed countries and 95.8% in developing countries (FAO 2007). Goats are highly adaptable to a broad range of climatic and geographic conditions and are more widely distributed than any other mammalian livestock. Goats are managed under every imaginable production system, including feral, transhumant, nomadic, extensive, intensive, and total confinement systems.

Use of Goats

Goats are exploited for diverse purposes, including meat production, cashmere and mohair fiber production, milk and cheese production, and skins for leather making. Specialty uses include brush and weed control, pack and draft use, animal experimentation (particularly as models of ruminant digestion and human heart disease and as transgenic animals), commercial antibody production, and companionship. Goat horn and bone are sometimes used for ornamental purposes and musical instruments, while goat skins are used for drum making.

Meat production is the major use of goats on a worldwide basis, particularly in Asia, Africa, the Middle East, and Latin America, and world goat meat production more than doubled between 1980 and 2000 (Morand-Fehr et al. 2004). In 2006, the seven leading goat meat producing nations in descending order were China, India, Pakistan, Sudan, Nigeria, Bangladesh, and Iran (FAO 2007a). A myriad of local and regional breeds exists around the world that are used mainly for meat. In recent years, more attention has been paid to selective breeding in goats for meat production, leading to the development of two highly efficient, purpose-bred meat goat breeds. These are the South African Boer goat (Mahan 2000) and the Kiko goat of New Zealand (Batten 1988), both of which have gained popularity in the United States, particularly in the southeast where commercial goat meat production has been expanding.

The major milking breeds of goats originated primarily in Europe. These breeds include the Saanen, Toggenburg, Anglo-Nubian, and Alpine breeds. The more recently developed La Mancha breed originated in the United States. The Jamnapari and Beetal breeds of India are also important dairy breeds that are well adapted to and becoming more widely distributed in the humid tropics. The use of goat milk to manufacture cheese is an important industry in France, Spain, and other European countries.

Angora goats, the source of mohair fiber, have traditionally been concentrated in a number of distinct areas, notably Turkey, where they originated, South Africa, Texas, Argentina, and some central Asian republics formerly in the USSR. Cashmere or Pashmina goats, which produce cashmere fiber, are found primarily in the mountainous regions of Central Asia, including parts of Tibet, China, Mongolia, Iran, Afghanistan, Kazakstan, Kyrgyzstan, and Tajikistan. Skins are usually a byproduct of goat slaughter for meat, but skins of certain goat breeds such as the Red Sokoto of Niger are prized for high-quality leather goods such as kidskin gloves and purses. Details of the various goat industries are beyond the scope of this veterinary text. The interested reader is referred to other sources (Gall 1981; Coop 1982; DeVendra and Burns 1983; Dubeuf et al. 2004; Morand-Fehr et al. 2004).

Current Interest in Goats

Worldwide interest in goats has continued to increase dramatically during the last decade. There is greater understanding of the importance of goats in agricultural systems in low-income countries. A number of humanitarian organizations, such as Heifer International and FARM-Africa, have recognized the value of using goats as a tool in rural development programs to improve the social and economic conditions of subsistence farmers and the rural poor. Methodologies for improved goat production in the tropics in support of rural development have been published (Peacock 1996).

There is also increased demand for goat products in developed countries, especially goat cheese, cashmere goods, and even goat meat. Demand for goat meat in the United States has exceeded domestic supply in recent years. In 2004, the United States imported 2,400 metric tons of goat meat, mostly from Australia (Ward 2006).

This expanding interest in goats has increased the demand for goat-related veterinary services in the areas of clinical medicine, research, and extension. In response to this need, interested veterinarians must familiarize themselves with goats as a species distinct from sheep and cattle, recognizing their often characteristic behavior, physiology, and response to disease.

Fortunately, a number of resources have become available to provide information in these areas. The International Goat Association (www.iga-goatworld.org/) sponsors a quadrennial international conference on goats and regularly publishes the peer-reviewed, international research journal, *Small Ruminant Research*, which reports research findings on all aspects of goat production including health, nutrition, genetics, physiology, and husbandry from all over the world. The American Sheep Industry Association regularly produces a similar, multidisciplinary research publication, *Sheep and Goat Research Journal*, which focuses specifically on small ruminant production in North America and is available on the Internet (http://www.sheepusa.org/).

The American Association of Small Ruminant Practitioners (AASRP) is an excellent resource for veterinary practitioners in North America. This member organization produces a regular newsletter, *Wool and Wattles*, full of current, relevant information on regulatory and clinical issues as well as an e-mail discussion forum for AASRP members. The AASRP Website (www.aasrp.org/) provides links to other useful resources for goat health and production. Another useful Web-based resource for veterinarians is Consultant, which generates differential diagnoses based on clinical signs entered by the user on a species basis, with goats recognized as a distinct species. It is available on the Internet at http://www.vet.cornell.edu/consultant/consult.asp. Finally, many state extension agencies now have much more information available on goat husbandry and production than they had in the past, and much of it accessible on the Internet.

Distinguishing Goats from Sheep

Source of Confusion

For those whose experience with sheep and goats is limited to the common European wool breeds of sheep and the European dairy breeds of goats, the notion that individuals of the two species could be confused may seem ridiculous. However, in tropical and subtropical regions, various breeds of hair sheep are common. These breeds are often maintained in mixed flocks with local breeds of goats, and may not be readily differentiated. The following information can help in distinguishing the two species.

Genetic Distinctions

Goats have 60 chromosomes and sheep have 54. Though very uncommon, fertile goat-sheep hybrids have been reported. These hybrids have 57 chromosomes. The phenomenon is discussed in Chapter 13.

Behavioral Distinctions

A major difference between sheep and goats is feeding behavior. Sheep are grazing animals, consistently feeding at ground level, while the goat is more of a browsing animal, readily feeding on shrubs, bushes, and trees. While both species are social, individual goats are less anxious than sheep when separated from the group. Goats are less tolerant of rain and more readily seek shelter in wet weather.

The males of both species will fight, buck goats by rearing up on their hind feet and coming down forcefully to butt heads, while rams back up and then charge forward to butt heads. The anatomic structure of the horns, frontal sinuses, and neck muscles of each species is appropriate to its method of fighting, minimizing the risk of injury to combatants (Reed and Schaffer 1972). When young bucks and rams are maintained together, the rams become dominant because they preemptively strike bucks in the abdomen while the male goats are still in the act of rearing up.

Whereas lambs are almost constantly at the side of ewes in early life, goats practice "lying out" or "planting" behavior with kids left in "camps" for a good part of the day while does feed.

Anatomic Distinctions

When wool is not obvious in sheep, other anatomic differences may be observed. Most goat breeds have an erect tail, while the tail of sheep always hangs down. The sheep has an upper lip divided by a distinct philtrum and the goat does not. Male goats, and to a lesser extent female goats, have beards, which are lacking in sheep. Goats do not have infraorbital, interdigital, or inguinal glands, while sheep do. Goats have sebaceous glands beneath the tailhead that sheep lack.

GOAT BEHAVIOR

General Characteristics

Goats exhibit some very distinct behavior patterns (Hafez 1975; Kilgour and Dalton 1984). Many aspects of goat behavior are conditioned by the circumstances in which the animals are kept. Many natural behavior patterns observed in free-ranging feral goats may be altered or not expressed at all under different degrees of confinement. Nevertheless, some behavior patterns are widely characteristic.

Goats tend to flock together in extended family groups. They have a strong hierarchical structure in the flock or herd. Both males and females will establish social dominance in their respective groups through head to head fighting. Goats use their horns to advantage when fighting to establish their social dominance. Therefore, all goats in a group should be either horned or hornless to avoid excessive bullying by horned goats.

When goats are accustomed to human contact, they will approach strangers rather than flee. When threatened or upset, they will turn and face an intruder and make a characteristic sneezing noise. In keeping with their browsing behavior, goats orally investigate everything in their environment. This includes veterinary equipment, paperwork, clothing, and jewelry brought within their reach. When drawing blood samples or writing health papers, it is essential to keep the paperwork in a safe place or it will be eaten or destroyed. Goats will chew on pen partitions and other structures made of wood, and a large group of goats can actually devour pen walls over a period of months. They will also eat the paint off walls, so lead paint should be avoided.

Goats are very agile and are excellent climbers. They are occasionally found in barn rafters, in trees, or on the hood of the veterinarian's vehicle, if allowed access. Providing a rock pile in paddocks or pastures can foster recreation and will help to control hoof overgrowth. Goats will stand on their hind legs and lean against fences, causing considerable damage over time. Broken limbs may occur if legs are caught in the openings of chain link fences. The goats' agility combined with their curiosity can be fatal if their heads get caught and they are strangled in fences, gates, doors, windows, or other structures. Backward curving horns contribute to this problem.

Goats are notorious for successfully undoing simple gate closures and latches. This is a common occurrence in accidental grain overload cases, so goat keepers must ensure that gates are securely fastened. Goats can easily jump fences designed for sheep and also will dig under fences that do not closely skirt the ground. Goat fencing should never have interior sloping support posts because goats will use them to climb out of the enclosure. Goats ignore barbed wire and therefore it should not be used because it can inflict serious damage. Thus, electric fencing has become popular for goat operations because the animals quickly learn to respect it.

Ingestive and Eliminative Behavior

A key to the adaptability of goats worldwide is their efficient browsing ability. This same efficiency, however, has given the goat notoriety as an important cause of desertification in some regions of the world. The reputation is not always deserved because overgrazing by numerous livestock species may be at fault, but only the goats are left surviving when vegetation is almost gone (Dunbar 1984). Goats may climb into trees to reach food when it is scarce. If permitted, they can girdle the bark from trees, thus killing them. Goats are used to clear brush to reclaim pasture land for sheep and cattle. When run simultaneously with sheep and cattle, they may improve pasture quality for these other species by contributing manure for fertilization, removing toxic plants such as oak to which they are more resistant than the other ruminant species, and eliminating brush to allow more sunlight for improved grass growth (Ward 2006).

Owners feeding goats in confinement often complain that the animals waste a good deal of hay, particularly leaving behind the nutritious leafy parts of good legume hay. This tendency can be countered to some extent by feeder designs that inhibit the goat from pulling hay out of the feeder and dropping it on the floor. Goats are also finicky about contaminated feed and water supplies and may refuse water containing fecal pellets or hay and grain in wet troughs that smell moldy.

In free-ranging feral and Angora goats, approximately 30% of the day is spent in feeding, usually divided into sunrise, midday, and sunset periods. One-third of this is grazing time, two-thirds browsing. About half the day is spent resting, 10% ruminating, and 12% traveling (Askins and Turner 1972; Kilgour and Ross 1980). In contrast, intensively managed Saanen milking goats eat for 20% of the day, ruminate 25%, travel 20%, sleep 11%, rest recumbent 14%, and rest standing approximately 8% of each day. They defecate on average 11.2 times and urinate 8.3 times daily (Pu, personal communication 1990).

Goats raise their tails to defecate and normally produce pelleted feces. Female goats squat to urinate. During the non-breeding season, males urinate on the ground with little or no extension of the penis beyond the prepuce. However, during the breeding season, the pattern of urination is markedly different and associated with sexual behavior as discussed below. Goats cannot be prompted easily to urinate by holding off their nares, as is done with sheep. This makes simple collection of a urine specimen problematic.

Sexual Behavior

In tropical and subtropical regions, estrus generally occurs year-round while in temperate regions goats are seasonally polyestrus, with breeding season triggered by decreasing day length. Breed factors may also play a role in this pattern because relocation of some indigenous breeds to new climatic zones does not result in a change of estrus pattern. Specific information on the frequency, signs, and patterns of estrus are provided in Chapter 13. Male sexual behavior reflects the pattern seen in does. Libido and sperm quality may be depressed during anestrous seasons. However, if females are brought into estrus by hormonal manipulation, bucks quickly respond out of season.

The obnoxious behavior and strong odor of bucks during breeding season are notorious. At least two factors contribute to buck odor. First, the aroused buck repeatedly urinates on himself, soaking his head, neck, and forequarters. He will sometimes take his erect penis into his mouth. Afterwards, the buck may yawn and demonstrate the flehmen reaction, curling his upper lip. Second, the buck possesses sebaceous scent glands on his head, caudomedial to the base of the horn, which during active rutting produce an odiferous compound identified as 6-trans nonenal (Smith et al. 1984). This compound may also be released from the sebaceous gland under the tail. It acts as a potent pheromone and the odor alone can induce estrus in the doe.

Bucks show active fighting behavior at the beginning of and during the breeding season to establish dominance. Veterinarians and owners should exercise caution when working around sexually active bucks. A full grown buck striking from the standing position can produce serious or fatal injury. For this reason, bucks of different sizes in confinement operations should be segregated so that smaller, younger bucks are not injured or killed. Do not turn your back to an unrestrained buck!

During courtship, the buck will sniff the urine of does and follow with the flehmen response. To display to does, a buck holds his head erect and high or he lowers his extended head and neck to the ground. He may also kick out at the doe with an extended forelimb, but rarely actually strike her. Courtship is accompanied by much frenzied vocalizing and flicking the tongue in and out. Sexually active bucks commonly lose weight during the breeding season.

Maternal Behavior

Free-ranging goats separate from the herd and hide to kid. Confined goats may attempt to conceal themselves. As parturition approaches, does become restless and paw at the ground, making rudimentary efforts to "nest build." Details of parturition and the recognition of dystocia are discussed in Chapter 13. Following parturition, the doe actively licks the kids, and this is considered to be critical to successful bonding. If does are frightened or disturbed at this point, or if licking is delayed longer than one hour, bonding may be impaired and kids may be abandoned or mothered less effectively.

Kids are precocial, standing and seeking the hairless udder shortly after birth. In free-ranging herds, there is a "lying-out" period of several days to several weeks when does may leave kids in sheltered areas for periods of two to eight hours while they feed. Does must be familiar with the geography to return successfully to their kids. Therefore, it is not advisable to move does to new grazing areas immediately before kidding. Does will respond to alarm calls from their distant kids and return to defend them if bonding is strong. Kids gradually begin to follow their dams, learning to browse and graze. The infrequent nursing pattern of young kids makes the goat adaptable to the twice-a-day feeding regimens that are often practiced under intensive management. If given boxes to hide in, kids raised in confinement will use them for the first week, coming out only to suckle the dam.

HANDLING GOATS

Group Considerations

Goats are highly adaptable and trainable animals. Feral goats captured in Australia and New Zealand may become used to handling in confinement within weeks, although if frightened suddenly they can clear sheep fences with ease. Dairy goats are readily trained into milking routines involving parlors and machine milking. Although Angora kids may scream the first time they are sheared, they get used to the procedure.

Goats used to human contact can be mustered by calling. Moving less tame goats on open range is similar to moving sheep. Dogs can be used, but they must be well trained. The flight distance of feral goats is eight to ten meters. Goats are more likely to turn and fight than sheep if provoked by a dog. Animals that break away from the group should be left to follow along rather than chased. The presence of sheep with the goats can actually facilitate flocking and driving, although on hills, goats tend to move upward and sheep downward. When collected in yards, anxious goats may pile up in a corner and some may suffocate, so they should be divided into small groups. When possible goats should be allowed to spend 24 hours in a handling facility before they are worked so they are more comfortable with their surroundings. Horned goats may be very wary of entering narrow races and gates. When working horned goats in close quarters, the danger of face and eye injuries to handlers is high, and protective eye wear should be used.

Individual Restraint

Tame goats will stop when caught by the gastrocnemius tendon. However, if a frightened or wary goat is actively fleeing or struggling, capture by the limb can lead to serious dislocations of joints or fractures of long bones, particularly in young animals. It is preferable to catch animals by hooking an arm around the neck or torso or by grabbing the collar, horns, beard, or, less desirably, the ears.

Goats used to human contact can be trained to lead. Goats that pull strongly against neck chains will commonly cough and, rarely, cause trauma to the trachea. Goats used to handling are usually easily restrained for examination, administration of medication, or routine sample collection. Such goats can be haltered or lead shanks can be tied to neck straps and then secured. Uncooperative goats can be straddled over the withers by a handler with the goat's hind end backed into a corner and the head held firmly by the handler (Figure 1.1). If a goat is horned, the horns should be held when restraining goats in close quarters to avoid injury to the handler. Bearded goats can be led by the beard and non-bearded goats by the ears, though some owners may object to the latter practice. For smaller, uncooperative goats, flipping the animal into lateral recumbency and then placing the handler's knee on the goat's neck may provide effective restraint.

Goats do not become passive when tipped up on the rump in the manner used for sheep, so this method of restraint is less useful; this is a problem regarding shearing. A modification of the technique to avoid struggling is to first tip up the goat, and then allow the head to fall backward between the handler's thighs so that the goat's back is resting on the handler's shins. This redistributes the goat's weight from the bony rump to the back, making it more comfortable for the goat. Tipping up the goat is useful for examining the prepuce and penis of male goats suspected of urolithiasis. In this case, the weight of the goat's upper body needs to be shifted forward to facilitate extension of the penis. Foot trimming is most easily carried out by raising the distal limbs of the standing goat.

Administering Medications

Oral Medications

Mass medication of feed and water is no more reliable in goats than in other species, because sick animals are likely to have reduced feed and possibly water intake. In addition, goats, being fastidious about water supplies, may detect a change in the odor or flavor of the water and refuse to drink it.

When drenching individual goats, the head should be held horizontally and not tilted up, reducing the chances of aspiration pneumonia. The drenching gun should be inserted at the commissure of the lips and the nostrils held off while the medication is quickly dispensed. To successfully administer boluses with a balling gun, the gun must be carefully worked over the base of the tongue before dispensing the bolus or the pill will be chewed and spit out. Put the gun into the mouth at the commissure of the lips to facilitate this process. Do not force the gun into the pharynx or traumatic injury can occur. Balling and drenching guns should be examined before use to ensure that they do not have sharp defects that could injure the goats. Passing a stomach tube in goats via the mouth is not particularly difficult if proper restraint and a suitable speculum are available. Commercially available sheep speculums work well with goats, as does a block of wood with a circular hole cut through it. Small diameter, well lubricated tubes can be passed through the nose to the stomach.

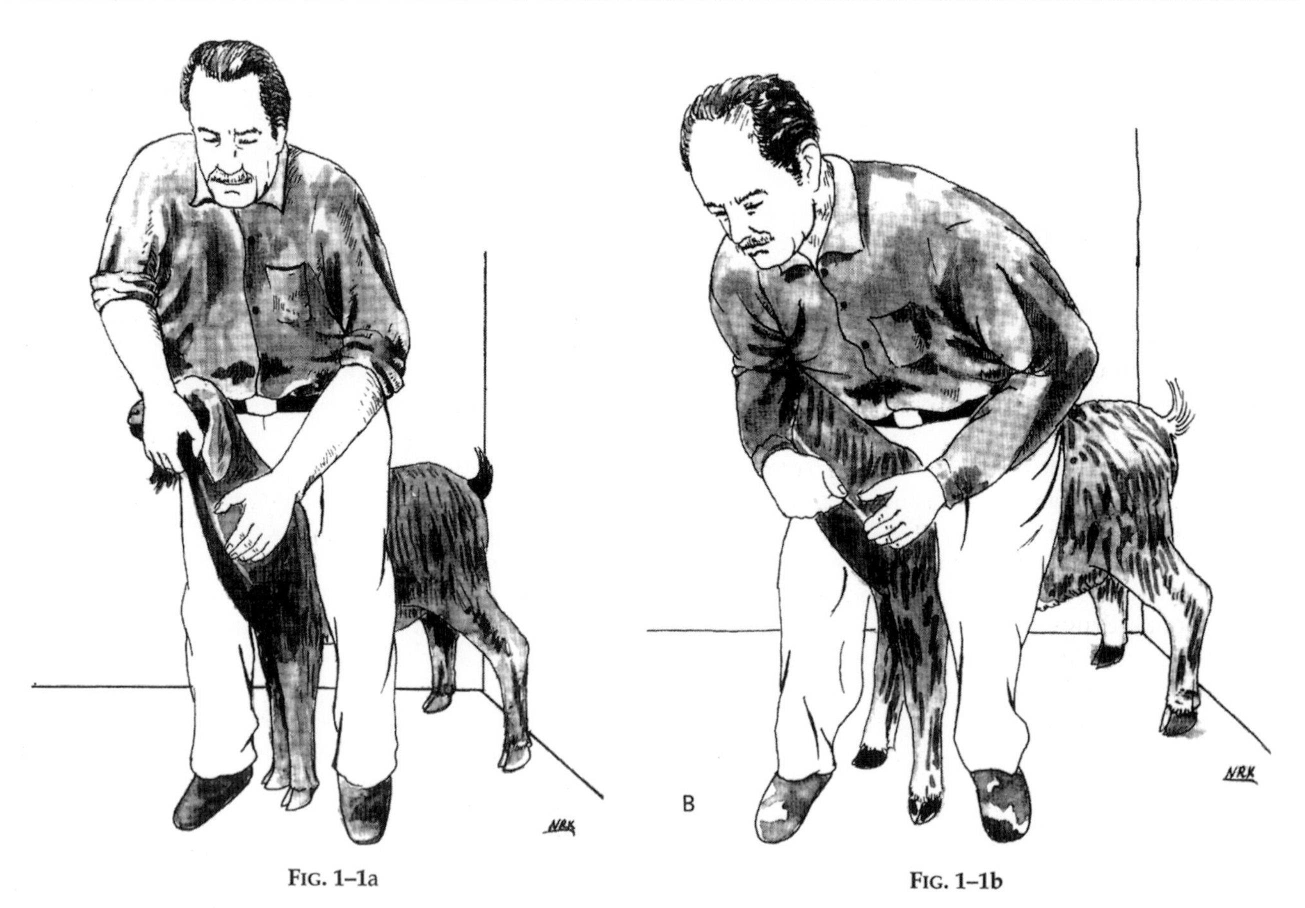

Figure 1.1. Useful restraint methods for intravenous blood sampling or medicine administration via the jugular vein of a goat. Backing the goat into a corner, as shown, improves control. In Figure. 1.1a, the goat is restrained so that an assistant, kneeling in front of the goat, can easily take the sample or give the medicine. In Figure. 1.1b, the goat is positioned with the head tucked under the handler's arm so that sampling or medicine administration can be accomplished by the handler alone. (Illustrations by Mr. Nadir Kohzad.)

Injections

Mass medication or vaccination using a common needle has long been practiced by some farmers and veterinarians. In the case of goats, as with other species, it is time to rethink this practice, particularly in light of the growing importance of caprine arthritis encephalitis virus (CAEV) in goats. This retrovirus may be transmissible by blood-contaminated needles. Certainly, in herds where the virus is known to exist, or attempts are under way to control it, it would be counterproductive and negligent to use common needles. Additional discussion of this important caprine disease is found in Chapters 4 and 5.

Another reason to use individual needles in conjunction with other good hygienic practices during vaccination is the tendency for goats to develop large swellings and even abscesses at injection sites after vaccination with clostridial, chlamydial, and paratuberculosis vaccines. If the veterinarian's technique is exemplary, he or she is unlikely to be held accountable for any problems that develop later.

If skins are marketed from a goat herd, the veterinarian should avoid injections of any kind in regions of the body that become part of the marketed skin, because defects can occur secondary to injection site reactions and devalue the skin. Therefore, the back and upper flanks should be avoided even though they are often convenient.

Intramuscular injections can cause difficulties in goats. The preferred site is in the neck, in a triangular region bounded by the vertebral column ventrally, the nuchal ligament dorsally, and the shoulder caudally. The triceps can also be used. If skin quality is not a consideration, the longissimus muscles over the back in the lumbar region may also be used. In all cases, the volume of drug administered in one site should not be greater than 5 ml. Needles should be 2 to 3 cm long and no larger than 18-gauge unless the medication is highly viscous. Shorter needles should be used for young kids.

The thigh muscles should be avoided as a site of intramuscular injection in adults and especially young goats. The muscle mass is small compared to other ruminants, and sciatic nerve damage is not uncommon. Owners should be counseled against using this site. Even when the nerve is not damaged, marked lameness can occur when irritating drugs such as oxytetracycline are given in the leg. Permanent muscle damage can also occur that devalues the carcasses of meat goats.

Subcutaneous injections are commonly given in the neck in the same region described for intramuscular injections, or on the chest wall about 5 cm behind the point of the elbow. Injections ahead of the shoulder should be avoided in show goats, because local reactions near the superficial cervical (prescapular) lymph node may be confused with caseous lymphadenitis. Needles should be 18- to 20-gauge. The risk of accidental intramuscular injection may be increased if long needles are used.

Intravenous drugs are given via the jugular vein generally using 2 to 3 cm long needles of 18- or 20-gauge. Blood samples can be taken from the jugular vein using an 18-gauge needle. Intradermal injections are given using 26-gauge, 1-cm long tuberculin needles. Intraperitoneal injections are rarely used except to treat neonates for hypoglycemia with glucose solutions or navel infections with aqueous based antibiotics. With the kid held hanging by the front legs, an 18- or 20-gauge needle is inserted perpendicular to the skin about 1 cm to the left of the navel no deeper than 1 cm.

When intramammary infusions are given, the teat should first be cleaned and swabbed with alcohol. As in cattle, single use teat cannulae should be used for each infusion with the cannula inserted into the teat only enough to gain entry into the teat cistern. For very small teat openings, sterile tomcat catheters can be used to infuse the teat.

CLINICAL EXAMINATION OF GOATS

A complete clinical examination consists of three major elements: history taking, physical examination, and inspection of the environment. Many diseases seen in individual goats are likely to represent potential herd problems; therefore, prompt diagnosis of clinical cases is essential so that, in addition to therapy, appropriate preventive measures can be introduced into the overall management program. In many caprine diseases, subclinical cases often exist in addition to the obvious clinical ones, and additional diagnostic testing may be required to identify them. The existence of subclinical infections and carrier states is a troublesome one for veterinarians performing prepurchase health examinations or writing health certificates for exportation or interstate travel. A list of such caprine diseases that the veterinarian must be aware of is given in Table 1.1.

History Taking

Very few diseases or health-related problems are randomly distributed in a flock or herd of goats; rather, they are concentrated in specific groups, usually by sex, function, production status, or age. Always establish early on what age, sex, breed, or group of goats is dying, showing signs of illness, aborting, or showing decreased productivity. If it is a mixed farm operation, the number of other types of livestock and their degree of contact with goats should be ascertained.

Detailed history should include a determination of the total flock or herd population and estimation of its breakdown by sex, age, breed, and pregnancy status. Having determined the total animal population, the population at risk, and the number of animals affected and dying, it is possible to determine rates of disease occurrence and case fatality rates. By counting cases,

Table 1.1. Goat diseases characterized by chronic infection or a carrier state.

Viral/prion	*Rickettsial*	*Bacterial*	*Protozoal*	*Unknown*
Caprine arthritis encephalitis Foot and mouth disease Scrapie	Chlamydiosis Coxiellosis (Q fever)	Caseous lymphadenitis Paratuberculosis Salmonellosis Listeriosis Brucellosis Melioidosis Tuberculosis Mycoplasmosis Staphylococcal mastitis	Toxoplasmosis	Udder warts in white goats

the investigator is also in a better position to determine the actual significance of a problem as compared to the farmer's perception of it. In some cases, the loss of a few animals may be insignificant compared to a more serious unrecognized problem such as endoparasitism or ectoparasitism.

Such an epidemiologically based history should aim to identify not only specific problems but also specific risk factors that appear to be associated with mortality, morbidity, or suboptimal performance. For example, when a primary complaint of kids developing diarrhea after weaning suggests coccidiosis, additional questions concerning the segregation of kids from adults, the manner that kids are fed, the design of feeders, the frequency and manner of barn cleaning, and details on the use of coccidiostats are necessary. In such cases, modification of management practices may halt the spread of disease.

Temporal relationships are important to note. Some diseases may occur seasonally, in association with abrupt weather changes, or in relation to specific events such as breeding, pregnancy, shearing, parturition, and lactation. For example, an unexpected cold snap or heavy rain right after shearing of Angora goats can increase pneumonia, abortion, and death rates, particularly if adequate shelter and supplemental feed have not been provided.

Localization of death or disease to specific areas on the premises is helpful. For example, if losses are seen only in certain areas of the farm, specific pastures, or particular barns, then suspicion of poisoning is increased.

Other important aspects of the history include questions pertaining to the actual ration being fed and its consumption, methods of feeding, changes in feeding, access to grazing, and water supply type and water availability.

If management interventions or preventive health procedures have been undertaken recently, they should be identified. Shearing, drenching, dehorning, spraying or dipping, castration, or vaccination can be associated with increases in morbidity and mortality. When range animals are mobbed for such procedures, sudden close confinement, temporary feed deprivation, and abrupt weather changes can predispose to outbreaks of conditions such as abortion, coccidiosis, salmonellosis, hypocalcemia, or starvation as a result of mismothering. When drugs or vaccines are used, the products and dosages, number of treatments, and method of administration should be determined, particularly because many goat farmers traditionally obtain their drugs and biologicals from nonveterinary sources.

If animals have been transported recently, dates, origins, means of transportation, and quarantine times should be determined. Information should also be collected on visits to shows or fairs and on the origin of purchased animals, be it other farms, stockyards, or specialized goat sales. If animals have come from out of state, the relevant health certificates should be examined and the disease situation in the state of origin reviewed.

Finally, the reliability of information obtained should be checked with the actual goat keepers if the owner is not involved with day-to-day management decisions. If the veterinarian has prior knowledge of the local disease patterns in goats, such knowledge should not be used to make hasty and possibly incorrect judgments.

Special Considerations for Range and Pastured Goats

Extensively managed animals may not be closely observed, and histories can be sketchy. With large flocks, it should be determined if the animals are managed as a single flock or in smaller, self-contained units. The seasonal pattern of grazing and the length of grazing periods should be noted. Pasture composition, seasonal stocking rates per acre, the degree of pasture subdivision, and length of resting periods between grazing should be established. Note if supplemental feeding is practiced and the types of feed used. This may be important in terms of meeting specific nutritional needs, and, in the case of silage, may be associated with diseases such as listeriosis or rumen acidosis. Inquiries should also be made about whether crops are fed or grazed, the type and stage of growth, and whether there is a recent history of fertilizer or herbicide application. Knowledge of local trace element deficiencies or excesses may be helpful.

The type of grazing, whether set stocked or rotational, may be relevant to some disease outbreaks, particularly to gastrointestinal helminthiasis. The presence of other livestock species and feral, predatory, or scavenging animals or birds should be established if relevant to the problem under investigation.

Special Considerations for Intensively Managed Goats

A complete history can usually be obtained from the owner or herdsman of intensively managed goats. The patterns of disease are also likely to be different, with pneumonia and enteric diseases of young goats assuming much greater significance than the foot rot, helminthiasis, predation, or toxic plant problems more often seen under grazing systems. Feed composition and intake are more regulated but the veterinarian must inquire about episodes of sudden changes, excesses, or deprivations in the feed and water supplies.

Under close quarters, the movement, mixing, or introduction of new animals is more likely to cause an outbreak of disease. Kidding is often assisted in intensively managed operations, and artificial kid rearing methods are commonly used. These procedures should be carefully reviewed when morbidity and mortality are concentrated in young kids. Weather, per se, should not adversely affect intensively managed animals. However, extremes in temperature may tax the ventilatory capacity of confinement buildings and extremely cold weather may freeze water supplies or incapacitate mechanized feeding equipment. Answers to questions about changes in dairy herd milking procedures or personnel may help to explain mastitis problems.

Special Considerations for Hobby Farms

Because hobbyists often have little previous agricultural or livestock experience, it might be helpful to practitioners to gauge the owners' knowledge and attitudes regarding basic animal husbandry before history taking. Some fundamental misunderstandings about the care and management of goats may be revealed, such as non-recognition of basic ruminant physiology and the need for roughage in the diet. In other situations, owners may know about basic husbandry and disease problems, but may have seemingly unorthodox ideas about management and treatment. A good deal of tact may be required to obtain a useful history and prescribe appropriate therapy while not offending the hobbyist's sensibilities.

In addition, hobby farmers often perceive goats more as companion animals than as livestock production units. While they may seek the expertise of a livestock clinician, they often expect the "bedside manner" of the companion animal practitioner. Therefore, the veterinarian who appears insensitive to the client's emotions or indifferent to pain of the goat or who emphasizes only the economic value of the animal may not be called to the farm again.

Special Considerations for Organic Goat Production

Consumer interest in organically produced food has grown considerably over the past twenty years or so and producers have responded by producing and marketing an expanding variety of foodstuffs certified as organic. Increasingly, this includes foods of animal origin. Goat owners may choose to raise their goats under organic conditions. Veterinary practitioners with such clients need to be aware of and familiar with the constraints on conventional therapy that are associated with organic livestock production, which is now strictly regulated by law (Karreman 2006).

In the United States, the Organic Food Production Act (OFPA) was signed into law in 1990, creating the framework for regulation and certification of organically produced foods of plant and animal origin. The OFPA created the National Organic Standards Board (NOSB) which reviews materials for consideration as acceptable for use in organic food production, including veterinary inputs used to maintain animal health. As a general rule, all natural materials are allowed for use in organic agriculture, unless specifically prohibited, while all synthetic materials are prohibited unless specifically permitted, following a successful petition process to the NOSB. The specific regulations of the National Organic Program are found in the United States Code of Federal Regulations at 7 CFR 205. These regulations became effective in 2002.

Vaccination is promoted as an organic livestock health care practice under 7 CFR 205, but the use of antibiotics and most anthelmintics is prohibited. Veterinarians must approach therapeutic interventions in organically raised animals differently than in conventionally raised animals, relying heavily on so-called natural treatments, including botanicals, acupuncture, homeopathy, etc. The standards of livestock health care practice which must be observed under the OFPA are given in 7 CFR 205.238. Veterinarians should be aware, however, that 7 CFR 205.238 considers the welfare of organically raised livestock by stipulating that an organic livestock producer may "not withhold medical treatment from a sick animal in an effort to preserve its organic status. All appropriate medications must be used to restore an animal to health when methods acceptable to organic production fail. Livestock treated with a prohibited substance must be clearly identified and shall not be sold, labeled, or represented as organically produced." The synthetic substances allowed for use in organic livestock production are found in 7 CFR 205.603. The full text of the regulations can be found at www.ams.usda.gov/nop/NOP/standards/FullRegTextOnly.html.

In Europe, organic production is regulated throughout the European Union (EU). EU regulation number 1804/99, which became effective in 2000, sets forth the rules for organic livestock production including animal health and veterinary interventions. All EU member states at a minimum comply with these rules, but some individual countries have included additional rules of their own. Specifications of the European and U.S. regulations have been compared (Nardone et al. 2004).

Special Considerations for Transgenic Goats

Production of transgenic animals using microinjection or nuclear transfer and the propagation of desirable animals using cloning are no longer just scientific research endeavors. They have become established production systems for the propagation and management of transgenic goats. It behooves veterinarians with active goat practice to be familiar with the basic techniques and health issues associated with transgenic goat production.

Transgenic technology began in 1980 when the first transgenic mouse was developed (Gordon et al. 1980).

The first transgenic goat was developed in 1989, producing rhtPA (recombinant human tissue plasminogen activator) in the milk (Ebert et al. 1991) as a potential human therapeutic agent. Since then, the field has markedly expanded with transgenic animals becoming commonplace within many programs and facilities.

The applications for transgenic animals are considerable and include not only the investigation of gene function but also the development of animal models, increased disease resistance through either transgene insertion or knock-out techniques, and production of recombinant, biopharmaceutical proteins in a number of biological fluids such as milk, blood, urine, and semen (Nieman and Kues 2003). In fact, distribution of the first transgenically derived human therapeutic recombinant protein from goat milk (ATryn®) was approved by the European Agency for the Evaluation of Medicinal Products in 2006 and by the Food and Drug Administration in the United States in 2009.

The two main techniques employed for making transgenic animals are microinjection and nuclear transfer (cloning). While microinjection was the first technology to be used in making large transgenic animals (Hammer et al. 1985), and specifically the goat (Gavin 1996), the process is inefficient with only a small percentage of the resulting animals being transgenic. Large animal nuclear transfer (Campbell et al. 1996; Wilmut et al. 1997) was developed later and provides for a near 100% transgenic rate when compared to microinjection. The cloning of the first transgenic goat soon followed (Baguisi et al. 1999; Keefer et al. 2001). There are other techniques for producing transgenic animals such as retroviral gene transfer and artificial chromosome insertion. However, these techniques have not been used yet in goats and are not mentioned further.

Most transgenic goats are maintained in USDA-APHIS-AC Licensed Research Facilities. Under the auspices of the Animal Welfare Act (AWA), these licensed facilities must maintain strict adherence to rules and regulations specifically governing animal care, health, and welfare (housing, lighting, feeding, veterinary care, and environmental enrichment at a minimum). Depending upon the type of research and the funding source, the National Institutes of Health (NIH) may also be involved through their Office of Laboratory Animal Welfare (OLAW) as government funding brings along its own slightly different set of rules and regulations for animals used in a research setting. A growing number of institutions are also striving for accreditation by the Association for the Assessment and Accreditation of Laboratory Animal Care, International (AAALAC-Int.), considered by many to set the gold standard for animal care in licensed research programs and facilities. Lastly, depending upon the intended use of any tissues/fluids from the transgenic animal, the FDA may also have regulatory oversight and impose its own set of rules and regulations.

The use of microinjection to produce a transgenic animal involves microinjection of the transgene into the pronucleus of a fertilized, one-cell embryo and then the transfer of surviving embryos to a surrogate mother. One of the first areas for possible concern, and for which observation and monitoring are appropriate, is the physical/mechanical effects on the nucleus/gene due to the actual microinjection process at the one-cell stage. If any negative impacts occur or gene functions are altered or impaired, one may see outcomes ranging from decreased pregnancy rates from transferred embryos to increased pregnancy loss, late term abortions, or possible physiological abnormalities at birth with clinical sequelae. However, years of experience now indicate that these phenomena, while possible, occurs at a very low incidence.

Regardless of the technique used to produce a transgenic goat, another possible concern involves endogenous gene function and potential transgene insertional site effects. The gene of interest inserts randomly into the genome following transgene introduction. Hence, there is a chance that an endogenous gene could be negatively impacted, leading to potential adverse physiological effects and a transgenic goat presenting with clinical signs of abnormal physiology or health. Therefore, appropriate post-parturitional monitoring of animal health is warranted for any transgenic founder animal.

Introduction of a transgene produces a goat that is hemizygous for that given transgene. Subsequent breeding within a lineage may be aimed at achieving a homozygous state for the transgene. Possible concerns may arise through this approach. First, inbreeding of related goats is the primary route to achieving a homozygous animal. Therefore, inbreeding coefficients need to be considered and animals need to be monitored for ill effects from this relatedness and for possible impacts on overall health and ability to thrive. Second, achieving a homozygous state may bring to light an insertional gene effect since both copies of an endogenous gene may now be affected thereby causing physiological or clinical issues that were not seen in the hemizygous state. Again, appropriate monitoring of animal health is warranted for the first homozygous animals produced. Lastly, the potential exists that breeding for the production of a transgenic homozygous animal will reveal a lethal outcome. A lethality issue may be suspected when: breedings of two hemizygous animals produce no detectable pregnancies; pregnancies do not hold to term with either resorptions or abortions; or, offspring succumb soon after birth. Thus, production of a homozygous transgenic animal may not always be possible and close animal health monitoring is warranted when homozygosity is pursued.

One additional set of concerns related to transgene effects is the possibility of systemic circulation of the recombinant protein being expressed and the potential health impacts arising from expression of pharmacologically active molecules. Depending on the tissue or fluid where the recombinant protein may be directed for expression (e.g., milk, blood, urine, semen, etc.), one must be vigilant for systemic effects as the protein usually will be found systemically due to leaky vasculature and normal lymphatic drainage. Therefore, the biological nature and function of the recombinant protein being introduced must be known so that any effects which may be exerted can be anticipated and recognized. Consideration must also be given to potential adverse health impacts if this is a new gene and novel protein not normally physiologically found in the genome or animal. Lastly, the quantity of the recombinant protein that is expressed and then found systemically in the transgenic animal must be considered. Even if the target protein is endogenous to the animal, it may be found at significantly higher levels than normal and may cause physiological effects that alter normal homeostasis.

As with any traditional goat agricultural production operation for meat, milk, or fiber, optimizing health and product output starts with a sound nutritional program. Relative to transgenic production, nutritional programs should consider the nature of the recombinant protein to be produced. Specifically, if the recombinant protein is novel to the physiological output of the goat's normal cellular machinery, or if quantities are above what is normally produced *in vivo*, then one may need to augment the diet. This modified or fortified diet may need to contain increased levels of vitamins, minerals, or specific amino acids. One should understand the normal cellular machinery and biochemical pathways involved in protein production to know if or what supplementation may be appropriate or necessary.

With the development of cloning technology, nuclear transfer has become the preferred method for producing transgenic goats and has greatly improved the overall efficiency of the process. However, the use of nuclear transfer has added some additional health concerns in a small percentage of animals.

Nuclear transfer starts by removing the maternal DNA from an unfertilized oocyte through enucleation. A full complement of genetic material is subsequently replaced by addition of a somatic cell (e.g. fetal or adult skin fibroblast cell) through a process termed reconstruction. Thereafter, *in vitro* techniques are used to fuse the oocyte and somatic cell and activate the couplet to begin dividing. Following a brief *in vitro* culture period, these newly developed cloned embryos are then transferred to recipient goats using traditional embryo transfer techniques.

With nuclear transfer, a decreased *in utero* fetal survival rate can be seen very early in pregnancy and has been well documented in many species (Campbell et al. 1996; Wilmut et al. 1997; Baguisi et al. 1999). This inability to thrive may be associated with inappropriate or inadequate reprogramming (Dean et al. 2001) of the nuclear/genetic material of the donor cell line or karyoplast and has been postulated to be at the level of the DNA (e.g., methylation pattern). An altered inheritance of cellular mitochondria (Wells 2005) has also been shown to occur in cloned embryos, adding to the possible causes for some of the abnormalities in homeostasis. Both of these phenomena may be directly linked to the small percentage of physiological problems seen *in utero* for some cloned animals such as abnormal placentation and/or organogenesis (Farin et al. 2006; Loi et al. 2006; Fletcher et al. 2007). Abnormal placentation can also lead to abnormal uterine fluid homeostasis and fluid retention in does carrying cloned embryos, which may warrant close clinical monitoring or intervention where appropriate. Other possible outcomes of abnormal placentation include: a tendency toward decreased pregnancy rates for animals receiving cloned embryos, an increased *in utero* loss rate through resorption, or an increased level of abortions if there is late term fetal loss.

The potential abnormal physiology with or without clinical presentations may continue after birth and into the neonatal and early prepuberal stages (Hill et al. 1999). Documented abnormalities in a few large animal species have been shown at the level of the renal, cardiac, respiratory, hepatic, hematopoietic, and immune systems. However, if the small percentage of animals, including goats, that present with these abnormal physiological entities can be clinically supported over time, as the animals grow, many of these abnormalities resolve and they can lead normal and healthy lives (Chavatte-Palmer et al. 2002).

The vast majority of transgenic and cloned animals are normal and healthy (Walsh et al. 2003; Enright et al. 2002; Tayfur Tecirlioglu et al. 2006) and subsequent generations of animals produced from first generation clones have not shown any of the health related issues seen in a small percentage of original clones (Wells 2005). In fact, passage through the germ line has been reported to reverse any abnormal patterns detected at the DNA level in first generation clones (Wells 2005).

PHYSICAL EXAMINATION

Inspection from a Distance

It is often useful diagnostically to observe a group of goats from a distance prior to disturbing them for "hands-on" examination. This is especially true at the time of the initial visit to identify the existence of common problems in the herd or flock. The animals should be observed at rest, while eating or drinking, and during spontaneous and forced movement. General impressions of body condition, mental attitude, and social hierarchy may be acquired and abnormal behaviors characteristic of certain diseases may be noted. Estimated prevalence of common disease problems such as kid pneumonia, diarrhea, and pinkeye can be roughly assessed, respectively, by counting coughers, stained hindquarters, and runny eyes. Other specific observations that might suggest commonly seen disease problems in goats are briefly discussed below. This is for illustration and is not meant to be comprehensive.

Individual goats that appear listless, separate themselves from the herd, or are not actively feeding when others are should be noted and later caught for careful examination as should animals in very poor body condition. Reluctance to feed may be due to a wide range of systemic diseases or localized conditions such as dental or pharyngeal problems, or the result of inadequate bunk space or bullying by dominant does.

Latent signs of respiratory disease or anemia associated with parasitism can be brought out by forced movement of a flock. Anemia is manifested by rapid fatigue, increased heart and respiratory rates, and sometimes collapse. Increased respiratory rate, dyspnea, and coughing indicate respiratory problems.

Signs of skin irritation or pruritus manifested as hair loss, fleece biting, or rubbing against fences or other solid objects usually suggest ectoparasitism, though scrapie, pseudorabies, and migrating *Parelaphostrongylus tenuis* are other possibilities. Goats scratching at their ears with their hind limbs or shaking their heads vigorously probably have ear mites.

Goats observed resting or walking on their knees often have chronic CAEV infection or sore feet. Any animals with abnormalities of gait or lameness after forced exercise should be carefully examined for evidence of arthritis, fractures, laminitis, and lesions of foot rot or foot scald.

A variety of clinical signs may be observed in goats with neurologic disease. Among the more common are ataxia, posterior paresis, circling, depression, head pressing, unilateral facial paralysis, and blindness. Details on carrying out a neurologic examination and differential diagnosis for signs of neurologic disease are provided in Chapter 5.

Straining while attempting to urinate, particularly in bucks and wethers, should suggest the possibility of urolithiasis or posthitis.

Cutaneous swellings or discharges may be observed. Draining abscesses associated with lymph nodes are highly suggestive of caseous lymphadenitis in the flock or herd. A high rate of subcutaneous swellings is often associated with injection site reactions in goats in response to certain adjuvanted vaccines or bacterins or when aseptic injection techniques are not followed.

When kids are left with does, careful observation of suckling behavior can indicate kids that are not successfully nursing. Their does should be examined particularly for signs of mastitis or other udder problems.

Direct Physical Examination of Individual Goats

A topographical approach to physical examination is presented here. Because of the small size of goats, rectal palpation is limited to insertion of a finger into the rectum to assess the pelvic structures and to determine the presence and character of feces. When economics permit, physical examination findings should be supplemented through use of appropriate imaging techniques, diagnostic procedures, and laboratory tests. When numerous individuals in a herd or flock show signs of disease, field necropsy examination may be the most effective way to establish or confirm a diagnosis.

General Inspection

Body condition, mental attitude, and the status of the superficial lymph nodes should be noted. The temperature, pulse, and respiration should be recorded. Fleece in Angora goats makes visual assessment of body condition difficult. Digital palpation of the ribs, spinous and transverse processes of the vertebrae, and the loin muscle may be necessary to evaluate condition. A word of caution about condition scoring in goats: scoring systems derived for sheep are not directly applicable to goats because goats as a species tend to deposit stored fat intra-abdominally rather than subcutaneously. Scoring systems for dairy goats combine palpation of the sternal and lumbar regions and are discussed in Chapter 19. In general, any palpable back fat in a dairy goat would classify her as obese. A scoring system applied to the Small East African goat in Zimbabwe showed a good correlation between a backbone condition score and changes in bodyweight (bw), with a 1-point change in condition score representing an average change of 12% in bw (Honhold et al. 1989).

Normally goats have an alert, attentive, and inquisitive mental attitude. A depressed attitude is characterized by dullness, separation from the flock, and indifference to handling. Depression is present in a wide variety of septic and toxemic conditions but is a particularly prominent sign in pregnancy toxemia and listeriosis. An anxious or apprehensive state is often associated with urethral obstruction in males, sudden blindness as may occur in polioencephalomalacia, or with persistent irritations such as flies and nasal myiasis. An attitude of extreme excitation is most often associated with neurological diseases such as tetanus and meningitis that may be accompanied by muscular rigidity, or encephalitic conditions such as pseudorabies and rabies.

Digital palpation of all superficial lymph nodes should always be a part of the physical exam because of the clinical importance of caseous lymphadenitis in goats. The mandibular, parotid, retropharyngeal, superficial cervical (prescapular), subiliac (prefemoral), and superficial inguinal (supramammary) lymph nodes should be inspected. Normal sized nodes may not be palpable in some of these locations but affected nodes should be readily evident. Any other swellings on the body surface should be noted. Temperature, pulse, and respiration should be measured when the animal is calm because the activity of catching the animal for examination may elevate all three parameters. When taking the goat's rectal temperature, an accumulation of brown, waxy material may be noted near the anus. This is the normal secretion of the sebaceous gland located below the base of the tail (Figure 1.2).

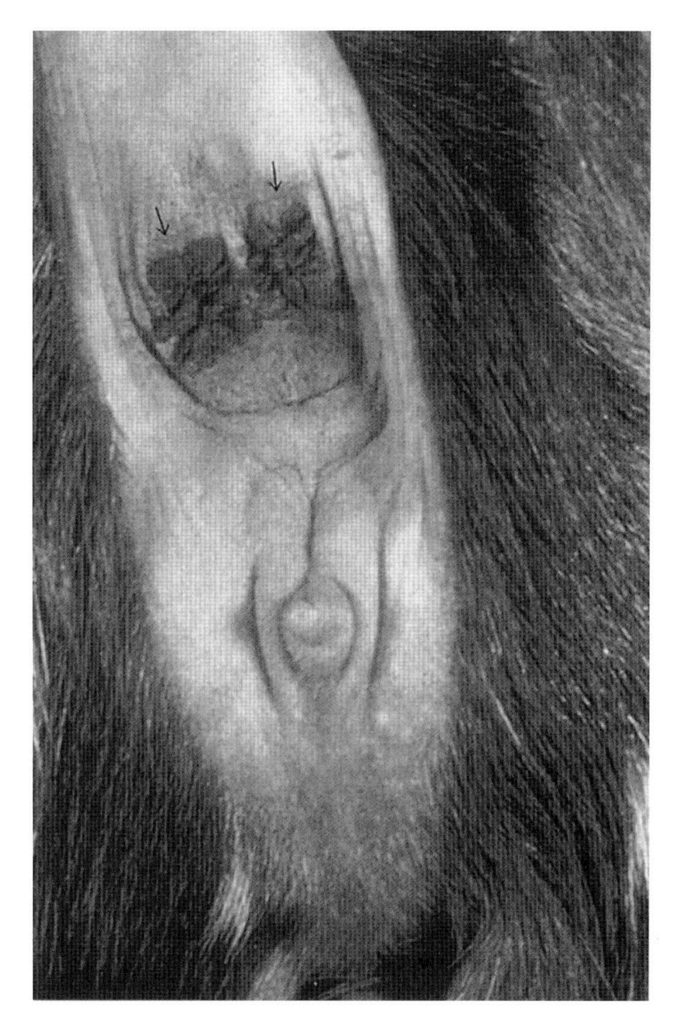

Figure 1.2. Typical waxy secretion found at the base of the tail of goats which is produced by the sebaceous glands in that area. This secretion should not be confused with diarrhea, vaginal discharge, or lochia. (Reproduced by permission of Dr. C.S.F. Williams.)

The normal body temperature of goats is usually reported in the range of 38.6° to 40°C (101.5° to 104°F). However, the body temperature of a normal Angora goat with a full fleece on a hot, humid day can reach 40.3°C (104.5°F) or higher, and goats of lighter bodyweight are more likely to have higher temperatures when exposed to sun than bigger goats (McGregor 1985). To accurately assess the febrile state of the patient, it is useful to record body temperatures in apparently normal herd mates.

The pulse can be measured by stethoscope over the heart or by digital palpation of the femoral artery. Normal pulse rate ranges from 70 to 90 beats per minute (bpm) in resting adults, but can be double that in young, active kids. Fetal heart rates up to 180 bpm have been recorded by ultrasound. It may be useful to assess respiratory rate both at rest and after exercise. Any abnormalities of respiration should also be noted, including flaring of nostrils, extension of head and neck, grunting, abdominal press, and so forth. Normal resting respiratory rate is 10 to 30 per minute in adults and 20 to 40 in kids.

Neonates should be inspected particularly for congenital defects. More commonly observed problems include brachygnathia, cleft palate, hydrocephalus, atresia ani, or rectovaginal fistula, and abnormalities of the genitalia associated with the intersex condition as discussed in Chapter 13. A list of congenital and inherited diseases is provided in Table 1.2. Not all of these, of course, will be evident at birth. Up-to-date information on inherited conditions of goats as well as other species is available through the Online Mendelian Inheritance in Animals (OMIA) database at http://omia.angis.org.au/.

Goat stature is quite diverse. Many small breeds of goats such as the Pygmy or West African Dwarf goat are in fact achondroplastic dwarfs. They appear disproportionate with short legs and normal size torsos. This may draw visual attention to the degree of abdominal distension present, which though quite pronounced, is usually normal. Dwarfism because of pituitary hypoplasia is also seen in goats. These small goats are proportionate in appearance; the Sudan goat is an example (Ricordeau 1981).

Examination of the Integument

In goats the character of the skin and haircoat is a good indicator of general health. A rough, dry, unglossy coat; excessive dander or flakiness; and failure to shed

Table 1.2. Congenital and inherited abnormalities in goats.

Known inherited conditions	*Known acquired conditions*	*Conditions of unclear status*
Afibrinogenemia in Saanen goats	Anthrogryposis and hydranencephaly caused by Akabane virus	Absence of hair
Beta mannosidosis in Nubian goats	Border disease	Atresia ani
Bipartite scrotum in Angora goats	Congenital copper deficiency	Atresia coli
Brachygnathia superior or inferior	Cyclopia due to *Veratrum californicum*	Cleft palate
Cryptorchidism in Angora goats	Freemartins	Congenital goiter of Boer goats
Excessive facial hair in Angora goats		Double or fused teats
Gynecomastia		Entropion
Hereditary goiter in Dutch goats		Hydrops
Inherited abortion in South African Angora goats		Patellar luxation
Intersexes associated with polled condition		Precocious milking
Myotonia congenita		Progressive paresis of Angora goats
N-acetylglucosamine 6-sulphatase deficiency in Nubian goats (mucopolysaccharidosis IIID)		Rectovaginal fistula
Recessive atrichosis		Skeletal malformations
Robertsonian translocation		Spastic paresis
Short tendons in Australian Angora goats		Sticky kid syndrome of Golden Guernsey goats
Sperm granulomas		Umbilical hernia
Supernumerary teats		
Testicular hypoplasia		

out in the spring are all suggestive of poor nutritional status, parasitism, or other chronic diseases. The hair or fleece should be parted and the skin examined for lice, ticks, fleas (in the tropics), nodules, swellings, crusts, eczema, necrosis, neoplasia, photosensitization, and sunburn and focal or regional alopecia. The differential diagnoses for these findings are discussed in Chapter 2.

Because many goats are used primarily for cashmere or mohair production, the veterinarian should know something about the nature of goat hair used in textiles. Detailed information on the subject is given in Chapter 2.

Examination of the Head

Many conditions can cause general asymmetry or focal swellings around the head and these abnormalities should be noted. The differential diagnoses for such swellings are discussed in Chapter 3.

Membranes

Inspection of the conjunctivae and mucous membranes of the mouth may reveal paleness due to anemia, icterus resulting from hemolysis or hepatic dysfunction, or hyperemia and congestion associated with acute febrile or toxemic states.

Oral Cavity

Evidence of brachygnathism, cleft palate, mucosal lesions, dental abnormalities, or dysphagia such as drooling, salivation, dropping food from the mouth, or accumulating food in the buccal space should be noted. The differential diagnoses for these signs are given in Chapter 10. Necrotic odors of the breath may occur. They may reflect necrotic stomatitis, alveolar periostitis, pharyngitis, or even pneumonia.

Thorough examination of the oral cavity requires good restraint, a speculum, a towel, and a penlight. All oral structures should be examined and the molar arcades digitally palpated for missing teeth from outside the mouth. If more direct examination of the teeth is required, extreme caution should be taken because the molars may have sharp, jagged edges and exert powerful grinding motion. Tranquilization is indicated, because fingers can be badly injured. Wearing gloves during oral examination is a wise precautionary measure, particularly if the goat shows neurologic signs.

Eyes

Facial hair covering the eyes is a heritable trait in Angora goats. Affected goats tend to do poorly on range because their ability to selectively browse is impaired. The body condition of such individuals should be noted as well as their prevalence in the flock. Blindness is initially assessed by testing the menace response, but facial nerve paralysis can render a sighted animal unable to blink. Intact pupillary light responses in a blind goat suggest a cerebrocortical lesion. Lacrimation and hyperemia of the conjunctiva, cloudiness of the cornea, and hypopyon in the anterior chamber should be noted if present. The differential diagnoses for these various findings are given in Chapter 6.

Nares

Both nostrils should be evaluated for symmetry of air flow. If nasal discharge is observed, determine if it is unilateral or bilateral and note its character. Collapse of a nostril may result from facial nerve paralysis. Crusting of the nares occurs when the sick animal does not clean the nostrils or it may be a sign of specific disease problems. The differential diagnoses for nasal discharge and crusting of the nares are given in Chapter 9.

Ears

Ear mites, if suspected, can be identified by collecting debris from the ear canal on a cotton swab and smearing it on a slide for examination.

Goats are often identified by tattoos inside the ear; tattoo numbers may have to be checked against health papers at shows and sales. It may be necessary to clean the inside of the ear with soap and water and use a powerful light source to backlight the tattoo to make it readable. Metal and plastic ear tags commonly tear out of goats' ears and their use should be avoided, especially in pet and show animals.

Ear tips may be lost on young goats due to prolonged exposure to freezing temperatures. Goats of the La Mancha breed lack a well-developed external ear. Only a vestigial pinna is present and is referred to as an elf (up to 5 cm, with some cartilage) or gopher (up to 2.5 cm, with little or no cartilage) ear. These animals are usually tattooed on the underside of the tail.

Horns

Goats may be horned or polled. Horn buds may be present at birth or become palpable within several days of birth. Generally, horned kids have two irregular whorls of hair over the location of the horn buds whereas hornless kids have a smooth poll with a single central symmetrical whorl of hair. It is important to establish and record which offspring are naturally polled because homozygous polled goats have a high incidence of infertility. The relationship of the polled trait and the intersex condition is discussed in detail in Chapter 13. Deformed horns, or scurs, are often seen on older goats as a result of incomplete removal of germinal horn tissue at the time of disbudding. Techniques for, and problems with, disbudding and dehorning are discussed in Chapter 18. The glands partially responsible for the characteristic odor of buck goats in the breeding season are located in skin folds just caudomedial to the horn buds.

Examination of the Neck

Traumatic injuries to the pharynx from balling guns and drenching equipment occur in goats. The throat should be palpated for swelling, heat, and pain associated with cellulitis from traumatic injury. A number of normal and abnormal structures and swellings in the neck must be differentiated on physical examination, including goiters, thymus, branchial cleft cysts, wattles, and abscesses. Their differentiation is discussed in Chapter 3. Thorough examination of the neck should include palpation of the jugular furrows for evidence of phlebitis, palpation of the esophagus for evidence of obstruction, and auscultation of the trachea. Prominent distension of the jugular vein, though possibly suggestive of congestive heart failure, is most commonly due to overly tight collars or neck chains in goats. This should be brought to the owner's attention if found.

Examination of the Chest

The extent and severity of respiratory disease is often difficult to assess in goats. To improve the chances of accurate diagnosis and prognosis, careful attention should be given to auscultation. When possible, the animal should be moved to quiet surroundings. The fleece in Angora goats should be parted to place the stethoscope in contact with the skin. The trachea and the lungs should be ausculted to identify the presence of referred sounds. Eliciting a cough by compression of the pharynx may clear the trachea or reveal the presence of bronchial exudate. Care should be taken to listen with a stethoscope placed well forward under the elbow and in front of the shoulder, otherwise cranial ventral pneumonias, which are common, may be overlooked. The intensity of identifiable sounds can be augmented by forced activity of the animal before auscultation or by placing a plastic bag or exam glove over the nares to increase the depth of respiration by rebreathing of carbon dioxide. Radiographic examination is indicated when questions about the severity of lung disease persist.

Normally the heart can be heard about evenly on both the right and left sides of the chest at the fourth or fifth rib space. Mediastinal abscesses may displace the heart, resulting in a shift in intensity of cardiac sounds. Muffling of the heart sounds because of pericarditis is uncommon in goats. Murmurs are rarely heard and are discussed in Chapter 8.

Examination of the Abdomen

The abdominal contour should be inspected to assess conditions such as bloat, advanced pregnancy in females, and ruptured bladder in wethers and intact males. Characteristic contours and their clinical significance are discussed in Chapter 10. Ballotment may help to detect abdominal fluid accumulations, pregnancy, or rumen impaction. Auscultation of the rumen in the left paralumbar fossa is essential. Normal rumen contractions occur at a rate of one to two per minute. Observation of cud chewing suggests normal rumen activity.

Examination of the Limbs

Locomotor problems are common in goats. Lameness and abnormalities of gait may result from neurological disease, conformational defects, muscular dysfunction, skeletal trauma, infectious and noninfectious arthritides, and diseases of the foot. Localization of the problem by careful physical examination is the first step in making an accurate diagnosis. Differential diagnoses of locomotor problems are discussed in detail in Chapter 4.

Overgrown hooves must be pared with shears or a hoof knife to adequately assess the health of the foot. Hyperemia and swellings at or above the coronary band should be noted. They may represent either local infections or systemic disease.

All joints should be carefully palpated. Distensions of the joint capsule, heat, pain, swelling or fibrosis of periarticular structures, limitations on the range of joint motion, and enlargement of bursae should all be noted. The degree of joint enlargement may not necessarily correlate with the severity of lameness.

The vertebral column and the long bones of the legs should be palpated for evidence of fractures in acutely lame or recumbent animals. A major goal of physical examination in recumbent goats is to differentiate musculoskeletal, metabolic, toxemic, and neurologic causes of recumbency. The differential diagnoses for recumbency are discussed in Chapter 4.

Examination of the Reproductive System

Mammary Gland

Careful examination of the udder is always warranted. Visual inspection may reveal weakness of the suspensory apparatus, slack halves, abnormal swellings, and discolorations of the skin. Digital palpation of the gland will identify udder edema, active inflammation, fibrosis, scarring, or abscesses in the parenchyma or teats. In gangrenous mastitis the udder skin may be blue-black and cold and in time the gland may slough if the animal survives. Patency of the teats should be assessed in lactating animals. Supernumerary teats may be present. Their identification and removal are discussed in Chapter 14.

The milk of lactating does should be observed on a black plate or strip cup to assess color, consistency, and the presence of clots or flakes. Bovine screening tests for subclinical mastitis such as the California Mastitis Test must be used cautiously in goats because normal goat milk tends to have higher cell counts. The somatic cell count issue and interpretation of test results are discussed in Chapter 14.

Vulva

Swelling and hyperemia of the vulva may be signs of heat or impending parturition, but may also be seen in herpes vulvovaginitis in conjunction with vesicles or scabs. Any vulvar discharges should be noted. As females come out of heat, the vulvar discharge, initially serous and mucoid, may become white and tenacious. This is often misinterpreted as a purulent discharge by the inexperienced observer. Often, there is a sanguinous discharge after termination of a pseudopregnancy. Speculum examination of the vaginal canal and cervix should be carried out when there is doubt about the source and nature of the discharge. Occasionally, otherwise normal does may have ectopic mammary tissue present at the vulva which may swell during lactation.

Does may show vaginal eversion or frank prolapse in advanced pregnancy or immediately post partum. After uncomplicated births, normal lochia may be discharged for a period of one to three weeks. It is reddish brown in color and odorless. Placentas are usually passed within four hours of parturition and are frequently eaten.

It is important to carefully examine the external genitalia of young does, particularly when there is a complaint of infertility, because of the high incidence of intersexes among polled goats. Malformations of the genitalia range from the clinically subtle, such as a slightly enlarged clitoris, to the overt, such as male phenotypes in genetically female individuals. Accurate record keeping may help to identify homozygous-polled individuals.

Scrotum

The scrotum and its contents should be palpated. Normally there is bilateral symmetry of all structures. A bipartite or split scrotum is a common congenital condition that some breeders consider a fault. The differential diagnoses for abnormalities of the scrotum, testes, and spermatic cord structures are given in Chapter 13. Semen samples can be collected for evaluation by electroejaculation or by use of an artificial vagina. These procedures are described in Chapter 13. Gynecomastia occurs in male goats and it is not extraordinary to detect distended teats anterior to the scrotum during physical examination, as discussed in Chapter 13.

Penis and Prepuce

Examining the penis of male goats, especially wethers, can be difficult and is not ordinarily attempted unless there is a history of urinary or breeding problems. Details on special examination and catheterization of the penis are given in Chapter 12.

The preputial opening should be routinely examined, particularly in wethers, for the presence of ulcerative posthitis. The preputial orifice may become occluded in this condition. Crystals or drops of blood may be noted at the orifice in cases of obstructive urolithiasis.

Examination of the Environment

An examination of the environment where goats are raised should include a detailed review of all feeds used, the feeding facilities, water sources and water delivery systems; the yards, pastures, range, or buildings where the animals are kept; and any mechanical or manual equipment used as part of the routine farm procedures. Too often, farmers attempt to make do with equipment and buildings that are inadequate for an expanding operation. Because of prolificacy, goat herds tend to expand faster than owners anticipate. Inadequate feeder space for does, a smell of ammonia in the air due to poor ventilation and/or soaked bedding, and overcrowded kid pens are three examples of common faults found on environmental inspection. Besides visual inspection of equipment, farmers could be asked to demonstrate how common procedures are carried out to detect if they are using inappropriate techniques.

Equipment used for treatment should be examined for its potential to cause injury. Poorly maintained syringes with either contaminated or overly long, large-gauge needles can result in injection abscesses or systemic infections. Drug and vaccine stocks should be examined to determine if they are appropriate, clean, unexpired, and maintained at proper temperatures. Storage facilities for these items should be properly secured. If the farmer blends his own feed or components, the techniques and constituents used should be examined, particularly when toxicities are suspected. Accidental inclusion of agricultural or other farm chemicals is not uncommon. Milking machines used for goats should also be examined to determine their efficiency and the milking procedures studied if it appears that mastitis is a significant problem. Finally, the facilities available and routinely used to dispose of any dead animals should be particularly noted to see that they are consistent with any legal requirements and do not serve as environmental contaminants or as a source of infection for the remainder of the flock or herd.

In recent years, in association with the expansion of international trade in livestock and livestock products and increasing concerns about bioterrorism, there has been a growing emphasis on food safety and biosecurity, with recognition that food safety encompasses all aspects of food production, from the farm to the table. As such, quality management assurance programs have grown in popularity as have procedures to ensure biosecurity to limit the introduction and spread of disease on and between farms. Environmental inspections should include an assessment of biosecurity and aspects of management and sanitation that can affect food quality.

Special Considerations for Range and Pasture Operations

The quality and quantity of pasture and the availability of supplementary or conserved feed should be assessed. This may require a specialized knowledge of pasture species, weeds, or other potentially toxic plants. A list of plants known to be poisonous to goats is provided in Chapter 19. If possible, animals should be observed while feeding. The source of water available both year-round and seasonally, its quality, and its quantity, should also be inspected. Feed and water samples should, if necessary, be collected for laboratory examinations.

On range or pasture, goats may congregate in certain shaded or sheltered areas, particularly during periods of high or low temperatures or precipitation, and after shearing. Provision of adequate shelter should be documented. Heat stress can be reduced by ensuring the animals have adequate shade and water when the livestock weather safety index is in the danger or emergency zone. Cold stress is particularly likely in recently shorn animals, and temporary shelter and extra feed are necessary for these animals. If shelter areas are limited or overused, buildup of infectious agents can occur, leading to increases in enteric and other diseases, especially in kids. This is aggravated by poor drainage under feeders and water troughs.

Fencing for these types of operations should also be inspected, particularly regarding its effectiveness in keeping goats in and keeping predators out.

Special Considerations for Confinement Operations

In semiconfinement operations adult animals and sometimes young stock are grazed on pasture during the warmer months but confined during the winter and early spring. As herds expand, there is a tendency for small pastures to be overused, with poor nutrition and increased parasitism as the result. Stocking rates should be noted and deworming history verified.

In confinement systems, the type of buildings used for housing should be evaluated for the following: available area (square feet or square meters) per adult breeding animal, type of flooring and bedding, degree of insulation, presence of supplemental heating if any, adequacy of natural or mechanical ventilation systems, source and availability of water, and the amount of trough or bunk space per goat. Requirements for goats are given in Chapter 9. The distribution of animals within buildings should be noted. Ideally, a separate kidding facility should exist and be hygienically maintained. Artificially reared kids should be in a separate facility from adult stock, and bucks should be housed separately from milking does. Methods and times of feeding for all groups within the herd should be noted. If other species of livestock are present, consideration should be given to them as possible sources of disease for goats.

Unfortunately, many confinement goat operations have both rodent and associated feline populations. Cats are a recognized source of *Toxoplasma gondii*, a major cause of abortion in goats. Farmers should be encouraged to seek alternate means of rodent control.

Special Consideration for Hobby Farms

The principles and procedures of environmental examination already described also apply to the hobby farm. Special considerations that occur are usually the result of inexperience on the part of the hobbyist. Medications, insecticides, and grain supplies may be inadequately secured, allowing access of inquisitive goats with resultant overdoses, poisonings, and/or grain overload. In the barn, overcrowding with inadequate feeder space is often observed along with fecal contamination of feed and water supplies.

In winter, lack of adequate ventilation in closed, overcrowded barns leads to outbreaks of pneumonia. Some owners consistently shut all windows and doors, believing that animals must stay warm in winter. These individuals need to be counseled on the beneficial effects of continuous air exchange on respiratory health. Pasture problems often involve disappearance of animals or predation due to inadequate fencing, bloat due to inadequate adaption to pasture, or parasitism due to placement of young stock on contaminated, overcrowded plots. The veterinarian should examine all elements of the ration being fed on the hobby farm to ensure that the hobbyist understands basic ruminant nutrition.

Field Necropsies and Slaughterhouse Checks

The economic value of most individual goats in commercial herds and flocks is such that most owners can be persuaded to have a necropsy undertaken of an ill or obviously moribund animal. This is an extremely useful adjunct to clinical examination, because necropsy can confirm the suspected diagnosis or suggest new avenues of investigation. All necropsies should be carried out following a systematic procedure with special regard to the likelihood of any zoonotic infections being transmitted and the safe and legal disposal of carcasses.

Necropsy of all or a random sample of young animals born dead or dying in the first two to three weeks of life is an extremely valuable service that veterinarians can provide to their clients. Categorization of deaths into preparturient, parturient, and postparturient causes can be done with a minimum of laboratory diagnostic techniques and immediately direct the owner to possible ways of reducing these losses.

Whenever possible, goats slaughtered for meat or culled from the herd or flock should be examined post mortem by a veterinarian as an inexpensive and worthwhile means of disease surveillance. Such inspections can provide information on the efficacy of parasite control measures; the presence of subclinical pneumonia; and the occurrence of injection site abscesses, visceral caseous lymphadenitis, and hydatid disease. Opportunities to perform routine slaughter checks on goats at an abattoir are uncommon in the United States because the goat meat industry is decentralized, though this may change as demand for goat meat continues to increase.

REFERENCES

Askins, G.D. and Turner, E.E.: A behavioural study of Angora goats on west Texas range. J. Range Mgmnt., 25:82–87, 1972.

Baguisi, A., et al.: Production of goats by somatic cell nuclear transfer. Nat. Biotech., 17:456–461, 1999.

Batten, G.J.: A new meat goat breed. International Goat Association. Prcdngs, IV International Conference on Goats, Brasilia, March 8–13, 1987, Volume 2, pp. 1330–1331.

Campbell, K.H.S., McWhir, J., Ritchie, W.A., and Wilmut, I. Sheep cloned by nuclear transfer from a cultured cell line. Nature, 380:64–66, 1996.

Chavatte-Palmer, P., et al.: Clinical, hormonal, and hematologic characteristics of bovine calves cloned from nuclei from somatic cells. Biol. Reprod., 66:1596–1603, 2002.

Coop, I.E., (ed): Sheep and Goat Production. Amsterdam, Elsevier Scientific Publ. Co., 1982.

Dean, W., et al.: Conservation of methylation reprogramming in mammalian development: aberrant reprogramming in cloned embryos. Proc. Natl. Acad. Sci. USA, 98:13734–13738, 2001.

Devendra, C. and Burns, M.: Goat Production in the Tropics. Slough, U.K., Commonwealth Agricultural Bureaux, 1983.

Dubeuf, J.-P, Morand-Fehr, P., Rubino, R.: Situation, changes and future of goat industry around the world. Small Rum. Res., 51:165–173, 2004.

Dunbar, R.: Scapegoat for a thousand deserts. New Scientist, 104:30–33, 1984.

Ebert, K.M., et al.: Transgenic production of a variant of human tissue-type plasminogen activator in goat milk: Generation of transgenic goats and analysis of expression. Bio/Tech, 9:835–838, 1991.

Enright, B.P., et al.: Reproductive characteristics of cloned heifers derived from adult somatic cells. Biol. Reprod., 66:291–296, 2002.

FAO: Livestock Units. In: ResourceSTAT Module of FAOSTAT, Food and Agricultural Organization of the United Nations, Rome, 2007. http://faostat.fao.org/site/405/default.aspx

FAO: Livestock Primary and Processed. In: ProdSTAT Module of FAOSTAT, Food and Agricultural Organization of the United Nations, Rome, 2007a. http://faostat.fao.org/site/526/default.aspx

Farin, P.W., Piedrahita, J.A., and Farin, C.E.: Errors in development of fetuses and placentas from in vitro-produced bovine embryos. Theriogenology, 65:178–191, 2006.

Fletcher, C.J., et al.: Somatic cell nuclear transfer in the sheep induces placental defects that likely preceded fetal demise. Reprod., 133:243–255, 2007.

Gall, C., (ed): Goat Production, London, Academic Press, 1981.

Gavin, W.G.: Gene transfer into goat embryos. Transgenic Animals–Generation and Use. L.M. Houdebine, ed. Amsterdam, Harwood Academic Publishers, 1996.

Gordon, J.W., et al.: Genetic transformation of mouse embryos by microinjection of purified DNA. Proc. Natl. Acad. Sci. USA, 77:7380–7384, 1980.

Hafez, E.S.E. (ed): The Behaviour of Domestic Animals, 3rd Ed. Baltimore, The Williams and Wilkins Co., 1975.

Hammer, R.E., et al.: Production of transgenic rabbits, sheep and pigs by microinjection. Nature, 315:680–683, 1985.

Hill, J.R., et al.: Clinical and pathological features of cloned transgenic calves and fetuses (13 case studies). Theriogenology, 51:1451–1465, 1999.

Honhold, N., Petit, H. and Halliwell, R.W.: Condition scoring scheme for Small East African goats in Zimbabwe. Trop. Anim. Health Prod., 21:121–127, 1989.

Karreman, H.J.: Organic Livestock Production: Veterinary Challenges and Opportunities, 2006 Convention Notes, 143rd AVMA Annual Convention, Honolulu, July 15–19, 2006.

Keefer, C.L., et al.: Generation of dwarf goat (*Capra hircus*) clones following nuclear transfer with transfected and non-transfected fetal fibroblasts and in vitro matured oocytes. Biol. Reprod., 64:849–856, 2001.

Kilgour, R. and Dalton, C.: Livestock Behaviour: A Practical Guide. Auckland, Methuen Publications Ltd. 1984.

Kilgour, R. and Ross, D.J.: Feral goat behaviour—a management guide. N.Z.J. Agric., 141:15–20, 1980.

Loi, P.L., et al.: Placental abnormalities associated with postnatal mortality in sheep somatic cell clones. Theriogenology, 65:1110–1121, 2006.

Mahan, S.W.: The improved Boer goat. Small Rum. Res., 36:165–170, 2000.

McGregor, B.A.: Heat stress in Angora wether goats. Aust. Vet. J., 62:349–350, 1985.

Morand-Fehr, P., et al.: Strategy for goat farming in the 21st century. Small Rum. Res., 51:175–183, 2004.

Nardone, A., Zervas, G., and Ronchi, B.: Sustainability of small ruminant organic systems of production. Livestock Prod. Sci., 90:27–39, 2004.

Nieman, H. and Kues, W.: Application of transgenesis in livestock for agriculture and biomedicine. An. Reprd. Sci., 79:291–317, 2003.

Peacock, C.: Improving Goat Production in the Tropics. Oxford, UK, Oxfam, 386 pp. 1996.

Pu, Jiabi, Chengdu, Sichuan, China, personal communication, 1990.

Reed, C.A. and Schaffer, W.M.: How to tell the sheep from the goats. Field Museum Nat. Hist. Bull., 43(3):2–7, 1972.

Ricordeau, G.: Genetics: breeding plans. In: Goat Production, C. Gall, ed. London, Academic Press, 1981.

Smith, P.W., Parks, O.W. and Schwartz, D.P.: Characterization of male goat odors: 6-trans nonenal. J. Dairy Sci., 67:794–801, 1984.

Tayfur Tecirlioglu, R., et al.: Semen and reproductive profiles of genetically identical cloned bulls. Theriogenology, 65:1783–1799, 2006.

Walsh, M.K., et al.: Comparison of milk produced by cows cloned by nuclear transfer with milk from non-cloned cows. Cloning and Stem Cells, 5:213–219, 2003.

Ward, M.L.: Cleaning up with goats. Beef Magazine. 42(12):46–47, August, 2006.

Wells, D.N.: Animal cloning: problems and prospects. Rev. sci. tech., Off. Int. Epiz., 24 (1):251–264, 2005.

Wilmut, I., et al.: Viable offspring derived from fetal and adult mammalian cells. Nature, 385:810–813, 1997.

2

Skin

NORMAL ANATOMY AND PHYSIOLOGY OF THE SKIN AND HAIR

The structure and function of the skin have been reviewed elsewhere (Scott 1988) and will not be discussed in detail here.

Skin

The epidermis can be divided histologically into four layers: stratum corneum, stratum granulosum, stratum spinosum, and stratum basale (Sar and Calhoun 1956). Goat skin is thickest on the forehead and dorsal aspect of the body. As in other species, the major histocompatibility system is involved in allograft rejection if skin grafting is attempted (van Dam et al. 1978).

Specialized Skin Structures

Wattles are specialized skin appendages sometimes found in the cervical region of goats. They contain a central cartilaginous core, smooth muscle, connective tissue, nerves, and blood vessels (Sar and Calhoun 1956). Wattles have no known function. Subcutaneous cysts associated with the base of the wattle are discussed in Chapter 3. The presence of wattles is determined by an autosomal dominant gene with complete penetrance but variable expression regarding location (neck, ear, face), size, and number (Lush 1926; Ricordeau 1981). In a study of Saanen goats in France, does with wattles were approximately 13% more prolific than does without wattles (Ricordeau 1967).

The skin caudomedial to the horns of buck goats contains branched sebaceous glands that produce lipids and chemicals that contribute to the buck odor (Van Lancker et al. 2005). The glands are also present but much smaller in female and castrated male goats (Bal and Ghoshal 1976). These glands and descenting procedures that destroy them are discussed in Chapter 18.

Hair and Shedding

Hair growth in goats resembles that in other land mammals (Shelton 1981; Scott 1988). Hair follicles are initiated prenatally by invagination of the epidermis into the dermis. Sweat and sebaceous glands and the arrector pili muscle develop in association with the follicle. The histologic anatomy of these structures has been reviewed by Scott (1988). The hair is produced by rapidly dividing cells in the bulb at the base of the follicle. During the active phase of the growth cycle (anagen), growth from the bulb is continuous. Anagen is followed by the resting phase (telogen) and then by molting. When growth resumes, the new fiber produced by the follicle helps to push out the old fiber. In goats not specifically selected for fiber production, fibers form brush ends and growth stops at about the time of the autumn equinox, and the follicles remain dormant until late spring (Ryder 1978).

Hair follicles in goats are grouped in bundles or clusters. Within each bundle are primary follicles (often a central and two laterals) and a variable number of secondary follicles. The primary follicles produce long, coarse guard hairs, while secondary follicles produce undercoat or down. In the Angora, secondary follicles have been modified to produce mohair. Goats adapted to tropical regions have little undercoat, while secondary fibers contribute to cold resistance in goats in cold climates.

The inheritance of coat color involves numerous genes. One possible interpretation of color in American goats has been proposed by Mitchell (1989). Several other papers have attempted to summarize various aspects of color inheritance in goats (Ricordeau 1981; Adalsteinsson et al. 1994).

FIBER PRODUCTION

Certain breeds of goats are kept specifically for fiber production. Anything that adversely affects the quality and quantity of fiber harvested, including skin diseases, can have severe economic consequences. Branding paint also damages the fleece, and thus range animals should be paint branded only on the ears or horns.

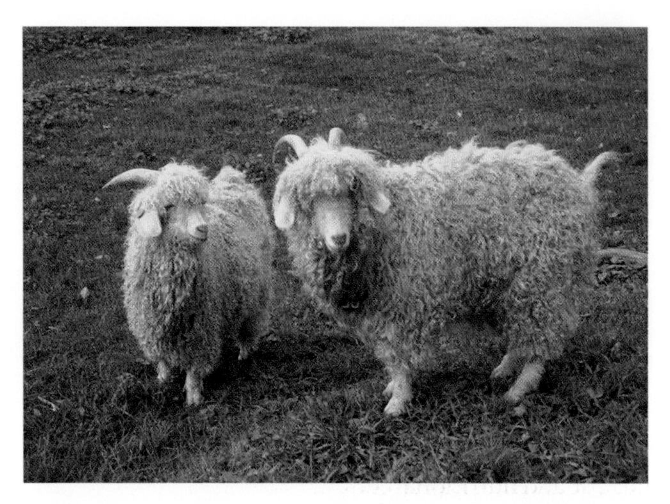

Figure 2.1. Angora goats, the source of mohair. (Courtesy Dr. M.C. Smith.)

Mohair

Mohair is the fleece of the Angora goat (Figure 2.1). The Angora evolved in Asia Minor many centuries ago, possibly a descendant of the wild goat of Persia. Mohair probably developed by elongation of the woolly undercoat of the primitive goat. Although the sultans of Turkey attempted to prevent exportation, populations of Angora goats reached South Africa and the United States in the mid-1880s. Currently, important production centers for mohair include South Africa, Texas, Turkey, Argentina, New Zealand, and Australia (Dubeuf et al. 2004).

Factors Affecting Mohair Quality

Mohair mainly consists of nonmedullated fibers that lack crimp. They arise mostly from secondary follicles and grow continuously, albeit at a lower rate in winter. These fibers are strong, elastic, and composed of keratin. Flat scales that hardly overlap give the fibers smoothness and luster (Margolena 1974). Different countries have different standards for fiber diameter, but the range is typically 24 to 46 microns. The fleece is typically harvested in two clips per year.

Kemp. At birth, goat fleece contains approximately 44% kemp, or medullated fibers from primary follicles, but this proportion drops to 7% by three months of age due to shedding of the kemp (Dreyer and Marincowitz 1967). Later in life, some primary follicles may produce fibers with discontinuous or no medullation. Kemp and colored fibers are generally undesirable fleece contaminants due to uneven dyeing. It has been proposed that shearing shortly before the spring and autumn equinoxes decreases the proportion of medullated fibers in the clip, because natural shedding of these fibers will have recently occurred (Litherland et al. 2000).

Perinatal Nutrition. In the developing fetus, a central and two (or more) lateral primary follicles are in place by ninety days of gestation (Wentzel and Vosloos 1974). The development of secondary hair follicles occurs later and is affected by nutrition during the fourth month of gestation through the first month after birth. Poor nutrition during these critical times probably will compromise the Angora goat's ability to produce mohair later in life (Eppleston and Moore 1990).

Age and Nutrition. Hair follicle density in the skin determines fiber density in the fleece and is under both genetic and nutritional control. Fiber diameter increases with age and bodyweight. Kids produce mohair with a fiber diameter of 28 microns or less at the first shearing, whereas the diameter of the fibers from adult goats varies from 36 to 46 microns. The mohair mass produced peaks at three to four years of age, but because the finer fibers are more valuable, the economic value of the fleece peaks somewhat sooner (van der Westhuysen et al. 1988).

Under nutrition results in reduced body growth and production of mohair as well as a reduction in fiber diameter (Russel 1992). Thus, finer, lighter fleece is produced during periods of drought or overstocking. A slightly coarser fleece may result from overfeeding, although published documentation of this is scarce. In one study in which Angoras were fed individually to maintain different bodyweights, fiber diameter increased 0.4 microns for each kilogram increase in bodyweight (McGregor 1986). Nutrition of Angora goats is discussed more in Chapter 19.

Stress Medullation. A reversible change from normal to medullated fibers occurs in a stress syndrome that seems to be comparable to wool break in sheep. Reported causes of stress-induced medullation include lactation for twins, transport, and hard work by bucks. The time period when the stress occurred can be demonstrated by immersing a full-length staple of fleece in kerosene in a black container. Kemp fibers and bands of medullation in mohair will show as white streaks due to air-filled cores. Normal mohair is almost invisible in kerosene (Ensor 1987).

Other possible causes of medullation have been reviewed (Lupton et al. 1991). Dietary protein and energy levels do not seem to be important in individually housed animals, but heredity may contribute. Selection should be based on objective evaluation of whole fleeces, not just mid-side samples, of Angora goats older than one year of age.

Freeze Loss

Whenever Angoras are shorn, even during summer months, they are vulnerable to exposure to wind, rain, and temperature changes. Angoras have minimal body fat and a small body size, with relatively greater surface area, as compared to sheep. Mortality can be very high in freshly shorn goats, especially if they have not had time to return to full feed before inclement weather arrives. Methods of limiting freeze loss include sheltering the animals for four to six weeks after shearing, shearing with a comb that leaves a longer stubble, and leaving a narrow strip of unshorn hair ("cape") along the backbone (Shelton 1981; Bretzlaff 1990).

Feeding of alkali-ionophore-treated grains (to avoid rumen acidosis, see Chapter 19) is helpful when shorn animals are exposed to severe weather. Individual recumbent animals may respond to intravenous or intraperitoneal glucose (van der Westhuysen et al. 1988).

Cashmere

Cashmere is a fine, soft fiber used to produce fashion-wear. It comes from the downy undercoat of certain goats (Figure 2.2). Originally, cashmere was combed from Pashmina goats in Central Asia (Mason 1984). Goat down (unmedullated, from secondary follicles) with a mean fiber diameter of 19 microns or less can be produced by many breeds. By comparison, the mean diameter of the guard hair outer coat is typically 60 to 90 microns. Latitude, and therefore photoperiod, appear to be more important than altitude as a factor influencing down production. Evidence of this is that most Australian cashmere production occurs near sea level (Couchman 1987). In spring-born kids, maximum secondary follicle development (as determined by skin biopsy or fiber measurements) is achieved by 20 weeks of age, permitting selection at that time (Henderson and Sabine 1991).

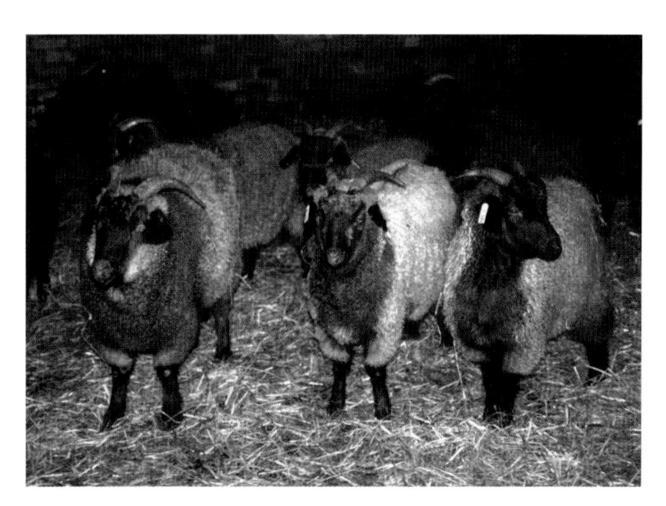

Figure 2.2. Cashmere goats from Mongolia. (Courtesy Dr. M.C. Smith.)

Cashmere goats have a three-phase annual cycle of fiber growth that is influenced by photoperiod, probably via melatonin (Klören and Norton 1995), and nutrition. The period of fiber growth typically coincides with summer in wethers and maiden does but is often delayed until autumn and early winter in lactating does (McDonald 1985). Next, fiber regression occurs and the root bulb of the fiber forms an enlarged brush end, which holds the fiber in the follicle. Finally, there is a follicle resting phase when no down is grown and improved nutrition has no direct effect on cashmere production. The fiber is shed (or the entire fleece may be cast simultaneously) when the fibers are lost from the secondary follicles. The fleece may be harvested by shearing just before it would be shed naturally, usually at the end of the winter. Freeze losses of shorn goats may occur. It may be several months before normal seasonal growth resumes (Betteridge et al. 1988). Chemical defleecing with mimosine has been investigated as a means of leaving the protective guard hairs on the goat (Luo et al. 2000).

Raw, or greasy, cashmere contains both guard hairs and down. Dehairing machinery removes the long guard hairs that remain after hand removal of most of the coarse hairs. Major suppliers of the raw fiber are China, Mongolia, Afghanistan, and Iran. The maximum guard hair content after dehairing is 0.5% for knitting and 3% for the weaving trade. Imported cashmere is sometimes contaminated with anthrax (*Bacillus anthracis*) spores (Hunter et al. 1989).

As with mohair, the finest cashmere fibers are produced under conditions of nutritional stress. In an Australian study, however, feeding enough energy to maintain or slightly increase body condition during summer and autumn maximized cashmere production. Fiber diameter of the total fleece averaged 1 micron larger for goats fed energy at 1.25 maintenance (M) compared with 0.8 M (McGregor 1988).

Cashgora

Cashgora is a coarse cashmere with more luster, mostly harvested from the progeny produced by crossing Angoras with feral goats in Australia and New Zealand. The current fiber diameter is 20 to 23 microns. Some breeders are attempting to stabilize the fleece type.

Pygora

Pygoras are a newly developed breed resulting from the crossing of purebred pygmy goats and purebred Angoras. Two such "first generation crossbreds" are mated to produce the actual pygora. Currently registration requirements include fleece evaluation. The soft undercoat resembles cashmere, comes in a variety of colors, and is often plucked or combed for sale to handspinners in the United States (Hicks 1988).

PRODUCTION OF SKINS

The annual worldwide production of goat skins was estimated at 200 million in 1983. Of these, 95% were produced in developing countries (Robinet 1984). The estimate for 1995 was 295 million pieces, with India, China, and Pakistan remaining important producers of goat leather products (Naidu 2000). The quality of the skins produced is influenced by breed, nutritional status of the goat, disease conditions affecting the skin, and traumatic injuries (e.g., from injections, thorns, and dog bites). Angora skins are considered to be unsuitable for leather production because of insufficient connective tissue (van der Westhuysen et al. 1988). Local drought conditions result in particularly weak skins. Mange, grubs, tick infestations, capripox and contagious ecthyma infections, and dermatophilosis decrease the value of goat skins. When the goat has been slaughtered, additional losses occur during flaying, drying, and storage. Humid weather predisposes to rotting while extremely arid conditions make cracking of the skins more likely.

Goat skins are used in local villages for water containers, tents, mats, and leather. Others are exported as cured skins, simple tanned skins, drum heads, or leather. Uses include footwear, garments, bookbinding, and luggage. The demand is expected to remain steady. Production could be most easily increased by limiting wastage (Holst 1987).

DIAGNOSIS OF SKIN DISEASE

The ideal approach to the diagnosis of skin disease is a logical progression from history, to an overall clinical examination of the goat, to a detailed examination of the skin, and finally to confirmatory testing or diagnosis by response to therapy. The experienced clinician often performs these steps subconsciously and in an abbreviated fashion. For instance, if contagious ecthyma has been diagnosed on the farm in past years and now three otherwise sleek and healthy kids have proliferative scabs restricted to the lips and muzzle, the prior probability that these kids also have contagious ecthyma is so high that no additional testing is justified. On the other hand, when the skin disease is unusual, chronic, or refractory to initial therapy, the entire sequence should be followed for best results.

History

Historical information to gather includes details on feeding and management, health history of the affected animals, date when signs were first noticed, and any apparent spread to others in the herd. It is also important to determine if there has been any contact, however brief, with goats or other ruminants from other farms, and what treatments have already been applied with what results (Jackson 1986).

Clinical Signs of Skin Disease

A reasonably short differential diagnosis list can usually be generated if close attention is paid to primary lesions (those directly reflecting the underlying disease). Primary lesions include papules, vesicles, pustules, and nodules. Secondary lesions such as scales, crusts, and alopecia are often the result of self-trauma or superimposed bacterial infections. Secondary lesions are less helpful for making a diagnosis, but may suggest the need for symptomatic therapy. Subcutaneous lesions are discussed in Chapter 3.

Papules

A papule (pimple) is a circumscribed solid mass less than 1 cm in diameter that is usually elevated and erythematous. Follicular papules suggest bacterial, fungal, or parasitic infection whereas papules without a hair follicle at the center are typical of allergy and ectoparasites. A large flat-topped lesion, usually arising from confluent papules, is termed a plaque.

Vesicles and Pustules

A vesicle is a papule-shaped fluctuant elevation containing serum. Vesicles are transient and suggest autoimmune, irritant, or viral etiologies. A pustule is a pus-filled vesicle and indicates infection if follicular in orientation but may be autoimmune (pemphigus) if non-follicular. Demodicosis is a common pustular disease in goats. Pox lesions (contagious ecthyma, capripox) follow a typical progression from papule, to vesicle, to pustule, to a crust or proliferative lesion.

Hyperkeratosis

Hyperkeratosis is an increased thickness of the stratum corneum. The term is often used in place of the more precise term orthokeratotic (anuclear) hyperkeratosis. Parakeratotic hyperkeratosis (often called parakeratosis) differs in that nuclei remain in the keratinized layer of the skin. Both of these conditions are common and nondiagnostic histologic findings in chronic skin diseases of many sorts. Diffuse parakeratosis suggests ectoparasitisms, seborrhea, zinc responsive disease, dermatophytosis, and dermatophilosis (Scott 1988). During physical examination, hyperkeratosis is used to refer to accumulations of adherent keratinized material.

Scales and Crusts

Scales (squames, flakes) are loose fragments of stratum corneum. Admixture with sebaceous and apocrine secretion makes the scales yellowish, greasy, and adherent. Crusts are solid adherent combinations of materials such as serum, blood, pus, keratin, microorganisms, and medications. They indicate that exudation has occurred and thus have multiple causes. Close examination (crust biopsy), however, may reveal diagnostic clues such as dermatophyte hyphae, *Dermatophilus*, or many acantholytic keratinocytes (pemphigus complex). Crusts are said to be pallisading when layers of keratin and exudate alternate, as is common in dermatophilosis and dermatophytosis. Bacterial colonies are to be expected in all crusts, whatever the cause, and have no diagnostic significance.

Alopecia

Spontaneous hair loss occasionally occurs in Angoras and more often in crossbreds, mainly at the end of winter. Shearing at an inappropriate time is thought to increase the risk of hair loss. Nutritional deficiencies or imbalances (such as high calcium with low zinc) have also been incriminated (van der Westhuysen et al. 1988). There are anecdotal reports that hair loss and scaling along the dorsal spine of adult goats resolve when an organic zinc supplement is added to the concentrate portion of the ration. Periorbital alopecia (with mild scaling) is often prominent in vitamin E or selenium responsive dermatosis and alopecic exfoliative dermatitis. There are also anecdotal reports of almost complete hair loss (early shedding) in dairy does that have been subjected to photoperiod manipulation for out-of-season breeding. Partial alopecia (hypotrichosis) is a nonspecific secondary lesion. Alopecia can be induced by self excoriation when pruritus is present or can be the result of grooming by pen mates (Figure 2.3).

Pruritus

Pruritus, or the semblance of itching, frequently leads to excoriations and other secondary lesions. If pruritus is severe, special consideration is given to the

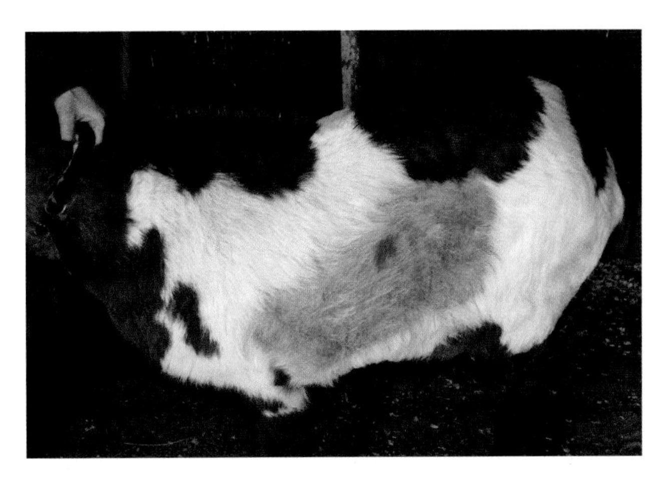

Figure 2.3. Alopecia on the side of a wether caused by grooming by its pen mate, a white-tail deer. (Courtesy Dr. M.C. Smith.)

possibility of sarcoptic or chorioptic mange. Other conditions that may be pruritic include lice, fleas, hypersensitivity to other insects such as *Culicoides*, zinc deficiency, pemphigus, and photosensitization. Occasionally, bacterial or fungal dermatitis is mildly pruritic. If vertically oriented linear excoriations develop, migration of *Parelaphostrongylus tenuis* through the spinal cord or dorsal nerve roots should be considered. Acute pruritus in a goat that dies very soon after clinical signs are noted is suggestive of pseudorabies (Baker et al. 1982). Extreme pruritus but with a longer clinical course has been reported in a single goat with confirmed rabies (Tarlatzis 1954). Pruritus was reported as a clinical sign in 11 of 20 goats in Great Britain with scrapie (Wooldridge and Wood 1991) and in more than 80% of 500 goats developing scrapie in Italy after infection via a contaminated contagious agalactia vaccine (Capucchio et al. 2001).

Erythema

Erythema, or reddening of the skin, occurs in many acute disease conditions and is thus not diagnostic. It is an early sign in photosensitization. When a chronic disease condition also has crusting and alopecia, response to therapy may be difficult to judge. Subsidence of a previously prominent erythema suggests improvement, even before hair regrowth is noted.

Pigmentary Changes

Few skin diseases in goats are associated with pigmentary changes. Decoloration of hair might occur with copper deficiency because a copper-containing enzyme is necessary for melanin production. Affected Toggenburg goats and repigmentation with copper supplementation have been reported (Lazarro 2007). Light-skinned Saanen goats normally develop large irregular areas of black pigmentation when exposed to sunlight. The color fades with confinement away from the sun.

Absence of Skin

Cutaneous asthenia, a congenital skin defect seen in sheep where the skin is abnormally fragile and easily torn, has apparently not been reported in goats. There is an anecdotal report of epitheliogenesis imperfecta, where a portion of the epidermis is absent, in a pygmy goat (Konnersman 2005b).

Body Localization as an Aid to Diagnosis

The entire body surface should be examined. The distribution of skin lesions over the body helps to arrive at a diagnosis. Listed here are some diseases found initially or most severely on the extremities of goats. These diseases are characteristically but not invariably found in the specified locations. Lesions present only on the ventrum may result from contact dermatitis or parasite invasion. Lesions present only on nonpigmented skin may be caused by photosensitization or sunburn.

Lips, Face, and Neck

- Contagious ecthyma
- Capripox
- Peste des petits ruminants
- Bluetongue
- Staphylococcal folliculitis
- Dermatophilosis
- Dermatophytosis
- Sarcoptic mange
- Zinc deficiency
- Pemphigus foliaceus
- Protothecosis

Ears

- Dermatophilosis
- Dermatophytosis
- Sarcoptic mange
- Ear mites
- Photodermatitis
- Squamous cell carcinoma
- Frostbite
- Pemphigus foliaceus

Feet

- Contagious ecthyma
- Foot and mouth disease
- Staphylococcal folliculitis
- *Dichelobacter* infection (foot rot)
- Dermatophilosis
- Sarcoptic mange
- Chorioptic mange
- *Pelodera* dermatitis
- *Besnoitia* dermatitis
- Zinc deficiency
- Contact dermatitis
- Pemphigus foliaceus

Udder

- Contagious ecthyma
- Staphylococcal folliculitis
- Zinc deficiency
- Hyperpigmentation from exposure to sun
- Neoplasia

Perineum

- Contagious ecthyma
- Caprine herpesvirus
- Staphylococcal dermatitis
- Ticks
- Neoplasia
- Ectopic mammary gland

Clinical Laboratory Examination

Simple observation allows identification of most of the clinical signs of skin disease, and thus many conditions can be diagnosed with reasonable certainty with just the findings of a physical examination. However, the repertoire of injured skin is limited, and the same sign (such as a pustule or crust) may occur in a variety of conditions of different etiologies.

Skin Scrapings

When searching for surface-dwelling ectoparasites such as lice and nits or chorioptic mange mites, a flea comb can be used to harvest scales and crusts or hair from extensive portions of the body. The collected sample is then placed in a petri dish or ziplock plastic bag for transport to good light or even a dissecting scope. After initial visual examination, the sample next undergoes a fecal flotation procedure. Mites and eggs come to the surface with centrifugation and can thus be concentrated and separated from the debris that would otherwise obscure their presence.

Repeated, deep scrapings using a scalpel blade dipped in mineral oil are usually necessary to identify sarcoptic mange mites or their eggs. A few drops of 20% potassium hydroxide solution are added to the sample, a coverslip is applied, and clearing of debris allowed to proceed for 15 to 30 minutes before microscopic examination. Larger samples may be processed by boiling 10 minutes in 10% potassium hydroxide solution, centrifuging, and performing a sugar flotation on the sediment.

Direct microscopic examination of hair and keratin is useful for demonstrating the presence of dermatophytes. Ectothrix infections of hair shafts often can be seen if the specimen is placed in mineral oil. Clearing in potassium hydroxide solution, as for mite identification, is another option.

Bacterial Examination

Skin lesions in goats are almost invariably heavily contaminated by bacteria, including *Staphylococcus aureus*. A culture is most meaningful, then, if material is aspirated from an intact pustule, nodule, or abscess. A punch biopsy obtained after careful disinfection of the skin surface is suitable for culture if intact pus-containing structures are absent. Routine inoculation onto a blood agar plate (aerobic) and into thioglycolate broth (anaerobic) is recommended. More immediate guidance can be derived by making a direct smear of an aspirate or deep aspect of a biopsy specimen and staining with new methylene blue, Gram's, or Diff Quik® (Harleco, Gibbstown, NJ) stain. Such a preparation should reveal bacteria within neutrophils and macrophages if they are pathogenic, rather than contaminant bacteria that will be extracellular and clumped in colonies. Gram-positive branching filaments are typical of dermatophilosis.

Fungal Culture

When ringworm is suspected, hairs should be plucked from the periphery of an active lesion after swabbing the area gently with 70% alcohol solution to discourage the growth of bacteria and saprophytic fungal contaminants. Sabouraud's dextrose agar (Sab Duet®, Bacti Labs, Mountain View, CA) is routinely used. Most strains of *Trichophyton verrucosum* require thiamine for growth; this can be supplied by adding 1 to 2 ml of injectable B-complex vitamins to the culture plate, but products containing alcohol should be avoided. The cultures are incubated at 86°F (30°C) with a pan of water in the incubator to maintain adequate humidity. Cultures should be checked every day for thirty days. Standard texts should be consulted for identification of fungal isolates (Scott 1988).

Biopsy for Histology

A biopsy should be performed if a skin disease appears to be unusual or severe and especially if there has been no response after three weeks of initial therapy.

Several areas are selected as having typical or primary lesions and marked by drawing a circle with a felt-tipped pen. The skin is prepared by clipping hair and injecting lidocaine subcutaneously at each chosen location. The skin must never be scrubbed. In very small kids, dilution of the lidocaine to 1% or 0.5% may be advisable. A 6-mm punch (Baker/Cummins, Miami, FL) is used to cut out a full thickness skin sample, which should be blotted flat, dermis side down, onto a small piece of a tongue depressor. The skin specimen quickly adheres to the wood; it can then be dropped upside down into a vial of 10% buffered formalin, where the wood will keep it suspended in the preservative. The skin defect is closed with absorbable suture. Consideration should be given to the tetanus vaccination status of the animal and tetanus antitoxin or toxoid given if indicated.

The testing laboratory should be consulted if electron microscopic examination is required (as for pox). Glutaraldehyde is usually the preferred fixative.

Immunofluorescence Testing

An autoimmune skin disorder (pemphigus foliaceus) may be suspected from clinical signs or after routine histologic examination of a skin biopsy specimen. If confirmation with direct immunofluorescence testing is desired, a new skin sample (with intact vesicles and pustules) should be procured and fixed with Michel's fixative, which is best obtained from the laboratory that will perform the testing. Glucocorticoids should not be administered for at least three weeks before testing to avoid false negative results (Scott 1988). Diffuse intercellular deposition of immunoglobulin is found in caprine pemphigus.

ETIOLOGIC DIAGNOSES

Readers who desire a more exhaustive reference list for any of the conditions described below should consult D.W. Scott's Large Animal Dermatology textbook (1988). Several review papers also discuss dermatologic diseases of goats (Smith 1981, 1983; Mullowney and Baldwin 1984; Scott et al. 1984a, 1984b; Manning et al. 1985; Jackson 1986) and many are illustrated in a recent text (Scott 2007).

VIRAL DISEASES

Contagious ecthyma and capripox viruses cause prominent skin lesions in goats. Virus infections involving other body systems also may have cutaneous manifestations. Warts (cutaneous papillomas) in goats have not been proven to be of viral origin and are discussed under neoplastic conditions.

Contagious Ecthyma

Contagious ecthyma is a contagious, zoonotic disease of goats and sheep (and camelids) that has several alternative names, including orf, soremouth, scabby mouth, and contagious pustular dermatitis. It has worldwide distribution.

Etiology and Epidemiology

The cause is an epitheliotropic parapoxvirus that enters the goat through skin abrasions (Mayr and Büttner 1990). The virus replicates in proliferating keratinocytes in the damaged epidermis (McKeever et al. 1988) and then causes a primary viremia to lymph nodes, bone marrow, and liver. In some cases, the virus then becomes generalized, with a second viremic phase, and spreads to the head, extremities, udder, genitals, lungs, and liver (Mayr and Büttner 1990). The morbidity in young kids often approaches 100%, while mortality from starvation and secondary infections may be as high as 20% (Van Tonder 1975) but is usually much lower.

Scabs that fall to the ground during resolution of lesions have long been incriminated as the source of infection to other animals months or even years later (McKeever and Reid 1986), and this is indeed possible if the environment remains dry. More recently, persistently infected carrier sheep, some of which are asymptomatic, have been demonstrated to be an important source of contagion (Lewis 1996). Presumably carrier goats also occur, and infection can be activated by stress (Mayr and Büttner 1990).

Clinical Signs

The incubation period is three to eight days (Mayr and Büttner 1990). Papules progress rapidly to vesicles, pustules, and scabs. Crusty, proliferative lesions typically form on the lips but can also affect the face, ears, coronary band, scrotum, teats, or vulva. In one outbreak, where exposure presumably occurred in contaminated pens at a show, lesions occurred on the neck, chest, and flanks of seven goats rather than on the lips or teats (Coates and Hoff 1990). In another case report, lesions were most common on haired skin of adult goats and the first crusty scabs noticed were on the caudal aspect of the hind legs (Moriello and Cooley 2001). The scabs frequently harbor secondary bacteria (such as staphylococci) or even screwworm maggots (Boughton and Hardy 1934). Sometimes large masses of granulation tissue develop under the scabs. Lesions regress in three or four weeks.

Most adult goats with lesions on the lips (Figure 2.4) continue to eat and milk well. Occasional goats, especially young kids exposed to other diseases or management deficiencies, will develop generalized lesions or severe secondary bacterial infections. Lesions on the teats of milking animals may compromise the health of the sphincter and predispose to bacterial mastitis. Associated pain may cause the doe to reject nursing efforts by its kid.

Severe generalized and persistent proliferative lesions have been seen in Boer goats and their crosses in the United States (Figure 2.5). Draining lymph nodes are markedly enlarged in these animals, and thymic atrophy is often present. Preliminary research has not proven whether this variation represents a viral strain difference or a difference in immune

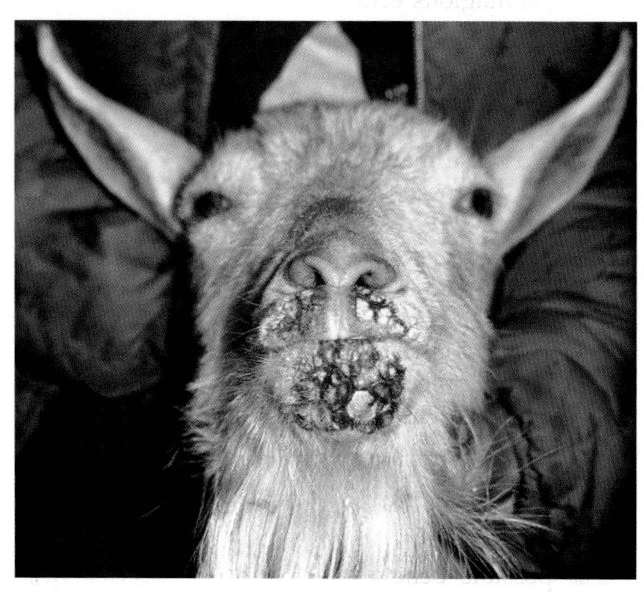

Figure 2.4. Healing crusts from contagious ecthyma on the muzzle of a mature doe. One large scab has fallen off, leaving healthy skin beneath. (Courtesy Dr. M.C. Smith.)

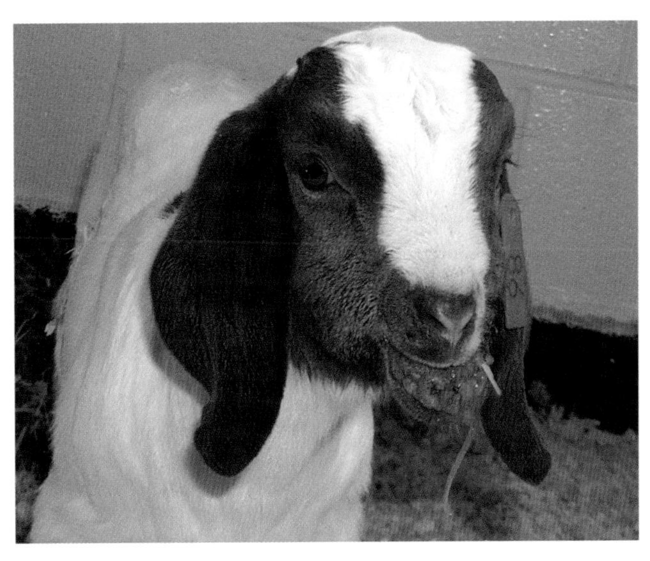

Figure 2.5. Severe contagious ecthyma lesions on the gums of a Boer kid. (Courtesy Dr. M.C. Smith.)

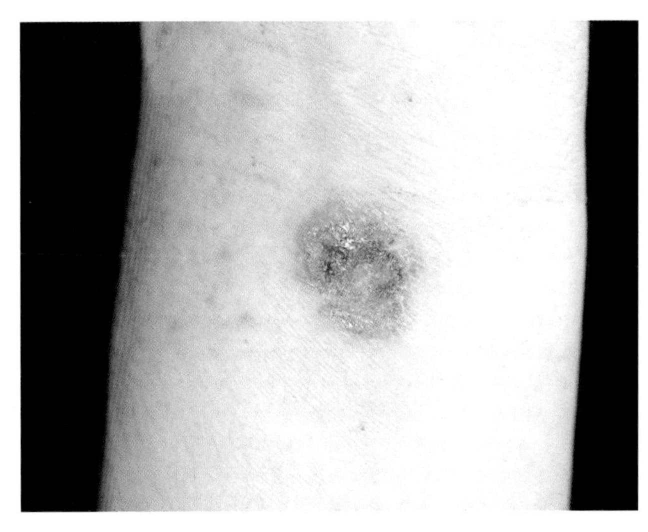

Figure 2.6. Orf (contagious ecthyma) lesion on the author's wrist. (Courtesy Dr. M.C. Smith.)

response of the affected Boer goats (de la Concha-Bermejillo et al. 2003; Guo et al. 2003). Close examination of many sheep and goats with a more typical presentation of contagious ecthyma often reveals a mild lymphadenopathy.

Diagnosis

Diagnosis is usually based on clinical signs alone, although electron microscopy or immunologic techniques to demonstrate antigen in scabs or serology could be used for confirmation or to rule out capripox infection (Robinson and Balassu 1981). In lambs experiencing contagious ecthyma, serum antibodies often do not appear until after reexposure (Mayr and Büttner 1990). Similarly, rural physicians usually make the diagnosis in their human patients on clinical signs alone, but urban dermatologists lacking experience with the disease may insist on biopsy for histologic or electron microscopic examination (Gill et al. 1990; Green et al. 2006). Skin biopsies of ruminants reveal ballooning degeneration of keratinocytes and eosinophilic cytoplasmic inclusions (Robinson and Balassu 1981; Scott 2007), although the inclusions are not always detectable (Housawi et al. 1993). The crusts consist of multiple layers of necrotic cellular debris and neutrophils. Histopathology helps to distinguish contagious ecthyma from the convalescent stages of peste des petits ruminants.

Therapy

The possible beneficial effects of treatment must be weighed against the danger of zoonotic infection (Figure 2.6). Any person handling an affected goat should wear gloves. Numerous products have been used topically, with anecdotal reports of faster healing. However, these products have been used with minimal consideration of meat and milk residues. These include kerosene mixed with lard, penetrating oil spray (WD-40®), and bismuth subsalicylate (Pepto-Bismol®). Systemic antibiotics are indicated if secondary bacterial infections are severe. An udder salve is indicated to keep scabs on the teats pliable. If painful, proliferative lesions within a kid's mouth cause feeding to decrease, the kid could be anesthetized and subjected to debridement (electrocautery after spray cryotherapy). This approach has been used in lambs with good results (Meynink et al. 1987).

Vaccination

Commercially available vaccines often are unattenuated live virus preparations (basically ground-up scabs) or are tissue culture strains, although the level of protection afforded by the latter appears to vary with the strain (Pye 1990). An autogenous vaccine can be made by crushing, in saline, a few grams of scabs between two spoons or with a mortar and pestle. The suspension is filtered through cheesecloth and a few drops of antibiotic solution such as penicillin/streptomycin are added to control bacteria (Bath et al. 2005). The skin in a hairless, protected area is lightly scarified and the virus suspension is rubbed in. Sites for vaccination include the inside of the ear pinna, the underside of the tail, or the axilla. Avoid the medial aspect of the thigh, because the infection can be spread to the lips by chewing and to the udder and teats by direct contact (Lewis 1996). Scabs appearing at the vaccination site in one to three days indicate a "take." Monitoring this reaction as evidence of continued vaccine viability permits owners to economize by freezing leftover vaccine for later use. If some animals in the herd develop vaccination scabs but others do not, a pre-existing immunity is probably responsible for absence of a take.

Where a newer, parenteral vaccine is available, subcutaneous vaccination with a live cell culture vaccine avoids postvaccinal disease or excretion of the virus. Use of this vaccine every six to twelve months has been recommended in noninfected herds, and in the face of an outbreak (Mayr and Büttner 1990).

In countries where capripox virus exists, vaccinating goats for capripox sometimes provides solid immunity against contagious ecthyma, whereas vaccination or natural infection with the contagious ecthyma virus provides no protection against capripox (Sharma and Bhatia 1958).

There are several controversies associated with vaccination. The first is whether to recommend vaccination in a herd that is not endemically infected. The vaccine, because it is unattenuated, will introduce the disease to such a herd. In herds in which buying or showing of goats occurs regularly, vaccination prevents the occurrence of an outbreak during the show season or in milking animals. It is important to vaccinate at least six weeks before the show season so that vaccine scabs will be gone before the first show. (Presumably this procedure would increase the prevalence of subclinical carriers at shows and thereby increase the risk to unvaccinated animals in attendance.) When soremouth has appeared on the premises, it may be desirable to vaccinate all as yet unaffected goats to limit the duration of the outbreak. A program of vaccination for all young kids often in conjunction with annual revaccination of late pregnant adults is then established. Disinfection of the pens after all lesions have cleared is recommended if the owner chooses not to follow a routine vaccination program. Suitable disinfectants include 5% creolin solution, formalin, detergents, and commercially available virucidal disinfectants (Mayr and Büttner 1990).

The occurrence of colostral immunity in vaccinated animals is disputed (Robinson and Balassu 1981). French enterprises that assemble kids from many sources, however, have found it advisable to pay a premium for kids from vaccinated dams. This is because vaccination of the dam seems to be more effective than vaccination of kids at birth in preventing adverse effects of the disease on the quality of kid skins (Faure 1988). In an experimental study in Mexico, kids born to dams vaccinated (virulent vaccine) in late pregnancy were challenged by skin scarification with virulent virus. Kids younger than forty-five days old resisted challenge, whereas kids older than forty-five days developed characteristic lesions (Perez 1989).

Work with sheep has suggested that vaccinating at the time of drying off is preferable to vaccinating later in pregnancy when lambs are to be raised by the ewes. Lymphocytes migrating to the udder at the end of lactation produce antibodies in the milk that may protect the lips and mouth of nursing lambs (Le Jan et al. 1978).

Capripox

The malignant pox diseases of sheep, goats, and cattle are not host-specific, although they show host preferences. Strains can be distinguished by restriction endonucleases but not by several serologic tests (Black 1986). Currently all strains are included in the Capripox genus of poxvirus.

Etiology and Pathogenesis

Capripoxviruses are distinct from parapoxviruses. They are acid-labile and sensitive to lipid solvents. Malignant sheep and goat pox infections occur in the Middle East, Far East, and Africa (Davies 1981). A benign form of goat pox has been reported from California (Renshaw and Dodd 1978) and Scandinavia (Bakos and Brag 1957) but the agents involved were not confirmed to be capripox viruses (Committee on Foreign Animal Diseases 1998). Skin lesions and scabs are major sources of virus. The virus resists desiccation and may survive in scabs for at least three months. Transmission is often through skin abrasions or by inhalation, with an incubation period of three to eight days. Viremia occurs, and the virus is carried to other sites in the skin, regional nodes, spleen, kidney, and lungs. The virus is excreted from skin lesions and in nasal exudates and milk. Night herding (congregating herds at night for protection) and stabling favor spread of the disease. Wild ungulates are not thought to serve as reservoirs.

Clinical Signs

The severity of signs varies with the strain of capripox. Young animals are most severely affected. Early signs include rhinitis, conjunctivitis, and pyrexia 104° to 107.6°F (40° to 42°C). The animals stand with arched back and are anorectic. Cutaneous lesions (reddish macules and papules, 0.5 to 1.5 cm diameter, Figure 2.7) and lesions on the external nares and lips and within the mouth appear one or two days later. Skin lesions persist for four to six weeks. In some outbreaks, vesicular lesions of the skin coalesce. Oral lesions on the tongue and gums tend to ulcerate. Regional lymph nodes may be enlarged up to eight times their normal size (Committee on Foreign Animal Diseases 1998). Animals that die frequently have lesions in the lungs and alimentary tract.

The hair is erect over skin lesions, the skin is thickened, and crusts of exuded serum form on the surface. Healing may leave an ulcer and then a permanent scar after the full skin thickness sloughs. Damage to hides causes important economic losses.

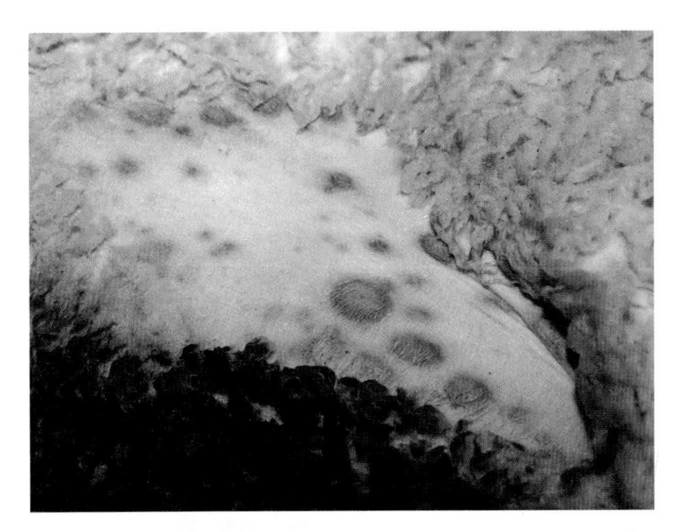

Figure 2.7. Early macules of capripox infection on the skin of an experimentally infected sheep. (Courtesy National Veterinary Services Laboratories, Ames, Iowa.)

When the disease first enters a susceptible flock, morbidity may be more than 75%, and 50% of affected animals die. Mortality may increase to 100% in kids or when superimposed on other virus infections such as peste des petits ruminants. The morbidity rate is lower in endemic flocks. Some animals convert serologically without development of clinical signs. European breeds are generally more severely affected than native breeds (Karim 1983; Kitching 1986).

There is also a nodular form ("stonepox") in sheep and goats that resembles lumpy skin disease of cattle (also caused by a capripox) (Patnaik 1986). Vesicles and pustules are absent and there is no cross-immunity with more typical strains of goat pox or with contagious ecthyma. The virus is present in blood and skin throughout the course of the disease, which is often fatal (Haddow and Idnani 1948).

In the benign goat pox form, vesicles and pustules develop from papules on the lips and udder (and sometimes on the perineum and inside of the thigh). Pock lesions heal in five to eight weeks, leaving behind permanent scars.

Goat pox, like contagious ecthyma, has been considered to be a zoonotic disease (Bakos and Brag 1957; Sawhney et al. 1972), but more recent authors dispute this (Committee on Foreign Animal Diseases 1998).

Diagnosis

Capripox is most likely to be confused with contagious ecthyma because lesions may be limited to the lips, oral mucous membranes, or udder. Electron microscopy (Hajer et al. 1988) and serologic tests (such as immunodiffusion and serum neutralization) readily differentiate capripox from the parapoxvirus of contagious ecthyma. Histopathology reveals large eosinophilic intracytoplasmic inclusions, vasculitis, thrombosis, and necrosis (Davies 1981).

Control

Import restrictions covering animals and animal products from endemic areas are required to avoid introduction of this disease to non-infected regions. Quarantine and slaughter of diseased and contact animals would be recommended if introduction occurred. A carrier state has not been documented to occur.

Prophylactic vaccination reduces morbidity in endemic (often nomadic pastoral) regions. Most trials have shown excellent cross-protection with various strains of sheep and goat pox (Davies 1981). Live, attenuated vaccines (using a mild strain) are preferred but difficult to distribute (Kitching 1986). An experimental subunit vaccine reduced the severity of signs without risking introduction of the disease (Carn et al. 1994). A recombinant capripoxvirus vaccine has been produced that protects goats against peste des petits ruminants as well as against capripox (Romero et al. 1995). Use of autogenous vaccines may increase the incidence of disease (Das et al. 1978). Contagious ecthyma vaccines do not protect against goat pox.

Miscellaneous Virus Infections

As already discussed under the heading of pruritus, goats with rabies or pseudorabies may show skin lesions that result from severe pruritus. These conditions are discussed in Chapter 5. Scrapie in goats (also discussed under neurologic diseases in Chapter 5) may be pruritic, as demonstrated by biting and rubbing at the legs, flanks, lumbar region, and neck, and by alopecia in these areas (usually without scab formation). The clinical course of scrapie may last three to four months (Hadlow 1961; Brotherston et al. 1968; Harcourt and Anderson 1974).

Peste des Petits Ruminants

Peste des petits ruminants (PPR) is a morbillivirus infection that causes serious losses in sheep and goats throughout its range (Committee on Foreign Animal Diseases 1998). The major clinical signs of stomatitis, enteritis, and pneumonia are described in the appropriate chapters. During early stages of the disease, the lips are edematous and brown scabs cover eroded and ulcerated epithelium. Goats that survive the acute phase of the disease may develop labial scabs that persist up to fourteen days; histologically, acanthosis and hyperkeratosis are evident. Necrotic epithelium is infiltrated with degenerating neutrophils. There is no papilliform proliferation or ballooning degeneration typical of contagious ecthyma, although lesions are grossly similar (Whitney et al. 1967; Abraham et al. 2005). Syncytial multinucleated giant cells and eosinophilic cytoplasmic inclusions may be seen in the epithelium (Çam et al. 2005). Goats that are vaccinated with inactivated vaccine (Nduaka and Ihemelandu 1975) or that are re-exposed to PPR after recovery from the virus also develop labial scabs that heal in about ten days (Ihemelandu et al. 1985). In these animals, histology reveals proliferation of macrophages and lymphocytes, suggesting an immune response.

Bluetongue

Bluetongue is a disease of sheep and cattle caused by an orbivirus that has at least twenty-four serotypes and is spread by *Culicoides* insects. Signs in sheep include fever, stomatitis, coronitis, and birth of lambs with congenital brain anomalies. Goats are susceptible to bluetongue in that viremia and fever occur and antibodies develop (Luedke and Anakwenze 1972; Backx et al. 2007), but overt clinical signs are rarely seen or described in goats in the United States. During an outbreak in cattle in Israel, two Saanen goats were found with swollen lips and marked salivation (Komarov and Goldsmit 1951). During the recent outbreak of bluetongue in northwestern Europe, a small number of goats developed edema of the lips and head, small scabs on the nose and lips suggestive of mild contagious ecthyma, and erythema of the udder skin (Dercksen et al. 2007). Goats may serve as a natural reservoir for the bluetongue virus (Erasmus 1975). Virus isolation and serology help to distinguish bluetongue from foot and mouth disease, rinderpest, and peste des petits ruminants. Bluetongue is discussed in detail in Chapter 10.

Caprine Herpesvirus

Experimental inoculation of kids with a herpesvirus isolate has produced vesicles, ulcers, and crusts on the muzzle and feet (Waldvogel et al. 1981). Ulcers also occurred in the mouth, esophagus, rumen, and intestines. In one naturally occurring outbreak, numerous foci of necrosis and hemorrhage were found in the skin of a single kid (Mettler et al. 1979). Any histologic finding of acidophilic intranuclear inclusion bodies in epithelial cells suggests the possibility of herpesvirus infection. The disease is discussed in Chapters 12 and 13.

Foot and Mouth Disease (FMD)

The picornavirus that causes FMD is a very important and exceedingly contagious disease of cattle in South America, Europe, Africa, and Asia, but is currently absent from the United States, Canada, and Australia. Signs in cattle include fever, stomatitis with vesicles and bullae, anorexia, agalactia, and a very prolonged convalescence. The disease in sheep and goats is usually mild, and only important in that these animals and meat from them may transmit the disease to cattle. However, during outbreaks of foot and mouth disease, other (often idiopathic) oral lesions can cause great concern to regulatory authorities, at least in sheep (Watson 2004). Lameness is often the most pronounced clinical sign in goats; vesicles or bleeding ulcers may be found in the interdigital space or at the coronary band (McVicar and Sutmoller 1968; Mishra and Ghei 1983). Goats are routinely vaccinated in endemic regions. The disease is discussed in detail in Chapter 4.

Vesicular Stomatitis

Vesicular stomatitis is a rhabdovirus disease primarily affecting horses, cattle, and swine, and limited to the Western Hemisphere. Typical signs in these species are oral vesicles and ulcers, salivation, coronitis, and teat lesions. Regulatory officials should be notified so that the disease may be differentiated from foot and mouth disease. The epidemiology is poorly understood, but may include insect vectors such as sand flies (*Lutzomyia*) and black flies (*Simulidae*) (Committee on Foreign Animal Diseases 1998). Goats are considered to be resistant, but according to unpublished reports, vesicular stomatitis in goats has been accompanied by vesicles at the commissures of the lips, which must be differentiated from early lesions of contagious ecthyma.

BACTERIAL DISEASES

Secondary bacteria, especially staphylococci, commonly invade almost any skin lesion on a goat. Thus, other etiologies should be ruled out before assuming that bacteria isolated from the surface of a lesion are causative. Other organisms, such as *Corynebacterium pseudotuberculosis* and *Dermatophilus congolensis*, are usually significant if present. Foot rot, an interdigital dermatitis caused by *Dichelobacter* and *Fusobacterium* spp., is discussed in Chapter 4.

Staphylococcal Dermatitis

Staphylococcal skin infections are common in goats and may be primary or secondary. The bacteria are also normal skin flora. In one Spanish study, 346 strains of staphylococci were isolated from axillary skin or udder of 133 healthy goats, and 21% of these isolates were coagulase-positive (*S. aureus* and *S. hyicus*) (Valle et al. 1991).

Etiology

Impetigo is a superficial pustular dermatitis that does not involve hair follicles. Staphylococcal folliculitis is an infection and inflammation of hair follicles (Scott 1988). The species involved often has not been reported. Staphylococcal species isolated from goats with skin disease include *S. intermedius*, *S. aureus*, *S. chromogenes*, and *S. hyicus* (Scott 1988; Andrews and

Lamport 1997; Mahanta et al. 1997). Species identification is not a good predictor of antibiotic sensitivity (Biberstein et al. 1984).

Clinical Signs and Diagnosis

The primary lesion is a nonfollicular or follicular papule that develops into a pustule. Lesions may enlarge or coalesce, discharge purulent or serosanguinous exudate, and become encrusted (furunculosis, Scott 2007). Alopecia and scaling are prominent in the chronic or healing stage. Multiple small pustules of impetigo frequently appear on the teats and udder (Figure 14.3) or perineum and underside of the tail. Because these pustules may be preceded by vesicles and followed by scabs, they may be confused with lesions of contagious ecthyma (Smith 1981). Direct smears show degenerate neutrophils with phagocytosed cocci (Scott 2007). When lesions remain localized they are relatively benign and self-limiting, except that lesions on the teats predispose to staphylococcal mastitis. Fly bites on the udder (fly worry) are said to resemble a staphylococcal infection but to be more pruritic (Matthews 1999).

In some goats, the infection becomes general, involving the skin of the abdomen, inner thighs, and even the neck and back. Other distributions are possible, especially if the staphylococci are secondary to another condition, such as chorioptic mange. Periocular alopecia and crusts comprise yet another possible manifestation (Scott 1988). Confusion with mycotic infections or nutritional deficiencies is possible.

A presumptive diagnosis is often based on inspection alone. Gram stains and cultures document the presence of staphylococci, while evaluation of skin biopsy specimens should help to rule out other diseases that might have been primary and still require therapy.

Treatment and Prevention

Localized lesions on the udder may be washed with an iodophor or chlorhexidine shampoo, dried, and then coated with an antiseptic or antibiotic ointment. Affected does should be milked last. Single service paper towels and attention to hand washing by the milker decrease the risk of spread to other does. Rubber gloves protect against transmission of infection to humans. Similar treatment of lesions around the tail is possible, but these seem to be less important and frequently heal spontaneously.

If a generalized infection is suspected, culture of the organism and determination of antibiotic sensitivity are recommended. Systemic antibiotic treatment (one to two weeks of therapy) may start with penicillin, pending results of sensitivity testing. As the concern over methicillin-resistant staphylococci increases in both veterinary and human medicine, it is very important for the practitioner to remember that many of the antibiotics used to control these infections in other species are forbidden by law in all sheep and goats in the United States, because of their status as food animals. Thus, no matter what the laboratory reports for a sensitivity pattern, chloramphenicol, fluoroquinolones such as enrofloxacin, and glycopeptides such as vancomycin are absolutely forbidden in all goats.

Autogenous bacterins may be tried for control of chronic or epizootic infections (Scott et al. 1984a), but bacterins have not received scientific evaluation in caprine dermatology.

Dermatophilosis

Dermatophilosis, also known as streptothricosis, is a common skin infection in goats worldwide. Cattle, sheep, horses, various wildlife species, and humans are also affected (Stewart 1972; Hyslop 1980).

Etiology

Dermatophilus congolensis is a Gram-positive, pleomorphic, facultative anaerobic actinomycete. It produces motile zoospores which invade the skin.

Pathogenesis

Dermatophilus congolensis may survive in soil or in dust on an animal's hair coat during dry weather. It is introduced into the epidermis following injuries of any sort, including those caused by tick bites and thorny vegetation. Its life cycle is activated by moisture (Bida and Dennis 1976). Outbreaks often occur during periods of heavy rain or high humidity (Mémery and Thiéry 1960; Yeruham et al. 2003).

Clinical Signs

Several localizations of the disease have been reported. Ears are commonly involved, especially in young kids (Larsen 1987). Tiny wart-like scabs first appear on the inner hairless surface of the ear pinna. They are easily rubbed off, exposing dry, circular, light-colored areas beneath. Raised scabs with matted hairs form on the external portions of the ears and are more tightly attached (Figure 2.8). The lesions are nonpruritic and benign and last two to three months in kids if not treated (Munro 1978).

Other affected areas of the body include the nose, muzzle, feet, scrotum, and underside of the tail (Mémery 1960; Yeruham et al. 2003; Loria et al. 2005; Scott 2007). These areas of skin frequently are exposed to moisture or mild abrasion from vegetation. Thick proliferative crusts may be mistaken for lesions of contagious ecthyma (sore mouth) (Tiddy and Hemi 1986). In fact, the simultaneous presence of both diseases has been reported in splenectomized kids (Munz 1969, 1976) and in Yaez goats, a cross between domestic goats and wild ibex (Yeruham et al. 1991). The dry

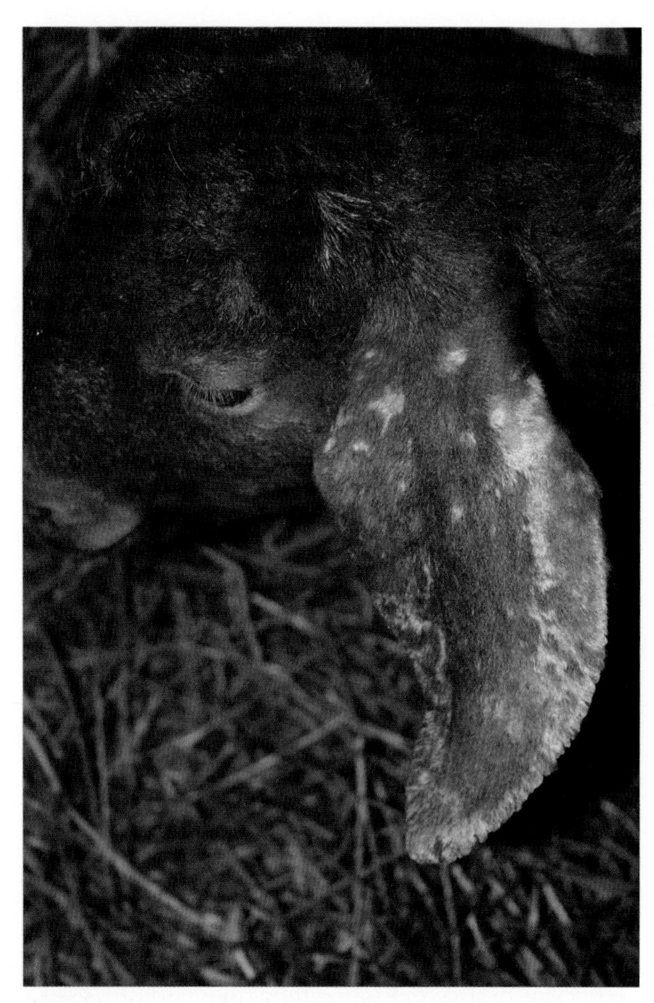

Figure 2.8. Dry scabs typical of dermatophilosis on the external surface and margin of the ear. (Courtesy Dr. M.C. Smith.)

crusts, scaling, and alopecia of healing or chronic lesions resemble ringworm. Secondary bacterial infections (e.g., staphylococci, corynebacteria, *Fusobacterium necrophorum*) are to be expected and may lead to pruritus or pain. Sometimes the entire dorsum of the goat is involved with lesions clinically resembling rain scald in horses; continuous exposure to wet weather presumably is an important etiologic factor (Bida and Dennis 1976; Scott et al. 1984a). Damage to hides can be extensive. Suppurative lymphadenitis has been reported in Beetal goats from which *D. congolensis* was demonstrated by smear and culture (Singh and Murty 1978).

Diagnosis

The diagnosis can be confirmed in several ways. When lesions are moist, an impression smear of the underside of a scab reveals Gram-positive branching filaments either unsegmented or in railroad track arrangements of two to eight parallel rows of cocci (Scott 2007). Giemsa or Diff Quik® stain may also be used. The organisms in smears also fluoresce under ultraviolet light after staining with acridine orange (Mathieson 1991). Fluorescent antibody techniques have been used for rapid identification of the organism in smears of exudate (Pier et al. 1964). In dry lesions, skin biopsy is necessary to demonstrate the organism. In addition to superficial exudate, there is hyperkeratosis and infiltration of the epidermis and hair follicles with neutrophils. Bacterial filaments in the biopsy sample are periodic acid Schiff (PAS) positive (Loria et al. 2005).

Culture of the organism by a diagnostic laboratory will also confirm the diagnosis, but this is best done under microaerophilic conditions with increased carbon dioxide (Scott 1988). Scabs are ground up in saline and cultured at once and also after twenty-four hours at room temperature. A medium that selects for Gram-positive organisms (such as colistin-nalidixic acid medium) is helpful. Tiny gray adherent colonies composed of branched mycelia may be visible after forty-eight hours and should then be subcultured; it is common for the original plate to be rapidly overgrown by contaminants.

Several serologic tests have been used to identify antibodies against *D. congolensis*. The purpose was to potentially monitor the prevalence of exposed animals. The tests have included passive hemagglutination (which showed 23% of slaughtered goats in a Nigerian study to be seropositive) (Oyejide et al. 1984) and radial immunodiffusion (Makinde 1980).

Therapy and Prevention

Penicillin-streptomycin was commonly recommended for dermatophilosis in individual animals in the past, but this product is no longer available in the United States. Tetracycline is also effective. Where feasible, shelter from the rain and bathing (iodophors, 2% to 5% lime sulfur) and grooming to remove crusts should be recommended. Improved nutrition and control of external parasites (especially ticks) are also desirable for treatment and prevention. Cleansing thick crusts with hydrogen peroxide will help to control secondary anaerobic infections. Brushes should be disinfected before being used on other animals. Goat handlers should also be warned that people are occasionally infected with this organism. Carrier animals appear to be the reservoir for the agent, but the organism can also survive for many months in the environment. Vaccination against dermatophilosis has not been successful (Bida and Dennis 1976), and recovery does not appear to provide immunity.

Corynebacterium pseudotuberculosis

Corynebacterium pseudotuberculosis is usually associated with lymph node enlargement (caseous lymphadenitis) and is discussed in detail in Chapter 3. However, small nodules and draining tracts in the skin sometimes occur in goats (Scott 2007) and may be a source of infection to others. Diagnosis is made by culture and by skin biopsy, which reveals a tuberculoid granulomatous reaction (Scott 1988). Affected animals should be isolated or culled.

Actinobacillosis, Actinomycosis, and Protothecosis

Actinobacillosis, a suppurative to granulomatous disease of sheep caused by *Actinobacillus lignieresii*, has not been well documented in goats. Diagnosis is based on demonstration of cheese-like granules less than 1 mm in diameter in pus or by aerobic or anaerobic culture of the organism. In direct smears, club-like bodies radiate from the center of the granules and crushing reveals small Gram-negative bacilli. Rinsing and culturing the granules, rather than simply swabbing a fistulous tract, is recommended to avoid overgrowth with secondary bacteria (Scott 1988). Treatment, at least for sheep, typically involves sodium iodide (20 mg/kg of sodium iodide as a 10% solution intravenously or subcutaneously) weekly for four to five weeks and streptomycin (20 mg/kg/day) for five to seven days.

A case of pyogranulomatous dermatitis has been reported on the udder of an aged dairy goat. A diagnosis of *Actinomyces* sp. was based on the appearance of the organism in Gram stained smears and the presence of sulfur granules. Raised knot-like lesions were yellowish brown or reddish black and abscesses extended into the parenchyma of the udder. Udder amputation was the proposed therapy but the goat died first (Hotter and Buchner 1995).

A single case of pyogranulomatous dermatitis around the nares caused by a *Prototheca* sp. has been reported from a mature goat in Brazil (Macedo et al. 2008). Ulcerated nodules contributed to inspiratory dyspnea and weight loss. Oval to spherical, nonbudded, walled sporangia typical of this algal-like organism that lacks chlorophyll were demonstrated in histologic section. Treatment was not attempted, but various antifungal agents are used to treat human and canine cutaneous protothecosis.

FUNGAL DISEASES

Ringworm and other fungal infections usually occur when nutrition or environmental conditions are inadequate. Crusting, alopecic skin disease should not be assumed to be of fungal origin without laboratory confirmation.

Ringworm

Etiology

A variety of dermatophytes have been cultured from ringworm in goats. These include *Microsporum canis* and *M. gypseum*, *Trichophyton mentagrophytes*, *T. schoenleinii* and *T. verrucosum*, and *Epidermophyton floccosum* (Philpot et al. 1984; Scott 1988).

Clinical Signs and Diagnosis

Lesions in goats consist of alopecia, scaling, erythema, and crusts. They typically involve the face, external ears, neck, or limbs, and may be annular in shape (Scott 2007). Pruritus is not usual, but has been reported (Chineme et al. 1981). Microscopic examination of hairs and keratin from the periphery of an active lesion (as described above) may reveal ectothrix invasion of hair shafts. Species identification requires culture and examination of both colony and microscopic morphology.

Treatment and Prevention

Young animals (Pandey and Mahin 1980) or those living in a dark, damp, dirty environment, or those with debilitating nutritional or infectious diseases are most at risk for developing ringworm. Management changes, then, may be required to control an outbreak in goats. Most cases of dermatophytosis in large animals regress spontaneously in one to four months. Thus, although oral griseofulvin has been reported to be effective in treating ringworm in goats at 25 mg/kg/day for three weeks (Chineme et al. 1981), this expensive therapy is usually not justified (Scott 1988).

Topical treatment does reduce contamination of the environment and the risk of spread to other animals or man. People handling infected goats should take precautions to avoid contracting the infection themselves. Lime sulfur (2% to 5%), iodophors, and 0.5% sodium hypochlorite as total body sprays daily for five days and then weekly are recommended for ringworm (Scott 1988). Captan (3%) is effective (Scott 1988), but not approved in the United States for food-producing animals. Topical thiabendazole paste or iodine ointments or products for athlete's foot (tinea pedis) can be used on small lesions. All in-contact animals should also be treated, and the environment disinfected with sodium hypochlorite if possible. Pens that have previously housed young cattle with ringworm should be thoroughly disinfected before goats are introduced.

Yeast Infections

Budding yeasts are occasionally present in large numbers in samples taken from goats with alopecia, scaling, and crusting (Scott 1988). In most instances they probably represent secondary opportunists (Reuter et al. 1987). A *Malassezia* (*Pityrosporum*) species was suspected in milking goats with annular lesion on the teats and udder, based on PAS-positive organisms seen in the epidermis (Bliss 1984). A *Malassezia* species, possibly *M. pachydermatis*, was isolated from an adult goat with chronic greasy, seborrheic lesions over the trunk but sparing the extremities (Pin 2004). The animal responded rapidly to weekly chlorhexidine-containing shampoo and topical enilconazole. In a third reported case, *Malassezia slooffiae* in hyphal and yeast forms was identified in the skin of an adult Pygmy goat with a one-month history of weight loss and extensive alopecia and crusting of the body and limbs (Uzal et al. 2007). Goats with yeast infections should be evaluated for chronic wasting diseases, with special attention given to possible nutritional deficiencies (e.g., protein, trace minerals).

Miscellaneous Fungal Infections

Peyronellaea glomerata, ordinarily a saprophyte on decaying vegetation, has been isolated from hyperkeratotic ear lesions on goats (Dawson and Lepper 1970). Brown septate hyphae were abundant in the stratum corneum in skin biopsies.

Several fungal species can produce mycetomas (granulomatous subcutaneous lesions with draining sinuses and granular fungal elements) in goats (Gumaa et al. 1978; Gumaa and Abu-Samra 1981). Proliferation of the periosteum of underlying bone may be marked.

Cryptococcus neoformans, a rare cause of pneumonia and mastitis in goats, has also caused ulcerated granulomas in the skin of the head of one goat and in the nasal passage of another goat in Australia (Chapman et al. 1990). The diagnosis was made by demonstrating the oval or budding encapsulated organisms in smears, histopathology samples, or culture.

PARASITIC DISEASES

Many external parasites, including lice, ticks, and mange mites, infest goats. Each is discussed separately, but there is an extensive overlap in the realm of therapy. For the convenience of the reader, some of the chemicals effective against external parasites are listed in Table 2.1 (Scott 1988; Bowman 2003).

Table 2.1. Some chemicals used for control of external parasites of goats.

Chemical	*Concentration and form*
Amitraz (L)	0.025%–0.05% spray
Coumaphos (L)	0.25% spray, 0.5% dust
Crotoxyphos (L)	0.25%–1% spray, 2% dust
Dichlorvos (L)	0.5%–1% spray
Eprinomectin (L)	0.5–1 mg/kg pour-on
Fenvalerate	0.05% dip
Fipronil	0.29% spray (not labeled for food animals)
Ivermectin	20–40 mg/100 kg subcutaneous injection
Lime sulfur (L)	2%–5% dip
Lindane	0.06% spray, 0.03% dip
Malathion	0.5% spray, 5% dust
Methoxychlor	0.5%–1% spray/dip, 5% dust
Permethrin (L)	0.05% spray, 0.5% spot treatment
Phosmet	0.15%–0.25% spray/dip
Trichlorfon	0.2% spray/dip

Note that many of these products are not licensed for goats in most countries. Chemicals designated by (L) are generally appropriate for dairy animals. Product labels should be read for instructions and safety precautions.

Lice

All species of goat lice complete their life cycle on the host and are quite host-specific. Eggs (nits) are attached to hairs and hatch in five to eighteen days. The nymphal stages look like tiny adults; young lice mature fourteen to twenty-one days after hatching. *Bovicola (Damalinia) ovis*, the sheep louse, can become established on goats, and thus goats may be a source for reinfesting sheep during louse control programs (Hallam, 1985).

Clinical Signs and Diagnosis

Bloodsucking lice (order Anoplura) have relatively narrow heads with piercing mouth parts. Two species have been reported from goats in the United States: *Linognathus stenopsis* (females 2.75 mm long, males 2.2 mm) and *Linognathus africanus* (distinguished by bulging posterolateral margins of the head; females 2.15 mm, males 1.65 mm). They are bluish-gray and infest both Angoras and the other breeds of goats (Price and Graham 1997). Blood loss and secondary bacterial skin infections may occur in addition to pruritus. Heavy infestations may kill kids.

Biting lice (order Mallophaga) have broader chewing mouth parts. They are pale, small (1 to 2 mm) and more difficult to see. They provoke rubbing and scratching and can also bite through the hairs, resulting in alopecia and moderate to severe damage to Angora fleeces, depending on the louse numbers. The yellowish, hairy *Bovicola (Damalinia) (Holakartikos) crassipes* and the red louse *Bovicola (Damalinia) limbatus* are common on Angora goats, while *Bovicola (Damalinia) caprae* is the slightly smaller biting louse usually found on meat or dairy goats in the United States. The same goat can be infested with more than one louse species at a time (Sebei et al. 2004). Certain goats appear to have a natural resistance to biting lice, as documented during efforts to cause experimental infestations (Merrall and Brassington 1988).

Diagnosis is by physical examination and demonstration of lice or nits directly or on material collected by plucking or combing. A flea comb works well to harvest material that can be placed in a ziplock bag for later examination with a dissecting microscope or hand lens. In one study, biting lice were concentrated in the withers area (where the goat had more difficulty grooming itself) while sucking lice were more prevalent over the brisket and shoulders (Merrall and Brassington 1988). Because lice are sensitive to elevated temperatures, their location on the body may vary with air temperature and exposure to sunlight. Populations are generally higher in winter than summer.

Therapy

Numerous insecticides are effective against goat lice (Moore et al. 1959; Bowman 2003), but nits are not killed. Resistance also may develop, and has been documented for permethrins (Levot 2000) but in some instances may be the result of product failure to reach the lice (Bates et al. 2000). Label directions should be followed to avoid contamination of milk and meat. Because nits are not killed by the initial therapy, treatment should be repeated at ten- to fourteen-day intervals if possible to remove young lice before they mature. Treating before kidding helps to prevent the normally rapid transfer of lice to newborn kids. In goat breeds that are shorn, and even in dairy breeds, the best results are obtained by treatment after removal of the fleece and attached nits.

Products used include crotoxyphos (1% in water spray or 3% dust), coumaphos (0.25% in water spray or 0.5% dust), dichlorvos, and fenvalerate. Pour-ons are more convenient than sprays or dips, and dusts are preferred to dips in cold weather. Coumaphos (Konar and Ivie 1988) and fenvalerate pour-ons may cause milk contamination. Newer permethrins appear to be both safe and effective, with no milk or meat withdrawal requirements. In India, flumethrin pour-on at 1 mg/kg provided complete louse control on goats for more than six weeks (Garg et al. 1998). Eprinomectin as a pour-on would be safe for lactating goats but is not approved in the United States. Ivermectin, also unapproved, at 20 mg/100 kg subcutaneously, is efficacious against sucking but not biting lice; it should not be used in lactating dairy goats and this dose is likely to select for resistant gastrointestinal parasites (see Chapter 10). For pets and young kids, rotenone, flea powders labeled for cats, and even flea collars may be more convenient that commercial livestock preparations. Note that extralabel use of pesticides is not sanctioned in the United States and agricultural products containing rotenone are being withdrawn from the market.

Insect hormones have been used experimentally to control lice (Price and Graham 1997). Three spray treatments of 0.1% synthetic juvenile hormone at two-week intervals controlled biting lice for four months (Chamberlain and Hopkins 1971).

Fleas

Dog and cat fleas (*Ctenocephalides* spp.) sometimes infest goats in tropical regions (Obasaju and Otesile 1980, Opasina 1983) and in the United States (Konnersman 2005b). In Greece, human fleas (*Pulex irritans*) cause long-term infestations of dairy goats (Christodoulopoulos and Theodoropoulos 2003; Christodoulopoulos et al. 2006). The wingless, laterally compressed, 2- to 4-mm-long adult insects suck blood and cause local irritation. Fleas frequently leave their hosts. Eggs are laid on the goat or on the ground. Clinical signs include restlessness, rubbing and chewing, excoriations, alopecia, nonfollicular papules, and crusts. The fleas are easiest to find when the goat is restrained on its back. Anemia and weight loss may occur in young or debilitated animals (Fagbemi 1982). Peripheral eosinophilia and infiltration of the skin by eosinophils suggest that an allergy to flea saliva may be involved in severe cases (Yeruham et al. 1997). Treatments suggested for lice are also appropriate for fleas, but the environment and all mammalian hosts must be treated.

Keds

Melophagus ovinus is a wingless blood-sucking fly (six legs) that infests both sheep and goats. The parasite is 6 to 7 mm long and easily seen, resembling a tick. The entire life cycle is completed on the host in five weeks or longer. The parasite causes skin irritation and blood loss, but damage to hides may have greater economic significance. Shearing removes many keds. The insecticides used for louse control are also effective against keds.

Biting Flies, Gnats, and Mosquitoes

Black flies (Simuliidae) may attack goats in swarms in the spring in areas of running water. Insecticides work poorly for repelling these pests, and stabling during the day may provide the most relief (Gnad and Mock 2001). Stable flies (*Stomoxys calcitrans*) and horse flies and deer flies (Tabanidae) also inflict painful bites. Residual topical permethrin products will provide some relief. *Culicoides* gnats are additional bloodsucking pests that swarm in the afternoon and evening. They are reported to cause significant skin lesions on small ruminants (Gnad and Mock 2001) but these lesions are not well described. Individual animals may become hypersensitized to the saliva of the gnats. *Culicoides* gnats are important vectors for bluetongue virus and bunyaviruses. Mosquitoes take blood meals from goats, as from other mammals. Control efforts are usually directed at eliminating stagnant water.

The diagnosis of insect hypersensitivity is usually presumptive in an animal that develops seasonal pruritus and self-excoriation (Figure 2.9). If insect

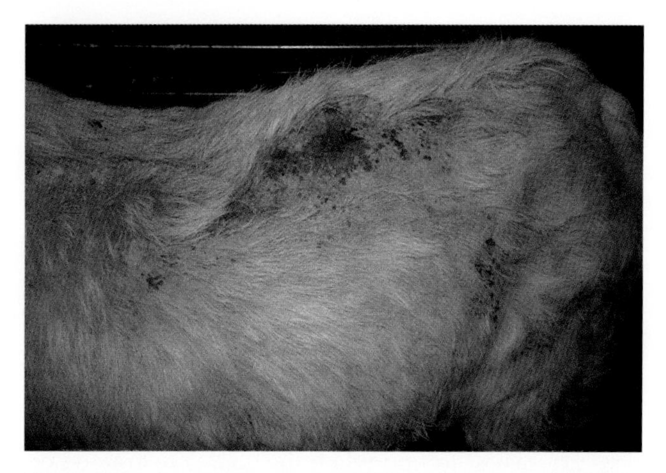

Figure 2.9. Apparent recurrent insect hypersensitivity in a buck that showed severe pruritus and self-excoriation in the early spring in New York. (Courtesy Dr. M.C. Smith.)

repellants and stabling do not control the signs, injectable dexamethasone can be used in nonpregnant goats.

Cutaneous Myiasis

The New World screwworms *Cochliomyia* (previously *Callitroga*) *hominivorax* in North, Central, and South America are the maggots of flies that must deposit their eggs in wounds or at body orifices rather than in dead carcasses. The species was eradicated from the United States in 1966 by the use of sterile males. The parasite is reportable in the United States and briefly entered Texas from Mexico in 1982; it also arrived on assorted imported animals and people in later years (Alexander 2006). One case involved a larva found on an Angora goat in Texas in 1998, following a hurricane (AVMA 1999). Shearing, dehorning, castration, and ear marking wounds and tick bites are common targets, as are the mouth and navel of newborns. As a complication to the presence of maggots in foul-smelling, pruritic lesions, toxemia or septicemia may kill the goat. Wounds should be debrided and treated with a topical insecticide such as malathion or coumaphos in ointment form. Fly repellents prevent repeat attacks, and antibiotics are indicated if the animal is systemically ill. Injectable avermectins have prevented establishment of screwworm larvae in wounds of calves (Alexander 2006). Dicyclanil, an insect growth regulator, shows promise for long-term prophylaxis of this and other forms of myiasis (Sotiraki et al. 2005).

Chrysomya bezziana is known as the Old World screwworm fly and has been documented to cause myiasis in goats on the Arabian peninsula (Spradbery et al. 1992; Abo-Shehada 2005). Although this fly has not yet been transferred to the Western Hemisphere, modern transportation certainly makes translocation possible.

Wohlfahrtia magnifica is an important cause of primary myiasis in Asia (Iran to Mongolia) and the Mediterranean area. Infestation of goats increases with age, and the body regions most commonly struck are the genitalia and the extremities (Ruiz-Martinez et al. 1991). Clinical signs include inflammation, pruritus, apathy, and weight loss (Ruiz-Martinez et al. 1987).

A variety of blowfly larvae (calliphorine myiasis) can be found in the same wounds that attract screwworms and are differentiated by close examination of larval anatomy. Bacterial activity (fleece rot, fecal contamination of skin, urine scald) also can make intact skin attractive to these flies. Foul-smelling ulcers are filled with maggots. Cleansing of the wound with a mild solution of pine oil is helpful, because most of the maggots will come out of their holes and drop to the ground. Insecticides, fly repellents, and antibiotics are applied as for screwworms.

Warbles

Przhevalskiana (*Hypoderma*) *silenus* is a warble fly that naturally infests goats in Mediterranean countries and Asia. *Hypoderma aeratum* is reported to parasitize goats in Cyprus, Crete, and Turkey, while *H. crossi* infests goats in the dry, hilly regions of India (Soulsby 1982). Recent authors have suggested that these are all one species (Otranto and Traversa, 2004). *Hypoderma bovis* and *H. lineatum* (warble flies of cattle) have not been documented to infest goats (Colwell and Otranto 2006).

Pathogenesis and Clinical Signs

Adult *P. silenus* flies lay eggs on the hairs of the legs and chest in spring. It is believed that the larvae migrate by a direct subcutaneous route to the back rather than passing through the esophagus or spinal cord (Otranto and Puccini 2000). First-stage larvae appear under the cutaneous trunci muscle, which becomes necrotic and infiltrated by neutrophils. The larvae penetrate the overlying muscle and skin and molt into the second instar. Larval debris and cellular infiltrates accumulate, and a wall of granulation tissue forms around each larva (Cheema 1977), which is typically 10 to 12 mm long. Third-stage larvae drop to the ground to pupate. As many as 150 larvae have been found in a single goat (Prein 1938). In a slaughterhouse survey in Turkey, 53% of 1,049 goats examined were infested with *P. silenus*. Larval numbers ranged from one to fifty-two per infested animal with an average of seven (Göksu 1976). Sometimes the hide has the appearance of a sieve. The holes in the hides cause tremendous losses in the fine leather industry in Iran, where 93% of goats in a slaughterhouse study were infested (Rahbari and Ghasemi 1997).

Therapy

Ivermectin, at dosages of 5 to 20 mg/100 kg, has been effective in killing all instars of the warbles (Tassi et al. 1987; Yadav et al. 2006). Even microdoses of ivermectin (0.5 mg/100 kg as injectable, 1 mg/100 kg as pour-on) are highly efficacious and result in minimal milk contamination (Giangaspero et al. 2003). Modern systemic insecticides are often not available in countries where this parasite abounds. Shepherds have been taught to remove warbles during the winter months.

Ticks

Ticks are important ectoparasites throughout the world.

Etiology

A discussion of the life cycles and identification of the many species reported to infest goats is beyond the scope of this book; readers should refer to standard parasitology texts (Soulsby 1982). Some important species are listed in Table 2.2 and species occurring in the United States have been reviewed by Gnad and Mock (2001). Soft ticks belong to the family Argasidae and feed repeatedly on their hosts. Hard ticks, family Ixodidae, have a shield on the dorsal surface and feed only once during each stage. Larval ticks have six legs, while nymphal and adult ticks have eight legs. Ticks are referred to as one-host, two-host, or three-host, according to whether they drop off the host to molt between larval and nymph stages and between nymphal and adult stages. Ticks are not especially host-specific (Scott 1988).

Clinical Signs and Diagnosis

The attachment site varies with the tick species (Baker and Ducasse 1968), and may show papules, pustules, or wheals initially, with crusts and ulcers forming secondarily. Demonstration of the tick will make the diagnosis, but skin biopsy to demonstrate embedded tick mouth parts may be necessary in persistent, nodular lesions. Secondary bacterial infections and myiasis are possible. Ticks such as *Amblyomma hebraeum* and *Rhipicephalus glabroscutatum* attach to feet, especially between the claws, and may predispose to foot abscesses (MacIvor and Horak 1987). Damage to hides is important. Other important consequences are blood loss and the transmission of very serious diseases such as anaplasmosis, babesiosis, heartwater, theileriasis, and tick-borne fever. Tick paralysis may also occur. Pituitary abscess has been associated with attachment of ticks beneath backswept horns of Boer goats in South Africa (Bath et al. 2005). These conditions are discussed elsewhere in this book.

Therapy

Simple extraction of the tick is recommended when ticks and goats are few. A device with a slit that is

Table 2.2. Some ticks of importance to goats.

Tick	*Distribution*	*Importance*
Argasidae: soft ticks		
Otobius megnini	North and South America, southern Africa, India	Causes irritation and blood loss in ears
Ornithodorus spp.	United States, Asia	Transmits Q fever, *Theileria*, and *Anaplasma*
Ixodidae: hard ticks		
Ixodes ricinus	Europe	Transmits tick-borne fever, louping ill, tick paralysis
Ixodes pilosus	South Africa	Does not cause paralysis
Ixodes rubicundus	South Africa	Tick paralysis
Boophilus decoloratus	Ethiopia	Transmits *Borrelia, Theileria*
Boophilus microplus	Tropics	Tropical cattle tick
Rhipicephalus appendiculatus	Africa	Attaches in ears and beneath tail; transmits Nairobi sheep disease
Rhipicephalus bursa	Africa and southern Europe	Transmits *Theileria ovis, Babesia ovis*
Rhipicephalus haemaphysaloides	India	Transmits tick-borne fever
Haemaphysalis punctata	Europe, North Africa	Transmits *Babesia motasi, Theileria*
Amblyomma hebraeum	Africa	Transmits heartwater
Amblyomma variegatum	Africa and Caribbean	Transmits heartwater
Amblyomma cajennense	North and South America	Tick paralysis (Brazil)
Dermacentor spp.	Worldwide	Sometimes causes tick paralysis

placed around the mouthparts and then rotated works better than tweezers and direct traction for manual removal (Zenner et al. 2006). A large variety of sprays, dips, and pour-ons (see Table 2.1) will reduce the population of ticks and provide temporary protection. The use of insecticides can be reduced by local spraying or hand-dressing of the body area (ear canal, perineum) where ticks are located (Baker and Ducasse 1968). Systemic ivermectin may also prevent complete engorgement (Wall and Shearer 2001). Residues in meat, milk, and the environment are a concern, as is the possible development of resistance of ticks to insecticides (Stampa 1964) and of gastrointestinal strongyles to ivermectin.

Control

Total eradication of a tick species is usually very difficult. A reduction in tick numbers is achieved by several applications of insecticide at two- to three-week intervals. Two- and three-host ticks require treatments throughout the tick season, while one-host ticks are more likely to be on the host and therefore killed with one or two treatments. Amitraz has been used as a pasture spray to decrease tick burdens (Harrison and Palmer 1981). In certain circumstances, burning the pasture or cultivating the land may aid in tick control.

Sarcoptic Mange

The mite that causes sarcoptic mange (scabies) in goats has been referred to as either *Sarcoptes rupicaprae* or a goat-specific strain of *Sarcoptes scabiei*. It tunnels through the epidermis and feeds on tissue fluids (Scott 1988). Experimental infection of desert sheep with a goat strain of *Sarcoptes scabiei* has been documented (Ibrahim and Abu-Samra 1987) and probably occurs naturally when the two species are raised together. Molecular analyses suggest that all sarcoptic mites belong to a single, heterogeneous species (Zahler et al. 1999). Human infection can occur from handling affected goats (Menzano et al. 2007).

Clinical Signs

The condition is reported to begin with the appearance of small pruritic nodules, especially on the head, several weeks after contact with another infested goat or chamois (Menzano et al. 2007). The skin disease seems to be self-limiting in some goats, while others develop extensive severe dermatitis around the eyes and ears and on the neck and thorax, inner thighs, udder, and scrotum. Hyperkeratosis and alopecia are accompanied by self-excoriation and restlessness. The thickened skin is wrinkled and fissured (Abu-Samra et al. 1981; Kambarage 1992) and may harbor a secondary bacterial infection. Severely affected goats lose weight and have prominent peripheral lymph nodes. Some deaths occur (Zamri-Saad et al. 1990; Menzano et al. 2007). The value of the hide is markedly decreased.

Diagnosis

Confirmation of the diagnosis usually requires deep scrapings at the margin of lesions; the mites are identified by the presence of long unjointed pedicels on the pretarsi. Even if no mites are seen in multiple scrapings, a biopsy report of eosinophilic dermatitis and tunnels should indicate a presumptive diagnosis of sarcoptic mange (Deorani and Chaudhuri 1965; Scott 1988). In some chronic cases, diagnosis is made by response to therapy. Local regulations may require reporting a positive diagnosis to government authorities.

Therapy

Treatment of lactating animals can be accomplished with repeated (perhaps five to ten) applications of lime sulfur solution every five to seven days. Two treatments of 0.05% amitraz seven to ten days apart are recommended for controlling scabies in dairy cattle in the United States, and should thus be safe for dairy goats. In nonlactating animals, many different parasiticides have been applied with some success, but relapses are common when treatment is discontinued (Jackson et al. 1983). Sprays often fail to adequately penetrate the long and thick hair coat of unshorn animals. Some animals may need antibiotics for secondary bacterial infections.

More recently, ivermectin (subcutaneously) has simplified treatment, especially because the inconvenience and stress of bathing a disgruntled goat in cold weather are avoided. A cleansing shampoo is recommended to remove crusts, even if ivermectin is given. However, excellent response, including disappearance of the crusts, was achieved in Saudi Arabia when goats were treated with ivermectin (1 ml of a 1% solution per adult of unspecified weight) twice, one week apart. Live mites were recovered from treated animals for at least two weeks, but all goats yielded negative skin scrapings three weeks after the second treatment (Wasfi and Hashim 1986). In another instance, three doses two weeks apart of subcutaneous ivermectin at 0.2 or 0.4 mg/kg were effective (Zamri-Saad et al. 1990). Three treatments fourteen days apart with topical moxidectin at 0.5 mg/kg were successful in clearing a severely infected Italian goat herd of the parasite; a higher dose, more appropriate for goats, might have been more rapidly effective (Menzano et al. 2007). For the lactating animal, a single topical application of eprinomectin (Eprinex® pour-on, Merial) at 1 mg/kg (twice the cattle dose) might be preferable, because milk residues remain below the limit established for dairy cows (Dupuy et al. 2001).

Chorioptic Mange

Some authors believe that the chorioptic mange mite of goats belongs to the species *Chorioptes bovis*, while others consider it to be host-specific and designate it as *C. caprae* (Scott 1988).

Epidemiology

The mite lives on the surface of the skin and feeds on epidermal debris. It may exist on nonclinical carrier goats and can also survive in the environment for as long as ten weeks (Liebisch et al. 1985). This accounts for sudden occurrence of mange lesions in closed herds. Mite populations are affected by the environment, with the highest mite numbers and most severe clinical signs in cold weather. In a New Zealand study of feral goats, the prevalence of chorioptic mites was 100% in the winter, although marked lesions were found on the legs of only five of 368 goats overall (Heath et al. 1983).

Clinical Signs and Diagnosis

The lesions (nonfollicular papules, crusts, alopecia, erythema, and ulceration) are most commonly or initially found on the lower limbs, with occasional spread to udder, scrotum, and perineal region (Scott 2007). Pruritus, as demonstrated by stamping or chewing at the limb lesions, may be obvious, or the alopecia and crusts may appear benign (Figure 2.10). Only rarely is the dermatitis caused by *Chorioptes* generalized (Dorny et al. 1994).

Diagnostic samples can be obtained with a flea comb or by skin scrapings; adding rotenone to the mineral oil used for collecting scrapings will prevent the escape of the mites on the way to the microscope (Scott 1988). The mites have short pedicels on their pretarsi. Zinc deficiency and bacterial skin infections are important differential diagnoses that may be present concurrently with mange.

Therapy

Treatment of chorioptic mange is sometimes very easy, but hypersensitivity of certain goats to the mites can lead to treatment failure and frustration. All in-contact goats should be treated simultaneously to eliminate the carrier state and the premises disinfected. Lime sulfur (four weekly, total body sprays or dips in 2% solution) is safe for lactating dairy goats. Crotoxyphos (0.25%), coumaphos (0.25%), trichlorfon (0.2%), amitraz (0.05%), and lindane (0.03%) must be applied at least twice at ten- to fourteen-day intervals. In one study, a single dip with fenvalerate (0.05%) killed all mites on Angora goats (Wright et al. 1988). Injectable ivermectin can be expected to kill many but not all of the mites, because of their superficial location. Topical application of ivermectin (0.5 mg/kg applied once to

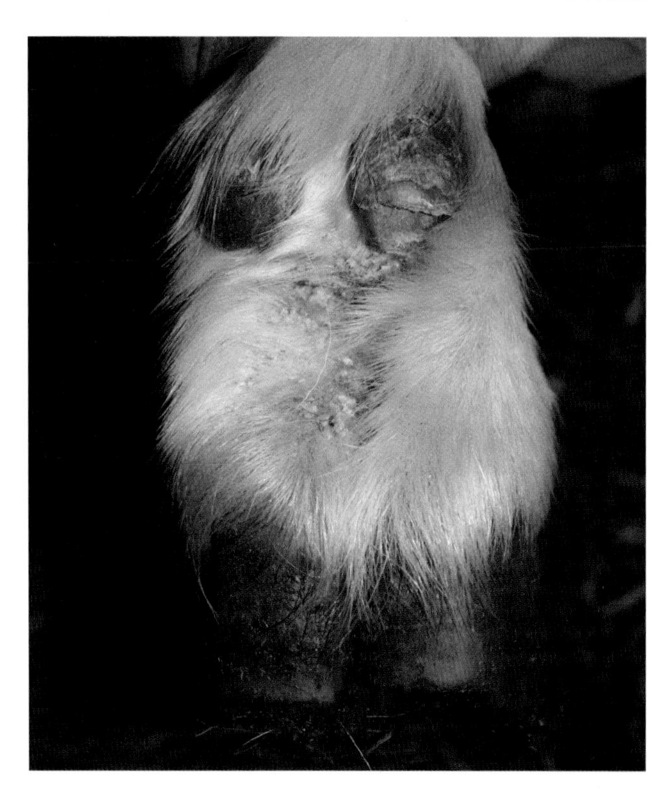

Figure 2.10. Mild crusting and scaling on the pastern of a goat with chorioptic mange. (Courtesy Dr. M.C. Smith.)

healthy skin) has been shown to be effective against *C. bovis* on cattle (Barth and Preston 1988). Fipronil (Frontline® Spray, Merial) has also been advocated for goats (Konnersman 2005b). National regulations concerning milk and meat residues should be respected. Using shampoo to remove crusts and shearing of mohair will improve efficacy of externally applied acaricides. Systemic antibiotics for secondary bacterial infections and judicious use of glucocorticosteroids in apparently allergic goats are indicated in select cases.

Psoroptic Mange

The classification of mites of the genus *Psoroptes* is currently unsettled (Scott 1988; Zahler et al. 1998; Bates 1999). The proposed role of ear mites in the transmission of mycoplasma infections is discussed in Chapter 9.

Etiology and Epidemiology

The most commonly reported ear mite of goats is the cosmopolitan *Psoroptes cuniculi*. Prevalence in necropsy studies appears to be high (twenty-one of twenty-four and eight of eighteen) (Williams and Williams 1978; Cook 1981). The mite can be found in the external ear canal of kids as young as ten days old, with most kids infested by the third week (Williams and Williams 1978). In feral goats in New Zealand, the infestation was often unilateral and was more common in winter and in older goats (Heath et al. 1983). When it causes body mange (in parts of the world where sheep are affected with psoroptic mange), the parasite is sometimes referred to as *P. caprae*. The mite has long, segmented pedicels and is often visible to the naked eye. It does not burrow but feeds on tissue fluids. Prolonged survival times (as long as twelve weeks) in the environment have been reported (Liebisch et al. 1985).

Clinical Signs and Diagnosis

Clinical signs of ear mite infestation include head shaking (Dorny et al. 1994) and scratching, sometimes with alopecia of the part of the ear repeatedly brushed by a hind foot. Occasional goats have flaky or scabby lesions or laminated crusts on the external ear or even on the poll, back, and pasterns (Littlejohn 1968; Munro and Munro 1980; Heath et al. 1983; Lofstedt et al. 1994), but most have no externally visible lesions. Otoscopic examination (tranquilization advised for adult goats) easily demonstrates the presence of the mite. A plug of yellowish wax is commonly found in the ear canal (Munro and Munro 1980; Cook 1981; Heath et al. 1983), and extracting some of this material with a cotton swab for examination is an alternative means of diagnosis. Palpation of the base of the external ear may elicit a crackling sound associated with exudate in the canal (Nooruddin and Mondal 1996). Rarely, otitis externa progresses to otitis media and interna with head tilt.

Body mange caused by *Psoroptes* resembles sarcoptic mange but is accompanied by less scab formation (Wasfi and Hashim 1986). Before sheep scab due to *Psoroptes ovis* was eradicated from Texas, Angora goats were noted to have a much more severe form of *Psoroptes cuniculi* infestation than was seen on dairy goats, as evidenced by serious damage to skin and hair (Graham and Hourrigan 1977). Skin scrapings should be collected from the margin of lesions. If the scrapings are collected into a ziplock bag or petri dish, the sample can be warmed to stimulate movement of the mites during later close examination. Reporting to regulatory authorities may be required.

Therapy

Treatment of ear mange is often foregone or limited to removal of any bells from goats showing clinical evidence of pruritus (to avoid continual disturbance of the owner). External lesions may be swabbed with an acaricide. Canine ear mite preparations may be used on goats with mites confined to the ear canal, but removal of crusts and debris is necessary and recurrence is likely (Munro and Munro 1980). The life cycle probably takes about three weeks, and several weekly treatments are advised (Littlejohn 1968). In nonlactating pet goats, two treatments with injectable or oral ivermectin one to two weeks apart (20 mg/100 kg) is a rational therapy (Lofstedt et al. 1994). Instillation of several drops of an ivermectin solution into each ear canal is also effective (Konnersman 2005b).

Body mange can be treated with routine acaricides (including amitraz; Harrison and Palmer 1981) as dips or sprays. Ivermectin (two injections one week apart) also has been found effective in treating psoroptic mange in goats (Wasfi and Hashim 1986).

Raillietia

A separate genus of ear mites of goats is *Raillietia* (Cook 1981; Lavoipierre and Larsen 1981). The feral goats that harbored only these mites showed no evidence of associated clinical disease, although ear irritation might be expected to occur. *Raillietia* mites tend to be larger than *Psoroptes*, and their longer legs originate from the anterior half of the body. The possible involvement of ear mites in transmission of mycoplasma infections is discussed in Chapter 9.

Demodectic Mange (Demodicosis)

Demodex caprae is a cigar-shaped mite that commonly inhabits the hair follicles and sebaceous glands of goats. It has a worldwide distribution. As in other hosts, demodectic mites have been found in the eyelids of goats with no visible lesions anywhere on the body (Himonas et al. 1975).

Epidemiology

Confinement housing and crowding seem to favor development of demodectic mange. The mites appear to survive only a few hours away from the goats, but infection via contact with contaminated feeders might occur. In fact, natural spread from one adult goat to another has not been documented. The appearance of nodules in certain goats in a herd but not in others may reflect the immune competency of the animal (Das and Misra 1972). This could be related to genetic factors, nutrition (e.g., selenium or protein deficiency), or stress (e.g., high production). It seems likely that goats are first infested as young kids but that lesions do not become detectable until many months later (Williams and Williams 1982).

Clinical Signs and Diagnosis

Portions of the body exposed to friction, such as the face, neck, shoulders, and sides, are commonly involved, whereas the ventral abdomen and udder remain free of nodules. Where animals with skin lesions have been followed, it has been observed that nodules are first detectable at ten to fifteen months of age (Euzeby et al. 1976). Initially the lesions are very small and only located by careful palpation (Smith 1961). However, defects may be readily detectable in

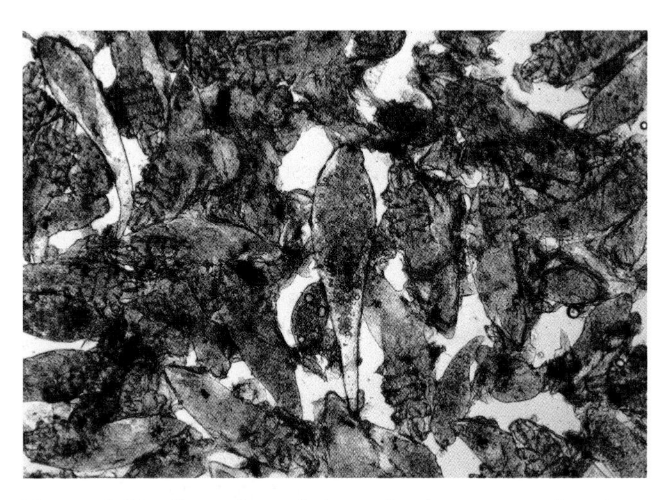

Figure 2.11. Cigar-shaped demodectic mange mites in a smear of exudate expressed from a skin nodule. (Courtesy Dr. M.C. Smith.)

hides at this stage or even earlier (Röhrer 1935). By eighteen to twenty months of age the nodules have enlarged to lentil or pea size, but because they remain painless they may not be noticed unless the goat is clipped (as for a show). Occasional animals demonstrate mild pruritus (Durant 1944), but this is a relatively rare finding.

Each nodule corresponds to a distended pilosebaceous follicle. Firm digital pressure will force out a ribbon of yellowish white paste from a central pore. Microscopic examination of this caseous material reveals numerous eggs, larvae, and mature mites (Figure 2.11). The diagnosis is thereby confirmed. The disease process peaks at about three years of age. Nodules may reach a diameter of 0.5 to 1.25 cm. At this time, the severely affected goat may be apathetic and unthrifty, and may lose weight or milk poorly. It is not clear if these signs are because of mange infestation or underlying (nutritional) problems. The nodules become smaller, firmer, and less numerous in older animals.

Therapy

Various treatments have been proposed. When only a few nodules are present, squeezing or incising each one to permit removal of its contents will result in a cure of the hair follicle thus treated. Iodine or other disinfectant is applied when the nodule is expressed to kill residual mites. Some goats carry several hundred discrete lesions. Others have a generalized dermatitis rather than the typical nodule form of the disease. For them, topical or systemic organophosphates, amitraz (0.025%), or weekly ivermectin or eprinomectin may be effective (Thompson and Mackenzie 1982; Strabel et al. 2003). Because the lesions resolve over weeks or months, documentation of a treatment effect is difficult. Nodules may remain long after the mites have died. In one instance, nodules reappeared after amitraz (twelve topical treatments) was discontinued (Brügger and Braun 2000). Because secondary bacterial infections are generally absent in undisturbed lesions, antibiotic therapy is not indicated.

Treatment is normally only undertaken in show animals, except when nutritional deficiencies exist. It has been suggested that severely affected animals should not be used for breeding because of a possible hereditary susceptibility to the disease (Scott 1988).

Free-living Mites

Trombiculid mite adults and nymphs are free-living. The larvae (chiggers, harvest mites) are reddish and six-legged. They attack the pasterns, muzzle, and ventrum of animals pastured in infested fields and woods or when contaminated forage is fed to housed animals. Clinical signs of irritation and pruritus, papules, edema, exudation, and ulceration may be expected. Skin scrapings to identify the larvae permit differentiation from other conditions such as chorioptic mange, staphylococcal dermatitis, and zinc deficiency. Mites may be absent in chronic cases. The condition is well reported in sheep (Wall and Shearer 2001) and is occasionally recognized in goats (Nooruddin et al. 1987). An insecticide dip or spray might give eventual relief.

Exposure to biting grain or forage mites such as *Tyroglyphidae* spp. may occasionally cause dermatitis in goats (Matthews 1999). Likewise, a pruritic goat housed with poultry, especially in late summer, might be being attacked at night by poultry mites (*Dermanyssus gallinae*) (Matthews 1999).

Rhabditic Dermatitis and Strongyloidiasis

Strongyloides papillosus larvae penetrate unbroken skin, enter capillaries, and travel in the blood to the lungs. Here they exit into air passages and travel up the trachea and down the gastrointestinal tract to the intestines. There are no histologic changes in the skin on first exposure, but pustular dermatitis is created as host resistance develops via repeated exposures. This is characterized by edema, inflammatory infiltration (neutrophils, eosinophils, lymphocytes, and giant cells), and destruction of the larvae. This condition is best described in sheep (Turner et al. 1960). Affected goats are reported to stamp, dance, and nibble at their feet, especially after a rain (Baxendell 1988). Warm, moist habitats for the larvae should be eliminated and the animal treated with an anthelminthic such as fenbendazole, levamisole, or ivermectin.

Pelodera (Rhabditis) strongyloides is a free-living soil nematode that can invade portions of skin in contact with moist ground and decaying organic matter (Scott 1988). Although not reported in goats, it could presumably cause pruritic dermatitis in goats housed under unsanitary conditions. Diagnosis is by scraping or skin biopsy and control by sanitation, including removal of dirty bedding. The hookworm (*Bunostomum*) is another nematode that could conceivably produce dermatitis while penetrating the skin. Additional conditions to be considered in the differential diagnosis include contact dermatitis, mange, and trombiculidiasis (chiggers).

Parelaphostrongylosis and Elaphostrongylosis

Parelaphostrongylus tenuis, the meningeal worm of the white-tail deer, commonly causes neurologic disease in goats in North America. Some paretic and nonparetic goats with *P. tenuis* infection have developed linear, vertically oriented skin lesions on the neck, shoulder, thorax, or flank (Smith 1981; Scott 1988, 2007). Owners report that the goat has excoriated these areas by biting or rubbing, as if responding to intense pruritus. Lesions are usually unilateral and alopecic, crusted, or scarred (Figure 2.12). One lesion may heal and another appear closer to the goat's head. One possible explanation is that migrating parasite larvae irritate dorsal nerve roots supplying individual dermatomes. The diagnosis of *P. tenuis*-induced dermatosis should be entertained when goats with linear pruritic lesions have been exposed to pastures frequented by deer. Neurologic deficits suggesting spinal cord damage and eosinophilia or increased protein in the cerebrospinal fluid lend additional support to the diagnosis. Treatment and control of this parasite are discussed in Chapter 5.

Goats in Norway have been affected with a very similar neurologic disease, in which the migrating parasite is *Elaphostrongylus rangiferi* and the natural host is the reindeer. In one herd pruritus was noted to precede the neurologic signs (Handeland and Sparboe 1991). When goat kids were experimentally infected with *E. rangiferi*, pruritus was common from four to ten weeks after infection (Handeland and Skorping 1993). The muscle worm of deer, *Elaphostrongylus cervi*, has been associated with neurologic disease of goats in Europe, but pruritic skin lesions have not been reported.

A differential diagnosis for this syndrome might be psychogenic self-mutilation (Yeruham and Hadani 2003). Examination of biopsy samples reveals only the skin damage induced by chewing or scratching. However, unless the spinal cord is also examined it will not be possible to rule out irritation to a nerve root supplying the affected skin.

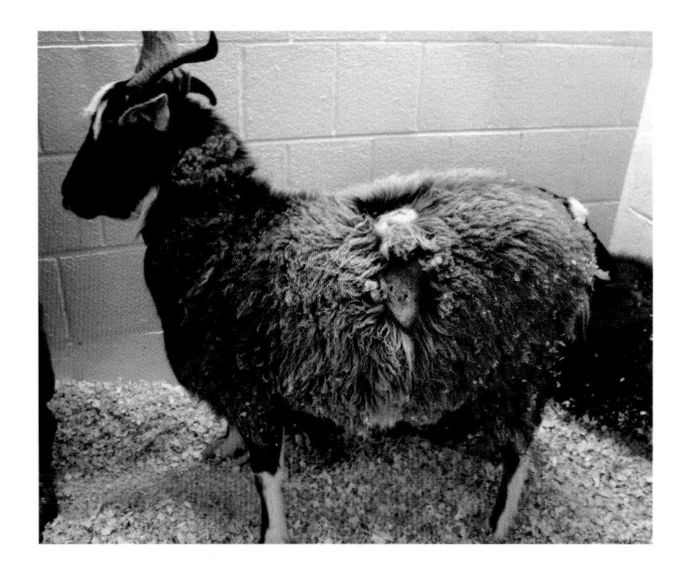

Figure 2.12. Vertically-oriented alopecic lesion on the side of a cashmere goat that had been pastured with white-tail deer, suggesting irritation of a dorsal nerve root by *P. tenuis*. (Courtesy Dr. M.C. Smith.)

Filarid Dermatitis

Several filarid worms are known to cause dermatitis in small ruminants. Insect vectors, especially flies, deposit larvae in skin wounds. Papular, alopecic, or crusty lesions develop, and are accompanied by pruritus. In Malaysia, a crusty dermatitis of the feet of goats has been ascribed to *Stephanofilaria kaeli* (Fadzil et al. 1973). In India, *Stephanofilaria assamensis* has been recovered from skin sores on goats (Patnaik and Roy 1968). Skin scrapings, and smears of blood oozing from the skin after the scrapings have been made, reveal adult parasites and microfilaria. Biopsy samples may be fixed in formalin or macerated and examined with a dissecting scope. Eosinophils predominate in the inflammatory reaction to the parasites. Trichlorfon has been efficacious for treating affected goats.

Elaeophora schneideri (a subclinical intra-arterial parasite of mule deer and black-tailed deer in the mountains of the western United States) occasionally infests sheep and elk. Transmission is by horseflies. Adult worms block arteries of the head, and microfilaria lodge in skin capillaries. Erythema, alopecia, ulcers, and crusts appear on the face and poll, and sometimes the abdomen and feet of sheep. Blindness, neurologic signs, and keratoconjunctivitis also may occur. The absence of documented caprine cases may reflect how rarely goats are grazed above 2,000 meters in the mountain ranges. However, the parasite has been reported in the southeastern United States, Texas, and the Pacific coast states, and goats are listed as occasionally infected (Haigh and Hudson 1993).

Besnoitiosis

In Africa and the Middle East, protozoal parasites of the genus *Besnoitia* cause a widespread dermatitis and alopecia in wild and domestic goats. Some workers believe that the organism infecting goats, termed *Besnoitia caprae*, is distinct from that infecting cattle, *B. besnoiti* (Njenga et al. 1995). Lesions may be especially severe on the scrotum and lower limbs. The skin is thickened to corrugated (hyperkeratosis), sometimes with hyperpigmentation and exudation (Oryan and Sadeghi 1997). Diagnosis is by demonstration in skin biopsy specimens of cysts (oval or spherical, average size 175 × 290 microns) containing bradyzoites and surrounded by a collagen capsule (Bwangamoi 1967; Cheema and Toofanian 1979). There is also a correlation with the presence of *Besnoitia* cysts in the scleral conjunctiva (Bwangamoi et al. 1989). No specific treatment is available. Control measures for goats have not been described but might include the use of a bovine tissue culture vaccine (Radostits et al. 2007) and avoiding feed contamination with cat feces. Biting flies possibly transmit the parasite.

NUTRITIONAL DISEASES

A goat subject to deficiencies in dietary energy or protein can be expected to have a dry, sparse hair coat and dry, thin, scaly skin. These changes are nonspecific because they occur with many chronic, wasting diseases. Copper deficiency, which is discussed in Chapter 19, has been associated with depigmentation of the hair coat (Lazzaro 2007). Certain trace mineral or vitamin deficiencies cause changes in the skin that have been described in more detail. Alopecia, possibly related to liver damage, has been produced by experimental feeding of *Aristolochia bracteata* in goats in Sudan (Barakat et al. 1983).

Zinc Deficiency and Zinc Responsive Dermatosis

It has been suggested that a practical level of dietary zinc in production diets is 45 to 75 ppm (McDowell et al. 1991). The National Research Council (2007) now admits that a previous recommendation of 10 ppm did not allow for poor absorbability, which can be estimated to be as low as 15%.

Etiology

Calcium excesses in the diet may contribute to a relative zinc deficiency. This might explain zinc-responsive dermatitis in nonlactating does or male goats receiving dairy rations or alfalfa. Zinc deficiency was recognized in two aged nonlactating does after their diet was switched to an alfalfa gruel to compensate for tooth loss (Singer et al. 2000). Other minerals which influence zinc absorption are selenium, copper, and cadmium (National Research Council 2007). Zinc is not stored in the body in an available form, so a daily dietary source is needed.

Some animals appear to have inadequate absorptive abilities (possibly genetically determined, Krametter-Froetscher et al. 2005), because dermatosis persists in the face of normal dietary concentrations of zinc and interfering minerals.

Second-generation goats on an experimental nickel-deficient diet developed zinc deficiency and associated parakeratotic skin changes (Anke et al. 1977). This is unlikely to occur with ordinary diets.

Clinical Signs

Clinical signs observed in goats with zinc deficiency include hyperemia and pruritus (inconstant) of the skin; alopecia; thick fissured crusts on the back legs, escutcheon, face, and ears; and dandruff-like scales over the rest of the body (Neathery et al. 1973; Nelson et al. 1984; Scott 1988; Krametter-Froetscher et al. 2005). Crusts commonly encircle the nares, eyes, and mouth. The hair of zinc-deficient goats has been described as greasy and matted (Groppel and Hennig 1971). Fiber break with loss of mohair can have serious economic consequences in Angoras (Schulze and Üstdal 1975). Weight loss may occur; clinical aspects of zinc deficiency unrelated to the skin are discussed further in Chapter 19.

Diagnosis and Treatment

Skin biopsies are important for demonstration of hyperkeratosis and parakeratosis and for ruling out other conditions with similar signs (e.g., mange, dermatophilosis). The diagnosis of zinc deficiency by laboratory tests is difficult. It appears that some goats may have a zinc responsive dermatitis, although plasma, liver, and even dietary zinc levels appear to be within normal ranges (Reuter et al. 1987). Serum levels less than 0.8 ppm might be associated with skin lesions. Lower serum zinc concentrations (0.54 ppm) have been recorded in goats from Florida herds with a history of seasonal dermatosis when compared with serum levels in other herds without such history (0.83 ppm) (McDowell et al. 1991). An Austrian report gives the normal caprine serum zinc range as 0.57 to 0.63 ppm (Krametter-Froetscher et al. 2005).

In many instances, the diagnosis is achieved by response to treatment. A rather arbitrary dose of 1 gram zinc sulfate orally per day has been used with good success; if marked improvement has not occurred after two weeks of therapy, other diagnoses should be pursued more vigorously. There is a published report of a single goat with skin lesions of lateral truncal alopecia and scaling improving in seven to ten days with institution of 14 grams zinc sulfate orally per day for six weeks. Signs reappeared two to three weeks after cessation of therapy (McDowell et al. 1991). In the Austrian report, two adult goats with onset of clinical signs during pregnancy responded to 1 gram zinc sulfate per day, whereas the response to 50 to 200 mg zinc oxide per day was less complete (Krametter-Froetscher et al. 2005). The efficacy of dietary zinc methionine for alleviating signs in goats has not been documented. A mineral supplement that includes zinc should be offered routinely, with additional zinc for animals with a suspected hereditary basis for the dermatosis. A slow-release bolus containing zinc, cobalt, and selenium is available in the United Kingdom (Matthews 1999). Dietary excesses of calcium should be corrected.

Iodine Deficiency

Diseases of the thyroid gland are discussed in detail in Chapter 3, and the role of iodine in caprine nutrition is discussed in Chapter 19.

Etiology

Certain soils (such as that found in much of the northern United States and the Himalayas) are deficient in iodine. Goitrogens (such as members of the Cruciferae family, see Chapter 3) may interfere with uptake of iodine by the thyroid gland. Additionally, inherited abnormalities of thyroid function have been recognized in inbred Dutch goats.

Clinical Signs

Adult goats with goiter caused by iodine deficiency generally show no skin changes (Kalkus 1920; Dutt and Kehar 1959). Likewise, clinical signs of hair loss or skin abnormalities were absent in one outbreak of goiter and cretinism in Angora kids ascribed to consumption of goitrogens during pregnancy (Bath et al. 1979). In iodine deficiency severe enough to cause stillbirth, however, newborn kids sometimes had a normal hair coat but often were hairless or covered with very fine hair (Kalkus 1920). Skin lesions have been reported in experimental hypothyroidism produced by administration of thiourea to kids. A rough hair coat and subcutaneous edema were noted clinically. Histologic changes included hyperkeratosis and plugging of hair follicles (Sreekumaran and Rajan 1977). Kids with hereditary goiters were similar to thiourea-treated animals in that they were sluggish and grew poorly. Again, the hair coat was sparse and the skin thick and scaly (Rijnberk 1977). It appears that goats with goiter may or may not have accompanying skin lesions, but that iodine deficiency should not be suspected as the cause of skin disease in the absence of goiters.

Treatment and Prevention

Iodine deficiency can usually be prevented by supplying an iodized salt or salt and mineral product (as the only source of supplemental salt). Excessive feeding of goitrogens should be avoided. Weekly application of an iodine-containing solution (such as 1 ml of tincture of iodine) to the skin will also meet the needs of the animal (Kalkus 1920).

Vitamin A Deficiency

Vitamin A is necessary for normal function of epithelial tissues, including the skin. Neurologic manifestations of deficiency are discussed in Chapter 5 and ocular manifestations in Chapter 6.

Etiology

Because beta-carotene, which is abundant in green-leaved plants, is converted into vitamin A after ingestion, deficiencies are unlikely when goats are fed good pasture or green hay. Grains (except yellow corn and green peas), roots (except carrots and sweet potatoes), and old or weathered hays are low in carotene. Cases of vitamin A deficiency in goats are most likely to occur in semi-arid environments (during the dry season or periods of drought) or when the diet consists of poor, old hay and grain other than corn. Experimental aflatoxicosis in goats has caused a gradual decrease in serum vitamin A levels (Maryamma and Sivadas 1973).

Colostrum is rich in vitamin A and usually supplies the needs of the kid until forage consumption begins. Colostrum-deprived kids can be expected to be deficient in vitamin A.

Clinical Signs and Diagnosis

Clinical signs relative to the skin include a rough, dry hair coat, patchy alopecia, and a generally unhealthy appearance (Majumdar and Gupta 1960; Caldas 1961; Dutt and Majumdar 1969). Hyperkeratosis (identified histologically) (Scott 1988) and plasma vitamin A levels less than 13 μg/dl, at least in sheep (Ghanem and Farid 1982), support the diagnosis, as do low levels of vitamin A in the liver (except for precolostral neonates).

Treatment and Prevention

Dietary supplementation, as discussed in the nutrition chapter, is preferable to injectable vitamin A. An excellent source is leafy alfalfa or alfalfa meal. Intramuscular or subcutaneous injection of vitamin A (3,000 to 6,000 IU/kg every two months) is appropriate for individual unthrifty goats or when daily oral supplementation is not possible. A single oral dose of 600,000 IU has proven effective in lambs for thirty-four weeks, and it is recommended that this be given two months after the start of the dry season (Ghanem and Farid 1982).

Massive overdose of vitamin A, as has been achieved in experimental feeding trials, results in a moderate hyperplasia of the dermis and seborrhea of the ventral abdominal and inguinal skin (Frier et al. 1974).

Vitamin E and Selenium Responsive Dermatosis

A nonpruritic dermatosis characterized by a dry, thin hair coat, general seborrhea and scales, and periorbital alopecia has been observed in kids and adult goats (Smith 1981).

In some instances, dietary selenium deficiency has been documented, and the response to injectable vitamin E/selenium has been dramatic. In other goats, diagnosis was based on negative skin scrapings and response to both injectable E/selenium and oral vitamin E (400 IU) given with vegetable oil daily for one month. Dietary supplementation with black oil sunflower seeds or wheat germ oil might be helpful because of vitamin E and fat content (Konnersman 2005b). Controlled therapeutic trials have not been conducted, and criteria for positively diagnosing the condition have not been established.

Zinc deficiency is an important differential. Skin biopsy results of goats with vitamin E and selenium responsive dermatosis have revealed orthokeratotic hyperkeratosis, whereas zinc responsive disease is characterized by parakeratotic hyperkeratosis (Scott 1988).

Selenium Toxicity

Hair loss in goats consuming *Astragalus* spp., especially involving the beard and flank region, has been linked to possible selenium excess (Reko 1928). This seems plausible because selenium toxicity from a variety of selenium-concentrating plants or from contaminated water causes loss of mane and tail hairs in horses. In another herd outbreak ascribed to consumption of a seleniferous (500 ppm) *Astragalus* spp., the only reported skin change in goats that died was a rough hair coat (Hosseinion et al. 1972). Selenium may substitute for sulfur in sulfur-containing amino acids in the hair and hoof (Scott 1988). This leads to alopecia and lameness, with cracks and deformities developing in horns and hooves (Gupta et al. 1982), as discussed in Chapter 4.

Sulfur Deficiency

A recently recognized condition of severe fleece eating in cashmere-producing goats and of sheep in one valley (Haizi area) in China has been ascribed to sulfur deficiency, possibly compounded by calcium and copper deficiency. Affected goats repeatedly bite bits of fleece off themselves or other animals in the flock, concentrating on the fiber over the hips, abdomen, and shoulder. Some animals are left with almost naked skin and may die of exposure. Skin is keratinized and hair follicles are reduced in size and number. Signs are alleviated by moving to another valley or by the arrival of lush spring grass. The sulfur content of the fiber in affected animals was low (2.4%) compared with a normal content of 4%. Medicated pellets containing aluminum sulfate prevented or treated the skin condition, although muscle atrophy and kidney lesions were not reversed (Youde 2001, 2002; Youde and Huaitao 2001).

Rule-outs for such a herd problem include external parasites, lack of dietary fiber, boredom, and accidental deposition of concentrates into the fleece during distribution of feed.

ENVIRONMENTAL INSULTS

The skin may be damaged by excessive exposure to light, cold, or irritants such as urine. Bites by poisonous snakes and spiders undoubtedly affect goats occasionally but are poorly documented.

Sunburn

Exposure to sunlight is associated with the development of skin tumors in white goats, as discussed below. Light-skinned animals exposed to bright sunlight (ultraviolet light, 290 to 320 nm) (Scott 1988) after a winter stabling period are also susceptible to sunburn, especially of the muzzle, perineum, and teats. Signs include erythema, edema, vesicles, ulceration, and crusts (Scott 2007). Prevention involves gradually increasing times of exposure to sunlight and applying sunblocking ointments or iodine teat dips after milking. Treatment is by temporary removal from the sun and use of soothing burn ointments. Contamination of milk should be avoided.

Photosensitization

In photosensitization, superficial layers of lightly pigmented skin are sensitized to ultraviolet light (320 to 400 nm) of wavelengths longer than those causing simple sunburn.

Etiology

There are several mechanisms by which a photodynamic agent may reach the skin and cause dermatitis if exposed to light (Galitzer and Oehme 1978). Certain toxins are ingested preformed, and are said to cause primary photosensitization. Examples include phenothiazine, fagopyrin (from buckwheat, *Fagopyrum esculentum*), hypericin (Bale 1978) (from *Hypericum* spp.) and furocoumarins (from *Ammi majus* and *Thamnosma texana*) (Ivie 1978; Scott 1988, 2007). Secondary, or hepatogenous, photosensitization occurs when the normal end product of chlorophyll degradation in the rumen, phylloerythrin, accumulates because of faulty liver excretion. Any severe liver disease could conceivably lead to photosensitization in goats consuming chlorophyll and exposed to sunlight, but toxic plants are most frequently incriminated. These include *Lantana* (Pass 1986), *Agave lecheguilla* (Mathews 1938; Burrows and Stair 1990), *Nolina texana* (Mathews 1940), *Panicum coloratum* (Muchiri et al. 1980), *Tribulus terrestris* possibly in association with the saprophytic fungus *Pithomyces chartarum* (Glastonbury and Boal 1985; Jacob and Peet 1987), and *Panicum coloratum* (Muchiri et al. 1980). Additional hepatotoxic plants are listed in

Chapter 11. An inherited congenital porphyria has been reported in other species, but apparently not in goats.

Clinical Signs

The clinical signs in goats with photosensitization vary, depending on the protection afforded the skin by long hair or pigmentation and whether liver disease is present. The head, udder, and vulva of white breeds exposed to sunlight initially develop erythema, edema, and intense pruritus. Photophobia is observed and the goats seek shade. Acutely there may be dyspnea or dysphagia. Eventually necrosis and sloughing of lips or teats may occur. Pigmented skin is unaffected. The entire dorsum may be involved in recently shorn animals. Liver function tests help to differentiate primary from secondary photosensitization.

Exudation of yellow, serous fluid from the skin surface and intense icterus of the entire carcass are reported in goats with hepatogenous photosensitization from *Tribulus terrestris*. This condition is called geeldikkop, which means "yellow thick head." Similar lesions have been produced experimentally by oral dosing of goats with sporidesmin. Feral and Angora cross goats were more resistant than Saanens, which in turn required two to four times as much sporidesmin as sheep to produce comparable liver lesions and clinical signs (Smith and Embling 1991).

Therapy and Prevention

Affected goats should be removed from the sun, and additional ingestion of hepatotoxic plants or toxins avoided. This may require moving or supplementing range animals. Laxatives might be helpful if ingestion has occurred recently, and antihistamines and antibiotics are given if much skin is destroyed. Affected skin is sprayed with methylene blue and fly repellents if housing is not possible. Selection for skin pigmentation will decrease the prevalence of photosensitization, but losses resulting from liver disease will continue unabated unless exposure to hepatotoxins is prevented.

Kaalsiekte

The South African bitterkarroo bush *Chrysocoma ciliata* (*C. tenuifolia*) produces skin disease in young kids and lambs if their dams consume large quantities of the plant pre partum. The toxin is excreted in milk, causing hair shedding and diarrhea (Steyn 1934). Kids develop pruritus when exposed to sunlight and lick off large patches of hair. Sequelae include death from exposure, a crusty dermatitis from sunburn, and abomasal hairballs. Supportive treatment (protection from sunburn and wind, laxatives to remove hairballs) should continue until hair returns. Keeping the does and ewes off the infested veld from one month before until one month after parturition will prevent the condition (Kellerman et al. 2005).

Frostbite

Special attention should be given to drying of the ears when kids are born in cold environments. Otherwise it is common for the ear tips to develop frostbite. If the initial edematous stage is not treated, the affected skin becomes necrotic and eventually sloughs. The ear tips are rounded and alopecic and the remaining pinna is of variable length. The feet of neonates and teats and scrotum of adults are also at risk of frostbite under extreme environmental conditions.

Ensuring that the extremities remain dry is important for prevention of such injuries. Immediate first aid involves rapid thawing in warm water 106° to 111°F (41°C to 44°C) (Scott 1988) or with a hair dryer. Beef calf producers report that freezing of the ear tips can be prevented by using stockinette or duct tape to keep the ears closely apposed to the warmer head during the first days.

Ergotism

Ergot toxicity (a mycotoxicosis caused by alkaloids produced by *Claviceps purpurea*) causes sloughing of the extremities in cattle, similar to frostbite, and is potentiated by exposure to cold. There is a single report of lameness and gangrenous necrosis with sloughing just above the coronary band in goat kids grazing on fescue parasitized by the fungus (Hibbs and Wolf 1982).

Urine Scald

During the breeding season bucks urinate on their face, beard, and front legs whenever sexually aroused. Although this habit heightens the doe-attracting aroma of the breeding male, it can lead to dermatitis in the areas that are continuously wet with urine. Clipping of long hair allows for faster drying of the skin. Skin lesions can be washed with a mild soap or vinegar solution (5 ml in 500 ml water, Konnersman 2005a) and then liberally coated with petroleum jelly, zinc oxide, or other water repellent ointment daily, until the end of the breeding season.

Similar skin care year-round may be required for intersexes or males after urethrostomy or bladder marsupialization if the perineum or inside of the thighs becomes wet during urination. Males on a high protein diet may develop posthitis and moist infections of the skin of the prepuce. In addition to general wound care, the ration should be corrected, as described in Chapters 12 and 19.

Other Contact Dermatitis Conditions

Caustic agents that cause stomatitis (see Chapter 10) may be expected to cause dermatitis as well, if applied to the external skin. There are various anecdotal reports of occasional skin irritation and hair loss following topical application of numerous parasiticides. If this occurs, the animal should be washed with warm water and a mild detergent to remove residual product.

Dehorning Paste

An alkaline paste is sometimes used by producers to disbud young kids. The paste eats through and destroys the skin from which horns would grow. Clipping hair and applying a ring of petroleum jelly may help contain the paste to the horn bud. Rubbing against other animals and pawing with a hind foot in response to local pain spread the paste and cause skin necrosis elsewhere on the body of the disbudded kid or other pen mates. Paste dehorning should be discouraged.

Milk

Some kids develop alopecia or even raw skin lesions (due to rubbing) on the lips and face where contact with milk or milk replacer has occurred. The condition has been termed "labial dermatitis" and can be prevented by washing or wiping the kid's face after each feeding (King 1984).

Decubital Sores

Emaciated or recumbent animals commonly develop full thickness skin necrosis over bony prominences such as elbows, hocks, and sternum. Deep, clean, dry bedding and frequent turning of the animal help prevent such lesions. Even with daily cleansing and drying of the sores, healing occurs very slowly, and only if underlying debilitating conditions are corrected. Sternal abscesses are discussed in Chapter 3.

Plant Awn Migration

The barbed seeds of numerous plants, especially grass awns, can penetrate the skin and migrate in the subcutaneous or deeper tissues. Nodules, abscesses, or draining tracts may develop (Scott 2007). An extensive discussion of potentially damaging plants in southern Africa (Kellerman et al. 2005) does not mention goats, but there is no reason to believe that they would not be affected.

NEOPLASIA

The most common skin tumors of the goat are cutaneous papilloma (warts), squamous cell carcinoma, and melanoma. Hemangioma, hemangiosarcoma, histiocytoma, mast cell tumor, and cutaneous lymphosarcoma have also been reported (Bastianello 1983; Manning et al. 1985; Roth and Perdrizet 1985; Allison and Fritz 2001; Bildfell et al. 2002; Konnersman 2005b). Ectopic mammary gland, which could be mistaken for a neoplastic condition, is discussed in Chapter 3.

Papilloma

Common warts probably occur much more frequently in goats than the caprine literature suggests. This is because those on the head or neck are benign and often self-limiting. If noticed at all, they are recognized as warts and because of a favorable prognosis, biopsy or treatment is not attempted. Favorable response to autogenous vaccine, after surgical removal of the largest warts, has been reported in a study with no untreated controls (Rajguru et al. 1988). The involvement of multiple animals in one closely confined herd has been taken as evidence for an infectious origin (Davis and Kemper 1936), although a wart virus has not been demonstrated in caprine papillomas.

Udder Warts

Warts on the udder have a different clinical course and are apparently limited to white goats (Saanens or Angoras) that have lactated at least once (Moulton 1954; Ficken et al. 1983; Theilen et al. 1985). The papillomas involve the white skin of both udder and teats and are typically multiple (Figure 14.5). They may either be flaky or form elongated cutaneous horns. Some transform into squamous cell carcinomas with wide base and ulcerated surface. The carcinomas may rarely metastasize to the supramammary lymph node. Additional discussion of these tumors is included in Chapter 14.

Carcinomas

Carcinomas of the skin also occur on other regions of the goat and without a preceding papilloma lesion. Again, white breeds in sunny climates are at risk. Angoras and Boer goats frequently develop carcinomas of the perineum (vulva and anus) (Thomas 1929; Curasson 1933; Hofmeyr et al. 1965; Yeruham et al. 1993). Ears, horn stumps, and muzzle (van der Heide 1963) may also be involved. The tumor may be sessile or pedunculated and becomes ulcerated as it enlarges. Detection often follows development of a foul-smelling exudate (Ramadan 1975). Possible origins for these tumors include squamous cells, basal cells, and sebaceous glands. Early surgical treatment is curative; otherwise affected animals should be culled. An affected ear can be easily amputated using local anesthesia and a Burdizzo emasculatome, placed on an angle to give a more cosmetically acceptable pointed shape to the remaining ear cartilage. Myiasis hastens the death of animals left untreated.

Melanomas

Melanomas appear to involve the same skin areas as the carcinomas, especially the vulva, perineum, and ear (Venkatesan et al. 1979; Bastianello 1983; Ramadan 1988). Indeed, it is sometimes unclear whether a given tumor is a pigmented basal cell carcinoma or a melanoma (Jackson 1936). In other instances, both clinical course (metastases to internal organs) and histologic findings are consistent with malignant melanoma (Sockett et al. 1984). The prognosis is poor, as metastases commonly occur to local nodes, liver, and lung. A breed predilection was demonstrated in the Sudan in a review of sixty-two affected goats; the gray or brown "American" goats originally imported from Syria were more commonly affected than the more numerous all black native Nubian goats (Ramadan 1988). The Angora goat has been proposed as a model for human melanomas, because both tumors and benign melanocytic lesions can be induced by exposure to sunlight (Green et al. 1996).

INHERITED OR CONGENITAL CONDITIONS

A possibly inherited absence of hair at birth has been reported in a buck kid and his sire (breed unspecified) (Kislovsky 1937). The sire developed a nearly normal fleece as it grew older, but the kid died young. Neither histology nor additional matings were performed.

"Sticky kid syndrome" is a congenital disease reported in purebred Golden Guernsey goats, and may be inherited as a recessive character. At birth the kids have a sticky and matted coat that does not dry normally. The coat remains harsh and sticky in older goats (Jackson 1986).

Kids, unlike lambs, do not appear to develop congenital changes in the hair coat when exposed in utero to border disease virus (Orr and Barlow 1978).

Wattle cysts, which are located subcutaneously in the cervical region, are discussed in Chapter 3.

MISCELLANEOUS CONDITIONS

Dermatologists in referral hospitals see a disproportionate number of goats with "uncommon" skin diseases that have not responded to empirical treatments, including antibiotics, parasiticides, and manipulations of the diet. Extensive diagnostic work-up has characterized and identified the cause of some of these conditions, but others remain perplexing. In particular, crusting lesions of Nubian goats, especially involving the ears and face, have frequently defied attempts to identify an etiology or an effective treatment.

Pemphigus

Pemphigus foliaceus is an autoimmune disease in which the affected individual (man, dog, cat, horse, or goat) develops auto-antibodies against the glycocalyx of keratinocytes. Reports of the condition in goats are few (Jackson et al. 1984; Scott et al. 1984; Valdez et al. 1995; Pappalardo et al. 2002). There is no evidence that the condition is hereditary.

Clinical Signs and Diagnosis

Clinical findings include vesicles or blisters, pustules, crusts, alopecia, and sometimes pruritus. The lesions may be generalized over the entire body or may be concentrated in or begin in a more restricted location, such as the perineal region, ventral abdomen, and groin (Jackson et al. 1984). Diagnosis requires full-thickness skin biopsies of lesions containing intact vesicles or pustules. Routine histology (formalin fixation) reveals intraepidermal acantholysis with formation of clefts, vesicles, or pustules. Cells of the stratum granulosum may be seen attached to the overlying stratum corneum (Scott 1988). These granular "cling-ons" may also be found in direct smears of intact vesicles, along with nondegenerate neutrophils and/or eosinophils (Scott 2007). Direct immunofluorescence testing (tissue in Michel's fixative; no glucocorticoids administered in the past three weeks) reveals intercellular deposition of immunoglobulin. Serologic testing (indirect immunofluorescence) is unreliable for the diagnosis of caprine pemphigus (Scott et al. 1987).

Treatment

Treatment of pemphigus may be attempted with high doses of systemic glucocorticoids (1 mg/kg prednisone or prednisolone IM twice daily for seven to ten days, then alternate morning therapy at reduced dosage). A long-acting corticosteroid injection (dexamethasone-21-isonicotinate 0.04 mg/kg IM) once every two months suppressed clinical signs in one goat (Pappalardo et al. 2002) but the potential risks are greater. Oral prednisolone is not used because of very low bioavailability in ruminants (Koritz 1982). In young or nonresponsive goats, chrysotherapy with aurothioglucose (1 mg/kg weekly until response is observed, then monthly) may be tried. This drug has been discontinued in the United States. Although adverse reactions to gold have not been reported in goats, hemograms and urinalyses should be monitored. Gold treatment was successful in one reported case (Scott et al. 1984) and unsuccessful in another (Valdez et al. 1995).

Alopecic Exfoliative Dermatitis, Psoriasiform Dermatitis

A nonpruritic, seborrheic skin condition affecting pygmy goats of all ages has been described in England. Hair loss, scaling, and crusting occur around the eyes, lips, chin, ears, ventrum, and perineum. Histology reveals a psoriasiform dermatitis, and the condition responds to steroids but recurs when treatment is stopped (Jefferies et al. 1987, 1991). There is orthokeratotic and parakeratotic hyperkeratosis (Scott 2007). A very similar condition has been studied in pygmy goats in the Netherlands (Kuiper 1989). The condition was not contagious and did not respond to administration of corticosteroids, zinc, vitamin A, or selenium. A hereditary basis was suspected.

Lichenoid Dermatitis

This idiopathic condition was reported in a two-year-old Boer buck in Israel (Yeruham et al. 2002). Pruritic flat-topped angular scaly papules were present in the skin over the entire surface of the goat. The lesions were 10 to 20 mm in diameter but coalesced into plaques on the head. Some lesions were fissured. Histologic findings included orthokeratotic hyperkeratosis, epidermal hyperplasia, and microabscesses. Poxviruses, dermatophytes, and granulomatous and neoplastic conditions were ruled out by histopathology. A photograph of a similar case from Belgium, which resolved spontaneously after several months, has been published by Scott (2007).

Allergy or Hypersensitivity

Occasionally a pruritic, alopecic to crusty condition is seen on the dorsal midline of pastured goats in spring and summer. No external parasites are found on the animal, and practitioners have implicated a hypersensitivity to the saliva of *Culicoides* spp. midges (Scott 2007). Stabling at dusk and dawn may limit exposure to the insects and a brief course of systemic corticosteroids may alleviate the pruritus.

Other cases of poorly explained pruritic skin disease have been observed and defied diagnostic efforts to determine the etiology. In one such instance, orthokeratotic hyperkeratosis and perivascular infiltration with eosinophils in a five-year-old wether with crusting on the back and neck suggested allergy, as did response to dexamethasone therapy, but skin testing and manipulation of diet and environment were unsuccessful (Humann-Ziehank et al. 2001).

REFERENCES

Abo-Shehada, M.N.: Incidence of *Chrysomya bezziana* screwworm myiasis in Saudi Arabia, 1999/2000. Vet. Rec., 156:354–356, 2005.

Abraham, S.S., et al.: An outbreak of peste des petits ruminants infection in Kerala. Indian Vet. J., 82:815–817, 2005.

Abu-Samra, M.T., Imbabi, S.E., and Mahgoub, E.S.: Mange in domestic animals in the Sudan. Ann. Trop. Med. Parasitol. 75:627–637, 1981.

Adalsteinsson, S., et al.: Inheritance of goat coat colors. J. Hered., 85:267–272, 1994.

Alexander, J.L.: Screwworms. J. Am. Vet. Med. Assoc. 228:357–367, 2006.

Allison, N., and Fritz, D.L.: Cutaneous mast cell tumour in a kid goat. Vet. Rec., 149:560–561, 2001.

Andrews, A.H., and Lamport, A.: Isolation of *Staphylococcus chromogenes* from an unusual case of impetigo in a goat. Vet. Rec., 140:584, 1997.

Anke, M., et al.: Der Einfluss des Mangan-, Zink-, Kupfer-, Jod-, Selen-, Molybdän- und Nickelmangels auf die Fortpflanzungleistung des Wiederkäuers. Wissenschaftliche Zeitschrift Karl-Marx-Universität Leipzig, Mathematisch-Naturwissenschaftliche Reihe 26(3):283–292, 1977.

AVMA: Screwworm returns to vex Texas. J. Am. Vet. Med. Assoc. 214:179, 1999.

Backx, A., et al.: Clinical signs of bluetongue virus serotype 8 infection in sheep and goats. Vet. Rec., 161:591–592, 2007.

Baker, J.C., Esser, M.B., and Larson, V.L.: Pseudorabies in a goat. J. Am. Vet. Med. Assoc. 181:607, 1982.

Baker, M.K., and Ducasse, F.B.W.: Tick infestation of livestock in Natal. The role played by goats as reservoirs of the economically important cattle ticks. J. So. Afr. Vet. Assoc. 39:55–59, 1968.

Bakos, K., and Brag, S.: Untersuchungen über Ziegenpocken in Schweden. Nord Vet.-Med. 9:431–449, 1957.

Bal, H.S., and Ghoshal, N.G.: The "scent glands" of the goat (*Capra hircus*). Anat. Histol. Embryol. 5:104, 1976.

Bale, S.: Poisoning of sheep, goats and cows by the weed *Hypericum triquetrifolium*. Refuah Vet. 35:36–37, 1978.

Barakat, S.E.M., Wasfi, I.A., and Adam, S.E.I.: The toxicity of *Aristolochia bracteata* in goats. Vet. Pathol. 20:611–616, 1983.

Barth, D., and Preston, J.M.: Efficacy of topically administered ivermectin against chorioptic and sarcoptic mange of cattle. Vet. Rec. 123:101–104, 1988.

Bastianello, S.S.: A survey of neoplasia in domestic species over a 40-year period from 1935 to 1974 in the Republic of South Africa. III. Tumours occurring in pigs and goats. Onderstepoort J. Vet. Res. 50:25–28, 1983.

Bates, P.G.: Inter- and intra-specific variation within the genus *Psoroptes* (Acari: Psoroptidae). Vet. Parasitol., 83:201–217, 1999.

Bates, P., et al.: Observations on the biology and control of the chewing louse (*Bovicola limbata*) of Angora goats in Great Britain. Vet. Rec., 149:675–676, 2000.

Bath, G.F., van Wyk, J.A., and Pettey, K.P.: Control measures for some important and unusual goat diseases in southern Africa. Small Rum. Res., 60:127–140, 2005.

Bath, G.F., Wentzel, D., and van Tonder, E.M.: Cretinism in Angora goats. J. S. Afr. Vet. Assoc. 50:237–239, 1979.

Baxendell, S.A.: The Diagnosis of the Diseases of Goats. Vade Mecum Series for Domestic Animals, Series B No. 9, University of Sydney Post-Grad. Foundation in Vet. Sci., Sydney, Australia, 1988.

Betteridge, K., et al.: Growth of fibre in cashmere producing goats. Sheep and Beef Cattle Society of the New Zealand Veterinary Association. In: Proceedings, Eighteenth Seminar, Lincoln, New Zealand, pp. 9–17, 1988.

Biberstein, E.L., Jang, S.S., and Hirsh, D.S.: Species distribution of coagulase-positive staphylococci in animals. J. Clin. Microbiol. 19:610–615, 1984.

Bida, S.A., and Dennis, S.M.: Dermatophilosis in northern Nigeria. Vet. Bull. 46:471–478, 1976.

Bildfell, R.J., Valentine, B.A., and Whitney, K.M.: Cutaneous vasoproliferative lesions in goats. Vet. Pathol., 39:273–277, 2002.

Black, D.N.: The capripoxvirus genome. Rev. Sci. Tech. Off. Int. Epiz. 5:495–501, 1986.

Bliss, E.L,: Tinea versicolor dermatomycosis in the goat. J. Am. Vet. Med. Assoc., 184:1512–1513, 1984.

Boughton, I.B., and Hardy, W.T.: Contagious ecthyma (sore mouth) of sheep and goats. J. Am. Vet. Med. Assoc. 85:150–178, 1934.

Bowman, D.D.: Georgis' Parasitology for Veterinarians. 8th Ed. St. Louis, Saunders, 2003.

Bretzlaff, K.: Special problems of hair goats. Vet. Clin. North Am. Food An. Pract. 6(3):721–735, 1990.

Brotherston, J.G., Renwick, C.C., Stamp, J.T., and Zlotnik, I: Spread of scrapie by contact to goats and sheep. J. Comp. Pathol. 78:9–17, 1968.

Brügger, M., and Braun, U.: Demodicosis in a Toggenburg goat. Schweiz. Arch. Tierheilkd., 142:639–642, 2000.

Burrows, G.E., and Stair, E.L.: Apparent *Agave lecheguilla* intoxication in Angora goats. Vet. Hum. Toxicol., 32:259–260, 1990.

Bwangamoi, O.: A preliminary report on the finding of *Besnoitia besnoiti* in goat skins affected with dimple in Kenya. Bull. Epizoot. Dis. Afr. 15:263–271, 1967.

Bwangamoi, O., Carles, A.B., Wandera, J.G.: An epidemic of besnoitiosis in goats in Kenya. Vet. Rec. 125:461, 1989.

Caldas, A.D.: Avitaminose A espontânea em caprinos. (Spontaneous avitaminosis A in goats.) O Biológico 27:266–270, 1961.

Çam, Y., et al.: Peste des petits ruminants in a sheep and goat flock in Kayseri province, Turkey. Vet. Rec., 157:523–524, 2005.

Capucchio, M.T., et al.: Clinical signs and diagnosis of scrapie in Italy: a comparative study in sheep and goats. J. Vet. Med. A, 48:23–31, 2001.

Carn, V.M., et al.: Protection of goats against capripox using a subunit vaccine. Vet. Rec., 135:434–436, 1994.

Chamberlain, W.F., and Hopkins, D.E.: The synthetic juvenile hormone for control of *Bovicola limbata* on Angora goats. J. Econ. Entomol. 64:1198–1199, 1971.

Chapman, H.M., et al.: *Cryptococcus neoformans* infection in goats. Aust. Vet. J., 67:263–265, 1990.

Cheema, A.H.: Observations on the histopathology of warble infestation in goats by the larvae of *Przhevalskiana silenus*. Zbl. Vet. Med. B. 24:648–655, 1977.

Cheema, A.H., and Toofanian, F.: Besnoitiosis in wild and domestic goats in Iran. Cornell Vet. 69:159–168, 1979.

Chineme, C.N., Adekeye, J.O., and Bida, S.A.: Ringworm caused by *Trichophyton verrucosum* in young goats: a case report. Bull. Anim. Health Prod. Afr. 29:75–78, 1981.

Christodoulopoulos, G., and Theodoropoulos, G.: Infestation of dairy goats with the human flea, *Pulex irritans*, in Central Greece. Vet. Rec., 152:371–372, 2003.

Christodoulopoulos, G., et al.: Biological, seasonal and environmental factors associated with *Pulex irritans* infestation of dairy goats in Greece. Vet. Parasitol., 137:137–143, 2006.

Coates, J.W., and Hoff, S.: Contagious ecthyma: an unusual distribution of lesions in goats. Can. Vet. J. 31:209–210, 1990.

Colwell, D.D., and Otranto, D.: Cross-transmission studies with *Hypoderma lineatum* de Vill. (Diptera: Oestridae): Attempted infestation of goats (*Capra hircus*). Vet. Parasitol., 141:302–306, 2006.

Committee on Foreign Animal Diseases: Foreign Animal Diseases. Richmond, VA, United States Animal Health Association. Revised, 1998.

Cook, R.W.: Ear mites (*Raillietia manfredi* and *Psoroptes cuniculi*) in goats in New South Wales. Aust. Vet. J. 57:72–74, 1981.

Couchman, R.C.: Cashmere production and utilization (a world overview). In: Proceedings, Fourth International Conference on Goats, Brazil, Vol. 1, pp. 153–167, 1987.

Curasson, M.G.: Le cancer cutané de la chèvre Angora. Bull. Acad. Vét. France 6:346–348, 1933.

Das, D.N., and Misra, S.C.: Studies on caprine demodectic mange with institution of effective therapeutic measures. Indian Vet. J. 49:96–100, 1972.

Das, S.K., Pandey, A.K., and Mallick, B.B.: A note on the natural goat pox outbreak in Garwal Hills of Uttar Pradesh. Indian Vet. J. 55:671–673, 1978.

Davies, F.G.: Sheep and goat pox. In: Virus Diseases of Food Animals. Vol II: Disease Monographs. E.P.J. Gibbs, ed. New York, Academic Press, 1981.

Davis, C.L., and Kemper, H.E.: Common warts (papillomata) in goats. J. Am. Vet. Med. Assoc. 88:175–179, 1936.

Dawson, C.O., and Lepper, A.W.D.: *Peyronellaea glomerata* infection of the ear pinna in goats. Sabouraudia 8:145–148, 1970.

de la Concha-Bermejillo, A., et al.: Severe persistent orf in young goats. J. Vet. Diagn. Invest., 15:423–431, 2003.

Deorani, V.P.S., and Chaudhuri, R.P.: On the histopathology of the skin lesion of goats affected by sarcoptic mange. Indian J. Vet. Sci. Anim. Husb. 35:150–156, 1965.

Dercksen, D., et al.: [First outbreak of bluetongue in goats in the Netherlands.] Tijdschr. Diergeneeskd. 132:786–790, 2007.

Dorny, P., et al.: Survey of the importance of mange in the aetiology of skin lesions in goats in peninsular Malaysia. Trop. Anim. Health Prod., 26:81–86, 1994.

Dreyer, J.H., and Marincowitz, G.: Some observations on the skin histology and fibre characteristics of the Angora goat (*Capra hircus angoraensis*). S. Afr. J. Agric. Sci. 10:477–500, 1967.

Dubeuf, J.P., et al.: Situation, changes and future of goat industry around the world. Small Rum. Res., 51:165–173, 2004.

Dupuy, J., et al.: Eprinomectin in dairy goats: Dose influence on plasma levels and excretion in milk. Parasitol. Res., 87:294–298, 2001.

Durant, A.J.: Demodectic mange of the milk goat. Vet. Med. 39:268–270, 1944.

Dutt, B., and Kehar, N.D.: Incidence of goiter in goats and sheep in India. Br. Vet. J. 115:176–178, 1959.

Dutt, B., and Majumdar, B.N.: Epithelial metaplasia in experimental vitamin A deficient goats. Indian Vet. J. 46:789–791, 1969.

Ensor, D.R.: Fibre types and their evaluation in goats. Proceedings, Seventeenth Seminar of the Sheep and Beef Cattle Society of the New Zealand Veterinary Association. Hamilton, NZ, May 27–29, pp. 35–37, 1987.

Eppleston, J., and Moore, N.W.: Fleece and skin characteristics of selected Australian Angora goats. Small Rum. Res. 3:397–402, 1990.

Erasmus, B.J.: Bluetongue in sheep and goats. Aust. Vet. J. 51:165–170, 1975.

Euzeby, J., Chermette, R., and Gevrey, J.: La démodécie de la chèvre en France. Bull. Acad. Vét. France 49:423–430, 1976.

Fadzil, M., Cheah, T.S., and Subramaniam, P.: *Stephanofilaria kaeli* Buckley 1937 as the cause of chronic dermatitis on the foot of a goat and on the ears and teats of cattle in West Malaysia. Vet. Rec. 92:316–328, 1973.

Fagbemi, B.O.: Effect of *Ctenocephalides felis strongylus* infestation on the performance of West African dwarf sheep and goats. Vet. Q. 4:92–95, 1982.

Faure, O.: Peau de chevreau, peau de chagrin? La Chèvre 164:14–17, Jan-Feb, 1988.

Ficken, M.D., Andrews, J.J., and Engeltes, I.: Papilloma-squamous cell carcinoma of the udder of a Saanen goat. J. Am. Vet. Med. Assoc. 183:467, 1983.

Frier, H.J., et al.: Formation and absorption of cerebrospinal fluid in adult goats with hypo- and hyper-vitaminosis A. Am. J. Vet. Res. 35:45–55, 1974.

Galitzer, S.J., and Oehme, F.W.: Photosensitization: a literature review. Vet. Sci. Commun. 2:217–230, 1978.

Garg, S.K., Katoch, R., and Bhushan, C.: Efficacy of flumethrin pour-on against *Damalinia caprae* of goats (*Capra hircus*). Trop. Anim. Health Prod., 30:273–278, 1998.

Ghanem, Y.S., and Farid, M.F.A.: Vitamin A deficiency and supplementation in desert sheep. 1. Deficiency symptoms, plasma concentrations and body growth. World Rev. Anim. Prod. 18:69–74, 1982.

Giangaspero, A., et al.: Efficacy of injectable and pour-on microdose ivermectin in the treatment of goat warble fly infestation by *Przhevalskiana silenus* (Diptera, Oestridae). Vet. Parasitol., 116:333–343, 2003.

Gill, M.J., Arlette, J., Buchan, K.A., and Barber, K.: Human orf. A diagnostic consideration? Arch. Dermatol. 126:356–358, 1990.

Glastonbury, J.R.W., and Boal, G.K.: Geeldikkop in goats. Aust. Vet. J. 62:62–63, 1985.

Gnad, D.P., and Mock, D.E.: Ectoparasite control in small ruminants. Vet. Clin. North Am. Food Anim. Pract., 17:245–263, 2001.

Göksu, K.: Hypodermatosis in Anatolian black goats. Istanbul Üniv. Vet. Fak. Dergisi, 1:45–52, 1975. Abstract 5102 of Vet. Bull. 46:683, 1976.

Graham, O.H., and Hourrigan, J.L.: Eradication programs for the arthopod parasites of livestock. J. Med. Entomol., 13:629–658, 1977.

Green, A., et al.: An animal model for human melanoma. Photochem. Photobiol., 64:577–580, 1996.

Green, G., et al.: Orf virus infection in humans—New York, Illinois, California, and Tennessee, 2004–2005. Morbid. Mortal. Wkly. Rep., 55(03):65–68, 2006.

Groppel, B., and Hennig, A.: Zinkmangel beim Wiederkäuer. Arch. Exp. Veterinärmed. 25:817–821, 1971.

Gumaa, S.A., and Abu-Samra, M.T.: Experimental mycetoma infection in the goat. J. Comp. Pathol. 91:341–346, 1981.

Gumaa, S.A., et al.: Mycetomas in goats. Sabouraudia 16:217–223, 1978.

Guo, J., et al.: Characterization of a North American orf virus isolated from a goat with persistent, proliferative dermatitis. Virus Res., 93:169–179, 2003.

Gupta, R.C., Kwatra, M.S., and Singh, N.: Chronic selenium toxicity as a cause of hoof and horn deformities in buffalo, cattle and goat. Indian Vet. J. 59:738–740, 1982.

Haddow, J.R., and Idnani, J.A.: Goat dermatitis: a new virus disease of goats in India. Indian Vet. J. 24:332–337, 1948.

Hadlow, W.J.: The pathology of experimental scrapie in the dairy goat. Res. Vet. Sci. 2:289–314, 1961.

Haigh, J.C., and Hudson, R.J.: Farming Wapiti and Red Deer. St. Louis, Mosby, 1993.

Hajer, I., Abbas, B., and Abu Samra, M.T.: Capripox virus in sheep and goats in Sudan. Rev. Elev. Méd. Vét. Pays Trop., 41:125–128, 1988.

Hallam, G.J.: Transmission of *Damalinia ovis* and *Damalinia caprae* between sheep and goats. Aust. Vet. J., 62:344–345, 1985.

Handeland, K., and Skorping, A.: Experimental cerebrospinal elaphostrongylosis (*Elaphostrongylus rangiferi*) in goats: I. Clinical observations. J. Vet. Med. B, 40:141–147, 1993.

Handeland, K., and Sparboe, O.: Cerebrospinal elaphostrongylosis in dairy goats in northern Norway. J. Vet. Med. B 38:755–763, 1991.

Harcourt, R.A., and Anderson, M.A.: Naturally-occurring scrapie in goats. Vet. Rec. 94:504, 1974.

Harríson, R., and Palmer, B.H.: Further studies on amitraz as a veterinary acaricide. Pestic. Sci. 12:467–474, 1981.

Heath, A.C.G, Bishop, D.M., and Tenquist, J.D.: The prevalence and pathogenicity of *Chorioptes bovis* (Hering, 1845) and *Psoroptes cuniculi* (Delafond, 1859) (Acari: Psoroptidae) infestations in feral goats in New Zealand. Vet. Parasitol. 13:159–169, 1983.

Henderson, M., and Sabine, J.R.: Secondary follicle development in Australian cashmere goats. Small Rum. Res. 4:349–363, 1991.

Hibbs, C.M., and Wolf, N.: Ergot toxicosis in young goats. Mod. Vet. Pract. 63:126–128, 1982.

Hicks, M.: Pygora—the new breed. Dairy Goat J. 66:404–405, 1988.

Himonas, C.A., Theodorides, J.T., and Alexakis, A.E.: Demodectic mites in eyelids of domestic animals in Greece. J. Parasitol. 61:767, 1975.

Hofmeyr, H.S., Joubert, D.M., Badenhorst, F.J.G., and Steyn, G.J. van D.: Adaptability of sheep and goats to a South African tropical environment. Proc. S. Afr. Soc. Anim. Prod. 4:191–195, 1965.

Holst, P.J.: The world production and utilization of goat skins. In: Proceedings, Fourth International Conference on Goats, Brazil, pp. 145–152, 1987.

Hosseinion, M., et al.: Selenium poisoning in a mixed flock of sheep and goats in Iran. Trop. Anim. Health Prod., 4:173–174, 1972.

Hotter, H., and Buchner, A.: Euteraktinomykose bei einer Ziege. Wien. Tierärztl. Mschr., 82:225–227, 1995.

Housawi, F.M.T., et al.: A close comparative study on the response of sheep and goats to experimental orf infection. J. Vet. Med. B 40:272–282, 1993.

Humann-Ziehank, E., et al.: Differential diagnostic, treatment trial and course of an allergic dermatitis in a goat. Tierärztl. Praxis G, Grosstiere/Nutztiere 29:356–360, 2001.

Hunter, L., Corbett, W., and Grindem, C.: Anthrax. J. Am. Vet. Med. Assoc. 194:1028–1031, 1989.

Hyslop, N.S.G.: Dermatophilosis (streptothricosis) in animals and man. Comp. Immunol. Microbiol. Infect. Dis. 2:389–404, 1980.

Ibrahim, K.E.E., and Abu-Samra, M.T.: Experimental transmission of a goat strain of *Sarcoptes scabiei* to desert sheep and its treatment with ivermectin. Vet. Parasitol. 26:157–164, 1987.

Ihemelandu, E.C., Nduaka, O., and Ojukwu, E.M.: Hyperimmune serum in the control of peste des petits ruminants. Trop. Anim. Health Prod. 17:83–88, 1985.

Ivie, G.W.: Toxicological significance of plant furocoumarins. In: Effects of Poisonous Plants on Livestock. R.F. Keeler, K.R. Van Kampen, and L.F. James, eds. New York, Academic Press, pp. 475–485, 1978.

Jackson, C.: The incidence and pathology of tumours of domesticated animals in South Africa. Onderstepoort J. Vet. Sci. Anim. Indust. 6:1–460, 1936.

Jackson, P.: Skin diseases in goats. In Practice 8:5–10, 1986.

Jackson, P.G.G., Lloyd, S., and Jefferies, A.R.: Pemphigus foliaceous in a goat. Vet. Rec. 114:479, 1984.

Jackson, P.G.G., Richards, H.W., and Lloyd, S.: Sarcoptic mange in goats. Vet. Rec. 112:330, 1983.

Jacob, R.H., and Peet, R.L.: Poisoning of sheep and goats by *Tribulus terrestris* (caltrop). Aust. Vet. J., 64:288–289, 1987.

Jefferies, A.R., Jackson, P.G.G., and Casas, F.C.: Alopecic exfoliative dermatitis in goats. Vet. Rec. 121:576, 1987.

Jefferies, A.R., et al.: Seborrhoeic dermatitis in pigmy goats. Vet. Dermatol., 2:109–117, 1991.

Kalkus, J.W.: A study of goiter and associated conditions in domestic animals. State College of Washington Agric. Expt. Station Bull. No. 156, July 1920.

Kambarage, D.M.: Sarcoptic mange infestation in goats. Bull. Anim. Hlth. Prod. Afr., 40:239–244, 1992.

Karim, M.A.: Pox among Sannen (sic) goats in Iraq. Trop. Anim. Health Prod. 15:62, 1983.

Kellerman, T.S., et al.: Plant Poisonings and Mycotoxicoses of Livestock in Southern Africa. Capetown, Oxford University Press, 2005.

King, N.B.: Skin diseases. In: Refresher Course for Veterinarians, Proceedings No. 73, Goats, The University of Sydney, The Post-Graduate Committee in Veterinary Science, Sydney, N.S.W., Australia, Update pp. 199–201, 1984.

Kislovsky, D.: Inherited hairlessness in the goat. J. Hered. 28:264–267, 1937.

Kitching, R.P.: The control of sheep and goat pox. Rev. Sci. Tech. Off. Int. Epiz. 5:503–511, 1986.

Klören, W.R.L., and Norton, B.W.: Melatonin and fleece growth in Australian cashmere goats. Small Rum. Res., 17:179–185, 1995.

Komarov, A., and Goldsmit, L.: A disease similar to blue tongue in cattle and sheep in Israel. Refuah Vet. 8:96–100, 1951.

Konar, A., and Ivie, G.W.: Fate of [14C]coumaphos after dermal application to lactating goats as a pouron formulation. Am. J. Vet. Res. 49:488–492, 1988.

Konnersman, M.: Diseases of the skin and hair coat in dwarf goats. Part 1. Forum Kleinwiederkäuer/Petits Ruminants, (10):11–16, 2005a.

Konnersman, M.: Diseases of the skin and hair coat in dwarf goats. Part 2. Forum Kleinwiederkäuer/Petits Ruminants, (12): 6–13, 2005b.

Koritz, G.D.: Influence of ruminant gastrointestinal physiology on the pharmacokinetics of drugs in dosage forms administered orally. In: Veterinary Pharmacology and Toxicology. Proceedings 2nd European Association for Veterinary Pharmacology and Toxicology, Toulouse. AVI Publ. Co., Inc., Westport CT, pp. 151–163, 1982.

Krametter-Froetscher, R., Hauser, S., and Baumgartner, W.: Zinc-responsive dermatosis in goats suggestive of hereditary malabsorption: two field cases. Vet. Dermatol., 16:269–275, 2005.

Kuiper, R.: A skin disease in dwarf goats. In: Goat Diseases and Productions, Second International Colloquium in Niort, France, Abstracts, p. 47, 1989.

Larsen, J.W.A.: An outbreak of mycotic dermatitis in goat kids. Aust. Vet. J. 64:160, 1987.

Lavoipierre, M.M.J., and Larsen, P.H.: A note on a new ear mite discovered in the auditory canal of California feral goats. Calif. Vet. 35(2):23–24, 1981.

Lazzaro, J.: Basic information on copper deficiency in dairy goats in southern California. Accessed October 15, 2007 at http://www.saanendoah.com/copper1.html.

Le Jan, C., et al.: Transfer of antibodies against the CPD virus through colostrum and milk. Ann. Recherche Vét. 9:343–346, 1978.

Levot, G.: Resistance and the control of lice on humans and production animals. Int. J. Parasitol., 30:291–297, 2000.

Lewis, C.: Update on orf. In Pract., 18:376–381, 1996.

Liebisch, A., Deppe, M., and Olbrich, S.: Untersuchungen zur Überlebensdauer von Milben der Arten *Psoroptes ovis*, *Psoroptes cuniculi* und *Chorioptes bovis* abseits des belebten Wirtes. (Experimental studies on the longevity of mange mites of the species *Psoroptes ovis*, *Psoroptes cuniculi* and *Chorioptes bovis* off the host.) Dtsch. Tierärztl. Wochenschr. 92:181–185, 1985.

Litherland, A.J., et al.: Effects of season on fleece traits of Angora does in the US. Small Rum. Res., 38:63–70, 2000.

Littlejohn, A.I.: Psoroptic mange in the goat. Vet. Rec. 82:148–155, 1968.

Lofstedt, J., et al.: Severe psoroptic mange and endoparasitism in a Nubian doe. Can. Vet. J., 35:716–718, 1994.

Loria, G.R., et al.: Dermatophilosis in goats in Sicily. Vet. Rec., 156:120–121, 2005.

Luedke, A.J., and Anakwenze, E.I.: Bluetongue virus in goats. Am. J. Vet. Res. 33:1739–1745, 1972.

Luo, J., et al.: Effects of mimosine on fiber shedding, follicle activity, and fiber regrowth in Spanish goats. J. Anim. Sci., 78:1551–1555, 2000.

Lupton, C.J., Pfeiffer, F.A., and Blakemen, N.E.: Medullation in mohair. Small Rum. Res. 5:357–365, 1991.

Lush, J.L.: Inheritance of horns, wattles, and color in grade Toggenburg goats. J. Hered. 17:73–91, 1926.

Macedo, J.T.S.A., et al.: Cutaneous and nasal protothecosis in a goat. Vet. Pathol., 45:352–354, 2008.

MacIvor, K.M. de F, and Horak, I.G.: Foot abscess in goats in relation to the seasonal abundance of adult *Amblyomma hebraeum* and adult *Rhipicephalus glabroscutatum*. J. So. Afr. Vet. Assoc. 58:113–118, 1987.

Mahanta, P.N., et al.: Identification and characterization of staphylococci isolated from cutaneous lesions of goats. J. Vet. Med. B, 44:309–311, 1997.

Majumdar, B.N., and Gupta, B.N.: Studies on carotene metabolism in goats. Indian J. Med. Res. 48:388–393, 1960.

Makinde, A.A.: The reverse single radial immunodiffusion technique for detecting antibodies to *Dermatophilus congolensis*. Vet. Rec. 106:383–385, 1980.

Manning, T.O., Scott, D.W., and Smith, M.C.: Caprine dermatology. Part III. Parasitic, allergic, hormonal, and neoplastic disorders. Comp. Cont. Educ. Pract. Vet. 7:S437-S452, 1985.

Margolena, L.A.: Mohair histogenesis, maturation, and shedding in the angora goat. Agric. Res. Service USDA Tech. Bull. 1495, 1974.

Maryamma, K.I., and Sivadas, C.G.: Serum vitamin A levels in experimental aflatoxicosis in the goat. Kerala J. Vet. Sci. 4:26–29, 1973.

Mason, I.L.: Goat. In: Evolution of Domesticated Animals. I.L. Mason, ed. London and New York, Longman, 1984.

Mathews, F.P.: Lechuguilla (*Agave lecheguilla*) poisoning in sheep and goats. J. Am. Vet. Med. Assoc. 93:168–175, 1938.

Mathews, F.P.: Poisoning in sheep and goats by sacahuiste (*Nolina exana*) buds and blooms. Texas Agric. Expt. Sta. Bull. 585, 1940.

Mathieson, A.O.: Mycotic dermatitis, ringworm and related infections. In: Diseases of Sheep. 2nd Ed. W.B. Martin and I.D. Aitken, eds. Oxford, Blackwell Scientific Publ. 1991.

Matthews, J.: Diseases of the Goat. 2nd Ed. Oxford, Blackwell Science, 1999.

Mayr, A., and Büttner, M.: Ecthyma (orf) virus. In: Virus Infections of Vertebrates. Vol. 3. Virus Infections of Ruminants. Z. Dinter and B. Morein, eds. New York, Elsevier Science Publ., 1990, pp. 33–42.

McDonald, B.: Cashmere growth cycle and skin histology. Australian Cashmere Goat Society, Cashmere Goat Note G1/1, July 1985.

McDowell, L.R., et al.: Mineral status comparisons in goats of Florida, with emphasis on zinc deficiency. Small Rum. Res. 5:327–335, 1991.

McGregor, B.A.: Liveweight and nutritional influences on fibre diameter of mohair. Proceedings, Aust. Soc. Anim. Prod. 16:420, 1986. Abstract.

McGregor, B.A.: Effects of different nutritional regimens on the productivity of Australian cashmere goats and the partitioning of nutrients between cashmere and hair growth. Aust. J. Exp. Agric. 28:459–467, 1988.

McKeever, D.J., Jenkinson, D.M., Hutchison, G., and Reid, H.W.: Studies of the pathogenesis of orf virus infection in sheep. J. Comp. Pathol. 94:317–328, 1988.

McKeever, D.J., and Reid, H.W.: Survival of orf virus under British winter conditions. Vet. Rec. 118:613–614, 1986.

McVicar, J.W., and Sutmoller, P.: Sheep and goats as foot-and-mouth disease carriers. In: Proceedings, U.S. Livestock Sanitary Assoc., 72:400–406, 1968.

Mémery, G.: La streptothricose cutanée. II. Sur quelques cas spontanés chez des caprins dans la région de Dakar. Rev. Élev. Méd. Vét. Pays Trop. 13:143–153, 1960.

Mémery, G., and Thiéry, G.: La streptothricose cutanée 1. Étude de la maladie naturelle et expérimentale des bovins. Rev. Élev. Méd. Vét. Pays Trop. 13:123–142, 1960.

Menzano, A., Rambozzi, L., and Rossi, L.: A severe episode of wildlife-derived scabies in domestic goats in Italy. Small Rum. Res., 70:154–158, 2007.

Merrall, M., and Brassington, R.J.: Lice on goats—Are they important? Sheep and Beef Cattle Society of the New Zealand Vet. Assoc., In: Proceedings, Eighteenth Seminar, Lincoln, New Zealand, pages 25–27, 1988.

Mettler, F., Engels, M., Wild, P., and Bivetti, A.: Herpesvirus-Infektion bei Zicklein in der Schweiz. Schweiz. Arch. Tierheilkd. 121:655–662, 1979.

Meynink, S.E., Jackson, P.G.G., and Platt, D.: Treatment of intraoral orf lesions in lambs using diathermy and cryosurgery. Vet. Rec. 121:594, 1987.

Mishra, K.C., and Ghei, J.C.: A severe outbreak of foot and mouth disease in local goats of Sikkim due to "A22" virus. Indian Vet. J. 60:410–412, 1983.

Mitchell, M.: Inheritance of coat color. Dairy Goat J. 67:494–496,533, 1989.

Moore, B., Drummond, R.O., and Brundrett, H.M.: Tests of insecticides for the control of goat lice in 1957 and 1958. J. Econ. Entomol. 52:980–981, 1959.

Moriello, K.A., and Cooley, J.: Difficult dermatologic diagnosis. J. Amer. Vet. Med. Assoc., 218:19–20, 2001.

Moulton, J.E.: Cutaneous papillomas on the udders of milk goats. N. Amer. Vet. 35:29–33, 1954.

Muchiri, D.J., Bridges, C.H., Ueckert, D.N., and Bailey, E.M.: Photosensitization of sheep on klein-grass pasture. J. Am. Vet. Med. Assoc. 177:353–354, 1980.

Mullowney, P.C., and Baldwin, E.W.: Skin diseases of goats. Vet. Clin. North Am. Large Anim. Pract. 6:143–154, 1984.

Munro, R.: Caprine dermatophilosis in Fiji. Trop. Anim. Health Prod. 10:221–222, 1978.

Munro, R., and Munro, H.M.C.: Psoroptic mange in goats in Fiji. Trop. Anim. Health Prod. 12:1–5, 1980.

Munz, E.: Gleichzeitiges Auftreten von Orf und Streptothrichose bei Ziegen und Schafen in Kenya. Berl. Münch. Tierärztl. Wochenschr. 82:221–240, 1969.

Munz, E.: Double infection of sheep and goats in Kenya with orf virus and *Dermatophilus*. In: Dermatophilus Infections in Animals and Man. D.H. Lloyd and K.C. Sellers, eds. London, Academic Press, 1976.

Naidu, A.S.: Recent advances in the production and use of goat skins. Proceedings, 7th International Conference on Goats, Tours, France, Vol 2, pp 627–630, May 2000.

National Research Council: Nutrient Requirements of Small Ruminants: Sheep, Goats, Cervids, and New World Camelids. Washington D.C., National Academies Press, 2007.

Nduaka, O., and Ihemelandu, E.C.: The control of pneumonia-enteritis complex in dwarf goats of Eastern States of Nigeria by the use of chloroform-inactivated tissue vaccine. Bull. Anim. Health Prod. Africa 23:343–348, 1975.

Neathery, N.W., et al.: Effects of long term zinc deficiency on feed utilization, reproductive characteristics, and hair growth in the sexually mature male goat. J. Dairy Sci. 56:98–105, 1973.

Nelson, D.R., et al.: Zinc deficiency in sheep and goats: Three field cases. J. Am. Vet. Med. Assoc. 184:1480–1485, 1984.

Njenga, J.M., et al.: Comparative ultrastructural studies on *Besnoitia besnoiti* and *Besnoitia caprae*. Vet. Res. Commun., 19:295–308, 1995.

Nooruddin, M., and Mondal, M.M.H.: Otoacariasis in Bengal goats of Bangladesh. Small Rum. Res., 1996; 19:87–90, 1996.

Nooruddin, M., et al.: Prevalence of skin diseases in Black Bengal goats. Bangladesh Vet., 4(1–2):5–9, 1987.

Obasaju, M.F., and Otesile, E.B.: *Ctenocephalides canis* infestation of sheep and goats. Trop. Anim. Health Prod. 12:116–118, 1980.

Opasina, B.A.: *Ctenocephalides canis* infestation of goats. Trop. Anim. Health Prod. 15:106, 1983.
Orr, M.B., and Barlow, R.M.: Experiments in border disease. X. The postnatal skin lesion in sheep and goats. J. Comp. Pathol. 88:295–302, 1978.
Oryan, A., and Sadeghi, M.J.: An epizooотic of besnoitiosis in goats in Fars province of Iran. Vet. Res. Commun., 21:559–570, 1997.
Otranto, D., and Puccini, V.: Further evidence on the internal life cycle of *Przhevalskiana silenus* (Diptera, Oestridae). Vet. Parasitol. 88:321–328, 2000.
Otranto, D., and Traversa, D.: Molecular evidence indicating that *Przhevalskiana silenus*, *P. aegagri* and *P. crossii* (Diptera, Oestridae) are one species. Acta Parasitol., 49:173–176, 2004.
Oyejide, A., Makinde, A.A., and Ezeh, A.O.: Prevalence of antibodies to *Dermatophilus congolensis* in sheep and goats in Nigeria. Vet. Q. 6:44–45, 1984.
Pandey, V.S., and Mahin, L.: Observations on ringworm in goats caused by *Trichophyton verrucosum*. Br. Vet. J. 136:198–199, 1980.
Pappalardo, E., Abramo, F., and Noli, C.: Pemphigus foliaceus in a goat. Vet. Dermatol., 13:331–336, 2002.
Pass, M.A.: Current ideas on the pathophysiology and treatment of lantana poisoning of ruminants. Aust. Vet. J. 63:169–171, 1986.
Patnaik, R.K.: Epidemic of goat dermatitis in India. Trop. Anim. Health Prod. 18:137–138, 1986.
Patnaik, B., and Roy, S.P.: Studies on stephanofilariasis in Orissa. II. Dermatitis due to *Stephanofilaria assamensis* Pande, 1936, in the Murrah buffalo (*Bos bubalis*) and the Beetal buck (*Capra hircus*) with remarks on the morphology of the parasite. Indian J. Vet. Sci. 38:455–462, 1968.
Perez, J.L.T.: Kids immunity to contagious ecthyma (orf) virus. Goat Diseases and Productions, 2nd International Colloquium in Niort, France, June 26–29, 1989. p. 135, Abstract.
Philpot, C.M., Westcott, G., and Stewart, J.G.: *Microsporum gypseum* ringworm. Vet. Rec., 114:22–23, 1984.
Pier, A.C., Richard, J.L., and Farrell, E.F.: Fluorescent antibody and cultural techniques in cutaneous streptothricosis. Am. J. Vet. Res. 25:1014–1020, 1964.
Pin, D.: Seborrhoeic dermatitis in a goat due to *Malassezia pachydermatis*. Vet. Dermatol., 15:53–56, 2004.
Prein, W.: *Hypoderma bovis* und *Oestrus ovis* bei Ziegen. Deutsche Tierärztl. Wochenschr. 46:33–35, 1938.
Price, M.A., and Graham, O.H.: Chewing and sucking lice as parasites of mammals and birds. United States Department of Agriculture, Agricultural Research Service Technical Bulletin, No. 1849, 1997.
Pye, D.: Vaccination of sheep with cell culture grown orf virus. Aust. Vet. J. 67:182–186, 1990.
Radostits, O.M., et al.: Veterinary Medicine: a Textbook of the Diseases of Cattle, Horses, Sheep, Pigs, and Goats. 10th Ed. New York, Elsevier Saunders, 2007.
Rahbari, S., and Ghasemi, J.: Study on economic aspects of goat grubs in Iran. Trop. Anim. Health Prod., 29:243–244, 1997.
Rajguru, D.N., et al.: A clinical report on cutaneous caprine papillomatosis. Indian Vet. J., 65:827–828, 1988.
Ramadan, R.O.: Squamous cell carcinoma of the perineum of the goat. Br. Vet. J., 131:347–350, 1975.
Ramadan, R.O., and El Hassan, A.M.: Malignant melanoma in goats: a clinico-pathological study. J. Comp. Pathol., 98:237–246, 1988.
Reko, V.A.: Der tropische Haarschwund bei Tieren. Ther. Monatsh. Vet. 2:76–78, 1928. Cited in Steyn, D.G.: Onderstepoort J. Vet. Sci. Anim. Indust. 3(2):359–473, 1934.
Renshaw, H.W., and Dodd, A.G.: Serologic and cross-immunity studies with contagious ecthyma and goat pox virus isolates from the western United States. Arch. Virol. 56:201–210, 1978.
Reuter, R., Bowden M., Besier, B., and Masters, H.: Zinc responsive alopecia and hyperkeratosis in Angora goats. Aust. Vet. J. 64:351–352, 1987.
Ricordeau, G.: Hérédité des pendeloques en race Saanen, différences de fécondité entre les génotypes avec et sans pendeloques. Ann. Zootech. 16:263–270, 1967.
Ricordeau, G.: Genetics: breeding plans. In: Goat Production. C. Gall, ed. New York, Academic Press, 1981.
Rijnberk, A.: Congenital defect in iodothyronine synthesis. Clinical aspects of iodine metabolism in goats with congenital goiter and hypothyroidism. Br. Vet. J. 133:495–503, 1977.
Robinet, A.H.: Les défauts des peaux de caprins exotiques et leurs remèdes. In: Les Maladies de la Chèvre, Niort (France), pp. 569–571, 9–11 October 1984.
Robinson, A.J., and Balassu, T.C.: Contagious pustular dermatitis (orf). Vet. Bull. 51:771–782, 1981.
Röhrer, H.: Demodicosis bei Ziegen. Tierärztl. Rundschau. 41:291–293, 1935.
Romero, C.H., et al.: Protection of goats against peste des petits ruminants with recombinant capripoxviruses expressing the fusion and haemagglutinin protein genes of rinderpest virus. Vaccine, 13:36–40, 1995.
Roth, L., and Perdrizet, J.: Cutaneous histiocytoma in a goat. Cornell Vet., 75:303–306, 1985.
Ruiz-Martinez, I. et al.: Myiasis caused by *Wohlfahrtia magnifica* in southern Spain. Isr. J. Vet. Med. 43:34–41, 1987.
Ruiz-Martinez, I., et al.: Myiasis caused by *Wohlfahrtia magnifica* in sheep and goats in southern Spain II. Effect of age, body region and sex on larval infestation. Isr. J. Vet. Med. 46:64–68, 1991.
Russel, A.J.F.: Fibre production from sheep and goats. In: Progress in Sheep and Goat Research. Oxon, UK, C.A.B. International, pp. 235–256, 1992.
Ryder, M.L.: Growth cycles in the coat of ruminants. Int. J. Chronobiol. 5:369–394, 1978.
Sawhney, A.N., Singh, A.K., and Malik, B.S.: Goat-pox: an anthropozoonosis. Indian J. Med. Res. 60:683–684, 1972.
Sar, M., and Calhoun, M.L.: Microscopic anatomy of the integument of the common American goat. Am. J. Vet. Res. 27:444–456, 1956.
Schulze, A., and Üstdal, K.M.: Mögliche Ursachen der Alopezie türkischer Angora-Ziegen. Berl. Münch. Tierärztl. Wochenschr. 88:66–73, 1975.
Scott, D.W.: Large Animal Dermatology. Philadelphia, W.B. Saunders Co., 1988.
Scott, D.W.: Color Atlas of Farm Animal Dermatology. Ames, Iowa, Blackwell Publishing, 2007.
Scott, D.W., Smith, M.C., and Manning, T.O.: Caprine dermatology. Part I. Normal skin and bacterial and fungal

disorders. Comp. Cont. Educ. Pract. Vet. 6:S190–S211, 1984a.

Scott, D.W., Smith, M.C., and Manning, T.O.: Caprine dermatology. Part II: Viral, nutritional, environmental, and congenitohereditary disorders. Comp. Cont. Educ. Pract. Vet. 6:S473–S485, 1984b.

Scott, D.W., Smith, M.C., Smith, C.A., and Lewis, R.M.: Pemphigus foliaceus in a goat. Agri-Practice 5:38–45, 1984.

Scott, D.W., Smith, M.C., Smith, C.A., and Lewis, R.M.: Pemphigus-like antibodies in the goat. Agri-Practice 8:9–10, 1987.

Sebei, P.J., et al.: Use of scanning electron microscopy to confirm the identity of lice infesting communally grazed goat herds. Onderstepoort J. Vet. Res., 71:87–92, 2004.

Sharma, R.M., and Bhatia, H.M.: Contagious pustular dermatitis in goats. Indian J. Vet. Sci. Anim. Husb. 28:205–210, 1958.

Shelton, M.: Fiber production. In: Goat Production. C. Gall, ed. New York, Academic Press, 1981.

Singer, L.J., Herron, A., and Altman, N.: Zinc responsive dermatopathy in goats: two field cases. Contemp. Top. 39(4):32–35, 2000.

Singh, V.P., and Murty, D.K.: An outbreak of *Dermatophilus congolensis* infection in goats. Indian Vet. J. 55:674–676, 1978.

Smith, B.L., and Embling, P.P.: Facial eczema in goats: The toxicity of sporidesmin in goats and its pathology. N.Z. Vet. J. 39:18–22, 1991.

Smith, M.C.: Caprine dermatologic problems: A review. J. Am. Vet. Med. Assoc. 178:724–729, 1981.

Smith, M.C.: Dermatologic diseases of goats. Vet. Clin. N. Am. Large Anim. Pract. 5:449–455, 1983.

Smith, H.J.: Demodicidosis in a flock of goats. Can. Vet. J. 2:231–233, 1961.

Sockett, D.C., Knight, A.P., and Johnson, L.W.: Malignant melanoma in a goat. J. Am. Vet. Med. Assoc. 185:907–908, 1984.

Sotiraki, S., et al.: Field trial of the efficacy of dicyclanil for the prevention of wohlfahrtiosis of sheep. Vet. Rec., 156:37–40, 2005.

Soulsby, E.J.L.: Helminths, Arthropods and Protozoa of Domesticated Animals. 7th Ed. Philadelphia, Lea and Febiger, 1982.

Spradbery, J.P., Khanfar, K.A., and Harpham, D.: Myiasis in the Sultanate of Oman. Vet. Rec. 131:76–77, 1992.

Sreekumaran, T., and Rajan, A.: Pathology of the skin in experimental hypothyroidism in goats. Kerala J. Vet. Sci. 8:227–234, 1977.

Stampa, S.: The control of the ectoparasites of Angora goats with Neguvon. Vet. Med. Rev. 1:5–15, 1964.

Stewart, G.H.: Dermatophilosis: A skin disease of animals and man, Part I and Part II. Vet. Rec. 91:537–544 and 555–561, 1972.

Steyn, D.G.: The toxicology of plants in South Africa. II. Alopecia (kaalsiekte) in kids and lambs caused by plant poisoning. Onderstepoort J. Vet. Sci. Anim. Indust. 3:434–467, 1934.

Strabel, D., et al.: Treatment with avermectins in two goats with demodicosis. Schweiz. Arch. Tierheilkd., 145:585–587, 2003.

Tarlatzis, C.B.: Un cas de rage prurigineuse chez la chèvre. Annales Méd. Vét. 98:87–89, 1954.

Tassi, P., Puccini, V., and Giangaspero, A.: Efficacy of ivermectin against goat warbles (*Przhevalskiana silenus* Brauer). Vet. Rec. 120:421, 1987.

Theilen, G., et al.: Goat papillomatosis. Am. J. Vet. Res. 46:2519–2525, 1985.

Thomas, A.D.: Skin cancer of the Angora goat in South Africa. 15th Annual Report of the Director of Vet. Services, Dept. of Agric., South Africa, pp. 661–761, 1929.

Thompson, J.R., and Mackenzie, C.P.: Demodectic mange in goats. Vet. Rec. 111:185, 1982.

Tiddy, R., and Hemi, D.: A scabby mouth-like condition in Saanen goat kids. N. Z. Vet. J. 34:119, 1986.

Turner, J.H., Shalkop, W.T., and Wilson, G.I.: Experimental strongyloidiasis in sheep and goats. IV. Migration of *Strongyloides papillosus* in lambs and accompanying pathologic changes following percutaneous infection. Am. J. Vet. Res. 21:536–546, 1960.

Uzal, F.A., et al.: *Malassezia slooffiae*-associated dermatitis in a goat. Vet. Dermatol., 18:348–352, 2007.

Valdez, R.A., et al.: Use of corticosteroids and aurothioglucose in a pygmy goat with pemphigus foliaceus. J. Am. Vet. Med. Assoc., 207:761–765, 1995.

Valle, J., et al.: Staphylococci isolated from healthy goats. J. Vet. Med. B, 38:81–89, 1991.

van Dam, R.H., Boot, R., van der Donk, J.A., and Goudswaard, J.: Skin grafting and graft rejection in goats. Am. J. Vet. Res. 39:1359–1362, 1978.

van der Heide, L.: Some cases of cutaneous carcinoma in goat and cow on Curaçao. Tijdschr. Diergeneesk., 88:510–512, 1963.

van der Westhuysen, J.M., Wentzel, D., and Grobler, M.C.: Angora Goats and Mohair in South Africa. 3rd Ed. Port Elizabeth, South Africa, NMB Printers, 1988.

Van Lancker, S., Van den Broeck, W., and Simoens, P.: Morphology of caprine skin glands involved in buck odour production. Vet. J., 170:351–358, 2005.

Van Tonder, E.M.: Notes on some disease problems in Angora goats in South Africa. Vet. Med. Rev. 1/2:109–138, 1975.

Venkatesan, R.A., Nandy, S.C., and Santappa, M.: A note on the incidence of melanoma on goat skin. Indian J. Anim. Sci. 49:154–156, 1979.

Waldvogel, A., et al.: Caprine herpesvirus infection in Switzerland: some aspects of its pathogenicity. Zbl. Vet. Med. B 28:612–623, 1981.

Wall, R., and Shearer, D.: Veterinary Ectoparasites: Biology, Pathology and Control. 2nd Ed. Oxford, Blackwell Science Ltd, 2001.

Wasfi, I.A., and Hashim, N.H.: Ivermectin treatment of sarcoptic and psoroptic mange in sheep and goats. World Anim. Rev. 59:29–33, 1986.

Watson, P.: Differential diagnosis of oral lesions and FMD in sheep. In Pract., 26:182–191, 2004.

Wentzel, D., and Vosloos, L.P.: Pre-natale ontwikkeling van follikelgroepe by die Angorabok. (Prenatal development of follicle groups in the Angora goat hair.) Agroanimalia 6:13–20, 1974.

Williams, J.F., and Williams, C.S.F.: Psoroptic ear mites in dairy goats. J. Am. Vet. Med. Assoc. 173:1582–1583, 1978.

Williams, J.F., and Williams, C.S.F.: Demodicosis in dairy-goats. J. Am. Vet. Med. Assoc. 180:168–169, 1982.

Whitney, J.C., Scott, G.R., and Hill, D.H.: Preliminary observations on a stomatitis and enteritis of goats in southern Nigeria. Bull. Epiz. Dis. Af. 15:31–41, 1967.

Wooldridge, M.J.A., and Wood, J.: Some aspects of scrapie epidemiology in the goat. Goat Vet. Soc. J. 12(2):4–7, 1991.

Wright, F.C., Guillot, F.S., and George, J.E.: Efficacy of acaricides against chorioptic mange of goats. Am. J. Vet. Res. 49:903–904, 1988.

Yadav, A., Khajuria, J.K., and Soodan, J.S.: Efficacy of ivermectin against warble fly larvae in goat. Indian Vet. J., 2006; 83:1133–1134, 2006.

Yeruham I., Elad, D., and Perl, S.: Dermatophilosis in goat in the Judean foothills. Rev. Med. Vet., 154:785–788, 2003.

Yeruham, I., and Hadani, A.: Self-destructive behaviour in ruminants. Vet. Rec., 152:304–305, 2003.

Yeruham, I., Rosen, S., and Perl, S.: An apparent flea-allergy dermatitis in kids and lambs. J. Vet. Med. A, 44:391–397, 1997.

Yeruham, I., et al.: Dermatophilosis (*Dermatophilus congolensis*) accompanied by contagious ecthyma (orf) in a flock of Yaez in Israel. Isr. J. Vet. Med. 46:74–78, 1991.

Yeruham, I., et al.: Perianal squamous cell carcinoma in goats. J. Vet. Med. A, 40:432–436, 1993.

Yeruham, I., et al.: Apparent idiopathic interface disease in a Boer billy goat. J. S. Afr. Vet. Assoc., 73:77–78, 2002.

Youde, H.: Preliminary epidemiological and clinical observations on shimaor zheng (fleece-eating) in goats and sheep. Vet. Res. Commun., 25:585–590, 2001.

Youde, H., and Huaitao, C.: Studies on the pathogenesis of shimao zheng (fleece-eating) in sheep and goats. Vet. Res. Commun., 25:631–640, 2001.

Youde, H.: An experimental study of the treatment and prevention of shimao zheng (fleece-eating) in sheep and goats in the Haizi area of Akesai county in China. Vet. Res. Commun., 26:39–48, 2002.

Zahler, M., et al.: Genetic evidence suggests that *Psoroptes* isolates of different phenotpes, hosts and geographic origins are conspecific. Int. J. Parasitol., 28:1713–1719, 1998.

Zahler, M., et al.: Molecular analyses suggest monospecificity of the genus *Sarcoptes* (Acari: Sarcoptidae). Int. J. Parasitol., 29:759–766, 1999.

Zamri-Saad, M., Hizat, A.K., and Kamil, W.M.: Effect of ivermectin on sarcoptic mange lesions of goats. Trop. Anim. Health Prod., 22:144–145, 1990.

Zenner, L., Drevon-Gaillot, E., and Callait-Cardinal, M.P.: Evaluation of four manual tick-removal devices for dogs and cats. Vet. Rec., 159:526–529, 2006.

3

Subcutaneous Swellings

Whether the owners in a locality refer to them as lumps, bumps, bunches, or something else, swellings beneath the skin on a short-haired goat are likely to attract attention and require diagnosis, if not a treatment. The diagnosis depends on both the physical characteristics of the lump and its exact anatomic location. Aspiration, along with culture or cytologic examination dictated by the nature of the aspirate, can usually provide a definitive diagnosis. However, after the practitioner gains experience with goats, aspiration is only occasionally required. Herd history, signalment of the animal, and physical examination findings give reasonable certainty in the diagnosis of numerous benign conditions. Aspiration, then, is limited to confirmation of diagnoses that might require some other action, often surgery, or that carry a grave prognosis.

SWELLINGS WITH UNRESTRICTED DISTRIBUTION

Certain conditions can cause local swelling over almost any part of the goat's body. They will be considered before conditions with a more regional distribution. Masses limited to the dermis or epidermis, joint distension, and changes involving the mammary gland and scrotum are discussed in other chapters.

Hematoma and Seroma

A fresh hematoma is easily diagnosed by aspiration of nonodorous, sterile, red fluid. A yellow sterile fluid containing few erythrocytes is present in a seroma or organized hematoma. Diagnostic aspiration, however, is not without risk. Even with very careful attention to skin preparation, the needle is likely to carry a few bacteria into the accumulated fluid. Unless the hole in the skin is offset from the point where the needle enters, a small tract will permit leakage of fluid and retrograde entry of more bacteria. It is hard to imagine better growing conditions for a bacterial culture than in whole blood or serum at body temperature.

The practitioner might choose to drain a fluctuating lump, whether it be hematoma, seroma, or abscess. This procedure should be delayed a week or more if a hematoma is suspected to avoid renewed bleeding when the pressure of containment is relieved. If the swelling is not over a large blood vessel and antibiotic residues in milk or meat are of no concern, then small fluid pockets may be drained through a needle and subsequently injected with penicillin or other antibiotic. A pressure bandage may prevent recurrence. Larger pockets must be opened widely and packed with gauze soaked in an antiseptic or provided with indwelling drains if proper healing is to occur. Seromas on the poll of breeding bucks, resulting from regular head bashing with other males, are best left totally alone.

Cellulitis and Abscess

Cellulitis is an acute, diffuse, edematous, suppurative inflammation of deep subcutaneous tissues or muscle. The swelling may be painful and accompanied by fever. The cause is often foreign body penetration or injection of irritant drugs. Aspiration for cytology and culture and sensitivity testing is warranted if the goat is systemically ill.

If encapsulation and abscess formation occur, signs of local inflammation (pain, heat) decrease (Figure 3.1). Given time, many abscesses "ripen" or develop a soft spot in the capsule where rupture is likely to occur. This helps to distinguish an abscess from a hematoma. The hematoma is initially fluctuant but later develops a firm capsule as the blood organizes and resorption begins. Abscesses usually heal rapidly when drainage is supplied. Lancing an abscess at its softest spot reduces both pain and hemorrhage associated with the surgical procedure. Another, more ventral location may be more appropriate for incision, however, to allow better drainage. Caseous lymphadenitis should be ruled out (by culture or with less certainty by absence of lymph node involvement in any animal in the herd) before the animal with a draining abscess is returned to the herd.

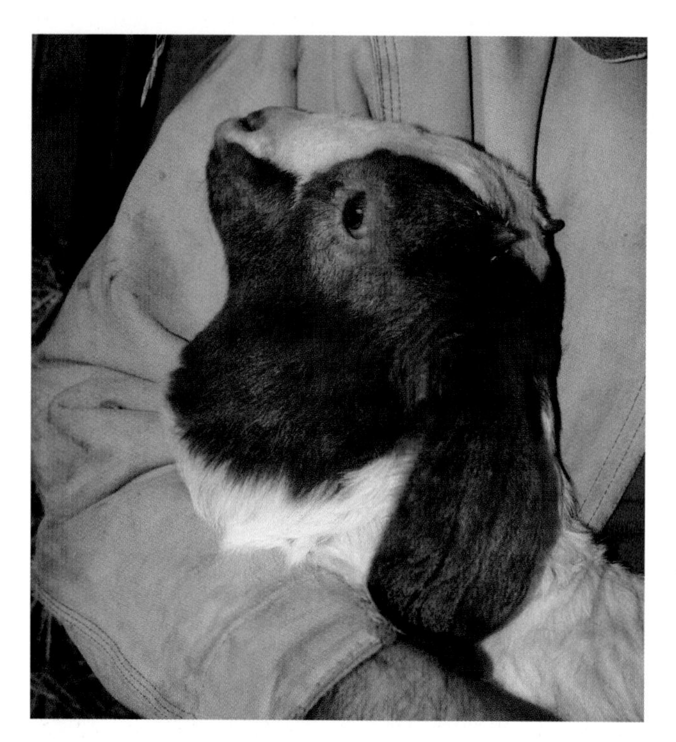

Figure 3.1. Large, thin-walled abscess in the upper neck of a one-month-old kid from which a *Streptococcus* sp. was cultured. (Courtesy of Dr. M.C. Smith.)

Emphysema

When crepitation is palpable in subcutaneous or deeper tissues, it is important to determine the origin of the air or other gas that is present. Air may be escaping from the respiratory tract (tracheal laceration, severe pulmonary emphysema) or it may be entering through sucking skin wounds (Tanwar et al. 1983). Attention to the primary problem should stop the inflow of air, and resorption will occur gradually over days or weeks.

A crepitant, painful swelling caused by infection of wounds with gas-forming clostridia such as *Clostridium chauvoei* may lead to death of the animal (van Tonder 1975). The condition can be diagnosed by cytologic examination of aspirates, anaerobic culture, or immunofluorescence testing. Aggressive treatment with systemic and intralesional penicillin is successful in early stages. Gangrenous tissues slough later if the animal survives. In regions where clostridial infections are common, multivalent clostridial vaccines (*C. chauvoei, C. septicum, C. novyi*) provide inexpensive protection.

Edema

Pitting edema without crepitation may occur in wounds infected with *Clostridium septicum* (malignant edema) or *C. novyi* (swelled head in bucks). Other causes include trauma without tissue infection, frostbite, hypoproteinemia (parasitism, kidney disease, paratuberculosis), and congestive heart failure. Udder edema is discussed in Chapter 14.

LYMPH NODE ENLARGEMENT

Although enlargement of one or more lymph nodes in a goat typifies caseous lymphadenitis, other etiologies may be involved. In particular, other bacterial infections may cause hyperplasia or abscessation of the regional node (Gezon et al. 1991). Lymph node enlargement is common in animals with joint infection, including caprine arthritis encephalitis virus infection. Skin diseases such as sarcoptic mange and contagious ecthyma are often accompanied by enlarged nodes. Finally, lymphosarcoma occasionally causes enlargement of external lymph nodes.

Caseous Lymphadenitis

Caseous lymphadenitis is a chronic contagious disease that mainly affects sheep and goats (Brown and Olander 1987; Williamson 2001) and is increasingly recognized in camelids (Anderson et al. 2004). The condition occurs worldwide and is well known in many regions of North and South America, Australia, New Zealand, Europe, and South Africa.

Etiology

Corynebacterium pseudotuberculosis (previously known as *C. ovis*) is the causative agent of caseous lymphadenitis. Its cultural characteristics are described under diagnosis. Horses are occasionally infected with the organism and may develop ulcerative lymphangitis or chronic abscess, but a different biotype from the one infecting sheep and goats is apparently involved (Aleman et al. 1996). Experimental intradermal inoculation of goats with strains of equine origin has caused abscesses at the injection site and in draining nodes but not in visceral locations (Brown et al. 1985). Most equine strains reduce nitrate to nitrite, whereas small ruminant strains do not.

Pathogenesis

The organism enters the goat's body through wounds or small breaks in the skin or mucous membranes and eventually becomes localized in a regional lymph node. Experimentally, tiny abscesses are detectable in lymph nodes by eight days after intradermal inoculation (Kuria et al. 2001). Cell wall lipid permits the organism to resist digestion by cellular enzymes, and *C. pseudotuberculosis* can survive as a facultative intracellular parasite, even in activated macrophages (Holstad et al. 1989). Sphingomyelin-specific phospholipase D exotoxin produced by the organism is largely responsible for its spread.

The incubation period until abscesses are noted in superficial lymph nodes is typically two to six months or longer (Ashfaq and Campbell 1980). These abscesses may rupture and drain spontaneously. The environment and curious herdmates thereby become contaminated, but the initially infected goat's abscess heals. It is common for one or more additional lymph nodes, following the lymphatic drainage pattern, to develop abscesses several months later. Experimental intradermic inoculation with small numbers of bacteria has demonstrated that spontaneous cures, without abscess rupture but accompanied by development of antitoxin titers, can occur (Langenegger and Langenegger 1988).

Internal (visceral) abscesses, especially in the lungs, may develop if the organism reaches the thoracic lymph duct or if it is inhaled. The association of internal abscesses with respiratory disease and wasting disease is discussed in other chapters. Other adverse economic effects of the infection in a herd include decreased market value of stock for sale and of hides from slaughtered goats. Milk production may be decreased.

Clinical Signs

The goat without internal abscesses typically shows no clinical signs other than enlargement and abscessation of one or more peripheral lymph nodes (Figure 3.2). Many of the external lymph nodes that may be involved in caseous lymphadenitis are pictured in Figure 3.3. Exactly which nodes are infected depends on the location of the wound that allowed entry of the organism into the body. Thus, most dairy goats (75% to 87%) with external abscesses have lesions on the head and neck (Ashfaq and Campbell 1979a, 1979b; Holstad 1986b; Schreuder et al. 1986) (parotid,

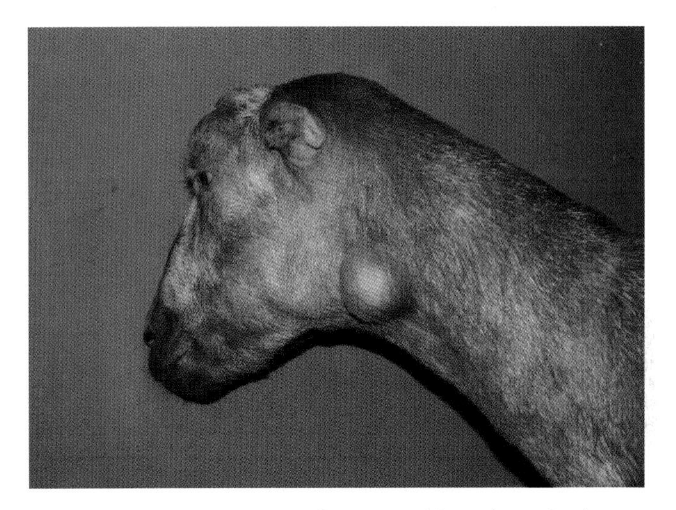

Figure 3.2. Abscessation of a parotid lymph node due to caseous lymphadenitis. (Courtesy of Dr. M.C. Smith.)

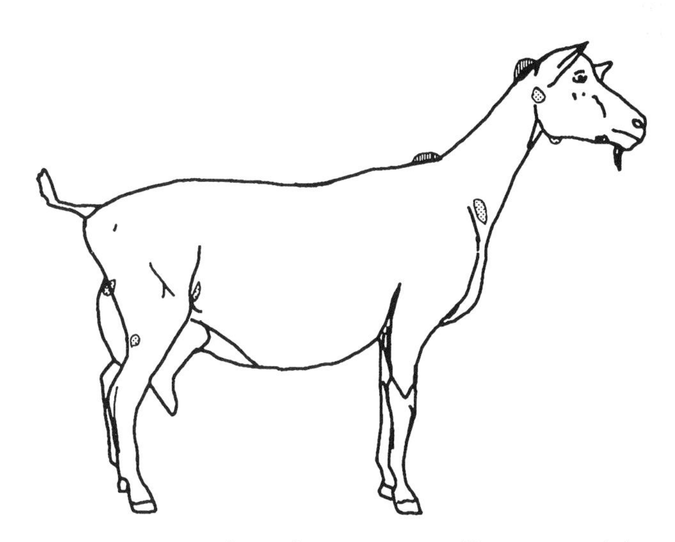

Figure 3.3. Location of common swellings caused by caseous lymphadenitis and caprine arthritis encephalitis. An abscess in the location of external lymph nodes (stippled) suggests caseous lymphadenitis. Enlargement of atlantal or supraspinous bursae (cross-hatched) may occur with CAE.

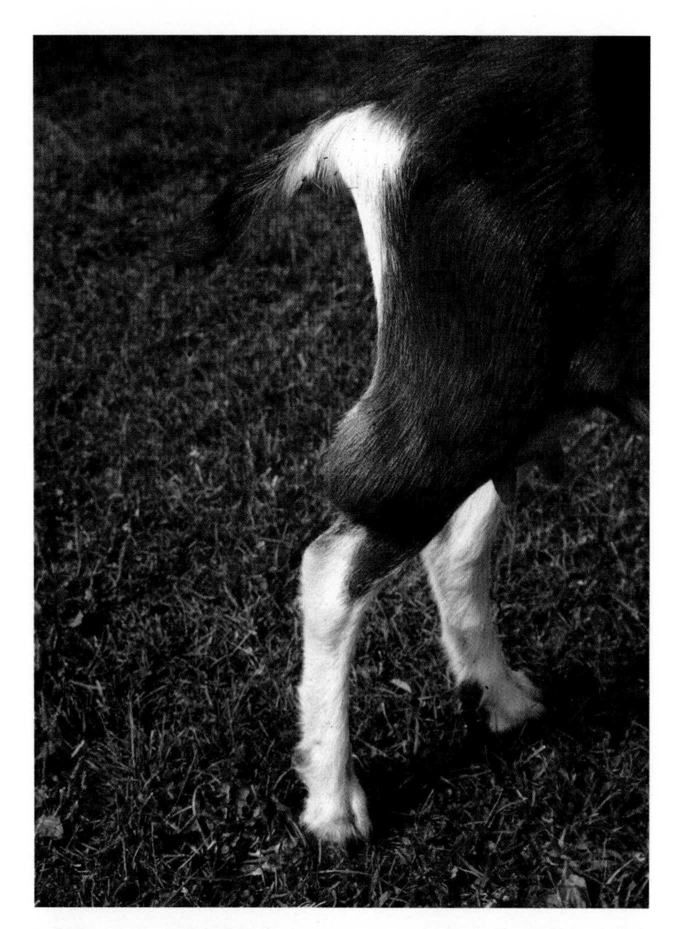

Figure 3.4. Abscessation of a popliteal lymph node. (Courtesy of Dr. M.C. Smith.)

mandibular, and superficial cervical "prescapular" nodes), presumably because injuries from thorns, splinters from wooden feeders, combat wounds, and scratching at lice most commonly occur here. Contact of these skin lesions with milking stands, feeders, or scratching posts contaminated by draining abscesses of other goats leads to infected nodes about the head and neck. By contrast, a popliteal lymph node (Figure 3.4) would only become enlarged if infection occurred in the distal hind limb. Mammary lymph node involvement can result from infection of skin lesions on the udder or from mastitis. Slaughterhouse studies typically show the highest prevalence in the prescapular node, among the nodes routinely inspected (Ghanbarpour and Khaleghiyan et al. 2005).

Diagnosis

Diagnosis of the condition is based on the presence of a firm to slightly fluctuant subcutaneous swelling in the anatomic location of a lymph node (Burrell 1981). In a herd with a history of caseous lymphadenitis, the clinical findings alone are considered presumptive evidence. When a herd history is lacking (no previous veterinary evaluation, assembled herd, individual purchased animal), then laboratory assistance may be indicated for confirming the diagnosis. A sample for culture is obtained by inserting a sterile needle through shaved, disinfected skin into the mass. If aspiration yields nothing, the needle is withdrawn and saline is flushed through the needle to obtain material for a stained smear or culture. Even when the point of skin penetration is intentionally offset from the point where the needle passes through the wall of the abscess, some pus can leak back and serve as a focus of infection to others in the herd. Thus, if pus is present, the lump and the goat should be handled as if caseous lymphadenitis were present (see below) until culture results become available. Cultures of pus from draining caseous lymphadenitis lesions are frequently overgrown by nonpathogenic organisms or secondary invaders such as *Proteus* species. However, other bacterial infections such as anaerobic *Staphylococcus aureus* (Alhendi et al. 1993) and *Arcanobacterium pyogenes* and neoplasia, including lymphosarcoma, must be ruled out if *C. pseudotuberculosis* is not isolated. The other conditions causing subcutaneous swellings, as discussed in this chapter and reviewed elsewhere (Williams 1980; Fubini and Campbell 1983), also should be considered in the differential diagnosis.

The pus in an abscessed node in a goat may be creamy white, yellowish, or greenish; it is typically odorless and is more pasty (less inspissated) than in sheep. A lamellar "onion ring" configuration as seen in sheep with this disease is rarely present in goats (Batey et al. 1986).

The organism (a facultative anaerobe) grows readily but slowly on blood agar (Brown and Olander 1987). The colonies are very tiny or invisible after twenty-four hours (Lindsay and Lloyd 1981), and a longer incubation period is recommended before declaring that no growth has occurred. The colonies are still tiny and button-shaped after forty-eight hours, but are surrounded by a narrow zone of hemolysis. The colonies can be easily moved around on the surface of the agar plate and splatter when placed in a flame, because of high content of lipid. The organism is catalase-positive whereas *Arcanobacterium pyogenes*, which also produces tiny colonies, is catalase-negative (Quinn et al. 2002). Gram-stained smears show Gram-positive or Gram-variable small coccoid rods. A longer rod form is sometimes seen in smears of pus.

Serologic tests such as the bacterial agglutination test and synergistic hemolysis-inhibition (SHI) test (Zaki 1968; Brown et al. 1985,1986b; Holstad 1986a) are valuable in identifying goats with early or internal forms of caseous lymphadenitis. The SHI test is commercially available in the United States, through the University of California, Davis, and several other laboratories, and has a sensitivity of 98% in goats (Brown and Olander 1987). However, in the same study population, 28% of goats with no demonstrable abscess were also SHI positive, indicating a lack of specificity.

Laboratory personnel report that a titer of 1:256 or greater correlates well with internal abscesses, but that occasionally an animal with a walled-off abscess tests negative. Experimental infections have not been detectable serologically until at least fifteen days after infection (Kuria et al. 2001), so purchased animals should be retested at the end of their quarantine period. Colostrally derived antibodies may cause false positive test results in kids under six months of age (Williamson 2001). Also, most tests have not been specific enough for current infection to justify their use in culling programs (Ellis et al. 1990). A decreasing titer on a retest taken two to four months after the first sample suggests that an active infection is not present. An ELISA test to detect antibodies against exotoxin and used for disease eradication in the Netherlands (Dercksen et al. 1996) has recently been improved to increase sensitivity to 94%, specificity of 98% (Dercksen et al. 2000).

Because the organism is a facultative intracellular pathogen, cell mediated immunity is involved in the immune response. Preliminary work with a commercially available bovine interferon gamma ELISA (Bovigam, Pfizer Animal Health) for cell mediated immunity to *C. pseudotuberculosis* has suggested that it is sensitive to prior infection and is unaffected by vaccination (Menzies et al. 2004). Caprine interferon gamma cross-reacts in the assay. This test may be useful to detect carriers in vaccinated herds, although it may not reflect the extent of the infection.

The increases in total serum proteins and gamma globulin that are reported for goats with caseous lymphadenitis (Desiderio et al. 1979) are also nonspecific. An intradermal allergic test using a water-soluble protein "lymphadenin" has been used to differentiate goats with abscesses from uninfected goats (Langenegger et al. 1986). Injections were made in the shoulder region and the maximum increase in skin-fold thickness occurred after forty-eight hours.

Surgical Treatment

Treatment of individual animals involves either draining or surgically removing the abscessed nodes. Ripened abscesses can be incised generously at a ventral point and the cavity flushed with dilute disinfectant. Because the infection is potentially zoonotic, people performing this procedure should wear gloves. The pus should be collected and burned and the goat should be kept strictly isolated until the lesion is completely covered by healthy skin, typically twenty to thirty days later (Ashfaq and Campbell 1980). Allowing an abscess to rupture in the main goat pen or returning the animal to the herd where herd mates will lick the wound will only serve to contaminate the environment and spread the infection. Stanchions, milking stands, and keyhole feeders in particular will become contaminated. The advantages of surgical removal of the encapsulated abscess are that the treated animal does not need to be quarantined afterward and spread to other nodes is less likely to occur, but veterinary expertise is required and there are dangers associated with anesthesia and dissection near large blood vessels and cranial nerves. Extirpation of abscessed parotid nodes is particularly dangerous, and treatment of a retropharyngeal abscess requires marsupialization.

An alternative but controversial treatment for carefully chosen abscesses is to inject them with 10% formalin at the point where the ripening abscess has become fixed to the overlying skin. A 16-gauge needle is used and approximately 20 ml of formalin is repeatedly injected into and withdrawn from the abscess until the cloudiness of the formalin/pus mixture in the syringe is no longer increasing; larger abscesses require a larger initial volume of formalin. This causes sloughing of the node within a few weeks but raises specters of meat or milk contamination or carcinogenesis in the minds of many veterinarians. Formalin is rapidly converted to formic acid, and formate is an intermediate in normal metabolism in the body. If the abscess is not fixed to the skin, formalin leaking out of the injected abscess will damage surrounding tissues as well as cause pain to the animal.

Antibiotic Therapy

In the past, long-term treatment with antibiotics or isoniazide of abscesses inaccessible to surgical management has not been rewarding. Antibiotic sensitivity testing is of little benefit, because most antibiotics do not penetrate into the abscessed lymph node and the organism itself may be intracellular. Administration of penicillin or tetracycline for a few days after spontaneous rupture or lancing of an abscess is suggested to prevent dissemination of the organism to other lymph nodes, but the value of this treatment has not yet been determined in controlled clinical trials.

Success in treating foal pneumonia caused by *Rhodococcus equi* with a combination of erythromycin and rifampin led to renewed interest in medical treatment of valuable sheep and goats. Pharmacokinetic data derived from other species suggest that an oral dose of 10 to 20 mg/kg rifampin s.i.d. might be appropriate (Sweeney et al. 1988; Frank 1990; Jernigan et al. 1991). A possible erythromycin dosage is 4 mg/kg administered intramuscularly or subcutaneously. Because erythromycin is highly irritating, a rifampin/penicillin combination might be preferable. Treatment should be continued for four to six weeks. Reports of the efficacy of rifampin in goats with caseous lymphadenitis are not yet available. One report of rifamyin at 10 mg/kg IM b.i.d. for ten days combined with long-acting oxytetracycline at 20 mg/kg IM every third day gave a promising reduction in the size of affected lymph nodes, though the animals were only followed for one month (Senturk and Temizel 2006). There is no information available for estimation of meat or milk withdrawals to avoid antibiotic residues after the use of rifampin.

More recently, azithromycin has become popular for treatment of rhodococcal pneumonia in foals because of good intracellular penetration and long half-life (Chaffin et al. 2008), and the pharmacokinetics of this antibiotic in goats have been studied (Carceles et al. 2005). Again, to date there is no information on efficacy, dose, or withdrawal times if azithromycin is used in goats with caseous lymphadenitis.

Herd Eradication and Control Programs

Eradication of caseous lymphadenitis from a herd is difficult. The owner must be willing to cull goats and sheep with multiple abscesses and forgo purchase of animals from infected herds. Introduction of the disease into the United Kingdom by imported goats has underscored the risks associated with an open herd status (Gilmour 1990; Lindsay and Lloyd 1991). Ideally, a negative serologic test should be required before purchase, even from a herd believed to be free of the disease. Newly acquired animals, including camelids, should be examined for lymph node enlargement at least monthly for one year or more after arrival. An eradication program based on culling of serologically positive animals was successful in fifty-three herds (approximately 13,000 adult goats) in the Netherlands (Dercksen et al. 1996).

Valuable infected animals may be kept isolated; their kids should be removed at birth and fed heat-treated or bovine colostrum to avoid transmission of the disease as the newborn searches for the udder. Commercial pasteurization is known to kill *C. pseudotuberculosis* in milk (Baird et al. 2005). Division of an enzootically infected herd into infected and apparently uninfected groups has also been proposed as a means of limiting spread (Mullowney and Baldwin 1984). The housing facilities should be free of nails, wire, and other objects that might induce breaks in the skin. Control of external parasites is very important because pruritic goats will rub themselves on nails and posts. Needles, tattooers, and surgical instruments should be sterilized between animals. Shearing equipment that has been used on another farm should likewise be disinfected.

All wounds should be treated promptly with a disinfectant, and the umbilical cords of kids should be dipped in iodine at birth. In infected herds of Angora or Cashmere goats, animals should not be dipped for control of external parasites during the two weeks immediately after shearing; topical pour-on insecticides can be substituted. Animals with chronic respiratory disease or wasting should be culled, or at least isolated from the herd. Natural transmission from lung lesions via discharge of pus into airways has been demonstrated in sheep (Ellis et al. 1987).

An environment contaminated with pus may be the source of new infections for weeks or months. Recovery of the organism from wood surfaces, straw, hay, and soil has been demonstrated by various researchers (Augustine and Renshaw 1986; Brown and Olander 1987). Thus, the isolation facilities used to contain a goat after rupture or lancing of an abscess should have a concrete floor. The bedding should be burned and the pen thoroughly cleaned (pressure washed) and disinfected between animals. In a successful herd eradication program in Norway, housing areas used by infected animals were left vacant for three months after disinfection and the upper 10 cm of soil in the paddocks was removed to decrease the risk of soil-borne infection (Nord et al. 1998).

Vaccination

Numerous studies using mice have evaluated immune responses to the organism. Cell-mediated immunity has been demonstrated to restrict bacterial proliferation. Neutralization of exotoxin (phospholipase D) produced by the organism is believed to limit spread from the primary site of infection.

The value of vaccination as an aid in controlling the disease in ruminants has been frequently questioned. A decrease in the prevalence of abscesses in the herd has often been noted where autogenous bacterins have been used, but concerned owners have simultaneously culled known infected goats and generally improved hygienic measures. As a note of caution, if not properly prepared and tested, an autogenous vaccine against this organism may contain enough free toxin to kill the vaccinated goat. The SHI test does not distinguish between naturally infected and vaccinated goats unless serial tests are compared, so test and cull is difficult to use once a vaccination program has been implemented. Likewise, vaccinated goats test falsely positive in an ELISA for antibodies against exotoxin and cell wall antigens (Sting et al. 1998).

A commercial vaccine (Glanvac®, Commonwealth Serum Labs, Melbourne, Australia) developed in Australia has been evaluated in goats (Anderson and Nairn 1984a, 1984b; Brown et al. 1986a). This product is a formalinized exotoxin with incomplete Freund's adjuvant. In one study, challenge by swabbing a live culture onto abraded skin revealed that either one or two doses of vaccine gave good protection; three of twenty vaccinated goats developed abscesses, as compared to ten of ten control goats (Anderson and Nairn 1984a). Colostrally derived immunity protected young kids against challenge (Anderson and Nairn 1984b). In enzootically infected herds, serologic titers in kids disappear by three to four months of age, only to reappear after exposure to the organism. Vaccination should probably be performed before four months of age (Holstad 1986c), but colostrally derived antibody may interfere when vaccination is begun before three months (Paton et al. 1991).

A different commercial vaccine (Case-Bac® and Caseous-DT®, Colorado Serum Co., Denver, CO) is available in the United States. This bacterin-toxoid preparation is only labeled for sheep, where its efficacy has been documented (Piontkowski and Shivvers 1998), but it has been used on goats. There are numerous anecdotal reports of adverse reactions including severe milk drop, lameness, anorexia, fever and depression for one to two days after vaccination in adult dairy goats in infected herds, but many owners and practitioners report that vaccination of young stock beginning at two or three months of age has been helpful in reducing disease prevalence. Vaccination should probably be continued for many years, because of the possibility that one or more members of the original herd remain carriers and shedders of the organism.

Field evaluation of crude filtrated *C. pseudotuberculosis* toxoid combined with whole killed cells has been disappointing in goats (Holstad 1989), whereas another experimental whole cell vaccine gave a nonstatistically significant trend for fewer cases in the vaccinated goats in a field trial in Canada (Menzies et al. 1991). A formalin-inactivated whole cell vaccine with aluminum gel phosphate adjuvant gave partial protection (estimated at 77%) in a field trial under extensive conditions in Brazil (Ribeiro et al. 1988). Whole cell preparations of the organism adjuvanted with mycobacterial components have been evaluated (Brogden et al. 1990). A modified live intradermal vaccine has been developed by EMBRAPA in the State of Bahia, Brazil.

Zoonotic Potential

Human lymphadenitis caused by *Corynebacterium pseudtotuberculosis* has been reported, especially from Australia (Peel et al., 1996; Mills et al. 1997). The course was often protracted and diagnosis delayed until a culture was performed. Recovery usually required surgical removal of the affected lymph node, with supplemental antibiotics. Owners, slaughterhouse workers, and veterinarians should handle infected animals and abscesses with caution.

Melioidosis

In tropical areas such as Southeast Asia, Malaysia, the Netherland Antilles, and parts of Australia, a zoonotic disease caused by *Burkholderia (Pseudomonas) pseudomallei* is seen in goats and must be differentiated from caseous lymphadenitis. The disease seen in humans has been reviewed recently (Cheng and Currie 2005).

Etiology

Burkholderia (Pseudomonas) pseudomallei is a Gram-negative bacillus with polar flagella that may show bipolar staining. It closely resembles *P. aeruginosa*. The organism may be cultured on sheep blood agar or MacConkey agar (up to four days at 37°C). Some strains are hemolytic.

Epidemiology and Pathogenesis

The organism resides in soil and contaminated water. Survival in soil for up to thirty months has been reported (Thomas and Forbes-Faulkner 1981). Infected animals, including rodents, pass the organism in feces. Spread from animal to animal by biting insects also occurs. Vertical transmission is possible, as natural and experimental infection of pregnant goats has led to infection of aborted and live born kids (Retnasabapathy 1966; Thomas et al. 1988a).

Clinical Signs

Initial bacteremia is followed by formation of abscesses and granulomas in superficial lymph nodes, lung, and other internal organs. Prescapular lymph nodes are commonly involved and contain grayish yellow, creamy pus (Sutmöller et al. 1957). Chronic mastitis (van der Lugt and Henton 1995), weight loss, polyarthritis, and meningoencephalitis are also reported.

Diagnosis and Control

The indirect hemagglutination test (positive at 1/40 or higher) is considered most suitable for screening, because it has a sensitivity of 98%. The 100% specific complement fixation test (positive at 1/8 or higher) is used for confirmation (Thomas et al. 1988b). Sensitivity of the complement fixation test is lowered (82%) in chronic infections. The final diagnosis is made by culture. Older lesions in goats are sometimes sterile (Thomas et al. 1988b).

Antibiotic treatment is ineffective. Infected goats are to be eliminated and the herd monitored by serologic testing (Baxendell 1984).

Other Infectious Agents

Goats with arthritis because of a variety of causes may have enlargement of the associated lymph node. Regional lymph node enlargement is a constant finding with caprine arthritis encephalitis virus infection (Robinson and Ellis 1986), which is a common cause of lameness and enlarged joints in dairy goats in North America, Europe, and Australia. The reader should refer to Chapter 4 for an in-depth discussion.

Dermatophilus congolensis, a Gram-positive organism that forms branching filaments in pus, has been isolated from abscessed superficial lymph nodes of Beetal goats. Other breeds housed with infected goats were not involved (Singh and Murty 1978). This organism more typically causes a superficial dermatitis. Goats with contagious ecthyma (soremouth) virus infection may have noticeable enlargement of lymph nodes draining the head. Mange can also cause marked lymph node enlargement. See Chapter 2 for discussion of skin diseases.

In regions where trypanosomiasis is endemic, *Trypanosoma brucei*, and to a lesser extent, *T. congolense* and *T. vivax*, cause a marked lymphadenopathy in goats. *Theileria* is another blood-borne parasite that causes enlargement of lymph nodes. These diseases are discussed in Chapter 7.

Infectious agents causing mastitis (including tuberculosis) may cause enlargement of the supramammary lymph nodes and are discussed in detail in Chapter 14.

Lymphosarcoma

Lymphosarcoma in goats is a neoplastic disease of unknown etiology. It has many similarities to sporadic or juvenile bovine lymphosarcoma. Neither the bovine leukemia virus nor antibodies against that virus associated with adult bovine lymphosarcoma have been found in goats with naturally occurring lymphosarcoma, although one experimentally produced goat case has been reported (Olson et al. 1981).

Lymphadenopathy of superficial nodes is not a consistent finding; only three of ten goats in one report were thus affected (Craig et al. 1986). In these animals, a lymph node aspirate yielding many lymphoblasts might confirm the diagnosis (Duncan and Prasse 1986). However, as least in cattle, fine needle aspirates have relatively low sensitivity for diagnosis of lymphosarcoma (Washburn et al. 2007).

Goats affected with lymphosarcoma are generally older than two years of age. They may have a variety of clinical signs, including high fever, emaciation, diarrhea, or dyspnea. The organs most frequently involved are liver, spleen, lungs, and lymph nodes, although the reproductive tract has also been involved (DiGrassie et al. 1997). Rapid deterioration occurs when clinical signs are noted, with death or euthanasia supervening in one week to two months in most cases. This is in contrast to the long and usually benign course of external caseous lymphadenitis.

Prominent Lymph Nodes of Normal Size

A distinction must be made between increased size and increased ease of palpation of lymph nodes. Animals that are emaciated because of malnutrition, parasitism, or chronic infectious diseases have very prominent nodes because subcutaneous fat is absent.

SWELLINGS INVOLVING THE HEAD

A number of specific conditions are limited to the head or neck. These are discussed below and some of them can be located with the aid of Figure 3.5.

Retention of a Cud in the Cheek

Contented goats frequently have a bulge in the cheek region during rumination. The swelling disappears as soon as mastication is complete or the goat is startled. If such a swelling persists and is found on careful digital examination to consist of a cud rather than a thickening of the cheek (abscess), neurologic dysfunction, a tooth problem, or some other condition interfering with mastication or swallowing should be suspected.

Tooth Problems

Absent, irregular, or abscessed teeth may lead to improper chewing and accumulation of feedstuffs or cuds between the dental arcade and the cheek. These problems are discussed below and in Chapter 10.

Facial Nerve Paralysis

Cud retention may indicate facial nerve paralysis, and thus should prompt a thorough neurological examination (see Chapter 5). Deviation of the philtrum, drooling, inability to blink, and drooping of the pinna may also be present. Conditions to be considered in differential diagnosis include traumatic injury to the facial nerve, otitis media, listeriosis, and other lesions involving the brain stem. Of these, listeriosis

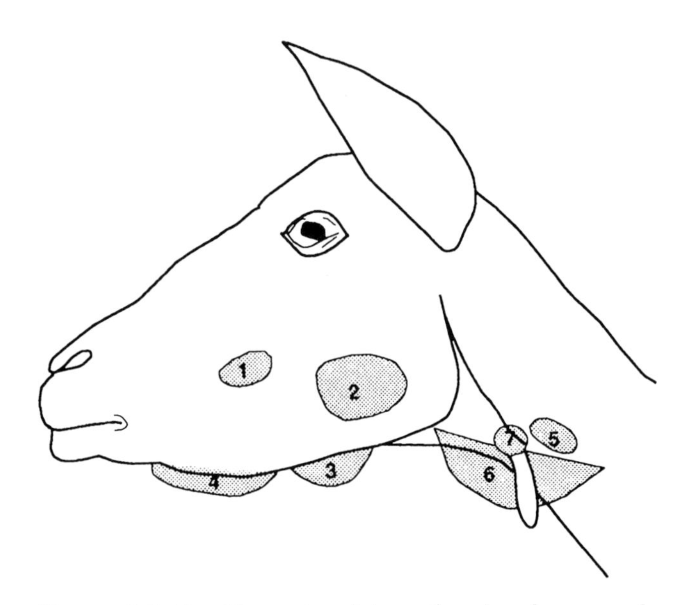

Figure 3.5. Swellings involving the head or neck: (1) cheek abscess or cud retention, (2) salivary mucocele, (3) tooth root abscess, (4) bottle jaw, (5) thyroid gland, (6) thymus gland, (7) wattle cyst.

should receive special consideration, because the disease is most apt to be successfully treated if clinical signs are limited to peripheral nerve dysfunction.

Salivary Mucocele

Painless swellings on the side of the face sometimes are cystic structures filled with saliva.

Anatomy and physiology

The parotid salivary glands of the goat are roughly rectangular and extend from the ear to the bifurcation of the jugular vein. Each parotid duct runs subcutaneously across the lateral surface of the masseter muscle near its ventral border. It empties into the mouth via the parotid papilla, which is opposite the upper fourth premolar or first molar (Habel 1975). The mandibular salivary glands are triangular in shape. They lie deep to the parotid gland and caudal to the mandibular lymph node, along the medial side of the angle of the mandible. The mandibular ducts, which are less accessible to injury than the parotid ducts, go to the medial side of each sublingual caruncle. The monostomatic ducts of the sublingual glands open on the lateral side of each sublingual caruncle. Sialography can be performed (Tadjalli et al. 2002). In addition to these major paired glands, there are diffuse layers of salivary gland tissue in the walls of the mouth and pharynx.

The salivary glands of ruminants secrete continuously. The saliva is slightly alkaline, because of its high concentration of bicarbonate. The physiologic function of saliva is discussed in Chapter 10.

Etiology

Blockage or rupture of a duct can lead to formation of a salivary mucocele. Forceful restraint of the head of young kids against a metal brace during disbudding has led to mucocele formation. It is also important to avoid damaging the glands or the parotid ducts in surgical operations involving the head and neck, in particular drainage or extirpation of abscessed lymph nodes.

Painless fluid-filled cysts have been reported on the side of the face or in the submandibular region of young Nubian goats. These cysts were found to be lined by pseudostratified columnar epithelium containing goblet cells. Parotid salivary gland duct epithelium appears similar, and thus these cysts were presumed to be developmental anomalies (Brown et al. 1989). Figure 3.6 shows a one-month-old Nubian kid that had fluid-filled cysts bilaterally at birth. These cysts, which appeared to be outpocketings of a salivary duct, were removed surgically and the ducts ligated.

Clinical Signs and Diagnosis

Aspiration of the soft, fluctuant, nonpainful swelling should yield a clear, watery or slightly blood-tinged mucoid fluid that is colorless and odorless. The pH level is higher than that of blood. Confusion with a tapeworm cyst over the mandible, as discussed below, might be possible (Ghosh et al. 2005).

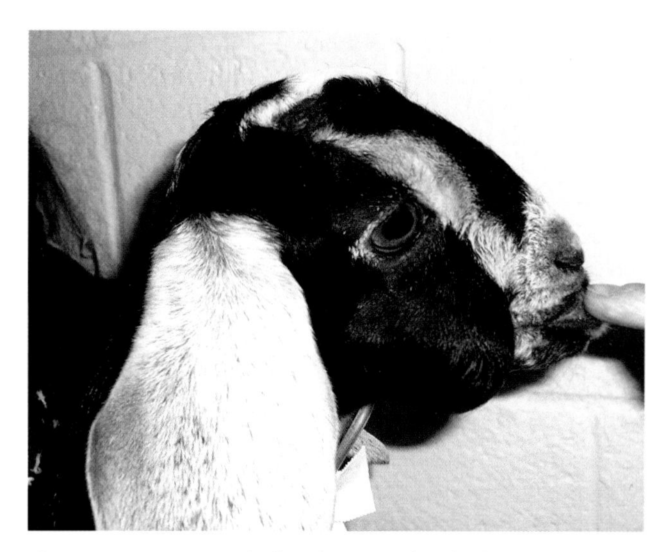

Figure 3.6. Congenital salivary gland duct cyst in a Nubian kid. (Courtesy of Dr. R.P. Hackett.)

Treatment

Salivary cysts can be excised, as long as the caudal portion is ligated to occlude the parotid salivary gland duct. Excision of the gland itself is not required (Brown et al. 1989). Such swellings should not be lanced, because a chronic fistula and continuous loss of saliva may result. The discharge is not only aesthetically displeasing; the loss of bicarbonate, which approaches 30 to 50 grams per day in experimentally cannulated sheep, can lead to life-threatening acidosis.

Abscess

Subcutaneous abscesses on the head, as elsewhere on the body, may involve a variety of organisms, including *Corynebacterium pseudotuberculosis*, *Arcanobacterium pyogenes*, *Escherichia coli*, and staphylococcal and streptococcal species (Ashfaq and Campbell 1979b). *Nocardia* has also been isolated from chronic subcutaneous abscesses on the face and elsewhere on the body (Jackson 1986). An anaerobic staphylococcus has been associated with a herd outbreak of subcutaneous abscesses involving the head in goats in the Sudan (El Sanousi et al. 1989).

From Biting Cheek

When an abscess is located in the cheek, exactly where upper and lower molar teeth meet, the possibility of a self-inflicted injury with contamination by bacteria in the oral cavity must be considered. Filing of exceptionally sharp points on the teeth may be justified to avoid recurrence. Manual restraint of a goat's head in such a way that skin of the cheek is forced between the molar arcades (as when teaching a kid to drink from a bucket) and tight halters should be avoided.

From Other Wounds

Wounds in the skin or oral mucosa may result from puncture by thorny vegetation or from grass awns. Bite wounds by predators or more dominant goats also offer a portal of entry for pyogenic organisms. In general, identifying the exact microorganism involved is not important, other than for ruling out caseous lymphadenitis. Draining and then flushing the abscess with dilute iodine usually provide adequate therapy. Systemic penicillin is given if the goat is systemically affected or the lesion is especially large.

Actinobacillosis is somewhat different in that *Actinobacillus lignieresii* causes multiple chronic, firm, nodular lesions, often with draining tracts in sheep. The lesions are located in soft tissues of the head or in the regional lymph nodes. The presence of small (less than 1 mm in diameter) granules in the pus is quite suggestive of actinobacillosis but unfortunately they are not often seen. Confirmation requires culture of the organism. Sulfonamides, streptomycin (not available in the United States), and sodium iodide have been recommended for treatment; penicillin is not effective. The occurrence of actinobacillosis in goats has not been documented. The condition is commonly seen in sheep flocks free of *C. pseudotuberculosis* and can be mistaken for caseous lymphadenitis, resulting in unnecessary culling if cultures are not performed.

From Dehorning

Dehorning represents a special wound that may become infected and eventually develop into an abscess beneath the eschar from heat cautery or the bandage or scab from surgical horn removal. This condition is discussed below under sinusitis.

Tooth Root Abscess

As a sequel to periodontal disease (perhaps from feeding coarse hay or hay containing grasses with barbed awns), foreign material gets between the tooth and gum and an abscess may form around the root of a molar tooth. In the authors' experience this occurs most often in the lower jaw and is accompanied by decreased hay consumption and difficulty cudding. The infection progresses until bony distortion of the ventral ramus is noted (Figure 3.7). The swelling is easily detected by comparing the thickness of the mandibles while palpating with the thumb and forefinger of each hand. This ventral swelling may break and drain pus. An oral exam (with xylazine tranquilization) should be conducted to identify obviously broken or loose teeth that need to be extracted. More typically,

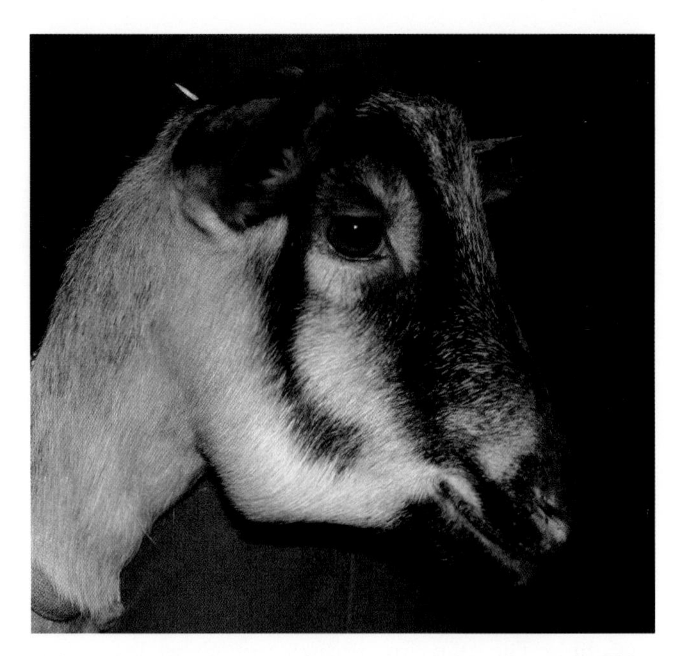

Figure 3.7. Tooth root abscess involving the mandible. (Courtesy of Dr. M.C. Smith.)

the tooth involved can only be identified with an oblique radiograph of the jaw. Some of these goats respond to repeated iodine flushing of the draining tract and three to four weeks of penicillin or florfenicol or some other antibiotic selected on the basis of culture and sensitivity. A pelleted hay product encourages feed consumption during the initial stages of therapy because extensive chewing is not required.

Although surgical extraction of the involved tooth has not been reported in the caprine literature, experience with other species suggests that this might be the preferred treatment if accomplished without fracture of the mandible. Oral extraction would be very difficult (if the tooth is not loose) because of poor exposure, and consideration should be given to osteotomy of the lateral mandibular plate, as is described for llamas and small exotic ruminants (Turner and McIlwraith 1989; Wiggs and Lobprise 1994; Niehaus and Anderson 2007). After the tooth is repelled into the mouth, a pack of dental acrylic will exclude food particles from the surgery site.

Actinomycosis

Lumpy jaw (*Actinomyces bovis*) apparently is very rare in goats (Baby et al. 2000; Seifi et al. 2003). Involvement of bone and presence of sulfur granules raises the suspicion of this infection. Treatment is as for actinobacillosis, with five to seven days of streptomycin if available (10 mg/kg twice or three times daily) combined with oral iodides as a possible protocol. Daily subcutaneous injections of oxytetracycline at 20 mg/kg can be substituted. Important conditions to consider in differential diagnosis are tooth root abscess, osteodystrophia fibrosa, and invasion of the jaw bones by lymphosarcoma (de Silva et al. 1985; Craig et al. 1986; Guedes et al. 1998; Rozear et al. 1998).

Osteodystrophia Fibrosa

A marked bilateral enlargement of the mandible has been reported in young (and occasionally adult) goats consuming mostly concentrate and thus having excessive phosphorus relative to calcium in the diet. The mandibles are soft (readily penetrated by a needle) and the cheek teeth are rotated so that the crowns are directed toward the tongue (Andrews et al. 1983). Demineralization is evident on radiographs (Singh 1995). In advanced cases, it may be impossible to open the mouth. Spontaneous fractures may occur. Feeding a good hay (such as alfalfa, which is high in calcium) and restricting the grain should prevent this condition, which is discussed in more detail in Chapter 4.

A similar mandibular (and maxillary) osteodystrophia fibrosa has been observed in four goats on a long-term (472 days) feeding trial with *Leucaena leucocephala*. The calcium to phosphorus ratio was more than 6:1. The kidney, thyroid, and parathyroid were histologically normal, and occurrence of the condition was not explained (Yates et al. 1987). Chronic renal disease might result in similar bone lesions.

Bottle Jaw

The presence of fluctuant pitting edema in the intermandibular space of goats that are not obviously in heart failure should arouse the suspicion of endoparasitism (see Chapter 10). The edema results from hypoproteinemia, which follows blood and plasma loss caused by nematode infestations of the gastrointestinal tract and liver failure in fluke infestation. Paratuberculosis also can cause severe enough hypoproteinemia to manifest as bottle jaw, as can renal disease. These conditions are discussed in Chapters 10, 11, and 12.

Swelled Head of Bucks

Fighting bucks may develop severe edematous infections of the head in regions where *Clostridium novyi* is prevalent. Other clostridia including *C. chauvoei*, *C. sordelli*, and *C. septicum* may be involved. The swelling begins near the horns and eyes but may extend down the face, neck, and chest. Tissues are full of yellow fluid and clostridia may be demonstrated on smear or anaerobic culture. Lymph nodes are swollen. The animal is lethargic and febrile. Death usually occurs within one to two days unless the swellings are opened surgically to allow oxygenation and massive doses of antibiotics (penicillin) are given. Photosensitization (see Chapter 2) might appear similar but does not spare the ears and is less rapidly fatal (King 1984). Bucks with a simple seroma on the poll from fighting will not be systemically ill.

Deformation of the Cranium

An abnormal profile of the cranial bones suggests hydrocephalus in the neonate and sinusitis or parasitic cyst in the older goat.

Hydrocephalus

Occasionally kids are born with an obvious doming of the skull and congenital hydrocephalus. This is usually sporadic, with no known predisposing cause, although some kids congenitally infected with Akabane virus (see Chapters 4 and 13) have hydrocephalus. The hereditary lysosomal storage disease of Nubians, beta mannosidosis, is also accompanied by deformation of the cranium, and is discussed in Chapter 5. Kids with hydrocephalus should be euthanatized if neurologic abnormalities are severe enough to interfere with nursing or locomotion.

Sinusitis

Except in neonatal kids, surgical dehorning invariably opens the frontal sinuses, into which hay and other foreign matter may easily fall. If a scab closes the opening before any infection present is eliminated, it is possible for an abscess to develop that may eventually lead to softening and distortion of overlying bone. A history of open dehorning within the last six months would be suggestive. Careful percussion may demonstrate a relative dullness over the affected sinus. Radiographic evaluation is recommended if there is any doubt that the swelling is over the frontal sinus rather than the cranial cavity or tooth roots. Drainage should be established and the sinus flushed daily, after removal of any foreign material or necrotic bone.

Enzootic intranasal tumor and lymphosarcoma, as discussed in Chapter 9, can invade the sinuses and cause bony distortion of the face. Digital pressure on softened bone causes expulsion of a seromucous exudate from the nostrils when an enzootic intranasal tumor is present (De las Heras et al. 1991). Decreased airflow is detectable through the nostril on the affected side. A dorsoventral radiograph reveals the space occupying nature of the tumor.

Coenurus Cerebralis (Gid)

Coenurus cerebralis is the larval form of the canine tapeworm *Taenia multiceps*. It can form cysts in the parenchyma of the brain or on its surface in sheep and goats. Blindness or various other neurologic signs occur, depending on the exact location of the cyst. The overlying skull may bulge and soften or even perforate. Where this sign is relied on for diagnosis it is reported to be common (Sharma and Tyagi 1975), although many affected animals show no outward changes in the skull. Insertion of an 18-gauge needle through the softened bone yields clear fluid under pressure, and sometimes the cyst can be extracted from the cranium by aspiration through a tube inserted via this needle. At least one goat has been cured by injecting Lugol's solution into the cyst. A more detailed discussion of this parasite is supplied in Chapters 5 and 6. The parasite may no longer be present in the United States.

SWELLINGS INVOLVING THE NECK AND CHEST

Caseous lymphadenitis, as already discussed, should always be considered when swellings are present in the region of cervical or prescapular lymph nodes. Many other conditions of varied etiology cause diffuse or localized swellings on the neck or chest.

Abscesses Other Than Caseous Lymphadenitis

Abscesses that do not respond to simple drainage should be reassessed (including radiographic examination) for possible presence of a foreign body such as a needle, plant fragment, or piece of necrotic bone. Abscesses in the neck and near the left elbow have been reported in goats that ingested sewing needles (Sharma and Ranka 1978; Tanwar and Saxena 1984).

Mycetomas, as discussed in Chapter 2, are chronic, subcutaneous, fungal-induced swellings, often with underlying periosteal reaction.

Tissue Necrosis ("Sterile Abscesses") Caused by Injections

A number of vaccines, including multivalent clostridial (Green et al. 1987), paratuberculosis (Holstad 1986d), caseous lymphadenitis, and foot and mouth disease vaccines, cause large, roughly spherical, firm, persistent swellings (granulomas). This occurs in most of the animals vaccinated and does not require contaminated vaccine or dirty needles to occur. A provisional diagnosis is based on the presence of such a tissue reaction in a site known to have been used previously for vaccination. No treatment is required in commercial animals unless local infection occurs. These swellings are of more concern in pets and show goats, where surgical extirpation of the lump may be requested by the owner. It is important to inject these animals in a cosmetically acceptable location, such as behind the shoulder or elbow, because a reaction can be expected from many adjuvanted, effective vaccines. In general, injections should not be given subcutaneously in the neck of a show animal. It is difficult for veterinarians writing health certificates to feel confident that goats with a nodular swelling in this region are free of caseous lymphadenitis.

Administering vaccines and antibiotics deep into musculature is not a satisfactory method of avoiding problems. The result, an often severe necrosis of muscle, is more difficult to observe but clearly painful to the goat. Tender, firm swellings, lameness, or reluctance to rise are common. When a site in the hind limb is used, sciatic nerve paralysis is also common, especially in young or emaciated animals with limited muscle volume. In addition, if the animal is to be used for meat, the muscle necrosis, which outlasts tissue residues by weeks or months, results in carcass damage that requires trimming or that escapes the notice of the meat inspector but is obvious and unappealing to the consumer.

Certain solutions are so irritating to tissue that they should not be administered subcutaneously or intramuscularly to goats. Some proprietary calcium preparations with phosphorus and dextrose included are noted for causing sloughing of tissue at the injection site. Failed attempts at intravenous injection may cause large swellings over the jugular vein where irritating drugs were mistakenly deposited in a perivascular location.

In animals kept for antibody production, it is normal to find numerous firm subcutaneous nodules where the adjuvanted antigen has been injected.

Wattle Cyst and Thyroglossal Duct Cyst

Wattles are reportedly caused by a dominant autosomal gene with complete penetrance but variable expression regarding the shape and location of the wattles (Ricordeau 1981). Occasionally, cysts occur unilaterally or bilaterally at the base of the wattle or at the site of previous wattle amputation. These cysts are certainly not rare but rarely are of enough concern to be reported in the literature. They are variously referred to as branchial cleft cysts (Williams 1980), dermoid cysts (Gamlem and Crawford 1977), or wattle cysts (Fubini and Campbell 1983). Wattle cysts are usually present at birth, although they may enlarge with time and become more noticeable later. They contain a thick or thin clear liquid and refill or become abscessed after aspiration. They can be excised intact under local anesthesia if care is taken to avoid the underlying jugular vein; excision may be necessary in show goats because of possible confusion with caseous lymphadenitis. Breed predilections reported in the literature may be biased by the prevalence of given breeds or family lines in certain regions.

Wattle cysts should be differentiated from thyroglossal duct cysts that are located on the midline, below the hyoid apparatus (Al-Ani and Vestweber 1986; Nair and Bandopadhyay 1990; Al-Ani et al. 1998). Thyroglossal cysts sometimes become quite large over time and can be removed surgically with due care.

Thyroid Gland and Goiter

Anatomy and Physiology

The thyroid of the goat is bilobed and located slightly behind the larynx. Right and left lobes, which lie lateral to the trachea, are joined by a thin isthmus that passes across the ventral aspect of the trachea (Reineke and Turner 1941). In young animals, the lobes of the thyroid gland are often embedded in thymic tissue. The isthmus becomes more fibrous (less glandular) and more caudally located with advancing age (Roy et al. 1975).

The thyroid gland forms several hormones by iodinating organic compounds that contain the amino acid tyrosine. Thyroxine (T_4) and 3,5,3-triiodothyronine (T_3), when formed, are stored in colloid within the acini of the thyroid gland until needed. The thyroid gland and its hormones control the metabolic rate of an animal by regulating cellular oxidation (Wilson 1975). Selenium is required for hepatic conversion of T_4 to T_3 (Köhrle 2000).

Goiter is an enlargement of the thyroid gland. In ruminants, goiter usually suggests attempted compensation for a hypothyroid state. Normally, low thyroxine and triiodothyronine output stimulates increased thyrotropin (thyroid-stimulating hormone) output, which leads to increased iodine uptake from the blood and hyperplasia of the gland. The enlarged gland may be able to compensate by increased iodine trapping.

Normal Thyroid Function Tests

Natural hypothyroid states other than goiters have not been reported in goats. If testing is done, it should be remembered that, at least in dogs, corticosteroid therapy and the terminal stages of nonthyroidal illnesses can both depress plasma T_4, possibly because of interference with T_4 binding by plasma proteins.

The thyroid function of goats has been investigated by researchers wishing to use the species as a model for the physiology of larger ruminants. For instance, uptake of radioiodine (^{131}I) has been studied in goats (Flamboe and Reineke 1959; Davis et al. 1966; Ragan et al. 1966). Thyroidectomy, as discussed below, has also been performed to study normal thyroid function.

Thyroid hormone level determinations are more accessible to practitioners, although caprine normals are not well established. Repeated serum thyroxine level determinations in twenty female and forty male goats of dairy breeds, from two weeks to six years of age, yielded a mean of 6.53 ± 0.03 (SE) μg/dl of thyroxine. The range was 2 to 17 μg/dl (Anderson and Harness 1975). Thyroid function tests were also performed on up to fifty-five pygmy goats from a laboratory colony (Castro et al. 1975). No sex differences were noted. Mean values recorded included: protein bound (organic) iodine, 8.1 ± 1.2 (SD) μg/dl; T_4, 7.2 ± 1.1 μg/dl; and cholesterol, 90 ± 29.7 mg/dl. Because values were within normal human ranges, the authors concluded that there was no evidence of thyroid malfunction.

As part of a study to establish normals for ten species, thyroid hormones were assayed in duplicate from ten goats (Reap et al. 1978). Average values (± standard deviation) and ranges were: T_4, 3.45 ± 0.47 (3 to 4.23) μg/dl and T_3, 145.9 ± 29.32 (88 to 190) ng/dl. The average thyroxine value for four young and four adult goats (breed not specified) was 4.25 μg/dl in another study (Kallfelz and Erali 1973). Thyroxine levels in Angoras in South Africa were found to fluctuate with no obvious seasonal pattern (Wentzel et al. 1979). In one study of dairy goats, the plasma thyroxine level decreased by approximately 30% during the first week of lactation, relative to the prepartum period (Emre and Garmo 1985).

The author has evaluated thyroid-stimulating hormone response in three normal adult dairy goats (M.C. Smith, unpublished data). Serum thyroxine concentrations approximately doubled four hours after intravenous injection of 5 IU of thyrotropin. A similar response was seen in 25 juvenile goats after receiving intravenous thyrotropin releasing factor at 1 μg/kg; T_3 increased a mean of 318% at one hour and T_4 increased a mean of 174% (97% to 227%) at four hours after stimulation (Reinemeyer et al. 1991). Baseline values in this study were 30 to 90 ng/dl T_3 and 3.1 to 6.1 μg/dl T_4.

Experimental Hypothyroidism

Thyroidectomy has been performed in the goat. Ectopic thyroid tissue can be destroyed by ^{131}I administration where surgical removal of the visible thyroid glands is not sufficient (Ekman 1965). Parathyroid function is maintained because a pair of external parathyroids is located separately from the thyroid glands, embedded in thymic tissue.

When adult goats underwent thyroidectomy, the major clinical sign was body weight gain. Does that received ^{131}I during pregnancy produced stillborn kids with no detectable thyroid glands. These does had reduced milk production. Goats that underwent thyroidectomy developed marked thickening and softening of the skin with local hair loss and they shivered intensely when exposed to cold (Andersson et al. 1967).

When young kids underwent thyroidectomy, growth stopped within one to two months, kids became lethargic, and the head developed a dish-faced appearance (Reineke and Turner 1941). Growth recommenced if iodinated proteins were fed.

Goats with hypothyroidism have also been created experimentally by daily oral feeding of thiourea (Sreekumaran and Rajan 1978) and by injection of methyl thiouracil or thiourea (Gupta et al. 1990). When young kids were thus treated, weight loss and myxedema (edema and gelatinous infiltration of subcutaneous tissue) developed (Sreekumaran and Rajan

1977). Skin changes in these kids are discussed in Chapter 2. When eight-month-old male goats were made hypothyroid with thiourea, plasma testosterone levels decreased to less than 12% of pretreatment levels (Gupta et al. 1991). Long-term feeding of *Brachiaria mutica* grass with high but sublethal nitrate concentration has resulted in abnormally small and firm thyroid glands and mild proliferation of the acinar epithelium (Prasad 1983).

Naturally Occurring Dietary Goiter

Enlargement of the thyroid gland is usually a nutritional disease.

ETIOLOGY. There are two major mechanisms by which diet can cause development of goiters in goats: iodine deficiency and feeding of goitrogens. In addition, experimental cobalt deficiency (and thus vitamin B_{12} deficiency) has produced elevated thyroxine levels accompanied by marked hypertrophy and hyperplasia of the thyroid gland (Mgongo 1981); however, in a later study thyroid function was not markedly impaired by cobalt deficiency (Mburu et al. 1994).

IODINE DEFICIENCY GOITER. "Endemic" goiter in goats has generally been recognized in the past in the same regions where human goiter occurred. Soils are deficient in iodine or do not release it readily to plants and drinking water. Iodine-deficient regions include the Great Lakes, Great Plains, Rocky Mountains, and Pacific Coast regions of the United States (Lall 1952); Switzerland; parts of Great Britain (Wilson 1975); and the Himalayas (Raina and Pachauri 1984). The availability of iodized salt has decreased the prevalence of this type of goiter in both the United States and Western Europe. Goiter remains common in the Himalayas, where supplementation is not as available (Singh et al. 2002).

Breeds of goats vary in sensitivity to iodine deficiency. The Boer goat, a rapidly growing meat breed from South Africa, seems to be especially susceptible. It is possible that selection for resistance to iodine deficiency would be selection for slow growth rate (van Jaarsveld et al. 1971). In the Himalayas, where caprine goiter was extensively studied, indigenous strains were apparently more resistant to iodine deficiency than were goats (Barbari or Alpine) purchased from outside regions (Rajkumar 1970). The Angora goat is apparently very susceptible to iodine deficiency (Kalkus 1920).

GOITROGENS. Goitrogens are compounds that interfere with the uptake of dietary iodine or with its metabolism in the formation of thyroxine (Bath et al. 1979; Cheeke 1998). Thiocyanate is a goitrogen present in many species of brassicas, members of the Brassicaceae (Cruciferae) family. Increasing dietary iodine will overcome the inhibitory effects of thiocyanate on selective concentration of iodine by the thyroid. Goitrin (thiooxazolidone) is a thiouracil-type goitrogen found in the seeds of rape, kale, and other *Brassica* spp. that blocks hormone synthesis; its action cannot be overcome by feeding additional iodine.

Thiourea is similar and also interferes with organic binding of iodine; it has been used to produce experimental hypothyroidism (Wilson 1975). Mimosine in *Leucaena leucocephala* is broken down metabolically to a goitrogen in ruminants (Hegarty et al. 1976; Prasad 1989) but this chemical can be detoxified by natural populations of rumen bacteria (Hammond 1995). See further discussion in Chapter 10. African pearl millet (*Pennisetum typhoides*) is goitrogenic for goats, although the toxin has not been identified (Abdel Gadir and Adam 1999).

CLINICAL SIGNS AND LABORATORY FINDINGS. The normal thyroid gland is 0.20% of body weight (Kaneko 1997). In goitrous regions, unsupplemented adults have marked enlargement of the thyroid, which is sometimes the size of an orange (Kalkus 1920). The goats otherwise look healthy. Reproductive performance may be decreased (Kategile et al. 1978). Humoral and cell-mediated immune responses may be decreased (Singh et al. 2006).

Affected kids have thyroid enlargement at birth (Figures 3.8 and 3.9), and enlargement of the kid's pituitary gland has also been described (Ozmen and Haligur 2005). They may be stillborn or are very weak and die within a few hours. Increased blood flow to the thyroid may cause a palpable thrill. Most of these kids are hairless or covered with very fine hair, while some have a normal hair coat (Kalkus 1920; Love 1942; Paliwal and Sharma 1979). It has suggested that multiple fetuses in a litter are more apt to be affected with dietary goiter than a single fetus (Ozmen and Haligur 2005).

In one outbreak in South African Angoras, believed to be caused by thiocyanate from heavily fertilized alfalfa pastures, kids were viable but abnormal from birth (Bath et al. 1979). They were short, blocky, obese, and inactive. The skull was broadened laterally and prognathia inferior was present in all cases. Goiters were easily palpated bilaterally. Mean thyroxine level for four goitrous goats was 3.1 µg/dl, whereas the mean of four normal goats was 5.9 µg/dl. Plasma cholesterol was five times higher (10.9 mmol/l versus 1.8 mmol/l) in goitrous than control goats. In another case report, does were fed on cabbages and the kids appeared normal except for goiters measuring as large as 7 cm by 4.5 cm (Lombard and Raby 1965). The largest goiters were associated with severe dyspnea and death, whereas less markedly affected kids grew poorly.

A study from an iodine deficient area of India evaluated 252 congenitally goitrous kids born to 574 does with goiter. Clinical signs included thyroid gland hypertrophy and palpable thrill, enlarged joints,

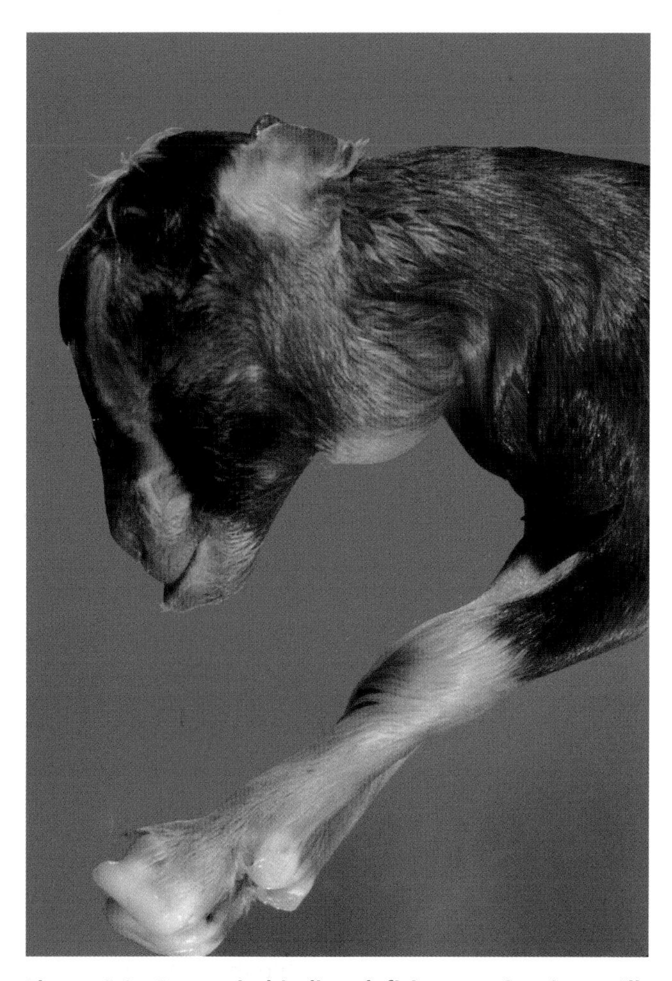

Figure 3.8. Congenital iodine deficiency goiter in a stillborn kid. (Courtesy of Dr. M.C. Smith.)

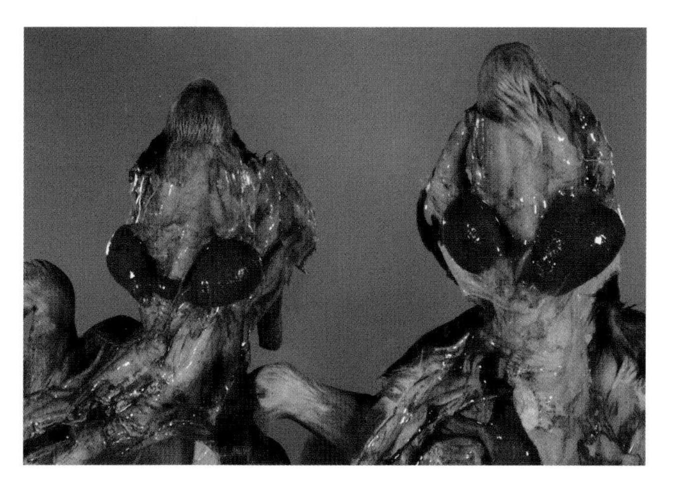

Figure 3.9. Goiters exposed in twin stillborn kids by reflecting the skin. (Courtesy of Dr. M.C. Smith.)

muscle contracture, an arched back and waddling gait, partial to complete alopecia, weakness, and lethargy. Hydrocephalus and prognathism were less common. Serum cholesterol was increased while T_3 and T_4 were decreased. The incidence of stillbirth in this study was 18% (Sing et al. 2003).

Diagnosis. Major differentials for a diagnosis of goiter include encapsulated abscesses and wattle cysts, which are unlikely to be bilateral and in the exact location of the thyroid. Thymic enlargement is more difficult to distinguish because the thyroid glands are normally embedded in the thymus. The kid with an enlarged thymus grows rapidly, has a healthy hair coat, and is active. As long as trace mineralized salt is available and no known goitrogens are being fed, the continued good health of the growing kid remains the ultimate diagnostic test to rule out goiter. Biopsy is not necessary, although normal thyroids contain acini lined by low cuboidal epithelium and filled with colloid, as opposed to the tall columnar epithelium, papillary infolding, and minimal colloid of goitrous glands (Love 1942; Roy et al. 1964). A hyperplastic goiter is transformed into a colloid goiter when the diet is improved or the lower iodine needs of an older animal are met, resulting in a gland that is still enlarged but has much colloid in the acini. Iodine content of the goitrous thyroid gland is reduced. Subclinical goiter is diagnosed when the glands appear to be normal size but are histologically hyperplastic.

Treatment and Prevention. The actual dietary iodine requirement for goats, as discussed in Chapter 19, is 0.8 mg/kg dry matter for lactating females and 0.5 mg/kg for the rest of the herd. Cruciferous plants increase the ration iodine requirement to approximately 2 mg/kg.

Iodine deficiency goiter is treated or prevented by supplying iodine to the goat, especially the pregnant doe. This can easily be done with iodized salt, assuming that no iodine-free salt source is available for the goats to satisfy their salt requirements. In a report from India, biochemical and hormonal values normalized in goitrous kids when colloidal iodine (I_2) was given orally at 0.1 mg/kg bodyweight for 100 days (Singh et al. 2003). Synthetic sodium thyroxine (0.2 mg/day orally to goats weighing 16 to 20 kg) also corrected many clinical signs of deficiency (Singh et al. 2006) but should not be necessary once the diet is corrected.

In the classic experiments of Kalkus (1920), oral daily potassium iodide (2 grains, 130 mg) or weekly application of 1 ml of tincture of iodine to the back throughout gestation were both successful in preventing goiter. Iodine treatment during the preceding pregnancy sometimes was enough to permit production of another normal kid. Adult goats with iodine deficiency goiter showed a decrease in thyroid size after treatment (Kalkus 1920; Welch 1928).

Congenital goiter caused by goitrogens is best avoided by not feeding the incriminated forages (especially brassicas) during pregnancy. Supplemental iodine can also be fed to the does (Heras et al. 1984).

Hereditary Goiter

Congenital goiter occurred spontaneously in an inbred strain of Dutch goats (mixed Saanen and dwarf goats). The trait was maintained and studied extensively as a model for thyroid defects in humans.

PATHOGENESIS. The condition was inherited as an autosomal recessive trait (Kok et al. 1987). Thyroglobulin, the normal precursor of the thyroid hormones T_3 and T_4, was not produced in the goat that was homozygous for this trait. As a consequence, the normal feedback mechanisms were impaired and continuous thyrotropin secretion led to development of a goiter. The responsible mutation in the thyroglobulin gene has been characterized (Rivolta and Targovnik 2006).

CLINICAL AND LABORATORY FINDINGS. Normal thyroids (both together) in this breed weighed 1 to 4 g, and goiters weighed 15 to 300 g. Plasma T_3 levels (9 to 36 ng/dl) and T_4 levels (less than 0.4 μg/dl) were substantially lower than normal goat T_3 (124 to 151 ng/dl) and T_4 (5.9 to 10.2 μg/dl) levels (de Vijlder et al. 1978). Histologically, the goitrous thyroid had hypertrophic and hyperplastic epithelium consistent with prolonged thyrotropin stimulation. Colloid was almost absent.

In addition to having enlargement of the thyroids, goitrous kids were sluggish and grew poorly. The hair coat was rough and sparse. If thyroxine replacement was not provided, the hair coat eventually disappeared almost completely and the skin became thick and scaly (Rijnberk 1977). Euthyroidism could be achieved with these goats using iodide supplementation (1 mg I^- per day orally). Other proteins were iodinated and then converted to T_3 and T_4 even though thyroglobulin still was not synthesized (van Voorthuizen et al. 1978).

CONGENITAL GOITERS IN OTHER BREEDS. Congenital goiters of possibly hereditary etiology have also been found in Boer goats (van Jaarsveld 1971). Except for the enlargement of the thyroid glands (average 37 g compared with the normal average 2 g), the kids appeared normal. Histologically, there was hypertrophy of the thyroid epithelium with absence of colloid. Normal iodoproteins were present, but the thyroglobulin polymers tended to dissociate into subunits. Congenital goiters (average 43 g compared with a normal average of 9 g) have also been suspected to be hereditary in Shami dairy goats (Al-Ani et al. 1998). An autosomal recessive hereditary goiter in goats in Inner Mongolia was controlled by removing known carriers and identifying other carriers in the herd using a goat-homologous assay for thyrotropin (Mei and Chang 1996).

Thymus

Young kids, especially if well fed, sometimes develop bilaterally symmetric swellings in the upper neck in the region of the thyroid gland (Figure 3.10). The swellings may first become noticeable as early as two weeks of age and regress spontaneously, often at about four months of age (Pritchard 1987) or somewhat later (Bertone and Smith 1985). The kid is otherwise healthy, with a good hair coat, and therefore is unlikely to be affected with severe iodine deficiency or goiter. Another subcutaneous swelling occurs at the thoracic inlet. Aspiration of either the cranial or caudal cervical masses, while not indicated, yields thymic tissue. The origin of the excessive thymic tissue might be remnants from embryologic development or accessory thymus; in any case, the glandular tissue involutes naturally and no treatment is needed. Owners should be warned of the potential for iodine toxicity if unnecessary supplements, such as kelp, are fed when no thyroid deficiency exists.

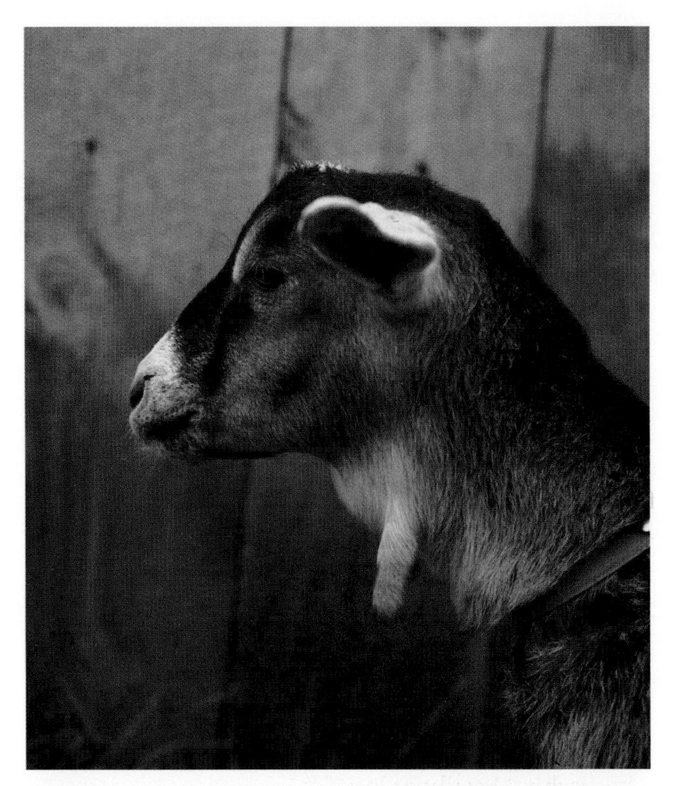

Figure 3.10. Enlarged thymus in the upper neck of a rapidly growing Nubian cross kid. (Courtesy of Dr. M.C. Smith.)

Tumors of the thymus occur in adult goats, and their presence as a space-occupying lesion or incidental finding in the thorax is discussed in Chapter 9. Less commonly, remnants of the cervical portion of the thymus become neoplastic. Diagnosis is by examination of a biopsy or aspirate, and treatment by surgical excision.

Thymic tissue may also be embedded within the thyroid gland of goats of any age (Roy et al. 1976), often in association with parathyroid tissue, but no clinical relevance has been reported for this histologic finding.

Phlebitis

Because the jugular veins are commonly used for venipuncture and administration of various medications, iatrogenic phlebitis may be expected to occur occasionally. Hematomas typically resolve quickly without treatment, whereas perivascular deposition of irritating drugs can lead to cellulitis or even abscessation. Conservative therapy, including application of hot compresses, is preferable to lancing a swelling so close to the jugular vein.

Atlantal Bursitis

Atlantal bursitis is a fairly specific but uncommon sign of caprine arthritis encephalitis virus infection. A fluctuant swelling is located underneath and extends on both sides of the ligamentum nuchae (Figure 3.11). The bursa often contains mineralized material, which can be demonstrated with a radiograph (Garry and Rings 1985). Histology shows hyperplasia of synovial cells and mononuclear cell infiltration (Gonzalez et al. 1987). An abscess can develop if aspiration is attempted. The supraspinous bursa may be similarly involved, as may be other bursae over the carpus, olecranon, or tuber ischii. Usually at least some degree of lameness is present by the time the atlantal bursa becomes noticeably distended.

Sternal Abscesses and Hygromas

Sternal abscesses were detected in seventy-two goats in a large antibody-producing herd over a sixteen-year period (Gezon et al. 1991). These abscesses were 3 to 15 cm in diameter and usually involved skin and subcutaneous tissues, but rarely invaded muscle or bone. Two of the goats, however, had osteomyelitis of the sternum. Bruises and abrasions of an area commonly exposed to manure were proposed as an explanation of the occurrence of the abscesses. Antibiotic therapy had little effect on the condition. The authors did not adequately report culture results, and thus no conclusions can be drawn from this study concerning bacteria present in unbroken sternal abscesses.

Sternal abscesses are, in the authors' experience, most common in goats afflicted with severe lameness, such as from arthritis associated with caprine arthritis encephalitis virus infection. Two hypotheses come to mind to explain this association. First, the lame goat spends more time in sternal recumbency and therefore may develop a hygroma or decubital sore. Second, the caprine arthritis encephalitis virus-induced arthritis might involve joints between sternebrae, with secondary bacterial infection. Successful treatment of these abscesses often requires surgical debridement. Radiographic evaluation for osteomyelitis or enlargement (and probable infection) of lymph nodes within the thoracic cavity are helpful in offering a prognosis and determining the extent of surgical debridement required. Goats that are markedly lame and emaciated or have extension of infection into the thorax will probably benefit little from treatment of a sternal abscess.

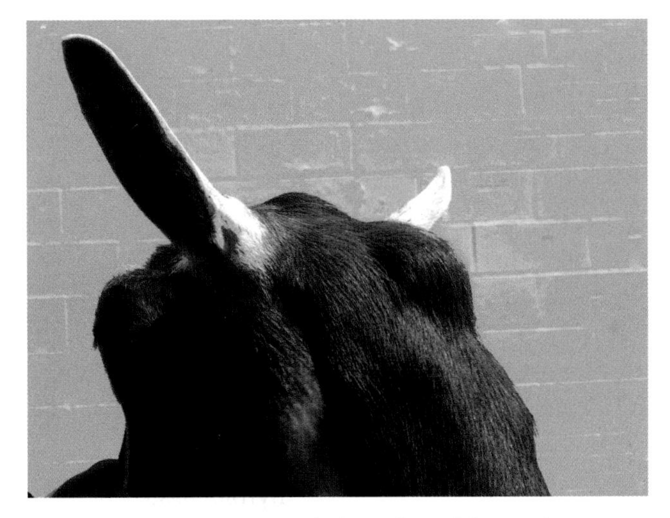

Figure 3.11. Distension of the atlantal bursa in a goat with clinical CAE arthritis. (Courtesy of Dr. M.C. Smith.)

Warbles

Larvae of *Przhevalskiana silenus*, a warble fly that migrates to the back region of goats in Mediterranean countries and Asia, are accompanied by localized inflammatory reaction and granulation tissue in the subcutaneous tissue. This parasite is discussed in Chapter 2. Although cattle warble fly larvae (*Hypoderma* spp.) could potentially invade goats, natural occurrence has not been documented and experimental infections with *Hypoderma lineatum* larvae did not progress to the development of subcutaneous warbles (Colwell and Otranto 2006).

Tapeworm Cysts

The intermediate form of the dog tapeworm *Taenia multiceps* (previously called *Multiceps multiceps* or *M. gaigeri*) forms cysts within the central nervous system (CNS) of sheep and goats, but also outside the CNS of goats, especially in muscle and subcutaneously (Verster 1969). Scolices are arranged in clusters and there are no internal or external daughter cysts. These cysts have been reported as the cause of large (approximately 15 cm in diameter) subcutaneous swellings distributed over the limbs and body of goats in the Sudan (Ramadan et al. 1973; Hago and Abu-Samra 1980) and India (Shastri et al. 1985). The cysts are fluctuating, cool, and covered with hairless skin. Depending on the cyst location, there may be interference with locomotion, feeding, or function of internal organs. Head shaking is commonly observed when cysts are near the base of the ear.

Several methods of treatment have been successful, including excision of the cyst, lancing the cyst and packing the cavity with gauze soaked in iodine, or aspirating all the fluid and infusing 0.5 to 1 ml of Lugol's iodine into the collapsed cyst (Nooruddin et al. 1996). When a herd outbreak occurs, as in a reported case involving forty-seven of 169 Black Bengal goats, emphasis should obviously be put on treating dogs for tapeworms and destroying the carcasses of dead goats to prevent consumption by the dogs or wild canids (Patro et al. 1997).

SWELLINGS INVOLVING THE ABDOMEN AND ESCUTCHEON

Alteration in the abdominal silhouette is discussed in detail in Chapter 10.

Umbilical Hernia

Umbilical hernia caused by the incomplete closure of the umbilical ring (in the absence of omphalitis) is rare in goats. A genetic predisposition has not been identified in this species (Hámori 1983). Nevertheless, prudence dictates that males that will be used extensively for breeding should be free of all recognizable congenital defects.

Goats with a swelling originating from the umbilical region should be examined by palpation while standing, and if necessary, in lateral recumbency. If the swelling is easily reduced with no tenderness or thickened stalk, then it is likely that it is a hernia unaccompanied by an abscess. In young female goats, wrapping the abdomen for two to four weeks with adhesive elastic tape may permit closure of the hernia ring to occur. If the defect is large, an internal abscess is suspected, or the patient is male, surgical repair is the preferred therapy. The goat is placed in dorsal recumbency and standard techniques appropriate for herniorrhaphy in calves are employed. Prosthetic mesh may be required to close large defects in the body wall (Fubini and Campbell 1983).

An alternative nonsurgical repair has been described using an elastrator castration band. The animal is lightly sedated and placed in dorsal recumbency. With all of the contents of the hernia sac replaced into the abdomen, two metal pins such as diaper pins are inserted through the skin on each side of the sac, so that they will sit close to the abdominal wall. An elastrator band is then placed around the hernial sac, between the pins and the body wall, where it causes sloughing of the skin and healing of the defect within two weeks (Navarre and Pugh 2002). Tetanus prophylaxis is imperative.

Umbilical Abscess

If palpation of an umbilical swelling reveals warmth, tenderness, or just an irreducible fluctuance, diagnostic aspiration is indicated. Omphalitis may result in abscessation of remnants of umbilical arteries, the umbilical vein, or the urachus. Ultrasonography may be useful for evaluation of the extent of internal involvement of an umbilical abscess. External abscesses are drained and systemic antibiotics are administered for one week or longer. If evidence of infection or concurrent hernia persists, surgical debridement and herniorrhaphy are recommended.

Abdominal or Flank Hernia

The abdominal wall of a goat is relatively thin. Muscle tearing and separation often occur from blunt trauma during fighting, shearing, or crowding through narrow doorways. Diagnosis of a unilateral flank hernia is usually obvious, although it is important to determine if a pregnant uterus is trapped in a subcutaneous location. When the hernia or stretching of the body wall is bilateral (as from doorways) it should be distinguished from pregnancy, hydrometra, obesity, or ascites by careful physical examination.

Small hernias may be surgically repaired, while hernias large enough to impede parturition are usually an indication for culling in a commercial herd. Tranquilization with xylazine and local anesthesia using a ring block of lidocaine (not to exceed 10 mg/kg) has been used for repair of abdominal hernias in goats (Al-Sobayil and Ahmed 2007). Either absorbable or nonabsorbable suture is satisfactory, with nonabsorbable (the authors used silk) favored in older animals or those with more longstanding hernias.

Ventral Hernia

Occasionally, trauma or extreme abdominal distention leads to rupture of the ventral abdominal muscles caudal to the umbilicus, as described in sheep (Arthur et al. 1989). This results in edematous swelling of the abdominal wall and dropping of the udder. Successful surgical repair has been reported in a goat (Misk et al. 1986). The late pregnant uterus can become trapped in the hernia in a subcutaneous location, making vaginal delivery difficult (Horenstein and Elias 1987). Successful surgical correction of such a "metrocele" at four months gestation has been reported (Radhakrishnan et al. 1993).

Ventral Edema of Angoras

Angora goats in South Africa, the United States, New Zealand, and England have developed severe edematous swelling ("swelling disease" or "water belly") of the ventral abdomen and chest and sometimes the limbs and submandibular region after shearing or other stress (Mitchell et al. 1983; Byrne 1994a, 1994b; Thompson 1994). As many as 15% of the herd may be affected. The swelling consists of clear, copious, nonclotting fluid and disappears spontaneously in a few days. Possible etiologies discussed in the literature include hypoproteinemia and change in capillary permeability, stress (via increased aldosterone secretion and sodium retention), and vitamin E deficiency. Research attempting to recreate the condition with parasitic infections or modify it with increased dietary protein has been inconclusive, but in general the smaller goats with lower plasma total protein concentrations are at higher risk (Snyman and Snyman 2005).

Hypoalbuminemia due to parasitism or paratuberculosis and edema caused by congestive heart failure must be ruled out in individual animals that do not recover rapidly. If sudden deaths occur in the herd, vitamin E status should be investigated (Byrne 1994a). Otherwise, no treatment is indicated except provision of feed and shelter for newly shorn animals.

Urethral Rupture

Bucks and wethers with urolithiasis may develop a ventral swelling (water belly) if the urethra ruptures and urine leaks into subcutaneous tissues. The swelling is edematous and cool; aspiration yields a watery fluid that may have an ammoniacal odor when heated. The fluid can be reabsorbed if the obstruction to normal urine flow is relieved. Localized skin sloughing may occur. Urolithiasis and its treatment are discussed in detail in Chapter 12.

Gangrenous Mastitis

The skin of the ventral abdomen anterior to the udder may become swollen and edematous because of vascular thrombosis in goats with gangrenous mastitis. Initially the swelling is cool; necrosis and sloughing may eventually occur. Gangrenous mastitis is discussed in Chapter 14.

Ectopic Mammary Gland

The embryonic mammary line of mammals extends from the pectoral region to the vulva. Although female goats usually develop only two functional glands in an inguinal location, milk-secreting tissue is occasionally located bilaterally in the lips of the vulva (Lesbouyries and Drieux 1945; Kulkarni and Marudwar 1972; Ramadan and El Hassan 1975; Smith 1986). As parturition approaches, the vulva enlarges, as does the udder. This vulvar swelling is firm and lobular (Figure 3.12), is separated from the skin, and does not subside promptly after parturition as physiologic edema would. Instead, the vulva remains distended for as long as three months, but eventually subsides as the glandular tissue becomes atrophied from the back-pressure of entrapped milk. The condition is merely a curiosity but can be confirmed by aspiration of a whitish fluid containing fat globules. The bilaterally symmetrical nature of the swelling also helps to differentiate ectopic mammary gland from an adenocarcinoma or other neoplasm (see Chapter 2).

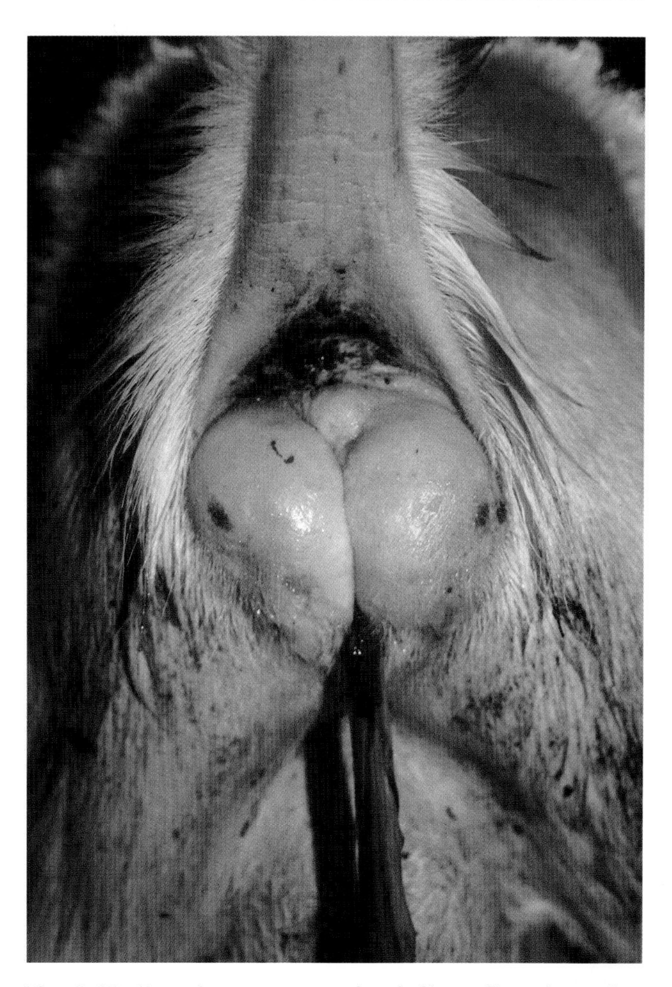

Fig. 3.12. Ectopic mammary gland distending the vulva of a mature Saanen doe one day after parturition. The doe also has a retained placenta. (Courtesy of Dr. M.C. Smith.)

Mammary gland development in the buck (gynecomastia) is discussed in Chapter 13.

REFERENCES

Abdel Gadir, W.S. and Adam, S.E.I.: Development of goiter and enterohepatonephropathy in Nubian goats fed with pearl millet (*Pennisetum typhoides*). Vet. J., 157:178–185, 1999.

Al-Ani, F.K. and Vestweber, J.: The embryologic origin of thyroglossal duct cysts. Vet. Med., 81:271–272, 1986.

Al-Ani, F.K., et al.: Occurrence of congenital anomalies in Shami breed goats; 211 cases investigated in 19 herds. Small Rumin. Res., 28:225–232, 1998.

Al-Sobayil, F.A., and Ahmed, A.F.: Surgical treatment for different forms of hernias in sheep and goats. J. Vet. Sci., 8:185–191, 2007.

Aleman, M., et al.: *Corynebacterium pseudotuberculosis* infection in horses: 538 cases (1982–1993). J. Am. Vet. Med. Assoc., 209:804–809, 1996.

Alhendi, A.B., et al.: An outbreak of abscess disease in goats in Saudi Arabia. Zentralbl. Veterinärmed A, 40:646–651, 1993.

Anderson, D.E., Rings, D.M., and Kowalski, J.: Infection with *Corynebacterium pseudotuberculosis* in five alpacas. J. Am. Vet. Med. Assoc., 225:1743–1747, 2004.

Anderson, R.R., and Harness, J.R.: Thyroid hormone secretion rates in growing and mature goats. J. Anim. Sci., 40:1130–1135, 1975.

Anderson, V.M., and Nairn, M.E.: Control of caseous lymphadenitis in goats by vaccination. In: Les Maladies de la Chèvre. Niort (France), 9–11 Octobre, pp. 605–609. 1984a.

Anderson, V.M., and Nairn, M.E.: Role of maternal immunity in the prevention of caseous lymphadenitis. In: Les Maladies de la Chèvre. Niort (France), 9–11 Octobre, pp. 601–604. 1984b.

Andersson, B., et al.: Studies of the importance of the thyroid and the sympathetic system in the defense to cold of the goat. Acta Physiol. Scand., 69:111–118, 1967.

Andrews, A.H., Ingram, P.L., and Longstaffe, J.A.: Osteodystrophia fibrosa in young goats. Vet. Rec., 112:404–406, 1983.

Arthur, G.H., Noakes, D.E., and Pearson, H.: Veterinary Reproduction and Obstetrics (Theriogenology). 6th Ed. London, Baillière Tindall, 1989.

Ashfaq, M.K. and Campbell, S.G.: Caseous lymphadenitis (abscesses) in goats in the United States. Dairy Goat J., 57(12):3, 76–77, 1979a.

Ashfaq, M.K. and Campbell, S.G.: A survey of caseous lymphadenitis and its etiology in goats in the United States. Vet. Med. Small Anim. Clin., 74:1161–1165, 1979b.

Ashfaq, M.K. and Campbell, S.G.: Experimentally induced caseous lymphadenitis in goats. Am. J. Vet. Res., 41:1789–1792, 1980.

Augustine, J.L. and Renshaw, H.W.: Survival of *Corynebacterium pseudotuberculosis* in axenic purulent exudate on common barnyard fomites. Am. J. Vet. Res., 47:713–715, 1986.

Baby, P.G., et al.: Actinomycosis in goat—a case report. Indian J. Vet. Med., 20:52, 2000.

Baird, G., Fontaine, M., and Donachie, W.: The effects of pasteurization on the survival of *Corynebacterium pseudotuberculosis* in milk. Res. Vet. Sci., 78(Suppl. A):18–19, 2005.

Batey, R.G., Speed, C.M., and Kobes, C.J.: Prevalence and distribution of caseous lymphadenitis in feral goats. Aust. Vet. J., 63:33–36, 1986.

Bath, G.F., Wentzel, D., and van Tonder, E.: Cretinism in Angora goats. J. S. Afr. Vet. Assoc., 50:237–239, 1979.

Baxendell, S.A.: Abscesses in goats. In: Refresher Course for Veterinarians, Proceedings No. 73, Goats, The University of Sydney, The Post-Graduate Committee in Veterinary Science, Sydney, N.S.W., Australia, pp. 373–375, 1984.

Bertone, J.J. and Smith, M.C.: Excessive cranial cervical thymic tissue in a Nubian kid. Comp. Contin. Educ. Pract. Vet., 7:S401-S404, 1985.

Brogden, K.A., et al.: Effect of muramyl dipeptide on immunogenicity of *Corynebacterium pseudotuberculosis* whole-cell vaccines in mice and lambs. Am. J. Vet. Res., 51:200–202, 1990.

Brown, C.C. and Olander, H.J.: Caseous lymphadenitis of goats and sheep: A review. Vet. Bull., 57:1–12, 1987.

Brown, C.C., et al.: Serologic response and lesions in goats experimentally infected with *Corynebacterium pseudotuberculosis* of caprine and equine origins. Am. J. Vet. Res., 46:2322–2326, 1985.

Brown, C.C., et al.: Use of a toxoid vaccine to protect goats against intradermal challenge exposure to *Corynebacterium pseudotuberculosis*. Am. J. Vet. Res. 47:1116–1119, 1986a.

Brown, C.C., et al.: Serodiagnosis of inapparent caseous lymphadenitis in goats and sheep, using the synergistic hemolysis-inhibition test. Am. J. Vet. Res., 47:1461–1463, 1986b.

Brown, P.J., Lane, J.G., and Lucke, V.M.: Developmental cysts in the upper neck of Anglo-Nubian goats. Vet. Rec., 125:256–258, 1989.

Burrell, D.H.: Caseous lymphadenitis in goats. Aust. Vet. J., 57:105–110, 1981.

Byrne, D.J.: Swelling disease of Angora goats. Vet. Rec., 134:507, 1994a.

Byrne, D.J.: Ventral oedema in exotic Angora goats. N. Z. Vet. J., 42:157–158, 1994b.

Carceles, C.M., et al.: Pharmacokinetics of azithromycin after intravenous and intramuscular administration to goats. J. Vet. Pharmacol. Ther., 28:51–55, 2005.

Castro, A., et al.: Normal functions of the thyroid gland of the pygmy goat. Lab. Anim. Sci., 25:327–330, 1975.

Cheeke, P.R.: Natural Toxicants in Feeds, Forages, and Poisonous Plants, 2nd Ed. Danville, IL, Interstate Publishers, Inc., 1998.

Cheng, A.C. and Currie, B.J.: Melioidosis: epidemiology, pathophysiology, and management. Clin. Microbiol. Rev., 18:383–416, 2005.

Colwell, D.D. and Otranto, D.: Cross-transmission studies with *Hypoderma lineatum* de Vill. (Diptera: Oestridae): Attempted infestation of goats (*Capra hircus*). Vet. Parasitol., 141:302–306, 2006.

Craig, D.R., Roth, L., and Smith, M.C.: Lymphosarcoma in goats. Comp. Contin. Educ. Pract. Vet., 8:S190-S197, 1986.

Davis, R.W., Kainer, R.A., and Flamboe, E.E.: The effects of an oxytetracycline preparation on the thyroid gland: a preliminary report. Am. J. Vet. Res., 27:166–171, 1966.

De las Heras, M., Garcia de Jalon, J.A., and Sharp, J.M.: Pathology of enzootic intranasal tumor in thirty-eight goats. Vet. Pathol., 28:474–481, 1991.

de Silva, L.N., et al.: Lymphosarcoma involving the mandible in two goats. Vet. Rec., 117:276, 1985.

de Vijlder, J.J.M., et al.: Hereditary congenital goiter with thyroglobulin deficiency in a breed of goats. Endocrinology, 102:1214–1222, 1978.

Dercksen, D.P., ter Laak, E.A., and Schreuder, B.E.C.: Eradication programme for caseous lymphadenitis in goats in the Netherlands. Vet. Rec., 138:237, 1996.

Dercksen, D.P., et al.: A comparison of four serological tests for the diagnosis of caseous lymphadenitis in sheep and goats. Vet. Microbiol., 75:167–175, 2000.

Desiderio, J.V., Turillo, L.A., and Campbell, S.G.: Serum proteins of normal goats and goats with caseous lymphadenitis. Am. J. Vet. Res., 40:400–402, 1979.

DiGrassie, W.A., Wallace, M.A., and Sponenberg, D.P.: Multicentric lymphosarcoma with ovarian involvement in a Nubian goat. Can. Vet. J., 38:383–384, 1997.

Duncan, J.R. and Prasse, K.W.: Veterinary Laboratory Medicine. Clinical Pathology. 2nd Ed. Ames, IA, Iowa State Univ. Press, 1986.

Ekman, L.: Thyroidectomy of the goat. Acta Physiol. Scand., 64:331–336, 1965.

El Sanousi, S.M., Hamad, A.A., and Gameel, A.A.: Abscess disease in goats in the Sudan. Rev. Élev. Méd Vét. Pays Trop., 42:379–382, 1989.

Ellis, J.A., et al.: Differential antibody response to *Corynebacterium pseudotuberculosis* in sheep with naturally acquired caseous lymphadenitis. J. Am. Vet. Med. Assoc., 196:1609–1613, 1990.

Ellis, T.M., et al.: The role of *Corynebacterium pseudotuberculosis* lung lesions in the transmission of this bacterium to other sheep. Aust. Vet. J., 64:261–263, 1987.

Emre, Z. and Garmo, G.: Plasma thyroxine through parturition and early lactation in goats fed silage of grass and rape. Acta Vet. Scand., 26:417–418, 1985.

Flamboe, E.E. and Reineke, E.P.: Estimation of thyroid secretion rates in dairy goats and measurement of I^{131} uptake and release with regard to age, pregnancy, lactation, and season of the year. J. Anim. Sci., 18:1135–1148, 1959.

Frank, L.A.: Clinical pharmacology of rifampin. J. Am. Vet. Med. Assoc., 197:114–117, 1990.

Fubini, S.L. and Campbell, S.G.: External lumps on sheep and goats. Vet. Clin. North Am. Large Anim. Pract., 5:457–476, 1983.

Gamlem, T. and Crawford, T.B.: Dermoid cysts in identical locations in a doe goat and her kid. Vet. Med. Small Anim. Clin., 72:616–617, 1977.

Garry, F. and Rings, D.M.: What is your diagnosis? J. Am. Vet. Med. Assoc., 187:641–642, 1985.

Gezon, H.M., et al.: Epizootic of external and internal abscesses in a large goat herd over a 16-year period. J. Am. Vet. Med. Assoc., 198:257–263, 1991.

Ghanbarpour, R. and Khaleghiyan, M.: A study on caseous lymphadenitis in goats. Indian Vet. J., 82:1013–1014, 2005.

Ghosh, R.C., et al.: Occurrence of *Coenurus gaigeri* cyst in a goat. Indian Vet. J., 82:90–91, 2005.

Gilmour, N.J.L.: Caseous lymphadenitis: a cause for concern. Vet. Rec., 126:566, 1990.

Gonzalez, L., et al.: Caprine arthritis-encephalitis in the Basque country, Spain. Vet. Rec., 120:102–109, 1987.

Green, D.S., et al.: Injection site reactions and antibody responses in sheep and goats after the use of multivalent clostridial vaccines. Vet. Rec., 120:435–439, 1987.

Guedes, R.M.C., Facury Filho, E.J., and Lago, L.A.: Mandibular lymphosarcoma in a goat. Vet. Rec., 143:51–52, 1998.

Gupta, P.S.P., Sanwal, P.C., and Varshney, V.P.: Induction of hypothyroidism in goats by parenteral administration of antithyroid drugs. Small Rumin. Res., 3:179–186, 1990.

Gupta, P.S.P., Sanwal, P.C., and Varshney, V.P.: Peripheral plasma testosterone levels in hypothyroid-induced male goats. Small Rumin. Res., 6:185–191, 1991.

Habel, R.E.: Ruminant digestive system. In: Sisson and Grossman's The Anatomy of the Domestic Animals. Vol. 1. R. Getty, ed. Philadelphia, W.B. Saunders Co., 1975.

Hago, B.E.D. and Abu-Samra, M.T.: A case of *Multiceps gaigeri* coenurosis in goat. Vet. Parasitol., 7:191–194, 1980.

Hammond, A.C.: Leucaena toxicosis and its control in ruminants. J. Anim. Sci., 73:1487–1492, 1995.

Hámori, D.: Constitutional Disorders and Hereditary Diseases in Domestic Animals. Developments in Animal and Veterinary Sciences 11. New York, Elsevier Scientific Publ. Co., 1983.

Hegarty, M.P., et al.: Mimosine in *Leucaena leucocephala* is metabolized to a goitrogen in ruminants. Aust. Vet. J., 52:490, 1976.

De las Heras, M., et al.: Bocio congenito en cabras asociado al consumo decoles. [Congenital goitre in goats fed cabbage.] Med. Vet., 1:41–44, 46–47, 1984. Abstract Number 3597 in Vet. Bull. 54:504, 1984.

Holstad, G.: *Corynebacterium pseudotuberculosis* infection in goats I. Evaluation of two serological diagnostic tests. Acta Vet. Scand., 27:575–583, 1986a.

Holstad, G.: *Corynebacterium pseudotuberculosis* infection in goats II. The prevalence of caseous lymphadenitis in 36 goat herds in northern Norway. Acta Vet. Scand., 27:584–597, 1986b.

Holstad, G.: *Corynebacterium pseudotuberculosis* infection in goats III. The influence of age. Acta Vet. Scand. 27:598–608, 1986c.

Holstad, G.: *Corynebacterium pseudotuberculosis* infection in goats V. Relationship between the infection and lesions resulting from vaccination against paratuberculosis. Acta Vet. Scand., 27:617–622, 1986d.

Holstad, G.: *Corynebacterium pseudotuberculosis* infection in goats IX. The effect of vaccination against natural infection. Acta Vet. Scand., 30:285–293, 1989.

Holstad, G., Teige, J. Jr., and Larsen, H.J.: *Corynebacterium pseudotuberculosis* infection in goats VIII. The effect of vaccination against experimental infection. Acta Vet. Scand., 30:275–283, 1989.

Horenstein, L. and Elias, E.: Ventral uterina (histerocoele) in the goat: a case report. Isr. J. Vet. Med., 43:86, 1987.

Jackson, P.: Skin diseases in goats. In Pract., 8:5–10, 1986.

Jernigan, A.D., et al.: Pharmacokinetics of rifampin in adult sheep. Am. J. Vet. Res., 52:1626–1629, 1991.

Kalkus, J.W.: A study of goiter and associated conditions in domestic animals. State College of Washington Agric. Expt. Stat. Bull., 156: July, 1920.

Kallfelz, F.A. and Erali, R.: Thyroid function tests in domesticated animals: Free thyroxine index. Am. J. Vet. Res., 34:1449–1451, 1973.

Kaneko, J.J.: Thyroid function. In: Clinical Biochemistry of Domestic Animals. J.J. Kaneko, J.M. Harvey and M.L. Bruss, ed. San Diego, CA, Academic Press, 1997.

Kategile, J.A., Mgongo, F.O.K., and Frederiksen, J.H.: The effect of iodine supplementation on the reproductive rates of goats and sheep. Nord. Vet. Med., 30:30–36, 1978.

King, N.B.: Clostridial diseases. In: Refresher Course for Veterinarians, Proceedings No. 73, Goats, The University of Sydney, The Post-Graduate Committee in Veterinary Science, Sydney, N.S.W., Australia, pp. 217–219, 1984.

Köhrle, J.: The deiodinase family: Selenoenzymes regulating thyroid hormone availability and action. Cell. Mol. Life Sci., 57:1853–1863, 2000.

Kok, K., et al.: Autosomal recessive inheritance of goiter in Dutch goats. J. Hered., 78:298–300, 1987.

Kulkarni, P.E. and Marudwar, S.S.: Unusual location of mammary glands in the vulval lips of she-goats. Vet. Rec., 90:385–386, 1972.

Kuria, J.K.N., et al.: Caseous lymphadenitis in goats: the pathogenesis, incubation period and serological response after experimental infection. Vet. Res. Commun., 25:89–97, 2001.

Lall, H.K.: A case of congenital goitre in kids. Indian Vet. J., 29:133–135, 1952.

Langenegger, C.H., Langenegger, J., and Costa, S.G.: Alèrgeno para o diagnèstico da linfadenite caseosa em caprinos. [An allergen for the diagnosis of caseous lymphadenitis in goats.] Pesq. Vet. Bras., 7(2):27–32, 1986.

Langenegger, J. and Langenegger, C.H.: Reprodução da linfadenite caseosa em caprinos com pequeno nùmèro de *Corynebacterium pseudotuberculosis*. [Reproduction of caseous lymphadenitis in goats by small numbers of *Corynebacterium pseudotuberculosis*.] Pesq. Vet. Bras., 8(1/2):23–26, 1988.

Lesbouyries and Drieux: Kystes galactogènes de la vulve chez une chèvre. Bull. Acad. Vét. France, 18:39–43, 1945.

Lindsay, H.J. and Lloyd, S.: Diagnosis of caseous lymphadenitis in goats. Vet. Rec., 128:86, 1991.

Lombard, C. and Raby, G.: Goitre congènital du chevreau dans la Vienne. Bull. Acad. Vét. France, 38:353–355, 1965.

Love, W.G.: Parenchymatous goiter in newborn goat kids. J. Am. Vet. Med. Assoc., 101:484–487, 1942.

Mburu, J.N., Kamau, J.M.Z., and Badamana, M.S.: Thyroid hormones and metabolic rate during induction of vitamin B_{12} deficiency in goats. N. Z. Vet. J., 42:187–189, 1994.

Mei, W. and Chang, Y.: Discovery, evidence, assay and elimination of hereditary goat goitre. VI International Conference on Goats, 2:753–754, 1996.

Menzies, P.I., Hwang, Y.T., and Prescott, J.F.: Comparison of an interferon to a phospholipase D enzyme-linked immunosorbent assay for diagnosis of *Corynebacterium pseudotuberculosis* infection in experimentally infected goats. Vet. Microbiol., 100:129–137, 2004.

Menzies, P.I., et al.: A field trial to evaluate a whole cell vaccine for the prevention of caseous lymphadenitis in sheep and goat flocks. Can. J. Vet. Res., 55:362–366, 1991.

Mgongo, F.O.K., Gombe, S., and Ogaa, J.S.: Thyroid status in cobalt and vitamin B_{12} deficiency in goats. Vet. Rec., 109:51–53, 1981.

Mills, A.E., Mitchell, R.D., and Lim, E.K.: *Corynebacterium pseudotuberculosis* is a cause of human necrotising granulomatous lymphadenitis. Pathology, 29:231–233, 1997.

Misk, N.A., Youssef, H.A., and Ali, M.A.: Ventral abdominal hernia at the level of the udder in a goat. Vet. Med. Rev., 2:200–202, 1986.

Mitchell, G., Hattingh, J., and Ganhao, M.F.: The composition of plasma and interstitial fluid of goats with swelling disease. J. S. Afr. Vet. Assoc., 54:181–183, 1983.

Mullowney, P.C. and Baldwin, E.W.: Skin diseases of goats. Vet. Clin. North Am. Large Anim. Pract., 6:143–154, 1984.

Nair, N.R. and Bandopadhyay, A.C.: Thyroglossal cyst in a goat. Indian Vet. J., 67:873 plus plate, 1990.

Navarre, C.B. and Pugh, D.G.: Diseases of the gastrointestinal system. In: Sheep and Goat Medicine D.G. Pugh, ed. Philadelphia, W.B. Saunders Co., 2002.

Niehaus, A.J. and Anderson, D.E.: Tooth root abscesses in llamas and alpacas: 123 cases (1994–2005). J. Am. Vet. Med. Assoc., 231:284–289, 2007.

Nooruddin, M., Dey, A.S., and Ali, M.A.: Coenuriasis in Bengal goats of Bangladesh. Small Rumin. Res., 19:77–81, 1996.

Nord, K., et al.: Control of caprine arthritis-encephalitis virus and *Corynebacterium pseudotuberculosis* infection in a Norwegian goat herd. Acta Vet. Scand., 39:109–117, 1998.

Olson., C., et al.: Goat lymphosarcoma from bovine leukemia virus. J. Nat. Cancer Inst., 67:671–675, 1981.

Ozmen, O. and Haligur, M.: Immunohistochemical observations on TSH secreting cells in pituitary glands of goat kids with congenital goitre. J. Vet. Med. Ser. A, 52:454–459, 2005.

Paliwal, O.P., and Sharma, A.N.: Congenital goitre in kids. Indian Vet. J., 56:154 and plate, 1979.

Paton, M.W., et al.: The effect of antibody to caseous lymphadenitis in ewes on the efficacy of vaccination in lambs. Aust. Vet. J., 68:143–146, 1991.

Patro, D.N., et al.: Incidence of generalised *Coenurus gaigeri* infection in a goat farm. Indian Vet. J., 74:68–69, 1997.

Peel, M.M., et al.: Human lymphadenitis due to *Corynebacterium pseudotuberculosis*; report of ten cases from Australia and review. Clin. Infect. Dis., 24:185–191, 1997.

Piontkowski, M.D. and Shivvers, D.W.: Evaluation of a commercially available vaccine against *Corynebacterium pseudotuberculosis* for use in sheep. J. Am. Vet. Med. Assoc., 212:1765–1768, 1998.

Prasad, J.: Effect of high nitrate diet on thyroid glands in goats. Indian J. Anim. Sci., 53:791–794, 1983.

Prasad, J.: A note on toxic effects of *Leucaena leucocephala* in goats: a clinical study. Indian J. Vet. Med., 9:151–152, 1989.

Pritchard, G.C.: 'Goitre' in goat kids. Vet. Rec., 121:430, 1987.

Quinn, P.J., et al.: Veterinary Microbiology and Microbial Disease. Oxford, Blackwell Science, 2002.

Radhakrishnan, C.; Balasubramanian, S., and Thilagar, S.: Repair of ventral metrocele (gravid) in a goat. Vet. Rec., 132:92, 1993.

Ragan, H.A., et al.: Application of miniature goats in ruminant research. Am. J. Vet. Res., 27:161–165, 1966.

Raina, A.K., and Pachauri, S.P.: Studies on the prevalence of goitre in goats in Tarai. Indian Vet. J., 61:684–688, 1984.

Rajkumar, S.S.: Incidence of goiter in goats. Indian Vet. J., 47:185–187, 1970.

Ramadan, R.O., and El Hassan, A.M.: Leiomyoma in the cervix and hyperplastic ectopic mammary tissue in a goat. Aust. Vet. J., 51:362, 1975.

Ramadan, R.O., Magzoub, M., and Adam, S.E.I.: Clincopathological effects in a Sudanese goat following massive natural infection with *Coenurus gaigeri* cysts. Trop. Anim. Health Prod., 5:196–199, 1973.

Reap, M., Cass, C., and Hightower, D.: Thyroxine and triiodothyronine levels in 10 species of animals. Southwest. Vet., 31:31–34, 1978.

Reineke, E.P. and Turner, C.W.: Growth response of thyroidectomized goats to artificially formed thyroprotein. J. Endocrinol., 29:667–673, 1941.

Reinemeyer, C.R., Bone, L.W., and Oliver, J.W.: Alteration in thyroid hormone and gastrin concentrations in goats infected with *Trichostrongylus colubriformis*. Small Rumin. Res., 5:285–292, 1991.

Retnasabapathy, A.: Isolation of *Pseudomonas pseudomallei* from an aborted goat fetus. Vet. Rec., 79:166, 1966.
Ribeiro, O.C., et al.: Avaliaçao de vacina contra linfadenite caseosa em caprinos mantidos em regime extensivo. [Evaluation of an inactivated vaccine against caseous lymphadenitis of goats kept under extensive management.] Pesq. Vet. Bras., 8(1/2):27–29, 1988.
Ricordeau, G.: Genetics: breeding plans. In: Goat Production. C. Gall, ed. New York, Academic Press, 1981.
Rijnberk, A.: Congenital defect in iodothyronine synthesis. Clinical aspects of iodine metabolism in goats with congenital goitre and hypothyroidism. Br. Vet. J., 133:495–503, 1977.
Rivolta, C.M. and Targovnik, H.M.: Molecular advances in thyroglobulin disorders. Clin. Chim. Acta, 374:8–24, 2006.
Robinson, W.F., and Ellis, T.M.: Caprine arthritis-encephalitis virus infection: from recognition to eradication. Aust. Vet. J., 63:237–241, 1986.
Roy, K.S., Saigal, R.P., and Nanda, B.S.: Gross histomorphological and histochemical changes in the thyroid gland of goat with age. I. Cross and biometric study. Anat. Anz., 137:479–485, 1975.
Roy, K.S., et al.: Gross, histomorphological and histochemical changes in the thyroid gland of goat with age. III. Occurrence of thymic tissue. Anat. Anz., 139:158–164, 1976.
Roy, S., Deo, M.G., and Ramalingaswami, V.: Pathologic features of Himalayan endemic goiter. Am. J. Pathol., 44:839–851, 1964.
Rozear, L., Love, N.E., and van Camp, S.L.: Radiographic diagnosis: pulmonary lymphosarcoma in a goat. Vet. Radiol. Ultrasound, 39:528–531, 1998.
Schreuder, B.E.C., ter Laak, E.A., and Griesen, H.W.: An outbreak of caseous lymphadenitis in dairy goats: first report of the disease in the Netherlands. Vet. Q., 8:61–67, 1986.
Seifi, H.A., et al.: Mandibular pyogranulomatous osteomyelitis in a Saanen goat. J. Vet. Med. A Physiol. Pathol. Clin. Med., 50:219–221, 2003.
Senturk, S. and Temizel, M.: Clinical efficacy of rifamycin SV combined with oxytetracycline in the treatment of caseous lymphadenitis in sheep. Vet. Rec., 159:216–217, 2006.
Sharma, H.N. and Tyagi, R.P.S.: Diagnosis and surgical treatment of coenurosis in goat (*Capra hircus*). Indian Vet. J., 52:482–488, 1975.
Sharma, K.B., and Ranka, A.K.: Foreign body syndrome in goats—report of five cases. Indian Vet. J., 55:413–414, 1978.
Shastri, U.V., Ghafoor, M.A., and Gaffar, M.A.: A note on a massive natural infection of *Coenurus gaigeri* cysts in a goat. Indian Vet. J., 62:615–616 and plate, 1985.
Singh, A.P.: Osteodystrophia fibrosa in a goat—a case report. Indian Vet. J., 72:191–192, 1995.
Singh, J.L., et al.: Prevalence of endemic goitre in goats in relation to iodine status of the soil, water and fodder. Indian Vet. J., 79:657–660, 2002.
Singh, J.L., et al.: Clinico-biochemical profile and therapeutic management of congenital goitre in kids. Indian J. Vet. Med., 23:83–87, 2003.
Singh, J.L., et al.: Immune status of goats in endemic goitre and its therapeutic management. Small Rumin. Res., 63:249–255, 2006.
Singh, V.P. and Murty, D.K.: An outbreak of *Dermatophilus congolensis* infection in goats. Indian Vet. J., 55:674–676, 1978.
Smith, M.C.: Neoplasms of the goat's reproductive tract. In: Current Therapy in Theriogenology 2. D.A. Morrow, ed. Philadelphia, W.B. Saunders Co., pp. 628–629, 1986.
Snyman, M.A. and Snyman, A.E.: The possible role of *Ostertagia circumcincta*, coccidiosis and dietary protein level in the development of swelling disease in Angora goat kids. J. S. Afr. Vet. Assoc., 76:63–68, 2005.
Sreekumaran, T. and Rajan, A.L.: Pathology of the skin in experimental hypothyroidism in goats. Kerala J. Vet. Sci., 8:227–234, 1977.
Sreekumaran, T. and Rajan, A.: Clinicopathological studies in experimental hypothyroidism in goats. Vet. Pathol., 15:549–555, 1978.
Sting, R., Steng, G., and Spengler, D.: Serological studies on *C. pseudotuberculosis* infections in goats using ELISA. J. Vet. Med. B., 45:209–216, 1998.
Sutmöller, P., Kraneveld, F.C., and van der Schaaf, A.: Melioidosis (pseudomalleus) in sheep, goats, and pigs on Aruba (Netherland Antilles). J. Am. Vet. Med. Assoc., 130:415–417, 1957.
Sweeney, R.W., et al.: Pharmacokinetics of rifampin in calves and adult sheep. J. Vet. Pharmacol. Ther., 11:413–416, 1988.
Tadjalli, M., Dehghani, S.N., and Ghadiri, M.: Sialography of the goat parotid, mandibular and sublingual salivary glands. Small Rumin. Res., 44:179–185, 2002.
Tanwar, R.K. and Saxena, A.K.: Radiographic detection of foreign bodies. Vet. Med., 79:1195–1197, 1984.
Tanwar, R.K., et al.: Subcutaneous emphysema in goats. Mod. Vet. Pract., 64:670, 1983.
Thomas, A.D. and Forbes-Faulkner, J.C.: Persistence of *Pseudomonas pseudomallei* in soil. Aust. Vet. J., 57:535–536, 1981.
Thomas, A.D., et al.: Clinical and pathological observations on goats experimentally infected with *Pseudomonas pseudomallei*. Aust. Vet. J., 65:43–46, 1988a.
Thomas, A.D., et al.: Evaluation of four serological tests for the diagnosis of caprine melioidosis. Aust. Vet. J., 65:261–264, 1988b.
Thompson, K.G.: Ventral oedema in exotic Angora goats. N.Z. Vet. J., 42:35–37, 1994.
Turner, A.S. and McIlwraith, C.W.: Techniques in Large Animal Surgery. 2nd Ed. Philadelphia, Lea and Febiger, 1989.
Van der Lugt, J.J., and Henton, M.M.: Melioidosis in a goat. J. S. Afr. Vet. Assoc., 66:71–73, 1995.
Van Jaarsveld, P., et al.: Congenital goitre in South African Boer goats. J. S. Afr. Vet. Med. Assoc., 42:295–303, 1971.
Van Tonder, E.M.: Notes on some disease problems in Angora goats in South Africa. Vet. Med. Rev., 1/2:109–138, 1975.
Van Voorthuizen, W.F., et al.: Euthyroidism via iodide supplementation in hereditary congenital goiter with thyroglobulin deficiency. Endocrinology, 103:2105–2111, 1978.
Verster, A.: A taxonomic revision of the genus *Taenia* Linnaeus, 1758 *s. str.* Onderstepoort J. Vet. Res., 36:3–58, 1969.
Washburn, K.E., et al.: Comparison of core needle biopsy and fine-needle aspiration of enlarged peripheral lymph nodes

for antemortem diagnosis of enzootic bovine lymphosarcoma in cattle. J. Am. Vet. Med. Assoc., 230:228–232, 2007.

Welch, H.: Goiter in farm animals. Univ. Montana Agric. Exper. Stat. Bull., 214, June 1928.

Wentzel, D., Viljoen, K.S., and Botha, L.J.J.: Seasonal variation in adrenal and thyroid function of Angora goats. Agroanimalia, 11:1–3, 1979.

Wiggs, R.B. and Lobprise, H.B.: Acute and chronic alveolitis/osteomyelitis ("lumpy jaw") in small exotic ruminants. J. Vet. Dent., 11:106–109, 1994.

Williams, C.S.F.: Differential diagnosis of caseous lymphadenitis in the goat. Vet. Med. Small Anim. Clin., 75:1165–1169, 1980. Reprinted in Dairy Goat J., 60:836–840, 1982.

Williamson, L.H.: Caseous lymphadenitis in small ruminants. Vet. Clin. North Am. Food Anim. Pract., 17:359–371, 2001.

Wilson, J.G.: Hypothyroidism in ruminants with special reference to foetal goitre. Vet. Rec., 97:161–164, 1975.

Yates, N.G., Hoffmann, D., and Seripto, S.: Mandibular osteodystrophy fibrosa in Indonesian goats fed leucaena. Trop. Anim. Health Prod., 19:121–126, 1987.

Zaki, M.M.: The application of a new technique for diagnosing *Corynebacterium ovis* infection. Res. Vet. Sci., 9:489–493, 1968.

4

Musculoskeletal System

Maintenance of musculoskeletal health is critical to the general well being of goats. Under extensive management systems, normal ambulation is essential for efficient and adequate food gathering and flight from predators. Agility and limb strength are especially important in hilly, rocky environments and during periods of food scarcity when goats will actually climb into trees to obtain feed. Successful breeding performance for male goats depends on sturdy, pain-free hind limbs for efficient mounting of does. For milking does, incorrect hind limb conformation and overgrown hooves can adversely affect udder health, and skeletal conformation is considered an important trait in linear appraisal systems for evaluating dairy goats.

This chapter presents clinically important background information relating to the musculoskeletal system, the differential diagnosis of musculoskeletal diseases on the basis of presenting sign, and detailed discussion of the primary diseases affecting the muscles, bones, and joints of goats. The reader is referred to Chapter 19 for additional background information on requirements and use of specific nutrients affecting bone and muscle health.

BACKGROUND INFORMATION OF CLINICAL IMPORTANCE

Anatomy and Physiology

A detailed review of the musculoskeletal anatomy of the goat is beyond the scope of this text and the information is available from other sources (Chatelain 1987; Constantinescu 2001; Popesko 2008). A representation of the caprine skeleton is given in Figure 4.1 and topographic muscular anatomy of the goat in Figure 4.2.

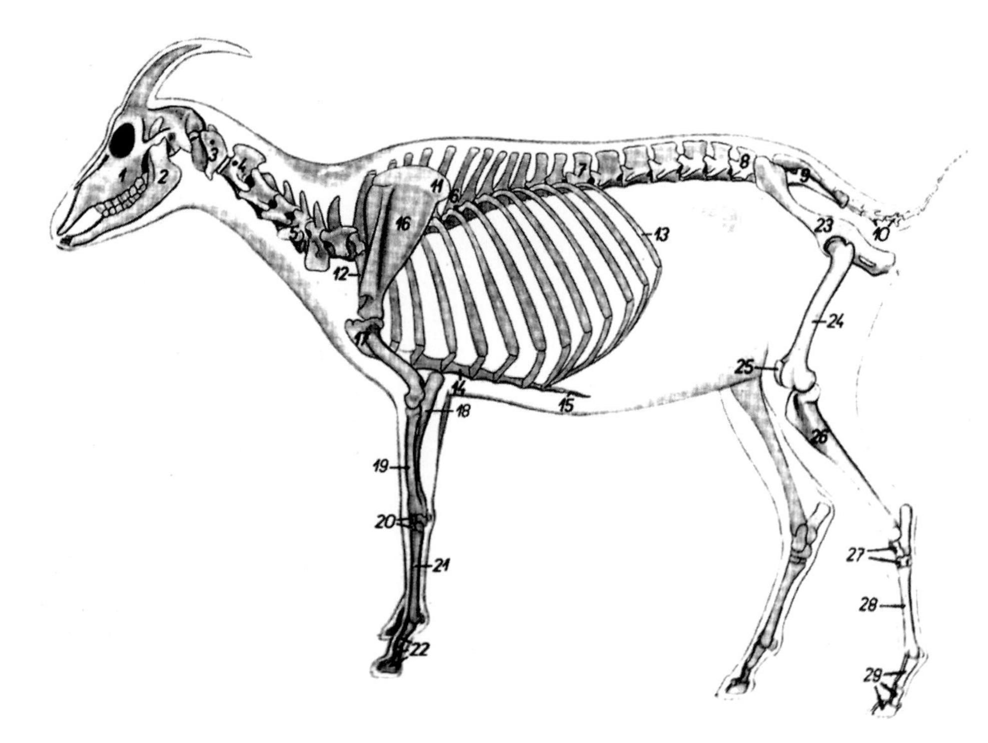

Figure 4.1. The caprine skeleton. 1. maxilla, 2. mandible, 3. atlas, 4. axis, 5. fifth cervical vertebra, 6. sixth thoracic vertebra, 7. thirteenth thoracic vertebra, 8. sixth lumbar vertebra, 9. sacrum, 10. coccygeal vertebrae, 11. cartilage of scapula, 12. first rib, 13. thirteenth rib, 14. body of sternum, 15. xiphoid cartilage, 16. scapula, 17. humerus, 18. ulna, 19. radius, 20. carpal bones, 21. third and fourth metacarpal bone, 22. bones of digits of thoracic appendage, 23. os coxae, 24. femur, 25. patella, 26. tibia, 27. tarsal bones, 28. third and fourth metatarsal bone, 29. bones of digits of pelvic appendage. (Reproduced with permission from Popesko P.: Atlas of Topographical Anatomy of Domestic Animals, new revised English edition, Vydavatelstvo Priroda, Bratislava, 2008, www.priroda.sk.)

Normal Skeletal Variations

Goats commonly have numerical variation in vertebrae. The normal vertebral formula is seven cervical, thirteen thoracic, six lumbar, five sacral, and seven to twelve coccygeal vertebrae. One survey of 185 goats revealed that 24% had numerical variation of vertebrae or the presence of structurally transitional vertebrae (Simoens et al. 1983). Common variations include twelve thoracic, five lumbar, and four or six sacral vertebrae. These variations are rarely, if ever, associated with clinical disease.

An extra sesamoid bone is infrequently found at the lateral head of the gastrocnemius muscle (Rajtova 1974). Floating ribs, with no connection to the costal arch, also occur infrequently (Hentschke 1980).

Bone Growth

There are several reports on epiphyseal closure times in growing goats (Dhingra and Tyagi 1970; Rajtova 1974; Ho 1975; Dhingra et al. 1978). The findings are widely disparate for numerous epiphyses; the reasons for these disparities are unclear. In the most recent study in Korean native goats, the distal humeral epiphysis fused at eight to twelve months; proximal radial epiphysis and distal tibial epiphysis fused at one year; and proximal and distal epiphyses of ulna and femur, proximal epiphyses of humerus and tibia, and distal epiphysis of radius fused at one year or later (Choi et al. 2006). Sexual dimorphism occurs in caprine bone growth. Males have longer and wider bones and later closure of epiphyses than females (Rajtova 1974).

The Parathyroid Glands

The parathyroid glands play an important role in the development and maintenance of normal bone through the action of parathyroid hormone on calcium and phosphorus metabolism (Hove 1981; Care and Hove 1982). Histologic evaluation of the glands can be a valuable aid in the diagnosis of metabolic bone disease. These glands may be difficult to locate in the goat because of small size and variable relationship to other tissues. There are usually two pairs, though accessory parathyroid tissue can occur.

The anterior pair are usually located deep in the anterior portion of the neck at the bifurcation of the

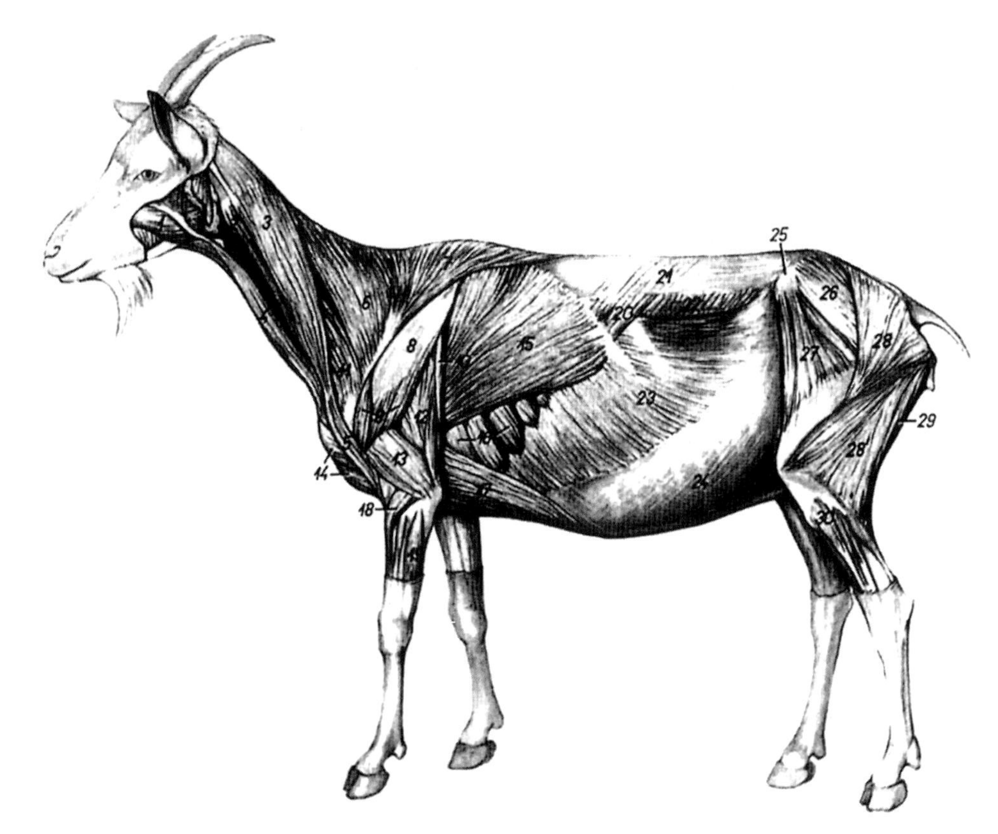

Figure 4.2. Topographic anatomy of the superficial caprine musculature. 1. masseter muscle, 2. brachiocephalic muscle, 3. cleido-occipital muscle, 4. sternomandibular muscle, 5. cleidobrachial muscle, 6. cervical part of trapezius muscle, 7. thoracic part of trapezius muscle, 8. aponeurosis of deltoid muscle, 9. deltoid muscle, 10. tensor fasciae antebrachii muscle, 11. omotransverse muscle, 12. long head of triceps brachii muscle, 13. lateral head of triceps brachii muscle, 14. superficial pectoral muscles, 15. latissimus dorsi muscle, 16. thoracic ventral serratus muscle, 17. deep pectoral muscle, 18. extensor carpi radialis muscle, 19. extensor carpi ulnaris muscle, 20. caudal dorsal serratus muscle, 21. thoracolumbar fascia, 22. internal oblique abdominal muscle, 23. external oblique abdominal muscle, 24. aponeurosis of oblique muscles of abdomen, 25. tuber coxae, 26. middle gluteal muscle, 27. tensor fasciae latae muscle, 28. gluteobiceps muscle (28–superficial gluteal muscle, 28′-biceps femoris muscle), 29. semitendinosus muscle, 30. peroneus longus muscle. (Reproduced with permission from Popesko P.: Atlas of Topographical Anatomy of Domestic Animals, new revised English edition, Vydavatelstvo Priroda, Bratislava, 2008, www.priroda.sk.)

common carotid artery. In the young goat, thymus is present at this site and the parathyroid gland may be recognized as a small reddish brown mass about 5 mm in diameter at the cranial pole of the thymus. Thymic tissue is atrophied in older goats, and the external parathyroid gland may be found caudal to the bifurcation of the common carotid artery. The posterior pair are usually located within the paired thyroid glands, most often in the middle portion on the medial aspect of the thyroid. The parathyroid tissue may be isolated in a distinct connective tissue capsule or mingled with thyroid tissue.

Conformation

There is increasing application of linear appraisal systems to generate sire summary information for the genetic improvement of dairy goats in breeding programs. The linear appraisal system is modeled after that used in dairy cattle and attempts to define a structural conformation consistent with functional durability as well as reproductive and productive efficiency. Type traits related to conformation that are included in linear appraisals are stature, rump angle, rump width, and rear legs (Wiggans and Hubbard 2001).

Skeletal conformation is also a significant component of dairy goat judging. Feet and legs are distinct structural categories subject to scoring. Recognized defects that reduce an animal's score include excessive spreading of the toes, shallow heels, turning out of the front feet or legs, rolled or turned-over claws, weak pasterns, winged-out shoulders or elbows, bowed or crooked forelimbs, straight stifles, rear limbs too close together (impinging on udder), turned-in hocks, and enlarged joints (Considine and Trimberger 1978). The selection and judging of meat goats also includes skeletal and conformational criteria (Martinez et al. 1991).

Clinical Pathology

The most commonly used clinical chemical parameters for assessment of bone in health and disease are serum alkaline phosphatase (AP), calcium, and inorganic phosphorus. Variations in these parameters associated with different metabolic and nutritional bone diseases of goats are summarized in Table 4.1. Serum vitamin D and magnesium levels are less frequently evaluated. For evidence of muscle damage, serum activities of creatine kinase (CK), aspartate aminotransferase (AST), and lactate dehydrogenase are most commonly measured. Reported values for these parameters in goats are given in Table 4.2. As discussed later, variation may occur with regard to age, breed, sex, and stage of production or pregnancy status.

Alkaline Phosphatase

In goats, as in other species, serum AP is higher in young animals compared with adults due to AP activity associated with the increased osteoblast function of growing bone (Castro et al. 1977; Sugano et al. 1980; Bogin et al. 1981). In healthy adults, most of the serum AP present is derived from liver, particularly bile duct epithelium. Tissue enzyme profiles in goats demonstrate that AP activity is fifty to one hundred times greater in kidney than in liver (Kramer and Carthew 1985). However, in renal disease, AP from tubular epithelium is released into the urine rather than the blood. There are now immunoassays available for measurement of bone-specific alkaline phosphatase that were developed for use in humans, validated in sheep, and successfully applied to goats (Liesgang et al. 2006).

There is considerable variation in serum AP activity between individual goats even within the same age group, resulting in a very wide range of reported normal values. In any individual healthy goat, however, serum AP levels usually remain constant (Kramer and Carthew 1985). More recently, measuring bone-specific alkaline phosphatase in Saanen does, it was shown that serum concentrations dropped progressively through pregnancy and reached their lowest point in the week following parturition. This reflects remodeling and calcium release from bone in response to skeletal demands of the fetus and early lactation (Liesegang et al. 2006, 2007). There is evidence that high and low AP enzyme levels in goats are heritable with the high level being genetically dominant (Lode 1970). Therefore, detection of a single high serum AP value in an individual goat may be difficult to interpret clinically. Increases in serum AP on serial samples within the same goat are a more reliable indication of bone or liver disease.

Calcium

The reported range of normal serum calcium in goats is fairly narrow. Nevertheless, within that range, significant differences have been noted with regard to age, breed, pregnancy status, and lactation status. Young goats tend to have higher serum calcium than mature goats (Bogin et al. 1981; Ridoux et al. 1981). In a French study, Saanen goats had higher mean serum calcium levels than Alpine goats (Ridoux et al. 1981). Mean serum calcium was significantly higher in black

Table 4.1. Clinical pathological changes associated with metabolic bone and muscle diseases in goats.

Disease	*Serum alkaline phosphatase*	*Serum calcium*	*Serum phosphorus*	*Other changes*
Rickets	Increased	Decreased	Decreased	Decreased serum vitamin D levels may also occur
Epiphysitis	Normal	Normal	Normal	Excessive calcium in ration likely
Fibrous osteodystrophy	Increased	Normal or decreased	Normal or increased	Excessive phosphorus in ration likely
Chronic fluorosis	Normal or increased	Normal or decreased	Normal or increased	Increased fluoride levels in bone
Enzootic calcinosis	Increased	Increased	Increased	Calcification of soft tissues
Hypervitaminosis D	Highly variable	Increased	Increased	Increased serum vitamin D_3 levels

Table 4.2. Some normal values for bone- and muscle-related enzymes and electrolytes in goat serum.

Parameter	*Unit*	*Goat description*	*Mean*	*± SD*	*Range*	*Reference*
Alkaline phosphatase	IU/l	F, pygmy, <1 year of age	87.7	29.2		Castro et al. 1977
	IU/l	F, pygmy, 1–2 years of age	79.5	34.6		Castro et al. 1977
	IU/l	F, pygmy, 2–3 years of age	28	14.2		Castro et al. 1977
	IU/l	F, pygmy, 4–6 years of age	15.1	11.2		Castro et al. 1977
	mU/ml	M, F, Israeli, 3–4 months of age	155	143		Bogin et al. 1981
	mU/ml	M, F, Israeli, 2–5 years of age	70	61		Bogin et al. 1981
	IU/l	M, F, Saanen × feral, all ages	960	1,666		Kramer and Carthew 1985
	IU/l	Adult goats from multiple farms	308	257.4		Stevens et al. 1994
Aspartate aminotransferase	U/l	General values			167–513	Kaneko et al. 1997
	IU/l	General values			43–142	Brooks et al. 1984
	IU/l	Adult goats from multiple farms	51.8	12.1		Stevens et al. 1994
Calcium	mEq/l	M, F, Pygmy, all ages	4.9	0.3		Castro et al. 1977a
	mg/l	Lactating Saanen, adult	100.8	8		Ridoux et al. 1981
	mg/l	Lactating Alpine, adult	94.6	7.2		Ridoux et al. 1981
	mg/dl	M, F, Israeli, 3–4 months of age	10.3	0.8		Bogin et al. 1981
	mg/dl	M, F, Israeli, 2–5 years of age	9.6	0.5		Bogin et al. 1981
	mEq/l	General values			4.5–5.8	Brooks et al. 1984
	mg/dl	Adult goats from multiple farms	9.7	0.7		Stevens et al. 1994
Creatine kinase	IU/l	F, Shiba, 2–6 months of age	28	39.1		Sugano et al. 1980
	IU/l	F, Shiba, 7–56 months of age	10.5	6.5		Sugano et al. 1980
	IU/l	F, Alpine, adult			14–62	Garnier et al. 1984
	IU/l	F, Saanen, adult	24	7		Boss and Wanner 1977
	IU/l	Saanen kids, 40–59 days old	48	22		Boss and Wanner 1977
	IU/l	Saanen kids, 240–259 days old	22	8		Boss and Wanner 1977
	IU/l	Adult goats from multiple farms	49.1	2		Stevens et al. 1994
Lactate dehydrogenase	IU/l	F, Pygmy, all ages	302.4	83.6		Castro et al. 1977
	IU/l	M, Pygmy, all ages	225.7	20.0		Castro et al. 1977
	mU/ml	M, F, Israeli, 3–4 months of age	238	35		Bogin et al. 1981
	mU/ml	M, F, Israeli, 2–5 years of age	190	34		Bogin et al. 1981
	IU/l	F, Alpine, adult			217–586	Garnier et al. 1984
	IU/l	Adult goats from multiple farms	176	50.6		Stevens et al. 1994
Magnesium	mEq/l	M, F, Pygmy, all ages	2.1	0.3		Castro et al. 1977a
	mg/dl	General values			2.8–3.6	Brooks et al. 1984
Phosphorus	mEq/l	M, F, Pygmy, all ages	4.8	0.9		Castro et al. 1977a
	mg/l	Lactating Saanen, adult	43.5	23.9		Ridoux et al. 1981
	mg/l	Lactating Alpine, adult	59.9	20.2		Ridoux et al. 1981
	mg/dl	M, F, Israeli, 3–4 months of age	9.3	0.5		Bogin et al. 1981
	mg/dl	M, F, Israeli, 2–5 years of age	7	1.4		Bogin et al. 1981
	mEq/l	General values			1.7–4.3	Brooks et al. 1984
	mg/dl	Adult goats from multiple farms	5.5	1.7		Stevens et al. 1994

M = male; F = female; SD = standard deviation

Bengal goats during pregnancy than during lactation. Levels were higher in early pregnancy than in late pregnancy but higher in late lactation than in early lactation (Uddin and Ahmed 1984).

Phosphorus

The range of inorganic phosphorus concentrations found in the serum of normal goats is often wider than calcium. Serum phosphorus levels are significantly higher in young animals than in mature animals (Boss and Wanner 1977; Bogin et al. 1981; Ridoux et al. 1981). The calcium-to-phosphorus ratio also is altered with age, reported as 1.1 in goats three to four months of age and 1.37 in goats two to five years of age (Bogin et al. 1981).

Breed differences have also been noted between Saanens and Alpines, with a lower mean serum phosphorus in the Saanen breed. Serum phosphorus concentration may be significantly higher during pregnancy than during lactation, but does not vary during different stages of pregnancy or lactation in contrast to calcium (Uddin and Ahmed 1984).

Magnesium

Serum magnesium levels have received less scrutiny in the goat than in other species. No variations of serum magnesium levels were noted as a function of age in goats three to four months of age compared with goats two to five years of age (Bogin et al. 1981). Similarly, no differences were noted in Saanen kids whose magnesium levels were measured every twenty days up to eight months of age. The mean serum magnesium ranged from 2.23 to 2.49 mg/dl (Boss and Wanner 1977).

Vitamin D

There is little published information on normal caprine serum or plasma levels of vitamin D and its metabolites in health or disease. Studies of vitamin D metabolism suggest that the conversion of vitamin D_3 to 25-(OH)D_3 is limited in goats compared with other farm animal species (Hines et al. 1986).

One comparative study of sheep, camels, and Sinai desert goats kept in direct sunlight in summer showed the goats to have lower mean plasma levels of 25-(OH)D_3 than either of the other species; 23.9 ± 5.7 ng/ml versus 40.7 ± 9.1 ng/ml for sheep and 443 ± 96 ng/ml for camels (Shany et al. 1978). Studies on the effects of pregnancy and lactation on bone metabolism in goats indicate that serum 1,25 dihydroxy Vitamin D levels peak in the first week of lactation under the influence of parathyroid hormone to stimulate active calcium transport in the intestine to help restore the serum calcium pool in the face of lactational demand (Liesegang et al. 2006). Serum vitamin D levels return to prepartum levels by one month post partum.

Creatine Kinase

Enzyme activity of creatine kinase (CK) in tissues other than cardiac and skeletal muscle is minimal in the goat, making CK the most reliable indicator of muscle damage (Kramer and Carthew 1985). Age differences have been observed in serum CK levels, with young, growing goats having higher concentrations than older goats (Sugano et al. 1980). Enzyme activity within muscle itself also decreases with age (Braun et al. 1987). No significant differences were observed in serum CK levels of adult female goats measured two weeks prepartum, three weeks post partum, and two months into lactation (Garnier et al. 1984).

The reported range of normal serum CK in goats is fairly narrow, yet the potential for elevation is enormous in the face of widespread muscle necrosis. Mild, nonpathologic increases in serum CK may be noted due to low level muscle damage after transport, fighting, poor venipuncture technique, or intramuscular injections, while in acute nutritional muscular dystrophy, serum CK levels may easily increase a hundredfold or more.

Aspartate Aminotransferase

Aspartate aminotransferase (AST) is found in muscle and is increased in the blood when myodystrophy occurs. It is less specific for muscle damage than CK, however, because it also occurs in high concentration in the livers of goats (Kramer and Carthew 1985). When evaluated alone, AST cannot be used to discriminate between muscle and liver disease.

Lactate Dehydrogenase

Serum lactate dehydrogenase (LDH) is a collection of LDH isoenzymes derived from a variety of tissues including liver and muscle. It is also present in high concentration in red blood cells, so hemolysis during handling of blood samples can artificially elevate serum LDH. It is not as reliable an indicator of muscle damage as is CK. Evaluation of isoenzymes of LDH would enhance the specificity for muscle, liver, and other tissue forms but this analysis is not routinely performed. The relative proportions of LDH isoenzymes in the serum of normal goats are LDH-1, 29% to 51%; LDH-2, 0% to 5%; LDH-3, 24% to 40%; LDH-4, 0% to 6%; and LDH-5, 14% to 36% (Brooks et al. 1984). Proportional increases in serum levels of LDH-3, LDH-4, and especially LDH-5 are indicative of skeletal muscle damage. An increase in LDH-5 was also noted in normal, healthy goat kids between birth and three weeks of age (Sobiech et al. 2005).

There is conflicting data on whether significant differences in serum LDH levels occur in relation to age (Castro et al. 1977; Bogin et al. 1981; Varshney et al. 1982). In adult females, the range of serum LDH levels may be higher during lactation than during pregnancy (Garnier et al. 1984). Females have significantly higher serum LDH levels than males (Castro et al. 1977). Normal serum LDH levels are generally lower in goats than in cattle or sheep. The LDH activity in muscle itself is significantly decreased in adult goats compared with kids (Braun et al. 1987).

Diagnostic Procedures

Imaging Techniques

Plain radiography can be extremely helpful in the diagnosis of skeletal disorders. The convenient size and relative cooperativeness of goats makes radiography a realistic option in caprine medicine. When necessary, goats can be sedated with xylazine or other sedatives to facilitate radiographic procedures. If sedated goats are made recumbent for radiographic procedures, care must be taken to avoid bloat and/or regurgitation. When possible, the animal should be fasted for twelve hours before sedation, the head placed lower than the body to facilitate drainage of ingesta out the mouth, and the left side should be dorsal to facilitate access to the rumen in case of bloat. Procedures for sedation are discussed in Chapter 17.

Reports of special radiographic procedures related to the caprine locomotor system are limited. Angiography of the caprine digit has been described (Burns and Cornell 1981). Bone scans using nuclear scintigraphy can help to identify localized areas of inflammation in the skeleton. Radiopharmaceuticals, however, are not approved for use in animals intended for the human food supply, so application may be limited to pet goats. The procedure has been done in goats using intravenous injection of 99m-technetium pyrophosphate followed by scanning three hours later with a rectilinear scanner (Milhaud et al. 1980). Good definition of ribs, joints, kidneys, and cervical vertebrae was achieved, while excessive accumulation of technetium in the urinary bladder interfered with visualization of the bony pelvis. Scintigraphy has been used in goats to quantitate the severity of joint inflammation in caprine arthritis encephalitis and has been found to correlate well with histopathological grading (Papageorges et al. 1991). Radiolabelled ^{99m}Tc-ciprofloxacin scintigraphy was also applied in the work-up of a case of acute hind limb paresis in a three-week-old goat that demonstrated suppurative vertebral osteomyelitis and diskospondylitis at necropsy (Alexander et al. 2005).

Electromyography

Normal electromyographic (EMG) responses of calves, sheep, and goats have been compared. Average action potentials of the superficial digital flexor muscle were 8.1 ms in the goat, 8.2 ms in the sheep, and 10.5 ms in the calf. The average peak potentials were 6.3 ms in the goat, 5.7 ms in the sheep, and 4.8 ms in the calf. Average amplitudes of the potentials were 322 uV in the goat, 253 uV in the sheep, and 337 uV in the calf. The proportion of biphasic and triphasic potentials was 93% in the goat, 92% in the sheep, and 85% in the calf (Mielke et al. 1981).

The EMG response can be used in the diagnosis of goats with myotonia congenita. Other applications of the EMG reported in goats include the diagnosis of ruminal adhesions to the abdominal wall (Cheong et al. 1987) and the identification of skeletal muscle denervation in swayback (Wouda et al. 1986).

Arthrocentesis and Synovial Fluid Analysis

Arthrocentesis and synovial fluid analysis can aid in the differential diagnosis of arthropathy. Strict asepsis should be observed during arthrocentesis. A 1.5-inch (3.8 cm) 18- or 20-gauge needle can be used to obtain fluid. Sedation facilitates the procedure.

The carpal joints are most often enlarged in goats with joint problems. The radiocarpal joint is distinct, while the midcarpal and carpometacarpal joints communicate. Access to these joints is improved when the carpus is flexed to a 90-degree angle. The extensor carpi radialis tendon running centrally over the anterior aspect of the carpus should be identified as a landmark. This may be complicated by the common occurrence of thick skin, callus, or hygroma on the carpi of goats. The radiocarpal joint is entered just lateral to the lateral edge of the extensor carpi radialis tendon, while the more distal midcarpal joint is entered medial to the medial edge of this tendon. The carpometacarpal joint is not accessible directly (Sack and Cottrell 1984).

The shoulder joint is approached laterally. The acromion and the notch in the proximal border of the greater tubercle of the humerus are used as landmarks. The needle is inserted into the joint distal to the midpoint between the two landmarks with the tip of the needle directed medial to the greater tubercle (Sack and Cottrell 1984).

The elbow joint is approached from the lateral aspect. The two landmarks are the lateral epicondylar crest of the humerus and the cranial border of the olecranon that together form an angle that points distally. The needle is inserted into the angle and directed mediodistally and slightly cranially into the olecranon fossa (Sack and Cottrell 1984). For aspiration of joint fluid from the stifle, the joint can be approached from the proximo-lateral side between the patella and the lateral patellar trochlea (Rørvik 1995). Approaches to other joints have not been described specifically in goats, but techniques described in cattle are generally suitable (Greenough et al. 1981).

Normal caprine synovial fluid should be clear and colorless to slightly yellow, free of particulate debris, and should not clot. Mean total protein has been reported as 1.84 ± 0.22 g/dl (Nayak and Bhowmik 1990). Total cell counts should be less than $500/mm^3$ (Crawford and Adams 1981). Monocytes and lymphocytes should predominate in normal synovial fluid and neutrophils should not exceed 10% of the total cell count. Abnormalities in synovial fluid reported in various caprine diseases are discussed throughout the chapter.

Muscle and Bone Biopsy

No special concerns have been identified for performance of muscle or bone biopsies in goats. The rib is commonly used for biopsy in the diagnosis of metabolic and nutritional bone disease. The costochondral junction is especially useful when rickets is suspected.

Regional Anesthesia

Intravenous regional anesthesia can be used successfully in goats to perform minor or major surgical operations on the distal forelimbs or hind limbs, including amputations (Babalola and Oke 1983). This procedure is described in Chapter 17.

Foot Trimming

Therapeutic and prophylactic foot trimming are important procedures in goats. Aggressive paring of the foot promotes healing in cases of foot rot, foot abscesses, and puncture wounds by allowing aeration and drainage of affected tissues. Corrective trimming also promotes normal comfort and conformation in cases of chronic laminitis.

Prophylactic trimming is required to maintain normal hoof structure and provide a strong base for support of the limbs. Overgrowth of the feet is particularly a problem in intensively managed goats, where normal wearing of the hoof associated with exercise is limited (Figure 4.3). Overgrown feet cause abnormal gait and undue stress on joints, tendons, and ligaments. Goats in confinement should have their feet trimmed a minimum of twice a year.

Pointed hoof shears or a hoof knife is appropriate equipment. Unlike sheep, goats resist being tipped on their rumps for foot trimming. The feet are simply lifted for trimming with the animal in a standing position. Large bucks and squirmy kids are often easier to trim if restrained in lateral recumbency by a knee placed on the neck. The basic steps of foot trimming are illustrated in Figure 4.4. They include removal of hoof wall that has overgrown the sole, shortening of the toe, and leveling of the sole and heel.

In the properly trimmed foot, the coronary band should be parallel to the weight bearing surfaces of the claws. Excessive shortening of the toe by trimming will cause the animal to "break forward" at the fetlock, while inadequate trimming of the toe causes the animal to rock backwards on the foot, reducing contact between the anterior sole and the ground, thus causing undue stretching of the flexor tendons.

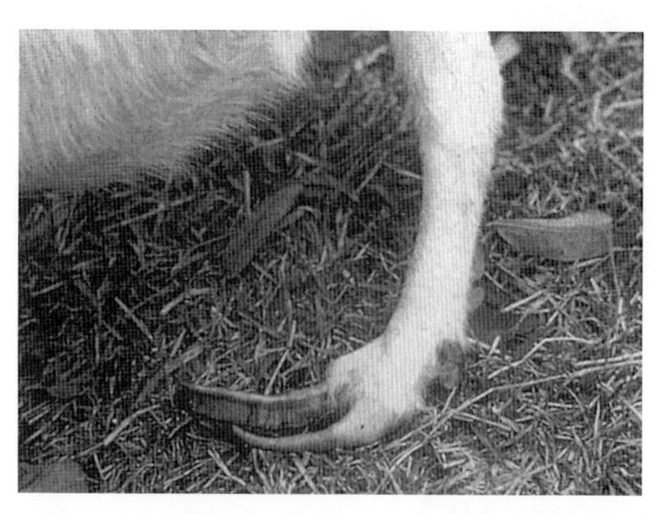

Figure 4.3. Severely neglected, overgrown foot of a goat. Such excessive growth is caused by continuous confinement and lack of exercise. (Reproduced by permission of Dr. C.S.F. Williams.)

DIAGNOSIS OF MUSCULOSKELETAL DISEASE BY PRESENTING SIGNS

This section is a guide to the differential diagnosis of musculoskeletal problems and attempts to include all possible diagnoses independent of geographic occurrence or relative incidence. Such information is included in subsequent discussions of the specific diseases later in the chapter or elsewhere in the text.

Abnormally Appearing or Sore Feet

Infectious causes of abnormally appearing or sore feet include foot scald, foot rot, foot abscess, foot and mouth disease, bluetongue, and dermatophilosis. In foot and mouth disease and bluetongue, which are most often subclinical in goats, oral lesions may be seen in conjunction with hoof lesions. Dermatophilosis, or mycotic dermatitis, can affect the feet and distal limbs as well as other areas of skin. This is also true of mange mite infestations, particularly chorioptic mange.

Metabolic and nutritional causes include zinc deficiency and laminitis. In zinc deficiency, hoof lesions are seen along with dermatitis. Acute and chronic forms of laminitis occur. In acute laminitis feet are predominantly sore and hot, while in chronic laminitis they are malformed and overgrown.

Chronic selenosis is the only reported toxic cause of abnormally appearing feet. Traumatic causes include overgrown hooves secondary to inadequate trimming, foreign bodies such as stones or wood chips lodged

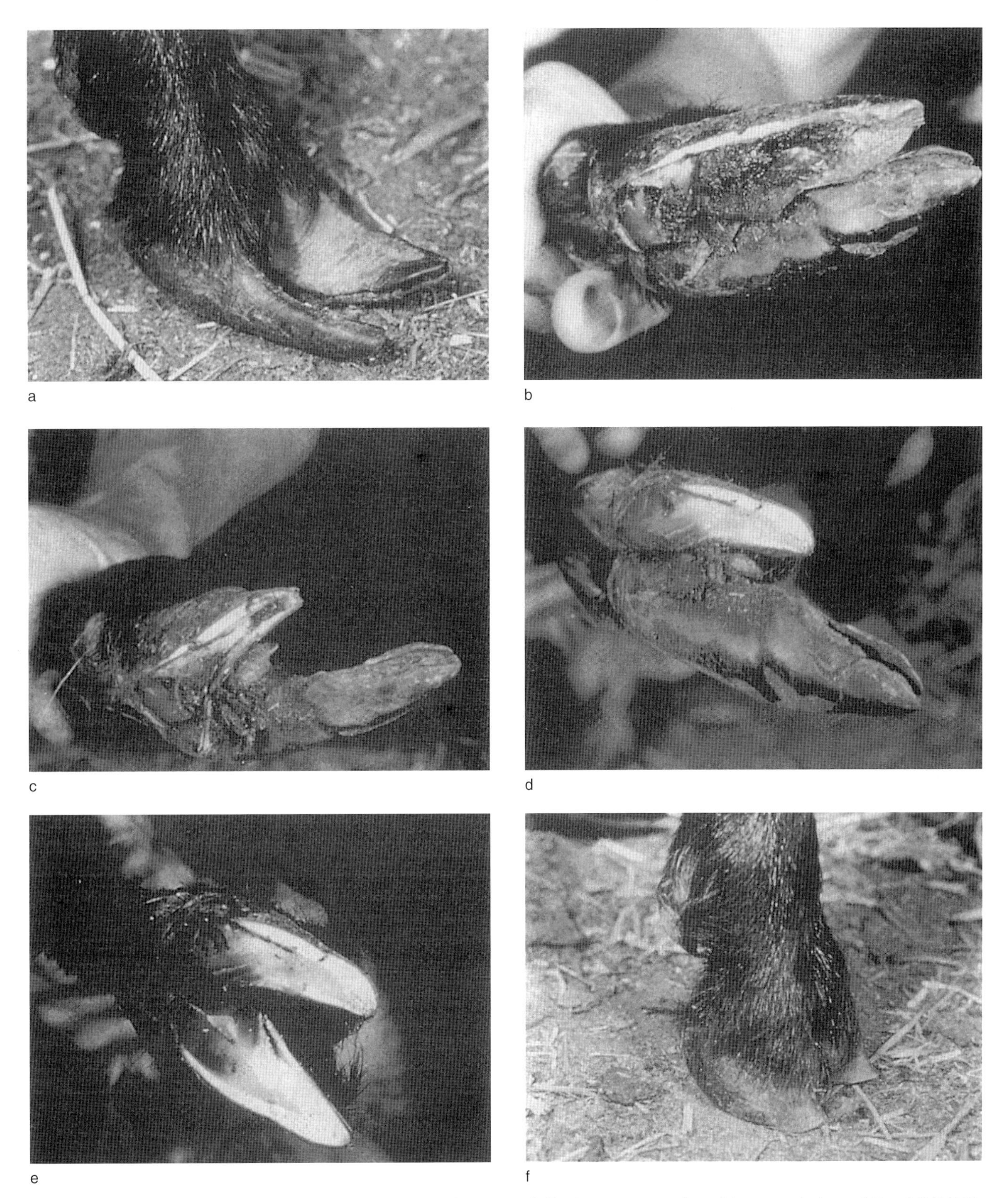

Figure 4.4. Procedure for proper foot trimming in the goat. (All pictures reproduced by permission of Dr. C.S.F. Williams.) a. Untrimmed goat foot prior to beginning. b. Overgrown wall covering sole is trimmed away, revealing debris packed between the wall and sole. c. Excessive toe growth is trimmed back. d. Sole is paired down to healthy fresh tissue. e. The same steps are repeated on the other claw of the foot. f. The completed, properly trimmed foot.

between the claws, bruising of the sole, and puncture wounds of the foot, especially those that lead to foot abscesses.

Swelling Around the Joints

Swollen joints usually imply arthritis. It is important to differentiate in the goat between true arthritides and periarticular or superficial swellings. Goats maintained in confinement, particularly on hard surfaces, develop a marked thickening of the skin, particularly over the carpi, hocks, and sternum, which can make the joint itself appear swollen. Goats are also prone to carpal hygromas. These are soft, fluctuant, periarticular swellings on the anterior aspect of the carpi. However, filling of the carpal bursa is also an early sign of arthritis caused by caprine arthritis encephalitis (CAE) virus infection and this must be differentiated from an uncomplicated hygroma.

Infectious causes of arthritis include the CAE virus, various *Mycoplasma* spp., and a variety of bacterial agents. Polyarthritis in neonates or young goats is usually bacterial or mycoplasmal in origin. Chlamydial arthritis is a well known cause of arthritis in sheep, but documentation of chlamydial arthritis in goats is lacking (Nietfeld 2001) despite the fact that it is sometimes cited as a cause of arthritis in the species. Similarly, erysipelothritic polyarthritis caused by *Erysipelothrix rhusiopathiae* is a well known endemic problem in young lambs, but its suggested occurrence in goats is poorly documented.

Nutritional and metabolic causes of swollen joints include rickets and so-called nutritional arthritis or osteopetrosis. Rickets is actually an enlargement or distortion of the improperly calcified epiphyses adjacent to a seemingly swollen joint. Nutritional arthritis, secondary to excessive calcium feeding, is reported primarily in bucks of dairy breeds.

Traumatic injury to the joints is common in goats because of their propensity to fight and to climb and explore. Swellings may occur secondary to avulsions of tendons and ligaments, dislocations, and hemarthrosis. Does in advanced pregnancy sometimes develop edematous swellings around and above the coronary bands, particularly on the hind limbs. This is presumably because of circulatory compromise and usually resolves with parturition. However, it may also be associated with pregnancy toxemia, as discussed in Chapter 19.

Degenerative osteoarthritis may be seen, especially in very old goats, or in goats with poor conformational characteristics, such as excessive straight-leggedness in the hind limb.

Stiff, Painful, or Abnormal Gait

Abnormalities of gait can be caused by neurologic dysfunction or musculoskeletal diseases. The differential diagnoses for neurologic causes of gait abnormality are given in Chapter 5. While most neurologic diseases cause some degree of paresis or ataxia, tetanus is noteworthy in producing a stilted, stiff gait, which suggests musculoskeletal pain. This is also true in the case of spastic paresis, a neurogenic disease that causes intermittent stiffening of the hind limbs. Similarly, peritonitis, pleuritis, or mastitis may cause sufficient pain on motion that affected animals show a guarded, stilted gait.

Regarding primary musculoskeletal diseases, any of the causes of painful feet or swollen joints identified above can contribute to development of a stiff, abnormal, or painful gait. Additional causes of muscle origin include nutritional muscular dystrophy in its early or mild stages, parasitic myositis involving tapeworm cysts of the muscle, and myotonia congenita, in which a stiff gait is intermittent and may be preceded by a generalized muscular contraction, causing the goat to fall down as seen in so-called "fainting goats." Enzootic calcinosis caused by ingestion of *Trisetum flavescens* or yellow oat grass can cause calcification of tendons and ligaments with a resulting painful gait.

Additional causes of skeletal origin include fibrous osteodystrophy associated with excessive phosphorus in the diet, and chronic fluorosis leading to abnormal bone growth and apparent bone pain. Copper deficiency in kids causes a primarily neurologic disease known as swayback or enzootic ataxia. However, affected kids may also have bone pain associated with abnormal osteogenesis and subsequent bone fragility.

Failure to Extend a Limb or Limbs

The differential diagnosis for failure to extend a limb or limbs varies markedly with the age of the affected animal. In newborn goats, arthrogryposis or persistent flexure of joints may be caused by congenital Akabane disease, inherited beta-mannosidosis in goats of the Nubian breed, possible congenital lupinosis, or contracted tendons associated with positional constraints *in utero* during fetal growth. An inherited tendon shortening also occurs in Australian Angora goats. In older kids, enzootic ataxia sometimes is accompanied by flexor contracture of the forelimbs.

In mature animals, ankylosis of joints in a flexed position is a common outcome of chronic CAE virus arthritis. The carpi are most often affected. However, any traumatic or infectious cause of arthritis may result in a reduced range of motion when chronic in nature. Dislocations or luxations may also cause pain on extension of joints, with animals favoring a flexed position.

When goats are recumbent from any cause, tendon contracture occurs rapidly. Initiation of regular physical therapy to manually straighten the front limbs is advisable if goats are expected to be recumbent more than twenty-four hours.

Non-weightbearing on a Single Limb

This refers to animals that are able to extend the affected limb, but are unwilling to bear weight on it. Differential diagnoses include fractures, dislocations, severe arthritis involving a single joint, puncture wounds of the foot, severe foot rot, foot scald, or foot abscesses. Fractures may be primarily traumatic in origin or may be predisposed by increased bone fragility such as occurs in rickets, fibrous osteodystrophy, copper deficiency, and chronic fluorosis. Osteomyelitis may also predispose to fracture or cause sufficient pain to result in non-weightbearing.

Bowed Limbs

Bowing of the forelimbs is seen primarily in metabolic bone diseases. Known causes include epiphysitis, rickets, and a condition known as bowie, or bentleg, associated with phosphorus deficiency. Bowing of the hind limbs may occur in zinc-deficient goats. Poor conformation in individual goats with weak attachments of the shoulder assembly may lead to winged out elbows and the appearance of bowed limbs.

Conditions Restricted to a Forelimb

Luxation of the scapulohumeral joint may be common in goats. One veterinary referral center reported on five cases seen over a twenty-six-month period. The affected limb is carried in a semiflexed position and abducted and rotated outward, with apparent pain on attempts at extension. The condition is successfully managed by surgical intervention to stabilize the joint (Purohit et al. 1985).

Carpal hygromas are common in goats maintained on rough, hard flooring. They must be differentiated from other causes of carpal swelling as discussed above in the section on swollen joints.

Conditions Restricted to a Hind Limb

Lateral luxation of the patella occurs in goats and is believed to be congenital, associated with hypoplasia of the lateral trochlear ridge. Progressive lameness occurs and the laterally displaced patella is palpable along with crepitus. Affected goats keep the stifle and hock flexed, because extension of the limb is difficult and painful when the patella is displaced. Successful surgical correction may be accomplished via trochlear sulcoplasty and desmotomy (Baron 1987).

Rupture of the gastrocnemius muscle belly above the tendon can occur in goats as in cattle, producing a palpable swelling on the caudal aspect of the hind limb above the hock and a characteristic hind limb position where the hock remains on the ground while the animal is standing (Figure 4.5). A similar stance was reported in a goat with a ruptured calcaneal tendon secondary to dog bite (Hunt et al. 1991). This case was successfully treated by tranposition of the tendon of the peroneus longus muscle.

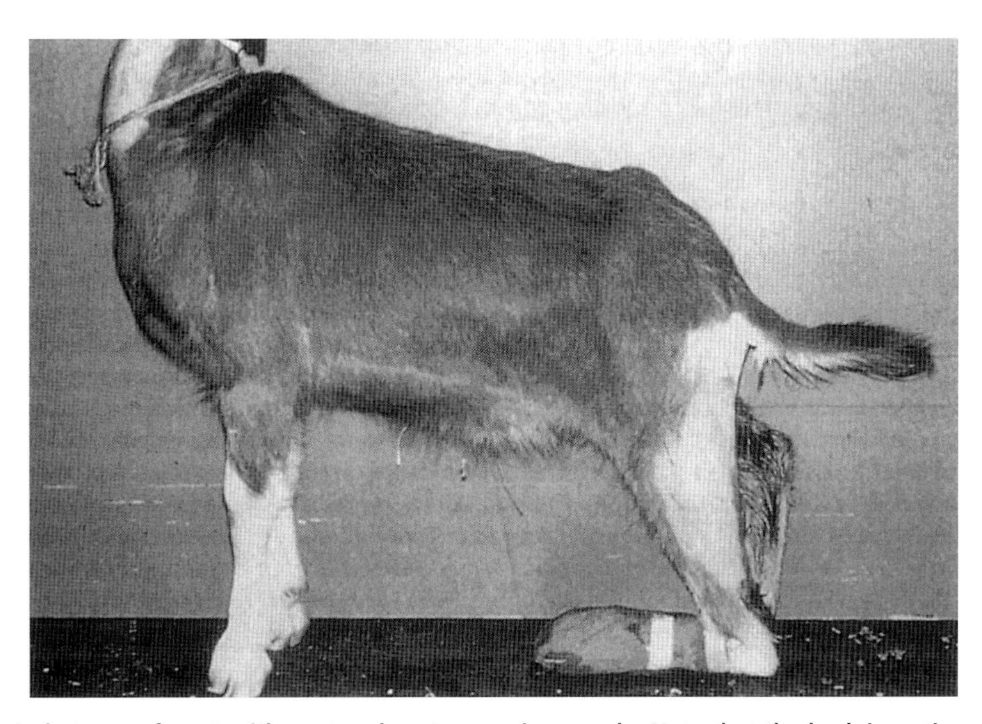

Figure 4.5. Typical stance of goat with ruptured gastrocnemius muscle. Note that the hock is resting on the ground while the animal is standing. (Courtesy of Educational Media, Cummings School of Veterinary Medicine at Tufts University, Mr. David Wilman, photographer.)

Spastic paresis, a progressive neurological disorder, manifests as intermittent episodes of muscular rigidity in the gastrocnemius muscle and hyperextension of one or both hind limbs. Affected goats may actually lift their hind ends off the ground during active episodes and walk only on the forelimbs if both hind limbs are affected simultaneously. The condition occurs in several breeds of cattle and is generally considered to be a genetic disorder with a complex manner of inheritance (Scarratt 2004). The condition is uncommon in goats and it is unclear if it also represents a genetic disorder in this species. In cattle, surgical treatments include tibial neurectomy or gastrocnemius tenotomy but there are no reports of treatment in goats.

Weakness and Recumbency

This clinical presentation encompasses a broad range of differential diagnoses, as weakness and recumbency can occur in a variety of neurologic and systemic diseases. Only primary muscle and skeletal problems are listed here.

Muscular diseases associated with weakness and recumbency include clostridial myositis, nutritional muscular dystrophy, ingestion of myodegenerative plants such as *Cassia roemeriana* or *Karwinskia humboldtiana,* and milk fever or hypocalcemia, a metabolic disease discussed in Chapter 19. Myotonia congenita can cause affected goats to be recumbent, but the effect lasts only approximately one minute.

Myasthenia gravis, a cause of profound muscle weakness in humans and dogs, has been reported in one veterinary text as occurring in the goat, but no primary reference is cited (Fraser 1986). A published review of this disease does not identify myasthenia gravis as a naturally occurring disease in goats (Lindstrom 1979) and a search of the literature as recently as 2007 produced no case reports in goats. However, myasthenia gravis has been produced experimentally using goats as an animal model by the induction of auto-antibodies to acetylcholine receptors. These antibodies block neuromuscular transmission (Lindstrom 1976).

Arthritis can be sufficiently painful to inhibit ambulation. Acute mycoplasma arthritis is especially associated with recumbency in goats. Severe hoof diseases, such as foot rot, chronic selenosis, and laminitis, can also keep goats recumbent.

Bone abnormalities can produce recumbency either through bone pain or secondary fracture. Metabolic bone diseases associated with recumbency include rickets and fibrous osteodystrophy. Traumatic fractures, especially those of the vertebral canal, must also be considered in goats unwilling to rise. Osteomyelitis can also predispose to fracture and recumbency, especially if involving the vertebrae.

SPECIFIC DISEASES OF THE MUSCULOSKELETAL SYSTEM

VIRAL DISEASES

Caprine Arthritis Encephalitis

First recognized in the early 1970s, caprine arthritis encephalitis (CAE) has emerged as a significant and costly disease of goats. Goats exposed to the causative lentivirus may remain subclinically infected or develop one or more of several clinical syndromes, which include arthritis, progressive paresis or other neurologic dysfunction, an induration of the udder with hypogalactia, chronic interstitial pneumonia, or progressive weight loss. Arthritis is the most common clinical presentation and is discussed here.

Etiology

The CAE virus is an enveloped, single-stranded RNA virus in the lentivirus genus of the family Retroviridae. Other lentiviruses, or slow viruses, include the maedi-visna (MV) virus of sheep, also known as the ovine progressive pneumonia or OPP virus, the equine infectious anemia virus, the bovine immunodeficiency virus, the feline immunodeficiency virus, the simian immunodeficiency virus, and types 1 and 2 of the human immunodeficiency virus (HIV) associated with acquired immunodeficiency syndrome (AIDS). Historically, CAE and MV viruses were considered to be similar but distinct viruses with strong host species predilection for goats and sheep respectively. However, recent phylogenetic studies indicate that these distinctions do not hold strongly, that genetic recombination occurs, and that there is evidence for cross species transmission. The two viruses are now classified together in the small ruminant lentivirus (SRLV) serogroup. The phylogenetic basis for this revision and its diagnostic and epidemiologic significance are discussed in more detail in the CAE-MV section of Chapter 5.

These are cell-associated viruses characterized by the presence of a magnesium-dependent, RNA-dependent DNA polymerase, or reverse transcriptase, which permits the production of proviral DNA from the viral RNA genome using the host cell machinery (Cheevers and McGuire 1988). Typical of lentiviruses in general, CAE virus infection is considered to be lifelong, and serum antibodies to the virus, if not of colostral origin, are considered synonymous with infection.

The CAE viral genome consists of three essential retroviral genes—*gag*, *pol*, and *env*—as well as the regulatory/accessory genes—*tat*, *rev*, and *vif*. The genome produces five structural proteins and four nonstructural proteins. The *env* gene encodes for the envelope glycoprotein gp135 or surface (SU) protein and the transmembrane protein. Antigenic variation in the

SU protein occurs as a result of *env* mutation and is responsible for the biological and serological variation of CAE virus isolates (Concha-Bermejillo 2003). The *pol* gene encodes for the viral enzymes reverse transcriptase, protease, endonuclease/integrase, and dUTPase involved in transcription and protein synthesis during viral replication. The molecular biology of CAE virus and other animal lentiviruses has been reviewed (Clements and Zink 1996).

The CAE virus can be identified from live animals *in vitro* by co-cultivation of concentrated leukocyte preparations derived from blood, milk, or synovial fluid with goat synovial membrane in cell culture. At necropsy, suspect tissues from joint, lung, or udder can be cultivated directly in tissue culture flasks and examined for cytopathic effect (CPE), which is manifested as development of refractile stellate cells and syncytia formation. When CPE is seen, presence of virus should be confirmed by immunolabelling or electron microscopy (OIE 2004). CAE virus is susceptible to heat, detergents, and formaldehyde.

Epidemiology

The neurologic form of CAE was the first to be described in the United States, in 1974 (Cork et al. 1974). The causative virus was first isolated from a case of arthritis in 1980 and the relationship of the two forms of the disease was recognized at that time (Crawford et al. 1980). The initial name of the disease, viral leukoencephalomyelitis of goats, was gradually replaced by the currently applied name, caprine arthritis encephalitis.

A global serologic survey reported in 1984 provided much initial information about the distribution of CAE virus in goats (Adams et al. 1984). The highest prevalence occurs in countries with long established, intensive goat dairying industries, namely Canada, France, Norway, Switzerland, and the United States. The seroprevalence exceeded 65% in all of these countries. In countries actively importing dairy goats, such as Kenya, Mexico, New Zealand, and Peru, the overall prevalence of CAE infection was often less than 10%. However, it was highest in imported dairy goats, next highest in local goats in contact with imported goats, and least prevalent or nonexistent in goats not having contact with imported goats. Indigenous African goat breeds tested in Somalia, Sudan, and South Africa were free of infection. The same pattern of prevalence in imported, contact, and indigenous goats was reported from Jamaica (Grant et al. 1988) and from Algeria (Achour et al. 1994).

In twenty-four states of the United States, 81% of 1,160 goats tested were positive for CAE virus infection (Crawford and Adams 1981) while a subsequent, larger survey in twenty-eight states reported only 31% of individual goats positive but 73% of herds positive (Cutlip et al. 1992). In Great Britain, 10.3% of herds tested and 4.3% of all goats tested were positive (Dawson and Wilesmith 1985). In New South Wales, Australia, 82% of 115 herds were infected. Among the five different dairy breeds tested, the prevalence varied from 26.8% to 43.4%, while the prevalence in Angora goats was only 4.8% (Grewal et al. 1986). In South Australia, prevalence in dairy goats tested over three years ranged from 18% to 45%, while the combined prevalence in Angora, Cashmere, crossbred, and feral goats was 0.1% (Surman et al. 1987). In most cases, Angora goats with serologic or clinical evidence of CAE infection have a history of contact with infected dairy goats. A New Zealand survey indicated a prevalence of 1.5%, with a distribution pattern associated with goats imported from Australia (MacDiarmid 1983).

Additional information continues to become available on the prevalence of CAE in different countries and regions. There are multiple reports from Europe. In Norway, fifty-one dairy goat herds distributed throughout the country were tested and 42% of animals and 86% of herds were positive (Nord et al. 1998). In Sweden, approximately 90% of the dairy goat herds, comprised mostly of the endangered native Swedish Landrace breed, were found to be infected with CAE (Lindqvist 1999). In Spain, where the disease was suspected but not yet confirmed, a survey of twenty-two dairy herds identified 77.3% of the herds and 12.1% of the individual goats tested as positive (Contreras et al. 1998). In Hungary, where 30% of goats tested were positive, the prevalence of infection was associated with purchase of breeding stock from farms that had imported purebred milking goats and an association was also made with large herd size (Kukovics et al. 2003). In a study from South Tyrol in Italy, 38% of herds and 23.6% of goats tested were positive, with goats older than twenty-six months having a significantly higher prevalence than younger goats. Goats born indoors had a significantly higher prevalence than those born outside, and dairy goats in commercial herds had a higher prevalence than dwarf goats kept as pets (Gufler et al. 2007).

In Latin America, Brazil has conducted numerous serosurveys of various size and design in different states and regions of the country. CAE is present in Brazil and, as in other places, is more common in imported or crossbred dairy goats than indigenous non-dairy breeds. One survey of dairy goat herds in Rio Grande Norte state revealed 57% of the herds with at least one positive goat (Souza e Silva et al. 2004). In Yucatan state of Mexico, seroprevalence was very low but all the animals identified as positive were exotic breed dairy goats which had been imported into the Yucatan (Torres-Acosta 2003).

From the Middle East, a Jordanian survey found that 23.2% of herds and 8.9% of goats sampled were positive for CAE (Al-Qudah et al. 2006). In Asia, Japan was presumed to be free of CAE, but a serosurvey reported in 2006 indicated a seroprevalence of 21.9% in goats from around the country as well as clinical disease in native Japanese Shiba goats, including arthritis, mastitis, and pneumonia (Konishi et al. 2006). More recent reports from Africa are limited. South Africa is reported to be "relatively free" of CAE and maintains strict import regulations to minimize risk while Kenya is reported to have eradicated the disease (Werling and Langhans 2004).

CAE virus can be transmitted vertically and horizontally. The main route of vertical transmission is from dam to kid via ingestion of virus-contaminated colostrum and milk. The main route of horizontal transmission is by direct or close contact with infected animals. Sexual transmission, though possible, plays a limited role in the spread of CAE. Risk factors associated with the transmission of CAE have been reviewed (Rowe and East, 1997; Blacklaws et al. 2004). The strong association of CAE virus infection with intensively managed dairy goats is due largely to management practices that facilitate transmission of the virus from does to kids in the perinatal period as well as horizontally between adults (East et al. 1987, 1993; Greenwood et al. 1995).

In the perinatal period, the major mode of transmission of CAE virus to kids is by direct suckling of their own infected dam or by consuming pooled milk or colostrum from other infected does. Virus may be present in colostrum and milk as free virus or incorporated into somatic cells. Even subclinically infected does can shed virus into colostrum and milk. Because common methods of identifying infected goats, such as the agar gel immunodiffusion (AGID) test, can produce false-negative test results, all colostrum and milk derived from does in known-infected herds is potentially suspect as a source of virus unless heat-treated or pasteurized, as discussed later.

Additional potential sources for infection of kids in the perinatal period include *in utero* infection, exposure to virus in birth fluids during kidding, licking of the kid by the doe after birth, or possibly aerosol transmission between a coughing doe and her kid. Experimental evidence for the presence of CAE virus *in utero* or in saliva, birth fluids, or aerosols is limited compared to what is known about the virus in milk and colostrum. However, epidemiological observations with CAE in goats as well as experimental evidence of the transmission of the maedi-visna virus from ewes to lambs suggest that these routes of transmission are possible and that CAE control programs should take them into account in order to succeed (Rowe and East 1997; Blacklaws et al. 2004).

To date, there are still no definitively documented cases of *in utero* infection of kids with CAE, although there are several indications that this is a possible route of infection. Some cesarean-derived or vaginally delivered kids raised in isolation have seroconverted in the first few months of life (Adams et al. 1983; East et al. 1993). There is also a report of uterine lesions in a goat with the arthritic and pneumonic forms of CAE infection (Ali et al. 1987). More recently, using PCR techniques, CAE virus-infected cells were detected in the uterus and oviducts of CAE virus-infected goats (Fieni 2003).

It is now evident that horizontal transmission also plays a significant role in the spread of CAE. An early indication of this related to international trade in livestock when it was observed that local goats became infected, seroconverted, or even manifested clinical disease when imported, infected purebred dairy goats were placed in their midst in countries not previously recording the disease. Another strong indication of horizontal spread is the common finding in many studies that seroprevalence increases with age in infected herds. Some seroconversion in goats less than one year of age may result from neonatal infections with delayed humoral response. However, it is highly unlikely that the majority of adult seroconversions are due to this, as in naturally and experimentally infected kids, an antibody response is usually detectable between three and ten weeks following exposure, though delays of up to eight months and possibly longer for seroconversion have been reported (Rimstad 1993).

Additional evidence has come from studies examining the spread of infection in known infected herds, which indicates that direct contact was involved in horizontal transmission. A California study examined the prevalence of seropositive goats in herds attempting to reduce CAE infection by feeding heat-treated colostrum and milk to kids. It was demonstrated that seroconversion still occurred in some of these kids later in life, particularly when CAE-positive adults were maintained in the herd (East et al. 1987). However, when seropositive animals in a herd were physically segregated from seronegative animals that had been raised on heat-treated colostrum and pasteurized milk, rates of seroconversion were three-fold lower than when seropositive animals remained commingled with seronegative animals (Rowe et al. 1992).

There are a number of possible ways that horizontal transmission can occur when infected and noninfected dairy goats are commingled. One important route is via milk in association with milking practices. Experimental intramammary transmission of virus has been reported (East et al. 1993; Lerondelle et al. 1995). In one study, direct contact for more than twelve months between uninfected and infected goats was necessary before horizontal transmission could be demonstrated under non-dairy conditions. However, when uninfected does were milked with infected does, 60% became infected in less than ten months (Adams et al. 1983). Rowe and East (1997) suggest a variety of mechanisms by which horizontal transmission might be effected via milk, including shared milking machines, the impact of backflowing milk against the teat end during machine milking, milk-contaminated hands or towels, aerosolization of milk during milking with subsequent inhalation or contamination of equipment, and spilled or open containers of milk licked or consumed by goats.

In addition to milk, the lungs of infected goats may be a source of aerosolized virus because the lungs are a target organ of CAE infection. Coughing may release virus into the air to be inhaled by nearby animals in confinement housing. Other lung infections may further exacerbate this risk because bacterial or other viral pneumonias stimulate an inflammatory response that may bring additional CAE virus-laden macrophages to the lungs and increase the frequency of coughing of inflammatory debris. There is good, indirect evidence that aerosol spread of CAE infection is important. In a French study, kids raised on treated colostrum and raw colostrum were maintained in varying degrees of separation and their rates of seroconversion monitored over time. With no separation at all, 34.7% of the kids receiving treated colostrum became seropositive. When separation by a hurdle was imposed, 28.4% seroconverted. When a wall separated them in the same building, 24.1% seroconverted, and when kept in totally separate buildings, only 16.4% seroconverted (Péretz et al. 1994).

Sexual transmission is a possible but unlikely factor in the spread of CAE infection. There are no reports of infection of does by infected bucks through mating or use of artificial insemination, although in one study, does were monitored for seroconversion for eighteen months following mating with or artificial insemination from infected bucks (Adams et al. 1983). There is a report, though, of CAE virus in the seminal fluid and non-spermatic cells of two of six bucks experimentally infected with the virus (Travassos et al. 1998). Virus-infected cells have also been identified in preputial swabs of several bucks and semen from the epididymis of an infected buck (Rowe and East 1997). In sheep, maedi-visna virus was not isolated from semen of experimentally infected rams until they were also superinfected with *Brucella ovis* and developed epididymitis with leukocytospermia (Concha-Bermejillo et al. 1996).

In a similar study, maedi-visna virus was found in epididymal tissues in rams coinfected with *B. ovis* and the virus (Preziuso et al. 2003). While the use of only noninfected bucks in breeding programs would be ideal, these observations and findings suggest that CAE virus-infected bucks may be used safely for breeding if some precautions are observed. Infected bucks should not commingle with does, but rather should be hand mated to does to limit their contact time. They also should be free of any concurrent disease of the genital tract that would possibly increase the presence of virus-infected inflammatory cells in the semen.

There are no reports of CAE transmission associated with embryo transfer. Nevertheless, while embryos with the *zona pellucida* intact could not be experimentally infected with CAE virus, those with the *zona pellucida* absent could be infected (Lamara et al. 2002) and supported productive replication of the CAE virus (Al-Ahmad et al. 2006). In another study, the presence of CAE-infected cells in oviductal washing fluid collected during embryo harvest from infected does was confirmed using a nested PCR for proviral DNA (Fieni et al. 2002). Embryos are considered safe as long as they are washed according to the International Embryo Transfer Society and are derived from seronegative flocks.

Iatrogenic transfer of CAE virus is also a consideration in horizontal transmission, though actual occurrences are not well documented. Since the virus is present in peripheral blood mononuclear cells, transfer of blood between animals by multiple use of needles for injection and the use of tattooing instruments without disinfection between animals are potential means of iatrogenic infection.

Finally, a number of behavioral traits were observed in CAE virus-infected dairy goat herds which were considered to contribute, at least potentially, to the spread of infection within the herds (Greenwood et al. 1995). These included teat sucking and biting by does, eye licking in hot weather, contact of the nose and mouth with vaginal and anal areas, nasal secretions present on muzzles of goats and in feed troughs, expulsion of milk into the environment when does lay on their udders, leaking of milk from udders before milking, drinking of milk in strip cups in the milking parlor, and drinking of urine and anal intercourse by bucks. While the risk associated with these different behaviors varies markedly, taken together they underscore the vigilance necessary for implementing successful control programs in infected herds.

Pathogenesis

Lentivirus infections are "slow virus" infections and are characterized by a high prevalence of inapparent infection, a prolonged but variable prepatent period, persistence of the virus in the host, multiple organ system involvement, and a chronic disease course with recurrent episodes of acute disease, such as is seen in the arthritic form of CAE (Cheevers and McGuire 1988). The pathogenic mechanisms of animal lentiviruses have been reviewed (Clements and Zink 1996).

Persistence of the virus in the host is facilitated by the ability of the lentivirus to sequester as provirus in host cells without the necessity of frequent multiplication. The CAE virus uses the monocyte/macrophage cell line as its principal host cell type. The virus remains inactive in monocytes and replication of virus is linked with maturation of monocytes to macrophages after they leave the bone marrow or blood and localize in tissue sites. This has been referred to as a "Trojan Horse" strategy whereby virus gains access to target tissues undetected in monocytes (Peluso et al. 1985). Activation of disease is associated with activation of virus translational activity in infected cells. The mechanisms by which lentiviral replication is first restricted and then subsequently expressed are complex and not yet completely understood, but the subject has been recently reviewed (Bertoni 2007). An important factor may be availability of viral transcription factors present in mature, tissue bound macrophages, but not present in circulating monocytes.

Infection of the goat with CAE virus induces both a strong humoral and cell mediated immune response, but neither is protective. In fact, caprine arthritis encephalitis is an immunopathological disease in which lesions result from an immune reaction to viral antigens, especially surface glycoproteins. This concept is supported by numerous observations including the fact that vaccinated goats develop more severe lesions when experimentally challenged than unvaccinated goats, that persistently infected goats develop acute arthritis when experimentally challenged, that the severity of joint lesions correlates with the presence of virus and antiviral antibody in the joint, and that the lesions occurring in CAE consist mainly of lymphocytes and macrophages (Adams et al. 1985; McGuire et al. 1986).

After kids consume colostrum or milk containing CAE virus-infected macrophages, these infected cells are taken up intact from the gut and enter the reticulendothelial system to establish infection in the kid (Narayan and Cork 1985). Subsequently, infected monocytes reach target tissues such as synovium, lung interstitium, choroid plexus, and udder where the activation of virus replication in conjunction with macrophage maturation induces the lymphoproliferative lesions that characterize CAE. Lungworms may possibly predispose to the pneumonic form of CAE in infected goats by inducing monocyte migration and macrophage proliferation in parasitized lung (Ellis et al. 1988).

Maternal antibody against CAE provides no protection against infection in suckling neonates and usually disappears within sixty to eighty-five days after suckling (Adams et al. 1983). Kids infected at birth can show an active antibody response as early as three to four weeks and usually by ten weeks (Ellis et al. 1986). When the antibody response develops, antibodies are present for life, although the serum concentration may wax and wane at different times or may be below the threshold of tests used to detect them.

Clinical Findings

In addition to subclinical infection, there are five known clinical forms of CAE in goats: arthritis, leukoencephalomyelitis, interstitial pneumonia, mastitis, and progressive weight loss. Arthritis, the most common form, is discussed here. The neurologic form is discussed in detail in Chapter 5 in association with maedi-visna. The respiratory form, a chronic progressive interstitial pneumonia of adult goats, is described in Chapter 9. It is sometimes also observed clinically in goats with the arthritic form. The udder form, an indurative viral mastitis with hypogalactia or agalactia noted at parturition in young does, is described further in Chapter 14. Progressive weight loss can occur as the sole clinical manifestation of CAE virus infection, or in conjunction with any of these other clinical forms. It is discussed in more detail in Chapter 15.

The arthritic form of CAE occurs in sexually mature goats, usually after the first year, most commonly in the second, but any time in adulthood. The onset may be insidious or acute and the clinical course varies considerably among individuals. All limb joints and the atlanto-occiptal bursa may be affected. The most common site is the carpal joint, the next most commonly involved joints are the tarsal, stifle, and fetlock joints; the atlanto-occipital bursa; and finally the coxofemoral joint. A single or multiple joints may be involved at any time in the course of disease.

Early signs of arthritis may be subtle. Joints may appear and feel normal but affected goats may have decreased ambulation and feeding activity, a reluctance or difficulty in rising, a stiff gait or abnormal posture after rising, and weight loss. Alternatively, affected goats early in the course of disease may present with an obvious, acute swelling in association with the joint but with little evidence of pain or restricted activity.

The most obvious swellings are on the anterior aspect of the carpus and are periarticular, associated with fluid accumulating in the carpal bursa. Such swellings may be up to 10 cm in diameter, and are fluctuant, cool, and not painful to the touch (Figure 4.6a). Fluid can be aspirated from these swellings for diagnostic purposes, but drainage only leads to refilling. The condition may remain at this stage of development in some animals for months or even years, or show periodic cycles of swelling, possible pain, and spontaneous improvement.

For many goats, however, the infection progresses steadily to a debilitating and painful arthritis. This is

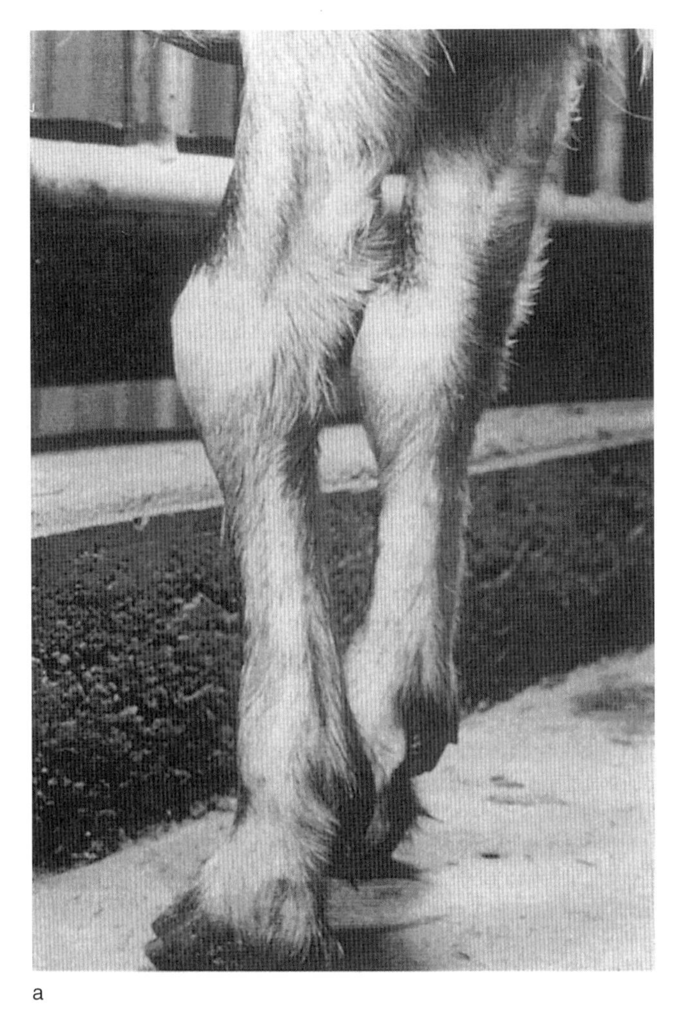

a

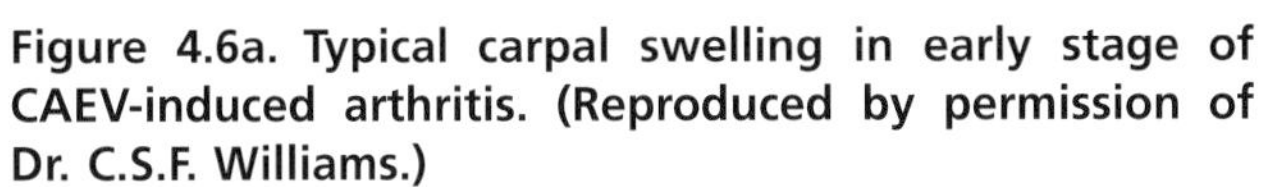

Figure 4.6a. Typical carpal swelling in early stage of CAEV-induced arthritis. (Reproduced by permission of Dr. C.S.F. Williams.)

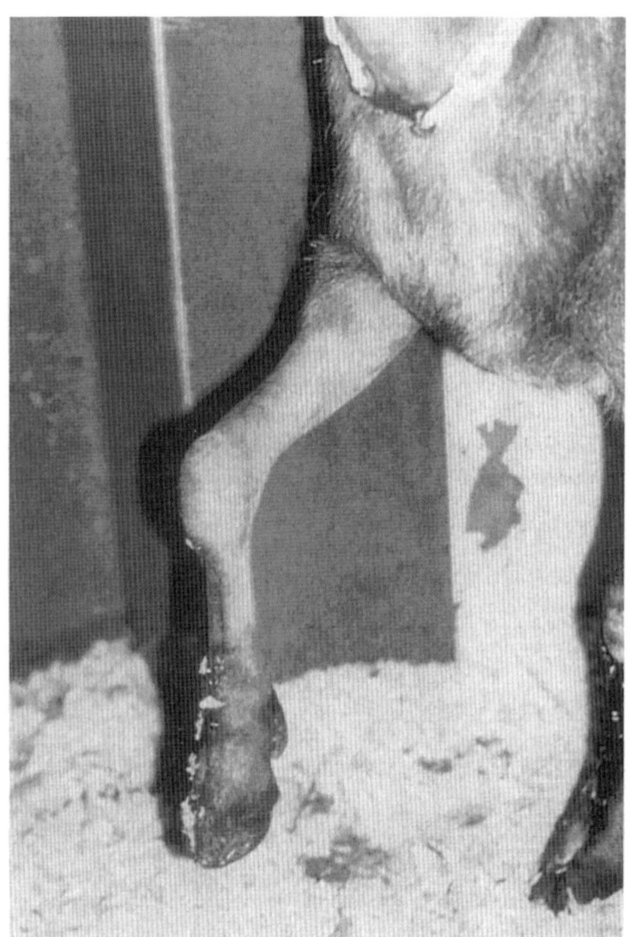

b

Figure 4.6b. Partial flexure contraction of the forelimb in a goat with progressive CAEV-induced arthritis of the carpus. (Courtesy of Dr. David M. Sherman.)

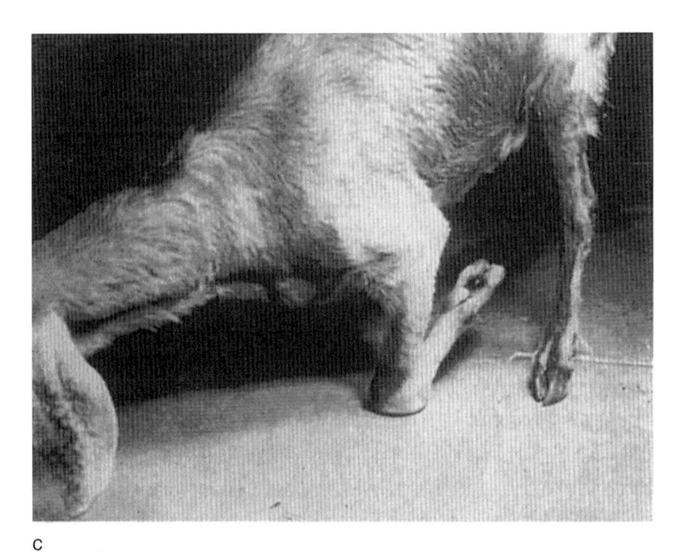

c

Figure 4.6c. Permanent kneeling due to ankylosis of the carpi in a goat with advanced CAEV arthritis of the carpi. (Reproduced by permission of Dr. C.S.F. Williams.)

Figure 4.6. Clinical progression of goats with carpal arthritis due to caprine arthritis encephalitis virus (CAEV).

usually accompanied by gradual weight loss and a rough hair coat. Fevers are not part of the disease process. The fluctuant swelling of the bursa gives way to a firmer swelling associated with inflammation and thickening of the joint capsule and surrounding structures, and the animal becomes increasingly reluctant to use the affected limb. Progressive mineralization of the joint capsule and soft tissues, exostoses of the bones, and collapse of the joint contribute to pain, a restricted range of motion, and finally ankylosis. When the carpus is involved, there is a marked tendency to carry the limb in a partially flexed position (Figure 4.6b). Ultimately, a permanent, severe flexion of the carpus may occur, and when both forelimbs are involved, the animal is forced to ambulate in a permanently kneeling position on the carpi (Figure 4.6c).

Involvement of the hind limbs usually results in less obvious swellings, but thickening of peri-articular structures may be palpable in the hock region. There is progressive reluctance to rise and increasing stiffness of gait. When the hips are involved the animal may develop a sufficiently painful and swaying gait to erroneously suggest neurogenic incoordination.

Clinical Pathology and Necropsy

Most diagnostic testing conducted relative to CAE is for the purpose of surveillance and implementation of control programs. As such, both clinically and subclinically infected animals must be identified. Isolation of the virus as a diagnostic tool is problematic in that virus concentrations in infected animals are low, particularly in subclinically infected animals and virus culture techniques are costly and time consuming. Since infection is lifelong and the presence of antibody signifies infection, serological methods for detection of antibody are preferable to virus isolation. The most commonly employed serological tests are the agar gel immunodiffusion test (AGID), the indirect ELISA (iELISA) and the competitive ELISA (cELISA). These are the prescribed tests for use in international trade to determine CAE infection status (OIE 2004). Additional, supplementary tests for detection of antibody are the radioimmunoprecipitation assay (RIPA), western blot (WB), and radioimmunoassay (RIA).

The AGID has been the most commonly used test for routine screening, providing good sensitivity and excellent specificity. Antigen for the prescribed AGID test is derived from whole virus that has been concentrated from culture supernatants and contains both the core antigen p28 and envelope antigen gp135. Detection of antibodies to both antigens improves the sensitivity of the test compared to using one or the other. While there is cross-reactivity of antibodies against the CAE and MV viruses, the sensitivity of the AGID test is improved if the CAE virus is used to detect CAE infection in goats.

There are more than thirty publications of ELISA tests for detection of SRLV infection with considerable variation in their performance relative to the AGID and relative to each other. A summary of all these SRLV ELISA test results has been published (Andrés et al. 2005). While early iterations of ELISA did not perform as reliably as the AGID, improvements in antigen development now make ELISA tests more sensitive and specific than AGID, and ELISA has become the preferred test for many laboratories and regulatory agencies. There are two main categories of ELISA assay in use—antibody detecting iELISAs, which use either whole virus or recombinant proteins/synthetic peptides as antigens, and cELISAs, based on the use of anti-viral monoclonal antibodies. For iELISAs overall, assays using whole virus antigen tend to be more sensitive than single recombinant antigen assays. However, if both a core antigen and an envelope antigen are included in the recombinant antigen assays, sensitivities and specificities are equivalent to whole cell antigen iELISAs (Andrés et al. 2005.)

In a recent report of a competitive ELISA using a monoclonal antibody binding to CAEV gp135 or SU glycoprotein, the sensitivity and specificity were recorded as 100% and 96.4%, respectively, as compared to RIPA (Herrmann et al. 2003). In the absence of a gold standard reference test to definitively establish CAE infection, RIPA, WB, and RIA are often used as reference tests to establish the comparative performance of various serologic methods with regard to sensitivity and specificity. They can also be used directly in serosurveillance but are generally considered too cumbersome and costly for high throughput testing.

The major limitation in the use of serosurveillance for control of CAE is the fact that delayed seroconversion is known to occur in CAE infection, as discussed earlier. With delays in seroconversion of eight months or longer following infection, some infected individuals will be missed in herd-wide testing programs. One potential solution to this problem is the detection of viral antigen by use of PCR techniques. A number of PCR protocols have been reported with most studies using peripheral blood mononuclear cells (PMBC) as the target cell for CAE virus detection. However, since only approximately one in a million leukocytes contain virus, PCR assays may fail to detect virus because the virus load is below the detection limit of the assay and some investigators have employed co-cultivation of PMBC with fibroblasts to increase virus load. Overall, PCR tests have tended to be less sensitive than many ELISA techniques (Andrés et al. 2005). Nevertheless, there are reports of PCR identifying CAE virus-infected goats prior to seroconversion without co-cultivation (Reddy et al. 1993; Rimstad et al. 1993).

In addition to testing of PBMC, PCR has been applied with equivalent results to semen, milk, and synovial fluid of goats. Currently, it is recommended that serology be combined with PCR for optimal detection of SRLV infection (Andrés et al. 2005).

Care must be taken in interpreting positive serology in the diagnosis of clinical cases of CAE. Because there are many causes of arthritis, pneumonia, and mastitis in goats, and because the majority of CAE-infected animals are subclinically infected, positive serology for CAE does not necessarily mean that the swollen joint, respiratory signs, or abnormal udder are due to CAE infection.

In the case of arthritis, arthrocentesis and examination of synovial fluid can support the diagnosis of CAE-induced arthritis. In active cases, the fluid is red to brown in color and has a low viscosity. Cell counts are elevated to the range of 1,000 to 20,000/mm^3 with mononuclear cells comprising more than 90% of the cell population. The majority are lymphocytes and the remainder are synovial cells and macrophages (Crawford and Adams 1981). Synovial biopsy can also be useful for histopathologic examination or for virus culture by explantation techniques. Examination of cells in synovial fluid using PCR techniques may also aid the diagnosis when lesions and clinical signs are consistent with CAE but serology is negative (Reddy et al. 1993).

A wide range of radiographic findings can be observed. In early cases, distension of bursae with fluid and other periarticular soft tissue swellings may be present. In advanced cases, CAE arthritis is characterized by more severe soft tissue changes including calcification of joint capsule and adjacent tendons, tendon sheaths, ligaments, and bursal contents (Figure 4.7). Early bony changes include mild periosteal reactions and periarticular osteophyte production. Later signs are more severe and include marked osteophyte production, breakdown of subchondral bone, collapse of joint spaces, and ankylosis (Crawford and Adams 1981).

At necropsy, affected goats are usually emaciated. Affected joints and adjacent bursae and tendon sheaths are usually enlarged. Foci of mineralization and/or necrosis as well as fibrous scar tissue may be visible in tendons and other periarticular structures. When the joint is opened a dramatic synovial proliferation is frequently observed. The synovial membrane appears brown and velvety and is thrown up into fingerlike projections. Cartilage surfaces can be roughened, ulcerated, or eroded depending on the severity of the case. "Rice bodies" are commonly found in the joint space, tendon sheaths, and bursae. Collapse of subchondral bone and ankylosis may also be noted (Crawford and Adams 1981).

Histologically, joint lesions are characterized by synovial hyperplasia with subsynovial mononuclear infiltrates, including lymphocytes, macrophages, and plasma cells. Multinucleated cells are occasionally observed. Fibrin deposition is common on synovial surfaces. There is necrosis and mineralization of synovial, perisynovial, and tendon collagen. The lesion of mononuclear infiltration seen in the synovium may also be seen in other target tissues such as udder and lung, even when there has been no clinical involvement of these organs. Similar mononuclear infiltrative lesions have also been observed in the uterus of a CAE virus-infected goat (Ali 1987) and the kidney of another (Dawson et al. 1983). Central nervous system lesions are described in Chapter 5, lung lesions in Chapter 9, and udder lesions in Chapter 14.

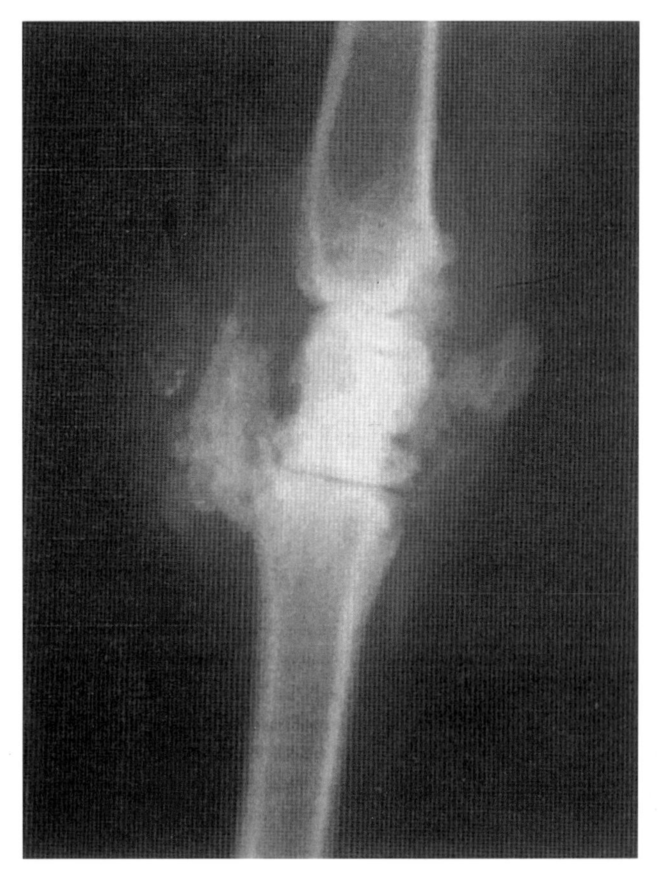

Figure 4.7. Radiographic changes in the carpus of a goat with advanced CAE arthritis. Note mineralization of extensor tendon and other soft tissue structures. (Courtesy of Cummings School of Veterinary Medicine at Tufts University.)

Diagnosis

A presumptive diagnosis of CAE arthritis is based on a combination of a history of CAE in the herd, positive serology and/or PCR, clinical signs consistent with the disease, synovial fluid abnormalities consistent with the disease, and typical histopathology on synovial biopsy or post mortem examination. All other traumatic, metabolic, and infectious causes of arthritis must be differentiated from CAE arthritis. Concurrent processes can occur, so cultures of synovial fluid for mycoplasma and bacteria are advised for definitive case assessment.

Treatment

There are no known treatments for any of the clinical forms of CAE. Animals with mild cases of the arthritic form of the disease can be made more comfortable by providing regular, correct hoof trimming, providing easily accessible feed and water, and by the long-term use of oral analgesics such as aspirin or phenylbutazone. Aspirin can be given at a dose of 100 mg/kg every twelve hours or phenylbutazone at a dose of 10 mg/kg once a day. Phenylbutazone must be avoided in goats producing meat or milk for human consumption. Additional nonsteroidal anti-inflammatory drugs are discussed in Chapter 17. Physical therapy could delay the progress of CAE arthritis, but there is no published evidence to support this.

Goats with advanced cases of arthritis, unable to extend the legs and forced to walk on their flexed carpi, should be euthanized. Such goats are less frequently encountered now than they were a decade ago because of increased awareness on the part of owners about CAE and more aggressive culling of advanced cases. Discovering such goats on a farm should alert the veterinarian to the need for client education concerning CAE.

Control

Attempts to prevent introduction of CAE into CAE-free countries or zones are based on import regulations that require validation of negative status in individual animals to be imported. The international standard suggested by the World Organization for Animal Health (OIE) is that animals be accompanied by an international veterinary certificate which attests that: the animals showed no clinical sign of CAE on the day of shipment, that animals over one year of age were subjected to a diagnostic test for CAE with negative results during the thirty days prior to shipment, or that CAE was neither clinically nor serologically diagnosed in the sheep and goats present in the flocks of origin during the past three years, and also that no sheep or goat from a flock of inferior health status was introduced into these flocks during that period. The prescribed serologic tests are AGID or ELISA (OIE 2007).

For countries, zones, or states where CAE is already present, testing and certification/accreditation programs may be implemented for control. Few countries, Switzerland being one (Perler 2003), have mandatory, nationwide regulatory control programs for CAE. Other countries, for example, New Zealand, France, and Sweden, have instituted voluntary testing and accreditation programs, usually in association with producer groups to encourage the establishment of CAE-negative herds and flocks (MacDiarmid 1985; Davidson 2002; Chartier 2008; de Verdier 2008). Australia has voluntary programs operating on the state and territory level (Animal Health Australia 2008). Such control programs usually involve annual or semiannual, herd-wide, serologic testing and removal of positive reactors from the herd.

At the farm level, efforts to eliminate CAE from herds known to be infected focus on three main areas: attempting to raise CAE-free kids by implementing kid-rearing techniques that reduce the risk of exposure to virus, periodic serologic testing of the herd, and culling or separating diseased and seropositive animals from healthy, seronegative animals.

Raising CAE-Free Kids. Modification of kid-rearing techniques is probably the most frequently implemented aspect of herd control programs. The goal is to eliminate exposure of kids to virus and is based on the assumption that most new infections in kids develop in an infected herd as a result of ingestion of virus-contaminated milk or colostrum. More stringent programs also remove kids from dams immediately at birth on the assumption that the potential exists for kids to be exposed to virus when they are licked and cleaned by their infected dams. Washing birth fluids off the kids immediately after birth has also been recommended.

To achieve this level of control, attendants need to be present at birth so kids can be removed from their dams before they are able to stand and suckle. To improve the chance of being present at kidding, timed induction of parturition with prostaglandins can be used as discussed in Chapter 13. Once kids are removed from the doe, they should be raised in separate facilities from adult animals, especially if infected adults are maintained on the farm, and they should never again be commingled with known-infected goats.

Ideally, kids removed from the dam should be fed heat-treated goat colostrum as an appropriate, CAE virus-free source of maternal antibodies to provide passive immunity against neonatal diseases. Pasteurization of colostrum at high temperature for short periods can denature protective immunoglobulins and causes the colostrum to gel, making it impossible to feed. As an alternative, heat treatment of colostrum at 132.8°F (56°C) for sixty minutes has been demonstrated experimentally to block transmission of virus and permit absorption of immunoglobulins (Adams et al. 1983).

Automated equipment for performing this task is now available but may not be affordable for many small herds. Owners of small herds can be advised to heat colostrum to 134.6°F (57°C) for ten minutes and then transfer it to a thermos flask that has been preheated with boiling water. The colostrum is then held in the closed thermos flask for sixty minutes to accomplish virus inactivation. It is essential that the temperature remain above 132.8°F (56°C) for the entire period (MacKenzie et al. 1987) and it should be verified by thermometer at the end of the holding period. Excess colostrum may be successfully frozen for later use to reduce labor expenditure.

Because heat treatment of colostrum is a laborious task, goat owners actively seek alternatives to this practice. Feeding no colostrum should be viewed as an unacceptable practice because this results in failure of passive transfer of immunity and puts kids at risk for other dangerous diseases. Feeding unpasteurized colostrum only from seronegative does is not without risk because false-negative serologic test results do occur. Administration of unpasteurized cow colostrum results in acceptable levels of circulating serum antibodies in kids, but the persistence and efficacy of such heterologous antibody in kids has not been documented. The practice is reported to be effective in raising orphan lambs. Of course, unpasteurized cow colostrum, while it does not contain CAE virus, may contain other organisms such as *Mycobacterium paratuberculosis* that are potentially infectious for goats. In addition, feeding of cow colostrum has occasionally been associated with hemolytic anemia in kids (Perrin and Polack 1988).

A number of products are being marketed as colostrum supplements for calves, lambs, or kids. Such products usually contain lyophilized colostrum or whey immunoglobulin concentrates. Many goat owners have seized upon these products as colostrum substitutes suitable for use in CAE control programs. However, it has been demonstrated that some of these products, when administered to kids as directed by the manufacturer, do not raise serum antibody levels above a level consistent with a diagnosis of failure of passive transfer of antibody (Sherman et al. 1990). Numerous anecdotal reports suggest a marked increase in the incidence of neonatal septicemia when some colostrum supplements have been used in place of colostrum (Scroggs 1989; Custer 1990).

Newer products on the market may be more reliable, but all such products should be used with caution and kids monitored for an increased occurrence of neonatal septicemia or other disease. Antibody levels in kid serum can be measured by a number of methods as discussed in the section on failure of passive transfer in Chapter 7.

After administration of heat-treated goat colostrum, kids must be raised on pasteurized goat milk, cow milk, or commercial milk replacer through weaning. Goat milk can be pasteurized by heating to 165°F (73.9°C) for fifteen seconds. The feeding of milk replacers to kids is discussed in Chapter 19.

PERIODIC SEROLOGIC TESTING. Submission of serum samples from all goats of breeding age and older for detection of antibody to CAE virus can be useful to establish the prevalence of disease, monitor progress in control programs, serve as a basis for creating infected and noninfected strings of goats in the herd, or identify animals for culling.

There is not universal agreement on the appropriate frequency of testing for herd control programs and the frequency of testing required varies between herds based on initial level of infection, size of herd, capacity to rigorously implement necessary management changes, and other epidemiological factors. It has been suggested, for example, that kids be tested monthly up to six months of age because of variability in the time of seroconversion following perinatal infection. This is not necessary if the kid-rearing interventions discussed above are assiduously practiced, but if management is lax, then such testing may be worthwhile to identify perinatally exposed kids and to underscore lapses in control practices. It should be noted that kids fed heat-treated colostrum from infected does will have false positive serologic tests for several months at least.

In general, goats should be tested at least annually, and preferably, semi-annually, because sensitivity of the serologic tests is not 100% and serum antibody levels may fluctuate in individual goats, as in late pregnancy when serum antibody levels may be reduced due to maternal transfer of antibodies from serum to colostrum. Timing a herd-wide test for the beginning of the breeding season is useful because the results can be used to advantage in making breeding, culling, and management decisions relating to CAE control well before kidding time.

CULLING OR SEPARATION. Kids raised CAE-free using the above protocols may still seroconvert after weaning as a result of horizontal transmission in herds where known-infected adults are allowed to remain and commingle in the herd (East et al. 1987). Herd owners attempting to eliminate CAE from their herds should be strongly encouraged to include aggressive culling of seropositive adults as an integral part of the control program. Otherwise, the efforts placed on rearing of CAE-free kids may, in many cases, be futile.

However, in many infected herds, particularly commercial milking herds where the need for milk and replacement does is high, there is frequently resistance to the notion of culling seropositive adults on economic grounds, even though kid rearing techniques are practiced to reduce the prevalence of CAE. In these cases, it is necessary to maintain two separate groups within the herd—a seropositive group and a seronegative group that are physically separated to the greatest extent possible. Separate buildings are ideal, but may be impractical. Solid wall separation is the next best option, but if that too is not possible, then the animals must be physically separated by a distance of at least 2 m with a double fence or barrier that allows no direct contact between individuals in the two groups.

Separate feeding, watering, grooming, and other such equipment should be maintained for each group, but if that is not possible, the equipment should be used first on seronegative animals and always washed and disinfected after using on seropositive animals. Seronegative goats should be milked first as a string before seropositive goats and considerable care must be taken to avoid contamination of surfaces, clothing, and equipment with milk from seropositive does in milking parlors where it might make contact with seronegative does the next time they are milked.

Other practical considerations for effective control programs are to avoid bringing goats to fairs and shows if possible, or at least avoid commingling goats either at the event or during transport to and from the event. No animals should be introduced into a herd attempting to eliminate CAE unless that animal comes from a known CAE-negative herd, or the individuals test negative and can be quarantined for six months and retested before entering the herd. Ideally, only seronegative bucks should be used for natural service, but if that is not possible, then the buck should be left with the doe only long enough to breed under observation to avoid unnecessary contact. Because the virus is present in peripheral blood monocytes in infected animals, the use of separate needles and syringes for each animal during treatment and vaccination is advised because iatrogenic transmission is at least theoretically possible. Similarly, tattooing of goats may involve blood contamination of the tattooing instrument, so disinfection with phenolic or quaternary ammonium compounds between uses is advised.

If sheep are kept on the same premises with goats and CAE control efforts are undertaken, sheep should be included in the testing program and subjected to similar segregation and management interventions for control. Recent evidence indicates that cross transmission of small ruminant lentivirus between the two species occurs (Shah et al. 2004, 2004a) and may adversely affect CAE control programs (Perler 2003).

Foot and Mouth Disease

Foot and mouth disease (FMD), also known as aphthous fever, is a highly contagious viral disease of wild and domestic, cloven-hoofed animals. Although it usually produces low mortality, it does produce high morbidity and represents a disease of extreme economic importance to animal industries worldwide through loss of productivity and constraints on trade in livestock and livestock products.

In the goat, FMD most often assumes a subclinical form, though clinical cases can and do occur. The major concern with caprine FMD is that subclinically infected goats may act as a source of infection for cattle in mixed livestock systems and through movement and international trade. Knowledge of the disease in small ruminants has been reviewed (Sharma 1981; Pay 1988; Barnett and Cox 1999; Kitching and Hughes 2002).

Etiology

FMD is caused by a nonenveloped, icosahedral, single-stranded RNA virus of the genus Aphthovirus, in the family Picornaviridae. There are seven immunologically distinct virus serotypes, each with numerous strains. The seven serotypes are identified as A, O, C, Asia 1, South African Territories (SAT) 1, SAT 2, and SAT 3. The development of immunity after natural exposure or vaccination is highly type-specific, and to a varying degree, strain-specific. Constant global surveillance of outbreaks is necessary to monitor changes in virus type prevalence so that appropriate type- and strain-specific vaccine formulations can be prepared and maintained. The global challenges of maintaining appropriate and sufficient vaccine banks and reserves for FMD has recently been reviewed (Paton et al. 2005).

The virus is cultivated *in vitro* on bovine thyroid, bovine kidney, or other suitable cell lines, and produces a cytopathic effect but no inclusion bodies. It is quite resistant to freezing and desiccation, but does not survive high temperatures or extremes in pH very well. Direct sunlight kills it, but organic debris protects it from the sun. It dies off rapidly in muscle tissue of infected animals, but can persist in offal, blood, and bone marrow. High relative humidity prolongs the life of aerosolized virus. Sodium hydroxide, acetic acid, sodium carbonate, and sodium hypochlorite are the most effective disinfectants. The commercial disinfectant Virkon®S, which contains multiple ingredients, has come to be widely used as a disinfectant in FMD outbreak control.

Epidemiology

Foot and mouth disease is one of the most highly regulated livestock diseases in the world, with extensive international efforts undertaken to control the spread of the virus through restricted movement of both live animals and animal products. FMD currently is enzootic in large areas of Africa, Asia, the Middle East, Eastern Europe, and South America. Areas free of FMD include North America, Central America, and the Caribbean, as well as Australia, New Zealand, Japan, and many islands of the Pacific.

At present, serotype O is geographically the most widely distributed FMD type in the world and a serotype O PanAsia lineage virus has been responsible for many FMD outbreaks over the last two decades. This lineage originated in India in 1990 and spread through the Middle East, Turkey, and Eastern Europe. It then moved eastward into the People's Republic of China in 1999 and then to Taiwan, South Korea, Japan, Mongolia, and far-east Russia. The virus then appeared in South Africa in late 2000 and in the United Kingdom in February 2001, where it produced a devastating outbreak of FMD. It spread from there to Ireland, France, and the Netherlands before being brought under control (Grubman and Baxt 2004). Goats are believed to have been involved in the spread of type O PanAsia, at least with regard to its introduction into Saudi Arabia when, in the 1990s, that country banned the importation of cattle from India due to concerns about rinderpest but continued to import Indian goats and sheep.

More than seventy species of wild and domesticated mammals are susceptible to FMD infection. Cattle and swine are seriously affected by FMD infection with high morbidity and overt clinical disease, but comparatively low mortality rates. In contrast, the disease in sheep and goats is less pronounced and often remains subclinical (O'Brien 1943; Nazlioglu 1972; Sharma 1981; Dutta et al. 1984). This is not always the case. In one Indian outbreak of FMD in goats due to virus type A22, morbidity was 82.5% and mortality 8.2% (Mishra and Ghei 1983).

Human infection very rarely occurs and the disease is generally not considered to be zoonotic. However, the virus can survive in the upper respiratory tract of people for twenty-four hours after exposure and be transmitted subsequently to animals. This has implications for effective disease control in the age of international jet travel.

Foot and mouth disease continues to be a threat to livestock worldwide, largely because the highly contagious virus is readily transmitted under a wide variety of conditions that are difficult to detect. Among these are: the shedding of virus by infected animals before the onset of clinical signs or during convalescence; the existence of subclinically infected, convalescent, or even vaccinated animals that can act as carriers; and the presence of virus in improperly processed products containing meat, milk, bone, blood, offal, or skin of infected animals. The potential for disease transmission via semen either during natural service or artificial insemination has not been investigated in goats, although it has been demonstrated to occur in cattle.

In enzootic regions, the primary mode of transmission is by close or direct contact between infected and susceptible animals. This can be via aerosolization of virus present in the secretions and excretions of the infected animal or by entry of virus through cuts and abrasions or mucous membranes. Wind or other mechanical vectors, including veterinarians on farm visits, can carry the infective virus long distances. Contaminated bedding, feed, and equipment can serve as a source of infection. Goats and sheep are less likely than cattle to become infected by long distance airborne virus because their lower respiratory volume makes it more difficult to take in infective doses of virus via aerosol (Kitching and Hughes 2002). Mechanical carriage of virus on humans and vehicles was considered a frequent factor in disease spread between flocks in the 2001 UK outbreak. In areas where pastoralism and communal grazing are common, as in many parts of Africa, south Asia, and the Middle East, infected small ruminants contaminate river water, ponds, pastures, shrubs, and other aspects of the environment, contributing to the dissemination and persistence of disease (Uppal 2004). In serosurveys in Morocco, transhumant and nomadic herds had a higher prevalence of FMD than stationary herds (Barnett and Cox, 1999).

It is now generally accepted that subclinically infected goats and sheep can play an important role in transmission of the disease to cattle, and small ruminants were deemed responsible for epizootics of FMD in cattle in Tunisia in 1989, Greece in 1994, Southeast Asia in 1999, and Turkey in 2001 (Kitching and Hughes 2002; Uppal 2004). In many parts of the world, sheep and goats are herded or managed together and traded in commerce together so it is often difficult to ascribe a specific role for goats in transmission or spread of FMD as distinct from sheep. However, there are also some documented situations in which goats are specifically identified as the source of new infections. A goat clandestinely brought from Turkey was deemed responsible for a type O outbreak in cattle in Bulgaria in 1991 (Kitching 1998). Goats have also been implicated in an outbreak of FMD in Kuwait with type Asia 1 when infected goats with this strain were imported from Bangladesh (Kitching and Hughes 2002). The index case for the FMD outbreak in the Netherlands in 2001 was a dairy goat/veal calf farm and the first clinical cases were seen in goats. It is believed that the infection was introduced with purchased, imported calves but because the calves on the premises were housed individually and the goats commingled freely, circulation and expression of the virus occurred first in the goats (Bouma et al. 2003).

Virus has been isolated from nasal secretions of healthy appearing goats forty-eight hours before the development of clinical FMD (Raghavan and Dutt 1974). Intranasal inoculation of goats with viruses of A, O, or C type produced a 100% infection rate, with virus present in the oropharynx for up to twenty-eight days in 87% of goats, and no cases of severe clinical disease. Lesions that did occur were mild enough to be overlooked by casual observation (McVicar and Sutmoller 1968). Animals in which virus can be recovered from the oropharynx beyond twenty-eight days post-infection are defined as carriers. The maximum duration of the carrier state in goats is reported to be four months, as compared to nine months in sheep and up to three and a half years in cattle (Alexandersen et al. 2003).

Some ruminant animals, including some goats, may become carriers when exposed to FMD virus, even if they are immune as a result of previous vaccination or recovery from infection. The percentage of animals that become carriers is variable and the infectivity titer of virus in oropharyngeal samples is usually low. Excretion is also intermittent and the titer declines over time. Development and persistence of the carrier state may be determined both by the animal species and the strain of virus involved (Alexandersen et al. 2003). In a review of the role of small ruminants in the transmission of FMD, it was concluded that sheep and goats are most likely to be involved with the transmission of FMDV during the early stages of either clinical or subclinical FMD infection rather than when they are carriers and the period of greatest risk of transmission is up to seven days after contact with the infection (Barnett and Cox 1999).

Host species susceptibility may also vary with virus type. For example, a devastating outbreak of FMD in pigs in Taiwan in 1997 with type O virus O/Taw/97 did not cause disease in cattle and goats on the same farms with affected pigs (Yang et al. 1999). That virus strain was related to others involved in earlier porcine FMD outbreaks in the Far East. However, in 1999, FMD occurred again in Taiwan, caused by a type O strain more closely related to type O strains circulating in the Middle East and India, and in the 1999 Taiwan outbreak, goats and cattle were clinically affected (Grubman and Baxt 2004).

The frequently mild clinical manifestations of FMD in small ruminants can lead to oversight or misdiagnosis and thereby contribute to the further spread of disease. For example, serotype O was introduced into Tunisia in 1989 in infected sheep and goats imported from the Middle East. Clinical signs were mild and lameness observed in these animals was initially thought to be due to bluetongue. Eventually the disease spread to cattle, at which time it was quickly identified as FMD due to the more obvious clinical manifestations in that species. However, by then the disease had time to disseminate and spread into Algeria and Morocco (Kitching 1998). In the UK in 2001, difficulty in accurately recognizing clinical FMD in sheep contributed to the dissemination of the disease through transport of unrecognized cases. However, it also contributed to the emergency destruction of many sheep flocks deemed clinically affected that subsequently turned out to be negative when test results were completed (Kitching and Hughes 2002).

Pathogenesis

Infection is most commonly initiated by inhalation of aerosolized virus or by direct entry of virus into abraded epithelium of the mouth or feet. After inhalation, multiplication occurs initially in the pharynx and, after direct entry, in the epithelium of the mouth or feet. After three to eleven days, a subsequent viremia ensues in susceptible animals. This is the febrile stage of the disease and lasts three to four days. Virus is found in most tissues and shed in all secretions and excretions during viremia. Young kids may die of viral myocarditis at this stage. In surviving goats, virus ultimately localizes in the epithelial cells of the buccal cavity and feet, and sometimes the teats. Virus multiplication in epithelium leads to hydropic degeneration and coalescence of fluid-filled cells to form enlarging vesicles up to 3 or more cm in diameter in cattle. The overlying epithelium becomes devitalized and the mechanical trauma of eating or walking causes sloughing of the tissue, exposing raw painful ulcers underneath. This leads to the signs of stomatitis and lameness characteristic of overt clinical disease.

Large, fluid-filled vesicles, such as those seen in cattle, are rarely observed in the mouths of goats and sheep. The thinness of the lingual epithelium in small ruminants causes superficial lesions to rupture early, leaving shallow erosions which usually heal within a few days. Lesions in the mouth of large and, to a lesser extent, small ruminants are most often seen on the dental pad and the tongue but may also be seen on the lips, gums, and cheeks, and sometimes on the hard palate (Alexandersen et al. 2003).

Clinical Findings

Subclinical infection is the most common outcome in goats exposed to FMD virus. In acute cases, initial, nonspecific signs of FMD may include dullness, inappetence, restlessness, increased heart and respiratory rates, shivering, and fever. Milking goats may become agalactic. Pregnant does may abort. Mortality, when it occurs, is most likely in neonatal kids. Mortality up to 55% in young kids has been observed even when older animals show no morbidity (Hedjazi et al. 1972). In such kids, peracute death from myocarditis often occurs with no other signs.

When goats do show specific signs of FMD, they are more often affected on the feet than in the mouth. Therefore, lameness is the most suggestive sign of caprine FMD and demands careful examination of the feet, though oral lesions and signs of stomatitis can and do occur. In a severe Indian outbreak of FMD in goats, 12.5% of cases had only oral lesions, 40% only foot lesions, and 47.5% both foot and oral lesions (Mishra and Ghei 1983). Similarly, in another Indian outbreak in a herd of 385 goats, 8.3% of cases had only oral lesions, 63.8% had only foot lesions, and 27.7% of cases had both foot and oral lesions. The overall morbidity rate was 16% and only one seven-day old kid died, for a mortality rate of 0.26%. All other affected animals recovered within a period of ten to fifteen days (Kumar et al. 2004).

Early in the course of clinical disease, vesicles may be found along the coronary band, in the interdigital space, and sometimes on the heels. Any or all of the feet may be involved. Over several days, vesicles rupture leaving behind painful ulcers. Lameness may grow more pronounced and the ulcers on the feet may become secondarily infected with bacteria. Animals may be reluctant to stand or move. Though uncommon, in extreme cases the hoof wall may separate at the coronary band and the hoof slough. Severely affected goats may succumb to starvation, dehydration, predation, septicemia, or secondary pneumonia. In uncomplicated FMD, or with supportive care, oral and foot lesions heal gradually over two to three weeks and goats return to normal, although some animals may remain thin for extended periods.

Early vesicle formation in the oral cavity can lead to signs of lip smacking and drooling. Hyperemic foci or small raised fluid-filled vesicles may occur in the mucosa of the lips, tongue, and palate, but are likely to rupture quickly due to the thin buccal epithelium in small ruminants. Rupture of oral vesicles exposes mucosal ulcers leading to mouth pain and a reluctance to eat, and produces lesions more easily confused with other, non-vesicular causes of stomatitis in small ruminants. Vesicles on the teats may also occur (Olah et al. 1976) as may vesicles on the prepuce.

Goats suspected of having FMD need to be inspected very carefully for vesicle formation. Vesicles in the mouth may be small and few in number and not lead to overt signs of stomatitis. Likewise, foot lesions may be mild, affect only one or more limbs, and produce minimal secondary signs. If actual fluid-filled vesicles are not observed, later lesions after vesicle rupture may look merely like abrasions due to trauma.

Clinical Pathology and Necropsy

A definitive diagnosis of FMD from field cases requires laboratory confirmation because the disease cannot be differentiated clinically from other vesicular diseases, including vesicular stomatitis which can occur, albeit rarely, in goats, and because in small ruminants, classical clinical signs as described in cattle may be minimal or absent. Due to the highly contagious nature of this disease and the need to initiate regulatory disease control plans in a timely fashion, laboratory diagnosis of any suspected FMD case is a matter of urgency. When FMD is suspected, regulatory authorities should be notified immediately and sample collection and shipment should be done by trained, authorized personnel according to strict standards of biosecurity with tests performed in a laboratory that meets the World Organization for Animal Health (OIE) requirements for Containment Group 4 pathogens (OIE 2007a).

The best samples to submit for laboratory diagnosis are epithelium from unruptured or freshly ruptured vesicles or vesicular fluid. If such samples are not available, which may commonly be the case in affected goats, blood and/or esophageal–pharyngeal fluid samples taken by probang cup can yield virus. Myocardium or blood can be submitted from fatal cases, but vesicles are preferred when available.

As prescribed by the World Organization for Animal Health (OIE), diagnosis of FMD is by virus isolation or the demonstration of FMD viral antigen or nucleic acid in tissue or fluid samples. Detection of virus-specific antibody can also be used for diagnosis, and antibodies to viral nonstructural proteins (NSPs) can be used to differentiate infection from vaccination. Detailed descriptions and reference sources for laboratory tests used in the diagnosis of FMD are found in the OIE Manual of Diagnostic Tests and Vaccines for Terrestrial Animals which is available in print and on the internet (OIE 2004a) and are outlined briefly here.

Virus isolation is best performed on cell culture systems using primary bovine (calf) thyroid cells or primary pig, calf, or lamb kidney cells. Other cell lines, such as BHK-21 (baby hamster kidney) and IB-RS-2 cells, may also be used but are generally less sensitive when there are low amounts of infectivity. Cytopathic effect (CPE) occurs in infected cell cultures in forty-eight hours. If none is seen, cell cultures are frozen and thawed and a new cell culture inoculated to check again for CPE.

For detection of viral antigens, an indirect sandwich ELISA technique has largely replaced complement fixation (CF) as the test of choice in recent years. The ELISA is more specific and sensitive than CF and not affected by pro- or anti-complement factors. This ELISA confirms the presence of FMD virus and the serotype. Different rows in multiwell plates are coated with rabbit antisera to each of the seven serotypes of FMD virus. Thus, the FMD viral antigens of different serotypes present are captured when sample suspensions are added to the wells. Guinea-pig antisera to each of the serotypes of FMD virus is then added to create the "sandwich" and this is followed by addition of rabbit anti-guinea-pig serum conjugated to an enzyme to reveal a color reaction that can be quantified by spectrophotometry.

Nucleic acid recognition tests, such as the reverse transcriptase-polymerase chain reaction (RT-PCR), are being used increasingly for virus detection. Agarose gel or real time RT-PCR can be used to amplify genome fragments of FMD virus in epithelium, milk, serum, and oropharyngeal samples. Specific primers have been designed to distinguish between each of the seven serotypes, and RT combined with real-time PCR has a sensitivity comparable to that of virus isolation.

Characterization of FMD strains is very important for tracking the spatial movement of FMD infection, identifying host species adaptations for particular strains, and developing suitable and effective vaccines. The molecular epidemiology of FMD is based on the comparison of genetic differences between isolates. Dendrograms showing the genomic relationship between vaccine and field strains for all seven serotypes based on sequences derived from the 1D gene, which encodes for the VP1 viral protein, have been produced. RT-PCR amplification of FMD virus RNA, followed by nucleotide sequencing, is the current preferred option for generating the sequence data for strain comparisons.

Serological tests for FMD are conducted for four main reasons: to certify individual animals prior to import or export, confirm suspected cases of FMD, substantiate the absence of infection, and demonstrate the efficacy of vaccination. To confirm mild cases or where epithelial tissue cannot be collected, as may often occur in small ruminants, the demonstration of specific antibodies to structural proteins (SPs) of FMD virus in animals known to be unvaccinated is sufficient for a positive diagnosis. The SP tests are serotype-specific and detect antibodies elicited by vaccination and infection. The virus neutralization test, the solid-phase competition ELISA, and the liquid-phase blocking ELISA for detection of antibodies to SPs are the prescribed tests of the OIE for use in international trade of livestock.

In addition to structural proteins, FMD virus also expresses eight non-structural proteins (NSPs) during viral replication. There is no viral replication in the host when killed virus vaccines are used for FMD control. Thus, tests for antibodies to some non-structural proteins of FMD virus are useful in providing evidence of previous or current viral replication in the host, independent of vaccination status. In contrast to structural proteins, NSPs are highly conserved and therefore are not serotype specific, so the detection of these antibodies is not serotype restricted. Unfortunately, some NSPs are produced during growth of vaccine virus in tissue culture and some traces of these NSPs may contaminate the final killed vaccine product and elicit a host immune response. The NSP 3D is most commonly associated with this contamination and therefore is not a good candidate antigen for NSP antibody tests.

Currently the non-structural polyproteins 3AB and 3ABC are the preferred antigens. Tests prescribed by OIE for detection of antibodies to NSPs include indirect ELISA and the enzyme-linked immunoelectrotransfer blot assay. The use of diagnostic techniques based on detection of antibodies to NSPs to distinguish FMD virus infection from vaccination has been recently reviewed (Clavijo et al. 2004).

A full necropsy should be conducted on suspect FMD cases that have died. At the time of necropsy, careful inspection of the feet, oral cavity, pharynx, and teats is required to determine the presence of vesicles or ulcerations consistent with a diagnosis of FMD. In addition, the so-called "tiger heart" lesion may be observed, especially in kids dying peracutely. This name refers to a striped appearance of the myocardium caused by the presence of necrotic, small gray foci and irregular streaks in the heart muscle. These same lesions may occasionally occur in skeletal muscle.

Microscopically, vesicular epithelial lesions include hydropic degeneration of cells in the *stratum spinosum*, disintegration of cells, and accumulation of fluid. Where vesicles have ruptured, ulcers will be noted and may be associated with suppurative inflammation if secondary bacterial infection has occurred. The heart lesion is one of focal coagulative necrosis accompanied by lymphocytic and sometimes neutrophilic infiltrates.

Diagnosis

Definitive diagnosis is based on isolation of virus from suspected cases of FMD. Because vesicular diseases of goats are uncommon, any vesicular lesion of the mouth, muzzle, oral cavity, feet, or teats should be considered as suspect for FMD, even in FMD-free countries, and reported to appropriate authorities immediately. Because vesicles are fragile and transient in goats, advanced cases may present with ulcers, or crusts over lesions that make the diagnosis less obvious. Therefore, FMD must be considered whenever there are signs of lameness and/or stomatitis, especially when the two signs occur together.

Diseases with the potential of producing both signs together in goats include bluetongue, vesicular stomatitis, pemphigus, and contagious ecthyma. Bluetongue and vesicular stomatitis rarely produce clinical disease in goats, though in the recent outbreak of bluetongue in Europe in 2006, goats in the Netherlands showed oral lesions and udder lesions (Dercksen et al. 2007). Pemphigus is unlikely to affect more than one goat in a herd. Lesions of contagious ecthyma are found primarily on the mouth but can be found in other locations as well, including the teats and legs, although overt lameness is unlikely. Ionophore toxicity is an important differential for the myocarditis lesion of FMD that causes sudden death in kids, as discussed in Chapter 8, as is nutritional muscular dystrophy as discussed later in this chapter.

Treatment

There is no specific treatment for FMD. However, supportive care can help facilitate recovery of affected animals. Such efforts include confinement, provision of easily masticated, high-quality feed and water, and the administration of antibiotics, or application of topical antiseptics to prevent or control secondary bacterial infections of ulcerative lesions. Foot baths using 5% potassium permanganate solution have also been recommended (Kumar et al. 2004). Depending on the regulatory protocols in effect, it may be required to destroy all animals involved in an epizootic, so consideration of treatment may become moot.

Control

Considerable international effort is made to restrict the global spread of FMD. The World Organization for Animal Health, based on the input of its member nations and technical experts, has produced recommended standards for trade in livestock and livestock products aimed at effective control. These recommendations are available in print or on the Internet in the Terrestrial Animal Health Code (OIE 2007b). Countries that are FMD-free, such as the United States, do not accept imports of livestock from FMD-enzootic countries. However, the importation of certain animal products is permitted but only from approved, inspected abattoirs and/or processing plants.

When outbreaks do occur in FMD-free countries, they are eradicated by stamping out procedures and zoo-sanitary measures, with or without the addition of ring vaccination of livestock around the outbreak locale. Countries that are FMD-free but that border enzootically infected countries may practice regular, annual "frontier" vaccination of livestock along the pertinent national boundaries to create buffer zones against incursion of infection.

In enzootic countries, FMD is controlled by restriction of livestock movement, isolation or slaughter of exposed and infected animals, ring vaccination around outbreak locales, or maintenance of a systematic national vaccination program. Effective vaccination depends on ongoing surveillance to ensure that all important, locally occurring strains of FMD virus are included in multivalent vaccines (Blaha 1989). Based on geography, livestock distribution, and other factors, some countries may maintain recognized FMD-free zones within their borders even when the whole country is not considered disease free. The same principles of movement control, surveillance, and vaccination apply for the maintenance of FMD-free zones, and export of livestock and livestock products are permitted from these FMD-free zones when international surveillance and testing standards are met.

Several disease control recommendations were made by the Permanent Commission on Foot and Mouth Disease of the OIE in 1972 specifically concerning goats and sheep (Anonymous 1972). Small ruminants brought to seasonal pasture grounds should be vaccinated against FMD at least once a year. If prophylactic vaccination campaigns are carried out in cattle, then goats and sheep should be vaccinated as well. When it is necessary to undertake ring vaccination of cattle after an outbreak, goats and sheep should be included in the vaccination scheme. Finally, veterinary supervision of goats and sheep should be intensified at markets and during movement to and from pasture grounds, because transhumance, or seasonal movement of livestock to different feeding grounds, has been associated with increased spread of FMD.

Despite these recommendations, inclusion of small ruminants in vaccination efforts is not widely practiced for several reasons. First, it is not proven that prophylactic vaccination of small ruminants is essential to eradicate the disease in cattle (Barnett and Cox 1999). In addition, there is some evidence that FMD in sheep and goats may be self-limiting (Anderson et al. 1976), although this depends on the strain of virus and the susceptibility of the small ruminants involved, e.g., indigenous breeds versus exotic imports.

Perhaps the most significant resistance to mass vaccination of small ruminants is related to the cost, particularly in developing countries with large populations of sheep and goats and limited veterinary service budgets for disease control. As a result, small ruminants tend to be vaccinated, if at all, only when they are in association with large numbers of cattle or swine. When sheep and goats are included in regular vaccination campaigns in countries where FMD is endemic, they are rarely vaccinated more than once a year (Kitching and Hughes 2002). In Israel, all susceptible species, i.e., cattle, sheep and goats, are vaccinated regularly every year. In the event of an outbreak, all the animals at the outbreak site and in the surrounding area are immediately revaccinated (Leforban 2002).

Killed vaccines are currently in widest use and are usually trivalent, containing strains A, O, and C. However, many FMD vaccines are produced locally to reflect prevalent serotypes and strains and therefore vary in composition, so blanket recommendations for vaccination cannot be made. Based on local production techniques, they may also vary in immunogenicity, purity, and efficacy. Standards for FMD vaccine production are provided by the World Organization for Animal Health (OIE 2004a) and development and performance of killed FMD vaccines has been reviewed (Barteling et al. 2002).

Killed vaccines can be effective in goats when given at one-third the dose volume applied to cattle, with immunity usually lasting from five to six months

(Sharma 1981). When cattle, sheep, and goats are vaccinated with inactivated FMD vaccines, sheep, and especially goats, respond with lower mean antibody titers than cattle (Polydorou et al. 1980; Garland 1981). Optimal responses are obtained when two primary vaccinations are given about two weeks apart followed by regular boosters at six-month intervals.

The choice of adjuvant used in vaccine may have an impact on goat response to vaccination. In a study comparing oil adjuvanted and aluminum hydroxide adjuvanted FMD vaccine, the oil adjuvant elicited superior immune response, the rapidity of development of response was quicker, and the persistence of antibody at higher concentrations was greater (Patil et al. 2002). Vaccinating goats for FMD at the same time other vaccines are given does not adversely affect the host response (Gogoi et al. 2004).

Public concerns of animal welfare sparked by images of the mass destruction of livestock in the UK during the FMD outbreak of 2001 have stimulated considerable discussion among scientists and regulatory policy makers on the use of vaccination to control FMD as a way of reducing the slaughter of animals. The topic is complex and beyond the scope of this presentation. More extensive discussions of the role of vaccination in FMD control are available elsewhere (LeForban 2002; Pluimers et al. 2002; Radostits et al. 2007).

There is considerable ongoing research to develop new and more effective FMD vaccines. Objectives include identification of antigens which might confer immunity across multiple serotypes, vaccine formulations that may stimulate more rapid and stronger protective responses, and vaccines which contain antigenic markers that can be used in serologic testing to distinguish between vaccinated and naturally infected animals. Recent developments in FMD vaccine technology have been reviewed (Barnett and Carabin 2002; Grubman and Baxt 2004; Grubman 2005). There is also interest in the use of antiviral compounds such as type 1 interferon which, if administered to animals at risk in an outbreak, can block the establishment of new infections (Grubman 2005).

Akabane Disease

Akabane virus infection is a cause of congenital arthrogryposis and hydrancephaly in kids, lambs, and calves in Asia, Africa, the Middle East, and Australia.

Etiology

Akabane virus is a helical, enveloped, single-stranded RNA bunyavirus in the Simbu group of the family Bunyaviridae. The virus can be cultivated in chick embryos or Vero cell or hamster lung cell cultures, and passaged in suckling mice. It is an insect-transmitted arbovirus. The principal vector is the biting midge *Culicoides brevitarsis* but some other *Culicoides* spp. and some species of *Aedes* and *Culex* mosquitoes are also known to carry the virus. Other arthropod-borne bunyaviruses in the Simbu group, the Aino and Peaton viruses, can also infect ruminants and cause congenital defects but there are as of yet no reports of clinical disease in goats with these two viruses. Antibodies to Tinaroo and Douglas viruses, non-pathogenic members of the Simbu group, have also been reported in goats (Cybinski 1984).

Epidemiology

The host range of Akabane virus includes goats, sheep, cattle, camels, horses, donkeys, and zebras, as well as other wild ruminants. Clinical disease has been observed only in goats, sheep, and cattle. Congenital arthrogryposis and hydrancephaly of domestic ruminants caused by the Akabane virus have been known in Australia and Japan for decades. Epizootics involving goats, cattle, and sheep have been reported from Japan (Inaba 1979) and Israel (Shimshony 1980). The virus infection is enzootic in Southeast Asia, extending northward to Japan and Korea, southward to northern and eastern Australia, and westward to the Middle East and eastern Africa. In Kenya, 50% to 90% of cattle sampled had serologic evidence of infection, while prevalence in goats and sheep was only 13% to 33% (Davies and Jessett 1985). New Zealand is free of infection (Oliver 1988). The infection is unknown in the Western Hemisphere, but in the United States another bunyavirus outside of the Simbu group, Cache Valley virus, has been associated with congenital arthrogryposis and hydrancephaly in sheep (Edwards et al. 1989). While there is serologic evidence of infection in goats, case reports in goats are rare (Edwards et al. 2003). The virus is discussed further in Chapter 13.

The geographic pattern of infection reflects closely the habitat of the arthropod vectors. In Australia, *Culicoides brevitarsis* is the only certain vector. Akabane virus has been isolated from *C. wadai* but no further studies have been carried out to confirm it as a vector (Animal Health Australia 2001). In Japan, *Culicoides oxystoma* may be the principal vector (Kurogi et al 1987), but the virus also has been isolated from the mosquitoes *Aedes vexans* and *Culex tritaeniorhynchus*. In the Middle East, the principal vector is *Culicoides imicola* (Brenner 2004). New infections with Akabane virus occur when weather conditions permit large populations of *Culicoides* to develop and expand or be carried by wind beyond their normal distribution limits (Al-Busaidy et al. 1988). Naive populations of livestock are then exposed.

Seroconversion occurs if these animals are nonpregnant, but no disease is observed (Sellers and Herniman 1981). If animals are pregnant, then abortions, stillbirths, or congenital defects are noted. Congenital defects are most likely when dams are infected in early gestation. Malformations in goat kids are common when infection occurs between days thirty and fifty of gestation and kids are normal when infection occurs during the last one hundred days of gestation (Kurogi et al. 1977; Shimshony 1980). Epizootics tend to occur at four- to six-year intervals, presumably when immune animal populations are replaced by younger, naive populations.

Neonatal losses can be severe. In the Israeli epizootic of 1969 to 1970, 563 kids were affected, representing up to 50% of the kids born in some herds. Goats appeared more susceptible than sheep, and male, twin kids were more often affected than female, single kids (Shimshony 1980).

Pathogenesis

Infection with Akabane virus does not result in clinical disease unless animals are pregnant. Virus is introduced to susceptible hosts through insect bites. A viremia usually of a two- to four-day duration ensues; in pregnant dams, the virus enters the placenta and fetus. The primary site of viral damage in the fetus is the developing neural tube. In calves, with a bovine gestation of nine months, the outcome of fetal infection depends on the stage of fetal development, with hydrancephaly alone occurring with early infection, hydrancephaly and arthrogryposis occurring in later infection, and arthrogryoposis occurring alone in still later infection. Goats have a shorter gestation and, as mentioned above, fetal malformations develop when infection occurs between days thirty and fifty of gestation, and both hydrancephaly and arthrogryposis may be seen together in affected kids.

In hydrancephaly, occlusion of the ependymal system leads to increased cerebrospinal fluid pressure and dilatation of the ventricles, resulting in progressive degeneration and thinning of the cerebral cortex. The cerebellum and brain stem are less frequently affected. Loss of mentation, blindness, and incoordination result from this process. In arthrogryposis, there is a marked diminution or disappearance of ventral horn cells in the spinal cord that leads to a neuromyodysplasia. The failure of normal muscle development in the limbs and along the vertebral column results in muscle dystrophy, tendon contracture, and permanently flexed or extended joints. The joints themselves are normal. Infected fetuses produce antibody to the Akabane virus, and serum samples obtained before the neonate's ingestion of colostrum can be used to diagnose infection.

Clinical Findings

Infection of nonpregnant goats is subclinical. Pregnant goats may remain healthy but abort or deliver stillborn kids. Veterinarians may first encounter Akabane disease when assisting a goat in labor, because dystocias are common when arthrogryposis is present. During epizootics, cattle and sheep in the practice area may also be delivering abnormal calves and lambs. Kids with arthrogryposis are usually born alive and at term. They are unable to rise and affected joints are rigidly flexed or extended. There is severe muscle wasting; there may be scoliosis or wry neck. With hydrancephaly, the kids may be dummies. They may be able to stand and walk if arthrogryposis is not concurrent, but the gait may be uncoordinated. These kids are usually blind and unaware of their surroundings. If a nipple or teat is placed in the mouth, they may suck.

Clinical Pathology and Necropsy

Umbilical and heart blood samples or thoracic fluid from aborted fetuses, or precolostral blood samples from live kids should be tested for antibody to Akabane virus. Serum neutralization titers of 1:2 or more are considered evidence of fetal infection and the mean titer of infected goats tested in Israel was 1:18 (Kalmar et al. 1975). Titers measured using the hemagglutination inhibition test correlate closely with serum neutralization test results (Furuya et al. 1980). AGID and ELISA tests are also in use. If aborted fetuses or precolostral serum in kids are not available, increased titers from paired serum samples in does or in surviving kids will indicate recent infection.

Gross necropsy findings of hydrancephaly are a marked thinning or total disintegration of the cerebral cortex. Occasionally, cerebellar hypoplasia is also observed. In arthrogryposis, the joints are inflexible due to tendon contracture and the muscle bundles surrounding the long bones may seem absent or significantly reduced in volume. The muscles may appear fibrotic and grayish-white. If tendons around the joints are cut, the joints move freely and there are no lesions on articular surfaces. Scoliosis, kyphosis, and torticollis may be observed.

Microscopically, there is muscular dystrophy with loss of striation and disappearance of muscle fibers with replacement by fat and connective tissue. Lesions in the spinal cord include a dilated central canal and ventral fissure, cavitation of the ventral gray horns with neuronal degeneration, and edema. In the cerebrum, there is hydrocephalus or more extreme hydrancephaly, subependymal gliosis, and generalized edema. Edema may also be prominent in the cerebellum, and Purkinje cell degeneration is common (Nobel et al. 1971).

Virus may be present in tissues of affected kids or aborted fetuses, especially in the central nervous system and muscles (Kurogi et al. 1977). However, virus isolation is not usually successful because neutralizing antibody is also present in the kid.

Diagnosis

Akabane disease is diagnosed on the basis of arthrogryposis and/or hydrancephaly in newborn kids and the identification of a positive antibody titer in those kids or aborted fetuses. The possibility remains that other bunyaviruses which produce similar congenital disease in cattle and sheep may be reported to do so as well in goats, but so far this has not been confirmed. Currently, the differential diagnosis for congenital arthrogryposis-hydrancephaly in goats is limited to beta mannosidosis, the inherited lysosomal storage disease that can produce arthrogryposis but not hydrancephaly and occurs only in Nubian or Nubian-crossbred goats. Bluetongue is an important consideration in sheep, but goats, while frequently seropositive for bluetongue, rarely develop clinical disease. If they do, adult animals are also likely to show signs.

Treatment and Control

There is no treatment for Akabane virus infection. Affected kids do not survive long without a good deal of nursing care. There is no practical way to control the insect vectors. However, effective killed vaccines have been developed and are used in Australia and Japan, where epizootics have previously occurred. Vaccination should be carried out in advance of the breeding season.

BACTERIAL DISEASES

Mycoplasma arthritis

Mycoplasma infections account for serious morbidity and mortality in goats throughout the world. Several distinct disease entities are recognized, notably contagious caprine pleuropneumonia, contagious agalactia, and infectious keratoconjunctivitis. However, mycoplasma infections are usually septicemic, and polyarthritis frequently occurs in these and other *Mycoplasma* spp. infections of goats.

Etiology

The study of caprine mycoplasmosis remains an active and dynamic field, with new species and strains being identified and old species and strains being renamed and reclassified. The frequent identification of new isolates coupled with historical problems of erroneous taxonomic identification of old isolates has produced some considerable confusion about the various causes of caprine mycoplasmosis. The current status of important mycoplasma infections in goats has been recently reviewed (Ruffin 2001; Al-Momani and Nicholas 2006).

Genera of the prokaryotic class Mollicutes that infect goats include *Mycoplasma*, *Ureaplasma*, and *Acholeplasma*. Species of importance in goats are identified in Table 4.3; the main pathogens are *Mycoplasma* spp. The first four *Mycoplasma* spp. listed in Table 4.3 belong to the so-called *M. mycoides* cluster, a group comprised of six species with shared biochemical, serological, genomic, and antigenic characteristics. Four of these species are pathogenic for goats. This soon may be reduced to three because, at the time of this writing, there is a proposal under consideration by the International Organization for Mycoplasmology to reclassify *M. mycoides* subsp. *mycoides* large colony (LC) type as *M. mycoides* subsp. *capri* on the basis of 16S rRNA

Table 4.3. *Mycoplasma* spp. isolated from goats.

Mycoplasma species	*Other hosts*	*Infected tissues*		*Associated diseases in goats*	*Pathogenicity*	*Geographic distribution*
		Primary	*Other*			
M. capricolum subsp. *capricolum*	Sheep	Joints	Udder, lungs, ears, urogenital tract, eyes; septicemia possible	Polyarthritis, mastitis, pneumonia, neonatal death, keratoconjunctivitis	High	Australia, India, Europe, United States, Egypt
M. capricolum subsp. *capripneumoniae* (formerly strain F38)	Goats only	Respiratory tract	Potential for septicemia	Contagious caprine pleuropneumonia (CCPP)	High	Currently Near East, Africa
M. mycoides subsp. *capri**	Goats only	Respiratory tract	Joints, ears	Pleuropneumonia, arthritis	Moderate	Africa, Middle East, western Asia, southern and eastern Europe

Table 4.3. *Continued*

Mycoplasma species	*Other hosts*	*Infected tissues*		*Associated diseases in goats*	*Pathogenicity*	*Geographic distribution*
		Primary	*Other*			
M. mycoides subsp. *mycoides* (large-colony type)*	Rare in sheep; very rare in calves	Respiratory tract	Udder, joints, eyes, ears, potential for septicemia	Pleuropneumonia, mastitis, arthritis, keratoconjunctivitis, neonatal death, abortion	Moderate	Europe, Africa, Asia, Australia, North America
M. agalactiae	Sheep	Udder	Joints, eyes, urogenital tract, ears, rarely lungs	Contagious agalactia (CA), arthritis, pneumonia, keratoconjunctivitis, vulvovaginitis	High	Europe, United States, former USSR, Asia, North Africa
M. arginini	Sheep, chamois, many others	Respiratory tract	Urogenital tract, joints, eyes	Pneumonia, arthritis, keratoconjunctivitis, vulvovaginitis	Very low or non-pathogenic	Worldwide
M. conjunctivae	Sheep, chamois	Eyes	Respiratory tract, rarely joints	Keratoconjunctivitis, pneumonia, arthritis	Moderate	Worldwide
M. ovipneumoniae	Sheep	Respiratory tract	Eyes, urogenital tract	Initiator of pneumonia	Low	Worldwide
M. putrefaciens	Goats only	Udder	Joints, ears	Mastitis, arthritis	Variable	United States, France, Australia
M. mycoides subsp. *mycoides* (small colony type)	Primarily cattle; very rare in goats	Respiratory tract	Joints	Pleuropneumonia, polyarthritis	Unknown	Africa
M. bovigenitalium (same as ovine/caprine M. serogroup 11)+	Primarily cattle and buffaloes; also sheep and goats	Reproductive tract	Udder, joints	Vulvovaginitis, cervicitis, endometritis, epididymitis, oophoritis, mastitis, arthritis	Variable with strain	Worldwide
Acholeplasma laidlawi	Many other hosts	Urogenital tract	Respiratory tract	No clinical disease produced	Non-pathogenic	Worldwide
Acholeplasma oculi	Sheep, cattle, horses, pigs	Eyes	Urogenital tract, lungs	Keratoconjunctivitis	Not well established	United States, United Kingdom, Japan, India
Ureaplasmas	Goat-specific strains exist	Urogenital tract	Respiratory tract	Vulvovaginitis	Not well established	Worldwide

*At the time of publication of this text, the International Organization for Mycoplasmology was considering action on combining *M. mycoides* subsp. *capri* and *M. mycoides* subsp. *mycoides* (large colony type) under the designation *M. mycoides* subsp. *capri* because they have been found to be identical in all but a few serological differences.

+At the time of publication of this text, it was proposed that *M. bovigenitalium* and ovine/caprine *Mycoplasma* serogroup 11 be combined under the designation *M. bovigenitalium* because of serological, structural, and genetic similarities (Nicholas et al. 2008).

sequencing which indicates a 99.9% phylogenetic similarity (Pettersson et al. 1996). The other two caprine pathogens in the *M. mycoides* cluster are *M. capricolum* subsp. *capricolum* and *M. capricolum* subsp. *capripneumoniae*.

Historically, there have been two forms of the species called *M. mycoides* subsp. *mycoides* in the *M. mycoides* cluster that shared similar immunologic and serologic characteristics but differed on the basis of colony morphology and specific biochemical tests (Cottew and Yeats 1978). The small colony (SC) type is the cause of contagious bovine pleuropneumonia (CBPP) and has been isolated from goats only rarely. The large colony (LC) type is principally a pathogen of goats and has a much wider geographic distribution. It only rarely infects cattle.

Reports of *M. mycoides* subsp. *mycoides* from diagnostic laboratories should clearly distinguish between these two organisms based on colony size and other discriminating factors to avoid confusion about the potential spread of CBPP to areas free from the disease, as CBPP is a highly regulated disease globally. This problem is less likely in the future as more sophisticated techniques such as PCR are applied for organism identification and because *M. mycoides* subsp. *mycoides* LC is likely to be reclassified and reported as *M. mycoides* subsp. *capri*, as mentioned above.

In addition to the established mycoplasmas identified in Table 4.3 as caprine pathogens, other mycoplasmas are reported from goats and new strains are continually being recognized. *M. bovis*, ordinarily a cattle pathogen, was isolated from a goat with pneumonia and found to be capable of causing caprine mastitis (Ojo and Ikede 1976). *M. bovigenitalium* has been isolated from the genital tracts of does with repeat breeding problems in India (Pathak et al. 1989), and recently it has been proposed that strains of the *Mycoplasma* ovine/caprine serogroup 11 be reclassified as *M. bovigenitalium* (Nicholas et al. 2008). The untyped strains G145 and A1343 have been isolated from goats in the United States (Al-Aubaidi 1972). Untyped strains identified as G, U, and V have been isolated from swabs of the ear canal of goats in Australia (Cottew and Yeats 1982). Several additional untyped strains have been isolated from ear swabs of California goats as well (DaMassa 1983).

Mycoplasmas are distinguished from other bacteria in that they do not have a rigid cell wall, and they possess only a cell membrane. They have the smallest genome of any free-living organism, but are capable of considerable phenotypic variation, producing variable surface proteins through complex genetic mechanisms which assist in evasion of the host immune system and adherence to host cells (Ruffin 2001). Mycoplasmas can be grown *in vitro* on culture medium but they are very fastidious and have numerous special growth requirements, including serum factors and yeast extracts. Many species produce characteristic spreading colonies with a "fried-egg" appearance. In general, these organisms are fragile away from the host and are rapidly inactivated by sunlight, dehydration, and heat, but are more resistant to cold. Effective disinfectants include formalin, phenols, cresols, peracetic acid, and iodophores. Procedures for the cultivation and differentiation of important caprine mycoplasmas have been reviewed (Nicholas and Baker 1998; Nicholas 2002).

Epidemiology

Arthritis caused by Mycoplasma in goats has been associated with numerous species. Major causes of importance include *M. agalactiae, M. capricolum, M. mycoides* subsp. *capri, M. mycoides* subsp. *mycoides* LC type, and *M. putrefaciens*. Minor causes include *M. arginini, M. conjunctivae*, and *M. mycoides* subsp. *mycoides* SC type.

M. agalactiae is the cause of contagious agalactia in goats and sheep and is discussed further in Chapter 14. Currently the disease is reported from Africa, Europe, Asia, and the Middle East, and is enzootic in much of the Mediterranean region. In the past, sporadic reports of *M. agalactiae* associated with arthritis and mastitis in individual goats have come from California (Jasper and Dellinger 1979; DaMassa 1983a). Goats are considered more susceptible than sheep. The highest incidence of disease is recorded in late spring and summer when does have kidded and are lactating. The morbidity can approach 100% and mortality ranges from 10% to 30%. The disease is characterized by the concurrent appearance of mastitis, arthritis, and keratoconjunctivitis, which are unlikely to be found together in a single animal, but are likely to be found throughout the herd. Respiratory involvement is minimal or absent. Transmission is by direct contact with infected animals or their discharges, including milk, urine, and lacrimal and nasal secretions. Introduction into the udder during milking is important in the spread of infection. Chronically ill or convalescent goats can sporadically shed the organism (Blaha 1989).

Contagious agalactia is considered by the World Organization for Animal Health (OIE) to be a transmissible disease of socio-economic importance within affected countries and also significant in the international trade of animals and animal products. As such it is regulated by governments in the international trade of livestock. Historically, *M. agalactiae* was recognized as the definitive etiologic agent of contagious agalactia. However, in recent years it has become clearer that *M. capricolum* subsp. *capricolum, M. putrefaciens*, and *M. mycoides* subsp. *mycoides LC* type (which may be identical to *M. mycoides* subsp. *capri*) also cause contagious agalactia syndromes in goats that are largely indistinguishable from classic contagious agalactia. Therefore, the OIE now recognizes all four organisms as causes of contagious agalactia for regulatory purposes (OIE 2004b). All four organisms frequently produce arthritis in goats in addition to mastitis, and they may also produce keratoconjunctivitis and/or pneumonia. The role of the various etiologic agents in contagious agalactia syndrome has been reviewed (Egwu et al. 2000).

M. capricolum subsp. *capricolum* has a worldwide distribution and is considered to be highly pathogenic, yet disease due to this organism has been reported only sporadically from diverse geographic locations, including California (Cordy et al. 1955), France (Perreau and Breard 1979), Spain (Talavera Boto 1980), Australia (Littlejohns and Cottew 1977), Egypt (El-Zeftawi 1979), India (Banerjee et al. 1979; Sikdar and Uppal 1983), and Morocco (Taoudi 1988). Morbidity and mortality in these reports are quite variable. Arthritis is the predominant sign in *M. capricolum* subsp. *capricolum* infection, but neonatal septicemia, pneumonia, keratoconjunctivitis, mastitis, and agalactia can also be seen. Transmission of *M. capricolum* subsp. *capricolum* occurs by direct contact with infected goats; inhalation of the organism from feces, urine, or respiratory discharges; and especially by ingestion of infected milk by sucking kids (DaMassa et al. 1983).

M. mycoides subsp. *mycoides* LC type, which may be identical to *M. mycoides* subsp. *capri* and soon renamed as such, has a worldwide distribution. It is a frequently reported caprine mycoplasma infection in the United States, particularly from eastern and western coastal states (DaMassa et al. 1983a; Kinde et al. 1994). Kids are more frequently and severely affected than adults. Though variable, mastitis may affect 25% to 33% of does, while morbidity and mortality rates may exceed 90% in kids on the same premises.

The most common clinical findings in adults are fever, mastitis, pleuropneumonia, and arthritis. In kids, arthritis, septicemia, and meningitis are more common. In addition, polyserositis, osteomyelitis, keratoconjunctivitis, abscesses, and abortion are also reported. Reports from France, California, and Israel suggest that morbidity and mortality are highest in intensive commercial goat dairy operations (Bar Moshe and Rapapport 1981; Perreau et al. 1981; DaMassa et al. 1983a; East et al. 1983). In an outbreak in a goat dairy in North Carolina in 1996, forty-seven of sixty-five kids (72.3%) either died or had to be euthanized due to polyarthritis and/or septicemia (Butler et al. 1998). Economic losses caused by decreased production, diagnosis and treatment costs, and death of replacement stock can be devastating in severe outbreaks.

Infected, lactating does can be asymptomatic carriers, with high numbers of organisms being shed in the milk. These does may become clinically ill themselves as a result of management, nutritional, or climatic stresses. The most explosive disease outbreaks occur among kids after the onset of kidding season. The principal mode of transmission to kids is the oral route via daily ingestion of infected colostrum and milk (DaMassa et al. 1983a). The mode of transmission among adults is not as clear. Direct contact is possible but not very efficient (Rosendal 1983). Transfer of infection during the milking process by introduction into the teat seems to play a larger role, particularly because improvement of sanitary procedures slows infection rates in known-infected herds (East et al. 1983). Infection may be introduced into a herd by the introduction of subclinically infected milking does (East et al. 1983). In New Zealand, an outbreak of polyarthritis in dairy calves due to *M. mycoides* subsp. *mycoides* LC type was linked to consumption of unpasteurized bulk goat milk from an affected dairy goat herd (Jackson and King 2002).

From a historical perspective, it is worth noting that *M. mycoides* subsp. *capri* was long considered to be the primary cause of contagious caprine pleuropneumonia (CCPP). Though the organism can indeed produce a pleuropneumonia, the causative agent of the classically described disease CCPP, which occurs exclusively in goats, is now known to be *Mycoplasma capricolum* subsp. *capripneumoniae*, and was formerly known as the *Mycoplasma F38* strain. While *Mycoplasma capricolum* subsp. *capripneumoniae* infects only goats, *M. mycoides* subsp. *capri* can also infect sheep and cattle experimentally.

M. putrefaciens infects goats in the United States, Europe, and the Middle East. It was first isolated from mastitic goats in California in 1955 and identified as a distinct species in 1974. It has been identified with arthritis in kids in Spain (Rodríguez et al. 1994), mastitis and arthritis in goats in France (Gaillard-Perrin et al. 1986), and mastitis and arthritis in goats in California. The potential for economic catastrophe with *M. putrefaciens* infection is pronounced. An outbreak in California in 1987 resulted in the destruction of an entire herd of 700 goats because of widespread mastitis, arthritis, and abortions (DaMassa et al. 1987).

The major mode of transmission of this organism among adults is by introduction through the teat due to poor hygiene during milking. For kids, the disease is spread by feeding of infected colostrum or milk. Stresses such as crowding, poor nutrition, and lack of shelter from wind and rain may predispose kids to clinical disease. Intensive dairy operations are likely to be hardest hit. A serologic survey in California indicated that Angora goats recently imported from Texas had a higher prevalence of infection than indigenous dairy breeds, but clinical disease caused by *M. putrefaciens* has not been recorded in Angoras

(Abegunde et al. 1981). In France, *M. putrefaciens* was identified as a cause of mastitis in a dairy goat herd and was treated with apparent success. However, at the beginning of the next lactation, *M. putrefaciens* could still be cultured from the udders, even though udders and milk were normal (Mercier et al. 2000).

All of the major mycoplasma species discussed above have been found in the ear canals and ear mites of normal goats. This represents an effective means for maintaining a carrier state and transmitting new infections to susceptible goats (Cottew and Yeats 1982; DaMassa 1983, 1990). In addition, all the species except *M. mycoides* subsp. *capri* have been isolated from the nasal and oral cavities and tonsils of clinically normal goats at necropsy (Cottew and Yeats 1981).

Among the minor causes of caprine mycoplasma arthritis, *M. arginini* is probably the least consequential. This ubiquitous organism causes minimal disease alone (Goltz et al. 1986) and is often isolated from clinically normal goats. It is frequently isolated in conjunction with other bacterial pathogens such as *Pasteurella* spp. from pneumonic lungs, and may serve as an initiator of bacterial pneumonia. There are occasional reports of *M. arginini* being isolated from the joints of arthritic goats (Barile et al. 1968; Al-Aubaidi et al. 1972), but the etiologic significance in arthritis is doubtful.

M. conjunctivae is found worldwide and associated primarily with keratoconjunctivitis in sheep and goats. However, it has the potential to become septicemic, and concurrent pneumonia and arthritis have been observed in at least one outbreak of keratoconjunctivitis caused by *M. conjunctivae* in a goat herd (Baas et al. 1977). The ocular disease is discussed in more detail in Chapter 6.

M. mycoides subsp. *mycoides* SC type is the cause of contagious bovine pleuropneumonia (CBPP). Although the disease is enzootic in cattle in many parts of Africa, and occurs sporadically in southern Europe with the last outbreak occurring in Portugal in 1999, the organism rarely infects goats. There are four published reports of caprine infection. The organism was isolated from joints of polyarthritic goats in New Guinea in 1955 and again from goats in Sudan and Nigeria in the 1960s. These represent, respectively, the O, P, and Vom strains (Cottew 1979). Most recently, it was isolated in Portugal from a ewe with mastitis and two goats with pneumonia (Brandao 1995). CBPP is a highly contagious disease and there is considerable effort to control its spread, particularly in Africa. There are concerns that goats may serve as a reservoir for *M. mycoides* subsp. *mycoides* SC type and thereby confound efforts to eradicate the disease in cattle (Sharew et al. 2005).

Mixed or concurrent mycoplasma infections causing arthritis and mastitis in goat herds can occur. An outbreak in a Saanen herd in Spain involved *M. agalactiae* and *M. putrefaciens* (Gil et al. 1999) while a large goat herd in California experienced arthritis, mastitis, and sudden death due to *M. agalactiae* and *M. mycoides* subsp. *mycoides* LC type (Kinde et al. 1994). Both organisms were producing disease in the herd, but no affected individual goat was infected with both agents.

Pathogenesis

Mycoplasmal arthritis in goats always occurs as a result of septicemia. Therefore, it frequently involves multiple joints and is accompanied by generalized malaise, fever, and evidence of infection at other organ sites. Septicemic goats may die without manifestation of localizing signs.

Experimental infections with *M. mycoides* subsp. *mycoides* (LC type) in goats suggest that vasculitis, coagulopathy, and thrombosis play significant roles in the pathogenesis of mycoplasma septicemia, leading to infarction and necrosis in numerous organs (Rosendal 1981; Bolske et al. 1989). Complement activation by *M. mycoides* subsp. *mycoides* LC type may also be an important initiator of inflammation (Rosendal 1984). The pathogenic mechanisms of *M. mycoides* subsp. *mycoides* SC type have recently been reviewed (Pilo et al. 2007) and may serve as a framework for understanding mycoplasma pathogenicity in general.

Unlike other bacterial species whose virulence is determined by factors such as toxins and invasins, the virulence factors of *Mycoplasma* species seem to be determined by intrinsic metabolic or catabolic pathway functions or by proper constituents of the mycoplasmal outer surface. In *M. mycoides* subsp. *mycoides* SC type, a few virulence determinants have been identified, including capsular polysaccharide, which may give the organism the capacity to persist and disseminate in the host. In addition, there are adhesion factors, immunomodulating factors, and toxic metabolic pathway products, which exert cytotoxic effects. One example of the latter is the production of large amounts of cytotoxic H_2O_2 facilitated by the organism's capacity to import and metabolize glycerol.

Clinical Findings

Mycoplasma arthritis may be seen in all ages and breeds of goats but is most common in young kids and yearlings in dairy goat breeds. In many instances, there is a history of purchased goats introduced into the herd some months before onset of disease. Arthritis rarely occurs alone in an outbreak of mycoplasmosis. Mastitis, abortion, agalactia, pneumonia, or keratoconjunctivitis may occur concurrently or precede the onset of arthritis. The presentation may vary with age or production group. For example, mastitis may occur in lactating does several months before arthritis is noted in kids. This underscores the importance of obtaining a thorough history. There is a tendency for disease incidence to increase around the kidding season.

Affected animals usually first show evidence of septicemia including fever of 104°F to 108.5°F (40°C to 42.5°C), anorexia, depression, weakness, and rough hair coat. One exception is in *M. putrefaciens* infection, where fever does not regularly occur (DaMassa et al. 1987). Some animals may die of septicemia without developing additional localizing signs. In most cases involving arthritis, lameness develops concurrently or within several days of the onset of fever but may precede the onset of joint swelling. Though a single joint may be affected, polyarthritis is the rule. Any diarthrodial joint may be involved but the carpi, tarsi, and stifle joints are most frequently affected, followed by the elbow and fetlock joints. The joints become swollen, hot, and painful. The pain is frequently so severe that affected goats refuse to bear weight on a single affected leg, or become persistently recumbent when multiple joints are involved. The clinical course is usually four to ten days and commonly ends in death if not treated. Occasional spontaneous recoveries occur, sometimes with complete resolution of joint swelling and lameness noted over several weeks. Morbidity and mortality are almost always higher in kids and yearlings than adults.

Goats with hot swollen joints should be carefully examined for indications of other organ system involvement, especially nasal discharges, increased lung sounds, corneal opacity or conjunctivitis, and mastitis or agalactia, all of which can occur in mycoplasmosis. Diarrhea is not usually associated with mycoplasmosis but has been reported in affected kids concurrently experiencing coccidiosis (East et al. 1983).

Clinical Pathology and Necropsy

Leukopenia with neutropenia is likely in the early stage of septicemia, and neutrophilic leukocytosis with hyperfibrinogenemia in the later stages. Synovial fluid analysis can be useful in diagnosing arthritic mycoplasmosis. While the volume of fluid may not be increased, the color is frequently yellow to red-brown, and cytologic examination reveals increased cellularity, particularly with increased numbers of neutrophils.

Diagnosis of mycoplasmosis requires isolation or identification of the organism or confirmation of serologic evidence of infection. Culture techniques are available for isolation of the organism, and have been improved in recent years, making culture a more reliable diagnostic method than in the past. Nevertheless, two species—*M. capricolum* subsp. *capripneumoniae*, the cause of CCPP, and *M. conjunctivae* are highly fastidious and remain more difficult to culture reliably.

The World Organization for Animal Health recommendations for preferred samples from living animals include: nasal swabs and secretions, milk from mastitic females or from apparently healthy females where there is a high rate of mortality/morbidity in kids, joint fluid from arthritic cases, and eye swabs from cases of ocular disease. Blood may yield mycoplasmas during the acute stage of the disease when there is mycoplasmaemia, but blood may also be taken for antibody detection from affected and non-affected animals. The ear canal can also be a productive source of pathogenic mycoplasmas, although the presence of nonpathogenic mycoplasmas in the ear canal may make confirmation difficult. At necropsy, samples should include: udder and associated lymph nodes, joint fluid, lung tissue taken at the interface of healthy and diseased lung and pleural/pericardial fluid. Samples should be dispatched quickly to a diagnostic laboratory in a moist and cool condition (OIE 2004b).

Biochemical tests still play an important role in differentiating isolates from culture, but identification of isolates can also be achieved using specific antisera in growth inhibition tests, film inhibition tests, the indirect fluorescent antibody (IFA) test, or a rapid dot immunobinding test. Polymerase chain reaction (PCR) assays have emerged as important diagnostic tools for identification of mycoplasmas. For instance, a set of PCR tests was developed that could detect all members of the *M. mycoides* cluster and distinguish *M. mycoides* subsp. *mycoides* LC type and *M. mycoides* subsp. *capri* from *M. capricolum* subsp. *capripneumoniae* and *M. capricolum* subsp. *capricolum* (Bashiruddin et al. 1994). Another PCR can specifically identify *M. capricolum* subsp. *capripneumoniae* (Woubit et al. 2004) and another specifically *M. agalactiae* (Tola et al. 1997). More recently, a new diagnostic test based on PCR of the 16S rRNA gene with *Mycoplasma*-specific primers and separation of the PCR product according to primary sequence using denaturing gradient gel electrophoresis (DGGE) allowed for the differentiation of sixty-seven *Mycoplasma* spp. of human and veterinary origin (McAuliffe et al. 2005).

PCR tests can be used directly on field samples when there is urgency in the need for a diagnosis, or they can be applied to organisms growing in culture. When used on field samples, false-negative results are possible.

Complement fixation tests, ELISA, and immunoblotting tests are used for serologic testing. ELISAs currently tend to be favored over complement fixation tests because of their greater sensitivity and ease of use for large scale testing (Nicholas 2002). Serologic tests are not generally used for the diagnosis of individual cases of mycoplasmosis, but can be valuable on a herd basis when acute and convalescent samples are obtained three to eight weeks apart. The application of diagnostic techniques for small ruminant mycoplasmosis has been reviewed (Nicholas and Baker 1998) and details of test methods recommended by the OIE for contagious agalactia syndrome and contagious caprine pleuropneumonia are available on the Internet (OIE 2004b, 2004c).

A variety of gross necropsy findings may occur in goats with septicemic mycoplasmosis. These include patchy or diffuse pneumonia; pulmonary congestion or edema; a watery, yellow or red-tinged hydrothorax; fibrinous pleuritis with adhesions to the chest wall; fibrinous pericarditis; serous or fibrinous peritonitis; meningitis; mastitis with firm, hyperemic glandular tissue; swollen, edematous lymph nodes; and fibrinopurulent arthritis.

In acute or peracute arthritis, synovial fluid is as described above. In advanced or severe cases, the affected joint is filled with a white to yellow fibrinopurulent exudate. There may be erosions of the articular cartilage; the joint capsule and periarticular tissues are hyperemic, thickened, and edematous; and fibrin tags may be noted extending up tendon sheaths.

Histologically, the joint lesion is characterized by necrosis of the synovium and joint capsule with fibrin covering the joint surfaces. There is congestion and edema of the subsynovial tissue with invasion of neutrophils into necrotic tissue and the joint spaces. Vasculitis and thrombosis may be observed with perivascular infiltrates of macrophages. Neutrophilic infiltration of adjacent bone marrow and foci of osteomyelitis may be present. Pneumonic and mammary lesions are described, respectively, in chapters 9 and 14. Other possible microscopic lesions observable in septicemic mycoplasmosis include myocardial and adrenal cortical necrosis, renal infarction, glomerulitis, enteritis, focal hepatic necrosis, focal splenic necrosis with depletion of white pulp, and lymphadenitis.

Diagnosis

Definitive diagnosis of mycoplasmosis of goats depends on isolation or identification of a known pathogenic *Mycoplasma* spp. from affected tissues. This is increasingly being accomplished with the aid of PCR. Veterinarians should suspect mycoplasma infection when arthritis occurs in conjunction with fever and generalized malaise, and when other localized infections such as pneumonia, mastitis, abortion, and keratoconjunctivitis occur in the herd or flock, either concurrently or historically. Mycoplasma infection should be considered even when a single case of arthritis is observed in a herd or flock as morbidity is not always high, and sporadic cases may precede a generalized outbreak. The differential diagnosis for caprine arthritis is given earlier in the chapter. The differential diagnoses for pneumonia, mastitis, abortion, and keratoconjunctivitis are discussed elsewhere in the text.

Treatment

The prognosis for recovery is generally poor in clinical mycoplasmosis involving arthritis, pneumonia, and mastitis, even with aggressive therapy. An extended course of parenteral antibiotic therapy is required, usually ranging from five to fourteen days. Complications of lameness from repeated injections are common. Because mycoplasmosis can spread rapidly through a herd or flock, all contact animals should be treated at the same time when the disease is identified in individual animals. Treatment, no matter how successful in controlling clinical disease, may not eliminate the carrier state. In fact, under some regulatory guidelines, treated animals are regarded as infected.

In general, *Mycoplasma* spp. are most often sensitive to tetracyclines, the macrolide antibiotics (tylosin, erythromycin, oleandomycin, spiramycin, tilmicosin), and tiamulin. The aminoglycosides, including spectinomycin, are sometimes effective, as are nitrofurans and chloramphenicol. Lincomycin has also been used successfully. Susceptibility of the various *Mycoplasma* spp. to these different antibiotics is variable, even within the same drug class, so that *in vitro* culture and sensitivity should be carried out whenever possible (Adler and Brooks 1982; Al-Momani et al. 2006). Antibiotics that inhibit cell wall peptidoglycan synthesis are not effective, and it is not unusual for owners to have treated mycoplasma infections unsuccessfully with penicillin before calling the veterinarian. There is also evidence that *Mycoplasma* spp. develop resistance to antibiotics. The *in vitro* susceptibility of various caprine mycoplasmas to a wide range of antibiotics has recently been reported (Al-Momani et al. 2006; Antunes et al. 2007).

A wide range of doses has been suggested for treatment of caprine mycoplasmosis, and antibiotic therapy is often met with less than satisfactory results. All the doses given here are for once daily intramuscular injection administered for at least five days: oxytetracycline at 15 mg/kg bw; streptomycin at 30 mg/kg bw, tiamulin at 20 mg/kg, and tylosin at doses of 5 to 44 mg/kg bw, but most commonly at 20 mg/kg. Spiramycin has been given at a loading dose of 50 mg/kg followed by daily doses of 25 mg/kg (Perreau 1979). More recently, the fluoroquinolone danofloxacin was reported to be highly effective in the treatment of CCPP when given at a dose of 6 mg/kg bw SQ once and repeated at forty-eight hours (Ozdemir et al. 2006).

Tiamulin was reported to be severely irritating at the injection site, producing general excitation in young goats (Ojo 1984). In poultry and swine, tiamulin given in conjunction with monensin produces a toxic myopathy (Pott and Skov 1981). Although not reported in goats, caution is advised when monensin is used as a coccidiostat at the time of tiamulin therapy. A combination of lincomycin at a dose of 5 mg/kg and spectinomycin at 10 mg/kg given intramuscularly once daily for 3 days produced recovery in 55% to 80% of treated goats and sheep with contagious agalactia in a field trial in Greece (Spais et al. 1981). Lincomycin used orally, however, has been associated with severe toxic reactions and high mortality in a large sheep flock in the United States (Bulgin 1988).

Control

Specific mycoplasmal diseases such as contagious agalactia and contagious caprine pleuropneumonia are of great regulatory concern to countries free of disease, and importation of goats from known infected countries is prohibited. Outbreaks are usually controlled by stamping out procedures. In enzootic regions, restrictions on animal movement, testing and culling of infected animals, and in some cases, vaccination are carried out. In France, vaccination for contagious agalactia is prohibited and control is based on test and slaughter.

A variety of vaccines are available and in use in various countries against *M. agalactiae, M. mycoides* subsp. *capri*, and *M. mycoides* subsp. *mycoides* LC type. In Europe, live mycoplasma vaccines are not acceptable and killed vaccines are used. Live vaccines may be more immunogenic but they also have been associated with transient infection and shedding of the organism, placing other animals at risk if they are not also vaccinated. An inactivated vaccine against *Mycoplasma capricolum* subsp. *capripneumoniae* to control CCPP is produced commercially in Kenya and is said to provide protection for one year (OIE 2004c).

There are several recommendations for controlling the introduction and spread of mycoplasmas in individual goat herds. Closed herds should be maintained where there is no history of mycoplasmosis, especially in commercial dairy operations. No animals should be purchased, and animals from the herd should not be brought to shows because of the risk of exposure to carrier animals.

When mycoplasmosis has occurred on the premises, management procedures should be evaluated, particularly in the areas of milking and kid rearing, and aggressive efforts made to reduce the risk of transmission (East et al. 1983; Rowe 2006). When mastitis has occurred, milk samples should be cultured from all lactating does, and infected, carrier does should be culled or at least managed as a separate string, housed and milked separately.

In the milking parlor, strict hygiene should be observed; a number of specific recommendations have been made (Rowe 2006). Does should be spray prewashed or pre-dipped and individual paper towels used to dry the udder. Post-milking teat dipping is also essential. Milkers should wear gloves and disinfect them between does. Teat cups should be back flushed or dipped in disinfectant between does, and thorough clean-up of the pipeline and milking equipment must be done after each milking. Does with elevated California mastitis test (CMT) reactions, elevated somatic cell counts (SCC), or clinical mastitis should be removed immediately from the milking string and a milk sample frozen for culture. Dairies should have weekly samples frozen from the tank for routine monitoring, and increase in SCC or increase in CMT on the dairy should be aggressively pursued.

Infected groups of kids should be culled to slaughter. Then, new kids should be separated from dams at birth and fed heat-treated colostrum prepared as described earlier in this chapter for control of caprine arthritis encephalitis virus infection. Kids should then be housed separately from adults and fed pasteurized milk or milk replacer. When these kids mature and reach their first lactation, the milk should be cultured and the doelings hand milked until a negative culture allows them to enter the milk string. Long-term surveillance by milk cultures should be continued in herds that have previously experienced mycoplasmosis. Regular herd-wide treatment of ear mite infestations is also advisable because of the potential role of these parasites in mycoplasma transmission. Systemic ivermectin is effective against *Psoroptes cuniculi*, but may not be effective against *Raillietia capra*. It should not be used in lactating does.

Bacterial Polyarthritis

Bacterial polyarthritis, also known as joint ill, occurs predominantly in neonates as a sequela to omphalophlebitis or bacteremia.

Etiology and Pathogenesis

A variety of bacteria have been isolated from joints of goats with arthritis. The most commonly reported isolates from kids include *Arcanobacterium* (*Actinomyces*) *pyogenes*, *Escherichia coli*, *Streptococcus* spp., and *Staphylococcus* spp., all common environmental contaminants that can gain entry into kids via the umbilicus (Guss 1977; Adams 1983; Nayak and Bhowmik 1988). More recently, *Streptococcus dysgalactiae* (Blanchard and Fiser 1994), *Pasteurella multocida* (Bhowmik and Dalapati 1995), and *Klebsiella pneumoniae* (Bernabé et al. 1998) have been reported as causes of caprine arthritis. Polyarthritis occurs secondary to bacteremia, when circulating bacteria localize in joints and produce a destructive inflammatory response. Underlying immunodeficiencies can predispose to the development of bacterial polyarthritis.

Historically, *Erysipelothrix rhusiopathiae*, a soil-borne pathogen, has been responsible for a high incidence of polyarthritis in young lambs after castration and tail docking, or as a result of navel infection. Improved hygiene and disinfection in lamb management have reduced the incidence of this disease and it is now considered to be of minor importance (Kimberling 1988). Some sources refer to *E. rhusiopathiae* polyarthritis as also occurring in kids (Guss 1977; Vaissaire et al. 1985). However, documented cases of infectious arthritis due to this organism in goats are scarce (Eamens et al. 1985). Similarly, texts or review articles sometimes refer to chlamydial arthritis in small ruminants. However, while the disease is well established in lambs, documentation of the condition in goats is lacking (Nietfeld 2001).

Epidemiology

Bacterial polyarthritis is most often seen in newborns and young kids after bacteremia. Factors that predispose these goats to bacteremia include kidding in contaminated environments, poor sanitation in housing, the development of omphalophlebitis after failure to disinfect the navel at birth, and failure of passive transfer of immunity via colostrum from the dam. Navel infection is not a prerequisite to bacteremia and polyarthritis. An outbreak due to *Klebsiella pneumoniae* occurred on a farm where navel disinfection was routine. It was postulated that infection occurred via the intestinal route in association with a recent switch to feeding artificial colostrum (Bernabé et al. 1998).

Bacterial polyarthritis is not restricted to young goats. An outbreak of infectious arthritis due to *Pasteurella multocida* affected twenty-two adult goats in a herd in India (Bhowmik and Dalpati 1995). Polyarthritis and limb edema with pain and reluctance to stand were seen in multiple adult Saanen does in a large California dairy goat herd. *Streptococcus dysgalactiae* was cultured from affected joints. While this organism is known to cause mastitis in cattle, mastitis was not a problem in this goat herd and the source of the infection was not identified. Interestingly, the herd was comprised of multiple dairy breeds but only Saanens were affected (Blanchard and Fiser 1994).

Clinical Signs

Affected kids have hot, swollen, painful joints, and may be reluctant to rise or walk. They usually have a fever in the range of 103°F to 105°F (39.4°C to 40.6°C). Carpi, stifles, and hocks are most often affected, but not exclusively. Any number of joints can be involved. Concurrent or previous episodes of diarrhea, pneumonia, or navel abscess are common. The umbilical stump should be palpated for evidence of omphalophlebitis.

Clinical Pathology and Necropsy

A neutrophilic leukocytosis or a leukopenia (in the case of Gram-negative sepsis) may be seen. Arthrocentesis reveals an abnormal, turbid, and flocculent synovial fluid with increased total protein and elevated cell counts consisting primarily of neutrophils (Nayak and Bhowmik 1990; Bhowmik and Dalapati 1995). Serum immunoglobulin levels are often low, reflecting the predisposing failure of passive transfer of colostral antibody. At necropsy, multiple joints may contain serofibrinous or purulent synovial fluid, and there is evidence of inflammation in the synovium and possibly cartilage erosion and hyperplasia of synovial villi. Evidence of infection may also be present in other organ systems, especially the lungs, gastrointestinal tract, and central nervous system. The umbilical remnant is often thickened and may contain focal abscesses.

Diagnosis

Bacterial polyarthritis and mycoplasma arthritis may occur in young goats under similar circumstances and with similar clinical presentations. Confirmation of the diagnosis and differentiation from mycoplasmosis depend on culture and identification of the causative agent.

Treatment

Successful therapeutic management of bacterial polyarthritis is difficult in goats, especially when economic constraints are present. Bacterial culture of affected joints and antibiotic sensitivity testing should be performed whenever possible. Joint lavage and intra-articular antibiotic therapy may be attempted in extremely valuable individuals. In most cases, practical therapy is limited to the parenteral administration of broad spectrum antibiotics and anti-inflammatory drugs. Little information is available about the concentration of various antibiotics in the joints of goats, and antibiotic selection is largely empirical. The prognosis for complete recovery in these cases is guarded.

Control

Bacterial polyarthritis is best managed by prevention. Extensively managed goats should have access to fresh, well-drained areas for kidding. For intensively managed goats, bedding should be changed frequently in kidding pens and pens disinfected regularly. Adequate and early ingestion of colostrum should be ensured. Umbilical cords should be left at least 4 cm long and dipped in disinfectant as soon after birth as possible. Tincture of iodine or strong (Lugol's) iodine solution are commonly used and effective. In problem herds, redipping navels on the second day may be helpful in controlling infection.

Osteomyelitis

Bacterial infections of the bone are infrequent in goats. When they occur, they most often result from

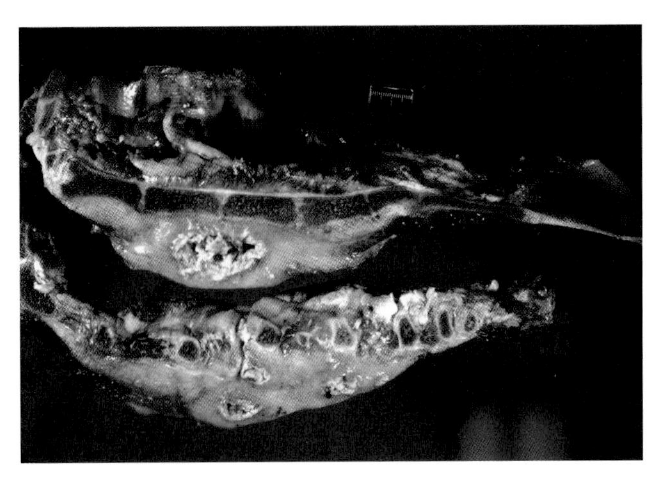

Figure 4.8. Cross section of the sternum of a goat showing a chronic abscess surrounded by much fibrous connective tissue, and with a tract penetrating the thorax. (Courtesy of Dr. M.C. Smith.)

septicemia or extension from local infections associated with puncture wounds or other types of trauma. The most common occurrence of osteomyelitis in goats involves the sternebrae secondary to skin trauma and chronic abscesses occurring in the soft tissues covering the sternum. These soft tissue lesions are associated with housing of goats on concrete or other hard surfaces with inadequate, wet, or unsanitary bedding and with prolonged sternal recumbency as is often associated with chronic CAE arthritis. If not treated early and aggressively, these infections become chronic and untreatable, leading to sternal osteomyelitis and possible extension into the chest, causing pleuritis and pneumonia (Figure 4.8). The prognosis is poor in these cases. Reports of successful treatment of osteomyelitis in goats with antibiotic therapy are lacking.

Other instances of osteomyelitis are sporadic. Infection of the femur has been reported in an eight-month-old Nubian buck secondary to septic gonitis. Lameness in the affected limb was severe. *Pseudomonas aeruginosa* was isolated from the stifle joint. The case was successfully managed by amputation of the affected limb (Ramadan et al. 1984).

Multifocal osteomyelitis due to *Corynebacterium renale* has been diagnosed in an eighteen-month-old French Alpine kid (Altmaier et al. 1994). The goat was lame on the right forelimb and radiographs revealed a fracture of the distal scapula associated with focal demineralization of bone and multifocal, lytic lesions in the ribs (Figure 4.9). At time of necropsy, osteomyelitis was confirmed and evidence of septicemia was present, with abscesses noted in intestine, lymph nodes, and liver.

An unusual multifocal *Rhodococcus equi* osteomyelitis of the skull and thoracic vertebrae has been recorded in a two-year-old Saanen doe in Australia. The clinical

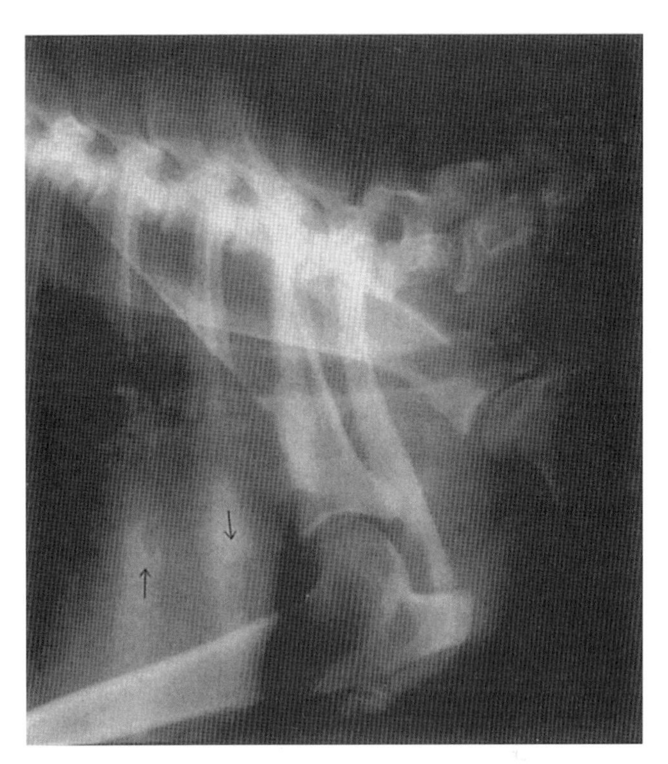

Figure 4.9. Radiographic evidence of osteomyelitis in the ribs of a goat (note arrows). (Courtesy of Cummings School of Veterinary Medicine at Tufts University.)

presentation was progressive posterior paralysis due to spinal cord involvement (Carrigan et al. 1988). Suppurative vertebral osteomyelitis and diskospondylitis have been reported in a three-week-old goat with acute hind limb paresis but the cause was not identified (Alexander et al. 2005).

Lyme Disease

Lyme disease or Lyme borreliosis is a tick-borne spirochetal disease of humans and animals originally described in people in Lyme, Connecticut, in 1977. The predominant clinical sign is arthritis. The disease is now known to occur in the northeastern, midwestern, and northwestern portions of the United States, as well as in Europe, Russia, China, Japan, and Australia, with a higher prevalence in forested regions. The causative agent is the spirochete *Borrelia burgdorferi* and it is transmitted mainly by *Ixodes* spp. ticks that normally complete their life cycle on deer and mice. Fragmentation of forest habitat and a concomitant increase in white-footed mouse (*Peromyscus leucopus*) populations relative to other small mammalian tick hosts is believed to be responsible for an increasing prevalence of the disease, at least in the United States (Ostfeld and LoGiudice 2003). Larval, nymph, and adult stages of *Ixodes* ticks are capable of transmitting the infection. While the different stages have different host feeding preferences among small and large mammals, all stages feed on and can infect humans. Risk of transmission is highest in spring and fall when nymphs and adults are most active.

Seroepidemiological studies on Lyme disease have been carried out around the world on various mammals and many of these surveys have included goats. The seroprevalence of antibodies to *B. burgdorferi* in goats has been reported as 5% in Bolivia (Ciceroni et al. 1997), 8.5% in France (Doby and Chevrier 1990), 17.2% to 19.4% in Slovakia (Travnieek et al. 2002), 18% in Egypt (Helmy 2000), 36.8% in Italy (Ciceroni et al. 1996), 48% in Bulgaria (Angelov et al. 1993), and between 19.1% and 61.3% in different provinces of China, with goats in mountainous regions having much higher seroprevalence than those in plains regions (Zhang et al. 1998; Long et al. 1999). A serosurvey of humans in the Canary Islands noted that male goat farmers had significantly higher seroprevalence than men of similar age who were not goat farmers and that the rate of seropositivity in goat farmers was three times higher than that of the general population. This suggests that goats may serve as a reservoir for human infection or that goat herders at pasture are more frequently exposed to infected ticks (Carranza et al. 1995). Assays for detection of antibody to *B. burgdorferi* currently in use include ELISA, the indirect immunofluorescent antibody test, and the western blot.

Clinical Lyme disease is well described in humans and dogs and also occurs in horses and cattle (Steere 1989). The disease in humans (Hengge et al. 2003) and in horses (Butler et al. 2005) has recently been reviewed. Cattle with acute Lyme disease show fever, a stiff gait, swollen joints, and decreased milk production. They may also show edematous lesions on the hairless skin of the udder and chronic weight loss (Radostits et al. 2007).

While goats and sheep commonly show serologic evidence of infection, definitive confirmation of clinical Lyme disease, manifested as arthritis, remains elusive in small ruminants. Two cases of suspected Lyme borreliosis in lambs were reported from Norway in 1992. The lambs were from flocks in a district heavily infested with *Ixodes ricinus* ticks and both had high serum IgG antibodies to *B. burgdorferi* by ELISA test, but attempts to isolate spirochetes were unsuccessful (Fridriksdottir et al. 1992). Presumptive cases of Lyme disease in goats and sheep were reported from endemic regions of Connecticut (Baldwin 1990). Putative signs in affected goats include depression, fever, pain in joints sufficient to preclude weight bearing, back pain, a bow-legged stance, an unsteady gait in the hind end, and a stiff neck. Ticks may be difficult to find on the animal because the infective nymphal stages are only pinhead size. Alternate day benzathine penicillin therapy carried out for twenty-one to twenty-eight days was reported as successful in these goats. In cattle, daily treatment with either penicillin or oxytetracycline for twenty-one days is recommended. A vaccine is now commercially available for use in dogs but is not approved or recommended for use in goats.

To date, the infective organism has not been isolated or identified from any presumed case of Lyme disease in goats. While affected animals had serologic evidence of infection, serologic surveys indicate that many individual animals with antibodies show no sign of clinical disease. Lyme disease may indeed occur in goats; however, definitive proof is still lacking. Presumptive diagnosis of Lyme disease should be made with caution and only in areas where the disease is known to occur in other animal species and only after other known causes of caprine arthritis, especially CAE and mycoplasmosis, have been definitively ruled out.

Confirmation of the presence of *B. burgdorferi* in affected tissues is still required for definitive diagnosis. Cultures are difficult to maintain and require several weeks to grow. Concentrations of organisms in affected organs or fluids may be very low, making culture problematic. However, alternatives to culture have become available for identifying the organism. PCR techniques can be used to identify *B. burgdorferi* in synovial fluid samples from affected joints or milk (Lischer et al. 2000) or from tissues at necropsy.

Clostridial Myositis and Myonecrosis

Blackleg and malignant edema (gas gangrene) are common, costly diseases of cattle and sheep caused by the "tissue invading" or "gas gangrene" group of clostridial organisms. In contrast, these clostridial diseases are uncommon in goats. One possible explanation is that the causative bacteria are soil-borne organisms that gain entry into livestock primarily through grazing of low lying, wet pastures. As browsing animals, goats may be less frequently exposed to clostridial spores in soil, though this hypothesis is unproven.

Etiology and Pathogenesis

Clostridium chauvoei, *C. septicum*, *C. sordelli*, and *C. novyi* are Gram-positive, rod-shaped, spore-forming, toxin-producing, anaerobic bacteria. They are ubiquitous in soil and persist for long periods under the protection of sporulation. They may also be present in the intestinal tract and liver of normal livestock without producing disease. Classical or true blackleg is caused by *C. chauvoei*. "False" blackleg, more appropriately referred to as malignant edema, is caused most often by *C. septicum*, but *C. novyi*, *C. sordelli*, *C. chauvoei*, and even *C. perfringens* have been isolated from lesions typical of malignant edema (Radostits et al. 2007).

The pathogenesis of blackleg is incompletely understood. It is thought that grazing animals ingest spores of *C. chauvoei* that cross the alimentary epithelium and are carried to muscle tissue via the lymphatics and blood. Spores remain dormant until local conditions in muscle favor bacterial multiplication. This might involve muscle trauma or circulatory disturbances that create anaerobic conditions. The proliferation of bacteria is accompanied by release of toxins that produce a necrotizing myositis and a fatal toxemia.

Malignant edema occurs when spores are introduced into tissue by penetrating wounds, which often result from routine management activities such as vaccinations, disbudding, castration, and especially shearing. Fighting and head butting among bucks can also facilitate introduction of spores and produce a type of malignant edema known as "swelled head." Tissue damage associated with wounds creates anaerobic conditions that allow bacterial proliferation. Toxins are released that produce severe localized inflammation and generalized, fatal toxemia. Local inflammation is often characterized by tissue necrosis with accumulation of edema and gas. Subcutaneous and connective tissue is often more directly involved than muscle, but muscle can be affected.

Epidemiology

Clostridial myositis has been reported infrequently in goats, mostly from southern Africa, Australia, and New Zealand. Angora or feral goats are most often affected, but this may reflect the preponderance of such goats in these locations rather than a breed predisposition. In the United States, it has been observed that blackleg and malignant edema are virtually unknown in goats, even where the diseases occur frequently in other animals on the same premises (Guss 1977).

A review of clostridial diseases in Australia indicated that classical blackleg due to *C. chauvoei* is virtually unreported and that goats may be less susceptible to the disease than sheep (King 1980). Mortality due to navel infections with *C. septicum* is also seen less frequently in kids than in lambs. More common is *C. novyi* infection in fighting bucks, leading to swelled head. The relationship of *C. novyi* infection to hepatic "black" disease in goats is discussed in Chapter 11.

In New Zealand, a group of 460 Angora and feral does were given intramuscular injections of cloprostenol to induce abortion. Fourteen of them (3%) died from *C. chauvoei* infection within six days after injection (Day and Southwell 1979). Gas gangrene after intramuscular injections with various medications is not uncommon in other livestock species.

In South Africa, the shearing of sheep is commonly associated with *C. chauvoei* infection, while shearing of Angora goats is not (Van Tonder 1975). It is presumed that the nature of the fleece and the relative absence of skinfolds and body pleats in goats produce fewer shearing wounds, with less secondary invasion of clostridial spores. When post-shearing clostridial infections do occur, they are more often caused by *C. septicum*. Gangrenous metritis caused by mixed clostridial infections with *C. septicum*, *C. novyi*, and/or *C. chauvoei* is the most common clostridial problem seen in Angora goats in South Africa. The condition is associated with the penning or kraaling of does during the kidding period (Bath et al. 2005). Morbidity is variable, but case mortality rates can approach 100% (Van Tonder 1975). In Namibia, spontaneous deaths of grazing adult cattle, sheep, and goats have been recognized as caused by *C. septicum* (Wessels 1972).

Clinical Signs

In blackleg, the clinical course is short and affected animals are usually found dead or recumbent and moribund. A sanguinous discharge from the nostrils or anus may be present. If there is a chance to observe animals early in the course of disease, lameness or a stiff gait may be noted when limb musculature is involved.

In malignant edema, which is associated with wounds or injections, there is usually heat, swelling, pain, and erythema at or around the wound site from twelve to forty-eight hours after introduction of the infection. As the infection progresses, skin becomes discolored and cold and subcutaneous gas may be identifiable as crepitus. Animals rapidly become weak and shocky and exhibit a high fever exceeding 106°F (41.1°C), and will die within hours.

Swelled head is seen primarily in group-housed bucks that fight. Large edematous swellings occur, usually beginning around the eyes and extending down the face and neck, sometimes to the chest. The swelling is quite disfiguring. The taut skin cracks and yellows, and edematous fluid seeps from the cracks. Affected bucks become extremely depressed and weak, with heads held low. They fall over and remain recumbent, dying within one to two days of onset of signs (King 1980).

Clinical Pathology and Necropsy

Impression smears and swabs taken from wound sites or subcutaneous aspirates may aid in the antemortem diagnosis of malignant edema or swelled head. Gram staining, fluorescent antibody testing, and anaerobic culturing can all be performed. In blackleg and many cases of malignant edema, necropsy is the primary approach to diagnosis. For bacteriologic confirmation, it is imperative that fresh necropsies be performed, preferably within one hour of death. Otherwise, clostridial organisms present in the alimentary tract or liver can invade tissues post mortem and produce false-positive diagnoses.

At necropsy, goats with blackleg may exhibit crepitant swellings over heavy muscle groups as well as gas bubbles in liver, kidney, and uterus and excessive accumulations of serosanguinous fluids in all body cavities (Pauling 1986). Goats with malignant edema may demonstrate generalized and advanced decomposition of the carcass, even when necropsy is performed shortly after death. There is a characteristic smell of clostridial decomposition and gelatinous infiltration of the pericardium. Pericarditis and myocarditis may be observed (Wessels 1972). In malignant edema and swelled head, there is marked accumulation of yellow or serosanguinous edema fluid in subcutaneous and intermuscular spaces, especially around wound sites.

Diagnosis

Definitive diagnosis of clostridial myositis in goats depends on confirmation of the presence of the causative clostridial organisms from tissues or wound sites of affected animals before or immediately after death. This can be accomplished by anaerobic culture, fluorescent antibody staining, or as has been recently reported, multiplex PCR (Sasaki et al. 2002).

When goats are found dead in the field, the differential diagnosis should include tympany, lightning strike, poisonings, and anthrax, especially because the latter condition is also associated with post mortem nasal and anal sanguinous discharges. If there is any suspicion of anthrax, the carcass should not be opened.

Treatment

Opportunities to treat blackleg are limited due to the rapid, fatal outcome. Individual cases of malignant edema, swelled head, or genital gas gangrene are more likely to be detected early enough for therapeutic intervention. In malignant edema and swelled head, the skin over affected regions should be liberally incised and serial fasciotomy performed on underlying muscles to allow aeration and drainage of infected tissues. Intravenous penicillin therapy at a dose of 20,000 IU/kg every six to eight hours should be initiated immediately and maintained until the patient is stabilized. The animal can then be placed on intramuscular procaine penicillin G for continued treatment. As animals are toxemic and often in shock, parenteral fluid therapy, steroids, and nonsteroidal anti-inflammatory drugs may also be indicated. The prognosis in advanced cases is always guarded.

Control

Vaccination in the face of an outbreak is indicated when blackleg or malignant edema occurs in a flock or herd. Numerous, multivalent clostridial vaccines manufactured throughout the world protect against the common causes of clostridial myositis. When vaccinating in the face of an outbreak, animals at risk should be treated with long-acting penicillin preparations at the same time that they are vaccinated to reduce losses while immunity develops.

Ideally, animals should be vaccinated routinely before outbreaks occur. However, the incidence of blackleg and malignant edema in goats is so low relative to sheep and cattle that widespread vaccination of goats may be difficult to justify economically except in those circumstances where the disease is predictably known to occur. When goats are routinely vaccinated against enterotoxemia caused by *C. perfringens*, use of multivalent clostridial vaccines may fit readily into the existing vaccination program. Where genital gas gangrene is known to occur, does should be vaccinated annually with appropriate multivalent clostridial vaccine three weeks before kidding. To control swelled head, bucks should be routinely vaccinated and housed separately to minimize fighting.

Foot Scald, Foot Rot, and Foot Abscesses

Infectious foot problems are not as widely reported in goats as in sheep but the pattern of disease is similar. Foot scald, also known as interdigital dermatitis, or benign foot rot, is defined as an infection confined to the interdigital epidermis with weakly virulent strains of *Dichelobacter (Bacteroides) nodosus*. Foot rot, also known as infectious foot rot or virulent foot rot, is defined as a co-infection of the interdigital epidermis with virulent strains of *D. nodosus and Fusobacterium necrophorum*, with extension of inflammation and infection into the horny and laminar structures of the foot. Foot abscess is an infection of the deep structures of the foot caused by bacteria other than *D. nodosus*, usually *Fusobacterium necrophorum* or *Arcanobacterium (Actinomyces) pyogenes*.

Etiology

Fusobacterium necrophorum, a Gram-negative anaerobic bacteria, is a common environmental organism that can colonize the interdigital epidermis when epithelial integrity is compromised and by itself can produce foot scald. *F. necrophorum* is also a copathogen with *Dichelobacter nodosus* in virulent foot rot. *F. necrophorum* can also be introduced into the deep structures of the foot by trauma and puncture wounds. *F. necrophorum* or *Arcanobacterium (Actinomyces) pyogenes* are the most common organisms associated with foot abscesses.

Dichelobacter (Bacteroides) nodosus is also a Gram-negative, anaerobic bacillus. In smears of exudate, it can be recognized by its characteristic morphology as a large, slightly curved rod with bulbous ends. It is an obligate anaerobe that is adapted to the interdigital epidermis of ruminants and survives only to a maximum of four days in the environment when passed in discharges from infected feet (Seaman and Evers 2006). Therefore, while the presence of *F. necrophorum* is required for virulent foot rot to develop, *D. nodosus* is considered the inciting pathogen because it must be introduced into a naïve herd or flock for foot rot to develop, whereas *F. necrophorum* is generally already present in the environment. Different strains of *D. nodosus* vary in their virulence based on their degree of keratolytic and elastolytic activity. The presence of proteases and elastases contribute to the invasiveness of horny hoof tissues. Caprine isolates of *D. nodosus* with high elastase activity were demonstrated to be virulent for sheep (Claxton and O'Grady 1986). The potential for cross-transmission of *D. nodosus* between goats and sheep must be taken into account when devising control programs.

Eight major serogroups of *D. nodosus* have been identified on the basis of agglutination responses to surface pili found on the organism. This is important regarding the efficacy of vaccination when vaccines comprised of pilus antigens are used because the degree of cross-protection varies between different serogroups.

Epidemiology

Foot scald, foot rot, and foot abscesses are most common in temperate regions of the world and occur most frequently in the spring and early summer in association with warm temperatures and heavy rainfall. The combination of wet pasture and warm temperatures (above 50°F [10°C]) facilitates transmission of the disease by softening and moistening the skin of the foot, thus predisposing to dermatitis and traumatic injury, and also by allowing the bacteria to persist away from the host for longer periods on pasture. In contrast, foot rot is rarely observed in hot, arid regions, even when large numbers of sheep or goats are maintained.

Other environmental and management factors predispose goats to infectious foot problems. These include wet, muddy yards or poorly drained pastures, overgrown hooves, overcrowding, the introduction of infected goats or sheep to a susceptible herd or flock, return of animals from shows or breeding stations, and turnout of goats onto contaminated pastures (Baxendell 1980). Goats are prone to excessive growth of the hoof when maintained in confinement. When the abaxial hoof wall overgrows the sole it may cause inward compression of the digits leading to excessive irritation of the interdigital skin (Claxton and O'Grady 1986). Dairy goat breeds are considered to be more susceptible to foot rot than fiber and meat goat breeds and some family lines of dairy goats are particularly prone to having "bad feet," requiring more frequent trimming (Skerman 1987). Heritability estimates have been reported in different breeds of goats regarding susceptibility to foot rot, suggesting that improved resistance is possible through selection (Banik and Bhatnagar 1983).

Transmission occurs by contact when infected and susceptible animals are commingled together at pasture under suitable conditions of moisture and temperature. The organism is present in discharges from animals with clinical lesions and can invade the damaged epidermis of the foot of susceptible goats. In sheep, the carrier state is known to be important in the spread of infection into susceptible flocks when carrier animals are newly introduced. This is also presumed to occur in goats. It has been reported that at least some strains of *D. nodosus* transmit readily between sheep and goats, so the risk of cross-species transmission must be considered and control efforts must be applied to both goats and sheep when the animals are kept together (Ghimire et al. 1996).

There may be differences in susceptibility between sheep and goats. In one study, few goats showed marked underrunning lesions of the hoof while sheep developed more severe lesions consistent with virulent foot rot when infected with the same strains. It was suggested that this might be because the *stratum corneum* of the interdigital skin is considerably thicker in goats than in sheep and therefore goats may be more resistant to maceration of the interdigital skin and subsequent invasion of *D. nodosus* (Ghimire et al. 1999).

Foot rot is less prevalent in goats than in sheep, and until 1985, confirmation that the condition in goats was caused by *D. nodosus* was notably lacking (Merrall 1985; Claxton and O'Grady 1986; Egerton 1989). Foot scald and, to a lesser extent, foot rot, are increasingly recognized as economic constraints on both fiber and milk goat production in the wetter regions of Australia and New Zealand (Anonymous 1987). While morbidity and mortality information for goats is scant, foot scald is cited by New Zealand goat farmers as the second most important disease of goats after enteric diseases (Merrall 1985).

Foot scald and foot rot can be important causes of economic loss in Angora goats in South Africa during periods of unusually wet weather (Van Tonder 1975). A seasonal prevalence of foot abscesses in Angora and Boer goats in South Africa is related to seasonal increases in populations of ticks with long mouth parts, notably *Hyalomma* spp., *Amblyomma* spp., and *Rhipicephalus glabroscutatum*. Adult ticks produce deep wounds in the interdigital space while feeding, and these wounds become secondarily infected, mostly by *Arcanobacterium (Actinomyces) pyogenes* (McIvor and Horak 1987; Bath et al. 2005). Foot rot occurs sporadically in dairy goats in the United States and Europe when they are maintained under conditions of poor management as described above (Guss 1977; Pinsent 1989).

Pathogenesis

The pathogeneses of foot scald, foot rot, and foot abscesses have not been expressly studied in goats. The development of these diseases is presumed to be similar to that described in sheep (Radostits et al. 2007). Wet conditions and softened hooves allow for infection of the interdigital skin and skin-horn junction with *F. necrophorum*. This can produce inflammation and hyperkeratosis and the relatively benign condition known as foot scald. However, the inflammation produced by *F. necrophorum* can facilitate the introduction of *D. nodosus* if that organism is present in the flock. In virulent foot rot, *D. nodosus* attaches to the foot with the aid of adherence pili and colonizes the interdigital epithelium. When these *D. nodosus* strains are virulent and keratolytic, the keratolytic activity allows invasion and underrunning of the horny hoof tissue. The interaction of *D. nodosus* and *F. necrophorum* causes marked inflammation and affected tissues are severely compromised, leading to necrosis. As a result, adherence of the hoof corium to the basal epithelium may be destroyed, resulting in detachment of the horny hoof from the underlying soft tissue. Treponemes are also associated with foot rot in sheep but their role in the pathogenesis of the disease remains uncertain (Egerton 2007).

Clinical Findings

There may be a mild lameness in foot scald. Careful inspection of the feet reveals erythema or swelling of the interdigital epidermis. There is usually little or no odor, and minimal underrunning of the horn at the coronet.

In foot rot, lameness can be quite pronounced when there is necrotic underrunning of the horn. Severely affected goats may walk on their carpi, and when all four feet are involved, may refuse to walk at all. In general, lesions of caprine foot rot are less severe than commonly seen in sheep (Claxton and O'Grady 1986). Swelling of the interdigital epidermis or possible separation of the hoof at the skin-horn junction may be noted. A small quantity of pus also may be visible at the coronet and detached horn can be readily pared or pulled off. The characteristic necrotic smell of foot rot may be detected.

Chronically affected animals may show a marked loss of body condition and decreased production. In addition, myiasis and tetanus are two possible sequelae of foot rot. Chronic cases may show hoof deformities after healing.

Foot abscesses may affect the heel or the toe. In contrast to foot rot and foot scald, only one foot may be involved, and only one claw of that foot. There may be a history of trauma or puncture. The foot is hot and swollen and very painful to the touch. The animal may carry the leg rather than bear weight. Swelling or draining pus may be present above the coronet.

Clinical Pathology and Necropsy

Gram-stained smears of exudate from underrun horn of affected feet can be used to identify the characteristic *D. nodosus* organisms in foot rot cases. Samples can be submitted for anaerobic culture. Serotyping of isolates can be important to determine the potential effectiveness of commercial vaccines. In early cases, evaluation of the virulence of isolates by measurement of proteolytic activity can be valuable in anticipating the severity of an impending outbreak. Radiography may be helpful in diagnosing goats with foot abscess and may assist in prognosis by identifying the presence of secondary osteomyelitis in the distal phalanx. At the time of necropsy, lesions are limited to the affected feet and reflect what is observed antemortem. Sagittal section of the distal limb may indicate the extent of foot abscesses and the occurrence of secondary osteomyelitis in the distal phalanx.

Diagnosis

Presumptive diagnosis of foot rot and foot scald is based on the onset of lameness, swelling at the interdigital space, and underrunning of the horn of the foot. Definitive diagnosis is based on culture of *D. nodosus* from lesions. Diagnosis of foot abscess depends on identifying a pus pocket in the deeper structures of the foot by paring of the sole or heel.

The differential diagnosis for the sudden onset of lameness in groups of goats should include foot and mouth disease and bluetongue. Lesions at the coronet may be seen in both diseases, but oral and muzzle lesions also occur in some affected individuals with bluetongue and FMD. Clinical bluetongue is rare in goats. Laminitis after grain engorgement can occur in groups of goats, but other signs such as diarrhea and bloat accompany or precede the lameness. Selenium toxicosis produces cracks in the hoof that become secondarily infected and may mimic foot rot except that the course is more chronic. The differential diagnosis for foot abscesses, when one leg is affected, include fractures, subluxations, and soft tissue injuries of the distal limb.

Treatment

Because of the highly contagious nature of foot scald and foot rot, recognition of even a single case of the disease calls for examination and potential treatment of all feet of all goats in the herd. As in sheep, several elements of therapy need to be considered, namely, paring of feet, use of antibacterial footbaths, topical or systemic antibiotic therapy, and vaccination, which can be used as an aid for control of outbreaks as well as for prevention. These various approaches can be used alone or in combination depending on the number of goats involved, their value and use, and the severity of the disease. A comparison of cost effectiveness of various treatments used in sheep has been reported (Salman 1988).

Paring of the feet is a critically important component of therapy in severe cases of foot rot, as removal of dead tissue exposes deep-seated *D. nodosus* organisms to oxygen and the antibacterial effects of subsequent footbaths or topical antibiotics. Paring feet is especially important in foot abscesses to find pus pockets and drain them to relieve pressure in the sore foot. Paring knives should be disinfected in 10% formalin between goats to avoid additional spread of infection.

Disinfectant footbaths are a useful way of treating large numbers of goats. However, goats are high jumpers and have a distinct aversion to walking in water. Footbath design, then, must be considered carefully. A circular bath with a central feeding trough is commercially available in New Zealand. This design encourages goats to wade into the bath to be rewarded with grain (Yerex 1986). Footbath solutions must be nonirritating if the owner expects the goats to enter the bath a second time. Zinc sulfate solutions of a 10% to 20% weight-to-volume ratio are both mild and effective, and are currently the solution of choice. The efficacy of the solution may be enhanced by addition of surfactants such as sodium lauryl sulfate at a concentration of 2% volume-to-volume ratio. In severe cases, one-hour foot soaks repeated weekly for three treatments may be required.

Formalin and copper sulfate footbaths are less desirable. A 5% formalin solution is an effective treatment but has several drawbacks including the production of irritating fumes, painful stinging of aggressively pared feet, hardening of the hoof, and the potential for permanently damaging the skin if concentrations are not strictly regulated. If formalin is used, the solution should be changed daily to ensure that evaporation has not resulted in excessive concentration. Goats stung by formalin footbaths are unlikely to enter them again voluntarily. Copper sulfate solution at a 10% weight-to-volume ratio is also effective but stains the hair or fleece blue-green and is potentially toxic if consumed. Splashing of solutions on the goats' bodies can be reduced by lining the footbath with wood chips, peat moss, or wool tags. After dipping, goats should be turned out on dry ground or slotted floors to permit drying of footbath solutions on hooves.

A number of topical disinfectants and antibacterials can be used after paring, in lieu of footbaths. Zinc sulfate, copper sulfate, copper naphthenate, the quaternary ammonium compound cetrimide (20% alcohol tincture), oxytetracycline, penicillin, and other compounds are available in different countries as paints, powders, or sprays for direct application to the hoof. Putting a bandage on the hoof after application may enhance healing. The feeding of zinc sulfate at a rate of 0.5 g/head/day for twenty-one days during the treatment period has also been recommended when the diet is known to be deficient in zinc.

Parenteral antibiotic therapy has also been used effectively in sheep. The *in vitro* effectiveness of beta-lactam antibiotics against caprine isolates of *Dichelobacter* spp. and *Fusobacterium* spp. has been reported (Piriz Duran et al. 1990). Azlocillin, mezlocillin, and piperacillin were most effective against the largest number of isolates. Penicillin G and ampicillin were almost as effective, and cefuroxime, cefoperazone, cefotaxime, cefoxitin, and imipenem were generally less effective. Current recommendations for antibiotic treatment in sheep are: a single IM dose of penicillin/streptomycin at 70,000 U/kg bw penicillin and 70 mg/kg dihydrostreptomycin, a single IM dose of erythromcycin at 10 mg/kg bw, a single IM dose of long-acting oxytetracycline at 20 mg/kg bw, or a single SQ dose of lincomycin/spectinomycin at 5 mg/kg bw lincomycin and 10 mg/kg bw spectinomycin (Radostits et al. 2007).

Treated animals should not be turned back into wet or muddy yards, nor should they be put out to pasture that has not been free of infected animals for at least seven days. Parings from trimmed feet should be considered as fomites and removed from the premises or burned. It is recommended that goats with foot rot be given tetanus antitoxin or reimmunized as the anaerobic environment of the affected foot may predispose to tetanus.

Vaccines are available against *F. necrophorum* and other vaccines are available against *D. nodosus*. In both cases, manufacturers indicate that vaccination can be helpful in the treatment of foot rot in sheep that are experiencing the problem as well as to prevent foot rot in herds not experiencing the problem. Neither vaccine is approved for use in goats in the United States.

Control

Premises with no history of foot rot or foot scald may remain free by maintaining completely closed herds. This means not purchasing any new stock and not taking animals to shows or breeding stations. Transport vehicles and common housing facilities can be contaminated with *D. nodosus* if not thoroughly cleaned and disinfected. If new animals are purchased, they should be from sources free of foot rot. Feet of purchased animals must be carefully inspected for lesions and if any doubt exists, the animals should be run through a foot bath or treated with parenteral antibiotics, quarantined for four weeks, and reexamined before joining the new herd.

When foot rot already exists on the premises, control is directed toward maintenance of proper hoof care, prophylactic use of footbaths, vaccination, and breeding programs.

Feet should be monitored for excessive overgrowth. Provision of rock piles for climbing and playing may help goats to naturally wear off excessive hoof growth. Regular trimming may be necessary to keep the hoof wall from overgrowing the sole and to keep toes from growing too long.

Use of walkthrough footbaths once a week during high-risk periods of wet, warm weather helps to control spread of infection. Zinc sulfate baths are preferred for repetitive use.

A commercial foot rot vaccine based on multiple pili of *D. nodosus* is available in Australia, New Zealand, the United States, and elsewhere for use in sheep. There are no controlled studies to evaluate efficacy in goats and anecdotal reports suggest that there are mixed results when vaccination is applied to goats (Merrall 1985; Skerman 1987). Antibody titers produced in goats are comparable to those of sheep (Skerman 1987). The vaccine is initially given twice at a thirty-day interval. The duration of immunity may only be twelve weeks so vaccination should be timed to precede those periods when transmission of the disease is most likely to occur (Egerton 2007).

The vaccine should be given subcutaneously but still may produce a sizable reaction at the injection site, particularly after the second injection. Owners should be so advised, particularly if show animals are involved. Commercial *D. nodosus* vaccines may contain up to ten different strains of the organism to represent the most common serogroups associated with foot rot, though inclusion of too many strains and their associated immunogenic pilus or fimbrial antigens may actually diminish the immune response. For *D. nodosus* vaccines to be effective, they must contain a strain or strains immunogenically related to those occurring in the affected flock. This was illustrated in Nepal, where an autogenous vaccine containing only two virulent serogroups isolated from local sheep and goats was more effective in reducing foot rot in both species than an imported, multivalent commercial vaccine in a controlled field study (Egerton et al. 2002).

A *Fusobacterium necrophorum* bacterin is also now available in the United States; it is approved for treatment and prevention of foot rot in sheep. Initial immunization requires two doses given three to four weeks apart IM or SQ and an annual booster dose.

The selection of goats with apparent resistance to foot rot for breeding programs is considered to offer long-range benefits to the goat industry for foot rot control. Culling goats with poor foot conformation is a good place to begin.

Control and eradication of foot rot is possible but it can be a long, complicated, and challenging process, and veterinarians need to work with producers so that this is understood. There is no magic bullet, and no single intervention will successfully eliminate the condition once established on a farm. Vaccination, for example, is more effective when carried out in association with hoof paring and/or foot bathing then when done alone. Additional details on eradication and control of foot rot in sheep, which serves as the model for goats, is available elsewhere (Egerton 2007).

PARASITIC DISEASES

Cestodiasis

Goats and sheep serve as intermediate hosts for the canid tapeworm *Taenia multiceps*. The cysts produced by the intermediate stage of the parasite are usually found in the brains of small ruminants and the resulting disease, coenurosis, or gid, is discussed in detail in Chapter 5. In goats more often than sheep, cysts may develop at sites outside the central nervous system, especially in the intermuscular fascia. Cases of goats affected in this way have been reported from the Sudan and India (Ramadan et al. 1973; Dey et al. 1988). Metacestodes in muscle connective tissue produce visible or palpable swellings in muscle masses, accompanied by discomfort, restricted gait, poor appetite, and general malaise. Cysts may number in the hundreds. They feel firm rather than fluctuant and may exceed 7 cm in diameter. They can be distributed all over the body, including the face, but are most common in the thighs and shoulders. Attempts to manage these cases by surgical removal of multiple cysts have not been particularly successful, but this may be due to the advanced debilitation of affected goats at the time of presentation. There is no other known effective therapy.

Muscle cysts may also occur in goats infected with metacestodes of *Taenia ovis*, though sheep are the principal intermediate host of this canid tapeworm. In the case of *T. ovis*, muscle is the primary site of metacestode formation, with cysts most commonly found in the heart, diaphragm, and masseter muscles. This canid tapeworm has a cosmopolitan distribution and is responsible for economic wastage through condemnation and trimming of small ruminant carcasses at slaughter.

Besnoitiosis

Infection with the protozoan parasite *Besnoitia* in goats is most commonly recognized as a granular conjunctivitis, as discussed in Chapter 6. However, *Besnoitia* infection can be generalized, producing respiratory disease, orchitis, and dermatitis, such as seen in goats in Iran (Bazargani et al. 1987). On post mortem examination, multiple small, white, gritty granules may be present in tissues of the musculoskeletal system, including ligaments, tendons, tendon sheaths, synovial membranes, and muscular connective tissue. These granules represent cysts containing large numbers of bradyzoites of *Besnoitia*.

Sarcocystosis

Sarcosystosis, also known as sarcosporidiosis, is a protozoal infection. The life cycle of *Sarcocystis* spp. involves predatory canids as definitive hosts and various species of livestock as intermediate hosts. The role of the goat as an intermediate host has been described (Collins and Charleston 1979; Collins et al. 1980; Dubey et al. 1984). *Sarcocystis* spp. affecting goats include: *S. capracanis*, with the dog, coyote, and fox as definitive hosts; *S. hircicanis*, with the dog as definitive host; and *S. moulei*, with the cat as definitive host. Muscle cysts containing host-specific *Sarcocystis* spp. have long been recognized in carcasses at slaughter plants and have been a cause of condemnation. Beyond that, the condition was thought to be incidental.

More recently, experimental studies have indicated that *Sarcocystis* spp. may produce a variety of clinical signs, including anemia, fever, vasculitis, myositis, abortion, chronic wasting, and sudden death in ruminants. The experimental disease in goats, produced by challenge with *Sarcocystis capracanis*, has been studied extensively (Collins et al. 1980; Dubey et al. 1981; Dubey 1981; Lopez-Rodriguez et al. 1986). It is hard to describe typical clinical signs in goats because the clinical response is clearly dose dependent, and a wide range of oral challenge doses of sporocysts has been used, from 4×10^3, which produced no clinical signs (Gomes et al 1992); to 7×10^4, which produced anemia, loss of appetite, and fever (Ivanov 1998); to 5×10^5, causing fever, loss of appetite, muscle tremors, and weakness (Dey et al. 1995). A dose of 1×10^4 sporocysts produced abortion in pregnant does (Juyal et al. 1989). In general, the most consistent signs of experimental infection are fever, which is often biphasic, anemia, and loss of appetite. At necropsy, streaky hemorrhage of skeletal muscles and petechiation of lymph nodes and serosal surfaces of abdominal viscera are prominent signs. Liver, kidneys, and spleen may also be swollen and friable (Wadajkar et al. 1995).

Despite the evidence for clinical disease in experimental work, cases of naturally occurring clinical caprine sarcocystosis have not been reported, save for one naturally occurring case of congenital sarcocystosis in a stillborn kid from a Saanen milking herd in Australia experiencing abortions (Mackie and Dubey 1996). Naturally occurring clinical disease has been confirmed in sheep. Sporozoan encephalomyelitis has been reported in the UK, affecting animals under one year of age. Clinical signs included ataxia, generalized tremors, compulsive nibbling, and hind limb paresis (Caldow et al. 2000; Sargison et al. 2000). Other manifestations in sheep without neurologic presentation include anemia, retarded growth, and reduced wool production. There is also a reported case of congestive heart failure and vegetative endocarditis associated with sarcocystosis in a young ram (Scott and Sargison 2001). Anticoccidial drugs such as amprolium and salinomycin may be effective in sarcocystosis.

Subclinical caprine infections with characteristic muscle cysts predominantly in esophagus, diaphragm, and heart, as well as other sites, are well documented around the world, usually from slaughterhouse surveys (Seneviratna et al. 1975; Chhabra and Mahajan 1978; Collins and Crawford 1978; Perez Garro et al. 1978; Barci et al. 1983; Saym and Ozer 1984; Dubey and Livingston 1986). Prevalence of subclinical infections may be greater than some survey reports suggest. A recent slaughterhouse survey from Iran detected grossly evident sarcocysts in twenty-eight of 169 goats by visual inspection. However, when impression smears of target tissues were examined microscopically, 168/169 had *Sarcocystis* spp. present and 169/169 were positive when tissues were subjected to pepsin digestion, centrifuged, and examined microscopically (Shekarforoush et al. 2005). Control of sarcocystosis requires separating dogs and goats, restricting access of goat offal to dogs, cooking meat fed to dogs, and burying dead goats.

NUTRITIONAL AND METABOLIC DISEASES

Nutritional Muscular Dystrophy

Nutritional muscular dystrophy (NMD), or white muscle disease, is the most common manifestation of selenium and/or vitamin E deficiency in goats. Suboptimal levels of these nutrients impair the animals' ability to control oxidative reactions in cells, which can result in extensive muscle necrosis. Cardiac muscle, the diaphragm, and other skeletal muscles may be affected, resulting in a wide range of clinical presentations that make accurate diagnosis a clinical challenge.

Etiology and Pathogenesis

Naturally occurring pro-oxidants, including hydrogen peroxide, superoxide radical, and hydroxyl ion, are generated through normal metabolic activities. These so-called reactive oxygen species can be toxic if allowed to accumulate. In particular, they can damage polyunsaturated fatty acids that are an integral part of cell membranes and the limiting membrane of cellular organelles through the process of oxidation. Muscle cells may be particularly prone to damage by oxidation because of their high metabolic activity. Both selenium and vitamin E participate in enzymatic reactions that control oxidative processes in cells of mammalian tissues via oxidation-reduction reactions.

Selenium is a cofactor of the enzyme glutathione peroxidase that reduces H_2O_2 to H_2O. The selenoprotein glutathione peroxidase is found in cells of numerous tissues, including muscle and red blood cells. While the enzyme activity in red blood cells is not directly related to the pathogenesis of nutritional myopathy, whole blood can be readily sampled and assayed for such activity as an indirect measure of selenium content in the body.

Vitamin E, or alpha tocopherol, also functions independently as an antioxidant, primarily protecting membrane polyunsaturated fatty acids against oxidation. Rather than reducing existing peroxides, it prevents their formation. The antioxidative role of vitamin E increases in importance with increased levels of polyunsaturated fats in the diet. Further details of the pathophysiology of selenium and vitamin E deficiency as they relate to cellular oxidation are available elsewhere (Van Metre and Callan 2001).

Dietary deficiencies of vitamin E and/or selenium can lead to reduced enzymatic activity and reduced protection of tissues from the adverse effects of peroxides. Muscle damage can be severe, with hyaline and granular degeneration of muscle fibers, necrosis, and replacement of muscle by proliferating connective tissue. Deficiency of only selenium or only vitamin E may not lead to clinical abnormalities if the other nutrient is available in abundant supply because their mechanisms of action, though distinct, may provide an adequate degree of physiologic cross-protection.

The location and severity of muscle damage dictates the various clinical manifestations observed in NMD. Sudden death may be observed when cardiac muscle is involved, or, if less acute, there may be signs of congestive heart failure. When the diaphragm is involved, there is labored respiration that may mimic pneumonia. When the limb muscles are involved, affected animals become stiff gaited initially or recumbent. Muscles of the thigh are most commonly affected. Involvement of the tongue or pharyngeal muscles may affect nursing and eating and suggest neurologic disease. Death may occur as a direct result of the effects of myopathy or due to secondary complications such as predation, starvation, exposure, or supervening infections, including inhalation pneumonia.

Epidemiology

Selenium deficiency is associated with selenium-deficient soils and the inadequate uptake of selenium by forages grown on those soils. Legumes are less able to extract soil selenium than grasses. Selenium-deficient areas in North America are discussed in Chapter 19 (Figure 19.3). In addition, the following countries have regions with selenium-deficient soils: most countries of Latin America, northern Europe, Australia, New Zealand, Indonesia, the Philippines, and China, and in Africa, Kenya, Sudan, Uganda, Swaziland, and South Africa (National Research Council 2007). In Australia, the disease in goats is associated with regions of high rainfall and acid soils and the application of superphosphate fertilizers (Baxendell 1988). Acidic soil pH and a high soil content of sulfates or phosphorus inhibit the absorption of Se by plants.

Vitamin E deficiency is independent of soil type and more closely reflects forage quality. Prolonged storage of feedstuffs results in degradation of vitamin E content. Housed goats fed stored feeds with no access to green feeds are more likely to experience deficiency. The feeding of excessive polyunsaturated fats in the diet may tax the ability of marginal or even adequate vitamin E levels to successfully perform their antioxidant function.

Numerous clinical syndromes of vitamin E/selenium deficiency are recognized in ruminants, horses, and pigs, (Radostits et al. 2007), as well as poultry. In goats, NMD is the most common disease manifestation and is recognized as a consequential caprine disease in the United States (Guss 1977), Australia (King 1980a), New Zealand (Thompson 1986), and some European countries (Tontis 1984; Roncero et al. 1989), as well as on the Mexican plateau, where it was identified as the main cause of death in extensively managed kids between eight and ninety days of age (Ramírez-Bribiesca et al. 2001). All breeds appear susceptible and the condition may develop under extensive or intensive management systems. In the former case, animals are grazing selenium-deficient pastures; in the latter, they are consuming feeds grown on selenium-deficient soils. The condition has been recorded in wild mountain goats *(Oreamnos americanus)* in Canada (Hebert and Cowan 1971) and in zoo goats (Biolatti and Vigliani 1980). Goats may be more susceptible to NMD than other ruminants, as cattle and sheep in New Zealand grazing the same areas as goats did not show the condition (Anonymous 1987a; Rammell et al. 1989).

Clinical disease is most common in young kids up to six months of age and less likely in adults. The selenium and vitamin E status of the dam is critical to the occurrence of NMD in her offspring. Stillborn and weak newborn kids have been attributed to nutritional muscular dystrophy in Australia (King 1980a). In parts of New Zealand, nutritional muscular dystrophy is the most common recognized cause of mortality in kids between one and nine weeks of age (Buddle et al. 1988). Mortality in New Zealand outbreaks is as high as 20% on some premises (Anonymous 1987a). Sudden, unaccustomed exercise is a common prelude to clinical muscular dystrophy in kids. This may occur when kids are turned out for cleaning of pens or put out to pasture for the first time.

In feeding trials with adult goats, selenium deficiency has been shown to impair reproductive performance and milk production. Conception rates were lower in selenium-deficient goats compared with control goats. Though no abortions were noted, kid survival rates were also reduced. During the first two months of lactation, selenium-deficient goats gave 23% less milk than control goats with relative reductions of 11% in milk fat content and 12% in milk protein content (Anke et al. 1989). A selenium-responsive dermatosis has been recognized in goats and is discussed in Chapter 2. Other clinical manifestations of vitamin E/selenium deficiency in adult goats have been suggested. These include fetal resorption, dystocia caused by decreased uterine tone, retained placenta, post partum recumbency, generalized ill thrift, and reduced semen quality.

Selenium deficiency may also increase susceptibility to infection in goats by reducing neutrophil function (Aziz et al. 1984; Aziz and Klesius 1986) and alter immune responses by inhibiting production of leukocyte migration inhibitory factor in caprine lymphocytes (Aziz and Klesius 1985). More is known about the effects of selenium and vitamin E on the immune responses of other domestic animal species and the subject has been reviewed (Finch and Turner 1996).

Clinical Findings

Nutritional muscular dystrophy is most often brought to the attention of veterinarians when previously healthy kids from three days to six months of age are found dead, recumbent, having difficulty rising, or exhibiting a stiff-legged gait. Faster-growing kids are more often affected. Recumbent kids are usually mentally alert but may be depressed. They may struggle to rise, and these efforts may be interpreted as convulsions or neurologic signs by the owner. If assisted to rise, they may be unable to stand or they may exhibit muscle tremors from the effort made, particularly in the hind limbs. Fever is a variable finding, usually associated with secondary infections. A history of unaccustomed exercise in the preceding few days can often be elicited. If untreated, kids with nutritional muscular dystrophy often will die within several days of the onset of signs.

Other clinical presentations may not immediately suggest nutritional muscular dystrophy but are consistent with localized muscle damage. The inability to nurse or swallow, with milk exiting through the nostrils or quidding of solid feed, may be seen when the tongue or pharyngeal muscles are involved. Dyspnea, increased respiratory rate, moist lung sounds, and coughing can occur when the diaphragm or left heart muscle is involved. Delivery of stillborn or weak, poorly suckling kids can be caused by severe *in utero* deficiencies of selenium or vitamin E. In this instance, a herd history may include complaints of dystocia and a high prevalence of retained placenta in adult does.

Clinical Pathology and Necropsy

Direct confirmation of selenium or vitamin E deficiency in the live animal can be obtained by measuring their concentrations in blood. In practice however, this is not commonly done because the assays are complex, expensive, and not widely available. Reference values for goats have been published (Van Metre and Callan 2001). Adequate selenium concentrations in caprine serum are reported from different laboratories to be 0.05 to 0.16 ppm or 80 to 100 ng/mL with values less than 60 ng/mL representing deficiency. For caprine whole blood the normal range for selenium is 0.15 to 0.25 ppm with less than 0.05 considered deficient. For vitamin E, 60 to 150 μg/dL in caprine serum is considered an adequate concentration. Experimental studies in goats indicate that plasma vitamin E concentrations less than 1.5 μmol/l in does and less than 1 μmol/l in kids increase the risk of myopathy (Jones et al. 1988).

An alternative but indirect method of determining selenium deficiency is to measure glutathione peroxidase activity in red blood cells from heparinized whole blood. Normal mean activity in goat kids has been reported as 113 IU activity/ml of red blood cells (Jones et al. 1988). When using this assay as an indicator of response to selenium therapy, it should be noted that there is a lag period of at least two weeks before parenterally administered selenium leads to measurable increases in glutathione peroxidase activity in whole blood. This is because selenium is incorporated into developing red cells in the bone marrow before their release into the blood and has no effect on cells already in circulation. Concerns have been raised about the glutathione peroxidase assay, including instability of the enzyme in storage even when samples are refrigerated, inconsistent expression of enzyme activity among laboratories, and wide variation in values between laboratories. As a result, use of the test has declined (Van Metre and Callan 2001).

Measurements of serum creatine kinase (CK) and serum aspartate aminotransferase (AST) are commonly used as indicators of muscle necrosis for making a presumptive diagnosis of nutritional muscular dystrophy. Creatine kinase is a muscle-specific enzyme. Mild to moderate elevations of serum CK may be seen secondary to trauma or prolonged recumbency from any cause, including birth, but marked elevations are seen in the acute phase of nutritional muscular dystrophy. Normal serum CK for goats is reported to be 49.1 ± 2 IU/l (Stevens et al. 1994), while other sources report a normal range of 14 to 62 IU/l (Garnier et al. 1984). Serum CK levels of 1,000 IU/l to more than 50,000 IU/l may be observed in NMD depending on acuteness and severity. Subclinically affected animals may also have elevations exceeding 1,000 IU/l. Serum AST will also be elevated, but AST is not muscle specific, so elevations of AST without concurrent elevations of CK may not indicate muscle damage. The serum half-life of CK is several hours, while the AST half-life is in days. Therefore, when both are increased, muscle damage is probably ongoing, whereas a decrease in CK with a persistent elevation of AST is more favorable, suggesting resolution of active muscle necrosis.

At necropsy, muscles of the limbs, diaphragm, heart, tongue, and pharynx should be carefully examined. Affected muscle appears white to gray, like cooked poultry, and stands out in contrast to adjacent, normal, red-brown muscle. The surface of the lesion may appear chalky when calcium has accumulated in degenerated muscle. The lesions in limb muscles are bilaterally symmetrical. Large muscle bellies may be abnormal, such as the semimembranosus muscles in the thighs, and patchy hemorrhage may occur in addition to pale discoloration (Figure 4.10). Especially in the heart and diaphragm, whitish yellow streaks or patches may be present within normal muscle masses. Heart lesions may extend through the myocardium to the endocardium and involve the papillary muscles as well. When the heart is involved, there may be evidence of congestive heart failure such as ascites, hydrothrorax, pericardial effusion, pulmonary edema or congestion, and/or a swollen, congested, friable liver. Fibrin tags have been observed on the liver surface (Thompson 1986). Aspiration pneumonia may be observed secondary to swallowing difficulties. Tongue

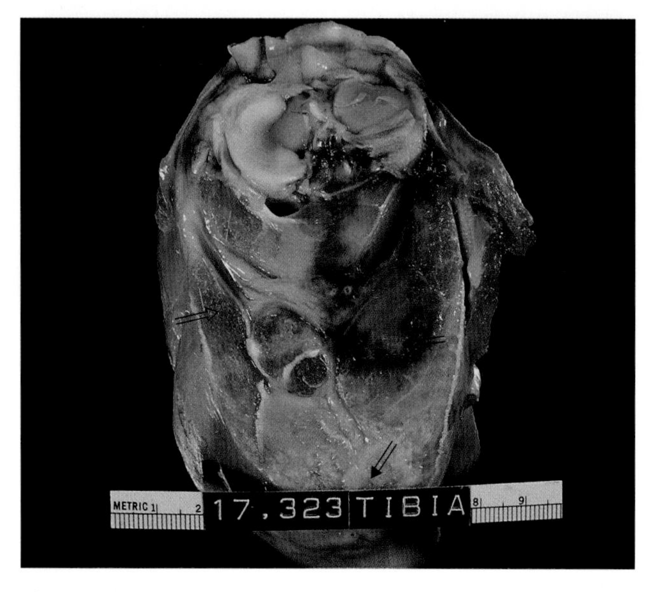

Figure 4.10. Gross post mortem lesions in the rear limb muscles of a goat with nutritional muscular dystrophy. Normal muscle is seen at the left (open arrow). The white chalky areas of muscle at the bottom of the picture are severely affected (black arrow). The lesion is demarcated by an area of hemorrhage (white arrow). (Courtesy of Dr. T.P. O'Leary.)

and pharyngeal muscles should be examined carefully in these cases.

Histologically, the muscle lesion is characterized by hyaline degeneration of striated muscle cells with coagulation necrosis, a pattern of degeneration referred to as Zenker's necrosis. Ultrastructural studies indicate that the lesion primarily involves the contractile components of the muscle cell cytoplasm.

Determination of selenium levels in liver at necropsy can give some indication of the severity of selenium deficiency. Normal liver selenium level in the goat has been reported at 1.00–4.80 ppm dry weight with concentrations of less than 0.40 ppm considered deficient (Van Metre and Callan 2001).

Diagnosis

Definitive diagnosis of nutritional muscular dystrophy depends on identification of typical muscle lesions in affected kids at necropsy or decreased levels of selenium and/or vitamin E in blood or tissues. A presumptive diagnosis in the field can be made on the basis of typical clinical signs, supportive laboratory findings, and a favorable response to treatment with parenteral administration of vitamin E and selenium.

When stillborn or weak kids are involved, other causes of infectious and noninfectious abortion must be considered, as discussed in Chapter 13. Sudden death in young kids may also be caused by gastrointestinal parasitism, especially haemonchosis and coccidiosis, colisepticemia, and enterotoxemia. Cases of nutritional muscular dystrophy may appear very similar to enterotoxemia when the heart muscle is involved because of the presence of pericardial and peritoneal effusions. Histologic examination of the heart is necessary for diagnosis. When dyspnea, coughing, and other signs of respiratory distress are observed, bacterial, viral, and verminous pneumonias must be considered.

Difficulties in swallowing in young goats may be associated with cleft palate or neurologic diseases such as listeriosis or polioencephalomalacia. When a stiff-legged gait is observed, tetanus must be considered. The differential diagnosis for recumbency in young goats includes musculoskeletal trauma, enzootic ataxia, and the neurologic form of caprine arthritis encephalitis. In enzootic ataxia and CAE virus infection, recumbency is usually preceded by a progressive ataxia that is characterized more by weakness than stiff leggedness, and with a more prolonged course.

Treatment

Parenteral administration of combination sodium selenite/alpha-tocopherol preparations is the treatment of choice in the acute phase of nutritional muscular dystrophy. Administration of both compounds together results in a higher rate of recovery in kids than either compound administered alone (Baran

1966). Combination products are marketed widely for administration either subcutaneously or intramuscularly. When dosage information is not specifically given for goats, one to two times sheep doses are appropriate. A recommended dose for sheep is 1 mg selenium as sodium selenite and 50 mg (68 IU) of alpha tocopherol/ 18 kg (40 pounds) of body weight, but label dosages can be followed for specific products (Van Vleet, 2005).

Affected goats usually respond favorably to a single treatment within twenty-four hours, though recovery may not be complete depending on the severity and extent of pre-existing muscle damage. Animals that do not respond may be retreated one time again at twenty-four hours. If no improvement is seen after the second treatment, then a poor prognosis must be offered, or an alternative diagnosis pursued. Excessive, repeated use of parenteral selenium can result in selenium toxicity. In some herd situations, vitamin E deficiency may play a greater role in the development of disease than selenium deficiency, and when combination products are not producing a desired therapeutic effect, administration of additional vitamin E or nutritional supplementation of vitamin E should be considered (Byrne 1992).

As nutritional muscular dystrophy indicates a nutritional deficiency, herd-wide administration of parenteral selenium/vitamin E preparations in the short term is justified at the time confirmed clinical cases are being treated in order to prevent additional cases. In the United States, recent reports of abortion in some sheep receiving parenteral injections have resulted in these products being disallowed for use in pregnant ewes. Abortions have not been reported in does, but caution should be exercised in using these products in pregnant does and clients advised of the risk. Alternatively for pregnant does, oral administration of selenium can be initiated, up to 0.3 mg Se/kg dry matter of the total ration.

Control

Selenium deficiency should be anticipated in goats in regions known to have selenium-deficient soils. Several approaches to correcting nutritional deficiency are possible, and the choice depends on economic, management, and regulatory factors. Feed supplementation with selenium is a desirable approach to control, though there may be regulatory constraints against the practice. In the United States, selenium supplementation of feed has been approved for use in sheep and beef for some time, but it was not until 2005 that allowance was made for goats. As of 2005, selenium can be supplemented in a complete ration for goats as selenium yeast at a level up to 0.3 ppm added selenium (FDA 2005). This is considered adequate to prevent occurrence of NMD.

Where feed supplementation is not permitted by regulation or is impractical, strategically timed parenteral administration of selenium/vitamin E preparations is an effective means of control during periods of high risk. Does can be given therapeutic doses of a combination preparation at the onset of breeding season and again four to six weeks before kidding, observing the caveats mentioned above in the treatment section regarding pregnant does. Kids should be given a therapeutic dose at birth and again at one month of age. In herds where clinical cases are observed in older kids, this can be repeated again at two or three months of age. Bucks should receive the preparation twice a year with the first administration timed to the onset of breeding season. Drenching forms of sodium selenite are available in some areas. This allows selenium administration to be conveniently incorporated into other preventive medicine activities such as parasite control. Sheep doses can be used.

Other control methods are being increasingly applied to cattle and sheep but have not been evaluated in goats. Injectable barium selenate, a repository form of selenium, maintains adequate selenium levels for as long as six months. Use of the preparation has been reported in goats in Spain. When given to dairy goats at a dose of 1 mg Se/kg bw fifteen days before breeding, seven- to eight-fold increases in glutathione peroxidase activity were still measurable at the time of kidding as compared to no change in untreated controls (Sánchez et al. 2007). However, it is not clear if increased selenium levels were present in milk, which would be a significant regulatory concern in the United States.

Orally administered selenium pellets can provide adequate levels for up to one year in sheep. A sodium selenite, four-month, constant-release bolus is approved for oral use in cattle in the United States, but not for small ruminants.

Topdressing of pasture with sodium selenate at a rate of 10 g/ha may be an economic alternative to individual animal treatment and will prevent selenium deficiency for as long as twelve months (Kimberling 1988). The risk of inadequate vitamin E in the diet still exists when these techniques are used, and vitamin supplementation is indicated, as discussed in Chapter 19. In contrast to selenium, vitamin E is reported to be nontoxic to goats (Ahmed et al. 1990).

Rickets

Rickets is a metabolic abnormality of growing bone. It is characterized by a failure of mineralization in newly formed bone matrix at the epiphyses of long bones. As such, it is a disease of young, growing animals. The condition is classically attributed to an absolute deficiency of vitamin D_2 arising from the housing of young stock in buildings devoid of sunlight or the provision of green feeds not cured in the sun. However, chronic deficiencies of either calcium or phosphorus in the face of adequate vitamin D can also produce the condition. Inadequate mineralization at the epiphyses leads to structural weakness and abnormal growth, particularly in the long bones, which will show enlargements at the end plates and deformation due to the stresses of weightbearing.

Clinical and subclinical rickets has been described in young goats (Yousif et al. 1986). Clinically affected animals show stiffness of gait, a tendency to remain recumbent, a bowing deformity of the forelimbs, swollen carpi, and enlargements of the costochondral junctions, a lesion commonly described as the rachitic rosary. Loosening of the shoulder blade attachments and a dropped withers have also been identified with caprine rickets, and may be the only signs seen (Guss 1977). Subclinically affected animals may show only signs of anorexia and a stunted growth rate.

The most consistent clinical pathologic finding in rickets is an elevation of serum alkaline phosphatase. Abnormalities in serum calcium and phosphorus levels are less consistent, though in at least one report, clinically affected goats had both hypophosphatemia (mean, 2.76 ± 0.15 mg/dl) and hypocalcemia (mean 7.05 ± 0.18 mg/dl), with a ratio of serum calcium to serum phosphorus consistently more than 2:1. Affected goats were also hypoproteinemic, and had decreased serum zinc, iron, copper, and magnesium levels compared with control goats (Yousif et al. 1986). Hypophosphatemia, hypocalcemia, hypovitaminosis D_3 and increased serum alkaline phosphatase were identified as the main biochemical abnormalities in two- to six-month old goats with rickets in Egypt (El-Sayed and Siam, 1992).

Radiographically, there is decreased density of affected bones, with widening and lipping of the nonmineralized growth plates. Antemortem biopsy of the costochondral junction or histologic examination of growth plates of long bones at necropsy confirms the failure of mineralization in the zones of provisional calcification in growth plates.

Successful treatment and control of rickets require accurate determination of the underlying cause through careful history taking, examination of housing and access to sunlight, and nutrient analysis of rations followed by correction of identified deficiencies. Nutrient requirements of vitamin D, calcium, and phosphorus are discussed in Chapter 19.

Epiphysitis

Epiphysitis is seen in young, rapidly growing goats that are fed excessive calcium. The lesion involves an unequal growth rate across the epiphyses of long bones, especially in the distal radial, distal metacarpal, and distal metatarsal epiphyses and can result in premature closure of the growth plate either axially or abaxially. The result is a clinically obvious valgus or varus angular deformity of the limb around the affected epiphyses.

The exact pathogenesis of the lesion and its relation to excessive calcium feeding are not completely understood. The condition is similar to that seen in rapidly growing, overconditioned foals with a calcium/phosphorus imbalance in the ration. In one published report involving a twelve-month-old pregnant Nubian doe, analysis of the total ration indicated a calcium-to-phosphorus ratio in the diet of 4.4:1 (Anderson and Adams 1983). The author has seen severe bilateral bowing deformity of the carpi in a twelve-month-old Saanen doe on a ration of alfalfa hay, a commercial goat chow supplemented with calcium, and free-choice dicalcium phosphate as a mineral lick (Figure 4.11).

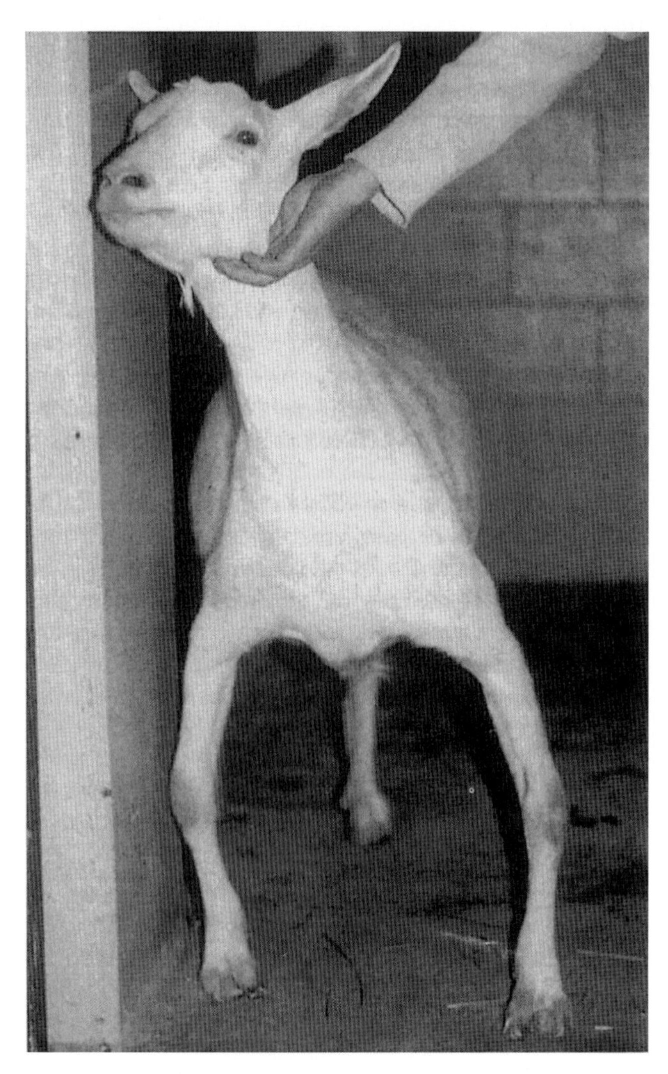

Figure 4.11. Bowing deformity of the forelimbs due to carpal epiphysitis associated with excessive calcium feeding in a yearling Saanen doe. (Courtesy of Dr. David M. Sherman.)

Elimination of the mineral and reduction of the goat chow in the diet resulted in some straightening of the forelimbs over the next two months.

Young, growing goats with painful epiphysitis may be reluctant to rise, have a stilted gait, or even walk on their knees. Overconditioned or pregnant goats may be especially painful due to the excessive burden of weight-bearing. Joints associated with affected epiphyses may appear swollen. Angular limb deformities may be pronounced, depending on the duration of the condition.

Serum calcium, phosphorus, and alkaline phosphatase levels are normal. Radiographs reveal an unequal growth rate across affected physes with lipping, or overgrowth, of new bone on the margins of the physeal plate.

Management of epiphysitis in young goats requires ration analysis and correction of excessive feeding of calcium. The normal calcium-to-phosphorus ratio in the diet should be in the range of 1.5:1 to 2:1. In active cases, use of nonsteroidal anti-inflammatory drugs such as flunixin meglumine, removal from hard surfaced flooring, and proper foot trimming may offer some clinical improvement.

Bentleg or Bowie

This is a condition most commonly seen in growing lambs grazed on pastures with phosphorus deficient soils, notably in South Africa, New Zealand, and Australia. Affected animals develop *genu valgum* (bentleg) or *genu varum* (bowie). The condition has also been reported in three- to four-month-old Saanen kids in New South Wales, Australia (Murphy et al. 1959). Affected kids developed a severely knock-kneed (*genu valgum*) appearance at the carpi and were also bent in at the fetlock with inward rolling on the medial claws. The condition was ascribed to an imbalance of calcium and phosphorus in the ration. In experimental trials, cases of bentleg were significantly reduced when a diet containing calcium and phosphorus in a ratio less than 1.4:1 was fed compared to a diet with a Ca:P ratio greater than 1.8:1 (Murphy et al. 1959). In New Zealand, mature does in late pregnancy are reported to experience bentleg (Merrall 1985).

Bentleg, at least in goats, may be a manifestation of epiphysitis associated with excessive calcium feeding. However, the roles of other mineral imbalances, including iron excess, copper deficiency, and manganese deficiency, as well as plant toxicities, in the pathogenesis of bentleg have not been completely clarified. The etiology of bowie or bentleg in lambs is still considered to be unknown, though supplementing the diet with phosphorus or topdressing pastures with superphosphate usually results in disappearance of the disease (Radostits et al. 2007).

Fibrous Osteodystrophy (Osteodystrophia Fibrosa)

Etiology and Pathogenesis

This bone disease is an example of nutritional secondary hyperparathyroidism that results from a chronic, sustained intake of excessive dietary phosphorus. Increased phosphorus intake leads to an analytically imperceptible hyperphosphatemia that suppresses serum calcium levels. The resulting hypocalcemia triggers an increased secretory response of parathyroid hormone. Parathyroid hormone mobilizes calcium from bone to restore normal serum calcium levels. In the face of chronic, excess phosphorus intake, this secondary hyperparathyroidism ultimately results in severe, generalized demineralization of bone and a fibrous reaction of the bony matrix.

Epidemiology

The condition is well known in goats (Carda Aparici et al. 1972; Naghshineh and Haghdoust 1973; Saha and Deb 1973; Andrews et al. 1983). It arises under circumstances of prolonged or monotonous feeding of rations with high phosphorus content. This often involves a diet high in grain and cereal hays with little or no access to leguminous forages or calcium-based mineral supplements. Bran feeding is a common factor in many cases. The condition was described in the 1930s in goats experimentally fed flaked maize and bran with a minimum amount of hay (Glock and Murray 1939). All breeds and ages of goats are susceptible when weaned.

Clinical Signs

The initial signs may be nonspecific and involve progressive lethargy, difficulty in eating and drinking, weight loss, and a preference for recumbency. Though all bones may be affected, there is a propensity for the mandibles to first show detectable abnormalities. There is a visible bilateral swelling of the mandibles, particularly over the rami, which may progress over several months and be quite pronounced (Figure 4.12a). These cases are frequently mistaken for lumpy jaw (actinomycosis) which is uncommon in goats. The jawbone may be palpably soft. The goat's ability to open the mouth widely may be restricted. Salivation may be present and the tongue may hang from the mouth. Disruptions of the dental arcades with displacement of individual teeth is common. Teeth may actually point horizontally instead of vertically. Affected animals may have a stiff or painful gait, or be recumbent, due to pathologic fractures that may spontaneously occur in dystrophic bones.

Clinical Pathology and Necropsy

Enlargement and rarefaction are evident and displacements of the teeth can be identified in radiographs

Figure 4.12. Clinical appearance and radiographic findings in fibrous osteodystrophy. (From Andrews et al. 1983; reproduced by permission of *Veterinary Record*.)

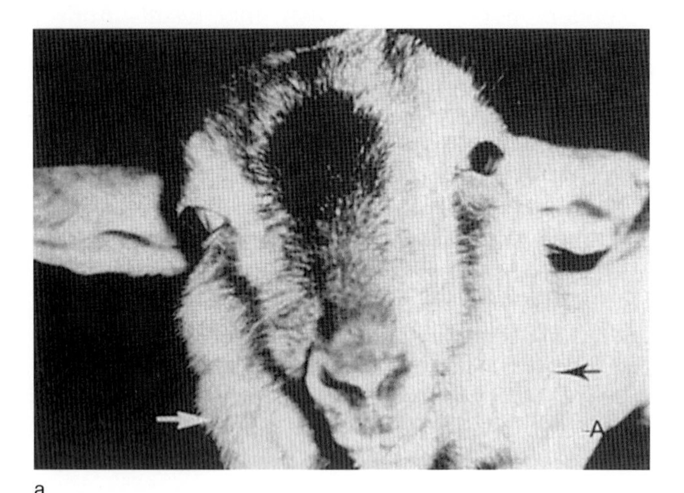

a

Figure 4.12a. Typical swelling of the face caused by mandibular distortions associated with fibrous osteodystrophy.

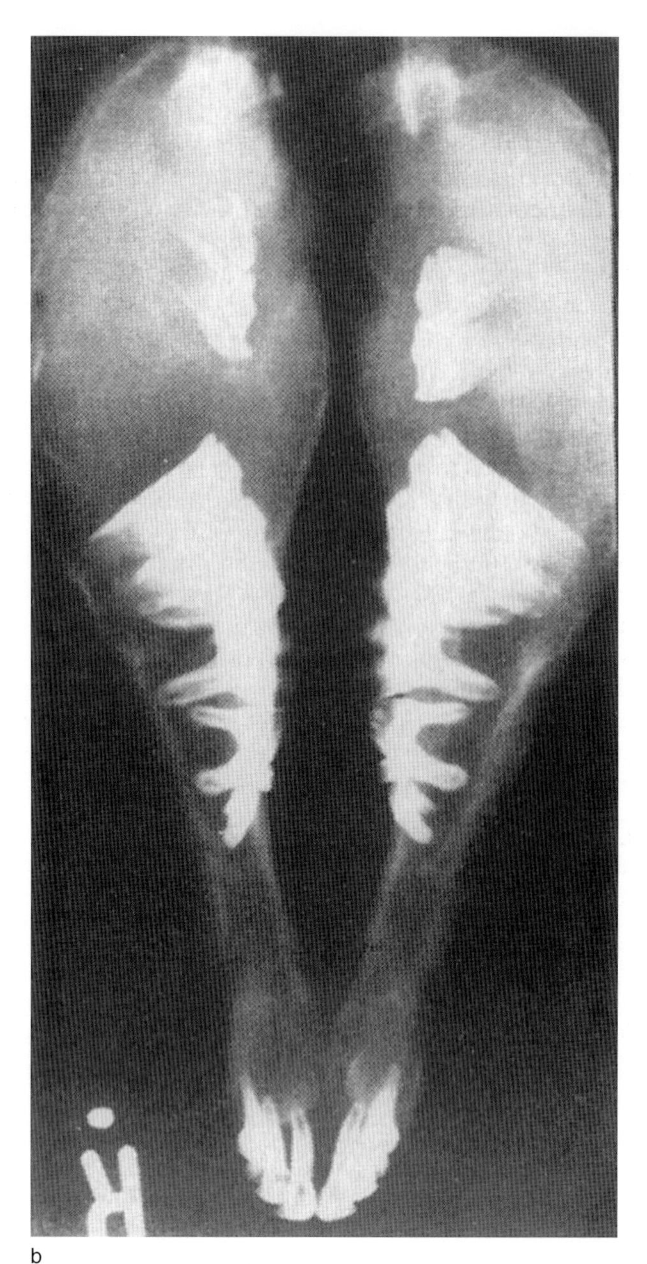

b

Figure 4.12b. Mandibular radiograph of the same goat. Note that in this advanced case, the occlusal surfaces of the teeth are directed medially.

of the mandible (Figure 4.12b). Fractures of long bones, especially incomplete fractures, may also be confirmed radiographically. Serum chemistry results are variable. Elevation of serum alkaline phosphatase is the most consistent abnormality. Hyperphosphatemia and hypocalcemia may also be noted but their absence does not rule out fibrous osteodystrophy.

At necropsy, affected bones are soft, and in severe cases, the mandibles can be cut easily with a knife. The gross enlargement and distortion of the mandibles are evident on cross section. Ribs are rubbery and flexible. Histologically, there is osteoporosis with marked demineralization of bony trabeculae surrounded by a loose fibrous connective tissue matrix. Hyperplasia of the parathyroid glands is present, principally involving increased numbers of light chief cells with extensive vacuolation and margination of cell nuclei (Carda Aparici et al. 1972).

Treatment and Control

Reversal of clinical lesions is possible, if recognized early, by dietary management involving reduction of phosphorus levels and correction of the calcium-to-phosphorus ratio. Additions of leguminous hay and/or ground limestone to the diet are practical ways of increasing calcium in the diet without increasing phosphorus content. For grain-fed small ruminants in Brazil, addition of 1% to 1.5% calcium carbonate to the grains improved the Ca:P ratio and prevented fibrous osteodystrophy (Riet-Correa 2004).

Osteopetrosis

Osteopetrosis has been described by one authority as a bony abnormality of adult male goats fed diets excessive in calcium (Guss 1977). It is postulated that such diets promote hypercalcitoninism and the excessive deposition of calcium into bone. The condition is believed to be similar to the disease ankylosing spondylitis that occurs in breeding bulls on high calcium diets. However, this has not been confirmed experimentally.

The condition is said to occur in mature dairy bucks that are fed rations formulated for lactating does on the same farm. Such rations usually contain calcium in excess of that required for a nonlactating, nongrowing male. Bucks show clinical signs only after they have ceased to grow and have been on the offending diet for many months. They develop proliferative calcification around the joints that leads to palpable enlargements, a stiff gait, and possible ankylosis with reduced range of motion in affected joints. Radiographs confirm the proliferative lesion. When bony proliferation is observed around joints in lame goats, caprine arthritis encephalitis virus infection must also be considered in the differential diagnosis, particularly if mineralization of tendons and joint capsule is also present.

There is no treatment, because the lesions are not reversible. Prevention is based on dietary management. Grass hay should serve as the basis of the diet, and calcium supplementation of the concentrate feed should not exceed 0.5%. If bucks are fed pure alfalfa hay, then no additional calcium supplementation should be offered, and addition of monosodium phosphate to the concentrate at a rate of 1% may be indicated.

Laminitis

Laminitis, or founder, is an aseptic inflammation of the sensitive laminae of the hooves. Acute and chronic forms occur in goats that result in lameness and possible deformities of the hoof.

Etiology and Pathogenesis

The causes and pathogenesis of laminitis in hoofed stock are not completely understood. The principal lesion appears to be vascular, associated with abnormal circulation within the corium, or dermis, of the hoof. Acute engorgement of vessels of the sensitive laminae leads to intense pain in the feet. Chronic circulatory dysfunction leads to both a breakdown of the connection between the corium and the hoof wall, allowing separation and rotation of the third phalanx within the hoof, and a distortion of new horny growth of the hoof.

Epidemiology

Laminitis in goats is seen more often in intensive management settings than extensive ones. Its occurrence following sudden ration changes, excessive feeding of grain, or overt cases of engorgement toxemia suggests lactic acidemia as a predisposing factor. Experimental induction of lactic acidosis in goats by overfeeding of grain resulted in lameness (Tanwar and Mathur 1983). The occurrence of laminitis after kidding in association with retained placenta, metritis, pneumonia, mastitis, and enterotoxemia suggests the action of bacterial toxins in the pathogenesis of the condition. Laminitis has also been observed after normal kidding, and in association with unspecified allergic conditions (Guss 1977). Chronic laminitis is more often recognized clinically in goats than acute laminitis.

Clinical Signs

Because acute laminitis often occurs in conjunction with other medical conditions such as grain overload that produce overt clinical signs, the presence of laminitis should not be overlooked. Affected goats may appear anxious and uncomfortable and grind their teeth from pain. Fever caused by underlying infectious diseases may be present. The goat may refuse to walk or even stand. The affected hooves are warm to the touch, particularly in the area just distal to the coronary band. Laminitis is almost always bilateral. The forelimbs are more often involved than the hind limbs, but all four feet can be affected. Goats with acute laminitis of the forelimbs may walk on their knees.

In chronic laminitis earlier episodes of acute laminitis may not have been seen, or recognized, so the onset may appear insidious. There is usually a vague lameness or an increasing tendency for animals to walk on their knees. The animal may stand with the hind limbs placed well forward under the torso. Though heat is not palpable in the feet in chronic laminitis, the conformation of the hoof becomes distorted. The hoof wall becomes thickened with a loss of distinction between the wall and sole, and the feet become characteristically overgrown in a "slipper foot" or "sled runner" shape with the unworn toes turned upward. This is due to rotation of the third phalanx causing convexity of the sole with the result that weight bearing is rocked back onto the heel (Pinsent 1989).

Clinical Pathology

There are no specific clinical laboratory abnormalities to support the diagnosis of laminitis, although the presence of lactic acidemia, endotoxemia, or a hemogram characteristic of inflammation may provide evidence of a likely underlying disease problem. Diagnostic radiography is rarely employed to confirm the diagnosis of laminitis in goats. The incidence of rotation of the third phalanx in caprine laminitis is unreported, and chronic laminitis is usually apparent from the gross appearance of the foot.

Diagnosis

The presumptive diagnosis of acute laminitis is based on a history of predisposing management and disease factors, an acute reluctance to walk or stand, and heat in the feet, especially the front feet. Foot rot and puncture wounds must be ruled out. In chronic laminitis, arthritis must be ruled out when goats walk on their knees. Chronic selenosis must be considered in regions where it occurs when the hooves appear abnormal in association with lameness. Simple neglect of routine foot trimming must also be considered.

Treatment

In acute laminitis, it is important to identify and aggressively treat any predisposing disease process, such as engorgement toxemia or toxic metritis, correcting lactic acidosis, dehydration, and bacterial toxemias when present. Therapy directed at the laminitis consists primarily of analgesics to reduce pain in the feet and keeping the animal mobile. Nonsteroidal anti-inflammatory drugs such as phenylbutazone and flunixin meglumine are particularly useful in this regard, because, as prostaglandin inhibitors, they probably also reduce the deleterious effects of endotoxins. Phenylbutazone can be given orally at a dose of 10 mg/kg once a day or flunixin parenterally at a dose of 1 mg/kg once a day with the treatment tapering off over several days. Phenylbutazone should be avoided in animals for milk or meat production because of residue concerns. Enforced exercise may be helpful in the acute phase to promote normal circulation. Affected goats should be fed only grass hay while they recover and then brought back onto richer feeds cautiously. The value of antihistamines in the treatment of acute laminitis remains unproven. The use of corticosteroids is controversial because they have been shown to induce laminitis in horses.

Management of chronic laminitis involves reduction of grain in the ration, avoidance of sudden ration changes, and frequent corrective foot trimming to approximate as normal a hoof conformation as possible. The foot is trimmed to reduce the height of the heel and to remove the convexity of the sole to minimize the downward pressure of the tip of the third phalanx. When separation of the white line has occurred, the abaxial hoof wall should be trimmed back to the top of the pocket; otherwise dirt and debris will pack in and deepen the lesion. When necessary, administration of analgesics may help to control pain and promote mobility. For long-term analgesic therapy, aspirin is useful because of low cost. Goats can be started at a dose of 100 mg/kg orally twice a day and titrated down to whatever lesser dose is needed to maintain comfort. Extended therapy at the starting dose could possibly lead to gastrointestinal ulceration or anorexia.

Control

To prevent laminitis in goats, abrupt feed changes should be avoided and grain feeding should be kept to a minimum. When high energy rations are indicated for milk or hair production, addition of buffers such as sodium bicarbonate to the diet should be considered to reduce the risk of lactic acidosis. Regular hoof trimming should be carried out.

Zinc Deficiency

Zinc deficiency in ruminants is most often recognized as a proliferative dermatitis (parakeratosis) as discussed in Chapter 2. Zinc also plays a role in the normal development of bone and hoof. Zinc is most concentrated in bone in the Haversian system and participates in the calcification of preosseous tissue either as an enzyme cofactor or as a metallic salt promoting crystal seeding during mineralization (Hidiroglu 1980). Dietary zinc requirements in goats are given in Chapter 19.

Zinc-deficient goats may display skeletal and hoof abnormalities in addition to dermatitis. Affected goats adopt an abnormal posture in which the back is arched and the feet are held closely together. Bowing of the hind limbs and swollen hocks may also be seen. The dermatitis may involve the coronets leading to inflammation of the hooves. Feet may be painful on palpation. Deep, transverse ridges may encircle the hoof wall. Zinc-deficient goats also show poor growth rates, decreased feed intake, loss of condition, excessive salivation, and testicular dysfunction (Neathery 1972). They may have impaired immune function, often dying of secondary pneumonic infections (Miller et al. 1964). Dwarfism has been reported in male goats in experimentally induced zinc deficiency. This was considered an indirect effect of zinc on pituitary function rather than a direct effect of zinc on bone development (Groppel and Henning 1971).

In experimental feeding trials, goats on limited zinc diets had mean plasma zinc levels in the range of 0.49 to 0.79 ppm, while the range in normal control goats was 0.83 to 1.1 ppm (Neathery 1972). In field cases of zinc deficiency in goats, plasma zinc levels in affected goats were in the range of 0.46 to 0.54 ppm (Nelson et al. 1984). Mean dry bone concentrations of zinc in goats on experimental zinc-deficient diets were 71 ppm, significantly less than the mean of 84 ppm in control goats (Groppel and Henning 1971). Hair samples can also be used to confirm zinc deficiency, with deficient goats having hair zinc concentrations less than 90 ppm (Neathery 1972).

Successful treatment of hoof and postural problems was reported with oral administration of 250 mg of zinc sulfate daily for four weeks (Nelson et al. 1984).

TOXICOLOGICAL DISEASES

Hypervitaminosis D

Vitamin D toxicity can result from excessive administration of parenteral or oral vitamin D. Such cases have been reported in cattle, horses, and pigs (Radostits et al. 2007). Excess vitamin D causes increased absorption of calcium from intestine, reabsorption from bone, and retention of phosphorus by the kidney. There is a tendency for thinning of bone and calcification of soft tissues to occur, especially muscle and vascular tissue, with multiple clinicopathologic consequences.

The risk to goats of iatrogenic vitamin D toxicity has been demonstrated experimentally (Singh and Prasad 1987). Goats given cholicalciferol injections weekly for two to eight months developed clinical signs of dullness, depression, rough hair coat, inappetence, diarrhea, polyuria, polydipsia, and reduced growth rate. Muscle weakness and a stiff gait were observed in some animals. Hypercalcemia and hyperphosphatemia were consistent findings. Serum alkaline phosphatase levels, however, were quite variable.

Enzootic calcinosis, caused by consumption of *Trisetum flavescens*, is discussed later in this chapter. It is considered to be a naturally occurring form of vitamin D toxicity, because the plant contains high levels of 1,25 $(OH)_2D_3$. It is reported in goats in Europe.

Fluorosis

Fluorosis in goats is a chronic intoxication caused by prolonged exposure to fluoride compounds in feed, water, and soils. The incorporation of excessive fluorine into the skeletal or dental matrices causes abnormal development of teeth and bone, especially in growing animals.

Etiology and Epidemiology

Animals may come into contact with fluorine in many ways. The element is found in high concentration in phosphate-rich soils in some regions of the world, particularly in North Africa. Although plants do not take up fluoride readily, grazing animals may ingest soil along with plants while feeding, thus increasing their exposure to fluoride. When vegetation does incorporate fluoride, a process enhanced by acid soils, then stems and leaves have higher concentrations than grains. Deep well water is a source of excessive fluoride in Australia and South America and volcanic ash is a source of pasture contamination in the Andes and in Iceland (Radostits et al. 2007).

Rock phosphate, rich in fluoride, is mined commercially for manufacturing fertilizers and mineral supplements for animal feeds. Unless these mineral supplements are specifically defluorinated before incorporation into animal feeds, they may provide dangerous levels of fluoride. Water and tailings from mining operations can be sources of excess fluoride to animals living nearby due to runoff or careless disposal. This occurs in many parts of North Africa. In west central Morocco, for instance, where phosphate mining is a major industry, fluorosis is recognized as an important clinical problem in human and livestock populations, and is known as darmous (Kessabi and Abdennebi 1985). Soils in endemic areas contain fluoride in the range of 1,450 to 4,085 ppm DM. Pasturage in these regions has fluoride concentrations in the range of 95 to 260 ppm DM; hay, 85 to 180 ppm DM; and barley grain, 11 to 18 ppm DM. Clear water has an average of 1.4 ppm fluoride. However, drinking water in these areas is often turbid, containing much soil and rock particulate matter, and the average fluoride concentration of turbid water is 14 ppm. Fluorosis is likely to develop in livestock when the long-term ration concentration of fluorine exceeds 100 ppm DM. In the wet season, grazing is identified as the major source of fluoride ingestion, while in the dry season, it derives from increased water consumption. In Egypt, chronic fluorosis has been reported in goats kept in the vicinity of a superphosphate factory emitting airborne hydrofluoric acid as a byproduct (Karram 1984).

Fluoride is also found frequently in ores processed for aluminum and iron. Smelting and milling operations release fluoride into the air, thus contaminating fields, crops, and water sources through settling of particulates. Animals grazing nearby can ingest sufficient deposited fluoride to develop toxicity as reported in goats near an aluminum smelter plant in India (Sahoo and Ray 2004). In Inner Mongolia in China, industrial fluoride pollution has a serious impact on cashmere goat production. The life span of goats may be reduced to two to three years due to impaired pasturing, mastication, and inanition resulting from teeth deformed by fluorosis (Wang et al. 2002).

Fluorine exposure from the sources discussed above involve inorganic fluoride compounds and toxicity usually arises from chronic exposure. Acute fluorine toxicity may also occur in livestock accidentally exposed to large doses of organic fluorides such as sodium fluoroacetate, which is used as a rodenticide and in predation control. Acute fluoride toxicity from such accidental poisoning has not been reported in goats, though they are presumably susceptible.

An unusual form of acute monofluoroacetate poisoning of goats in South Africa occurs after ingestion of the plant *Dichapetalum cymosum*, also known as gifblaar, which accumulates monofluoroacetate. The clinical manifestation is usually rapid death due to heart failure, as discussed in Chapter 8.

Pathogenesis

Chronic fluorosis results from prolonged but not necessarily continuous ingestion of excessive fluoride compounds. Tolerance levels for goats have not been reported, but safe ration concentrations for breeding ewes up to 60 ppm and for feeder lambs up to 100 ppm have been established (Osweiler et al. 1985). In experimental studies involving daily administration of sodium fluoride, the response of goats appears to be similar to that of sheep (Milhaud et al. 1983). Fluorides are readily absorbable from the digestive tract, though the availability and digestibility of fluorides varies with the source. In goat studies, fluoride was 75% available from sodium fluoride, 65% from ground raw rock phosphate, 34% from defluorinated phosphate, and 38% from dicalcium phosphate (Clay and Suttie 1985).

Though fluorine accumulates in all tissues, the manifestations of chronic fluorosis are referable to fluorine accumulation in hard tissues, namely, bone and teeth (Milhaud et al. 1980).

Fluorine can be incorporated into bone throughout the life of the animal, but accumulates in teeth only during development. Therefore the presence or absence of lesions in teeth erupting at different ages gives some indication of the duration and onset of exposure to fluoride. The effect of excessive fluoride on developing teeth is to impair normal mineralization of the preenamel, predentine, and precementum matrices. There is evidence that high fluoride interferes with normal collagen synthesis to produce imperfect collagen or even noncollagenous protein, which alters the tooth matrix structure and results in abnormal tooth morphology (Wang et al. 2003). Affected teeth are softer, appear mottled, and wear more quickly. Typical staining of affected teeth results from oxidation of exposed organic material in the tooth. Affected animals may have difficulty drinking cold water, and due to excessive tooth wear, may have difficulty in prehension and mastication. These animals grow poorly and are underconditioned as a result of impaired feed intake.

The adverse effects on bone include disruption of osteogenesis, acceleration of bone remodeling, development of exostoses and sclerosis, and osteoporosis. An important underlying mechanism for abnormal bone development in fluorosis is the impact of fluoride on collagen metabolism leading to structural changes in collagen fibers that affect the extracellular matrix of bone. Recently it was reported that at the molecular level, collagen gene expression is altered in goats with fluorosis (Li et al. 2006, 2007). Animals with skeletal fluorosis may have visible swellings on bones and exhibit a stiff and painful gait or intermittent lameness. Chronic fluorosis can also produce anemia in affected livestock through accumulation in the bone marrow and suppression of erythropoiesis.

Clinical Findings

Signs of chronic fluorosis may be nonspecific and include anorexia, a stiff gait, a history of intermittent lameness, emaciation, a rough, dry hair coat, and pale mucous membranes suggesting anemia. Morbidity rates can be high, especially in endemic areas. Careful observation of animals while they eat and drink may reveal difficult mastication or mouth pain. Specific examination of the teeth and palpation of the skeleton are necessary to correlate these general findings with a diagnosis of fluorosis. Incisors are most easily examined. Affected teeth show streaky or splotchy yellow to brown to black staining, and have a mottled chalky appearance to the enamel surface (Figure 4.13). Teeth may be worn beyond expectation

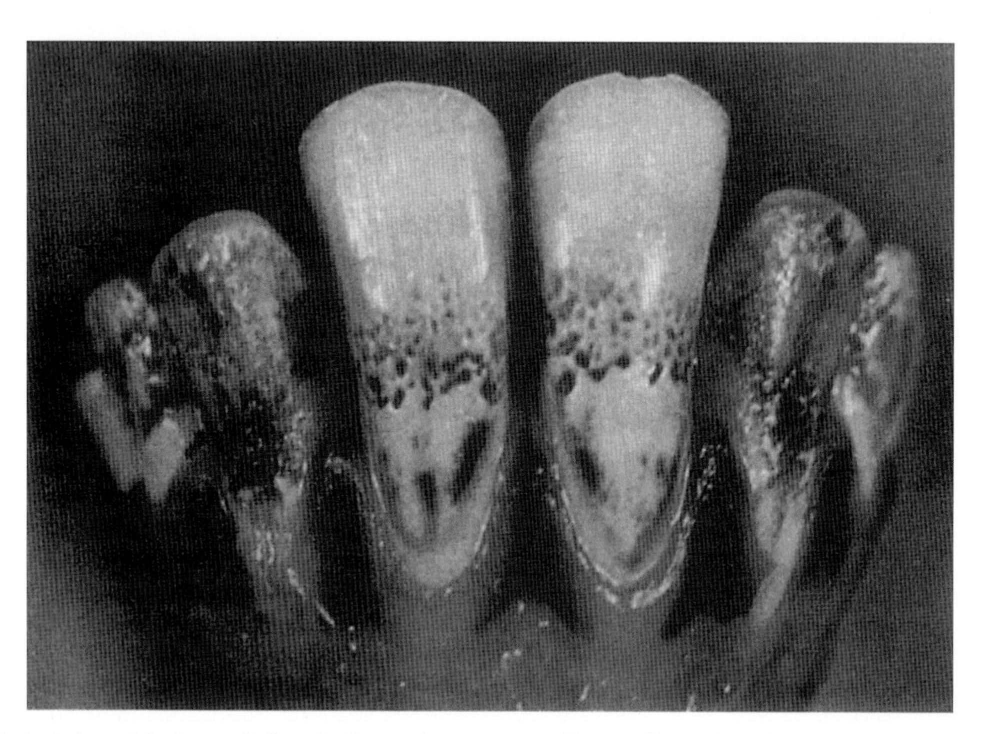

Figure 4.13. Typical dental lesions of chronic fluorosis. Note mottling and staining. (From Milhaud et al. 1980a.)

for the age of the animal, and some individual teeth may be prematurely lost. The number of teeth involved will vary depending on when exposure to fluorides began. However, pairs of teeth, for example, corner incisors, are bilaterally affected because they developed at the same time.

Palpation of the skeleton may reveal a general thickening of bones or focal swellings caused by exostoses, particularly on the mandibles, ribs, and metacarpal and metatarsal bones. Overt lameness or recumbency may be due to either bone pain or fractures occurring secondary to fluorotic changes in bone. Rib fractures are common in smaller does that have been mounted by large bucks at breeding.

Clinical Pathology and Necropsy

Normal plasma fluorine levels in goats have been reported in the range of 0.09 to 0.22 mg/l, while goats with signs of chronic fluoride intoxication have concentrations of 0.6 to 1.1 mg/l (Milhaud et al. 1980a). Urine fluoride levels of more than 15 ppm suggest chronic fluorosis in cattle, but diagnostic levels in goats have not been reported.

Anemia may be documented in the hemogram of goats with chronic fluorosis (Karram et al. 1984). In other species, serum calcium and phosphorus levels are usually within normal limits but serum alkaline phosphatase is often elevated. In experimental chronic fluorosis in goats, serum alkaline phosphatase levels were normal, as were serum calcium and phosphorus levels (Milhaud et al. 1980). In a naturally occurring field outbreak, affected goats were hypocalcemic and hyperphosphatemic, but alkaline phosphatase was not measured (Karram 1984).

Radiographically, the severity and extent of detectable lesions depends on the duration, degree, and onset of exposure to fluoride. In the jaws, maxillary borders become hazy and irregular. Bone structure becomes more porous with reduced density of cancellous bone. Compact or cortical bone is thinned. Molar and premolar tooth roots become less opaque and less substantial and abnormal tooth wear is apparent. In long bones, increased porosity and decreased density are also noted. Physeal cartilage of the metatarsal and metacarpal bones becomes hazy and double lines are noted at the growth plate. Osseous bridging across the growth plate may also be seen and joint spaces may be narrowed. Pseudoarthroses may be seen when rib fractures are present. Periosteal hyperostosis is a consistent finding in advanced, severe chronic fluorosis in cattle, but was not reported in experimental chronic fluorosis of goats (Milhaud et al. 1980).

At necropsy, the carcass may be in poor flesh. There are no gross or histologic lesions in soft tissues. Bones may be brittle and have a chalky white appearance with a roughened, irregular surface. They may be thicker and heavier than normal. Mandibles and metatarsal and metacarpal bones are most commonly affected. Fluorotic molars and premolars may show staining, mottling, chalkiness, and excessive wear similar to affected incisors. The staining, which involves the organic matrix of the tooth, cannot be scraped off, in contrast to superficial food staining. Microscopically, bones may show varying degrees of osteopetrosis or osteoporosis depending on the type, intensity, and duration of fluoride exposure. When fluorosis is suspected, bone should be analyzed for fluoride content. Mandible, rib, metatarsal, and metacarpal bones are most commonly submitted. In normal goats, fluorine concentration in these bones is reported to be less than 17.5 ppm/fat-free dry matter (Milhaud et al. 1983).

Diagnosis

Presumptive diagnosis is based on a history of chronic exposure to fluorides, lameness or stiff gait, characteristic dental lesions, and consistent radiographic findings. Fibrous osteodystrophy, which occurs on high phosphorus diets, may produce lameness, jaw swelling, and disruption of normal dental alignment, but mottling and chalkiness of teeth are absent. Diagnosis is most challenging in the early stages when ill thrift or stiff gait may be the only presenting complaints. Definitive diagnosis requires confirmation of increased fluoride levels in bone samples taken by biopsy or at necropsy.

Treatment and Control

There is no specific treatment for chronic fluorosis beyond removal of animals from the fluoride source, which is difficult when the source is industrial or environmental. Attempts should be made to identify all sources of fluorine and their relative danger. When possible, management should allow young, growing stock access to the least contaminated pastures, feeds, and water supplies to reduce the incidence of dental fluorosis. Turbid water sources should be allowed to settle and clear water only offered to goats. Water can be pretreated with slaked lime at a rate of 500 to 1,000 ppm and allowed to settle for six days. When fluoride exposure is unavoidable, daily feeding of aluminum salts such as aluminum sulfate, aluminum chloride, or calcium aluminate can help reduce fluorine absorption and its toxic effects. A dose of 30 g/head/day has been recommended in cattle, but no dosages have been found for goats.

When mineral supplements are fed to goats, raw rock phosphate and superphosphate should be avoided or at least checked for fluorine levels before use. Defluorinated phosphate supplements are recommended. Suitable products should have a phosphorus-to-fluorine ratio of 100:1 or more (Osweiler et al 1985).

Extensively defluorinated products, however, are generally more expensive due to increased refining costs and may not be attractive to producers.

In parts of China, where industrial fluorosis is a major problem for grazing goats, a number of interventions have been attempted to reduce the problem, including: removal of goats from high to low fluoride areas, use of stored green grass in the dry season as fodder, trimming of affected teeth, and mineral supplementation. However, the best results for controlling the wearing down of affected teeth was to supply supplemental protein-rich feed to goats in high fluoride areas (Wang et al. 2002).

Chronic Selenium Poisoning

Chronic selenium poisoning is characterized by deformation and sloughing of the hooves with marked lameness and secondary emaciation in grazing animals resulting from decreased locomotion.

Etiology and Epidemiology

Chronic selenium poisoning of livestock occurs mostly in regions of the world where soil selenium levels are high. Seleniferous soils are found in the Rocky Mountains and Great Plains of North America, parts of Australia and India, as well as Israel, Ireland, New Zealand, portions of the former Soviet Union, and elsewhere. Plants growing on seleniferous soils absorb selenium and prolonged consumption of these plants by livestock leads to toxicosis. Indicator or converter plants, such as *Astragalus* spp., require selenium for growth and contain particularly high concentrations. Though often unpalatable, livestock will eat these plants under conditions of deprivation or overgrazing. Facultative plants may also absorb selenium from the soil but do not require it for growth. Grains such as corn, when grown on seleniferous soils, may contain toxic levels of selenium. More detailed information on seleniferous soil characteristics and soil-plant interactions is available elsewhere (Dhillon and Dhillon 2003).

Chronic selenium poisoning associated with prolonged ingestion of indicator plants assumes two clinical forms. The first, alkali disease, is characterized by weight loss and musculoskeletal abnormalities and is presented here. The second, blind staggers, is characterized by signs of neurologic dysfunction. In recent years the role of selenium in blind staggers has been called into question and the theory proposed that this condition is actually a manifestation of polioencephalomalacia resulting from excessive sulfur intake (O'Toole et al. 1996). Blind staggers is discussed further in Chapter 5.

Chronic selenium poisoning may also occur when selenium supplements are improperly mixed into feeds at excessive amounts. Experimental studies demonstrated that goats fed sodium selenite at a rate of 6 mg/kg bw daily became sick and died within four to nineteen days after feeding began. Goats fed 3 mg/kg bw daily showed no adverse effects after ninety days (Pathak and Datta 1984). Acute selenium poisoning has been produced experimentally in goats. Single oral doses of sodium selenite in the range of 40 to 160 mg/kg bw killed goats in a matter of hours. Repeated daily doses in the range of 5 to 20 mg/kg bw produced signs of inappetence, diarrhea, hind limb weakness, arching of the back, weight loss, recumbency, and death over a period of days to several weeks (Ahmed et al. 1990a).

Clinical Signs

Chronic selenosis seen in grazing goats in India appears clinically similar to the disease as seen in cattle and buffalo (Gupta et al. 1982). Animals introduced into seleniferous regions of Punjab develop signs within six months after arrival. All ages and both sexes are affected. The earliest signs are visible cracks in the horns and hooves, with irregular new growth at the coronary bands. The cracks gradually deepen and separate the older distal segments of the hoof from the new growth above. Hooves become deformed and elongated. Infection often occurs in the deep cracks of the hoof wall. The foot emits a necrotic odor and becomes extremely painful as pus accumulates. Affected goats have increasing difficulty standing, move with a staggering gait, or exhibit overt lameness. Severely affected animals remain recumbent. Impairment of locomotion drastically reduces feed intake and goats become weak, depressed, and emaciated. Decreased conception and increased abortion rates are also seen. Death is by inanition, predation, or secondary infection.

Clinical Pathology and Necropsy

Necropsy lesions are not particularly helpful in the diagnosis of alkali disease, but tissue samples should be collected to determine selenium levels. Specific toxic tissue levels have only infrequently been reported in goats. In other herbivores, levels of selenium in liver and kidney in the range of 4 to 25 ppm are found in chronic poisoning. Affected hoof tissue has selenium levels in the range of 8 to 20 ppm (Osweiler et al. 1985). In goats with selenium toxicosis from eating maize grown on seleniferous soils in China, blood Se concentrations greater than 0.2 µg/g were an indicator of early Se toxicity. Overt signs of Se poisoning appeared when blood and hair values were over 0.5 and 0.3 µg/g, respectively (Hou et al. 1994). Mean liver and kidney concentrations of selenium in these affected goats were 20.46 ± 0.89 µg/g and 20.96 ± 1.21 µg/g respectively, while liver and kidney selenium concentrations in control goats were 0.50 ± 0.16 μg/g and 8.92 ± 2.20 μg/g, respectively.

Treatment and Control

There is no effective treatment for selenium poisoning. Some practical recommendations for rangeland management have been offered to aid in control (Davis et al. 2000). Soils should be tested to identify high selenium content and livestock fenced out of the worst affected areas. Avoid overgrazing so as not to oblige livestock to consume seleniferous plants. Practice rotational grazing to limit the length of time animals spend on soils with high selenium levels. Graze animals on pastures with higher selenium concentrations only in the fall and winter, when grasses are more mature and have lower selenium content. Practice weed control because broadleaf plants are greater selenium accumulators than grasses. Unless soil sulfate levels are already high, selenium uptake by plants can be reduced by applying sulfur or gypsum to soil because sulfur is competitive with selenium in plant uptake. Avoid use of phosphate fertilizers which themselves may have a high selenium content and can also enhance selenium uptake in plants by displacing selenium bound to soil. When economically feasible, supplementary feeding with feedstuffs derived from nonseleniferous regions is the best method to dilute the uptake of selenium in chronically exposed animals. Feeding of supplemental copper and sulfur in a mineral mix can be beneficial in counteracting a high selenium diet as can an increase in the overall protein content of the diet.

Plants Toxic to the Musculoskeletal System

Senna (Cassia) roemeriana

Ingestion of *Senna* (*Cassia*) *roemeriana* (twin leaf senna) has caused death due to skeletal myopathy in grazing cattle and sheep in the southwestern United States and northern Mexico. Experimental feeding of the dried plant to adult Spanish goats at a rate of 5 or 7 g/kg bw for an average of twenty-four days resulted in toxic effects related to muscle damage. After about two weeks of intake, affected goats demonstrated decreased appetite, weight loss, increased heart and respiratory rates, and progressive weakness of the hind limbs, leading to recumbency. Elevations in serum creatine kinase as high as 43,800 IU/l were also detectable after two weeks. At necropsy, muscles were pale, especially in the hindquarters. There were also pericardial and pleural effusions and pulmonary edema in some goats. Histologically, affected muscle shows necrosis and fragmentation of myofibers with infiltration of necrotic sarcoplasm by neutrophils and macrophages (Rowe et al. 1987). In naturally occurring cases, nutritional muscular dystrophy would be the principal differential diagnosis.

Karwinskia humboldtiana

This shrub is indigenous to the southwestern United States and northern Mexico and is responsible for coyotillo poisoning, or limberleg, in livestock. The condition, which principally causes a neuropathy, is discussed in more detail in Chapter 5. However, it has been demonstrated that the fruits of *K. humboldtiana* can produce widespread skeletal and cardiac muscle degeneration in addition to neuropathy (Dewan et al. 1965). The lesion in skeletal muscle is one of hyaline degeneration, similar to that seen in nutritional muscular dystrophy. At least some of the incoordination and weakness observed in limberleg may be due to muscle damage in addition to neurologic dysfunction.

Trisetum flavescens

In alpine regions of Europe, a condition of livestock known as enzootic calcinosis is ascribed to the ingestion of *Trisetum flavescens*, or yellow oat grass, at pasture or in harvested forages. The plant contains high concentrations of 1,25-dihydroxycholicalciferol, the active metabolite of vitamin D. This metabolite markedly increases the intestinal absorption of calcium by herbivores. Chronic ingestion results in calcification of selected soft tissues, notably the great vessels, heart, lungs, tendons, and ligaments. A reluctance to walk and constant shifting of weight from leg to leg are common signs of tendon and ligament involvement. Further information on the cardiac effects of enzootic calcinosis are available in Chapter 8.

Enzootic calcinosis has been recorded in milk goats in Switzerland on a farm where yellow oat grass comprised 8% to 34% of the herbage on various fields (Kessler 1982). Twelve goats died over a three-year period. Affected goats showed progressive wasting, decreased milk production, increased heart and respiratory rates, and altered locomotion. Serum calcium, phosphorus, and alkaline phosphatase levels are increased in affected goats (Wanner et al. 1986). Evidence of calcification of soft tissues should be sought at necropsy. Paratuberculosis of goats also produces chronic wasting and calcification of the aorta, and this must be ruled out.

Delaying harvesting of *T. flavescens* reduces the toxic effect of the plants because young plants have greater vitamin D activity. Silage made with yellow oat grass is more toxic than hay.

A similar syndrome of soft tissue calcification caused by increased vitamin D activity occurs with ingestion of *Solanum malacoxylon* by herbivores in the Caribbean, South America, and Hawaii and from *Cestrum diurnum* ingestion in the southern United States. Reports of toxicity in goats from either of these plants were not found.

Lupinosis

Several forms of lupine toxicity occur in livestock and all are poorly documented in goats. The neurologic and hepatopathic forms are mentioned briefly in their respective Chapters, 5 and 11. In calves, a congenital skeletal form also occurs and is known as "crooked calf disease" in the western United States. The development of skeletal deformities results from transplacental transfer of a lupine alkaloid, anagyrine, during the second month of gestation. There is circumstantial evidence from California that the condition also may occur in developing goat fetuses whose dams consume *Lupinus latifolius* during pregnancy. Arthrogryposis, torticollis, and scoliosis are the characteristic signs. In addition, similar skeletal deformities have been observed in a human infant in California whose mother drank local goat milk during pregnancy, though a definitive causal link was not established (Kilgore et al. 1981).

INHERITED AND CONGENITAL DISEASES

Myotonia Congenita

Myotonia congenita is an inherited disease of goats that manifests as transient tetanic spasms of the skeletal musculature initiated by visual, tactile, or auditory stimuli. The condition represents an involuntary persistence of a voluntary muscle contraction. Goats affected are commonly known as fainting goats, fainters, or wooden-legged goats. Caprine myotonia congenita is used as an animal disease model for studies of human myotonia congenita, also known as Thomsen's disease.

Etiology and Pathogenesis

Caprine myotonia congenita appears to be inherited as an autosomal dominant gene with incomplete penetrance. Two classes of affected goats exist regarding clinical signs: mild and severe. The mildly affected goats are assumed to be heterozygous and severely affected goats homozygous for the responsible gene. Breeding studies argue against the condition being sex-linked.

Only voluntary striated skeletal muscles are involved in this disease. The defect appears to be at the level of the muscle fiber membrane and may be caused by a reduced number of chloride channels in myotonic fibers (Bryant and Owenburg 1980). This leads to a reduction in chloride conductance with decreased accommodation, increased membrane excitability, and abnormal repetitive muscle firing (Bryant et al. 1968; Adrian and Bryant 1974). The myotonic discharge may be triggered by any sustained depolarization such as a burst of nerve impulses in response to surprise, noise, or handling. The disease is characterized by a generalized, sustained tetanic contraction of skeletal muscles lasting for several seconds to approximately one minute. For reasons unclear, withholding water from myotonic goats for up to three days results in disappearance of the myotonic response. Reintroduction of water is accompanied by return of myotonia (Hegyeli and Szent-Gyorgyi 1961). The condition is also exacerbated by cold exposure and ameliorated by exercise (McKerrell 1987).

Epidemiology

Caprine congenital myotonia was first recognized in goats in Tennessee in the 1880s and was first described in the veterinary literature in 1904 (White and Plaskett 1904). Such goats were favored because they did not wander or easily escape confinement. They also became popular as an amusement. Recognition of these goats as a model for human myotonia congenita received growing attention in the 1930s (Kolb 1938).

Veterinarians may encounter myotonic goats in research herds maintained for studies of human myotonia congenita. The goats are also maintained as pets or curiosities, and their popularity as such seems to have grown in recent years, at least when gauged by media publicity. A few breeding herds exist to supply the research and pet markets and there are at least two breed registries for fainting goats. These animals are also being used increasingly as meat goats because of the heavy muscling that occurs in their hindquarters. Both males and females can be affected. Crossbreeding of a myotonic goat and a nonmyotonic breed of goat can produce a myotonic offspring.

Clinical Findings

The myotonic condition is not usually recognized in affected goats younger than two weeks of age and is clearly recognizable by six weeks. Younger goats may show some slight stiffening during handling. Buck kids tend to show more pronounced signs than females. Episodes of myotonia congenita can be triggered by visual, auditory, or contact stimuli such as the sudden appearance of strangers, clapping, or handling for vaccinations. Mildly affected goats develop maximal rigidity in the hind limbs. They visibly stiffen and when running away exhibit a "bunny hopping gait" caused by impaired mobility of the hind limbs. Severely affected goats show general muscular rigidity, stiffen, and fall over. Hyperextension of muscles can be so severe that recumbent animals involuntarily roll over on their backs with legs extended in the air. Some animals may temporarily stop breathing because of rigidity of thoracic muscles. Affected animals maintain a normal sensorium even during the tetanic episodes that may last up to a minute. Upon recovery from each episode, the goat will be stiff gaited for a short period and then return to normal. Affected goats become conditioned to intentional repeated stimulations and the veterinarian is less likely to be able to induce a myotonic episode as the examination progresses. The condition persists for life.

Clinical Pathology and Necropsy

There are no detectable abnormalities in hematology or clinical chemistry. Routine necropsy and histologic examination reveal no lesions. Electromyographic studies of the live animal may be helpful in diagnosis. Affected goats produce a distinctive response characterized by an audible "divebomber" sound typical of the persistent, high frequency discharge of muscle associated with a hyperexcitable muscle cell membrane (Steinberg and Botelho 1962). Myotonic goats have some characteristic ultrastructural abnormalities. Mitochondria from myotonic fibers have an altered lipid composition (Harris 1983). Isomyosins from myotonic fibers have a characteristic distribution with increased fast isomyosins (Martin et al. 1984).

Diagnosis

The presumptive diagnosis is based on the characteristic pattern of intermittent, sustained muscle stiffening in response to external stimuli in goats with a history of myotonic lineage. When the background of goats is unknown, electromyography tests can support the diagnosis. Tetanus is a progressive condition in which muscular rigidity becomes persistent rather than intermittent. The author has seen a pygmy goat with intermittent rigid collapse that, on necropsy, had extensive lesions of CAE virus infection in the cerebrum.

Treatment and Control

Goats with myotonia congenita are not usually treated. In humans, the condition is managed by daily administration of quinine sulfate or procainamide. Because fainting goats are often bred with the goal of maintaining the defect for research purposes, control is not an appropriate topic of discussion. Intentional breeding of these goats for amusement purposes should be discouraged on humane grounds.

Various Congenital Skeletal Abnormalities

Achondroplastic dwarfism is a breed characteristic of pygmy and dwarf goats. Akabane virus infection is discussed earlier in the chapter as an infectious cause of congenital skeletal deformity. Lupinosis is also discussed above as a possible phytotoxic cause. Ingestion of *Veratrum californicum* by does during gestation also has the potential of producing hypoplasia of metatarsal and metacarpal bones in kids in addition to the more commonly known sign of cyclopia (Binns et al. 1972). There are numerous reports of spontaneous congenital skeletal deformity in goats of unknown etiology. Hemivertebra of the fourth thoracic vertebra causing spinal injury and hind limb weakness was seen in a two-month-old Saanen cross kid and presumed to be hereditary (Rowe 1979). Increased limb length with knuckling of unknown cause was recognized in an Osmanabadi kid as a cause of dystocia (Kulkarni and Deshpande 1987). Tibial agenesis has been reported in a newborn Toggenburg kid (Giddings 1976). Radial agenesis and ulnar hypoplasia occurred in two Saanen kids from the same kidding (Baum et al. 1985). Complete absence of a forelimb at birth has also been observed in a West African Dwarf goat (Onawunmi et al. 1979). Lateral luxation of the patella secondary to a hypoplastic lateral trochlear ridge may be congenital in goats, though the condition is usually not observed until goats are older than one year of age (Baron 1987). Various other sporadic congenital deviations of the forelimbs and hind limbs have also been described (Koch et al. 1957).

An inherited condition of short tendons occurs in 0.03% to 4.5% of Australian Angora goats. Severely affected kids may die, but milder cases are correctable by splinting or plaster casting. The trait is transmitted as a recessive autosomal allele (Baxendell 1988). An inherited metacarpal gait has been reported in Saanen goats in Iran (Bazargani and Khavary 1976). Believed to be a recessive, sex-linked trait, only males of twins of different sexes were affected at birth. These animals walked on their metacarpi and died within a few weeks of age.

TRAUMATIC DISEASES

Predation

Predation can be a serious constraint on goat production. It is generally associated with death loss, particularly of neonates. However, nonfatal maiming of older goats occurs in certain situations, particularly those involving domestic dogs. Predation is discussed in the present chapter because musculoskeletal trauma is a common outcome in these instances.

Epidemiology

The subject of predator/prey relationships involving livestock is very complex and is fraught with economic, ecologic, ethical, and sociologic issues. For a more complete discussion of predation in general, the reader is referred to other sources (Gaafar et al. 1985; Rollins 2001; Shelton 2004).

Predation of goats is reported as a problem in Australia, the United States, and widely throughout the tropics. In Australia, predator importance varies with the type of goat involved and their geographic location, but is generally recognized as a major cause of kid mortality (Holst 1986). Feral goat kids are lost to foxes, dingoes, feral pigs, and hunters. Milk goats, more likely kept in semirural or suburban areas, are preyed upon primarily by domestic dogs. Angora kids are lost to foxes, eagles, and urban and wild dogs. In Southern Australia, fox predation occurs in Cashmere goat flocks. Attacks are nocturnal and kids are the primary target. Nevertheless, kid losses caused by predation by foxes may be less than those caused by mismothering and pregnancy wastage (Long et al. 1988).

In the United States, predation of hair goats and dairy goats has been studied. In south Texas, attacks on Angora goats were caused primarily by coyotes and secondarily by bobcats. Dramatic reductions in kid crop were attributable to predation, though aggressive predation control had little effect on reducing losses. Adult goats were not preyed upon until kids were decimated. It was concluded that in areas of high coyote density, intense local predator control would be insufficient to prevent heavy kid losses (Guthery and Beasom 1978). In 1999, in Arizona, New Mexico, and Texas, three major goat-producing states, 61,000 goats and kids were lost to predators, with losses valued at $3.4 million (Howery and DeLiberto 2004).

On eighty-four goat farms located in rural and semirural areas of Louisiana, domestic dogs were the most commonly recognized predators (Hagstad et al. 1987). Attacks occurred most commonly during periods of reduced light. Of those attacked, 80% were killed outright or required slaughter while 20% survived or recovered. Four management factors were identified as reducing the likelihood of attacks: penning of goats at night, the use of a night light, keeping goats near an occupied residence, and the presence of a dog belonging to the owner. Anecdotal reports from around the United States support the finding that domestic dogs allowed to run free at night are largely responsible for attacks on dairy goats. However, dairy goat owners in New England are increasingly complaining about attacks on kids by a growing coyote population.

Predation is cited as a cause of lost productivity throughout the tropics and housing goats at night is suggested as the most basic means of reducing losses (Devendra and Burns 1983). In a central Mali study, 17% of deaths in goats were ascribed to "lost" kids presumably taken by predators. Uncontrolled domestic dogs and lax herding practices were considered responsible (Traore and Wilson 1988). In West Timor, Indonesia, goat herders identified predation by dogs and pigs as the third largest cause of kid death after navel infection and enteritis (Gatenby 1988).

Domestic dogs are more likely than wild predators to maim rather than kill goats, because the pursuit of goats begins more as a game than as an earnest attempt at food acquisition. Domestic dogs often form packs that can wreak havoc in a flock or herd of goats with limited routes of escape. Far more goats are injured than could possibly be consumed as food. Goats and sheep make relatively easy targets for dogs because of their small size and nonaggressive behavior.

Clinical Signs and Diagnosis

Evidence of predation is variable. Predation is often assumed when young kids are lost in areas where predators are endemic. Owners and herders may actually witness acts of predation or the presence of predators near flocks or herds. In the aftermath of an unobserved predator attack, evidence may suggest the type of predator involved (Guthery and Beasom 1978; Squires 1981; Long et al. 1988). Coyotes, for example, most often attack young kids and devour them completely. The presence of coyote spoor containing mohair in the vicinity of livestock areas may be the only circumstantial evidence that coyotes are involved. Foxes may partially bury a carcass, and rather than devouring it completely, may slash open the abdomen and consume the entrails. When only small pieces of the carcass remain, and there is wide scattering of blood, pigs are the likely predators. Two to four, deep, focal penetrations of the skull, rib cage, or abdomen suggest killing by eagles. Primarily predation must be differentiated from scavenging of animals dead of other causes. In predation, there is extensive hemorrhage and free blood around the site of wounds while in scavenging, such as caused by crows, there is no hemorrhage and little free blood. Evidence of crow scavenging includes removal of eyes or tongue and evisceration through the anus or umbilicus.

In dog attacks, flesh wounds are common on the flanks and hindquarters, indicative of a chase, and carcasses may show no evidence of consumption. Animals surviving attack may show varying degrees of injury from superficial skin and muscular trauma to severe trauma with extensive blood loss and shock. Injuries may include crushing fractures of bones and visceral damage caused by deep bites. All bites can lead to secondary infection. While flesh wounds are relatively obvious, bites penetrating the abdomen and thorax should not be overlooked due to the threat of secondary peritonitis or pyothorax.

Treatment

The approach to management of goats after a predator attack depends a great deal on economics. When pet goats or valuable show or breeding stock are attacked and survive, aggressive medical therapy can be economically justified. Treatment of shock or blood loss with fluids, blood transfusion, and corticosteroid therapy is indicated. Broad-spectrum, parenteral antibiotic therapy should be initiated immediately and maintained for at least ten days in cases of severe attack. Surgical interventions to manage visceral trauma may be immediately necessary, though orthopedic interventions can usually wait until patients are stabilized. If animals are brought for veterinary attention shortly after attack, primary closure of skin and flesh wounds can be attempted. These should be left open or drains installed if it appears that much necrotic muscle will develop in wounds. Topical insecticide sprays should be used when fly strike is a potential problem. Affected animals should be kept in clean, warm, dry surroundings and fed a high-quality forage during convalescence. Tetanus prophylaxis is indicated.

In commercial flocks, treatment of individual survivors may be economically constrained and the veterinarian should help the owner to minimize economic losses subsequent to dog attacks where large numbers of animals may be involved. Some suggestions made for the care of sheep flocks after predator attack are applicable to goats as well (Dille 1985).

It may be possible to shear hair goats and salvage the fleece. Hides may also be salable if not severely damaged. If fresh, carcasses may be sold as feed for animal consumption, for example, to mink farms. Carcasses can also be used as bait to trap predators where trapping is allowed or used as evidence to derive compensation from owners of dogs involved in attacks. There may be government compensation in some places for losses to predators.

Live animals that are seriously wounded and unlikely to recover can be butchered for human consumption, unless there is a cause for suspecting rabies in the attacking animals. Animals with elevated or subnormal temperatures should not be butchered. Areas around bite wounds should be liberally trimmed. Animals unable to walk after attack and animals with evidence of penetration of body cavities by bite wounds should be considered for emergency slaughter.

Control

At the flock or herd level, losses to predation may be controlled in a number of ways. Active destruction of predators through trapping, poisoning, or shooting may be subject to local regulation and may or may not be economically justified when the costs of predator control are weighed against losses. Each situation should be evaluated on its merits. When domestic dogs are involved, stock owners must be sure that local ordinances controlling unleashed dogs are adequate and rigidly enforced. Poison baits for controlling predators have been withdrawn from use in the United States sine 1972 and other methods, such as trapping, snaring, M-44 sodium cyanide ejectors, gas cartridges for denning coyotes, and livestock protection collars have been restricted or eliminated by ballot initiatives in some states (Andelt 2004).

As predator control options have become more restricted, the use of livestock guarding animals has emerged as a cost effective and humane approach to protecting small ruminants from predation and their use has been recently reviewed (Andelt 2004). A number of dog breeds selectively developed in Europe and Asia to protect livestock from bears have become popular as guarding dogs for small ruminant flocks in the United States. These include the Great Pyrenees, Akbash, Anatolian Shepherd, and Komondor breeds, as well as the Maremma and Shar Planinetz breeds. Guard dogs in the United States are reported to be effective against coyotes, black bears, grizzly bears, and mountain lions, but may not be effective against wolves (Andelt 2004). Donkeys and llamas are also used as herd guardians with the advantage that they eat what the goats eat and thus do not require separate feeding as do dogs. Llamas are particularly effective against dogs, coyotes, and foxes because they are naturally aggressive toward canids. Intact males may try to breed ewes, so female llamas or geldings are preferred. Fencing is a costly and often inefficient means of predator control, though in Australia, dingo-proof fencing has been helpful to sheep farmers.

At a minimum, where predators are a problem, surveillance of the flock should be increased during kidding times and goats confined to a restricted kidding area when management conditions permit. Goats should be kept in a pen at night and the holding area should be illuminated. Control is improved if the holding area is near an occupied residence.

Fractures

Fractures are common in goats, though epidemiologic data on prevalence and predisposing factors is limited.

Epidemiology

Environmental hazards are often implicated in the occurrence of fractures. All forms of gating, fencing, and penning material should be evaluated carefully for the likelihood of goats catching limbs or necks in structural spaces before the material is used. The curiosity and climbing instincts of goats ensure that they will find a way to become entangled whenever possible. In the author's experience, chain link fences especially predispose to limb fractures in intensively managed goats. The animals stick their legs through the fence and then, if frightened or crowded by other goats, are unable to extricate the limb. Fracture secondary to struggling is a likely outcome. Trauma from dog attacks is another common cause of limb bone fractures in goats in the United States. Preexisting bone diseases such as osteomyelitis, chronic fluorosis, fibrous osteodystrophy, or rickets can predispose to fractures.

Two surveys from India give differing perspectives on the occurrence of caprine fractures. In Hisar, most fractures occurred in goats between one and three years of age. In order of decreasing frequency, fractures were observed in femur, tibia, metacarpus or metatarsus, phalanx, humerus, radius, and ulna (Singh et al. 1983). The prevalence of femoral fractures was attributed to free ranging goats around villages being hit from behind by vehicles with bumpers at thigh level. In Ranchi, fractures occurred most commonly in goats younger than six months of age. The most commonly involved bones were, in descending order of frequency, metacarpus, metatarsus, femur, tibia, radius and ulna, humerus, and phalanx. Forelimb and hind limb fractures occurred with approximately equal frequency. The occurrence of fractures was believed to be predisposed by soil calcium and phosphorus deficiencies and the hilly terrain in the region. Causes of fracture identified by history included slipping while grazing on hillsides (54%), playing or gamboling (24%), automobile accidents (18%), and trapping of limbs in wire enclosures (4%) (Dass et al. 1985).

Clinical Signs and Diagnosis

Fractures are usually identifiable by an acute onset of lameness, deviation of limbs, and/or palpable crepitus. Fractures secondary to nutritional deficiency rather than trauma are less likely to displace or be recognized on physical examination. Radiographic studies help to define the nature of the fracture and suggest therapeutic approaches.

Treatment

In young kids, simple splinting of distal limb fractures is frequently adequate and economically advantageous. Toothbrushes and split sections of PVC pipe are examples of splints that permit closed fractures of young kids to heal within three weeks. Adults may require five to six weeks to heal. The reader is referred to textbooks of large animal surgery for discussions of surgical repair of fractures. Suffice it to say here that numerous approaches to successful fracture management have been reported in goats including compression plating of radial and ulnar fractures (Bacher and Potkay 1975) and full limb casting of tibial fractures followed by application of a Robert Jones bandage (Mbiuki and Byagagaire 1984). Use of plaster casting alone was found to be an unsatisfactory method of managing radial and ulnar fractures (Buchoo and Sahay 1987).

When fracture repair and return to normal function are complicated by osteomyelitis or permanent nerve damage, limb amputation has been demonstrated to be a reasonable salvage operation in goats (Misk and Hifny 1979). The pelvic limb can be disarticulated at the hip or stifle, or amputated at the mid femoral level. Treated goats show excellent adaptation to three-legged locomotion.

Control

When fractures occur more than sporadically in a given herd or flock, underlying problems of structural hazards or nutritional deficiencies must be considered as predisposing to an increased incidence of skeletal trauma. Careful attention must be paid to calcium, phosphorus, and vitamin D levels in the ration.

NEOPLASTIC DISEASES

Primary and metastatic neoplasms of bone and muscle are rare in goats. There are reports of an osteochondrosarcoma in the rib and sternum of a goat (Cotchin 1960), an osteogenic sarcoma at a previously repaired fracture site in the humerus of a ten-year-old Toggenburg wether, and an osteoma of the mandible in a ten-year-old female Toggenburg-cross goat that resulted in dislocation of the jaw (Steinberg and George 1989).

Several nonbony tumors have been reported to secondarily affect the mandible or maxilla of goats, resulting in visible distortion of the face, dislocation of teeth, dysphagia, or stridor if the maxillary sinus is involved. These include oral adenocarcinoma (Lane and Anderson 1983), ossifying fibroma (Pritchard 1984), nasal papillary adenoma (Pringle et al. 1989), and lymphosarcoma (Craig et al. 1986). The latter has also been found to infiltrate the marrow of long bones.

REFERENCES

Abegunde, T.O., Adler, H.E., Farver, T.B. and DaMassa, A.J.: A serologic survey of *M. putrefaciens* infection in goats. Am. J. Vet. Res., 42:1798–1801, 1981.

Achour, M.H., Azizen, S., Ghemmam, Y. and Mazari, B.: Caprine arthritis-encephalitis in Algeria. Rev. Élev. Méd. Vet. Pays Trop., 47(2):159–161, 1994.

Adams, D.S.: Infectious causes of lameness proximal to the foot. Vet. Clin. N. Am. Large Anim. Pract., 5:499–509, 1983.

Adams, D.S., et al.: Transmission and control of caprine arthritis-encephalitis virus. Am. J. Vet. Res., 44:1670–1675, 1983.

Adams, D.S., et al.: Global survey of serological evidence of caprine arthritis-encephalitis virus infection. Vet. Rec., 115:493–495, 1984.

Adams, D.S., et al.: The relationship between caprine arthritis-encephalitis virus expression and clinical disease. In: Slow Viruses in Sheep, Goats, and Cattle. Report EUR 8076. J.M. Sharp and R. Hoff-Jorgnesen, eds. Luxembourg, Commission European Communities, pp. 227–231, 1985.

Adler, H.E. and Brooks, D.L.: Mycoplasma infections—the cause of arthritis, mastitis, and pneumonia of dairy goats in the United States. Proc., 3rd Internat. Conf. Goat Prod. Dis., Scottsdale, Dairy Goat Publ. Co., pp. 212–216, 1982.

Adrian, R.H. and Bryant, S.H.: On the repetitive discharge in myotonic muscle fibres. J. Physiol., 240:505–515, 1974.

Ahmed, K.E., Adam, S.E.I. and Idris, O.F.: Vitamin E is non-toxic to goats. Vet. Hum. Toxicol., 32:572, 1990.

Ahmed, K.E., Adam, S.E.I., Idrill, O.F. and Wahbi, A.A.: Experimental selenium poisoning in Nubian goats. Vet. Hum. Toxicol., 32:249–251, 1990a.

Al-Ahmad, M.Z.A., et al.: Cultured early goat embryos and cells are susceptible to infection with caprine encephalitis virus. Virology, 353(2):307–315, 2006.

Al-Aubaidi, J.M.: Biochemical characterization and serological classification of caprine and ovine mycoplasma with special reference to the antigenic relationships of *M. mycoides* var. *capri* and *M. mycoides* var. *mycoides*. D.Sc. Thesis, Cornell University, Ithaca, N.Y., 1972.

Al-Aubaidi, J.M., Taylor, W.D., Bubash, G.R. and Dardiri, A.H.: Identification and characterization of *Mycoplasma arginini* from bighorn sheep *(Ovis canadensis)* and goats. Am. J. Vet. Res., 33:87–90, 1972.

Al-Busaidy, S.M., Mellor, P.S. and Taylor, W.P.: Prevalence of neutralizing antibodies to Akabane virus in the Arabian peninsula. Vet. Microbiol., 17:141–149, 1988.

Alexander, K., Drost, W.T., Mattoon, J.S. and Anderson, D.E.: ^{99m}TC-ciprofloxacin in imaging of clinical infections in camelids and a goat. Vet. Radiol. Ultrasound, 46(4):340–347, 2005.

Alexandersen, S., Zhang, Z., Donaldson, A.I. and Garland, A.J.: The pathogenesis and diagnosis of foot-and-mouth disease. J. Comp. Pathol., 129:1–36, 2003.

Ali, O.A.: Caprine arthritis-encephalitis related changes in the uterus of a goat. Vet. Rec., 121:131–132, 1987.

Al-Momani, W. and Nicholas, R.A.J.: Small ruminant mycoplasmoses with particular reference to the Middle East. CAB Reviews: Perspectives in Agriculture, Veterinary Science, Nutrition and Natural Resources. 1:004, 11 pp, 2006.

Al-Momani, W., et al.: The *in vitro* effect of six antimicrobials against *Mycoplasma putrefaciens*, *Mycoplasma mycoides* subsp. *mycoides* LC and *Mycoplasma capricolum* subsp. *capricolum* isolated from sheep and goats in Jordan. Trop. Anim. Health Prod., 38(1):1–7, 2006.

Al-Qudah, K., Al-Majali, A.M. and Ismail, Z.B.: Epidemiological studies on caprine arthritis-encephalitis virus infection in Jordan. Small Rumin. Res., 66(1/3):181–186, 2006.

Altmaier, K.R., et al.: Osteomyelitis and disseminated infection caused by *Corynebacterium renale* in a goat. J. Am. Vet. Med. Assoc. 204(6):934–937, 1994.

Andelt, W.F.: Use of livestock guarding animals to reduce predation on livestock. Sheep Goat Res. J., 19:72–75, 2004.

Anderson, E.C., Doughty, W.J. and Anderson, J.: The role of sheep and goats in the epizootiology of foot-and-mouth disease in Kenya. J. Hyg, Camb., 76:395–402, 1976.

Anderson, K.L. and Adams, W.M.: Epiphysitis and recumbency in a yearling prepartum goat. J. Am. Vet. Med. Assoc., 183:226–228, 1983.

Andrés, D. de, et al.: Diagnostic tests for small ruminant lentiviruses. Vet. Microbiol., 107(1/2):49–62, 2005.

Andrews, A.H., Ingram, P.L. and Longstaffe, J.A.: Osteodystrophia fibrosa in young goats. Vet. Rec., 112:404–406, 1983.

Angelov, L., et al.: Study of the epizootiology of Lyme borreliosis in Bulgaria. Infectology 30(5):12–14, 1993.

Animal Health Australia. The history of bluetongue, Akabane and ephemeral fever viruses and their vectors in Australia. Animal Health Australia, Deakin, ACT, Australia, p. 40, 2001. http://www.animalhealthaustralia.com.au/programs/adsp/namp/

Animal Health Australia. Animal Health in Australia Report 2007, Chapter 2, Terrestrial Animal Health, Canberra, Australia, p. 30, 2008. http://www.animalhealthaustralia.com.au/aahc/programs/adsp/nahis/ahia.cfm

Anke, M., et al.: The effect of selenium deficiency on reproduction and milk performance of goats. Arch. Anim. Nutr., 39:483–490, 1989.

Anonymous: Recommendations XIII Conference of OIE Permanent Commission on Foot and Mouth Disease. Disease Bulletin OIE, 77:1381–1388, 1972.

Anonymous: Foot problems frustrate goat farmers. N.Z. Goat Health Prod., 1(2):1–2, 1987.

Anonymous: White muscle disease in kids. Goat Health Prod., 1(1):1–2, 1987a.

Antunes, N.T., et al.: *In vitro* susceptibilities of field isolates of *Mycoplasma mycoides* subsp. *mycoides* large colony type to 15 antimicrobials. Vet. Microbiol., 119:1, 72–75, 2007.

Aziz, E.S. and Klesius, P.H.: Depressed neutrophil chemotactic stimuli in supernatants of ionophore-treated polymorphonuclear leukocytes from selenium-deficient goats. Am. J. Vet. Res., 47:148–151, 1986.

Aziz, E.S. and Klesius, P.H.: The effect of selenium deficiency in goats on lymphocyte production of leukocyte migration inhibitory factor. Vet. Immunol. Immunopathol., 10:381–390, 1985.

Aziz, E.S., Klesius, P.H. and Frandsen, J.C.: Effects of selenium on polymorphonuclear leukocyte function in goats. Am. J. Vet. Res., 45:1715–1718, 1984.

Baas, E.J., Trotter, S.L., Franklin, R.M. and Barile, M.F.: Epidemic caprine keratoconjunctivitis: Recovery of *Mycoplasma conjunctivae* and its possible role in pathogenesis. Inf. Immun., 18:806–815, 1977.

Babalola, G.O. and Oke, B.O.: Intravenous regional analgesia for surgery of the limbs in goats. Vet. Q., 5:186–189, 1983.

Bacher, J.D. and Potkay, S.: Compression plating of radial and ulnar fractures in the goat. Vet. Rec., 96:538–539, 1975.

Baldwin, C.H.: Lyme disease in sheep and goats: a practitioner report. Large Anim. Vet. Rep., 1:51, 1990.

Banerjee, M., Singh, N. and Gupta, P.P.: Isolation of Mycoplasmas and Acholeplasmas from pneumonic lesions in sheep and goats in India. Zbl. Vet. Med. B, 26:689–695, 1979.

Banik, S. and Bhatnagar, D.S.: Note on the inheritance of foot rot, mastitis and utero vaginal disorders in native, exotic, and their two/three crossbred adult goats. Asian J. Dairy Res., 2:184–186, 1983.

Bar Moshe, B. and Rapapport, E.: Observations on *Mycoplasma mycoides* subsp. *mycoides* infection in Saanen goats. Isr. J. Med. Sci., 17:537–539, 1981.

Baran, S.: White muscle disease in kids and treatment with selenium, vitamin E, and vitamin C. Vet. Fak. Derg. Ankara Univ., 13:135–156, 1966.

Barci, L.A.G., do Amaral, V., Santos, S.M. and Reboucas, M.M.: *Sarcocistose caprina*: Prevalencia em animais provenientes do estado da Bahia-Brasil, com identificação do agente etiologico. Biológico (São Paulo), 49(4):97–102, 1983.

Barile, M.F., et al.: Isolation and characterization of *Mycoplasma arginini*: spec. nov. (33351). Proc. Soc. Exp. Biol. Med., 129:489, 1968.

Barnett, P.V. and Carabin, H.: A review of emergency foot-and-mouth disease (FMD) vaccines. Vaccine, 20(11/12):1505–1514, 2002.

Barnett, P.V. and Cox, S.J.: The role of small ruminants in the epidemiology and transmission of foot-and-mouth disease. Vet. J., 158(1):6–13, 1999.

Baron, R.J.: Laterally luxating patella in a goat. J. Am. Vet. Med. Assoc., 191:1471–1472, 1987.

Barteling, S.J.: Development and performance of inactivated vaccines against foot and mouth disease. Rev. sci. tech. Off. int. Epiz., 21(3):577–588, 2002.

Bashiruddin, J.B., Taylor, T.K. and Gould, A.R.: A PCR-based test for the specific identification of *Mycoplasma mycoides* subspecies *mycoides* SC. J. Vet. Diagn. Invest., 6(4):428–434, 1994.

Bath, G.F., Wyk, J.A. and Pettey, K.P.: Control measures for some important and unusual goat diseases in southern Africa. Small Rumin. Res., 60(1/2):127–140, 2005.

Baum, K.H., Hull, B.L. and Weisbrode, S.E.: Radial agenesis and ulnar hypoplasia in two caprine kids. J. Am. Vet. Med. Assoc., 186:170–171, 1985.

Baxendell, S.A.: Foot problems in goats. In: Proceedings, Refresher Course for Veterinarians, Post-Graduate Committee in Veterinary Science, University of Sydney, 52:351–352, 1980.

Baxendell, S.A.: The Diagnosis of the Diseases of Goats. Sydney South, Post-Graduate Committee in Veterinary Science, 1988.

Bazargani, T.T. and Khavary, H.: Inherited metacarpal gait in kids. J. Vet. Fac. Univ. Tehran, 31:82–86, 1976.

Bazargani, T.T., Charagozlou, M.J. and Ebrahimi, A.: A survey on besnoitiosis in goats in Baft, Kerman. J. Vet. Fac. Univ. Tehran, 41:40–44, 1987.

Bernabé, A., et al.: Polyarthritis in kids associated with *Klebsiella pneumoniae*. Vet. Rec., 142(3):64–66, 1998.

Bertoni, G.: Caprine arthritis encephalitis complex. In: Recent Advances in Goat Diseases, M. Tempesta, ed. International Veterinary Information Service, Ithaca, NY, 2007. http://www.ivis.org/advances/Disease_Tempesta/bertoni/chapter.asp?LA=1

Bhomik, M.K. and Dalapati, M.R.: Infectious arthritis in goats caused by *Pasteurella multocida*. Indian J. Vet. Pathol., 19(1):26–29, 1995.

Binns, W., Keeler, R.F. and Balls, L.D.: Congenital deformities in lambs, calves and goats resulting from maternal ingestion of *Veratrum californicum*: hare lip, cleft palate, ataxia and hypoplasia of metacarpal and metatarsal bones. Clin. Toxicol., 5:245–261, 1972.

Biolatti, B. and Vigliani, E.: Sulla miocardiodistrofia nelle caprette tibetane e nel dromedario. Nuovo Prog. Vet., 35:1127–1128, 1980.

Blacklaws, B.A., et al.: Transmission of small ruminant lentiviruses. Vet. Microbiol., 101(3):199–208, 2004.

Blaha, T.: Applied Veterinary Epidemiology. Amsterdam, Elsevier, 1989.

Blanchard, P.C. and Fiser, K.M.: *Streptococcus dysgalactiae* polyarthritis in dairy goats. J. Am. Vet. Med. Assoc., 205(5):739–741, 1994.

Bogin, E., Shimshony, A., Avidar, Y. and Israeli, B.: Enzymes, metabolites and electrolytes levels in the blood of local Israeli goats. Zbl. Vet. Med. A, 28:135–140, 1981.

Bolske, G., Engvall, A., Renstrom, L.H.M. and Wierup, M.: Experimental infections of goats with *M. mycoides* subspecies *mycoides* 1c type. Res. Vet. Sci., 46:247–252, 1989.

Boss, P.H. and Wanner, M.: Klinisch-chemische Parameter im Serum der Saanenziege. Schweiz. Arch. Tierheilk., 119, 293–300, 1977.

Bouma, A., et al.: The foot-and-mouth disease epidemic in The Netherlands in 2001. Prev. Vet. Med., 57(3):155–166, 2003.

Brandao, E. Isolation and identification of *Mycoplasma mycoides* subspecies *mycoides* SC strains in sheep and goats. Vet. Rec., 136(4):98–99, 1995.

Braun, J.P., Bezille, P., Raviart, I. and Rico, A.G.: Distribution de l'alanine et de l'aspartate aminotransferases, de la gamma-glutamyl transferase, de la lactate deshydrogenase, des phosphatases alcalines et de la creatine kinase dans les principaux organes de chèvres adultes et de chevreaux. Ann. Res. Vet., 18:389–392, 1987.

Brenner, J.: Congenital bovine abnormalities outbreaks of large scale in Israel. Isr. J. Vet. Med., 59(1/2):7–11, 2004.

Brooks, D.L., Tillman, P.C., Niemi, S.M.: Ungulates as laboratory animals. In: Laboratory Animal Medicine. J.G. Fox, B.J. Cohen, and F.M. Loew, eds. Orlando, Academic Press, 1984.

Bryant, S.H. and Owenburg, K.: Characteristics of the chloride channel in skeletal muscle fibers from myotonic and normal goats. Fed. Proc., 39:579, 1980.

Bryant, S.H., Lipicky, R.J. and Herzog, W.H.: Variability of myotonic signs in myotonic goats. Am. J. Vet. Res., 29:2371–2381, 1968.

Buchoo, B.A. and Sahay, P.N.: Clinico-radiographic evaluation of compression osteosynthesis for radial and ulnar fractures in goats. Indian J. Anim. Sci., 57:703–705, 1987.

Buddle, B.M., et al.: A goat mortality study in the southern North Island. N. Z. Vet. J., 36:167–170, 1988.

Bulgin, M.S.: Losses related to the ingestion of lincomycin-medicated feed in a range sheep flock. J. Am. Vet. Med. Assoc., 192:1083–1086, 1988.

Burns, J. and Cornell, C.: Angiography of the caprine digit. Vet. Radiol., 4:174–176, 1981.

Butler, A.B., Anderson, K.L. and Lyman, R.L.: Mycoplasmal polyarthritis and septicemia in a goat herd. Large Anim. Pract., 19(6):23–25, 1998.

Butler, C.M., Houwers, D.J., Jongejan, F. and Kolk, J.H.: *Borrelia burgdorferi* infections with special reference to horses. A review. Vet. Q. 27(4):146–156, 2005.

Byrne, D.J.: Vitamin E deficiency in a flock of Angora goats. Goat Vet. Soc. J., 13(2):55–62, 1992.

Caldow, G.L., Gidlow, J.R. and Schock, A.: Clinical, pathological and epidemiological findings in three outbreaks of ovine protozoan myeloencephalitis. Vet. Rec., 146(1):7–10, 2000.

Carda Aparici, P., Gallego Garcia, E. and Rodriguez Sanchez, E.: Contribucion al estudio de la osteodistrofia fibrosa (la

osteodistrofia fibrosa en la cabra). Zootechnia, 21:425–446, 1972.
Care, A.D. and Hove, K.: The simultaneous, direct measurement of the secretion rates of parathyroid hormone and calcitonin in the conscious goat. J. Physiol., 330:21P, 1982.
Carranza, R., Borobio, M.V., Pascual, F. and Perea, E.J.: Seroprevalence of antibodies against Lyme borreliosis in the healthy population of the island of Lanzarote. Med. Clin. 104(1):38, 1995.
Carrigan, M.J., Links, I.J. and Morton, A.G.: *Rhodococcus equi* infection in goats. Aust. Vet. J., 65:331–332, 1988.
Castro, A., et al.: Serum biochemistry values in normal pygmy goats. Am. J. Vet. Res., 38:2085–2087, 1977.
Castro, A., et al.: Serum electrolytes in normal pygmy goats. Am. J. Vet. Res., 38:663–664, 1977a.
Chartier, C.: Personal communication. Director, Agence Française de Sécurité Sanitaire des Aliments, Laboratoire d'études et de recherches caprines Niort, France, April, 2008.
Chatelain, E.: Atlas d'Anatomie de la Chèvre. Paris, Institut National Recherche Agronomique, 1987.
Cheevers, W.P. and McGuire, T.C.: The lentiviruses: maedi/visna, caprine arthritis-encephalitis, and equine infectious anemia. Adv. Virus Res., 34:189–215, 1988.
Cheong, J.T., Cheong, C.K. and Nam, T.C.: Electromyographic diagnosis of ruminal adhesions to the abdominal wall in Korean native goats. Korean J. Vet. Res., 27:335–337, 1987.
Chhabra, M.B. and Mahajan, R.C.: *Sarcocystis* spp. from the goat in India. Vet. Rec., 103(25):562–563, 1978.
Choi H.J., et al.: A radiographic study of growth plate closure compared with age in the Korean native goat. Kor. J. Vet. Res., 46(3):285–289, 2006.
Ciceroni, L., et al.: Antibodies to *Borrelia burgdorferi* in sheep and goats. Alto Adige-South Tyrol, Italy. Microbiologica 19(2):171–174, 1996.
Ciceroni, L., et al.: Serological survey for antibodies to *Borrelia burgdorferi* in sheep, goats and dogs in Cordillera Province, Bolivia. J. Vet. Med. Ser. B., 44(3):133–137, 1997.
Clavijo, A., Wright, P. and Kitching, P.: Developments in diagnostic techniques for differentiating infection from vaccination in foot-and-mouth disease. Vet. J., 167(1):9–22, 2004.
Claxton, P.D. and O'Grady, K.C.: Foot rot in goats and characterisation of caprine isolates of *Bacteroides nodosus*. In: Foot rot in Ruminants, Proc. Workshop, Melbourne, 1985. D.J. Stewart, J.E. Peterson, N.M. McKern, and D.L. Emery, eds. Glebe, N.S.W., CSIRO Division Animal Health/Australian Wool Corp., pp. 119–123, 1986.
Clay, A.B. and Suttie, J.W.: The availability of fluoride from NaF and phosphorus supplements. Vet. Hum. Toxicol., 27:3–6, 1985.
Clements, J.E. and Zink, M.C.: Molecular biology and pathogenesis of animal lentivirus infections. Clin. Microbiol. Rev., 9:1, 100–117, 1996.
Collins, G.H. and Charleston, W.A.G.: Studies on *Sarcocystis* species. IV. A species infecting dogs and goats; development in goats. N. Z. Vet. J. 27:260–262, 1979.
Collins, G.H. and Crawford, S.J.S.: *Sarcocystis* in goats: prevalence and transmission. N. Z. Vet. J., 26:288, 1978.
Collins, G.H., Sutton, R.H. and Charleston, W.A.J.: Studies in *Sarcosystis* species V: A species infecting dogs and goats; observations on the pathogenicity and serology of experimental sarcocystosis in goats. N. Z. Vet. J., 28:156–158, 1980.
Concha-Bermejillo, A. de la: Caprine arthritis-encephalitis: an update. Sheep Goat Res. J., 18:69–78, 2003.
Concha-Bermejillo, A. de la, Magnus-Corral, S., Brodie, S.J. and DeMartini, J.C.: Venereal shedding of ovine lentivirus in infected rams. Am. J. Vet. Res., 57(5):684–688, 1996.
Considine, H. and Trimberger, G.W.: Dairy Goat Judging Techniques, Scottsdale AZ, Dairy Goat Journal Publishing Co. 272 pp., 1978.
Constantinescu, G.M.: Guide to Regional Ruminant Anatomy Based on the Dissection of the Goat. Iowa State University Press, Ames, 243 pp., 2001.
Contreras, A., et al.: Caprine arthritis-encephalitis in an indigenous Spanish breed of dairy goat. Vet. Rec., 142(6):140–142, 1998.
Cordy, D.R., Adler, H.E. and Yamamoto, R.: A pathogenic pleuropneumonia-like organism from goats. Cornell Vet., 45:50–68, 1955.
Cork, L.C., et al.: Infectious leukoencephalomyelitis of young goats. J. Inf. Dis., 129:134–141, 1974.
Cotchin, E.: Tumors of farm animals. Vet. Rec., 40:816–823, 1960.
Cottew, G.S.: Caprine-ovine mycoplasmas. In: The Mycoplasmas. II: Human and Animal Mycoplasmas. J.G. Tully and R.F. Whitcomb, eds. New York, Academic Press, pp. 103–132, 1979.
Cottew, G.S. and Yeats, F.R.: Subdivision of *M. mycoides* subsp. *mycoides* from cattle and goats into two types. Aust. Vet. J., 54:293–296, 1978.
Cottew, G.S. and Yeats, F.R.: Occurrence of mycoplasmas in clinically normal goats. Aust. Vet. J., 57:52–53, 1981.
Cottew, G.S. and Yeats, F.R.: Mycoplasmas and mites in the ears of clinically normal goats. Aust. Vet. J., 59:77–81, 1982.
Craig, D.R., Roth, L. and Smith, M.C.: Lymphosarcoma in goats. Comp. Cont. Educ. Pract. Vet., 8:S190–S197, 1986.
Crawford, T.B. and Adams, D.S.: Caprine arthritis-encephalitis: clinical features and presence of antibody in selected goat populations. J. Am. Vet. Med. Assoc., 178:713–719, 1981.
Crawford, T.B., Adams, D.S., Cheevers, W.P. and Cork, L.C.: Chronic arthritis in goats caused by a retrovirus. Science, 207:997–999, 1980.
Custer, D.M.: Shortcut to disaster. United Caprine News, 13(10): 6–9, 1990.
Cutlip, R.C., Lehmukuhl, H.D., Sacks, J.M. and Weaver, A.L.: Prevalence of antibody to caprine arthritis-encephalitis virus in goats in the United States. J. Am. Vet. Med. Assoc., 200(6): 802–805, 1992.
Cybinski, D.H.: Douglas and Tinaroo viruses: two Simbu group arboviruses infecting *Culicoides brevitarsis* and livestock in Australia. Australian J. Biol. Sci., 37(3):91–97, 1984.
DaMassa, A.J.: Preliminary report: prevalence of mycoplasmas and mites in the external auditory meatus of goats. Calif. Vet., 37:10–13, 17, 1983.

DaMassa, A.J.: Recovery of *M. agalactiae* from mastitic goat milk. J. Am. Vet. Med. Assoc., 183:548–549, 1983a.

DaMassa, A.J.: The ear canal as a culture site for demonstration of mycoplasmas in clinically normal goats. Aust. Vet. J., 67:267–268, 1990.

DaMassa, A.J., Brooks, D.L., Adler, H.E. and Watt, D.E.: Caprine mycoplasmosis: acute pulmonary disease in newborn kids given *M. capricolum* orally. Aust. Vet. J., 60:125–126, 1983.

DaMassa, A.J., Brooks, D.L. and Adler, H.E.: Caprine mycoplasmosis: widespread infection in goats with *M. mycoides* subsp. *mycoides* (large-colony type). Am. J. Vet. Res., 44:322–325, 1983a.

DaMassa, A.J., Brooks, D.L. and Holmberg, C.A.: Caprine mycoplasmosis: an outbreak of mastitis and arthritis requiring the destruction of 700 goats. Vet. Rec., 120:409–413, 1987.

Dass, L.L., et al.: Incidence of fractures in goats in the hilly terrain of Chhotanagpur. Indian Vet. J., 62:766–768, 1985.

Davidson, R.M.: Control and eradication of animal diseases in New Zealand. N. Z. Vet. J., 50(3,Suppl.):6–12, 2002.

Davies, G. and Jessett, D.M.: A study of the host range and distribution of antibody to Akabane virus (genus bunyavirus, family Bunyaviridae) in Kenya. J. Hyg., 95:191–196, 1985.

Davis, J.G., et al.: Preventing Selenium Toxicity. Natural Resources Series Fact Sheet 6.110. Colorado State University Extension Service, Fort Collins, CO. November 2000. 2pp. http://www.ext.colostate.edu/pubs/natres/06110.pdf

Dawson, M. and Wilesmith, J.W.: Serological survey of lentivirus (maedi-visna/caprine arthritis-encephalitis) infection in British goat herds. Vet. Rec., 117:86–89, 1985.

Dawson, M., et al.: Isolation of a syncytium-forming virus from a goat with polyarthritis. Vet. Rec., 112:319–321, 1983.

Day, A.M. and Southwell, S.R.G.: Termination of pregnancy in goats using cloprostenol. N. Z. Vet. J., 27:207–208, 1979.

Dercksen, D., et al.: First outbreak of bluetongue in goats in the Netherlands. Tijdschr. Diergeneeskd. 132(20):786–790, 2007.

Devendra, C. and Burns, M.: Goat Production in the Tropics. Slough, U.K., Commonwealth Agricultural Bureaux, 1983.

de Verdier, K.: Personal communication. Department of Animal Health and Antiobiotic Strategies. National Veterinary Institute (SVA), Uppsala, Sweden. April, 2008.

Dewan, M.L., Henson, J.B., Dollahite, J.W. and Bridges, C.H.: Toxic myodegeneration in goats produced by feeding mature fruits from the coyotillo plant *(Karwinskia humboldtiana)*. Am. J. Pathol., 46:215–226, 1965.

Dey, P.C., et al.: A brief note on massive infection of *Coenurus gaigeri* cysts in a Desi goat. Indian Vet. J., 65:166, 1988.

Dey, S., Gupta, S.L. and Singh, R.P.: Clinico-haematologic findings in caprine sarcocystosis. Indian J. Anim. Sci., 65(1):44–46, 1995.

Dhillon, K.S. and Dhillon, S.K.: Distribution and management of seleniferous soils. Adv. Agron., 79:119–184, 2003.

Dhingra, L.D. and Tyagi, R.P.S.: A study of the prenatal ossification centers and epiphyseal ossification in the limbbones of the goat. Ceylon Vet. J., 18:111–118, 1970.

Dhingra, L.D., et al.: Studies on the fusion of epiphysis of limb bones of female goat *(Capra hircus)*. Haryana Vet., 17:85–91, 1978.

Dille, S.E.: Care of the flock after a predator attack. Proc. Regional Symp., Am. Assoc. Sheep Goat Pract., Univ. Minn. College Vet. Med., pp. 191–194. Feb. 27, 1985.

Doby, J.M. and Chevrier, S.: Serological survey of *Borrelia burgdorferi* antibodies in 602 goats in Brittany. Rec. Med. Vet., 166(8–9):799–804, 1990.

Dubey, J.P.: Abortion and death in goats inoculated with *Sarcocystis* sporocysts from coyote feces. J. Am. Vet. Med. Assoc., 178:700–703, 1981.

Dubey, J.P. and Livingston, C.W.: *Sarcocystis capracanis* and *Toxoplasma gondii* infections in range goats from Texas. Am. J. Vet. Res., 47:523–524, 1986.

Dubey, J.P., Speer, C.A., Epling, G.P. and Blixt, J.A.: *Sarcocystis capracanis*: Development in goats, dogs, and coyotes. Int. Goat Sheep Res. 2:252–265, 1984.

Dubey, J.P., Weisbrode, S.E., Speer, C.A. and Sharma, S.P.: *Sarcocystosis* in goats: Clinical signs and pathologic and hematologic findings. J. Am. Vet. Med. Assoc., 178:683–699, 1981.

Dutta, P.K., Sarma, G. and Das, S.K.: Foot-and-mouth disease in sheep and goats. Indian Vet. J., 61(4):267–270, 1984.

Eamens, G.J., Turner, M.J. and Catt, R.E.: Serotypes of *Erysipelothrix rhusiopathiae* in Australian pigs, small ruminants, poultry, and captive wild birds and animals. Aust. Vet. J., 65:249–252, 1985.

East, N.E., et al.: Milkborne outbreak of *M. mycoides* subspecies *mycoides* infection in a commercial goat dairy. J. Am. Vet. Med. Assoc., 182:1338–1341, 1983.

East, N.E., et al.: Modes of transmission of caprine arthritis-encephalitis virus infection. Small Rumin. Res., 10(3):251–262, 1993.

East, N.E., Rowe, J.D., Madewell, B.R. and Floyd, K.: Serologic prevalence of caprine arthritis-encephalitis virus in California goat dairies. J. Am. Vet. Med. Assoc., 190:182–186, 1987.

Edwards, J.F., Livingston, C.W., Chung, S.I. and Collisson, E.C.: Ovine arthrogryposis and central nervous system malformations associated with in utero Cache Valley virus infection: spontaneous disease. Vet. Pathol., 26:33–39, 1989.

Edwards, J.F., Angulo, A.B., and Pannill, E.C.: Theriogenology question of the month. J. Am. Vet. Med. Assoc., 222:1361–1362, 2003.

Egerton, J.R.: Foot rot of cattle, goats, and deer. In: Foot rot and Foot Abscess of Ruminants. J.R. Egerton, W.K. Yong, and G.G. Riffkin, eds. Boca Raton, CRC Press, Inc., pp. 47–56, 1989.

Egerton, J.R.: Diseases of the feet. In: Diseases of Sheep. 4th Ed. Aitken, I., ed. Wiley-Blackwell, pp. 273–281, 2007.

Egerton, J.R., et al.: Eradication of virulent foot rot from sheep and goats in an endemic area of Nepal and an evaluation of specific vaccination. Vet. Rec., 151(10): 290–295, 2002.

Egwu, G.O., Ball, H.J. Rodriguez, F. and Fernadez, A.: *Mycoplasma capricolum* subspecies *capricolum*, *Mycoplasma mycoides* subspecies *mycoides* LC and *Mycoplasma mycoides* subspecies *capri* in "Agalactia Syndrome" of sheep and goats. Vet. Bull., 70(4):391–402, 2000.

Ellis, T.M., Carman, H., Robinson, W.F. and Wilcox, G.E.: The effect of colostrum-derived antibody on neonatal transmission of caprine arthritis-encephalitis virus infection. Aust. Vet. J., 63:242–245, 1986.

Ellis, T.M., Robinson, W.F. and Wilcox, G.E.: The pathology and aetiology of lung lesions in goats infected with caprine arthritis-encephalitis virus. Aust. Vet. J., 65:69–73, 1988.

El-Sayed, R.F. and Siam, A.A.: Clinical and biochemical aspects associated with rickets in young goats. Assiut Vet. Med. J., 27, 540:162–167, 1992.

El-Zeftawi, N.M.N.: The role of mycoplasmatales in diseases of sheep and goats in Egypt. Thesis, University of Cairo, Egypt, 1979.

Fieni, F., et al.: Presence of caprine arthritis-encephalitis virus (CAEV) infected cells in flushing media following oviductal-stage embryo collection. Theriogenology, 57(2):931–940, 2002.

Fieni, F., et al.: Presence of caprine arthritis-encephalitis virus (CAEV) proviral DNA in genital tract tissues of superovulated dairy goat does. Theriogenology, 59(7):1515–1523, 2003.

Finch, J.M. and Turner, R.J.: Effects of selenium and vitamin E on the immune responses of domestic animals. Res. Vet. Sci., 60(2):97–106, 1996.

FDA: FDA permits the use of selenium yeast in sheep and goat feed. CVM Update. United States Food and Drug Administration, Center for Veterinary Medicine, Rockville MD, March 8, 2005.

Fraser, C.M., ed.: The Merck Veterinary Manual. 6th Ed. Rahway, Merck and Co., 1986.

Fridriksdottir, V., Øvernes, G. and Stuen, S.: Suspected Lyme borreliosis in sheep. Vet. Rec., 130(15):323–324, 1992.

Furuya, Y., Shoji, H., Inaba, Y. and Matumoto, M.: Antibodies to Akabane virus in horses, sheep and goats in Japan. Vet. Microbiol., 5:239–242, 1980.

Gaafar, S.M., Howard, W.E. and Marsh, R.E. (eds): Parasites, Pests and Predators. Amsterdam, Elsevier, 1985.

Gaillard-Perrin, G. Picavet, D.P. and Perrin, G.: Isolation of *Mycoplasma putrefaciens* in two herds of goats showing symptoms of agalactia. Rev. Méd Vét., 137(1):67–70, 1986.

Garland, A.J.M., et al.: The 1975 foot-and-mouth disease epidemic in Malta. III. serological response of cattle, sheep, goats and pigs to type O vaccine. Br. Vet. J., 137:507–512, 1981.

Garnier, F., Benoit, E., Jacquet, J.P. and Delatour, P.: Enzymologie sérique de la chèvre: valeurs usuelles de CPK, LDH, ICDH et SDH. Ann. Recherche Vét., 15:55–58, 1984.

Gatenby, R.M.: Goat husbandry in West Timor, Indonesia. Small Rumin. Res., 1:113–121, 1988.

Ghimire, S.C., Egerton, J.R. and Dhungyel, O.P.: Characterisation of *Dichelobacter nodosus* isolated from foot rot in sheep and goats in Nepal. Small Rumin. Res., 23(1):59–67, 1996.

Ghimire, S.C., Egerton, J.R. and Dhungyel, O.P.: Transmission of virulent foot rot between sheep and goats. Australian Vet. J., 77(7):450–453, 1999.

Giddings, R.F.: Tibial agenesis in a Toggenburg kid. J. Am. Vet. Med. Assoc., 169:1306–1307, 1976.

Gil, M.C., et al.: Outbreak of acute mastitis and arthritis in goats caused by both *Mycoplasma agalactiae* and *M. putrefaciens*. ITEA Prod. Anim. 20(1):393–395, 1999.

Glock, G.E. and Murray, M.M.: Preliminary observations on the effects of a low calcium diet on goats and kids. J. Comp. Pathol. Ther., 52:229–248, 1939.

Gogoi, M., Phukan, A. and Sarma, D.K.: Immune response of goats vaccinated simultaneously with FMD and enterotoxaemia vaccines and with or without levamisole injection. Indian J. Anim. Sci., 74(4):357–359, 2004.

Goltz, J.P., Rosendal, S., McCraw, B.M. and Ruhnke, H.L.: Experimental studies on the pathogenicity of *Mycoplasma ovipneumoniae* and *Mycoplasma arginini* for the respiratory tract of goats. Can. J. Vet. Res., 50:59–67, 1986.

Gomes, A.P.M., Vogel, J., Pacheco, R.G. and Botelho, G.G.: Clinical aspects of sarcocystosis in goats. Arq. Univ. Fed. Rur. Rio de Janeiro. 15(1):1–6, 1992.

Grant, G.H., Johnachan P.M., Oliviera, D. and Pitterson, S.: Seroprevalence of caprine arthritis encephalitis in the Jamaican goat population. Trop. Anim. Health Prod., 20:181–182, 1988.

Greenough, P.R., MacCallum, F.J. and Weaver, A.D.: Lameness in Cattle. 2nd Ed. Philadelphia, J.B. Lippincott Co., 1981.

Greenwood, P.L., North, R.N. and Kirkland, P.D.: Prevalance, spread and control of caprine arthritis-encephalitis virus in dairy goat herds in New South Wales. Aust. Vet. J., 72(9):341–345, 1995.

Grewal, A.S., et al.: Caprine retrovirus infection in New South Wales: virus isolations, clinical and histopathological findings and prevalence of antibody. Aust. Vet. J., 63:245–248, 1986.

Groppel, B. and Henning, A.: Zinkmangel beim Wiederkäuer. Arch. Exp. Veterinärmed., 25:817–822, 1971.

Grubman, M.J.: Development of novel strategies to control foot-and-mouth disease: marker vaccines and antivirals. Biologicals, 33(4):227–234, 2005.

Grubman, M.J. and Baxt, B.: Foot-and-mouth disease. Clin. Microbiol. Rev. 17(2):465–493, 2004.

Gufler, H., et al.: Serological study of small ruminant lentivirus in goats in Italy. Small Rumin. Res., 73:169–173, 2007.

Gupta, R.C., Kwatra, M.S. and Singh, N.: Chronic selenium toxicity as a cause of hoof and horn deformities in buffalo, cattle and goat. Indian Vet. J., 59:738–740, 1982.

Guss, S.B.: Management and Diseases of Dairy Goats. Scottsdale, Dairy Goat Journal Publ. Corp., 1977.

Guthery, F.S. and Beasom, S.L.: Effects of predator control on Angora goat survival in south Texas. J. Range Manage., 31:168–173, 1978.

Hagstad, H.V., Hubbert, W.T. and Stagg, L.M.: A descriptive study of dairy goat predation in Louisiana. Can. J. Vet. Res., 51:152–155, 1987.

Harris, A.S.: Morphologic, compositional, and functional investigations of mitochondria isolated from skeletal muscle of normal goats and goats with myotonia congenita. Dis. Abstr. Int., 44:120B, 1983.

Hebert, D.M. and Cowan, I.M.: White muscle disease in the mountain goat. J. Wildl. Manage., 35:752–756, 1971.

Hedjazi, M., Ansari, H. and Nadalian, M.Gh.: Etude clinique de quelques enzooties de fièvre aphteuse chez les agneaux et chevreaux à la mamelle en Iran. Rev. Méd. Vét., 123:1085–1088, 1972.

Hegyeli, A. and Szent-Gyorgyi, A.: Water and myotonia in goats. Science, 133:1011, 1961.
Helmy, N.: Seasonal abundance of *Ornithodoros* (*O.*) *savignyi* and prevalence of infection with *Borrelia* spirochetes in Egypt. J. Egypt Soc. Parasitol. 30(2): 607–619, 2000.
Hengge, U.R., et al.: Lyme borreliosis. Lancet Infect. Dis., 3(8):489–500, 2003.
Hentschke, P.W.: The goat skeleton in relation to basic conformation. Dairy Goat J., 58:27–29, 1980.
Herrmann, L.M., et al.: Competitive-inhibition enzyme-linked immunosorbent assay for detection of serum antibodies to caprine arthritis-encephalitis virus: diagnostic tool for successful eradication. Clin. Diagn. Lab. Immunol., 10(2):267–271, 2003.
Hidiroglou, M.: Zinc, copper and manganese deficiencies and the ruminant skeleton: a review. Can. J. Anim. Sci., 60:579–590, 1980.
Hines, T.G., et al.: Vitamin D_3 and D_3 metabolites in young goats fed varying amounts of calcium and vitamin D_3. J. Dairy Sci., 69:385–391, 1986.
Ho, C.C.: Radiographic study of the Taiwan goat. I. The extremities—radiographic fusion of ossification centers. J. Chin. Soc. Vet. Sci., 1:31–36, 1975.
Holst, P.J.: Personal communication. Agricultural Research Station, Cowra, New South Wales, Australia, 1986.
Hou, J.W., Qi, Z.Y., Liu, B.F., and Dong, Q.G.: The variation in selenium content of wool, blood and tissues of goats poisoned by feeding on natural high-selenium feeds. Acta Vet. Zootech. Sinica 25:5, 400–405, 1994.
Hove, K.: A permanent preparation allowing measurements of secretion of parathyroid hormone in conscious goats. J. Endocr., 90:295–306, 1981.
Howery, L.D. and DeLiberto, T.J.: Indirect effects of carnivores on livestock foraging behavior and production. Sheep Goat Res. J., 19:53–57, 2004.
Hunt, R.J., Allen, D., Jr. and Thomas, K.: Repair of a ruptured calcaneal tendon by transposition of the tendon of the peroneus longus muscle in a goat. J. Am. Vet. Med. Assoc., 198(9):1640–1642, 1991.
Inaba, Y.: Akabane disease: an epizootic congenital arthrogryposis-hydranencephaly syndrome in cattle, sheep and goats caused by akabane virus. Jpn. Agric. Res. Q., 13:123–133, 1979.
Ivanov, A.: Studies on some features in the biology of the sarcocysts in goats. Bulg. J. Vet. Med., 1(2):89–94, 1998.
Jackson, R. and King, C.: *Mycoplasma mycoides* subspecies *mycoides* (Large Colony) infection in goats—a review with special reference to occurrence in New Zealand. Surveillance, 29(3):8–12, 2002.
Jasper, D.E. and Dellinger, J.D.: Isolation of exotic mycoplasma from goats. Proc. Ann. Meet. Am. Assoc. Vet. Lab. Diag., 22:119–124, 1979.
Jones, D.G., Suttle, N.F., Stevenson, L.M. and Hay, L.: Observations on the diagnostic significance of plasma alpha-tocopherol (vitamin E) estimations in goats. In: Animal Clinical Biochemistry: The Future. J.D. Blackmore, ed. Cambridge, Cambridge University Press, pp. 340–345, 1988.
Juyal, P.D., Ruprah, N.S. and Chhabra, M.B.: Experimentally induced *Sarcocystis capracanis* infection in pregnant goats. Indian Vet. Med. J., 13(3):200–202, 1989.
Kalmar, E., Peleg, B.A. and Savir, D.: Arthrogryposis-hydranencephaly syndrome in newborn cattle, sheep and goats-serologic survey for antibodies against Akabane virus. Refuah Vet., 32:47–54, 1975.
Kaneko, J.J., Harvey J.W., and Bruss, M.L.: Appendixes. In: Clinical Biochemistry of Domestic Animals. 5th Ed., J.J. Kaneko, J.W. Harvey and M.L. Bruss, eds. San Diego, Academic Press, 1997.
Karram, M.H., Amer, A.A. and Ibrahim, H.A.: Aplastic anaemia in caprine fluorosis. Assiut Vet. Med. J., 12:167–171, 1984.
Karram, M.H.: Studies on fluorosis in goats in Assiut province. Assiut Vet. Med. J., 11:233, 1984.
Kessabi, M. and Abdennebi, E.H.: Contribution a l'étude épidémiologique du darmous. Maghreb Vet. 1:37–42, 1985.
Kessler, J.: Goldhaferbedingte Kalzinose beim Kleinwiederkäuer. Mitt. Schweiz. Landwirtsch., 30:179–184, 1982.
Kilgore, W.W., Crosby, D.G., Craigmill, A.L. and Poppen, N.K.: Toxic plants as possible human teratogens. Calif. Agric., 35:6, 1981.
Kimberling, C.V.: Jensen and Swift's Diseases of Sheep. 3rd Ed. Philadelphia, Lea and Febiger, 1988.
Kinde, H., DaMassa, A.J., Wakenell, P.S. and Petty, R.: Mycoplasma infection in a commercial goat dairy caused by *Mycoplasma agalactiae* and *Mycoplasma mycoides* subsp. *mycoides* (caprine biotype). J. Vet. Diagn. Invest., 6(4):423–427, 1994.
King, N.B.: Clostridial diseases. In: Proceedings, Refresher Course for Veterinarians, Post-Graduate Committee in Veterinary Science, University of Sydney, 52:217–219, 1980.
King, N.B.: Metabolic Diseases. In: Proceedings, Refresher Course for Veterinarians, Post-Graduate Committee in Veterinary Science, University of Sydney, 52:203–208, 1980a.
Kitching, R.P.: A recent history of foot-and-mouth disease. J. Comp. Pathol., 118(2):89–108, 1998.
Kitching, R.P. and Hughes, G.J.: Clinical variation in foot and mouth disease: sheep and goats. Rev. Sci. Tech. Off. Int. Epiz., 21(3):505–512, 2002.
Koch, P., Fischer, H. and Schumann, H.: Erbpathologie der landwirtschaftlichen Haustiere. Berlin, Paul Parey, 1957.
Kolb, L.C.: Congenital myotonia in goats. Bull. Johns Hopkins Hosp., 63:221–237, 1938.
Konishi, M., et al.: Epidemiological survey and pathological studies on Caprine arthritis-encephalitis (CAE) in Japan. Bull. Natl. Inst. Anim. Health, 113, 23–30, 2006.
Kramer, J.W. and Carthew, G.C.: Serum and tissue enzyme profiles of goats. N. Z. Vet. J., 33:91–93, 1985.
Kukovics, S., et al.: Presence of CAEV infection in the Hungarian goat industry as an effect of livestock import. Bulet. Univ. Stiinte Agric. Med. Vet. Cluj-Napoca, Ser. Zooteh. Bioteh., 59:42–48, 2003.
Kulkarni, G.B. and Deshpande, B.B.: A case record of congenital anomaly in kid having longer limbs with knuckling. Livestock Adviser, 12:39–40, 1987.
Kumar A., Barua, S., Rana, R. and Vihan, V.S.: Epidemiological features of foot and mouth disease (O type) in goats. Vet. Pract. 5(2):134–137, 2004.

Kurogi, H., et al.: Experimental infection of pregnant goats with Akabane virus. Natl. Inst. Anim. Health Q., 17:1–9, 1977.

Kurogi, H., Akiba, K., Inaba, Y. and Matumoto, M.: Isolation of Akabane virus from the biting midge *Culicoides oxystoma* in Japan. Vet. Microbiol. 15(3):243–248, 1987.

Lamara, A., et al.: Early embryonic cells from in vivo-produced goat embryos transmit the caprine arthritis-encephalitis virus (CAEV). Theriogenology, 58(6):1153–1163, 2002.

Lane, M.V. and Anderson, B.C.: Adenocarcinoma of the mouth of a goat. J. Am. Vet. Med. Assoc., 183:1099–1100, 1983.

Leforban, Y.: How predictable were the outbreaks of foot and mouth disease in Europe in 2001 and is vaccination the answer? Rev. Sci. Tech. Off. Int. Epiz., 21(3):549–556, 2002.

Lerondelle, C., Greenland, T., Jane, M. and Mornex, J.F.: Infection of lactating goats by mammary instillation of cell-borne caprine arthritis-encephalitis virus. J. Dairy Sci., 78(4): 850–855, 1995.

Li W.T., et al.: Effect of industrial fluoride pollution on COL2A1 gene expression in rib cartilage of Inner Mongolia cashmere goats. Fluoride, 39(4):285–292, 2006.

Li W.T., et al.: Quantification of rib COL1A2 gene expression in healthy and fluorosed Inner Mongolia cashmere goats. Fluoride, 40(1):13–18, 2007.

Liesegang, A., Risteli, J. and Wanner, M.: The effects of first gestation and lactation on bone metabolism in dairy goats and milk sheep. Bone, 38(6):794–802, 2006.

Liesegang, A., Risteli, J. and Wanner, M.: Bone metabolism of milk goats and sheep during second pregnancy and lactation in comparison to first lactation. J. Anim. Physiol. Anim. Nutr., 91(5/6):217–225, 2007.

Lindqvist, A. Caprine arthritis encephalitis should be eradicated from Swedish dairy goats. Svensk Vet., 51(13):654–658, 1999.

Lindstrom, J.: Autoimmune response to acetylcholine receptors in myasthenia gravis and its animal model. Adv. Immunol., 27:1–50, 1979.

Lindstrom, J.: Immunological studies of acetylcholine receptors. J. Supramol. Struct., 4:389–403, 1976.

Lischer, C.J., Leutenegger, C.M., Braun, U. and Lutz, H.: Diagnosis of Lyme disease in two cows by the detection of *Borrelia burgdorferi* DNA. Vet. Rec., 146(17):497–499, 2000.

Littlejohns, I.R. and Cottew, G.S.: The isolation and identification of *Mycoplasma mycoides* subsp. *capri* from goats in Australia. Aust. Vet. J., 53:297–298, 1977.

Lode, T.: Genetic dominant serum alkaline phophatase activity in goats. Acta Vet. Scand., 11:181–185, 1970.

Long, J., Mawson, P., Hubach, P. and Kok, N.: Fox attacks on Cashmere goats. J. Agric. West. Aust., 29:104–106, 1988.

Long, J., Lin T. and Li, W.B.: Investigation on human and animal Lyme disease in Shanggao County of Jiangxi Province. Chin. J. Vector Biol. Control, 10(1):45–47, 1999.

Lopez-Rodriguez, R., Hernandez, S., Navarrete, I. and Martinez-Gomez, F.: Sarcocistosis experimental en la cabra (*Capra hircus*). II. Signos clinicos e indices de eritrocitos. Rev. Iber. Parasitol., 46(2):115–122, 1986.

MacDiarmid, S.C.: Survey suggests low prevalence of caprine arthritis encephalitis. Surveillance, N. Z., 10:4–8, 1983.

MacDiarmid, S.C.: The first year of the CAE flock accreditation scheme. N. Z. Vet. J., 33(12):217, 1985.

MacKenzie, R.W., Oliver, R.E., Rooney, J.P. and Kagei, H.: A successful attempt to raise goat kids free of infection with caprine arthritis-encephalitis virus in an endemically infected goat herd. N. Z. Vet. J., 35:184–186, 1987.

Mackie, J.T. and Dubey, J.P.: Congenital sarcocystosis in a Saanen goat. J. Parasitol., 82(2):350–351, 1996.

Martin, A.F., Bryant, S.H. and Mandel, F.: Isomyosin distribution in skeletal muscles of normal and myotonic goats. Muscle Nerve, 7:152–160, 1984.

Martinez, E.E., Paschal, J.C., Craddock, F. and Hanselka, C.W.: Selection, Management and Judging of Meat-Type Spanish Goats. Publication B-5018. Texas Agricultural Extension Service, The Texas A&M University System, College Station, Texas, 1991.

Mbiuki, S.M. and Byagagaire, S.D.: Full-limb casting: a treatment for tibial fractures in calves and goats. Vet. Med., 79:243–244, 1984.

McAuliffe, L., et al.: 16S rDNA PCR and denaturing gradient gel electrophoresis: a single generic test for detecting and differentiating *Mycoplasma* species. J. Med. Microbiol. 54(8):731–739, 2005.

McGuire, T.C., et al.: Acute arthritis in caprine arthritis-encephalitis virus challenge exposure of vaccinated or persistently infected goats. Am. J. Vet. Res., 47:537–540, 1986.

McIvor, K.M. de F. and Horak, I.G.: Foot abscess in goats in relation to the seasonal abundance of adult *Amblyomma hebraeum* and adult *Rhipicephalus glabroscutatum* (Acari: Ixodidae). J. S. Afr. Vet. Assoc., 58:113–118, 1987.

McKerrell, R.E.: Myotonia in man and animals: confusing comparisons. Equine Vet. J.: 19:266–267, 1987.

McVicar, J.W. and Sutmoller, P.: Sheep and goats as foot and mouth disease carriers. U.S. Livestock Sanitary Assoc. Proc., 72:400–406, 1968.

Mercier, P., Coutineau, H., Lenfant, D. and Decoux, V.: Agalactia caused by *Mycoplasma putrefaciens* in a goat herd. Point Vét., 31(208):345–348, 2000.

Merrall, M.: Lameness in goats. In: Goat Husbandry and Medicine, Publication 106, Massey University, Palmerston North, NZ, pp. 66–77, 1985.

Mielke, H., Arndt, H., Kreher, G.: Vergleichende elektromyographische Untersuchungen an Kälbern, Schafen und Ziegen. Archiv. Exp. Veterinärmed., 35:307–335, 1981.

Milhaud, G., Enriquez, B. and Riviere, F.: Fluorosis in the sheep: new data. In: Veterinary Pharmacology and Toxicology. Y. Ruckebusch, P.L. Toutain, and G.D. Koritz, eds. Westport, AVI Publishing Co., 1983.

Milhaud, G., Mathieu, E., Chary, J.F. and Parodi, A.L.: Etude expérimentale de la fluorose caprine. II. Etude du squelette, discussion générale. Rec. Med. Vet., 156:211–218, 1980.

Milhaud, G., Zundel, E. and Crombet, M.: Etude expérimentale de la fluorose caprine. I. Protocole expérimental, comportement des animaux, lésions dentaires. Rec. Méd. Vét., 156:37–46, 1980a.

Miller, W.J., Pitts, W.J., Clifton, C.M. and Schmittle, S.C.: Experimentally produced zinc deficiency in the goat. J. Dairy Sci., 47:556–569, 1964.

Mishra, K.C. and Ghei, J.C.: Target sites of aphthovirus infection in Sikkim local goats. Indian Vet. Med. J., 7:227–228, 1983.

Misk, N.A. and Hifny, A.: Amputation of the pelvic limb in goats. Assiut Vet. Med. J., 6:219–228, 1979.

Murphy, W.J.B., McBarron, E.J. and Doyle, P.W.: Bent leg in goats. Aust. Vet. J., 35:524–529, 1959.

Naghshineh, R. and Haghdoust, I.S.: A case of osteodystrophia fibrosa in a goat. J. Vet. Fac. Univ. Tehran, 29:87–91, 1973.

Narayan, O. and Cork, L.C.: Lentiviral diseases of sheep and goats: chronic pneumonia, leukoencephalomyelitis and arthritis. Rev. Inf. Dis., 7:89–98, 1985.

National Research Council: Nutrient Requirements of Small Ruminants. Washington D.C., National Academies Press, pp. 134–137, 2007.

Nayak, N.C. and Bhowmik, M.K.: Caprine bacterial arthritis. Kerala J. Vet. Sci., 19:80–82, 1988.

Nayak, N.C. and Bhowmik, M.K.: Caprine bacterial arthritis: Physical, biochemical and cytologic properties of synovial fluid. Indian Vet. J., 67:1016–1020, 1990.

Nazlioglu, M.: La fièvre aphteuse chez les moutons et les chèvres. Bull. Off. Int. Epiz., 77:1281–1284, 1972.

Neathery, M.W., et al.: Effects of long term zinc deficiency on feed utilization, reproductive characteristics, and hair growth in the sexually mature male goat. J. Dairy Sci., 56:98–105, 1972.

Nelson, D.R., et al.: Zinc deficiency in sheep and goats: three field cases. J. Am. Vet. Med. Assoc., 184:1480–1485, 1984.

Nicholas, R.A.J., et al.: Proposal that the strains of the *Mycoplasma* ovine/caprine serogroup 11 be reclassified as *Mycoplasma bovigenitalium*. Int. J. Syst. Evol. Microbiol., 58(1):308–312, 2008.

Nicholas, R.A.J.: Improvements in the diagnosis and control of diseases of small ruminants caused by mycoplasmas. Small Rumin. Res., 45(2):145–149, 2002.

Nicholas, R.A.J. and Baker, S.E.: Recovery of mycoplasmas from animals. In: Mycoplasma Protocols, Miles R.J. and Nicholas R.A.J., eds., Humana Press, Totowa, pp. 37–44, 1998.

Nietfeld, J.C.: Chlamydial infections in small ruminants. Vet. Clin. N. Am. Food Anim. Pract., 17(2):301–314, 2001.

Nobel, T.A., Klopfer, U. and Neumann, F.: Pathology of an arthrogryposis-hydranencephaly syndrome in domestic ruminants in Israel—1969/70. Refuah Vet., 28:144–151, 1971.

Nord, K., Rimstad, E., Storset, A.K. and Løken, T.: Prevalence of antibodies against caprine arthritis-encephalitis virus in goat herds in Norway. Small Rumin. Res., 28:115–121, 1998.

O'Brien, T.F.: Notes on the behaviour of the foot-and-mouth virus during the 1941 epizootic in Eire. Vet. Rec., 55:341–343, 1943.

O'Toole, D., Raisbeck, M., Case, J.C. and Whitson, T.D.: Selenium-induced "blind staggers" and related myths. A commentary on the extent of historical livestock losses attributed to selenosis on western US rangelands. Vet. Pathol., 33:104–116, 1996.

OIE: Manual of Diagnostic Tests and Vaccines for Terrestrial Animals. Chapter 2.4.4/5, Caprine arthritis/encephalitis and maedi-visna. 5th Edition. Office International des Epizooties, Paris, 2004. http://www.oie.int/eng/normes/mmanual/A_00071.htm

OIE: Manual of Diagnostic Tests and Vaccines for Terrestrial Animals. Chapter 2.1.1, Foot and Mouth Disease. 5th Edition. Office International des Epizooties, Paris, 2004a. http://www.oie.int/eng/normes/mmanual/A_00024.htm

OIE: Manual of Diagnostic Tests and Vaccines for Terrestrial Animals. Chapter 2.4.3, Contagious Agalactia. 5th Edition. Office International des Epizooties, Paris, 2004b. http://www.oie.int/eng/normes/mmanual/A_00070.htm

OIE: Manual of Diagnostic Tests and Vaccines for Terrestrial Animals. Chapter 2.4.6, Contagious Caprine Pleuropneumonia. 5th Edition. Office International des Epizooties, Paris, 2004c. http://www.oie.int/eng/normes/mmanual/A_00072.htm

OIE: Terrestrial Animal Health Code. Chapter 2.4.4, Caprine arthritis encephalitis. 16th Edition. Office International des Epizooties, Paris, 2007. http://www.oie.int/eng/normes/mcode/en_chapitre_2.4.4.htm

OIE: Terrestrial Animal Health Code. Chapter 1.4.5, International Transfer and Laboratory Containment of Animal Pathogens. 16th Edition. Office International des Epizooties, Paris, 2007a. http://www.oie.int/eng/normes/mcode/en_chapitre_1.4.5.htm

OIE: Terrestrial Animal Health Code. Chapter 2.2.10, Foot and Mouth Disease. 16th Edition. Office International des Epizooties, Paris, 2007b. http://www.oie.int/eng/normes/mcode/en_chapitre_2.2.10.htm

Ojo, M.O. and Ikede, B.O.: Pathogenicity of *M. agalactiae* subsp. *bovis* in goat mammary gland. Vet. Microbiol., 1:19–22, 1976.

Ojo, M.O.: In vitro and in vivo activities of tiamulin against caprine mycoplasmas. In: Les maladies de la chèvre, Les Colloques de l'INRA, No. 28. P. Yvore and G. Perrin, eds. Paris. Institut National de la Recherche Agronomique. 1984. pp. 287–293.

Olah, M., et al.: Klinicka slika i diferencijalna dijagnostika slinavke i sapa kod ovaca i koza. Vet. Glasnik, 30:239–245, 1976.

Oliver, R.E.: Akabane disease. Surveillance, N.Z., 15:12, 1988.

Onawunmi, D.A., Smith, O.B. and Munyabuntu, C.M.: Deformed goat birth. Vet. Rec., 105:359, 1979.

Ostfeld, R.S. and LoGiudice, K.: Community disassembly, biodiversity loss, and the erosion of an ecosystem service. Ecology, 84(6):1421–1427, 2003.

Osweiler, G.D., Carson, T.L., Buck, W.B. and Van Gelder, G.A.: Clinical and Diagnostic Veterinary Toxicology. 3rd Ed. Dubuque, Kendall Hunt Publishing Co., 1985.

Ozdemir, U., et al.: Effect of danofloxacin (Advocin A180) on goats affected with contagious caprine pleuropneumonia. Trop. Anim. Health Prod., 38(7/8):533–540, 2006.

Papageorges, M., et al.: Quantitative Tc-99m-MDP joint scintigraphy in a lentivirus-induced arthritis of goats. Vet. Radi., 32:2, 82–86, 1991.

Pathak, D.C. and Datta, B.M.: The effects of oral administration of sodium selenite on clinical signs and mortality. Indian Vet. J., 61:845–846, 1984.

Pathak, R.C., Singh, P.P. and Kappoor, S.G.: Prevalence and pathogenicity of *Mycoplasma bovigenitalium* in goats. 2nd

Internat. Colloq. Niort, Goat Diseases Prod., p. 62, Abstr. 1989.
Patil, P.K., et al.: Immune responses of goats against foot-and-mouth disease quadrivalent vaccine: comparison of double oil emulsion and aluminum hydroxide gel vaccines in eliciting immunity. Vaccine. 20:2781–2789, 2002.
Paton, D.J., et al.: Selection of food and mouth disease vaccine strains—a review. Rev. Sci. Tech. Off. Int. Epiz., 24(3): 981–993, 2005.
Pauling, B.A.: Clostridial diseases and vaccination of goats. Proc. 16th Seminar, Sheep and Beef Cattle Soc., N.Z. Vet. Assoc., Palmerston North, pp. 56–72, 1986.
Pay, T.W.F.: Foot and mouth disease in sheep and goats: a review. Foot Mouth Dis. Bull., 26:2–13, 1988.
Peluso, R., et al.: A Trojan horse mechanism for the spread of visna virus in monocytes. Virology, 147(1):231–236, 1985.
Péretz, G., Bugnard, F. and Calavas, D.: Study of a prevention programme for caprine arthritis-encephalitis. Vet. Res., 25(2/3):322–326, 1994.
Perez Garro, C., Rodrigues Osorio, M., Gomez Garcia, V. and Gonzales Castro, J.: Prueba de latex y hemaglutinacion indirecta para el diagnostico de la sarcosporidiosis. Rev. Iber. Parasitol., 38(3/4):793–804, 1978.
Perler, L.: Swollen knees eradicated on Swiss goats. Annual Report 2003. Swiss Federal Veterinary Office. SVFO Magazine, 2:16–17, 2004. http://www.bvet.admin.ch/shop/00008/00047/index.html?lang=en
Perreau, P.: Les mycoplasmoses de la chèvre. Cah. Méd. Vét., 48:71–85, 1979.
Perreau, P. and Breard, A.: La mycoplasmose caprine à *M. capricolum*. Comp. Immun. Microbiol. Infect. Dis., 2:87–97, 1979.
Perreau, P., Breard, A. and Le Goff, C.: Mycoplasme caprine à *Mycoplasma mycoides* subsp. *mycoides* en France. Bull. Acad. Vét. France, 52:575–581, 1981.
Perrin, G. and Polack, B.: Bovine colostrum warning. Vet. Rec., 122:240, 1988.
Pettersson, B., et al.: Phylogeny of the *Mycoplasma mycoides* cluster as determined by sequence analysis of the 16S rRNA genes from the two rRNA operons. J. Bacteriol., 178(14):4131–4142, 1996.
Pilo, P., Frey, J., Vilei, E.M.: Molecular mechanisms of pathogenicity of *Mycoplasma mycoides* subsp. *mycoides* SC. Vet. J., 174(3):513–521, 2007.
Pinsent, P.J.N.: The care and diseases of the goat's foot. Br. Goat Soc., 82:72–73, 1989.
Piriz Duran, S., Valle Manzano, J., Cuenca Valera, R. and Vadillo Machota, S.: Susceptibilities of *Bacteroides* and *Fusobacterium* spp. from foot rot in goats to 10 beta-lactam antibiotics. Antimicrob. Agents Chemother., 34:657–659, 1990.
Pluimers, F.H., et al.: Lessons from the foot and mouth disease outbreak in the Netherlands in 2001. Rev. Sci. Tech. Off. Int. Epiz., 21(3):711–721, 2002.
Polydorou, K., et al.: Investigations on foot and mouth disease vaccine in Cyprus 1972–1975. Bull. Off. Int. Epiz., 92:863–873, 1980.
Popesko P.: Atlas of Topographical Anatomy of Domestic Animals, new revised English edition, Vydavatelstvo Priroda, Bratislava, 2008.
Pott, J.M. and Skov, B.: Monensin-tiamulin interactions in pigs. Vet. Rec., 109:545, 1981.
Preziuso, S., et al.: Association of maedi visna virus with *Brucella ovis* infection in rams. Eur. J. Histochem., 47(2), 151–158, 2003.
Pringle, J.K., Wojcinski, Z.W. and Staempfli, H.R.: Nasal papillary adenoma in a goat. Can. Vet. J., 30:964–966, 1989.
Pritchard, G.C.: Ossifying fibroma in a goat. Goat Vet. Soc. J., 5:31, 1984.
Purohit, N.R., Choudhary, R.J., Chouhan, D.S. and Sharma, C.K.: Surgical repair of scapulohumeral luxation in goats. Mod. Vet. Pract., 66:758–759, 1985.
Radostits, O.M., Gay, C.C., Hinchcliff, K.W. and Constable, P.D.: Veterinary Medicine. A textbook of the diseases of cattle, horse, sheep, pigs and goats. 10th Ed., Edinburgh, Saunders Elsevier, 2007.
Raghavan, R. and Dutt, N.S.: A note on isolation of foot and mouth disease virus from the nasal secretion of apparently healthy goats. Indian J. Anim. Sci., 43:789, 1974.
Rajtova, V.: Die postnatale Entwicklung des Extremitätenskeletts bei Schaf und Ziege. Anat. Histol. Embryol., 3:29–39, 1974.
Ramadan, R.O., Ismail, O.E. and Shour, N.A.: Localized osteomyelitis and septic gonitis in a goat. J. Vet. Orthopedics, 3:31–35, 1984.
Ramadan, R.O., Magzoub, M. and Adam, S.E.I.: Clinicopathological effects in a Sudanese goat following massive natural infection with *Coenurus gaigeri* cysts. Trop. Anim. Health Prod., 5:196–199, 1973.
Ramírez-Bribiesca, J.E., Tórtora, J.L., Hernández, L.M. and Huerta, M.: Main causes of mortalities in dairy goat kids from the Mexican plateau. Small Rumin. Res., 41(1):77–80, 2001.
Rammell, C.G., Thompson, K.G., Bentley, G.R. and Gibbons, M.W.: Selenium, vitamin E and polyunsaturated fatty acid concentrations in goat kids with and without nutritional myodegeneration. NZ. Vet. J. 37(1):4–6, 1989.
Reddy, P.G., Sapp, W.J. and Heneine, W.: Detection of caprine arthritis-encephalitis virus by polymerase chain reaction. J. Clin. Microbiol., 31(11):3042–3043, 1993.
Ridoux, R., Siliart, B. and Andre, F.: Paramètres biochimiques de la chèvre laitière I. Determination de quelques valeurs de reference, Rec. Méd. Vét., 157:357–361, 1981.
Riet-Correa, F.: Mineral supplementation in small ruminants in the semiarid region of Brazil. Ciencia Veterinaria nos Tropicos. 7(2/3):112–130, 2004.
Rimstad E., et al.: Delayed seroconversion following naturally acquired caprine arthritis-encephalitis virus infection in goats. Am. J. Vet. Res., 54(11):1858–1862, 1993.
Rodríguez, J.L., et al.: Polyarthritis in kids associated with *Mycoplasma putrefaciens*. Vet. Rec., 135(17):406–407, 1994.
Rollins, D.: Interpreting physical evidence of predation on hoofstock and management alternatives for coping with predators. Vet. Clin. N. Am. Food Anim. Pract., 17(2):265–282, 2001.
Roncero, V., Redondo, E., Gasquez, A. and Duran, E.: Estudio histopatologico de la miodistrofia nutricional enzootica en los pequenos rumiantes. Med. Vet., 6:363–370, 1989.
Rørvik, A.M.: Methods and errors in measurements of synovial fluid volume in stifles with low volume and high

viscosity synovial fluid. An experimental study in goats. Acta Vet. Scand., 36:2, 213–222, 1995.
Rosendal, S.: Experimental infection of goats, sheep, and calves with the large colony type of *M. mycoides* subsp. *mycoides*. Vet. Pathol., 18:71–81, 1981.
Rosendal, S.: Susceptibility of goats and calves after experimental inoculation or contact exposure to a Canadian strain of *M. mycoides* subsp. *mycoides* from a goat. Can. J. Comp. Med., 47:484–490, 1983.
Rosendal, S.: Pathogenetic mechanisms of *M. mycoides* subsp. *mycoides* septicemia in goats. Isr. J. Med. Sci., 20:970–971, 1984.
Rowe, C.L.: Hemivertebra in a goat. Vet. Med. Small Anim. Clin., 74:211–214, 1979.
Rowe, J.D.: Control programmes for chronic goat diseases. Proceedings, No. Amer. Vet. Conf., Large Animal, Vol. 20, Orlando, FL, 7–11 Jan, 2006. The North American Veterinary Conference, Gainesville, FL, pp. 290–293, 2006.
Rowe, J.D. and East, N.E.: Risk factors for transmission and methods for control of caprine arthritis-encephalitis virus infection. Vet. Clin. N. Am. Food Anim. Pract., 13(1):35–53, 1997.
Rowe, J.D., et al.: Cohort study of natural transmission and two methods for control of caprine arthritis-encephalitis virus infection in goats on a California dairy. Am. J. Vet. Res., 53(12):2386–2395, 1992.
Rowe, L.D., Corrier, D.E., Reagor, J.C. and Jones L.P.: Experimentally induced *Cassia roemeriana* poisoning in cattle and goats. Am. J. Vet. Res., 48:992–997, 1987.
Ruffin, D.C.: Mycoplasma infections in small ruminants. Vet. Clin. N. Am. Food Anim. Pract., 17(2):315–332, 2001.
Sack, W.O. and Cottrell, W.: Puncture of shoulder, elbow, and carpal joints in goats and sheep. J. Am. Vet. Med. Assoc., 185:63–65, 1984.
Saha, A.C. and Deb, S.K.: Osteodystrophia fibrosa in goat. Indian Vet. J., 50:14–17, 1973.
Sahoo, N. and Ray, S.K.: Fluorosis in goats near an aluminum smelter plant in Orissa. Indian J. Anim. Sci., 74(1):48–50, 2004.
Salman, M.D., et al.: An economic evaluation of various treatments for contagious foot rot in sheep, using decision analysis. J. Am. Vet. Med. Assoc., 193:195–204, 1988.
Sánchez, J., Montes, P., Jimenez, A. and Andres, S.: Prevention of clinical mastitis with barium selenate in dairy goats from a selenium-deficient area. J. Dairy Sci., 90(5):2350–2354, 2007.
Sargison, N.D., et al.: Unusual outbreak of sporozoan encephalomyelitis in Bluefaced Leicester ram lambs. Vet. Rec., 146(8):225–226, 2000.
Sasaki, Y., Kojima, A., Kikuchi, E. and Tamura, Y.: Multiplex PCR for direct detection of pathogenic clostridia in bovine clostridial infections. J. Vet. Med., 55(11):889–893, 2002.
Saym, F. and Ozer, E.: Dogu anadolu'da kecilerde sarcosporidiosis'in yayilisi uzerinde arastirmalar. [Incidence of goat sarcosporidiosis in East Anatolia]. A.U. Vet. Fak. Derg., 31:316–323, 1984.
Scarratt, W.K.: Cerebellar disease and disease characterized by dysmetria or tremors. Vet. Clin. N. Am. Food Anim. Pract., 20(2):275–286, 2004.
Scott, P.R. and Sargison, N.D.: Extensive ascites associated with vegetative endocarditis and *Sarcocystis* myositis in a shearling ram. Vet. Rec., 149(8):240–241, 2001.
Scroggs, P.: Diary of a tragedy. Dairy Goat J., 67:793, 795, 799, 817, 1989.
Seaman, J. and Evers, M.: Foot rot in sheep and goats. Primefacts, Primefact #265, New South Wales Department of Primary Industries, Australia, December 2006, 8 pp. http://www.dpi.nsw.gov.au/__data/assets/pdf_file/0015/102381/footrot-in-sheep-and-goats.pdf
Sellers, R.F. and Herniman, K.A.J.: Neutralizing antibodies to Akabane virus in ruminants in Cyprus. Trop. Anim. Health Prod., 13:57–60, 1981.
Seneviratna, P., Atureliya, D. and Vijayakumar, R.: The incidence of *Sarcocystis* spp. in cattle and goats in Sri Lanka. Ceylon Vet. J., 23:11–13, 1975.
Shah, C., et al.: Phylogenetic analysis and reclassification of caprine and ovine lentiviruses based on 104 new isolates: evidence for regular sheep-to-goat transmission and worldwide propagation through livestock trade. Virology, 319:12–26, 2004.
Shah, C., et al.: Direct evidence for natural transmission of small-ruminant lentiviruses of subtype A4 from goats to sheep and vice versa. J. Virol., 78(14):7518–7522, 2004a.
Shany, S., Yagil, R. and Berlyne, G.M.: 25-hydroxycholecalciferol levels in camel, sheep and goat. Comp. Biochem. Physiol., 59B:139–140, 1978.
Sharew, A.D., Staak, C., Thiaucourt, F. and Roger, F.: A serological investigation into contagious caprine pleuropneumonia (CCPP) in Ethiopia. Trop. Anim. Health Prod., 37(1):11–19, 2005.
Sharma, S.K.: Foot and mouth disease in sheep and goats. Vet. Res. J., 4:1–21, 1981.
Shekarforoush, S.S., Razavi, S.M., Dehghan, S.A. and Sarihi, K.: Prevalence of *Sarcocystis* species in slaughtered goats in Shiraz, Iran. Vet. Rec., 156(13):418–420, 2005.
Shelton, M.: Predation and livestock production perspective and overview. Sheep Goat Res. J., 19:2–5, 2004.
Sherman, D.M., Arendt, T.D., Gay, J.M. and Maefsky, V.A.: Comparing the effects of four colostral preparations on serum Ig levels in newborn kids. Vet. Med., 85:908–913, 1990.
Shimshony, A.: An epizootic of Akabane disease in bovines, ovines and caprines in Israel, 1969–1970: epidemiologic assessment. Acta Morphol. Acad. Sci. Hung., 28:197–199, 1980.
Sikdar, A. and Uppal, P.K.: Isolation and identification of *M. capricolum* from pashmina goats. Indian J. Anim. Sci., 53:528–531, 1983.
Simoens, P., De Vos, N.R., Lauwers, H. and Nicaise, M.: Numerical vertebral variations and transitional vertebrae in the goat. Zbl. Vet. Med. C. Anat. Histol. Embryol., 12:97–103, 1983.
Singh, A.P., Mirakhur, K.K. and Nigam, J.M.: A study on the incidence and anatomical locations of fractures in canine, caprine, bovine, equine and camel. Indian J. Vet. Surg., 4:61–66, 1983.
Singh, S.K. and Prasad, M.C.: Hypervitaminosis D in goats: clinicobiochemical studies. Indian J. Vet. Pathol, 11:7–13, 1987.

Skerman, T.M.: Footscald and foot rot in goats. Proc. 17th Seminar, Sheep and Beef Cattle Soc., N. Z. Vet. Assoc., Wellington, pp. 65–70, 1987.

Sobiech, P., Pomianowski, A. and Snarska, A.: Activity of LDH isoenzymes in goat kids during the first life period. Ann. Univ. Mariae Curie-Skodowska. Sectio DD, Med. Vet. 60:153–157, 2005.

Souza e Silva, J. de, Castro, R.S., Melo, C.B. and Feijo, F. M.C.: Serological determination of the caprine arthritis encephalitis virus in dairy goat herds from Rio Grande Norte State, Brazil. Ciencia Vet. Trop., 7(1):26–35, 2004.

Spais, A.G., Argyroudis, S. and Sarris, K.: Field evaluation of a combination of lincomycin and spectinomycin for the treatment of contagious agalactia of sheep and goats. Bull. Hellenic Vet. Med. Soc., 32:290–298, 1981.

Squires, V.: Livestock Management in the Arid Zone. Melbourne, Inkata Press, 1981.

Steere, A.C.: Lyme disease. New Eng. J. Med., 321:586–596, 1989.

Steinberg, H. and George, C.: Fracture-associated osteogenic sarcoma and mandibular osteoma in two goats. J. Comp. Pathol., 100:453–457, 1989.

Steinberg, S. and Botelho, S.: Myotonia in a horse. Science, 137:979–980, 1962.

Stevens, J.B., et al.: Hematologic, blood gas, blood chemistry, and serum mineral values for a sample of clinically healthy adult goats. Vet. Clin. Pathol., 23(1):19–24, 1994.

Sugano, S., et al.: The clinical values for chemical constituents of blood in normal miniature Shiba goats. Exp. Anim., 29:433–439, 1980.

Surman, P.G., Daniels, E. and Dixon, B.R.: Caprine arthritis-encephalitis virus infection of goats in South Australia. Aust. Vet. J., 64:266–271, 1987.

Talavera Boto, J.: Estudio sobre la agalaxia contagiosa de la oveja y de la cabra en Espana. I.N.I.E. Serie: Higiene y sanidad animal. No. 4, 1980. Ministerio de Agricultura, Instituto Nacional de Investigaciones Agrarias, Espana.

Tanwar, R.K. and Mathur, P.D.: Studies on experimental rumen acidosis in goats. Indian Vet. J., 60:499–500, 1983.

Taoudi, A., Karib, H., Johnson, D.W. and Fassi-Fehri, M.M.: Comparaison du pouvoir pathogène de trois souches de *M. capricolum* pour la chèvre et le chevreau nouveau-né. Rev. Élev. Méd. Vet. Pays. Trop., 41:353–358, 1988.

Thompson, K.G.: Some diseases of importance in goats as seen by animal health laboratories. Proc. 16th Seminar, Sheep and Beef Cattle Soc., N. Z. Vet. Assoc., Palmerston North, pp. 39–45, 1986.

Tola S., et al.: Detection of *Mycoplasma agalactiae* in sheep milk samples by polymerase chain reaction. Vet. Microbiol., 54:17–22, 1997.

Tontis, A.: Zum Vorkommen der nutritiven Muskeldystrophie (NMD) bei Zicklein in der Schweiz. Schweiz. Arch. Tierheilk., 126:41–46, 1984.

Torres-Acosta, J.F.J., et al.: Serological survey of caprine arthritis-encephalitis virus in 83 goat herds of Yucatan, Mexico. Small Rumin. Res., 49:207–211, 2003.

Traore, A. and Wilson, R.T.: Livestock production in central Mali: environmental and pathological factors affecting morbidity and mortality of ruminants in the agropastoral system. Prev. Vet. Med., 6:63–75, 1988.

Travassos, C., et al.: Detection of caprine arthritis encephalitis virus in white blood mononuclear cells and semen of experimentally infected bucks. Vet. Res., 29(6):579–584, 1998.

Travnieek, M., et al.: Seroprevalence of anti-*Borrelia burgdorferi* antibodies in sheep and goats from mountainous areas of Slovakia. Ann. Agric. Environ. Med. 9(2):153–156, 2002.

Uddin, M.M. and Ahmed, S.U.: Effect of pregnancy and lactation on serum calcium and phosphorus level of black Bengal goat. Bangladesh J. Agric. Sci., 11:111–114, 1984.

Uppal, P.K.: Foot and mouth disease in small ruminants—An issue of concern. Report of the Session of the Research Group of the Standing Technical Committee, Appendix 29. European Commission For The Control Of Foot-And-Mouth Disease (EUFMD), Chania, Greece, October 11, 2004. http://www.fao.org/ag/againfo/commissions/docs/greece04/App29.pdf

Vaissaire, J.: et al.: *Erysipelothrix rhusiopathiae*: agent du rouget dans les différentes espèces animales. Bull. Acad. Vét. France, 58:259–265, 1985.

Van Metre, D.C. and Callan, R.J.: Selenium and vitamin E. Vet. Clin. No. Am. Food Anim. Pract., 17(2):373–402, 2001.

Van Tonder, F.M.: Notes on some disease problems in Angora goats in South Africa. Vet. Med. Rev., 1/2:109–138, 1975.

Van Vleet, J.F.: Myopathies and Myositides, In: Merck Veterinary Manual, 9th Ed. C.M. Kahn, ed. Merck and Co., Whitehouse Station, NJ, pp 947–957, 2005.

Varshney, V.P., Pande, J.K. and Sanwal, P.C.: Studies on some biochemical components of the blood serum in immature and mature male goats. J. Vet. Physiol. Allied Sci., 1:29–33, 1982.

Wadajkar, S.V., Shastri, U.V. and Narladkar, B.W.: Caprine sarcocystosis: clinical signs, gross and microscopic pathology. Indian Vet. J., 72(3):224–228, 1995.

Wang J.D., et al.: Effect of high fluoride and low protein on tooth matrix development in goats. Fluoride 35(1):51–55, 2002.

Wang, J.D., Guo, Y.H., Liang, Z.X. and Hao, J.H.: Amino acid composition and histopathology of goat teeth in an industrial fluoride polluted area. Fluoride. 36(3):177–184, 2003.

Wanner, M., Kessler, J., Martig, J. and Tontis, A.: Enzootische Kalzinose bei Ziege und Rind in der Schweiz. Schweiz. Arch. Tierheilk., 128:151–160, 1986.

Werling, D. and Langhans, W.: Caprine arthritis-encephalitis, In: Infectious Diseases of Livestock, Vol 1, 2nd Ed. J.A.W. Coetzer and R.C. Tustin, eds. Cape Town, South Africa, Oxford University Press, pp. 741–746, 2004.

Wessels, T.C.: Sudden deaths from *Clostridium septicum* infection in the Gobabis district. J. So. Afr. Vet. Assoc., 43:420, 1972.

White, J.B. and Plaskett, J.: "Nervous," "stiff-legged" or "fainting goats." Am. Vet. Rev., 28:556–560, 1904.

Wiggans, G.R. and Hubbard, S.M.: Genetic evaluation of yield and type traits of dairy goats in the United States. J. Dairy Sci., 84 (Elect. Suppl.): E69-E73, 2001.

Woubit, S., et al.: A specific PCR for the identification of *Mycoplasma capricolum* subsp. *capripneumoniae*, the causative agent of contagious caprine pleuropneumonia (CCPP). Vet. Microbiol., 104(1/2):125–132, 2004.

Wouda, W., Borst, G.H.A. and Gruys, E.: Delayed swayback in goat kids, a study of 23 cases. Vet. Q., 8:45–56, 1986.
Yang, P.C., Chu, R.M., Chung, W.B. and Sung H.T.: Epidemiological characteristics and financial costs of the 1997 foot-and-mouth disease epidemic in Taiwan. Vet. Rec. 145:731–734, 1999.
Yerex, D.: The Farming of Goats. Fiber and Meat Production in New Zealand. Carterton, N.Z., Ampersand Publ. Assoc. Ltd., 1986.
Yousif, M.A., El-Attar, H.M., Mahmoud, A.R.M. and El-Magawry, S.: Clinical and subclinical rickets in goats in relation to some blood parameters. Assiut Vet. Med. J., 17:89–94, 1986.
Zhang, D.R., Lin T. and Li Q.: Investigation on the seroepidemiology of Lyme disease in Anhui province. Chin. J. Vector Biol. Control, 9(4): 265–267, 1998.

5

Nervous System

Information on the prevalence of neurologic disease in goats is limited. One American survey indicated that neurologic disease was diagnosed in 5% of all goat cases at necropsy (Lincicome 1982). Despite this low number, neurologic diseases are an important aspect of caprine practice. Diseases such as rabies and listeriosis represent serious potential zoonoses and demand accurate diagnosis. Certain nervous diseases of goats, such as organophosphate toxicities or pseudorabies, can result in high morbidity or mortality rates on individual farms despite a low general prevalence. Still others, such as polioencephalomalacia or neonatal meningoencephalitis, suggest management problems and the need for client education. Diseases such as scrapie need to be recognized and reported so that appropriate regulatory intervention can be initiated. Finally, accurate diagnosis and management of neurologic disease in goats can be a stimulating and satisfying clinical challenge for the veterinarian.

Most of the neurologic diseases of goats are presented in this chapter, with some exceptions. Pregnancy toxemia, hypomagnesemia, and milk fever are primarily nutritional diseases and are discussed in Chapter 19. Cowdriosis or heartwater produces both neurologic and cardiac signs and is essentially a vasculitis. It is discussed in detail in Chapter 8. The neurologic aspects of caprine arthritis encephalitis (CAE) are discussed in this chapter in conjunction with maedi-visna, a closely related retroviral disease. However, CAE is covered in more detail in Chapter 4, because arthritis is the most common presenting sign. Finally, the causes of hepatoencephalopathy are discussed in Chapter 11.

BACKGROUND INFORMATION OF CLINICAL IMPORTANCE

Anatomy and Physiology

An atlas of the caprine brain in twenty-three transverse sections has been published (Yoshikawa 1968). The gross anatomy of the caprine central nervous system (CNS) and peripheral nerves has been described elsewhere and compared with sheep and cattle (Dellmann and McClure 1975; Godhinho and Getty 1975; Ghosal 1975). Published studies on the neurophysiology of goats are uncommon and no neurophysiological attributes of clinical importance unique to the species have surfaced.

Thalamic melanosis has been reported frequently as an incidental finding at post mortem in goats with brown hair coats and occasionally white coats, but has no clinical significance (Bestetti et al. 1980). One anomaly of the goat that could affect the clinical evaluation of the nervous system is a high frequency of variation in vertebral body numbers and the occurrence of transitional vertebrae (Simoens et al. 1983). This variation can complicate the technique of cerebrospinal fluid collection at the lumbosacral site and confuse interpretation of spinal radiographs and myelography. Details concerning vertebral anomalies are given in Chapter 4.

Neurologic Examination

The small size and reasonably cooperative nature of goats facilitate the performance of a thorough neurologic examination. A consistent, systematic approach should be taken. Protocols and procedures for neurologic evaluation of small ruminants have been published and are similar to those used in small animal medicine (Brewer 1983; Constable 2004). The examination must always include assessments of five major factors: mental status and behavior, cranial nerve functions, postural reactions, locomotion, and spinal reflexes. A summary of the types of signs associated with lesions in different regions of the CNS is given in Table 5.1 and details of the evaluation of cranial nerve function are given in Table 5.2.

Cerebrospinal Fluid Analysis

Analysis of cerebrospinal fluid (CSF) can be used to diagnostic advantage in caprine medicine (Smith 1982). Two sites, the atlanto-occipital and the lumbosacral site, are routinely used for collection of CSF from the subarachnoid space. Heavy sedation or general anesthesia of the goat is required to accomplish an atlanto-occipital tap. Several methods have been recorded, including use of intravenous diazepam (5 to 10 mg total dose), intramuscular xylazine at a dose of 0.1 mg/kg bw, intravenous thiopental sodium at a dose of 15 mg/kg, or inhalation anesthesia with halothane (Brewer 1983; Chandna et al. 1983). The lumbosacral tap may be accomplished using tranquilization or, if the risks of medication are high, manual restraint. A lumbosacral CSF tap without chemical restraint is best attempted only in comatose, paralyzed, or severely paretic goats. Because abnormal CSF is not necessarily homogeneous in character, the site of collection should be closest to the suspected lesion to maximize the value of the sample. Regardless of the site selected, the procedure should be done using strict aseptic techniques to avoid iatrogenic meningitis.

For atlanto-occipital puncture, the goat is laid in lateral recumbency. The head is flexed at a right angle to the cervical spine and positioned so that the head and neck are in a single plane parallel to the ground or table. This extreme flexion of the neck may compromise air movement through the trachea, particularly when a flexible tracheal tube is in place. The site of skin penetration is on the dorsal midline at the point of intersection with an imaginary line connecting the anteriormost aspects of the wings of the atlas. Ideally, a styletted, 2.5-inch (6.4 cm), 20-gauge spinal needle should be used, but an ordinary 1.5-inch (3.8 cm) 20- or 22-gauge disposable needle can be used if necessary (Brewer 1983). The needle should be directed toward the lower jaw as it penetrates the skin. The usual depth to the subarachnoid space is 1- to 1.5-inch (2.5 to 3.8 cm), but the needle should not be passed the full depth without stopping frequently to remove the stylette and check the progress. The advancing needle should remain perpendicular to the dorsal midline to avoid hemorrhage from entering the paravertebral venous sinuses.

The CSF should rise readily up the needle when the subarachnoid space is reached and the stylette removed. The fluid may be allowed to drip into a collecting tube, or aspirated gently with a syringe. If it runs forcefully from the needle, this may suggest increased CSF pressure and rapid egress or aspiration of fluid could result in caudal herniation of the brain. A manometer can be attached to the needle hub via a three-way stopcock to record CSF pressure. If CSF pressure is not increased, up to 0.22 ml of CSF/kg of bw may be extracted safely. On average, the total volume of CSF in adult goats is 20 to 25 ml, 8 to 12 ml of which is in the ventricles (Pappenheimer et al. 1962).

Table 5.1. Clinical signs associated with lesions in different regions of the nervous system.

Region of nervous System	*Clinical signs possibly observed*
Autonomic nervous system	Miosis or mydriasis, salivation, increased or decreased gut motility, changes in fecal and urinary continence, muscle twitching
Cerebrum	Changes in mental status, mania, hyperexcitability, hysteria, depression, nonresponsiveness, coma Changes in behavior, convulsions, opisthotons, head pressing, teeth grinding, constant chewing or vocalizing, yawning, inability to chew, blindness with normal pupillary responses Changes in gait, compulsive walking or circling, contralateral proprioceptive deficits
Cerebellum	Incoordination with no accompanying weakness, hypermetria in all limbs, base-wide stance, possible intention tremors, loss of menace response (also involves cranial nerves, cerebrum, and brain stem)
Vestibular system	Ipsilateral head tilt, circling, hemiparesis with staggering gait, resting nystagmus
Brain stem	Ipsilateral weakness, incoordination, spasticity, proprioceptive deficits
Cranial nerves	Deficits in vision, smell, hearing, or swallowing; changes in tone, motor control, or sensation of facial structures; abnormal eyeball position; carriage of head or balance
Spinal cord C1 to C6	Incoordination and weakness in affected limbs with loss of proprioception, potentially all four limbs affected, usually worse in rear limbs, reflexes are hyperactive in all affected limbs, skin sensation diminished in affected dermatomes
Spinal cord C7 to T2	Incoordination and weakness in affected limbs with loss of proprioception, forelimb deficits often equal rear limbs deficits, hyporeflexia of forelimbs, hyperreflexia of hind limbs, loss of skin sensation in affected dermatomes
Spinal cord T3 to L3	Incoordination, weakness and loss of proprioception in one or both hind limbs, hind limb reflexes hyperactive, forelimbs normal in all respects, loss of skin sensation in affected dermatomes
Spinal cord L4 to S2	Incoordination, weakness and loss of proprioception in one or both hind limbs, hyporeflexia of hind limbs, forelimbs normal in all respects, loss of skin sensation in affected dermatomes
Spinal cord S1 to S3	Distended bladder and loss of anal and tail tone; caprine spinal cord ends at spinal cord S_3 and the subarachnoid space extends to the second caudal vertebra
Peripheral nerves	Deficits of extension, flexion, or adduction; muscle atrophy in a single limb; localized loss of skin sensation on affected portions of limb; possible hyporeflexia
Neuromuscular junctions	General weakness, muscle twitching, or tremors

C = cervical spinal segment, T = thoracic spinal segment, L = lumbar spinal segment, S = sacral spinal segment.

For a lumbosacral tap, the animal is restrained in lateral recumbency and the spine markedly flexed with the plane of the midline parallel to the supporting surface. The puncture site is located on the dorsal midline where it intersects an imaginary line connecting the anteriormost aspects of the two *tuber sacrale*. There is frequently a palpable depression in the skin at this point. A local skin block of the puncture site with lidocaine is advised if the goat is not sedated. The occurrence of transitional lumbosacral vertebrae may make it difficult to identify and penetrate the lumbosacral space in goats. If frequent attempts are met with failure, the tap should be attempted in the L5–L6 intervertebral space. This is accomplished by palpating the two caudalmost dorsal spinous processes identifiable cranial to the sacrum and passing the needle between them on the midline, just anterior to the more caudal spinous process. The L4–L5 space can be used similarly.

A technique for placement of a styletted, stainless steel cannula in the third ventricle of the goat under anesthesia has been described (Mogi et al. 2003). This allows for repeated collection of CSF during research studies requiring multiple samples over time.

Some interpretation of the CSF is possible without laboratory support. Normal CSF is clear and colorless. Cloudiness suggests inflammation caused by increased cells or protein. Xanthochromia, or yellow discoloration, suggests earlier presence of blood in the CSF frequently associated with trauma. Increased CSF pressure may be recorded in cases of polioencephalomalacia, hydrocephalus, or other causes of cerebral edema. Reagent test strips designed for urinalysis may be applied to CSF in the field (Brewer 1983). Protein content more than 1+ is abnormal, blood should not be present, and the absence of glucose may suggest bacterial meningitis.

Table 5.2. Evaluation of cranial nerve function in goats.

Activity, condition, or test response observed in normal goats	*Cranial nerves and other components of nervous system responsible for normal activity, condition, or response*
Goat can see	II, cerebrum, connecting pathways, eye
Normal menace response (eyelids close in response to noncontact threatening gesture)	II, VII, cerebrum, cerebellum, brain stem
Bilaterally similar pupil size	II, III, sympathetic nervous system, brain stem
Normal pupillary light response	II, III
Eyes normally positioned in head	III, IV, VI, VIII
Eyeball retracts when cornea is touched	III, V, VI
Jaw tone and nostril sensation are normal	V
Eyelids close when canthus is touched	V, VII
Ear twitches when inside of ear is touched	V, VII, X
Lips retract when probe is introduced into commissure of lips	V, VII
Nostrils held symmetrically and move normally	VII
Ears held in normal position	VII
Eyelids held open normally	III, VII, sympathetic nervous system
Goat responds to sound	VIII
Head is held in normal position	VIII, cerebrum
Eyeballs drop slightly and evenly when head is tilted upward	VIII
Normal vestibular nystagmus is seen when head is turned to side, fast component is toward turned side	III, IV, VI, VIII, brain stem
No spontaneous nystagmus is observed	VIII
Swallowing and tongue movement are normal	IX, X, XII
Tongue tone is normal	XII

I = olfactory n., II = optic n., III = oculomotor n., IV = trochlear n., V = trigeminal n., VI = abducens n., VII = facial n., VIII = vestibulo-cochlear n., IX = glossopharyngeal n., X = vagus n., XI = spinal accessory n., XII = hypoglossal n.

Normal laboratory values reported for cellular and chemical constituents of caprine CSF are given in Table 5.3. Glucose levels in the CSF are normally 60% of those in blood. When xylazine is used to sedate goats for a CSF tap, glucose concentration in the CSF may double within thirty minutes of administration (Amer and Misk 1980).

Imaging Techniques

Plain radiography is useful to identify bony lesions that may affect the integrity of the brain and spinal cord. Myelography can aid in identification and localization of intramedullary and extramedullary lesions of the spinal cord and meninges. Preparation and positioning of goats for myelography are similar to that described above for the CSF tap, and procedures and applications for myelography of goats at both the atlanto-occipital and lumbar sites have been described (Chandna et al. 1978; Rowe 1979; Chandna et al. 1983). Cerebral angiography has been used in goats to assist in the diagnosis and surgical treatment of coenurosis (Sharma et al. 1974). Scintigraphy with radiolabelled ^{99m}Tc-ciprofloxacin was used as a diagnostic aid in a case of vertebral osteomyelitis and diskospondylitis in a three-week-old goat with acute hind limb paresis (Alexander et al. 2005). Image quality was best four hours after injection of the radiolabelled drug.

A topographic study of the cranioencephalic structures of the goat using computed tomography (CT) has been reported (Arencibia et al. 1997), though the use of CT in clinical practice has been limited in goats. CT has been used as a diagnostic aid in a case of paraplegia in an adult Boer goat (Levine et al. 2006). The scan revealed the presence of diskospondylitis and a compressive myelopathy. CT was also employed in the diagnosis of a glioma in the right frontoparietal cortex of the brain of an adult male goat that presented with a one-week history of circling (Marshall et al. 1995).

Magnetic resonance imaging (MRI) has been used to identify spinal cord compression due to a mass in the lumbar region of an adult goat with paraparesis (Gygi et al. 2004). At necropsy the mass was determined to be a lymphosarcoma. MRI has also been used to identify lesions in the thoracolumbar region of the spinal cord as an aid in diagnosing the neurological form of caprine arthritis encephalitis (CAE) in a five-

Table 5.3. Selected normal values for constituents of cerebrospinal fluid of goats.

Constituent	*Unit*	*Mean*	*Range (or ± standard deviation)*	*Reference*
Aspartate aminotransferase	IU/l	79.8	(±27)	Aminlari and Mehran 1988
Calcium	mg/dl	4.6*		Kaneko 1980
	mg/dl	9**	5.5 to 14.5	Cissik et al. 1987
Chloride	mEq/l		116 to 130	Cissik et al. 1987
Glucose	mg/dl	56		Fletcher et al. 1964
	mmol/l	1.8	(± 0.8)	Aminlari and Mehran 1988
Lactate dehydrogenase	IU/l	8.9	(±9.3)	Aminlari and Mehran 1988
Magnesium	mg/dl	2.4	1.7 to 3.2	Cissik et al. 1987
Pandy test***		negative	negative	Brooks et al. 1964
pH			7.3 to 7.4	Brooks et al. 1964
Phosphorus	mg/dl	11.6		Brooks et al. 1964
Potassium	mEq/l	3		Kaneko 1980
Sodium	mEq/l	131		Kaneko 1980
Specific gravity		1.005	1.004 to 1.008	Fletcher et al. 1964; Brooks et al. 1964
Total protein	mg/dl	12	0.0 to 45	Smith 1982; Kaneko 1980; Brooks et al. 1964
	mg/dl	29.6	(±15.1)	Aminlari and Mehran 1988
Urea	mg/dl		5 to 6.2	Brooks et al. 1964
White blood cells****	#/mm^3		0 to 9	Smith 1982; Fletcher et al. 1964

*Characteristics of goats not specified.

**Pregnant does only, n = 20.

***The Pandy test is a semiquantitative precipitation test that identifies the presence of globulin in the cerebrospinal fluid. Normally, there is no globulin present.

****Cells normally present may be lymphocytes, macrophages, or intact neutrophils. Red blood cells are not found in the normal caprine cerebrospinal fluid.

month-old goat with posterior paresis (Steiner et al. 2006). Most recently, the use of MRI was reported as an aid in the diagnosis of polioencephalomalacia in a two-month old Boer goat kid, identifying bilateral symmetric high-water-content lesions of the fronto-parietal cortex (Schenk et al. 2007).

Electroencephalogram (EEG)

The normal EEG of goats has been recorded in varying states of consciousness and in reference to rumination (Sugawara 1971; Bell and Itabisashi 1973). The EEG of goats also has been recorded under experimental disease conditions including urea poisoning (Itabisashi 1977) and Bermuda grass-induced tremors (Strain et al. 1982), as well as in a clinical case of partial epilepsy in an adult Nubian doe (Olcott et al. 1987) and in a group of goats with putative *Solanum viarum* toxicity (Porter et al. 2003).

Several physiological studies have also included recordings of the EEG in goats (Sugawara et al. 1989; Bergamasco et al. 2005, 2006). Determination of the bispectral index of the EEG was reported to be useful in monitoring the depth of isoflurane anesthesia in goats (Antognini et al. 2000). The use of visual-evoked brainstem potentials (VEP) and electroretinograms (ERG) in the clinical assessment of polioencephalomalacia in a goat has been reported. The ERG was normal but the VEP was abnormal in the acute phase of disease when the goat was clinically blind. At one year post treatment, vision was restored and the VEP showed an almost normal recording (Strain et al. 1990).

DIAGNOSIS OF NEUROLOGIC DISEASE BY PRESENTING SIGNS

It is unusual for a goat to show a single, isolated sign of neurologic disease, and multiple signs may be exhibited serially or simultaneously during the course of disease. Therefore, in the following discussion of diagnosis of neurologic disease by presenting sign, the same disease may show up repeatedly under different headings as a possible cause of clinical signs. When using this list, you may start with the most predominant sign of the case at hand and then refer to the detailed discussion of the disease elsewhere in the text. The potential causes of a given sign are not presented by frequency of occurrence because this can vary considerably with geography and type of management. Instead, they are presented by etiologic grouping.

Signs of Altered Mental State or Behavior

Excitability, Mania

Signs of excitation or mania include behaviors such as excessive bleating, resistance or overreaction to touch or handling, hyperesthesia, obvious fear or aggression, frenzy, aimless running, compulsive walking, head pressing, constant chewing, teeth grinding, or fluttering of the eyelids.

Infectious causes include rabies, pseudorabies, Borna disease, cowdriosis, scrapie, and bacterial meningoencephalitis. Thermal meningoencephalitis secondary to hot iron horn bud removal also occurs. Possible parasitic causes include coenurosis (gid), aberrant *Oestrus ovis* larval migration into the brain (false gid), trypanosomosis, and *Strongyloides papillosus*.

Metabolic causes include polioencephalomalacia, pregnancy toxemia, and hypomagnesemic tetany. Hepatoencephalopathy secondary to liver disease can produce hyperesthesia or head pressing.

Toxic agents that can cause excitation in goats include organophosphates, chlorinated hydrocarbons, cyanide, nitrates, urea, nitrofurans, and the coyotillo plant *(Karwinskia humboldtiana)*.

Levamisole or ivermectin given parenterally at therapeutic doses by injection may result in a transient excitatory reaction in some goats. Affected goats run around frantically after injection, throwing their heads in the air. Virtually all return to normal within several minutes and there is no residual effect. This is presumed to be caused by local irritation at the site of injection. In contrast, actual overdosing with levamisole can produce true neurotoxicity with excitatory signs.

Coma

Infectious causes include meningoencephalitis, pseudorabies, and enterotoxemia. Metabolic causes include polioencephalomalacia, pregnancy toxemia, and milk fever. Hepatoencephalopathy secondary to liver disease may result in coma, as can uremia.

Toxic causes include milkweed *(Asclepias)* poisoning; oxalate poisoning; salt poisoning; and organophosphate, carbamate, or chlorinated hydrocarbon insecticide toxicities.

Head trauma with subdural hemorrhage can result in coma. It is the nature of goats to frequently butt heads but this does not preclude the possibility of occasional serious injury.

Signs of Cranial Nerve Deficits

See Table 5.2.

Ocular Abnormalities

The differential diagnoses for abnormalities of pupillary function, blindness, ocular position, lid function, and sensation associated with the cranial nerves are discussed in Chapter 6.

Facial Nerve Paralysis

Characteristic signs include ear droop, eyelid droop, slack facial muscles with accumulation of feed in the buccal space, collapsed nostril, and drooling.

Infectious causes include CAE, listeriosis, brain abscess, otitis media, or otitis interna. Rupture of the tympanic membrane secondary to ear mite infection with *Psoroptes cuniculi* has resulted in facial nerve paralysis and signs of vestibular disease (Wilson and Brewer 1984). Trauma to the facial nerve, which is superficial along much of its course, can also occur.

Dysphagia

Potential neurologic causes of difficult swallowing include rabies, CAE, bacterial meningoencephalitis, and listeriosis. The numerous, non-neurologic causes of dysphagia are discussed in Chapter 10. Gloves should be worn when examining a goat that presents with difficulty in swallowing due to the risk of rabies.

Head Tilt

Persistent tilting of the head (one ear higher than the other) indicates vestibular dysfunction. Infectious causes of head tilt in goats include CAE, listeriosis, brain abscess, otitis media, and otitis interna.

Parasitic causes include cerebral nematodiasis caused by *Parelaphostrongylus tenuis*, *Elaphostrongylus* spp. or *Setaria digitata*, coenurosis (gid), or rupture of the tympanic membrane secondary to ear mite infection (Wilson and Brewer 1984).

Lymphosarcoma infiltrating the pituitary gland and producing a head tilt has been reported in a goat. Lymphosarcoma is discussed in Chapter 3. A choroid plexus carcinoma in a goat also produced a head tilt.

Deafness

On clinical examination, evaluation of deafness is difficult and interpretation subjective. However, deafness has been identified in neonatal kids with congenital beta mannosidosis. Otitis can also lead to deafness.

Signs of Involuntary Activity

Muscle Tremors

Some goats naturally tremble or shiver due to fear during an examination. This must be differentiated from nervous dysfunction. Infectious causes of tremors include rabies, scrapie, CAE, border disease, Borna disease, and bacterial meningoencephalitis. Tremors may also be an early sign of tetanus. Metabolic and nutritional causes include hypoglycemia, polioencephalomalacia, hypomagnesemic tetany, hepatoencephalopathy, and enzootic ataxia or swayback.

Toxicologic causes include plant poisoning with bitterweed or rubberweed (*Hymenoxys* spp.), neem tree (*Azadirachta indica*), coyotillo (*Karwinskia humboldtiana*), tropical soda apple (*Solanum viarum*), *Ipomoea carnea*, and possibly Bermuda grass hay (*Cynodon dactylon*), as well as cyanide poisoning, nitrate poisoning, oxalate poisoning, salt poisoning, boron ingestion, organophosphate, carbamate or chlorinated hydrocarbon insecticide poisonings, urea poisoning, levamisole overdose, and diesel fuel consumption. A hereditary cause of muscle tremors is beta mannosidosis.

Convulsions (Seizures)

Infectious causes include pseudorabies, Borna disease, enterotoxemia, tetanus, bacterial meningoencephalitis, and cowdriosis (heartwater).

Parasitic causes can include coenurosis (gid) and aberrant *Oestrus ovis* migration into the brain (false gid). Metabolic causes include polioencephalomalacia, hypomagnesemic tetany, pregnancy toxemia, hypoglycemia, and hepatoencephalopathy.

Toxic causes include the poisonous plants bitterweed or rubberweed (*Hymenoxys* spp.) and milkweed (*Asclepias* spp). Non-phytogenic poisonings include organophosphate, carbamate, and chlorinated hydrocarbon insecticides, levamisole overdose, dinitro herbicides, and pentachlorophenol wood preservatives. Lead and salt poisonings are potential causes of convulsions but are poorly documented in goats.

Lidocaine in sheep produces convulsive signs at an approximate dose of 6 mg/kg intravenously and circulatory collapse at a dose of 37 mg/kg intravenously (Morishima et al. 1981). Overdosing is most likely to occur in small kids when lidocaine is used as a local anesthetic.

Partial epilepsy of unknown cause has been reported as a cause of convulsions in an adult Nubian doe (Olcott et al. 1987).

Nystagmus

Infectious causes include rabies, CAE, listeriosis, brain abscess, and otitis. Parasitic causes include cerebrospinal nematodiasis with either *Parelaphostrongylus tenuis*, *Elaphostrongylus* spp., or *Setaria digitata* and coenurosis (gid). Metabolic causes include polioencephalomalacia.

Toxic causes include locoism caused by consumption of locoweeds (*Astragalus* spp.) and possibly salt poisoning. Hereditary beta mannosidosis causes nystagmus in affected newborn kids.

Pruritus

Primary dermatologic diseases are the most common cause of itching in goats, as discussed in Chapter 2. Pruritus of neurogenic origin tends to be more severe and animals frequently itch to the point of self-mutilation. All the neurogenic causes of pruritus in goats are of infectious or parasitic origin and include rabies, pseudorabies, scrapie, *Parelaphostrongylus tenuis*, and *Elaphostrongylus* spp.

Gait Abnormalities

Circling

Circling in goats may be cerebral or vestibular in origin. Animals with circling caused by cerebral disease usually have other abnormalities of behavior or mental status to suggest cerebral involvement. Signs associated with circling caused by vestibular lesions are usually more localized and may be limited to head tilt, nystagmus, hemiparesis, and other specific cranial nerve deficits such as facial nerve paralysis.

Infectious causes of circling include rabies, CAE, Borna disease, listeriosis, brain abscess, otitis media or interna, and cowdriosis (heartwater).

Parasitic causes can include cerebrospinal nematodiasis with either *Parelaphostrongylus tenuis*, *Elaphostrongylus* spp. or *Setaria digitata*, trypanosomosis, coenurosis (gid), and aberrant *Oestrus ovis* migration into the brain (false gid).

Metabolic and nutritional causes are limited to polioencephalomalacia.

There is a report of neoplasia as a cause of circling. This was in an adult goat with a glioma in the cerebrum (Marshall et al. 1995).

Toxic causes include plant poisonings with *Burttia prunoides*, or selenium accumulating *Astragalus* spp., as well as chlorinated hydrocarbon insecticide toxicity and nitrofuran overdose.

Hypermetria

A high stepping gait with overflexion of joints has been reported in coenurosis (gid), coyotillo (*Karwinskia humboldtiana*) poisoning, and enzootic ataxia. The author has observed pronounced hypermetria in an adult Saanen buck that, on necropsy, had a focal meningioma impinging on the anterior cervical spinal cord.

Ataxia (incoordination)

Ataxia or incoordination in goats most frequently suggests spinal cord lesions, but cerebellar, vestibular, and occasionally cerebral lesions can produce ataxia. Signs include a staggering gait, swaying or weaving from side to side, difficulties with abduction or adduction of the limbs, crossing of legs when standing or walking, general unawareness of placement and position of feet, and pivoting on the inside limb when circled. When paresis accompanies ataxia, it can be difficult to differentiate the effects of the two processes.

Infectious causes include rabies, scrapie, CAE, listeriosis, bacterial (or thermal) meningoencephalitis, brain abscess, and cowdriosis (heartwater).

Parasitic causes include cerebrospinal nematodiasis with either *Parelaphostrongylus tenuis*, *Elaphostrongylus* spp., or *Setaria digitata*; coenurosis (gid); aberrant *Oestrus ovis* migration into the brain (false gid); tick paralysis; trypanosomosis; and possibly *Strongyloides papillosus*.

Metabolic and nutritional causes include milk fever, polioencephalomalacia, hypomagnesemic tetany, and enzootic ataxia.

Toxic causes include plant poisonings resulting from ingestion of coyotillo *(Karwinskia humboldtiana)*, locoweeds (*Astragalus* spp.), guajillo *(Acacia berlanderi)*, cycad palms (*Cycas, Zamia, Microzamia*, and *Bowenia* spp.), milkweed (*Asclepias* spp.), larkspur (*Delphinium* spp.), fool's parsley *(Aethusa cynapium)*, tropical soda apple (*Solanum viarum*), *Ipomoea carnea*, maize contaminated with the fungus *Diplodia maydis*, and possibly rye grass and Bermuda grass hay *(Cynodon dactylon)*. The incoordination occurring with *Astragalus* spp. consumption may be due either to locoism or selenium toxicosis.

In addition to plant toxicities, incoordination can be seen with bromide, lead, salt, oxalate, urea, cyanide, or nitrate poisonings; organophosphate, carbamate, or chlorinated hydrocarbon insecticide intoxications; diesel fuel consumption; and nitrofuran or levamisole overdosage.

Neoplastic causes of ataxia have been reported sporadically. Lymphosarcoma associated with the brain or meninges has resulted in incoordination (Craig et al. 1986). A choroid plexus carcinoma in a goat also produced ataxia.

Congenital or hereditary causes include congenital vertebral or spinal abnormalities such as hemivertebra (Rowe 1979). There is a report of atlanto-axial malarticulation in two young Angora goats which led to spinal cord degeneration at the level of the atlanto-axial joint resulting in ataxia (Robinson et al. 1982).

Diseases of unknown etiology that can produce incoordination include polyradiculoneuritis and caprine encephalomyelomalacia.

Postural Abnormalities

Opisthotonos

Opisthotonos is a backward arching of the head and neck caused by spasm of extensor muscles. It may be observed in standing or recumbent animals. The list below includes those diseases in goats for which observation of opisthotonos has been specifically reported. However, opisthotonos may be observed during convulsions and the list of causes of convulsions should be consulted when the two signs are seen together.

Infectious causes include rabies, CAE, enterotoxemia, tetanus, brain abscess, and bacterial (or thermal) meningoencephalitis.

Disseminated toxoplasmosis is rare in goats and only one report has identified clinical signs of encephalitis, including opisthotonos, torticollis, and paresis (Fatzer 1974). Nevertheless, evidence of brain involvement may be common on necropsy of stillborn kids or fetuses (Nurse and Lenghaus 1986). Trypanosomosis is another potential protozoal cause of opisthotonos.

Metabolic and nutritional causes include hypomagnesemic tetany and polioencephalomalacia. Toxic causes include plant poisonings by bitterweed or rubberweed (*Hymenoxys* spp.), locoweeds (*Astragalus* spp.), salt poisoning, and chlorinated hydrocarbon toxicity.

Paresis (Weakness)

Neurogenic impairment of motor function leading to weakness may result from lesions of the brain stem, spinal cord, peripheral nerves, or neuromuscular junctions. Tetraparesis, paraparesis, hemiparesis, or involvement of a single limb may occur. Signs can include difficulty in rising, dragging of one or more limbs, trembling when standing, difficulty in standing for long periods, and collapse or buckling of the limbs. When hemiparesis is present, leaning, falling or rolling to one side may be noted. Careful observation and thorough neurologic examination are necessary to distinguish ataxia from paresis when both are present.

Infectious causes of paresis include rabies, CAE or visna, listeriosis, and botulism. Parasitic causes include cerebrospinal nematodiasis with either *Parelaphostrongylus tenuis*, *Elaphostrongylus* spp., or *Setaria digitata*; coenurosis; and tick paralysis.

Metabolic and nutritional causes include milk fever, pregnancy toxemia, and enzootic ataxia or swayback. Toxic causes include plant poisonings by coyotillo *(Karwinskia humboldtiana)*, locoweeds (*Astragalus* spp.), carpetweed *(Kallstroemia hirsutissima)*, milkweed (*Asclepias* spp.), tropical soda apple (*Solanum viarum*), *Ipomoea carnea*, and maize contaminated with the fungus *Diplodia maydis*. Toxic causes other than plant poisoning include salt poisoning, bromide intoxication, boron toxicity, organophosphate and carbamate insecticide poisoning, and pentachlorophenol toxicity.

Neoplastic causes of paresis are uncommon but reports include lymphosarcoma sporadically associated with the brain or meninges (Craig et al. 1986) and malignant melanoma metastasized to the vertebral canal (Sockett et al. 1984).

Congenital or inherited causes include hydrocephalus and progressive paresis of Angora goats. Caprine encephalomyelomalacia, a disease of unknown etiology, can also produce paraparesis or tetraparesis.

Paralysis

Paralysis is the complete loss of motor function in any part of the body. Many of the conditions that cause paresis progress to paralysis. Regarding the limbs, tetraplegia, paraplegia, or hemiplegia may be observed. Paralysis of the limbs may be flaccid or spastic depending on the location of the lesions. The former is associated with hyporeflexia and the latter with hyperreflexia.

Infectious causes include rabies, pseudorabies, CAE or visna, Borna disease, botulism, and brain abscess. Parasitic causes include cerebrospinal nematodiasis with either *Parelaphostrongylus tenuis*, *Elaphostrongylus* spp. or *Setaria digitata*, and tick paralysis.

Metabolic causes include milk fever and enzootic ataxia or swayback. Toxic causes include mycotoxicosis caused by consumption of maize contaminated with the fungus *Diplodia maydis* and organophosphate or carbamate insecticide toxicity.

Congenital or hereditary causes include hydrocephalus and congenital malformations of the vertebral canal or spinal cord, such as hemivertebra, and progressive paresis of Angora goats.

Trauma is the usual cause of peripheral nerve injuries leading to paralysis. While injury may occur to any of the peripheral nerves, the most common peripheral nerve dysfunction in goats is damage to the sciatic nerve from mechanical injury caused by poor intramuscular injection technique or the introduction of irritating medications on or near the nerve. The problem may be aggravated by the secondary development of abscesses. Typical signs of sciatic nerve injury include flaccid carriage of the entire hind limb with the dorsum of the hoof dragging on the ground during walking and a loss of skin sensation over most if not all of the limb. A case of hind limb paralysis caused by a metastatic malignant melanoma of the sciatic nerve has also been reported (Sockett et al. 1984).

Radial nerve paralysis related to trauma occurs in goats. Signs include flaccid carriage of the forelimb with a dropped elbow and an inability to extend the carpus and fetlock joints. The limb is dragged on ambulation. Skin sensation loss occurs on the anterior aspect of the pastern, fetlock, and digit. Restoration of limb use in a goat with radial paralysis by transplantation of the *flexor carpi radialis* tendon has been described (Batcher and Potkay 1976).

Trauma to the vertebral column can lead to paralysis by damage to the spinal cord. Vehicular injuries and fighting between goats are the most common causes of vertebral trauma, but fractures of the vertebrae may be predisposed by the presence of abscesses or osteoporosis associated with rickets.

Caprine encephalomyelomalacia, a disease of unknown etiology, can also produce paraplegia or tetraplegia.

SPECIFIC DISEASES OF THE NERVOUS SYSTEM

VIRAL AND PRION DISEASES

Rabies

Though the occurrence of rabies in goats is infrequent, rabies should not be left out of the differential diagnosis of caprine neurologic disease for two reasons: one, rabies is a consistently fatal zoonotic disease, and two, the signs of rabies are highly variable and may mimic other neurological conditions.

Etiology

Rabies virus is a bullet-shaped, enveloped, single-stranded, negative-sense, non-segmented, RNA virus in the genus Lyssavirus of the family Rhabdoviridae. The viral genome encodes for five proteins: nucleoprotein, phosphoprotein, matrix protein, glycoprotein, and an RNA polymerase. The Lyssaviruses are neurotropic viruses, well adapted to replication in the mammalian nervous system. There are seven genotypes in the genus Lyssavirus based on sequencing of the nucleoprotein (N) gene. In addition to the rabies virus (genotype 1), they include: Lagos bat virus (genotype 2), Mokola virus (genotype 3), Duvenhage virus (genotype 4), European bat virus 1 (genotype 5), European bat virus 2 (genotype 6), and Australian bat virus (genotype 7), all of which have demonstrated capacity to be animal and human pathogens causing encephalitis.

With the exception of rabies virus, which occurs essentially worldwide, these Lyssaviruses have distinct but sometimes overlapping geographic distributions. Australian bat virus is found solely in Australia. The European bat viruses are distributed among insectivorous bats in Eurasia. Lagos bat virus, Duvenhage virus, and Mokola virus have not been encountered outside of Africa (Markotter et al. 2006). Neutralizing antibody to Mokola virus has been identified in goats in Nigeria (Kemp et al. 1972; Nottidge et al. 2007).

Within the rabies virus genotype, virus variants associated with particular host species and geographic areas are recognized. They can be identified by reactions with panels of monoclonal antibodies or by genetic analysis of nucleotide substitutions (Rupprecht et al. 2002). In the continental United States, for example, there are three distinct rabies virus variants infecting skunks, found in California, the upper Midwest and the lower Midwest, while a raccoon adapted variant predominates on the eastern coast.

Two gray fox adapted variants are found focally in Arizona and Texas and separate variants adapted to red foxes and arctic foxes are found in Alaska. In addition, however, there are numerous independent reservoirs of rabies variants in insectivorous bats whose overlapping ranges essentially make the entire United States enzootic for rabies (Blanton et al. 2006).

The rabies virus grows in tissue culture, embryonating chicken eggs, and suckling mice. It has a short survival time outside the mammalian host and it becomes non-viable in dried saliva within a few hours. It is a relatively fragile virus, readily inactivated by ultraviolet irradiation and common disinfectants. For this reason, thorough cleansing and disinfection of bite wounds immediately following their occurrence is a very important and useful aspect of rabies prophylaxis.

Epidemiology

Several countries, islands, and regions are rabies-free, including Antarctica, Australia, New Zealand, Scandinavia, Great Britain, Cyprus, Japan, Papua New Guinea, and Hawaii. However, in much of the world, rabies is still endemic. In Europe and North America, most reported rabies is sylvatic, occurring primarily in wildlife reservoirs such as foxes, skunks, raccoons, and insectivorous bats. In much of Asia, Africa, and the Middle East, rabies is still largely urban, with dogs and cats comprising the majority of cases. In Latin America, rabies is an important problem, especially in dogs and cattle, with bites by vampire bats the primary source of livestock infection. Though Australia is still considered to be free of rabies, the related Lyssavirus, Australian bat virus, was identified in the mid-1990s and has produced fatal encephalitis in humans. To date, there is no evidence of infection or spillover of Australian bat virus into terrestrial mammal populations.

Rabies remains a serious zoonotic disease worldwide, particularly in developing countries of Asia, the Middle East, and Africa, where comprehensive programs to control rabies in dogs may be lacking and access to or awareness of post exposure prophylaxis is limited. Worldwide, there are an estimated 55,000 human deaths due to rabies each year (WHO 2007). India alone accounted for up to 60% of the world's rabies cases annually during the 1990s, although improved public education and greater availability of post exposure prophylaxis has improved the situation somewhat in recent years (Sudarshan et al. 2007). In the developing countries, domesticated dogs continue to be the major reservoir of rabies and dog bites the major cause of human cases. Dog bites are most likely the major cause of goat cases as well.

Goats are moderately susceptible to rabies, in the same category with sheep, cattle, and dogs (Crick 1981). While epizootics in goats are uncommon, goat rabies does occur sporadically in all enzootic regions. In the United States in 2005, for example, there were 6,418 cases of rabies reported in animals. Wild animals accounted for 5,923 (92.3%) of these cases and domestic animals, 494 (7.7%). Only six of these domestic animal cases occurred in goats (Blanton et al. 2006). In forty-one countries of Europe, including the Russian Federation, Ukraine and Turkey, there were 9,831 rabies cases documented in 2005. Wildlife accounted for 5,806 (59.1%) and domestic animals 3,980 (40.5%) of these cases (WHO 2007a). Goats and sheep, reported together, accounted for only 123 of the domestic animal cases.

In the United States, the principal reservoirs of sylvatic rabies are raccoons (*Procyon lotor*) on the east coast, skunks (mainly *Mephitis mephitis*) in the Midwest and California, and foxes (mainly *Vulpes vulpes*) along the Texas-Mexico border. However, insectivorous bat reservoirs have major public health significance. From 1900 through 2005, forty-eight human rabies cases were confirmed in the United States, with ten infections originating outside the country. Of the remaining thirty-eight cases, thirty-five (92.1%) were infected with bat rabies variants (Blanton et al. 2006).

In Europe, the principal reservoir is the red fox (*Vulpes vulpes*). The raccoon dog (*Nyctereutes procyonoides*) has been growing in significance in recent years, especially in the Baltic states of northeastern Europe as the raccoon dog population migrates westward from Asia (Holmala and Kauhala 2006). Oral rabies vaccination campaigns targeting red foxes have been extremely effective, with many countries of western and central Europe declaring rabies free status in recent years. The continued expansion of the raccoon dog population in Europe therefore is a major concern.

In tropical portions of Mexico and in northeastern Brazil, cases of goat rabies have been associated with vampire bat bites (Batalla et al. 1982; Silva and Silva 1987; Shoji et al. 2006). In Nigeria, where rabies continues to be a serious problem in humans and dogs, and goat populations are high, only eight goat cases were documented nationwide over thirty-three years. All were presumed associated with dog bites except one attributed to a genet bite (Okoh 1981). In Bombay, India, 3% of 265 animal rabies cases diagnosed in 1981 and 1982 were goats maintained in urban settings and bitten by dogs (Jayarao et al. 1985).

Pathogenesis

All mammals are susceptible to rabies infection. Though rabies can be transmitted rarely by aerosol infection of mucous membranes, rabies virus is most likely introduced into the goat by the bite of a rabid animal whose saliva is infected with the virus. Replication of the virus occurs initially in muscle at the site of introduction and the infection may remain localized at the initial site for many days. The virus then enters local nerves and moves centripetally up nerve trunks to the CNS. Variations in incubation times and clinical presentation are largely a function of the distance the virus must migrate to the central nervous system and whether it first reaches the brain or spinal cord. When an animal is bitten on the face, the incubation time tends to be shorter and the clinical presentation is one of encephalitis. When an animal is bitten on the hind limb, there is a longer incubation period and the early clinical signs suggest an ascending myelitis. Wherever it first reaches the CNS, the virus continues to replicate and extend throughout the brain and spinal cord. At the same time, it begins to move centrifugally back down nerve trunks to nerve endings. In this manner, virus becomes present in saliva via nerve endings in the salivary gland. Hematogenous spread of rabies is extremely rare.

When canine-derived virus was injected into the masseter muscles of experimental goats, incubation periods for clinical rabies ranged from fourteen to twenty-four days (Umoh and Blenden 1982). Immunofluorescence studies indicated that virus was abundant in brain tissues, but little or no virus was evident in distal sections of cranial nerves. Whether this low concentration of virus in peripheral nerves was a function of the experimental design or an indication that goats may not shed virus extensively during clinical rabies is unclear. No documented cases of human rabies resulting from exposure to goats could be found in the literature during preparation of this text.

Clinical Findings

Clinical reports of rabies in goats are rare. A ten-year retrospective of rabies in South Africa identified eighteen cases of caprine rabies. The furious form appears more commonly than the dumb form in goats. Aggressive behavior was the most common sign, occurring in 83% of the cases. Excessive bleating was observed in 72% of cases, salivation in 29%, and paralysis in only 17%. In no cases were hydrophobia, straining, pica, or circling observed (Barnard 1979). The clinical course is usually between one and five days and always results in death.

In experimental caprine rabies, early signs observed in nineteen goats were variable and included hyperexcitability, apparent blindness, anxiety, aggressiveness with piloerection, pruritus with self-mutilation, salivation, frothing, depression, standing off in corners, shaking of the head, and fine tremors, especially in the thighs. Later signs included frothy salivation, which was common, incoordination, staggering, circling, torticollis, extensive muscle tremors, protrusion of the tongue, and inability to eat. Terminally, goats showed posterior paralysis, lateral recumbency, paddling, nystagmus, and pupillary dilatation. Many goats had food hanging from the mouth (Umoh 1977).

In a separate report of experimental caprine rabies involving two male goats three to four months of age infected with a fox-derived isolate in the masseter muscle, both goats initially showed an exacerbation of sexual behavior, priapism, and aggressiveness followed progressively by incoordination, recumbency, opisthotonos, and myoclonia. The two goats died three and five days after onset of signs (Gomes et al. 2005).

Clinical Pathology and Necropsy

Laboratory confirmation of rabies antemortem is difficult. Immunofluorescent staining of corneal scrapings or hair follicles in skin biopsies taken during clinical disease is confirmatory if positive, but false-negative results occur (Umoh and Blenden 1982).

Gross lesions are minimal at necropsy. There may be evidence of trauma caused by maniacal behavior. The meninges and brain may be congested and edematous. Histologically, neuronal degeneration with swelling and necrosis may be present throughout the brain with a striking absence of inflammatory response. The most significant finding is Negri bodies in the cytoplasm of neurons, particularly in the hippocampus and in Purkinje cells. This finding has been considered diagnostic for rabies in the past, but false-positive interpretations may occur.

Currently, immunofluorescence staining of brain sections is routinely carried out for rapid, accurate diagnosis of rabies, and the direct fluorescent antibody (DFA) test remains the gold standard in rabies diagnosis. Impression smears of hippocampus, medulla, cerebellum, or gasserian ganglion are the preferred samples. Smears from brain stem, thalamus, and pons may also be diagnostic. If brain samples are submitted they should be fresh or glycerol preserved, because formalin fixation impairs performance of the DFA test. Peroxidase conjugate may be used on sections of formalin-fixed tissue for immunohistochemical tests in lieu of the DFA test.

Not all countries have the laboratory capacity to run the DFA test because it requires expensive, specialized fluorescent microscopes, so alternative test methods may be used. For example, the use of an avidin-biotin dot ELISA has been reported for detection of rabies antigen from the brains of suspect animals, including goats, with results comparable to the DFA test (Jayakumar et al. 1995) Immunohistochemistry including immunoperoxidase staining is also used.

The most definitive, but cumbersome, diagnostic test is intracerebral inoculation of mice with brain, spinal cord, or salivary tissue of suspect cases. When positive, weanling mice develop rabies and virus can be identified by immunofluorescence in their brains. Cell culture in neuroblastoma cell lines with confirmation by fluorescent antibody testing is now available as an alternative to mouse inoculation (OIE 2007).

Diagnosis

Regardless of the species of animal affected, rabies is one of the most difficult diseases to diagnose clinically because of the diversity of potential presentations. Veterinarians working in rabies endemic countries should always consider rabies in the differential diagnosis when goats show any behavioral change or neurologic abnormality. Potentially, rabies can mimic all of the various neurologic diseases of goats. As has been so aptly stated, rabies is an unpredictable disease—the only characteristic feature is that it is uncharacteristic in its presentation (Rupprecht et al. 2002). Every reasonable attempt should be made to arrive at a definitive diagnosis other than rabies while the goat is alive. If the animal dies undiagnosed, it is incumbent upon the veterinarian to pursue a postmortem diagnosis of rabies.

Treatment and Control

There is no treatment for rabies. The zoonotic potential of rabies must always be considered when dealing with suspect cases. Such cases should be isolated and human contact kept to a minimum. Gloves and masks should be worn during examination or when performing necropsies and hands washed thoroughly afterward with disinfectant soaps. When the suspicion of rabies is high, euthanasia should be recommended to expedite a definitive diagnosis at necropsy. A careful history of human contact should be documented and all people potentially at risk should be apprised of the situation and referred to physicians for post-exposure counseling in the event that the suspect animal is confirmed as positive.

With regard to post-exposure prophylaxis for goats exposed to rabies, the information available suggests that it is unreliable and should not be attempted. Repeated vaccination alone or with administration of antisera prolonged the incubation period for as long as 174 days in experimentally infected goats, but in no case did it prevent development of clinical disease (Umoh and Blenden 1981).

Based on incubation times reported in experimental caprine rabies, goats with suspect exposure should be strictly isolated and observed for at least one month in anticipation of the possible development of clinical rabies. Given the limited amount of information available on rabies in goats, it is possible that the incubation period for goats might exceed one month. Therefore, any goat showing clinical signs consistent with rabies during (or after) the observation period should be euthanized and submitted for necropsy diagnosis.

Vaccination of goats in endemic areas may be possible according to local regulations. However, there is currently no vaccine specifically approved for use in goats in the United States, though several killed rabies vaccines derived from cell cultures are approved in the country for use in cattle and sheep. The lack of an approved vaccine for goats is a source of great frustration for American goat owners and the veterinarians who serve them (de la Concha-Bermejillo et al. 1998). In sheep and cattle, the vaccine is given initially at three months of age or older and then repeated annually or, in sheep, triennially depending on the product used.

According to data from the Food and Agriculture Organization, rabies vaccination in goats is permitted in approximately twenty countries worldwide including Brazil, India, Nepal, and the former Soviet Union (FAO 1989). The use of modified live rabies vaccines not approved for use in goats is strongly discouraged or prohibited.

Complete control of rabies depends on national and international efforts. Beyond vaccination there is little that individual herd or flock owners can do to control rabies except to know the likely reservoirs in their areas and minimize goat contact with them through housing, fencing, or animal control measures.

Pseudorabies

This acute fatal viral disease, also known as Aujesky's disease, infectious bulbar paralysis, or mad itch, is primarily a disease of swine and is reported only sporadically in goats. Clinical signs include peracute death or hyperexcitability, intense pruritus, convulsions, and terminal coma. Reported cases of caprine pseudorabies have invariably included direct or indirect contact with pigs.

Etiology

The causative agent is a double stranded DNA, enveloped, alphaherpesvirus. It is known by several names including pseudorabies virus (PRV), porcine herpesvirus type 1 (PHV-1), and most recently, suid herpesvirus type 1 (SuHV-1). The virus is quite stable. It can survive in saliva, carcasses, and clean, damp bedding for several months in winter, and several weeks in summer. Free, unprotected virus can persist for one to two weeks. However, the virus can be inactivated by a number of disinfectants including sodium hypochlorite, formalin, peracetic acid, phenolics, and quaternary ammonium compounds.

Epidemiology

The virus is extremely well adapted to domestic swine, which serve as the agent reservoir. Adult pigs usually show only mild disease when infected, though abortions or early embryonic death can occur in pregnant sows. Affected piglets may show signs of neurologic disease and high mortality. Typical of the herpesviruses, latent infections and a carrier state occur in infected, recovered swine that can shed the virus in saliva and nasal discharges. All other susceptible species, including goats, cattle, sheep, dogs, and cats are essentially dead-end hosts. They develop acute neurologic disease and die quickly.

In reported cases of caprine pseudorabies, the goats have been housed with or in fence contact with pigs (Herweijer and De Jonge 1977; Baker et al. 1982). The pigs may be latent carriers that shed virus but show no evidence of infection. Other potential sources of exposure include transport vehicles in which infected swine have recently been hauled as well as modified live virus vaccines. Pseudorabies has occurred in sheep that were given parenteral medication using an uncleaned syringe previously used to vaccinate pigs for pseudorabies.

Transmission of virus is by inhalation or via skin abrasions. Morbidity can be high, with 80% of exposed goats contracting the disease in an outbreak in the Netherlands (Herweijer and De Jonge 1977). The mortality rate is 100%.

Pathogenesis

The incubation period is one to four days. When the virus is introduced through the skin, it enters peripheral nerves and produces the characteristic localized pruritus that is observed in some cases of ruminant pseudorabies ("mad itch"). The virus then moves centripetally and enters the CNS, producing a rapidly fatal encephalitis or myeloencephalitis. With inhalation of the virus, signs of encephalitis occur without a prodrome of pruritus.

Clinical Findings

All ages, breeds, and sexes can be affected. Goats may be found dead with no warning. Alternatively, they may show signs of intense rubbing or licking and even self-mutilation associated with severe, localized neurogenic pruritus (Figure 5.1). In cases where pruritus does not occur, initial signs may include agitation or excitation, repeated lying down and rising, hysterical bleating, profuse sweating, and convulsions. Fevers as high as 106.7°F (41.5°C) may be recorded. These excitatory signs give way to recumbency, paralysis with bloat and dyspnea, coma, and finally death. The clinical course may be only several hours up to twenty-four hours.

Clinical Pathology and Necropsy

While serology is useful in the identification of infected swine, it has no application in caprine pseudorabies because goats become clinically ill and die before an antibody response can develop. At time of necropsy, attempts should be made to isolate the virus from brain tissue. There are no obvious gross necropsy findings, but there are histologic lesions of severe, focal, nonsuppurative encephalitis and myelitis. Eosinophilic intranuclear inclusion bodies typical of herpesviruses may be found in degenerating neurons. Immunofluorescence and immunoperoxidase methods can be used to confirm the identity of the SuHV-1 in infected brain tissue.

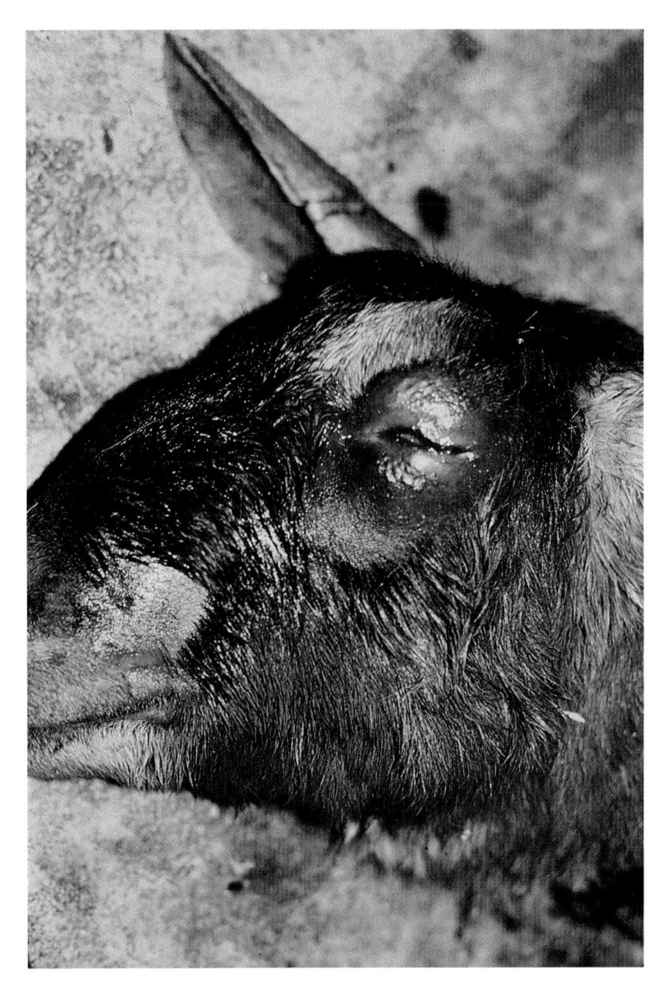

Figure 5.1. Periorbital alopecia and inflammation due to excessive rubbing of the face from pruritus due to pseudorabies infection in a goat having fence line contact with pigs. (From Baker et al. 1982. Reproduced by permission of the Journal of the America Veterinary Medical Association.)

Diagnosis

When pruritus is present, primary dermatologic conditions, particularly ectoparasites, must be ruled out. Scrapie, rabies, and cerebrospinal nemotodiasis can also produce neurogenic pruritus in goats. When encephalitic signs predominate, consider also rabies, heartwater, polioencephalomalacia, and hypomagnesemia. The acute nature of the disease also suggests poisonings, notably cyanide, nitrates, urea, organophosphates, and chlorinated hydrocarbons.

Treatment and Control

There is no treatment for pseudorabies. Control depends on recognizing the risks of commingling goats with pigs whose pseudorabies status is unknown. If pigs must be housed with goats, the pigs should be serologically negative for pseudorabies before purchase. National regulatory programs to eradicate pseudorabies in commercial swine greatly reduce the risk of goats contracting the disease. In the United States, a pseudorabies eradication program was initiated in 1989, and by 2004 all fifty states were declared free of pseudorabies in commercial swine.

Pseudorabies is not considered a public health risk. However, there have been some putative reported cases of pseudorabies from Europe in people exposed to cats. Antibodies to pseudorabies virus were documented in these individuals (Mravak et al. 1987). Therefore, veterinarians and others working directly with the virus or with pseudorabies infected animals or carcasses should observe appropriate safety precautions.

Scrapie

Scrapie is an infectious, contagious, degenerative neurologic disease that occurs naturally only in sheep and goats. It belongs to the group of diseases known as transmissible spongiform encephalopathies (TSEs) which are believed to be caused by abnormal proteins known as prions. Prions are unique as infectious agents in that they contain no genetic material. Other TSEs include bovine spongiform encephalopathy (BSE) of cattle; chronic wasting disease of deer and elk (CWD); transmissible mink encephalopathy of farmed mink (TME); and several diseases of humans including Kuru, Creutzfeldt-Jakob disease (CJD), and variant Creutzfeldt-Jakob disease (vCJD).

Scrapie is characterized by an extended incubation period of months to years. When clinical signs ultimately develop, they may include weight loss, incoordination, changes in mental status, progressive debilitation, and pruritus. Historically, clinical reports of scrapie in goats have been far less common than in sheep, but the disease has become a major concern for the goat industry because goats are now regularly included in regulatory surveillance and control programs for TSEs, including scrapie. Veterinarians, and the goat owners they serve, must be aware of the details of these control programs because they can affect management and commercial aspects of goat production.

Interest in and knowledge of scrapie have increased dramatically in the last twenty years as a result of the emergence of bovine spongiform encephalopathy (BSE), a TSE that is transmissible to humans. BSE has numerous clinicoepidemiological similarities to scrapie and this has sparked concerns that BSE could also occur in small ruminants and therefore needs to be differentiated from scrapie. As a result, better tools are now available for the diagnosis of scrapie, there is a clearer understanding of the pathogenesis, and because of active surveillance programs, there is also more epidemiological knowledge about scrapie in goats. Despite similarities to BSE, scrapie of sheep and goats is not considered to be transmissible to humans.

Etiology

The generally accepted cause of scrapie and other TSEs in animals is the expression of the abnormal form of a naturally occurring, cellular protein called PrP^c. This protein is found in cells throughout the body but is of clinical and diagnostic interest primarily in the nervous system and the lymphoreticular system. It is a membrane glycoprotein bound to the outer surface of neurons, lymphocytes, and other cells. The normal function of PrP^c is not completely known, but it may be involved in copper transport and homeostasis (Waggoner et al. 1999) and neuro-protection, signal transduction, or circadian rhythm regulation (Huber et al. 1999). The structure and pathobiology of prions and the diseases they cause in animals and humans have been reviewed (Prusiner 1998; Aguzzi and Heikenwalder 2006; Aguzzi 2006)

Through mechanisms not fully understood, the development of scrapie is associated with abnormal replication of normal host prion protein, PrP^c (also referred to in the literature as PrP^{sen}) to produce a prion protein of modified structure, PrP^{Sc} (also referred to in the literature as PrP^{res} or PrP^d), the accumulation of which occurs simultaneously with degeneration of nervous tissue and other manifestations of disease. This process is complex, with several factors involved: exposure of the animal to abnormal, exogenous forms of the PrP protein PrP^{Sc} which induce abnormal replication of PrP^c in the host; variations in the strain of PrP^{Sc} encountered; and variations in the genetic composition of the animals exposed to PrP^{Sc}. Together these factors can influence host susceptibility to the production of abnormal endogenous PrP^{Sc} following exposure, the incubation period for manifestation of disease, and the severity of disease. The details of these interactions are currently topics of active research.

PrP^c protein is comprised of 210 amino acids. Structurally, it contains a highly flexible N-terminal domain and a structured C-terminal domain consisting of three helices with α-helical folding and a short β-sheet. The molecule contains two N-glycosylation sites and the naturally occurring protein may be comprised of mono-, di-, or non-glycosylated forms. The fully glycosylated form has a molecular weight of 33 to 35 kDa. The ratio of the three forms in tissue extracts of PrP^{Sc} is referred to as the glycotype. Differences in patterns of glycosylation are one tool used to differentiate various strains of the scrapie prion.

In scrapie, as in most other TSEs, the key factor in the pathogenesis of the disease is the conversion of normal PrP^c protein into an isoform, PrP^{Sc}, which is characterized by insolubility and partial resistance to degradation by proteases. The isoform demonstrates important secondary structural change as compared to the normal PrP^c protein. This is manifested as aberrant folding of the protein molecule that results from one of the three normal α-helices being replaced by β-sheet or β-helix structure. The conversion from PrP^c to PrP^{Sc} has been described as a stabilization of a proto-β-helical motif by a neighboring PrP^{Sc} molecule and subsequent extension to form the complete β-helix (Wille et al. 2002).

The agent produces no detectable immune response in the host and the absence of scrapie-induced antibody is a major obstacle to detecting the disease in live animals. However, monoclonal antibodies against various components of the PrP^{Sc} molecule are now being routinely produced and these have proven to be most valuable in the laboratory, particularly with regard to identifying various prion strains and the development of rapid immunoassays for detecting the prion protein in tissue.

In recent years, it has become apparent that so-called atypical strains of scrapie exist which have different molecular characteristics and produce different histopathologic lesion patterns than the scrapie prion which produces classical scrapie. The first of these atypical strains was reported from Norway in association with five clinical cases of atypical sheep scrapie with unusual clinical and pathologic features, the first of which was seen in 1998. The strain has been designated as Nor98. Among its unusual features are the fact that it produced disease in sheep with genotypes ordinarily associated with resistance to scrapie; an atypical distribution of lesions in the brain, with a notable absence of lesions at the level of the obex; the absence of detectable PrP^{Sc} in lymphoid tissues using immunohistochemistry and ELISA; and a distinctive molecular PrP^{Sc} profile on western blot assay which indicates a glycotype that is distinct from classical scrapie strains and the prion strain producing BSE (Benestad et al. 2003). In 2007, the first sheep in the United States, originating from Wyoming, was confirmed with the Nor98 strain of scrapie through slaughter surveillance (USDA 2007).

There is also evidence for the existence of other atypical scrapie strains in European sheep in addition to the Nor98 strain (Buschmann et al. 2004; DEFRA 2005). Furthermore, by 2005, France had reported six atypical scrapie cases in goats to the European Commission, and a case of atypical scrapie in a Swiss goat was reported in 2007 that included a comprehensive description of the neuropathic and biochemical characteristics of the atypical prion (Seuberlich et al. 2007). The existence of such strains and their behavior may have significant implications for scrapie surveillance programs and the overall strategies for control of the disease as discussed further below.

Scrapie prions are very resistant to physical and chemical destruction and are believed to persist on pastures for months and possibly years when excreted by infected sheep or goats. Standard disinfectants do not destroy prions. Recommended disinfection procedures include deactivation with 2% sodium hydroxide solution, steam sterilization at 132°C for one hour, or incineration.

Epidemiology

Most nations where small ruminants are raised have never reported scrapie to the OIE, the world regulatory body for animal health. However, it is unclear whether these countries are actually free of the disease or if the disease exists undetected or unreported due to the lack of active surveillance programs and a lack of recognition by farmers of the clinical picture of scrapie. An informative overview on the epidemiology of scrapie with an extensive bibliography has been published by the OIE (Detwiler and Baylis, 2003).

Scrapie is enzootic in many countries of Europe, including the UK, as well as in Iceland, the United States and Canada. It also has been reported in Australia, New Zealand, India, South Africa, Kenya, Brazil, and Colombia as a result of sheep importations from the United Kingdom from the 1930s through the 1970s. Australia and New Zealand subsequently eliminated the disease in the 1950s and have remained free through surveillance and strict importation rules. South Africa's last reported case was in 1972.

Recent studies from Iceland suggest that iron and manganese content of soils and forages may influence the occurrence of scrapie in that country. Forages from scrapie-afflicted farms had significantly higher iron concentrations and Fe/Mn ratios than forages from scrapie-free farms. It was speculated that manganese may in some manner inhibit absorption of prions from the gut and that high iron levels suppress manganese in the diet and thereby facilitate absorption of prions (Gudmunsdóttir et al. 2006).

In recent years, as a result of increased surveillance associated with bovine spongiform encephalopathy in the European Union, information on the occurrence of caprine scrapie is improving (European Commission, 2006). Between 2002 and 2005 inclusive, for all twenty-five EU member countries, a total of 420,299 goats were tested for scrapie and 1,669 (0.4%) were positive. These goats included healthy animals at slaughter as well as animals dead on farm and suspect clinical cases. In comparison, 1,511,375 sheep were tested during this same period and 8,930 (0.6%) were positive. It is noteworthy that large scale data collection suggests that the prevalence of scrapie infection in the goat population is not that different from the sheep population. The conventional wisdom has long been that scrapie, at least clinical scrapie, occurs less frequently in goats than sheep. A different perspective may emerge as more active surveillance of sheep and goats expands and continues. It is also noteworthy that one goat from France, tested in 2002 through this active surveillance effort, was ultimately diagnosed with BSE instead of scrapie. A second BSE suspect goat was identified from the UK in 2005 with the final diagnosis pending at the time of this writing. All other goats and sheep in the EU program that tested positive for TSEs were positive for scrapie.

Increased surveillance in Europe has also increased the discovery of atypical scrapie cases in small ruminants. From the initiation of the surveillance program in 2002 through 2004, 325 atypical scrapie cases were detected and reported to the European Commission, 319 in sheep and six in goats. Countries reporting atypical cases included Spain, Portugal, the United Kingdom, Germany, France, the Netherlands, Sweden, Ireland, Finland, Belgium, and Norway (European Food Safety Authority 2005). All six affected goats were from France. There are concerns that even greater numbers of atypical cases may be occurring but are not being detected because most surveillance programs limit sampling and examination of neurologic tissue to the caudal brainstem and possibly cerebellum, while in some atypical scrapie cases these areas may be free of lesions which instead are in more rostral areas of the brain not being sampled. Furthermore, some of the approved screening tests for BSE which are in use in scrapie surveillance do not consistently detect the atypical strains so that unless a full complement of screening tests is performed, atypical scrapie cases may be missed (Seuberlich et al. 2007).

Reports of naturally occurring clinical scrapie in goats are uncommon. It is not clear if this is due to a comparatively low incidence or failure to recognize the disease in goats. Naturally occurring caprine scrapie was reported in France in 1942 (Chelle, 1942), the United States in 1969 (Hourrigan et al. 1969), Canada in 1975 (Stemshorn 1975), Switzerland in 1982 (Fankhauser et al. 1982), Cyprus in 1989 (Toumazos and Alley 1989), and the UK on several occasions through the 1960s and 1970s (MacKay and Smith 1961; Brotherston 1968; Harcourt and Anderson, 1974). More recently, clinical caprine scrapie has been reported from Italy in 1998 (Capucchio et al. 1998), Greece in 2002 (Billinis et al. 2002), and Finland in 2002 (Government of Finland, 2002). In the United States, from 1990 to 2007, there were nineteen cases of caprine scrapie confirmed by regulatory authorities. The distribution of these cases was five in California; three in Colorado; two each in Washington, South Dakota, and Ohio; and one each in Wyoming, Nebraska, Illinois, Michigan, and New Hampshire (USDA 2007a).

In the majority of caprine cases occurring worldwide, there is a history of contact between affected goats and infected sheep, though direct contact with sheep does not appear to be an absolute prerequisite for caprine infection. In the Canadian report, five years had elapsed between the last case of ovine scrapie on a property and the first case in goats, although sheep remained on the farm (Stemshorn, 1975). In one report from the UK, there was no discernible contact of four affected Saanen goats with scrapie-infected sheep (Harcourt and Anderson, 1974). Wood et al. (1992) reported on twenty caprine scrapie cases seen at the U.K. Central Veterinary Laboratory since 1975. In at least seven of those cases, it was established that there had been no direct or indirect contact with sheep.

Iatrogenic transmission is also possible. Outbreaks of scrapie involving goats in Italy between 1997 and 1999 were linked to vaccination of goat and sheep herds with a *Mycoplasma agalactia* vaccine for contagious agalactia. The vaccine had been prepared from ovine CNS, lymph node, and mammary tissues which apparently contained the scrapie prion (Agrimi et al. 1999; Caramelli et al. 2001).

It is generally accepted that the principal method of natural transmission from sheep to goats is horizontal via direct contact with infected placentas or by indirect contact with pastures or bedding contaminated by such placentas (Pattison et al. 1972). The presence of the infective agent PrP^{Sc} has been confirmed in placentas of infected sheep (Tuo et al. 2001). Experimental attempts to transmit scrapie to progeny indicate that vertical transmission is unlikely to occur by sexual contact or transplacental infection (Pattison 1964). Goat-to-goat transmission, if it occurs, is also most likely by the horizontal route (Hadlow et al. 1980).

The role of semen and embryo transfer in the spread of scrapie requires further investigation, particularly because of significant implications for international trade. To date, various research studies have given mixed indications regarding the importance of embryos in transmission. Semen appears unlikely to be involved in transmission but more studies are warranted. The role of various body fluids in horizontal transmission of the disease also requires further investigation because current information appears paradoxical. The infective agent has not been identified in feces, saliva, colostrum, or milk, yet it has been found in gut tissue, salivary glands, and blood. This suggests that the infective agent may be in the various secretions derived from those sources, but the tools currently available for detection are not sensitive enough to detect it (Detwiler and Baylis, 2003).

Pathogenesis

Experimentally, the disease has been produced in goats by subcutaneous and intracerebral inoculation of the agent and by feeding of fetal membranes from infected sheep (Pattison 1957; Pattison et al. 1972;

Hadlow et al. 1974). In naturally occurring scrapie, it is most likely that oral ingestion of the infective prion initiates new infections. Following ingestion, the portal of entry for the scrapie agent may be the Peyer's patches of the ileum (Heggebø et al. 2000) from which it is transported via blood or lymphatics to other sites in the lymphoreticular system (LRS), including tonsil, spleen, and retrophyaryngeal and mesenteric lymph nodes. Presence in the gut associated lymphoid tissues likely facilitates access of the infective agent to the enteric autonomic nerves which may in turn provide access to the CNS, though the precise mechanisms for neuroinvasion in the CNS remains an area of active research. Replication in the LRS continues for weeks to months before infectivity can be detected in the brain and it may be years before there is clinical manifestation of disease.

In experimentally infected goats, inoculated intracerebrally or subcutaneously, the infective agent is disseminated to a variety of tissues in different levels of concentration, based on subsequent mouse inoculation assays conducted with titrations of various tissues (Hadlow et al. 1974). Brain and spinal cord had the highest levels of infectivity. Moderate levels were found in retropharyngeal, superficial cervical and subiliac lymph nodes, spleen, tonsil, and adrenal gland. Low levels were found in cerebrospinal fluid, sciatic nerve, pituitary gland, nasal mucosa, ileum, proximal colon, distal colon, liver, thymus, mediastinal and bronchial lymph nodes, and parotid salivary gland. No infectivity was found in blood clot, submaxillary salivary gland, thyroid, heart, lung, kidney, skeletal muscle, bone marrow, pancreas, ovary, and saliva.

Once the infective agent has reached the brain, it induces the normal cellular form of PrP to undergo a conformational change, resulting in increased β-sheet folding and subsequent appearance of PrP^{Sc}, often as scrapie-associated fibrils in the nervous tissue. The exact mechanisms of this process at the molecular level are currently an area of active research. The net result of this protein misfolding and fibril accumulation is a progressive degeneration of nervous tissue characterized by a sponge-like pattern of vacuolation, which leads to the general description of scrapie and other TSEs as spongiform encephalopathies. The brain lesions of scrapie are described further below in the section on necropsy findings.

Susceptibility to disease and the incubation period are now known to be genetically controlled in sheep and goats, though less is currently known about the latter species. The genetics of scrapie in sheep and goats has recently been reviewed (Baylis and Goldmann, 2004). The mammalian PrP gene, depending on species, is composed of two or three exons with the entire open reading frame (ORF) contained in the last exon. The gene that codes for PrP protein in goats and sheep has an ORF of 256 codons in length, with post-translational processing resulting in a mature PrP^{c} protein of 210 amino acids. Polymorphisms occur in the protein coding region of the PrP gene that are known to be associated with susceptibility to scrapie and the incubation period of the disease in sheep. Such relationships are also likely in goats, but currently are less well defined.

At present, three specific ovine PrP polymorphisms are definitively known to affect the development of the disease in exposed sheep. These occur at codons 136, 154, and 171 and are expressed as A136V, R154H, and Q171R/H, respectively. The amino acid valine (V) instead of alanine (A) is encoded at 136, histidine (H) instead of arginine (R) at codon 154, and arginine (R) or histidine (H) instead of glutamine (Q) are incoded at position 171. There are numerous additional polymorphisms in sheep that have been identified in recent years in the PrP gene but their effects on the elaboration of scrapie are not yet fully established.

Unfortunately, knowledge about the genetics of goats relative to scrapie lags behind that of sheep. This is due in part to the fact that naturally occurring scrapie in goats is less common in sheep and infected herds have been less available for relevant genetic studies. Nevertheless, a number of polymorphisms have been identified in scrapie-infected goats from herds representing different breeds, though no definitive picture has yet emerged as to the significance of these various polymorphisms relative to the susceptibility to scrapie in goats or whether their importance extends beyond the specific breeds studied.

Polymorphisms in the caprine PrP gene that were identified in the review of Baylis and Goldmann (2004) included W102G, T110P, G127S, I142M, H143R, R154H, P168Q, R211Q, Q220H, and Q222K. Association with disease was noted for three of these polymorphisms, namely I142M, H143R, and R154H, and according to Baylis and Goldmann (2004), may also be expected for P168Q and Q222K. Polymorphism I142M in particular is associated with scrapie incubation period in response to various prion strains (Goldmann et al. 1996). Additional polymorphisms have been noted for the gene expressing caprine PrP and previously recognized polymorphisms have been reconfirmed in different breeds. Billinis et al. (2002) reported additional polymorphisms for V21A, L23P, and G49S in goats in Greece. For the Ionica breed of goats in Italy, Vaccari et al. (2006) reported polymorphisms for G37V, T110P, H143R, R154H, Q222K, and P240S, with the suggestion that the polymorphism at codon 154 is associated with resistance to classical scrapie and susceptibility to atypical scrapie, while the presence of lysine (K) at codon 222 is associated with resistance to classical scrapie.

Two additional polymorphisms not previously reported in goats were identified in Italian goats by Acutis et al. (2006), namely L133Q and M137I. In addition, they also noted a protective role against scrapie in goats for the glutamine to lysine mutation at codon 222 (Q222K). Zhang et al. (2004) evaluated five Chinese breeds of goats for PrP polymorphisms. All breeds possessed the R154H polymorphism and they also identified a previously unreported polymorphism in two of the breeds, I218L. The known polymorphisms of the PrP gene in goats and their possible roles in modulating scrapie infection are summarized in Table 5.4.

Even in sheep, where the role of genetics is better established, there are still many unanswered questions on the pathogenesis of the disease as it relates to genotype. Notably, in 2005, it was reported that sheep homozygous for A136/R154/R117, the known scrapie-resistant PrP genotype, were infected with the strain Nor98 prion protein and that their infection was transmissible to transgenic mice (Le Dur et al. 2005). Additional evidence that atypical strains can produce scrapie in sheep with genotypes known to confer resistance to classical scrapie has since been reported (Arsac et al. 2007). This raises concerns about the ultimate effectiveness of scrapie eradication programs based on genetic selection and also about the role of different agent strains on the pathogenesis of scrapie. It is known that phenotypically distinct strains of prions occur and that they can be distinguished by specific characteristics such as the distribution of spongiform changes they induce in the brain, the molecular profile of protease resistant PrP^{Sc}, and the fraction of PrP^{Sc} that is detected after treatment with proteinase K.

Clinical Signs

Naturally occurring clinical scrapie has been seen only in adult goats from two to eight years old. The clinical presentation may vary. Typically, the clinical course is slowly progressive over one to six months. The onset of signs is insidious, often beginning with a loss of inquisitiveness and the development of an irritable disposition which often first manifests as a resistance in lactating does to being milked. Early on, affected goats often show a characteristic posture of carrying the rear limbs forward so that the rump is elevated and the withers are held low. In addition the tail is held up, cocked forward over the rump, and the ears are frequently pricked forward suggesting heightened alertness (Pattison et al. 1959). Restlessness increases and goats become hypersensitive to handling. Affected goats may attempt to flee, bleat uncon-

Table 5.4. Currently known polymorphisms of the caprine PrP gene and their possible effects on modulation of scrapie infection in the goat.

Caprine PrP gene polymorphism	*Possible role in caprine scrapie*	*References*
V 21 A	?	Billinis et al. 2002
L 23 P	?	Billinis et al. 2002
G 37 V	?	Agrimi et al. 2003
G 49 S	?	Billinis et al. 2002
W 102 G	?	Goldmann et al. 1998
T 110 P	?	Agrimi et al. 2003
G 127 S	?	Goldman et al. 2004
L 133 Q	?	Acutis et al. 2006
M 137 I	?	Acutis et al. 2006
I 142 M	Incubation period	Goldmann et al. 1996
H 143 R	Susceptibility	Goldmann et al. 1996; Bilinis et al. 2002
R 154 H	Susceptibility	Billinis et al. 2002; Zhang et al. 2004
P 168 Q	?	Billinis et al. 2002
R 211 Q	?	Goldman et al. 2004
I 218 L	?	Zhang et al. 2004
Q 220 H	?	Billinis et al. 2002
Q 222 K	Resistance	Agrimi et al. 2003; Acutis et al. 2006
P 240 S	?	Goldmann et al. 1996

? = role unknown, A = alanine, G = glycine, H = histidine, I = isoleucine, K = lysine, L = leucine, M = methionine; P = proline, Q = glutamine, R = arginine, S = serine, T = threonine, V = valine, W = tryptophan. In these polymorphisms for specific codons, the expected amino acid to be produced is identified to the left of the codon number and the actual amino acid produced as a result of the polymorphism is identified to the right of the number.

trollably, or stiffen with muscular rigidity when handled. Left alone, they may hold the head down and stomp as if bothered by imaginary flies. Fine tremors may be observed.

Pruritus is a prominent and often dramatic sign in sheep. The name of the disease derives from the act of sheep scraping themselves raw on inanimate objects in response to the intense itching they experience. Pruritus is also a predominant sign of scrapie in goats but is often less severe than observed in sheep. Some goats may show localized pruritus, particularly over the withers or tail head. Horned goats may lean their heads back and scratch this area persistently with the horn tips or scratch, dog-like, with their hind limb if the itchy spot is reachable.

Over time, hyperesthesia may give way to drowsiness or seeming drunkenness. Incoordination becomes more pronounced with increased stumbling and falling and increased difficulty in rising. Other signs may include teeth grinding, salivation or slobbering, regurgitation of rumen contents, and impaired vision. Weight loss may become marked and anorexia develops in the terminal stages (Figure 5.2). Affected animals eventually become prostrate and die if not destroyed first. Fever does not occur in the course of the disease.

Clinicians and goat owners should recognize that the clinical presentation in individual goats may vary considerably. One documented case of scrapie in a goat showed no signs other than listlessness, progressive weight loss, and premature cessation of milk production (Harcourt and Anderson, 1974). In another confirmed case, the only apparent clinical sign was regurgitation of rumen contents (Wood et al. 1992).

Clinical Pathology and Necropsy

There are no consistent hematological, biochemical, or gross pathological changes in animals with clinical or preclinical scrapie that are diagnostic of the disease. However, genotyping has become an important tool in identifying sheep that are susceptible or resistant to scrapie. To date, this testing is not applicable to goats because genetic polymorphisms that impart resistance or susceptibility have not been worked out to the extent that allow for genotyping of goats to be used as an effective disease management tool.

Scrapie has been known as a disease of small ruminants for more than 250 years, yet it is only in the last decade or so that new laboratory tests have started to become available for confirmation of the disease. One major obstacle has been a lack of understanding about the nature of the causative agent and the inability to culture it *in vitro* or identify it *in vivo*. A second important obstacle is that prion infection produces no detectable host humoral immune response so that no serologic tests for detection of antibodies have been possible. While serologic tests remain unavailable, scientists now are able to produce monoclonal antibodies to specific components of the PrP^{Sc} protein, and this has become a tremendously useful tool for better characterizing the scrapie agent and for identifying PrP^{Sc} in tissues through the use of immunobiological tests such as immunohistochemistry and electrophoresis followed by immunoblotting.

Before the application of these techniques, diagnosis of scrapie was limited to histologic examination of affected brain tissue to identify characteristic lesions

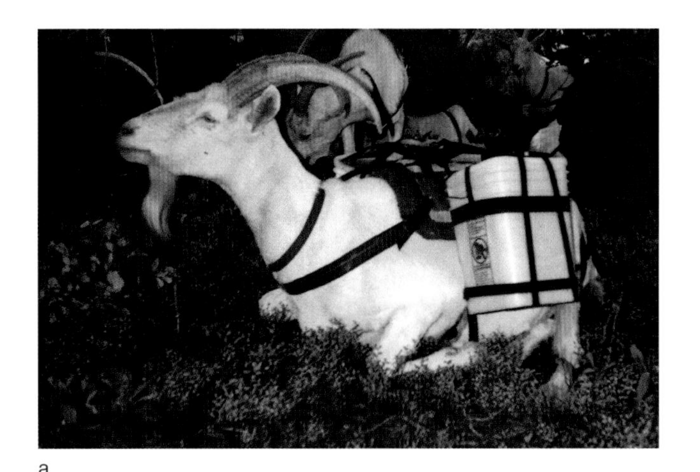

a

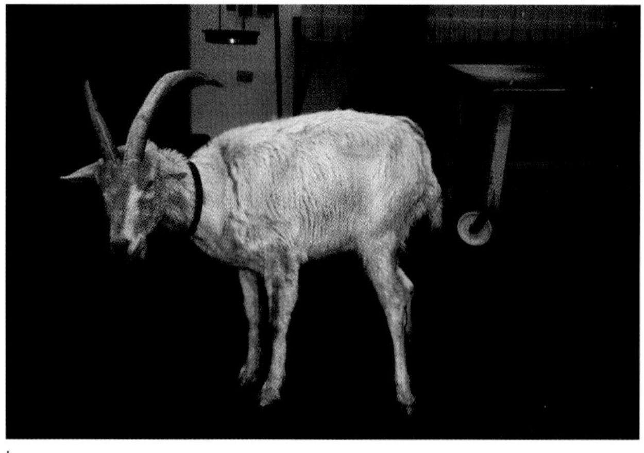

b

Figure 5.2. Clinical progression of a laboratory-confirmed case of scrapie in a Saanen wether goat. Figure 5.2a shows the goat robust and healthy prior to the onset of clinical signs, and actively working as a pack goat. Figure 5.2b shows the same goat in an advanced state of debilitation and emaciation five months later at seventy-one months of age. In addition to the apparent weight loss, the goat developed fearful behavior, difficulty swallowing, and pruritus, with hair loss over the face and forequarters. The goat herd from which this animal came had no history of association or contact with sheep. (Courtesy of Dr. David M. Sherman).

and confirmation of infectivity by inoculation of mice with tissues taken from suspect cases, a cumbersome procedure that can take one to two years to yield results. Fresh brain homogenates also could be examined by transmission electron microscopy to detect scrapie-associated fibrils (SAFs) (Cooley et al. 1999). The diagnostic procedures currently available for scrapie and their appropriate use have been reviewed (OIE 2004; Gavier-Widen 2005).

Immunohistochemistry (IHC) can be used to detect the presence of PrP^{Sc} in formalin fixed tissues. IHC techniques can be applied to biopsy materials taken from live animals or from sections of tissue obtained at necropsy. IHC has been used in live animals to detect PrP^{Sc} from tonsil, lymphoid tissue in the third eyelid (nictitating membrane), and rectal mucosa.

Immunoblotting by the western blot technique is performed on fresh tissues. It is used in regulatory surveillance and monitoring programs to screen for TSEs, including scrapie. Reference laboratories use Western blot to distinguish different strains of scrapie prion and to differentiate PrP^{Sc} from that of the prion causing bovine spongiform encephalopathy (BSE). These differentiations are based on conformational differences that may be revealed by immunoblotting using peptide-specific antibodies to the flexible tail of the disease-specific PrP^{Sc}.

In addition to the western blot assay, there are now several commercially available immunoassays using ELISA and other techniques that can be used as rapid screening tests in TSE surveillance programs (Moynagh et al. 1999). They were initially approved for use in screening cattle for BSE in 1999, but in 2002, the EU expanded their use to include screening of goats and sheep for scrapie. Since that time, additional rapid tests are being developed and evaluated (Deslys and Grassi 2005). Tests currently in use in the EU are an indirect ELISA, a colorimetric sandwich ELISA, a chemiluminescent sandwich ELISA, and a western blot assay.

The approved immunoassays are being applied primarily for confirmatory post mortem diagnosis of scrapie using CNS tissues or lymphoreticular tissues. The OIE (2004) recommends that tests to confirm the presence of PrP^{Sc} in tissue be performed in addition to histological examination of brain sections in suspect cases to minimize the risk of false negative results. Vacuolation of neurons is the most consistent histopathological finding in animals with scrapie. However, individual scrapie cases and at least one experimental sheep scrapie inoculum are recorded in which neuronal vacuolation is virtually undetectable by light microscopy, indicating that a clinical diagnosis of suspected scrapie cannot be absolutely refuted by a failure to find significant vacuolar changes in the brain.

The presence of the scrapie agent in lymphoreticular tissue has offered the opportunity for the diagnosis of scrapie in live animals because some lymphoreticular tissues, such as found in tonsil and third eyelid (nictitating membrane), can be readily obtained from the live animal by non-invasive means. O'Rourke et al. (2000) described the technique for antemortem biopsy of nictitating membrane by using topical anesthetic and a restraint apparatus. This technique is now in use by USDA APHIS for antemortem diagnosis in the U.S. scrapie control program. Schreuder et al. (1998) have described the procedure for tonsillar biopsy in anesthetized sheep for collection of palatine tonsil for preclinical diagnosis of scrapie.

Through use of tonsillar biopsy, preclinically affected animals were identified one and a half years before clinical signs normally appear in sheep of known genotypes with predictable incubation periods. While this represents a significant breakthrough in the antemortem diagnosis of scrapie, techniques that depend on identification of the scrapie agent in lymphoreticular tissue must be used with caution. This is because there is a significant potential for false negative results, as the presence of PrP^{Sc} in such tissues of infected animals depends on the age of the animal, its genotype, the strain of the scrapie agent involved, and possibly other factors yet unknown. In the study of Schreuder et al. (1998), for example, there was a difference in the presence of PrP^{Sc} in animals between three and a half months of age and four months of age. Similarly, Monleón et al. (2005) compared the presence of PrP^{Sc} in CNS tissue and lymphoreticular tissue at post mortem in sheep of a specific genotype in a known infected herd and reported that in some preclinical cases, the agent was present in tonsil and lymph node but not in brain while in some advanced and terminal clinical cases, the reverse was true with the agent present in brain but not in tonsil or lymph node.

Additional, new, non-invasive tests are now being evaluated that may further improve the prospects for antemortem diagnosis. These include detection of prion protein in the buffy coat fraction of blood taken from preclinical, scrapie-infected sheep using immunocapillary electrophoresis (Yang et al. 2005; Jackman et al. 2006), identification of PrP^{Sc} by western blot in rectal biopsies taken from live sheep without the use of anesthesia (Espenes et al. 2006; Gonzalez et al. 2006), and identification of PrP^{Sc} in placentas of infected sheep (Race et al. 1998). It may be necessary to evaluate these tests specifically in goats to assess their value in the ante-mortem diagnosis of caprine scrapie.

Histologic examination of the CNS still remains a critical element in the definitive diagnosis of scrapie. At necropsy, gross findings, if present at all, are limited to evidence of cachexia, and dermabrasion if pruritus is a component of the clinical picture. Sections from the entire brain and spinal cord should be examined histologically. The principal lesion is a progressive degeneration of the gray matter. The most consistently affected part of the brain is the tegmentum and its connections (Zlotnik 1961). Lesions are most constant in the thalamus, midbrain, cerebellar cortex, and medulla oblongata and are uncommon in the cerebral cortex and spinal cord (Hadlow 1961). They are characterized by neuronal degeneration and shrinkage with vacuolation as well as astrocyte hypertrophy.

Vacuolation of neurons is considered the most significant finding. Vacuolated neurons are observed on histologic section of the medulla only rarely in clinically healthy goats, while vacuoles are seen in large numbers in the medulla of goats with advanced scrapie (Pattison et al. 1959). There is a notable absence of inflammatory response. The spongiform appearance of the brain classically described in sheep is less commonly observed in goats (Hadlow et al. 1980). Other tissues are not affected histologically.

In a more recent study of goat natural scrapie cases, vacuolation was detected in some instances as far forward as the neocortex and striatum (Wood et al. 1992). Widespread spongiform changes in the midbrain, thalamus, and basal ganglia, but not cortical regions, were found in goats infected by intracerebral challenge with BSE (Foster et al. 1993).

With regard to sampling, a 3 to 10 gm sample of cervical spinal cord and/or medulla caudal to the obex is best for possible detection of PrP^{Sc} by western blotting or for detection of scrapie-associated fibrils (SAFs) by transmission electron microscopy. That sample should be unfixed and frozen. The rest of the brain should be fixed in neutral buffered 10% formol saline for histological examination. If necessary, the immunoassays as well as electron microscopic examination for scrapie associated fibrils can be conducted on autolyzed brain tissue.

The OIE (2004) cautions that the absence of lesions is clearly not evidence of the absence of scrapie infection, because infection can exist in the absence of either clinical signs or pathological changes. For this reason, immunohistochemistry on tissue sections and/or immunoblotting/ELISA methods on fresh tissues to demonstrate accumulation of PrP^{Sc} should be carried out in parallel with routine histology in suspected cases. This is also recommended where lesions are mild in severity and considered equivocal. Where a rapid differential diagnosis is required by histopathological examination, and tissues have been fixed for less than one week, PrP^{Sc} detection should also be used to resolve possible uninterpretable observations.

Diagnosis

Clinical diagnosis of scrapie is presumptive on the basis of slowly progressive neurologic disease in an adult goat and is confirmed by identification of characteristic lesions histologically in the CNS and the presence of PrP^{Sc} by immunohistochemistry or immunoblotting in nervous or lymphoreticular tissue. In some cases, mouse inoculation studies may be carried out using tissue from suspect cases to confirm the diagnosis.

If chronic pruritus is a component of the clinical picture in goats, differential diagnoses should include lice, mange, paraelaphostrongylosis, elaphostrongylosis, and primary or hepatic photosensitization. If the onset of pruritus is rapid and the course of disease short, then pseudorabies and rabies should be considered. When tremors and progressive incoordination are the predominant signs, CAE, pregnancy toxemia, enzootic ataxia, parelaphostrongylosis, elaphostrongylosis, gid, spinal cord abscesses, Borna disease, and the dumb form of rabies should be ruled out. However, none of these conditions are likely to be as slowly progressive as scrapie. Unexplained weight loss with no other localizing signs can be consistent with scrapie in goats. The differential diagnosis of unexplained weight loss is discussed in Chapter 15.

Treatment

There is no treatment for scrapie. Even if therapeutic options were available, there would likely be little or no opportunity to use them because scrapie is becoming a reportable and highly regulated disease worldwide. Suspect cases are increasingly likely to be euthanized for diagnostic purposes by the appropriate authorities. Nonetheless, concerns about TSEs in human beings have prompted research into possible therapeutic regimens that in principle could be applicable to animals with scrapie. Obstacles and opportunities for treatment of TSEs have been reviewed (Liberski 2004; Weissmann and Aguzzi 2005).

Control

Control of scrapie at the herd level involves improved awareness of the disease among producers, implementation of appropriate management practices to minimize risk of infection, and in the case of sheep, genotyping of animals to develop a herd that is genetically resistant to infection with the scrapie agent. Unfortunately, the latter option is not yet available to goat farmers because specific genotypes that confer resistance to scrapie in goats have not yet been definitively identified or established.

Goat owners need to be educated about the insidious nature of scrapie and be able to recognize the potentially varied clinical signs of disease. In terms of improved management, the risk of scrapie can be reduced in herds by minimizing outside purchases of stock and reducing opportunities for horizontal transmission. Sheep and goats should not be commingled when the infection status of sheep is unknown. During kidding season, placentas and other fetal membranes should be found and removed immediately. Bedding should be changed in kidding pens between kiddings and the soiled bedding burned or buried. Any animals showing tremors, incoordination, or pruritus should be isolated from the herd and a definitive diagnosis attempted. There are currently no vaccines available for controlling scrapie.

At the national level, strong regulatory programs need to be established and enforced. Once scrapie becomes endemic in a country, it is difficult to eliminate. However, as the experience of Australia and New Zealand in the 1950s demonstrated, if scrapie is recognized early on and aggressive stamping out measures are instituted, the disease can be eliminated and strict border controls and importation requirements can keep it out. The scrapie status of many sheep- and goat-producing countries in the world remains unknown at present due to the absence of active surveillance programs. From 2001 to 2003, the United States Department of Agriculture (USDA) conducted the Scrapie Ovine Slaughter Surveillance Study (SOSS) on healthy, mature market sheep to determine the national prevalence of the disease, which was determined to be 0.2% (USDA 2004). Goats were not included in that national study. However, a goat prevalence study was initiated by USDA in May 2007 and by September 30, 2007 1,515 goats were tested for scrapie. All were negative (USDA 2007a).

In the United States, several approaches to sanitary control have been implemented since 1952. They have been modified in response to changing views on, and understanding of, the factors involved in scrapie transmission. Historically, these approaches have included depopulation of infected flocks, source flocks, and exposed flocks; slaughter of infected animals and all their blood relations regardless of flock of origin; slaughter of female blood relations and lateral contact sheep; and until recently slaughter of female blood relations only. None of these approaches was completely successful.

In October 1992, as a result of a negotiated rulemaking process between government, industry, and producer groups in the United States, a new Voluntary Scrapie Flock Certification Program was enacted as part of the National Scrapie Eradication Program. This voluntary program allowed flocks to be certified as scrapie-free after a five-year period. Voluntary participation involves careful animal identification and record keeping, constraints on animal movement and purchase, and regular monitoring of flocks by APHIS veterinarians. The program applies to goats and sheep.

In 2001, APHIS announced the accelerated National Scrapie Eradication Program (NSEP) with the stated goal of eliminating scrapie in the nation's sheep and goat flocks by 2010 and having official OIE recognition of the United States as being scrapie free by 2017. The key elements of the accelerated NSEP, which encompasses the Voluntary Scrapie Flock Certification Program, include identifying pre-clinical infected sheep through live-animal testing and active slaughter surveillance; making it possible to effectively trace infected animals to their flock/herd of origin through new identification requirements; and providing effective cleanup strategies that allow producers to stay in business, preserve breeding stock, and remain economically viable.

To facilitate effective clean-up strategies, USDA/APHIS provides indemnity for high-risk, suspect, and scrapie-positive sheep and goats, which owners agree to destroy; scrapie live-animal testing; genetic testing; and testing of exposed animals that have been sold out of infected and source flocks/herds. While the program applies to both sheep and goat flocks, genetic testing currently is not applied to goats because the genetics of goat susceptibility and resistance to scrapie are not as well understood as in sheep. More detailed information about the national scrapie eradication program, targeted to veterinarians and producers, is available online at http://www.aphis.usda.gov/vs/nahps/scrapie/eradicate.html.

Scrapie has been a notifiable disease within the European Union since January 1993. Active surveillance programs for scrapie in sheep and goats were legislated in the EU in 1998, and in 2001, regulation (EC) No. 999/2001 of the European Parliament established rules for the prevention, control, and eradication of certain transmissible spongiform encephalopathies in the European community, including scrapie. Genotyping of confirmed positive sheep was mandated in this legislation and rules governing the import and export of sheep and goats and their products were spelled out.

Until 2003, it was left to member states to determine what to do with herds and flocks from which scrapie had been confirmed. However, Commission Regulation (EC) No. 260/2003 set community-wide rules for the compulsory disposition of known positive flocks and herds. All animals in goat flocks must be destroyed. In sheep flocks, there is an option to genetically test and cull susceptible genotypes only. In 2004, the UK adopted a Compulsory Scrapie Flocks Scheme in place of their voluntary scheme to harmonize with the new European approach. EU regulations concerning control of TSEs change regularly to accommodate new knowledge and tools. All TSE legislation of the EU is available at http://ec.europa.eu/food/food/biosafety/bse/chronological_list_en.pdf.

Scrapie control remains a subject of active research and much policy debate. The occurrence of atypical scrapie cases in sheep with genotypes considered resistant for classical scrapie, such as ARR/ARR, casts doubt on the ultimate success of scrapie eradication programs that depend on genetic selection of sheep as the basis of control. Their effectiveness remains to be determined.

Bovine Spongiform Encephalopathy

BSE, like scrapie in goats and sheep, is one of the prion-associated diseases classified as a transmissible spongiform encephalopathy (TSE). BSE was first recognized as a disease of cattle in the United Kingdom in 1986. Then, in 1996, it was reported that a new, fatal, human TSE, called variant Creutzfeldt-Jakob disease (vCJD), was thought to be associated with the consumption of contaminated animal products derived from BSE-infected cattle. Thus, BSE became a zoonotic disease, a major public health concern, a catastrophe for cattle farmers, and the focus of enormous international media attention.

There are two reasons for including a discussion of BSE in this textbook of caprine medicine. First, because BSE can be produced in goats by experimental inoculation, and second, because in 2005, a naturally occurring case of BSE was confirmed in France in a goat tested at slaughter in 2002 through the TSE surveillance program of the European Commission.

The identification of this BSE-positive goat has significant implications for the goat industry worldwide. It raises questions, not yet fully answerable, about whether or not a potentially fatal zoonotic disease could be transmitted to humans through the consumption of goat-derived products. This will no doubt result in increased research related to the occurrence of BSE in goats and its potential for transmission to humans. It also will likely lead to more stringent regulatory controls on trade in live goats and goat products. Therefore, veterinarians and the goat producers they serve need to be aware of BSE as a possible disease in goats.

A comprehensive presentation of what remains primarily a bovine disease is beyond the scope of this book. The discussion here is limited to what is relevant and known about the disease in goats and its implications for the goat industry. A more detailed review of BSE in cattle can be found elsewhere (Prince 2003).

Etiology and Pathogenesis

The etiologic agent of the TSEs has yet to be fully characterized. The predominant theory for the causative agent is believed to be the result of an abnormal folding of a naturally occurring, cell membrane-associated, prion protein called PrP^{C}, which is a ubiquitous protein found in cells throughout the host animal. The abnormal conformation of this cellular protein is triggered by the introduction into the host animal of an infectious form of the PrP protein, known as PrP^{Sc}, but also referred to in the literature as PrP^{res} or PrP^{d}. It is proposed that during the infectious process this abnormal isoform of the prion protein binds to and changes the normal PrP^{C} three-dimensional conformation, with at least a portion of the PrP^{C}-associated α-helical structure assuming the form of β-sheets which is characteristic of PrP^{Sc}. In many cases the accumulation of this abnormal PrP^{Sc} in the grey matter of the brain leads to a histologically apparent degeneration characterized by sponge-like vacuolation of affected brain tissue that gives the disease its descriptive name. Alternate theories on the pathogenesis of TSEs also persist; for example, that the wall-less bacterium *Spiroplasma* may be a transmissible agent of TSEs (Bastian 2005).

It is now well documented in sheep that the genotype of the host animal plays some role in the animal's susceptibility or apparent resistance to scrapie infection. Results of experimental infection of sheep with BSE indicate that these genetic factors may also influence the ovine response to BSE, though a recent study demonstrated that sheep with the most scrapie resistant genotype ARR/ARR could be orally infected with BSE and have significant amounts of PrP^{Sc} in their spleens (Andréoletti et al. 2006). As discussed in the scrapie section of this chapter, genotype of goats may also play a role in modulating the response to scrapie infection but the details of this relationship are less well documented at this time and there is little or no evidence concerning the role of genotype in experimental caprine BSE infection. Genetic factors play little if any role in the susceptibility or resistance of cattle to BSE infectivity.

Epidemiology

BSE was first recognized in cattle in the United Kingdom in 1986. It manifested as a neurological disease with characteristic behavioral changes that led to the popular name of "mad cow" disease. While the cause of the disease was unknown, epidemiological studies strongly suggested that the disease was being spread through the feeding of concentrate feed that contained animal protein by-products derived from ruminants. It was hypothesized that removing ruminant protein from cattle feed supplements would lead to a reduction of disease occurrence and in fact, this turned out to be correct (Wilesmith et al. 1992; Anderson et al. 1996). A ban on feeding ruminant-derived meat and bone meal (MBM) to cattle in the UK was instituted in 1988. Following that ban, the UK epizootic peaked in 1992 with 37,280 confirmed cases and has declined steadily since, with only 225 cases confirmed in 2005 and 114 in 2006 (OIE 2007a).

No other food-producing animals manifested signs of BSE during the course of the UK BSE epizootic, though there are still ongoing investigations concerning the presence of BSE in sheep and goats. In zoological parks, some exotic ruminants that likely received prion-contaminated livestock feed became infected with a TSE. These included greater kudu, nyala, eland, gemsbok, and oryx. Similarly, twenty captive exotic felids, including cheetahs, lions, ocelots, pumas, and tigers developed TSEs, most likely from being fed meat or offal from BSE-infected cattle. In addition, eighty-nine domestic cats diagnosed with feline spongiform encephalopathy (FSE) in the UK were associated with the BSE epizootic (DEFRA 2007). Several other countries have also detected cases of FSE. These include Norway, Liechtenstein, France, Portugal, Italy, and Switzerland.

Unfortunately, livestock feeds containing MBM had also been exported to other countries, as had infected livestock from the UK, and ultimately, additional cases of BSE were found in numerous countries in Europe and elsewhere, though never to the extent that occurred in the UK By the end of 2006, twenty-four countries had reported at least one case of BSE. This includes twenty countries in Europe as well as Israel, Japan, Canada, and the United States (OIE 2007a). As a result, the European Union and many other nations have also instituted bans on feeding ruminant-derived protein to ruminant livestock. In Europe, problems with cross contamination of feed for ruminants and non-ruminants has prompted the bans to include prohibiting the feeding of most animal proteins to food-producing animals. As experimental studies and field observations indicate that horizontal transmission does not occur from cow to cow, the feed ban is the most effective tool there is to control the spread of the disease in livestock. Studies have also been done to determine whether BSE can be transmitted by frozen cattle semen and frozen cattle embryos. This does not appear to be a risk. Similarly, researchers were unable to transmit BSE via goat embryos (Foster et al. 1999).

The first human death due to vCJD occurred in a nineteen-year old British man in 1995 and by 1996 the likely link between BSE and vCJD was acknowledged. It became accepted that consumption of bovine meat products which were contaminated with nervous tissue of infected cattle was the most likely route of transmission of BSE prions to humans in cases of vCJD. As a result, the European Union and other countries with BSE-infected cattle instituted new restrictions on the bovine slaughter industry to exclude so-called specified risk materials (SRM) from meat products derived from slaughter plants.

The SRM are tissues with the potential to contain significant amounts of BSE infectivity in infected animals. This SRM restriction was not instituted in the United States until 2004, since the first bovine case of BSE in the country was only diagnosed in 2003. This intervention appears to have had the desired effect of limiting the occurrence of vCJD. The annual incidence of vCJD in the UK peaked in 2000 and has declined since. From 1995 through June of 2007, 162 human cases of vCJD were reported in the UK; twenty-two in France; four in Ireland; three in the United States; two in the Netherlands; and one each in Canada, Italy, Saudi Arabia, Japan, Portugal, and Spain (National Creutzfeldt Jakob Disease Surveillance Unit 2007). All three affected individuals diagnosed in the United States had lived outside the country for extended periods—two in the UK and one in Saudi Arabia.

The origin and character of the infective prion initially consumed by cattle to produce the epizootic of BSE in the UK has never been established. One of the original theories is that the infective prion was originally the scrapie prion introduced into the food chain via infected sheep tissues and that the prion was somehow transformed into a unique species-specific agent affecting cattle. An alternate theory is that a spontaneous mutation of normal bovine prion with the capacity for infectivity entered the animal food chain via affected slaughter cattle from whom meat and bone meal was derived. This theory is now being examined in greater depth since the finding of atypical manifestations of BSE in cattle (Biacabe et al. 2004; Casalone et al. 2004; Brown et al. 2006) and the reported capacity of one atypical BSE prion strain to undergo transformation after serial passage in mice to produce a neuropatholological and molecular disease phenotype that was indistinguishable from that of mice infected with the class BSE prion strain (Capobianco et al. 2007). Regardless of the origin, the prion that produces classical BSE can be differentiated from various strains of the scrapie prion due to advances in laboratory techniques now available for characterization of prion proteins. It remains to be seen if the atypical strains of BSE currently being identified will confound this laboratory capacity for differentiation.

The clinicopathological similarities of BSE and scrapie have spurred research on prion diseases in small ruminants, including investigations on the potential of sheep and goats to become infected with BSE. Successful experimental infections have demonstrated that both sheep and goats are susceptible to BSE infection and can manifest clinical disease. The first experimental transmission of BSE to goats was reported by Foster et al. (1993). Six goats were inoculated with brain homogenates of known BSE-infected cows either intracerebrally or orally. Three of three Anglo-Nubian goats challenged intracerebrally developed clinical signs of BSE 506 to 570 days after challenge and two of three goats challenged orally developed the disease 941 and 1,501 days after challenge (Foster et al. 1993, 2001). This indicated that the presumed natural route of infection, i.e., oral ingestion, could produce BSE in goats.

The results of such studies, and the general concern of the zoonotic potential of TSEs, spurred the establishment and/or expansion of active surveillance programs for the presence of BSE and scrapie in cattle, sheep, and goats. The European Commission was particularly active in implementing such programs. Beginning in 2002, the EU countries started to test sheep and goats in large numbers for TSEs. The samples included healthy animals sent to slaughter, animals culled as part of ongoing scrapie eradication programs, reported suspect TSE cases, and other suspect animals such as fallen stock or animals which had died on farm. With regard to goats, the EU countries tested 54,444 in 2002, 63,022 in 2003, 36,115 in 2004, and 265,489 in 2005 (European Commission, 2003, 2004, 2005, 2006). In contrast, through 2006, approximately 800 goats in the United States were tested at slaughter for TSEs, though goat slaughter surveillance activities were increased in 2007.

On January 28, 2005, the EC announced that an apparently healthy two-and-a-half-year-old goat slaughtered in France in October, 2002 and tested under the active TSE surveillance system had been confirmed as a positive case of BSE. As a precaution, the French authorities culled the entire herd of origin; no animals or animal products were allowed to enter the human or animal food chains. All other of the approximately 300 adult goats in the herd were tested, with no detectable evidence of a TSE found. Samples from the one positive goat were sent from France to the OIE Reference Laboratory for BSE, the Veterinary Laboratories Agency at Weybridge, UK, for further assessment. Mouse inoculation studies conducted at Weybridge confirmed this to be the first known case of naturally occurring BSE in a goat (Eloit et al. 2005).

In February of 2005, UK authorities announced that samples from a goat which had initially tested positive for scrapie in 1990 had been reevaluated as part of a research effort to assess newer, more sensitive testing methods for discriminating scrapie from BSE in goats (DEFRA 2005a). The case is now being considered as a possible suspect BSE case, but at the time of this writing, final confirmation is pending the outcome of ongoing transmission studies (Jeffrey et al. 2006).

These two cases, one confirmed and one suspect, establish that naturally occurring BSE can occur in the goat. However, many questions remain unanswered about the origin of these infections, the risk that BSE may spread through goat populations, and whether goats and goat products may act as a source of infection for vCJD in humans.

The confirmed BSE-positive French goat was born before the EU initiated its extensive animal protein feed ban in 2001, so the possibility exists that oral consumption of the BSE prion in contaminated feed was the source of exposure for this goat. Similarly, the UK goat was born in 1987, before the 1988 U.K. feed ban on meat and bone meal. Even before the emergence of these two reports, there was considerable concern among experts that BSE would be identified in small ruminants, though the focus of concern was more on sheep than goats due to the greater numbers of sheep in Europe and the greater economic value of the sheep industry (Schreuder and Somerville 2003).

The Scientific Steering Committee (SSC) of the European Commission issued an opinion on the risk of infection of sheep and goats with the BSE agent in 1998 (European Commission 1998). In summary, the committee believed that the transmission of the BSE agent to small ruminants was possible and if it occurred, it would likely be through the same mechanism by which cattle were infected, namely by consumption of concentrate feed containing prion-contaminated animal protein. Because the route was likely to be the same, the geographic distribution of small ruminant cases would also likely be the same, with the occurrence in small ruminants reflecting the occurrence in cattle. It was also recognized that dairy goats were more likely to have consumed contaminated concentrate feed with a possible higher risk of exposure to prion contamination than sheep and goats kept for other purposes. By 1998, it was already clear that the feed ban on animal protein in the UK had effectively dampened the BSE epizootic in cattle there, with fewer cases being reported each year. While it might be assumed that the risk of infection in small ruminants would subside in a similar fashion, the SSC expressed concern that it was not known if BSE in small ruminants would behave like scrapie in sheep, where there is evidence of lateral transmission, or like BSE in cattle, where transmission is limited to feed sources.

In BSE of cattle, there is no indication that the disease is transmitted either horizontally or vertically between animals. Virtually all bovine cases are presumed to derive from direct consumption of contaminated feed. In contrast, scrapie can be transmitted between small ruminants, either directly or indirectly. Horizontal transmission has been demonstrated in both sheep and goats, and in sheep, the possibility of vertical transmission has not been completely ruled out (Detwiler and Baylis 2003). Thus, if BSE were to behave like scrapie in small ruminants, the infection could continue to be maintained in sheep and goat populations and continue to spread despite the feed ban.

One study has shown that BSE appears to be able to spread from infected dams to lambs, though it was not clear if this occurred *in utero* or in the perinatal period (Bellworthy et al. 2005). The fact that only one goat and no sheep have been confirmed with BSE since the SSC issued their opinion in 1998 suggests that BSE has not been widely circulated or maintained in small ruminant populations at highest risk. The increase in active surveillance for TSEs in small ruminants which began in the EU in 2002 will help to clarify the status of BSE in the small ruminant populations of those countries which had the most bovine BSE. However, there is an important caveat. It is possible that serial passage of natural BSE may change the biochemical signature of the prion, making it very difficult, if not impossible, to distinguish it from scrapie (Ronzon et al. 2006).

The other major concern is the possible risk to humans of BSE occurring in small ruminants. The issue is whether or not the controls now in place to protect humans from zoonotic prion infection from bovine products are sufficient to protect humans from BSE in small ruminants. Again, this depends on whether or not BSE in small ruminants behaves like scrapie in small ruminants or like BSE in cattle. The distribution of prions in host tissues is the key factor for consideration in this regard. Several studies have now been completed on the experimental infection of sheep with BSE (Foster et al. 1993, 2001; Jeffrey et al. 2001; Bellworthy et al. 2005a). These studies indicate that experimental BSE in sheep behaves like scrapie, with a wide distribution of PrP^{d} (another designation of PrP^{sc}) in tissues of the lymphoreticular system and the enteric nervous system in the preclinical stages of infection. Among the PrP^{d} positive tissues identified were submandibular, retropharyngeal, prescapular, mesenteric, ileocecal, and mediastinal lymph nodes; tonsil; and spleen. In the enteric system, PrP^{d} was identified in association with lymphoid tissue or enteric nervous tissue in the large and small intestine. Of interest was the observation of PrP^{d} in the abomasum (Jeffrey et al. 2001). This PrP^{d} was found in macrophages associated with focal inflammatory lesions presumed to be induced by gastrointestinal parasites.

The notion that PrP^{d}-laden macrophages can be drawn to sites of infection as part of the inflammatory response is both intriguing and alarming. It suggests the possibility that, in cases of mastitis, even subclinical mastitis, macrophages containing PrP^{d} could be drawn to the udder and thereby be present in milk. In fact, this process has been observed in mastitic sheep with scrapie (Ligios et al. 2005). Clearly, classification of milk as a specified risk material would have devastating consequences for dairying in small ruminants. The fact that prions are not destroyed by standard methods of pasteurization does not help matters. A recent study reported that normal PrP^{c} protein could be identified in store-bought, pasteurized cow, sheep, and goat milk in Switzerland with the use of a new technology that binds prions in bodily fluids with high affinity and specificity (Franscini et al. 2006). The finding of normal PrP^{c} in this context is not surprising, and further studies are warranted to determine if abnormal prion protein can be detected in milk using similar technologies.

The risk potential of transmitting TSEs via milk in sheep and goats to humans needs to be specifically addressed through vigorous research so that zoonotic disease control policy can be properly based on science. A similar concern derives from reports that experimental BSE in sheep can be transmitted via blood transfusion to other sheep, even when the donor sheep are in the preclinical stages of infection (Houston et al. 2000; Sisó et al. 2006). The presence of infectivity in blood in naturally infected sheep and goats, if it were confirmed to occur, could have dire implications for the marketing of all small ruminant-derived food products intended for human consumption.

A cautionary note on the research to date is warranted. Some experimental transmissions of BSE have involved routes of infection, e.g., intracerebral, or large challenge doses not likely to occur under conditions of natural infection. In addition, because of the considerable time and expense involved in conducting transmission and infectivity studies in prion diseases, very few animals have been involved in these reported experiments. The largest number of sheep involved in any of these studies was sixty and the largest number of goats was six.

Initially, at least in sheep, it appeared that the genetic polymorphisms known to affect susceptibility and resistance to scrapie seemed to also hold for susceptibility and resistance to experimental BSE (Bellworthy et al. 2005a). However, more recent research calls this assumption into question. Scrapie resistant sheep of the ARR/ARR genotype have been experimentally infected with BSE (Andréoletti et al. 2006; Bencsik and Baron 2007). In one report, ARR/ARR sheep so infected were still clinically normal for up to six years after infection, suggesting that these sheep may even serve as silent carriers for BSE (Ronzon et al. 2006). In goats, similar to the situation with scrapie, the role of genetics remains uncertain for BSE infection.

So, while research findings to date suggest cause for concern regarding the potential for small ruminants to contract BSE, transmit it horizontally, and possibly infect humans, much more research needs to be done to develop precise quantitative risk assessments. As recently as 2006, investigators reporting on the accumulation of PrP^{d} in the brains of goats experimentally infected with BSE acknowledged that the distribution of PrP^{d} in the peripheral tissues of such goats remains undocumented (Jeffery et al. 2006). The most pressing question at present is whether or not the increase in active surveillance of sheep and goats in the EU for naturally occurring TSEs, along with the improved laboratory capacity to distinguish scrapie from BSE, will reveal additional cases of BSE in goats and sheep.

Clinical Findings and Diagnosis

Because the only known case of BSE in a goat was identified in a healthy animal at slaughter through the EC active surveillance program, there are no descriptions of the clinical signs of naturally occurring BSE in the goat. Clinical BSE has been produced in goats by experimental infection and signs of the experimentally induced disease have been described (Foster et al. 1993, 2001). These descriptions should be understood in the context in which they were produced. The routes of infection and dosages of infective material used under experimental conditions may not produce the clinical manifestations of the disease as likely to be seen under natural circumstances, particularly with regard to the temporal course of clinical disease, which appears relatively short when compared to natural BSE in cattle or natural scrapie in goats and sheep.

Foster et al. (1993, 2001) reported that three goats inoculated intracerebrally with a brain homogenate from BSE-infected cattle developed clinical disease between 506 and 570 days post inoculation. Two of three goats dosed orally developed clinical disease at 941 and 1,501 days, respectively, and a third remained healthy at 1,720 days post challenge. All three intracerebrally inoculated goats and one of the orally dosed goats developed sudden and pronounced ataxia which progressed so acutely, once manifest, that each of these goats had to be euthanized within six days after the onset of ataxia for reasons of welfare. The other orally dosed goat that developed clinical signs did not show signs of ataxia. Rather, it simply became lethargic and lost weight over a period of three weeks before it was culled. None of the five affected animals developed pruritus, a sign characteristic of scrapie, the more common TSE of small ruminants.

Given the uncertainty of the clinical presentation of BSE in goats at this time, and given the serious regulatory concerns associated with all TSEs in ruminant animals, it is prudent for veterinary practitioners to consider both of the TSEs, scrapie and BSE, in the differential diagnosis of neurological disease in goats, particularly chronic or progressive neurological disease. It is reasonable to assume that were clinical BSE to occur naturally in goats, it would appear similar to BSE in cattle or scrapie in goats and sheep.

In cattle with natural BSE, the onset of disease is insidious and the course is long. The predominant clinical signs are neurological in nature and include apprehension, hyperesthesia, and ataxia, the latter progressing to the point at which affected animals may be unable to rise. It is important to note that clinical signs of the TSEs may be very subtle and often go unnoticed until near the end stage. The clinical disease in cattle is described in more detail elsewhere (Radostits et al. 2007). The clinical signs of scrapie in goats are described in this chapter in the discussion of scrapie, along with the likely differential diagnoses for consideration in both scrapie and BSE.

Clinical Pathology and Necropsy

There are no consistent hematological, biochemical, or gross pathological changes in animals with clinical or preclinical BSE that are diagnostic of the disease. BSE produces characteristic spongiform lesions in selected regions of the brain similar to those described for scrapie (Foster et al. 2001). However, in small ruminants, discriminatory tests such as immunohistochemistry and western blot using certain antibodies are required to determine if the characteristic lesions are due to scrapie or BSE (OIE 2004a). In those clinical cases where practitioners suspect that TSEs may be involved, regulatory authorities must be notified so that suitable samples of brain tissue can be collected for analysis if deemed necessary. Detailed descriptions of the necropsy techniques for collecting appropriate tissue samples for diagnosis of TSEs in goats and sheep are available on the Internet (Canadian Food Inspection Agency 2005; USDA 2007b).

A three-tiered testing program is currently in effect in the EU to identify BSE in small ruminants. Brain tissue from sheep and goats is first screened in active surveillance programs for TSE using approved rapid screening tests that can identify proteinase K resistant prion fragments in samples, but cannot distinguish between BSE and scrapie. As of February, 2006, the EC had approved eight such rapid tests under EC Regulation No. 253/2006 for use with ovine and caprine samples. These include two sandwich immunoassays, three chemiluminescent assays, a conformational dependent immunoassay, a western immunoblot assay, and an immunocapture assay (European Commission, 2006a). The second tier of testing involves application of discriminatory tests to TSE-positive samples, such as immunohistochemistry or a modified western immunoblotting technique. The third phase is confirmatory testing, which involves inoculation of inbred or transgenic mice with BSE suspect material and then conducting discriminatory tests on the brains of inoculated mice.

Mouse inoculation studies are laborious and take upwards of a year or more for the mice to develop disease and for final tests to be completed. Such delays can hamper prompt, effective regulatory action. Not surprisingly then, the development of new discriminatory methods for quickly differentiating BSE and scrapie in small ruminants is an area of active research. New approaches include evaluation of the molecular size and glycosylation pattern of the prion protein accumulated in the brain of affected animals as well as epitope mapping studies using monoclonal antibodies directed at different portions of the prion molecule with comparative analysis of the ratios of antibody binding (Lezmi et al. 2004; Thuring et al. 2004). Jeffrey et al. (2006) reported that in goats with experimental BSE, intra-neuronal PrP^d was labeled only by antibodies recognizing epitopes located C-terminally of residue His99, whereas in scrapie cases, PrP^d was also detected by antibodies to epitopes located between residues Trp93 and His99.

With regard to the French goat confirmed with BSE, Eloit et al. (2005) reported that the animal was first identified as a TSE case through the EU active surveillance program in 2002. It was subsequently subjected to further testing at four separate, independent labs using additional western blot and ELISA assays. The results obtained at all the labs were convergent and the French goat sample results were indistinguishable from results of samples derived from goats and sheep experimentally infected with BSE. The French goat sample was subsequently inoculated into four strains of wild type and transgenic mice used to assay BSE infectivity. The inoculated mice developed disease with incubation times compatible with those resulting from inoculation with experimental ovine BSE. The mice also produced a histological lesion profile in the brain identical to the lesion profile characteristic of experimental ovine BSE. Finally, western blot profiles produced by brain samples from inoculated mice showed that the French goat profile was again indistinguishable from those obtained with experimental ovine BSE. The suspect caprine BSE case from the UK was identified by application of immunohistochemical epitope mapping of archived brain tissue samples of caprine TSE cases diagnosed originally as scrapie (Jeffrey et al. 2006). Results of mouse inoculation studies are pending at the time of this writing.

Treatment and Control

There is no treatment for BSE. Even if therapeutic options were available, there would likely be little or no opportunity to use them because the disease is reportable and highly regulated worldwide. Suspect cases would be euthanized for diagnostic purposes by the appropriate authorities. Nonetheless, concerns about TSEs in humans have prompted research into possible therapeutic regimens which in principle could be applicable to animals with TSEs, including BSE. Obstacles and opportunities for treatment of TSEs have been reviewed (Liberski, 2004; Weissmann and Aguzzi, 2005).

Different countries have different specific regulations for the control of BSE, but the basic principles apply in all cases. The key element in controlling the spread of BSE has been the ban on feeding ruminant-derived meat and bone meal to ruminant animals, which was later expanded in some countries to a ban on the use of most animal-derived protein in the rations of all farm animal species. The global prevalence of BSE in cattle has progressively decreased since these measures were adopted, first in the UK in 1988 and then elsewhere. In addition, countries without BSE strive to keep it out by establishing import restrictions on live ruminants and a varying array of ruminant products, including, in some cases, semen and embryos of cattle, sheep, and goats. BSE-free countries may also establish surveillance programs to ensure that the disease has not been introduced despite import regulations.

Countries with BSE have instituted stamping out measures to help control the disease. Initially, in countries other than the UK, herds containing BSE-confirmed animals were depopulated. As it became clearer that horizontal or vertical transmission did not occur in cattle, depopulation was limited to birth cohorts of BSE-confirmed animals on the assumption that they were most likely exposed to the offending feed at an early age. In addition, active surveillance programs have been implemented to detect new cases of BSE and track the overall prevalence in countries with BSE. Active surveillance programs usually include sampling a sub-population of healthy animals at slaughter, as well as suspect BSE cases, fallen or "downer" animals, and animals that have died on the farm. Scrapie eradication programs in many countries, including the United States, have been intensified as a result of concerns about BSE and these initiatives dovetail nicely with efforts to detect or eliminate TSEs in small ruminant populations.

The establishment of a zoonotic link between BSE in cattle and variant CJD in humans around 1996 resulted in additional control measures to prevent the transmission of infective prions to humans through the food chain. The identification of specified risk materials (SRM) to be removed from the human food supply during slaughter and meat processing has been the main intervention. SRM are tissues that are removed from the carcass because they pose a potential increased risk of carrying infective prions due to the predilection of infective prions for nervous and lymphoreticular tissue. As a precaution, the UK took measures to remove certain of these high-risk tissues from food in 1990. Again, there may be variation between countries in the tissues selected and the age of the animals included, but in general, for cattle, SRM include brain, eyes, skull, spinal cord with dorsal root ganglia, tonsils, vertebral column, intestines, and mesentery. Because the distribution of BSE in small ruminants may be more similar to that of scrapie in small ruminants than BSE in cattle, the list of SRM for sheep and goats may encompass a wider range of tissues and a different age range. For example, the EU does not designate the spleen as an SRM for cattle, but removal of spleen is required for all ages of sheep and goats. It should be noted that if BSE were to be confirmed as a disease of sheep under natural conditions, the current SRM bans for both sheep and goats would likely become more stringent.

Initially, efforts to monitor and control BSE in goats and sheep were a secondary concern of regulatory agencies facing the daunting challenge of controlling this dangerous new disease in cattle. However, two things prompted a greater focus on BSE in small ruminants. The first was the link between BSE and vCJD which demonstrated the risk that products of animal origin could be a source of TSEs for humans. The second was the confirmation of the case of BSE in the goat from France in 2005. Because Europe was the source of most of the world's BSE cases in cattle, the vCJD cases in humans, and the single goat with BSE, it is not surprising that the strongest and quickest regulatory response with regard to small ruminants came from the European Union.

In May 2001, the European Parliament approved EC Regulation No. 999/2001 (European Commission 2001), laying down rules for the prevention, control, and eradication of certain transmissible spongiform encephalopathies. This comprehensive legislation addressed numerous key issues: establishment of a national status category for countries relative to the presence of TSE based on quantitative risk analysis; establishment of active surveillance programs for TSEs in sheep and goats (scrapie and BSE) with minimum sample sizes identified for each member state; identification of specified risk materials for small ruminants and cattle; establishment of regulatory procedures for the diagnosis of TSE and destruction of sheep and goat flocks confirmed with either scrapie or BSE along with guidelines for compensation of owners; rules for import and export of live animals, semen, embryos, and animal products relative to TSE status of importing and exporting countries; identification of TSE reference laboratories; and identification of approved sampling and laboratory methods.

The enhanced surveillance of sheep and goats for TSE which began in earnest in 2002 has already had two significant consequences. It demonstrated that the prevalence of scrapie in both sheep and goats is higher than previously suspected, and it led to the identification of the BSE-positive goat from France.

Identification of the caprine BSE case led to an immediate response from the EC regarding concerns that goat products could serve as a source of TSE infection for humans. The European Food Safety Authority ordered its Scientific Panel on Biohazards to conduct a risk assessment of goat meat and goat meat products with regard to BSE and report by June 2005. The panel noted that very little is known about the behavior of BSE in goats because information from experimental caprine infections is extremely limited at present. The panel also noted that it is possible that the tissue distribution of BSE in goats, both clinically and preclinically, could be similar to that of scrapie, indicating a wider distribution than found in BSE of cattle. More goat-specific experimental studies were called for, particularly to assess tissue distribution of infective prions in the preclinical stages of disease. The panel also pointed out that there was presently limited information available about the consumption patterns of goat meat by consumers in the EU, and such information would be necessary to undertake a truly quantitative risk analysis (Scientific Panel on Biological Hazards 2005).

Nevertheless, the panel concluded that a "qualitative risk assessment (RA) on goat meat could be made considering the existing risk management (RM) measures in place since 2001 and the results of the recently increased level of surveillance in goats and the discriminatory testing. For such a qualitative RA on goat meat, account is taken of a number of facts including that the goat found positive was born before the feed ban in 2001, and that currently, goats slaughtered for human consumption at a young age and born after the introduction of the feed ban, would present a lower risk than the adult population. Also other risk management measures in place (e.g. Specified Risk Material [SRM] list, rendering) contribute to the further reduction of the risk to the consumer. Moreover, the initial results of increased testing and discriminatory testing have not indicated any additional suspect BSE cases in goats or sheep. Therefore, the current risk in terms of BSE, related to the consumption of goat meat and goat meat products is considered at this time to be small for goats born after the feed ban, i.e. in 2001 and later." (Scientific Panel on Biological Hazards 2005).

Since the panel issued this statement, however, three unusual TSE cases in sheep, two from France and one from Cyprus, have been identified by routine surveillance for which testing to date could not definitively rule out BSE. Samples from these sheep have been submitted for discriminatory testing using the mouse bioassay test but the results of these tests are not available at the time of this writing (European Commission 2006b).

With regard to goat milk and goat milk products, the EC drew on an earlier opinion of the Scientific Panel on Biological Hazards (2004). Again, the panel cautioned that little specific information is available about the distribution of BSE infectivity in experimentally infected goats and that more studies are required to make quantitative risk assessments. They pointed out that prion infectivity could potentially cross the blood/milk barrier in the case of inflammation of the mammary gland (Scientific Panel on Biohazards 2004). Nevertheless, the EU advised no change in current consumption of goat milk or cheese as long as milk is not derived from TSE-positive goats, and that goats are healthy and without mastitis.

The true risk of BSE from goat-derived products remains to be quantitatively determined. It appears that at present, regulatory authorities are hopeful that the BSE-positive French goat and the BSE-suspect UK goat represent the end, not the beginning, of detection of BSE cases in small ruminants. This hopeful position is bolstered by the facts that both animals were born before feed bans were fully in place and both came from countries where BSE in cattle was common. Furthermore, since the confirmation of the French goat case, hundreds of thousands of goats have been tested for TSEs in Europe and no additional cases have been found. In 2006 alone more than 200,000 goats were tested, and in 2005, 153 scrapie-suspect goat samples were subjected to discriminatory testing with no cases of BSE detected (European Commission 2006).

However, only time, additional research, and an active ongoing surveillance program will determine if BSE in goats is a problem with serious consequences for the goat industry. In the meantime, goat producers and veterinarians should consider the possibility of BSE in all cases of neurological disease of goats and report suspect cases to regulatory authorities.

Caprine Arthritis Encephalitis (CAE) and Maedi-Visna (MV)

Caprine arthritis encephalitis (CAE) is a disease of goats caused by a retrovirus belonging to the small ruminant lentivirus (SRLV) serogroup. There are five main clinical presentations for CAE, namely, arthritis, which is predominant, mastitis, pneumonia, a neurological form, leukoencephalomyelitis, and progressive weight loss. The focus of the discussion here is the neurological form of the disease. A second small ruminant lentivirus, known as maedi-visna virus (MVV), affects sheep and produces similar clinical conditions in that species, with the pneumonic form being predominant.

In the past, some cases of neurological disease in goats were attributed to infection with MVV. Clinically and histopathologically, these cases were strongly suggestive of CAE but occurred at a time when relatively little was known about the CAE virus (CAEV) and its relationship to MVV. The neurological disease of goats caused by small ruminant lentiviruses is described below and new relevant information about the relationship of CAEV and MVV is presented. The arthritic, pneumonic, and mastitic forms of CAE are discussed further in Chapters 4, 9, and 14, respectively.

Etiology

CAEV and MVV are viruses in the family *Retroviridae* in the genus *Lentivirinae*. The lentiviruses are also known as slow viruses because they cause persistent infections that slowly manifest as progressive, clinical disease. More detailed information about the physicochemical, genetic, and immunological aspects of the SRLV is available in the main discussion of CAE in Chapter 4.

The lentiviruses are classified into five serogroups reflecting the hosts with which they are associated. CAEV and MVV belong to the SRLV serogroup and cause maedi-visna in sheep and caprine arthritis encephalitis in goats. The other serogroups include the cattle serogroup associated with bovine immunodeficiency disease, the equine serogroup associated with equine infectious anemia, the feline serogroup associated with feline immunodeficiency disease, and the primate serogroup which contains the simian immunodeficiency virus (SIV) and the human immunodeficiency virus (HIV). The latter is responsible for acquired immunodeficiency syndrome or AIDS in people.

The close relationship of the small ruminant lentiviruses to HIV has spurred a great deal of research in the last twenty years on CAEV and MVV. Though neither is zoonotic, the diseases they cause, CAE and maedi-visna, have served as models for the study of AIDS. As a result of this heightened interest, the veterinary community now has a better understanding of the small ruminant lentiviruses, their relationship to each other, and the diseases they produce.

MVV is the prototype small ruminant lentivirus, first described in the 1950s, whereas CAEV was first described in the 1970s. Historically, MVV and CAEV have been considered as distinct viral entities with well defined host specificity for sheep and goats, respectively. However, ongoing advances in phylogenetic analysis and studies of cross-transmission now indicate that the two viruses may be more closely related than previously thought.

Zanoni (1998) reported phylogenetic studies of small ruminant lentiviruses based on available sequence data for fragments of their *env*, *pol*, and *gag* genes and their long terminal repeats (LTR). The results indicated that at least six different clades could be differentiated with no clear separation of SRLV strains derived from goats (CAEV) or sheep (MVV). The first clade consisted of the prototype Icelandic visna virus and related MVV strains. The second clade included North American ovine lentivirus strains, the third SRLV from Norway, and the fourth SRLV from France. The fifth clade notably included the prototype North American CAEV strain, CAC-CO, as well as CAEV strains from France and Switzerland along with North American ovine lentivirus strains. The sixth clade included French SRLV. Based on this phylogenetic analysis, in which there was no clear resolution of clades according to host species origin, it was concluded that the SRLV may cross the host species barrier with ease and it was hypothesized that all the SRLV strains derive originally from MVV.

More recently, Shah et al. (2004) reported additional phylogenetic studies using a larger number of virus isolates and longer sequences of the *gag* and *pol* genes. Though the specifics of the classification system that emerged differed from that of Zanoni (1998), a key observation was reconfirmed—namely, that the SRLV do not segregate phylogenetically according to host specificity. In this more recent analysis, four of nine designated subtypes of SRLV contained both sheep and goat isolates. It was also noted that Swiss strains in the so-called B1 subtype differed no more from French, Brazilian, or United States strains than from each other, suggesting virus propagation through international livestock trade. Furthermore, isolates in subtypes A3 and A4 were derived from both goats and sheep. This was documented from specific herds where there was contact between the two species, providing further evidence for interspecies transmission of the SRLV (Shah et al. 2004, 2004a). In a separate study, phylogenetic evidence of transmission of SRLV subtype B1 from goats to sheep in mixed flocks was also reported (Pisoni et al. 2005).

Epidemiology

MV was first described in South Africa as a chronic respiratory disease of sheep in 1915. It was later reported from the United States in 1923 and subsequently in Iceland where it was first recognized in the respiratory form (maedi is Icelandic for dyspnea) and then later in the neurologic form (visna is Icelandic for wasting), which occurred only in flocks of sheep with the respiratory form of the disease (Clements and Zink 1996). Intensive epidemiological, pathological, and virological studies in Iceland in the 1950s led to the recognition and characterization of the respiratory and neurological forms of the disease as being due to a single, slow virus infection (Sigurdsson 1954; Sigurdsson and Palsson 1958; Sigurdsson et al. 1952, 1957, 1960, 1962). Respiratory disease is the dominant manifestation of MVV infection. In North America, the disease is known as ovine progressive pneumonia, in France as *la bouhite*, in South Africa as Graaff-Reinet disease, and in Holland as *zwoegerziekte*. MVV in sheep has been reviewed elsewhere (Pépin et al. 1998). MV occurs in most major commercial sheep producing countries except Australia and New Zealand. However, those countries do have CAE in their goat populations. The status of MV in many developing countries is unknown because surveillance programs are lacking.

Sporadic occurrences of a neurological disease in goats characterized by granulomatous encephalomyelitis were recorded in West Germany in 1969 and 1978 and Sweden in 1981 (Stavrou et al. 1969; Weinhold and Triemer 1978; Sundquist et al. 1981). At the time, these were considered to be putative cases of visna or a visna-like disease of goats. The German reports each involved a single goat herd and the Swedish report involved multiple herds in north and central Sweden. In all these cases, a neurologic disease syndrome occurred in adult, dairy breed goats, characterized clinically by progressive paresis and histologically by two key features—granulomatous encephalitis and demyelination. In the later West German report, neutralizing antibodies to sheep visna virus were identified in affected goats (Weinhold and Triemer 1978). A visna-like virus was isolated from the Swedish goats (Sundquist 1981). Notably, the virus isolated from the Swedish goats formed syncytia in tissue culture but was not cytopathic. This is characteristic of CAEV, whereas MVV viruses usually produce syncytia and a cytopathic effect (Quérat et al. 1984).

While the neurologic form of CAE (viral leukoencephalomyelitis) is most common in young goats between two and six months of age, clinical cases do occur beyond this limited age range, extending well into adulthood (Norman and Smith 1983). Therefore, the occurrence of these putative visna cases in adult dairy goats is not inconsistent with CAE. In addition, adult goats with the arthritic form of the disease commonly show histologic evidence of neurologic involvement at necropsy. While CAE virus rarely induces neutralizing antibody, such antibody may develop over time (Ellis et al. 1987).

Given the better understanding of the phylogenetic relationship of some MVV and CAEV isolates and the growing evidence for cross species transmission, it is most likely that these early cases of putative visna in adult dairy goats in Europe were actually CAE (Andrésdóttir et al. 2005).

New evidence on cross species transmission of SRLV also has implications for control programs. Switzerland has a national CAE control program based on testing, culling, and indemnification that has been very effective in reducing the infection in goats from more than 50% of the Swiss goat population in the 1980s to about 0.3% in 2003 (Perler 2004). However, it has been observed that some herds participating in the program, which had been seronegative for extended periods, inexplicably became positive again. Recent investigations indicate that these herds often contain sheep or have a history of contact with sheep. Shah et al. (2004, 2004a) specifically demonstrated that virus obtained from goats in the control program that were commingled with sheep was phylogenetically related to the virus obtained from sheep. This means that for CAE control programs to be fully effective, strict segregation of goats and sheep must be a core element of the program.

Pathogenesis

While knowledge has increased considerably, some aspects of the pathogenesis are still unknown.

Additional information on the transmission and early stages of infection with CAEV is provided in Chapter 4 in the section on caprine arthritis encephalitis. The pathogenesis of neurological disease caused by SRLV in goats and sheep has been recently reviewed (Andrésdóttir et al. 2005) and is summarized as follows.

Cells of the monocyte lineage in the bone marrow and spleen are the primary targets of CAEV. Replication in these cells is restricted until the monocytes differentiate into macrophages, which appears to be regulated at the transcriptional level. The mechanism by which infected macrophages cross the blood-brain barrier and enter the CNS is not fully understood. It most likely occurs via the bloodstream with monocytes crossing non-specifically in their capacity as immune surveillance cells, or it may be in response to signals from activated T cells in response to inflammation or other infections. Other possibilities for introduction include lentivirus infection of brain capillary epithelial cells or choroid plexus with subsequent release of virus to the brain. Once in the brain, virus may infect a variety of cell types including lymphocytes, plasma cells, macrophages, endothelial cells, pericytes, fibroblasts, and choroidal epithelial cells. However, replication may be limited to macrophages. Different strains of SRLV show varying neurotropism and varying neurovirulence, and the two attributes appear to be independent.

Very few cells in infected brains are found to contain viral DNA. This suggests that lesions are not due to viral replication but rather the induction of an immune inflammatory response. One possible initiator is the tat protein produced by SRLV, certain peptides of which have experimentally produced microgliosis, astrocytosis, and neuronal loss in rodents. Goats and sheep produce a strong humoral and cell mediated immune response to SRLV infection. The host immune response likely plays a significant role in the development of lesions; experimentally, administration of immunosuppressive drugs almost abolished early lesions of visna in sheep. The host immune response is likely directed against virus induced antigens rather than host antigens and amplification of the immune response by infection results in a large influx of macrophages and lymphocytes and secretion of cytokines which contribute to the development of the lesions described below in the section on necropsy.

Infection with CAEV is lifelong. How and why the infection remains dormant for long and variable periods of time is not fully understood. For example, it is interesting that the neurologic form of CAE occurs more commonly in young animals while visna in sheep is more common in adults. Strain differences and variations in neurotropism and neurovirulence as well as host factors may play a role.

Clinical Findings

In the neurologic form of CAE, the majority of affected animals are dairy breed kids between one and six months of age, though older goats also can be affected. The disease develops slowly over a period of weeks and is characterized by a progressive paresis and paralysis of the limbs, suggesting principally a spinal cord involvement. The hind limbs are almost always affected, but tetraparesis is common and asymmetric limb involvement may also occur. Kids may initially show some knuckling and inappropriate placement when standing and incoordination when walking, particularly in the hind limbs (Figure 5.3a). Gradually, the animal may have increased difficulty rising and then be unable to rise at all (Figure 5.3b).

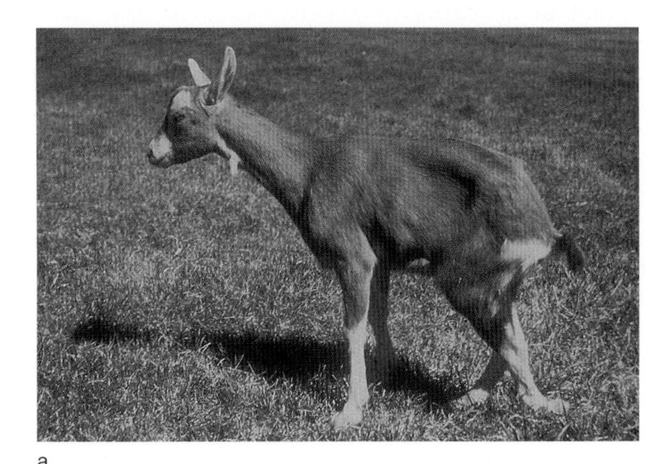

a

Figure 5.3a. Lack of proprioception manifested by cross-legged rear limb stance and knuckling of hind foot.

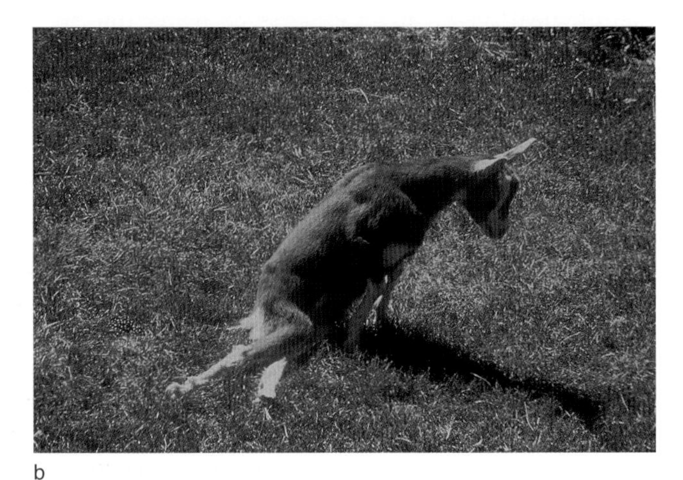

b

Figure 5.3b. More advanced stage with inability to stand on hind limbs.

Figure 5.3. Progressive paresis in a kid with the nervous form of caprine arthritis encephalitis virus (CAEV) infection. (Both photos courtesy of Dr. Linda Collins Cork.)

Reflexes and muscle tone are likely to be increased, but are sometimes found to be decreased if the gray matter of the spinal cord is involved. When the hind limbs are more affected than the forelimbs, which is common, the goat may pull itself around on the ground with the forelimbs. At least in the early stages of disease, many affected kids remain bright and alert and continue to eat and drink despite locomotor difficulties. Eventually, affected kids usually succumb to pneumonia, exposure, or other secondary disease problems if not euthanized first. Rarely, recoveries have been reported.

Clinical signs of CAE are not always limited to locomotor deficits. In a retrospective of thirty cases, additional neurologic signs were observed in more than 50% of the cases. These signs included depression, blindness, abnormal pupillary response, nystagmus, opisthotonos, head tremor, head tilt, torticollis, circling, facial nerve deficits, and dysphagia. A variable increase in body temperature was also noted in the majority of cases (Norman and Smith 1983).

Clinical Pathology and Necropsy

Serology, using AGID or ELISA tests, may be helpful in establishing the presence of retroviral infection. However, identifying antibody does not confirm that clinical disease is caused by retrovirus, because animals can be subclinically infected with CAEV yet have neurologic disease due to other causes. Conversely, serum antibody levels may fall below the sensitivity threshold of the agar gel immunodiffusion (AGID) test, resulting in false negative results. Polymerase chain reaction assays on peripheral blood mononuclear cells from whole blood samples may be useful to identify the presence of viral antigen in suspect animals that are seronegative.

The CSF may suggest a viral encephalomyelitis without indicating the definitive cause. Total protein content and white blood cell counts tend to be mildly to moderately increased. In most cases, the increase in cellularity is caused by lymphocytes and monocytes, but increased neutrophils have also been observed. Median CSF total protein concentration in cases of CAE has been reported as 80 mg/dl and median white blood cell counts as 26.5/mm^3 (Smith 1982; Norman and Smith 1983). The hemogram is variable and of little diagnostic value.

At necropsy, gross lesions, when present, are limited to cloudiness of the meninges, focal brownish discoloration of the white matter in the brain and spinal cord and the ventricular surfaces, and/or swelling of the spinal cord. Microscopic lesions described in adult goats in Germany and Sweden initially presumed to have visna or visna-like disease (Stavrou et al. 1969; Dahme et al. 1973; Griem and Weinhold 1975; Sundquist et al. 1981) were similar to those described for the neurologic form of CAE (Cork et al. 1974; Norman and Smith, 1983). The lesions are similar to those originally described in sheep with visna (Sigurdsson et al. 1962).

Histologically, SRLV infections are characterized by a multifocal, mononuclear inflammatory leukoencephalomyelitis accompanied by extensive demyelination. The inflammatory response is principally perivascular and is comprised of aggregates of lymphocytes, macrophages, and plasma cells. In all cases, areas of inflammation are ringed by areas of increased astrocytes and microglia. Demyelination of nearby axons is a prominent finding. Axons are destroyed and there is general malacia in severely affected areas. In general, lesions are distributed periventricularly and periaqueductally and extend into the white matter along vessels. In severe cases, lesions may be found in adjacent gray matter. Lymphocytic infiltration of the meninges and the choroid plexus is a common finding.

Early reports of caprine visna and CAE suggested a possible difference in the two diseases based on location of lesions in the CNS, with CAE less likely to involve the brain and more likely to involve selected regions of the spinal cord (Cork et al. 1974). However, later studies of CAE demonstrated that brain lesions are common, occurring in as many as 60% of cases either with or without concurrent spinal cord lesions and that spinal cord lesions are widely distributed and not often restricted to the cervical or lumbar regions (Norman and Smith 1983). Mononuclear inflammatory responses similar to those described in the CNS may also be found in the joints, lungs, and other tissues of goats with CAE.

Diagnosis

Currently the presumptive diagnosis of the neurologic form of CAE is based on a history of other forms of CAE in the herd, e.g., arthritis or mastitis, characteristic clinical signs, evidence of antibody in the affected goat, and typical neuropathology at time of necropsy. Definitive diagnosis of any CAE infection depends on *in vitro* cultivation of virus from affected tissues.

The predominant sign in neurologic disease caused by CAEV is progressive paresis and paralysis. In young kids, the differential diagnosis must include enzootic ataxia due to copper deficiency, vertebral body or spinal cord abscesses, congenital abnormalities of the spinal cord or vertebral column, and cerebrospinal nematodiasis. If the onset is reported to be acute because early signs of paresis were overlooked, then enzootic muscular dystrophy, spinal trauma, tick paralysis, and polyradiculoneuritis also must be ruled out. Multiple conditions may be concurrent as in the reported cases of CAE and enzootic ataxia occurring in goat kids in the northeastern United States (Lofstedt et al. 1988).

In adult goats, cerebrospinal nematodiasis, abscesses, possible delayed organophosphate neurotoxicity, and scrapie must be considered in the differential diagnosis. Unlike in sheep, intense pruritus is not commonly reported in caprine scrapie and therefore the condition may look more like an SRLV infection than it would in sheep.

When lesions suggestive of brain involvement are observed, polioencephalomalacia and listeriosis should then also be considered in the differential diagnosis. In all cases, rabies should be considered because it can also present as an ascending paralysis.

Treatment and Control

There are no known treatments for retroviral infections of small ruminants in veterinary medicine. In the case of CAE, the control methods described in Chapter 4 for the arthritic form of the disease also apply to the neurologic form.

Border Disease

Border disease, also known as "hairy shaker" disease in lambs, is an infectious, contagious viral disease of sheep and goats. It causes abortions, infertility, stillbirths, weak lambs and kids, and a characteristic pattern of tremors, or shaking, in newborn lambs and kids. In lambs, it also produces a characteristic hairy appearance to the fleece and histologic changes in the skin. These skin changes are not seen in affected kids.

Etiology

Border disease is caused by a pestivrus. The pestiviruses are enveloped, single-stranded, positive sense, RNA viruses in the family *Togaviridae*. The pestivirus genus includes four related species responsible for livestock diseases: border disease virus (BDV), bovine virus diarrhea virus-1 (BVDV-1), bovine virus diarrhea virus-2 (BVDV-2), and classical swine fever (hog cholera) virus (CSFV). The viruses share physical, chemical, and biological properties including a shared common soluble antigen. Cross-species infections are known to occur as antibodies against pestivirus have been identified in more than forty ruminant species (Hamblin and Hedger 1979).

Definitive classification of the pestiviruses is currently a work in progress. Recent phylogenetic analysis of the pestiviruses based on the N^{pro} gene encoding for the non-structural protein N^{pro} indicate that indeed, these viruses do not segregate according to their traditional classifications based on host species origin (e.g., bovine versus porcine versus ovine) (Becher et al. 1997). Based on this analysis, three pestivirus isolates derived from goats were classified in the BVDV-1 genotype rather than the BDV genotype traditionally associated with border disease in sheep and goats. BVDV-1 was subsequently isolated from goat kids from mixed sheep and goat flocks in Italy with signs consistent with border disease while BVDV-2 was identified in sheep from those flocks (Pratelli et al. 2001). More recently, an isolate from goats with border disease type signs in the Republic of Korea was classified in the BVDV-2 genotype, again on the basis of phylogenetic analysis of the N^{pro} gene (Kim et al. 2006).

Additional phylogenetic analysis of pestivirus isolates indicated that the BDV genotype could be further divided into four subgroups: BDV-1, BDV-2, BDV-3, and BDV-4 (Becher et al. 2003; Arnal et al. 2004). Subsequent to that, a pestivirus isolated from caprine fetuses in a mixed sheep and goat herd in central Italy experiencing abortions was characterized phylogenetically as a BDV, but based on its N^{pro} sequence, could not be included in one of the existing subgroups. Therefore, an additional new BDV subgroup was proposed (De Mia et al. 2005). At present, it would seem that goats may be infected with different species and genotypes of pestivirus and manifest clinical disease consistent with a diagnosis of border disease.

Epidemiology

The incidence of border disease in goats and its impact on the goat industry are unclear. The disease in sheep occurs in North America, Europe, Australia, and New Zealand. In contrast, naturally occurring, clinical border disease in goat kids has been reported only sporadically. While the disease was first described in sheep in 1959, the first naturally occurring case of border disease in a goat herd was not reported until 1982, from Norway (Løken et al. 1982). However, there was a report of a pestivirus isolated from the lungs of four-week-old kid with pneumonia in Australia the previous year (Fraser et al. 1981). Since then there has been little additional documentation of clinical border disease in goat flocks, save for some reports of goat cases along with sheep cases in mixed flocks in Italy (Pratelli et al. 1999; De Mia et al. 2005). These goat related cases may have involved BVDV virus as well as BDV virus.

Despite the relative lack of clinical reports, serologic surveys performed on goats in Canada (Elazhary et al. 1984; Lamontagne and Roy 1984), the United States (Fulton et al. 1982), Austria (Krametter-Frötscher et al. 2007), Norway (Løken 1989), Nigeria (Taylor et al. 1977), Chile (Celedon et al. 2001), and Brazil (Flores et al. 2005) indicate the presence of antibodies to BVDV or BDV in the range of 3% to 16% of goats tested. The significance of antibody responses in goats is not clear. They may merely represent an exposure to sheep with BDV, cattle with BVDV, or actual caprine infection. It is clear at least that the exposure of goats to pestivirus has a wide geographic distribution.

It is possible that clinical border disease in goats is frequently unrecognized because of a different disease pattern in goats than sheep. In experimental caprine infection, early abortion, fetal resorption, and mummification occur more commonly than in sheep, while the delivery of live, weak, term kids, or kids with tremors, occurs less commonly. In a New Zealand study, border disease was implicated or suspected in 23% of caprine abortions (Orr et al. 1987; Orr 1988). In an episode of naturally occurring caprine border disease in Norway, only one shaker kid was identified, but 43% of does in the herd were seropositive, a considerably higher percentage than observed in general field surveys (Løken et al. 1982). An outbreak of border disease affecting five goat herds was reported from Norway in which the source of infection was an orf vaccine contaminated with pestivirus (Løken et al. 1991). There was notable reproductive failure with barrenness, abortion, and birth of weak or dead kids, but no live offspring showed characteristic signs of border disease, though lambs present in one flock did show neurologic signs.

Pathogenesis

Horizontal and vertical transmission of the virus occurs. Horizontal transmission is believed to be by ingestion or aerosol inhalation of virus. The fetus is infected transplacentally. The outcome of intrauterine and fetal infection depends to a great extent on the time of infection, although virus strain variation and breed factors are believed to also play roles. In an experimental challenge of goats, infection at forty days of gestation resulted in no live kids born, infection at sixty days resulted in 11% live kids born, and infection at one hundred days in 73% live kids born (Løken and Bjerkås 1991).

Intrauterine infection produces a more severe placentitis in goats than in sheep and this may account for more frequent fetal death and less frequent delivery of full term shaker kids when compared with sheep (Barlow et al. 1975; Huck 1973). Fetuses infected *in utero* can result in birth of immunotolerant kids if infection occurs as late as one hundred days of gestation. Healthy appearing kids as well as shaker kids born to infected does can carry and shed the virus, serving as a source of new infections (Løken and Bjerkås 1991).

Goat fetuses and kids from experimentally infected does all show some characteristic CNS lesions, regardless of whether they show clinical signs of tremors after birth. Goat kids, however, do not have the characteristic dermal follicular changes associated with the hairy fleece in affected lambs (Orr and Barlow 1978).

Clinical Findings

Shaker kids and lambs show muscle tremors right from birth. These rhythmic tremors are most prominent in the hindquarters but may extend up the trunk and neck. The general impression is one of jerkiness. Affected young have difficulty rising and when they do, they have an awkward gait. Nursing is difficult and affected young may become quickly hypothermic and hypoglycemic. They appear weak, listless, and depressed if not attended to. The long bones of the limbs may feel finer than usual, and the head appears narrowed and exaggeratedly convex in the frontal area. No abnormalities of the hair coat or skin occur in affected goats (Orr and Barlow 1978). Does show no clinical signs other than a history of barrenness, abortion, stillbirth, or fetal mummification.

It is possible that clinical manifestations may vary depending on the specific pestivirus species or genotype infecting goats. For example, a border disease-like syndrome occurring in the Republic of Korea since 1998 included diarrhea and a high mortality rate in addition to the expected signs of abortions, stillbirths, and kids with neurologic signs. Laboratory investigations revealed that the causative agent was bovine viral diarrhea virus genotype 2 (BVDV-2) (Kim et al. 2006).

Clinical Pathology and Necropsy

Seroconversion against pestivirus antigens in association with abortion in a herd is suggestive of border disease. In the one reported field outbreak in Norway, 90% of does with serum neutralizing antibodies to the BVD virus had titers of 1:500 or more (Løken et al. 1982). In affected kids, absence of antibody does not rule out border disease, due to the possible development of *in utero* immunotolerance. For definitive diagnosis of border disease in abortion cases, it is recommended that formalin fixed fetal brain, fresh fetal kidney and liver, and maternal serum be submitted for histology, virus isolation, and serology (Orr 1988).

No gross lesions are observed at necropsy of affected kids. Histologic lesions in the CNS are characterized by pronounced hypomyelinogenesis, hypergliosis, and vasculitis, particularly in the white matter of the cerebrum and cerebellum. There is perivascular gliosis and infiltration of vessel walls with lymphocytes and histiocytes. Corpora amylacea are also noted. In aborting does, there is a marked placentitis with necrotizing caruncülitis. Virus may be isolated from uterine contents or vaginal discharges. Fetuses may be autolyzed, mummified, or grossly normal, but may show reduced numbers of myelinated fibers in the ventral spinal tracts histologically.

Diagnosis

Diagnosis is based on a history of reproductive failure, occurrence of newborn shaker kids, and laboratory confirmation of infection. The differential diagnoses for reproductive failure and abortion are discussed in Chapter 13. Hypoglycemia, septicemia, or meningitis may produce convulsions in newborn kids that could be mistaken for border disease shakers. When kids have difficulty rising, the following should be considered: nutritional muscular dystrophy, congenital vertebral malformations, spinal trauma, and swayback.

Treatment

There is no specific treatment. Supportive care to ensure regular feeding promotes kid survival, but the overall herd status must be considered with regard to the advisability of keeping potential carrier animals in the herd.

Control

All does that abort, regardless of cause, should be isolated from the herd. The border disease virus is present in vaginal discharges after abortion or kidding. In general, goats should be maintained separately from cattle and sheep. Does producing shaker kids should be culled on the presumption that they themselves are infected. Elimination of infection from the herd based on serologic testing is problematic because some nonreactors may in fact be persistently infected, immunotolerant shedders of the virus. In sheep, total depopulation with repopulation from virus-free flocks is suggested as the only possible means of disease eradication (Radostits et al. 2007).

The use of BVDV vaccine has been suggested in sheep flocks suffering annual outbreaks of border disease, but this pattern of disease has not been reported in goat herds. If vaccines are used, vaccine failures may occur because different strains of BVDV and BDV virus may not be cross-protective.

Louping-ill

Louping-ill, also known as ovine encephalomyelitis, is an acute, non-contagious, encephalomyelitis caused by the louping-ill virus (LIV), an enveloped, positive sense, single-stranded RNA virus in the genus *Flavivirus*. LIV is included in the tick borne encephalitis virus complex (TBEV) that also includes Kyasanur Forest disease virus and Alkhurma virus. Phylogenetic studies have been conducted on LIV (Gao et al. 1997; McGuire et al. 1998). The disease is documented to occur only in Scotland, England, Wales, Ireland, and Norway. There is also evidence of infection of sheep and goats with two additional Flaviviruses that have been recognized in Europe: the Greek goat encephalomyelitis virus (Papa et al. 2008) and the Spanish sheep encephalomyelitis virus that can cause disease similar to louping-ill (Gould et al. 2003).

The LIV is maintained primarily in populations of sheep, red grouse, and mountain hares on tick-infested moors or pastures. It is transmitted by the three-host tick vector *Ixodes ricinus*, which can transfer the virus transtadially but not transovarially. The virus may also be transferred by blood-contaminated needles, instruments, and contact with infected tissues.

Clinical disease occurs most commonly in sheep, but other animals are sporadically reported to be affected, including goats, dogs, horses, cattle, pigs, farmed red deer, and most recently llamas (Macaldowie et al. 2005). Louping-ill has serious zoonotic potential; the virus can produce fatal meningoencephalitis in humans. Because of the zoonotic risk, veterinarians and producers should observe proper safety precautions when handing sick animals or carcasses.

In sheep, the clinical signs include fever during the initial viremic stage followed by neurologic signs once the virus enters the CNS. These include fine muscle tremors, ataxia, nibbling motions, weakness, and collapse, with death occurring one to three days following onset of signs. During the course of the disease, the sheep may walk with jerky, stiff, almost bouncy movements, which account for the name louping-ill. There is one report of suspected louping-ill occurring in a goat recently arrived on the Scottish island of Islay (Gray et al. 1988). The suspect goat showed fever, trembling, forelimb weakness, and retching, became recumbent, and died. It had a high reciprocal hemagglutination inhibition antibody titer to the louping-ill virus and had characteristic histologic lesions in the brain.

Goats can be experimentally infected but appear to be more resistant than sheep (Reid et al. 1984). All challenged does became viremic and shed the virus in their milk for up to nine days after challenge. This resulted in infection of suckling kids with more severe clinical disease. These findings suggest that subclinically infected dairy goats could potentially transmit louping-ill to people consuming unpasteurized milk.

Confirmation of the disease requires histologic examination of the brain, virus isolation from CNS tissue, and serology using serum neutralization or hemagglutination inhibition assays. Recently, the use of TaqMan® reverse transcription polymerase chain reaction was reported to identify the virus in clinical specimens. The technique was faster than cell culture and identified virus in some specimens which gave negative cell culture results, presumably due to antibody interference (Marriott et al. 2006).

There is no specific treatment, but some affected animals may recover with nursing and supportive care. An inactivated tissue culture vaccine, which can be given to sheep, goats, and cattle, is in use in the U. K. A single dose should be administered four weeks before turn out to tick-infested pastures. Immunity is considered to last for at least two years.

Borna Disease

Borna disease is a non-suppurative viral polioencephalomyelitis which historically has affected horses and sheep in central Europe. Recent studies suggest that the virus is more widely distributed than previously thought, that species other than horses and sheep may be infected, and that the disease also may be an emerging zoonosis, though the latter point remains controversial. Goats can be infected experimentally (Ihlenburg 1962) and there is evidence that naturally occurring caprine cases have occurred, though rarely. Several reviews of progress in the understanding of Borna disease and the controversies surrounding it have been published (Ludwig and Bode 2000; Staeheli et al. 2000; Dauphin et al. 2002; Dürrwald et al. 2006).

Etiology

The causative virus is now identified as Borna disease virus in the newly created family *Bornaviridae* in the order Mononegavirales. It is an enveloped, single-stranded, negative sense RNA virus measuring 100 to 130 nm in diameter. Several unique aspects of the virus led to the creation of the new *Bornaviridae* family as summarized by Dauphin et al. (2002). Borna disease virus is the only negative, non-segmented, single-stranded RNA animal virus with a nuclear site of replication and transcription. Its genome compaction is overcome by the overlapping of ORF and transcription units and by post-transcriptional RNA splicing. The virus is characterized by strict neurotropism. It is noncytolytic and has a low rate of replication and persistence in the CNS. Unlike the majority of other RNA viruses, the Borna disease virus genome sequence is extremely stable over time.

Epidemiology

The disease has been known for almost two centuries in horses in southwestern Germany and the name is associated with the town of Borna in Saxony where the disease later emerged and peaked in the 1890s. The disease is also recognized to affect sheep. Reports of the disease in those two species remained localized to Germany for most of the history of the disease until it spread through the Rhine valley to Switzerland, Austria, and Liechtenstein starting in the 1970s. In this enzootic region of central Europe, horses and sheep remain the principal species affected, but there have also been confirmations in small numbers of cattle, donkeys, dogs, deer, rabbits, South American camelids, and goats. The goat cases were recorded in Switzerland, two from a single premises in 1987 and a single case in 1995 (Caplazi et al. 1999). The diagnoses were retrospective by immunohistochemistry. No clinical descriptions were provided.

In the 1960s, there were reports of a neurologic condition in the Middle East. It was first described as Near East Equine Encephalitis but then later proposed as Borna disease based on clinical and histopathological similarities, including the presence of Joest-Degen bodies in the brains of affected horses, a characteristic of Borna disease (Daubney 1967). Two cases of putative Borna disease in goats in Lebanon were included in those reports (Daubney 1967). It now appears unlikely that these were truly cases of Borna disease (Rott et al. 2004).

Contemporary understanding of Borna disease suggests that the cases described were caused by a virus other than Borna disease virus because Borna disease virus does not produce a cytopathic effect in cell culture. Moreover, the lesion profile described is not consistent with the histopathology of classical Borna disease, and the inclusion bodies initially identified as Joest-Degen bodies may in fact have been multiple nucleoli, which occur quite often in large neurons (Ehrensperger, personal communication 2007).

More recently, Borna disease virus has been reported to be responsible for disease occurrences in ostriches in Israel (Malkinson et al. 1993), cats in Sweden (Lundgren and Ludwig 1993), and horses in Japan (Taniyama et al. 2001) and Iran (Bahmani et al. 1996). The virus appears to have a much more cosmopolitan distribution that goes beyond the enzootic region of central Europe. In 2006, subclinical infections were reported in Chongqing goats in China based on detection of Borna disease virus p24 gene in brain tissue and peripheral blood mononuclear cells (Zhao et al. 2006)

Borna disease has also been considered as a possible cause of neurologic and psychiatric disease in humans in various countries including the United States, Japan, and Germany (Rott et al. 1991). The role of Borna disease virus in human disease remains controversial and the evidence for and against has been recently reviewed (Chalmers et al. 2005; Dürrwald et al. 2007).

In the enzootic region of central Europe, Borna disease historically has a seasonal occurrence with a peak in the spring. This has led to the presumption that an agent reservoir exists, most likely in wildlife populations, though considerable efforts have been undertaken to identify such reservoirs without definitive success. Most recently it has been suggested that the bicolored, white toothed shrew (*Crocidura leucodon*) may serve the role of agent reservoir (Hilbe et al. 2006).

Knowledge of the transmission of Borna virus is incomplete. The virus is shed in nasal, salivary, and conjunctival secretions and inhalation and ingestion are considered to be important routes of transmission. Viral RNA and proteins are also found in peripheral blood mononuclear cells so blood-borne infection may be possible. However, some efforts to demonstrate horizontal transmission from horse to horse or sheep to sheep have been unsuccessful (Staeheli et al. 2000). Infected animals develop an antibody response but it is not protective. The role of carrier animals in transmission remains unclear.

Clinical Findings

Clinical findings in goats are not well documented. In other species, the clinical presentation reflects neurologic disease, but specific signs may vary between affected animals and include behavioral changes, paresthesia, motor dysfunction, incoordination, paralysis, and death. In sheep, disturbances of sensory function are more pronounced than signs of motor dysfunction, which are more predominant in horses. However, head pressing, staggering, and ataxia are reported in sheep as the clinical course progresses over a period of four to ten days (Ludwig and Bode 2000).

In the putative cases of caprine Borna disease reported from Lebanon, the clinical findings included fever, anxiety, bleating, salivation, champing of the jaws, partial facial paralysis, fine tremors, head pressing, circling, paraplegia, convulsions, and death (Daubney 1967).

Clinical Pathology and Necropsy

Serologic tests can be applied to blood or cerebrospinal fluid. Western blot, ELISA, and immunofluorescence assay (IFA) have been applied with the latter considered to be the most sensitive. Antibody levels may be low in acute clinical cases of Borna disease so serological tests must have a high sensitivity. Antibodies may be undetectable in subacute and chronic cases (Dauphin et al. 2002). For these reasons, efforts to identify virus or viral antigen should also be pursued.

Virus isolation in cell culture can be attempted from the brain tissues of affected animals but the number of infectious particles may be low, leading to false negative results. Immunohistochemistry may be more rewarding. Reverse transcriptase-polymerase chain reaction is now being used to detect virus in blood and brain tissue.

Gross lesions are non-specific and may include mild leptomeningitis, congestion of cerebral vessels, and hemorrhage between the cerebrum and cerebellum. Histological changes are consistent with viral encephalitis and are characterized by perivascular and parenchymal infiltration of lymphocytes in affected portions of the brain. Characteristic inclusion bodies, known as Joest-Degen bodies, may be present in the nuclei of infected neurons but their presence is variable.

Diagnosis

A presumptive diagnosis may be made on the basis of encephalitic signs in goats in countries or regions where Borna disease is enzootic, with the realization that the disease is quite rare in goats and that there are more common causes of caprine encephalitis. Definitive diagnosis is by laboratory confirmation. Other possible causes of acute encephalitic signs in goats include rabies, pseudorabies, polioencephalomalacia, bacterial meningoencephalitis, and possibly CAE.

Treatment and Control

There is no treatment for Borna disease and the prognosis for recovery is guarded. In species other than goats, affected animals sometimes recover spontaneously but then relapse. The disease does not occur commonly in goats and specific control measures directed toward goats are not formulated. Given the possible zoonotic potential of Borna disease and other conditions such as rabies that may appear like Borna disease, proper precautions should be taken when handling clinical cases or during necropsy.

West Nile Encephalomyelitis

West Nile encephalomyelitis is caused by West Nile virus (WNV), a mosquito-borne flavivirus. WNV can infect numerous species of mammals, birds, and even some reptiles, but causes clinical, neurologic disease mainly in horses and humans. To date there are no confirmed cases of the disease in goats from anywhere in the world, though antibodies to WNV are readily detectable in goats in those regions where WNV is present and circulating through mosquito populations. This indicates that goats can be infected with WNV following the bite of mosquitoes and that they mount an immune response but their likelihood of developing clinical disease is very low. Therefore, a diagnosis of West Nile encephalomyelitis should not be made in a goat with neurologic disease based solely on the presence of antibody to WNV in a single serum sample. A four-fold rise in titer between acute and convalescent serum samples taken ten to fourteen days apart and initiated at the onset of disease would be far more convincing, but other causes of neurologic disease in goats should nevertheless be ruled out.

Etiology and epidemiology

West Nile virus is a single-stranded RNA virus in the genus *Flavivirus* and is a member of the Japanese encephalitis virus serocomplex. Members of this group of flaviviruses have a close antigenic relationship, which accounts for serologic cross-reactions that occur in laboratory diagnosis. These viruses include WNV, Japanese encephalitis, St. Louis encephalitis, Murray Valley encephalitis, and Kunjin virus (Petersen and Marfin 2002).

WNV is an arbovirus and is maintained in a primary enzootic cycle involving *Culex* spp. mosquitoes and wild birds of many species. Migratory birds may carry the infection to new locations and infection may become established in those locations if there are suitable mosquito hosts present. In temperate regions, mosquitoes hatch in the late spring and feed on birds through the spring and summer so that the virus population in birds and mosquitoes is much amplified by late summer/early autumn. At that time, certain populations of mosquitoes which serve as "bridge vectors" also feed on humans and horses and other mammals, as well as on birds, creating a secondary cycle that can lead to clinical disease in humans and horses and possibly other animals. Humans, horses, and other mammals, however, do not produce sufficient viremia in response to WNV infection to pass the virus back to mosquitoes and are therefore dead-end hosts. The primary bird/mosquito cycle is required to maintain the WNV reservoir.

The name of the virus derives from the fact that it was first isolated from a woman with fever in the West Nile district of Uganda in 1937. The first documented disease epidemic in humans associated with WNV occurred in Israel in 1951 (Bernkopf et al. 1953). The virus became recognized or established in many countries of Africa, the Middle East, western Asia, and southern Europe in subsequent years, affecting horses as well as humans. In 1999, the disease was introduced to North America with the first cases recognized in birds in New York City. By 2005, the virus was present in *Culex* spp. mosquitoes and/or wild bird populations in all forty-eight of the continental United States and most states had reported human and/or equine cases. The disease is now widespread in Mexico and Canada as well. It is not clear how the disease was introduced into North America.

Among the domestic animals, horses and other equids are the most likely to exhibit clinical disease following infection, and among domestic poultry, geese and very young chickens are most likely to become ill. Farmed alligators have been definitively diagnosed with West Nile encephalitis in Georgia and Florida (Miller et al. 2003; Jacobson et al. 2005). Clinical illness in ruminants is rare and experimental infection of ruminants is not consistently achieved (McLean et al. 2002). There have been no reported cases in goats, even from countries such as Israel which has a reasonably large goat population and where the virus has been endemic for more than fifty years (Zamir 2007). A case of West Nile encephalitis in a six-month-old sheep from Nebraska was confirmed by reverse transcriptase polymerase chain reaction (RT-PCR) assay in 2002 (Callan and Van Metre 2004) and a second two-year-old sheep from Missouri was confirmed with West Nile encephalitis by similar methods the same year (Tyler et al. 2003). In camelids, eight of seventeen alpacas demonstrating neurologic signs were confirmed as having West Nile encephalitis by PCR in Colorado in 2003 (Callan and Van Metre 2004).

While there are no reported clinical cases in goats, there are numerous reports of goats with circulating antibody to WNV. Countries where serologic surveys have revealed WNV antibody-positive goats include Romania with 3.2% of goats sampled testing positive (Topica et al. 1971), Greece with 8.7% (Koptopoulos and Papadopoulos 1980), Pakistan with less than 5% (Go 1990), India with 6.75% (Mall et a1. 1995), and Nigeria with 18% (Olaleye et al. 1990). Antibody to WNV has also been identified in goats in the United States (Bowen 2007). This data underscores the fact that goats are regularly exposed to WNV in enzootic countries. The lack of clinical case reports suggests that they are either resistant to infection or that the low level viremia associated with ruminant species is unlikely to result in clinical manifestation of disease. There are concerns, however, that more virulent strains of WNV are emerging and the disease patterns in mammalian species may change in the future as a result (McLean et al. 2002).

Clinical Findings

Because there are no reported confirmed cases in goats, no reliable clinical findings can be reported for this species. In humans, the most common presenting signs are fever, weakness, nausea, vomiting, and changes in mental status or confusion (Petersen and Marfin 2002). In horses, a retrospective study of 569 cases indicated the following signs present, in decreasing order of frequency: incoordination, muscle tremors, twitching of the face or muzzle, weakness or paralysis of limbs, caudal paresis, recumbency or difficulty rising, lip droop, teeth grinding, fever, circling, and blindness. Of the 569 horses, 345 (61%) recovered, 126 (22%) died, and ninety-eight (17%) had an unknown outcome (Schuler et al. 2004).

In the two reported cases in sheep, both animals presented in recumbency of five to seven days duration. One sheep showed muscle fasciculation as well as hyperesthesia with brief muscle spasms and extensor rigidity when touched. It also exhibited tonic clonic convulsions of short duration on presentation. These convulsions became more frequent and severe and the animal was euthanized (Tyler et al. 2003). The second sheep was mentally depressed, unable to stand, and exhibited spontaneous nystagmus as well as muscle fasciculation. It too was euthanized (Callan and Van Metre 2004).

Clinical Pathology and Necropsy

There are no reports of laboratory or necropsy findings in goats with West Nile virus encephalitis. In other species, CSF analysis may reveal an elevated protein and increased cellularity comprised of lymphocytes and large mononuclear cells.

At necropsy, in other species gross lesions in the CNS are limited to focal hemorrhage in the brain or spinal cord on cut section. Histologically, there is mild to moderate, multifocal, lymphocytic polioencephalomyelitis with perivascular cuffing, microgliosis, and some neuronal degeneration in severely affected areas (Cantile et al. 2001).

Diagnosis

In horses, the most commonly affected domestic mammal, diagnosis of WNV is currently based on observation of compatible clinical signs such as ataxia, paresis, paralysis, hyperesthesia, muscle fasciculation, seizures, or fever, and on one or more of the following: virus isolation or reverse transcriptase–polymerase chain reaction (RT-PCR) detection of WNV from tissue, blood, or cerebrospinal fluid; a four-fold increase in plaque reduction neutralization test (PRNT) antibody titers between paired serum samples taken two weeks apart (in temporal association with clinical signs of disease); detection of IgM antibody to WNV by IgM-capture ELISA; or a neutralizing titer of more than 1:10 by PRNT in a single serum sample (Kleiboeker et al. 2004).

As the intensity of viremia and the strength of the antibody response may differ in goats relative to horses, it is not clear that these same diagnostic criteria would apply to goats. The most reliable criterion for goats would likely be documentation of a four-fold rise in titer between two serum samples, one taken at the start of clinical disease and the other ten to fourteen days later.

A necropsy should be performed with histopathologic examination of the CNS in goats that die with neurologic signs, as much to rule out other important diseases as to rule in WNV infection. The differential diagnosis should at least include rabies and listeriosis in any goat, pregnancy toxemia in pregnant females, and caprine arthritis encephalitis in young goats. If other conditions are ruled out and WVN is still under consideration, then immunohistochemistry and/or PCR techniques on brain and spinal cord should be conducted to identify WNV antigen.

Treatment and Prevention

There is no specific treatment for WNV encephalitis. Affected animals may recover, so efforts to provide supportive and nursing care are justified to ensure proper nutrition and hydration and to prevent injuries associated with incoordination or prolonged recumbency. Efforts to control mosquitoes around goats and goat barns may be justified. Commercial WNV vaccines are available for use in horses, but they are not approved for use in goats or other ruminants. Given the absence of reports of confirmed clinical disease in goats, there is no apparent economic justification for the use of WNV vaccines in goats.

BACTERIAL DISEASES

Listeriosis

Listeriosis is an important infectious disease of goats most commonly associated with neurologic disease, but also capable of causing septicemia and abortion. The organism can be shed in the milk of healthy-appearing carrier goats as well as in the milk of sick goats. The zoonotic potential of listeriosis from milk and dairy products is a growing concern.

Etiology

Listeria monocytogenes is a motile, aerobic and facultative anaerobic, small, Gram-positive rod. It produces a narrow zone of beta hemolysis on blood agar. It is capable of growth over a wide pH range of 5.5 to 9.6 and a temperature range of 37.5°F to 113°F (3°C to 45°C), but optimal growth occurs at pH 7 to 7.2 and a temperature range of 68°F to 104°F (20°C to 40°C). Isolation of the organism from tissues and organic materials such as animal feeds can be difficult, so dispersion of tissues in a blender, cold enrichment of samples, subculturing from tryptose phosphate enrichment broth, and use of selective media such as trypaflavine nalidixic acid serum agar have been recommended (Dijkstra 1984). Newer selective plating media are now available, including polymixin acriflavine LiCl cetazidime esculin mannitol (PAL-CAM) and Oxford agar, which isolate *Listeria* on the basis of esculin hydrolysis, as well as chromogenic media, which allow rapid visualization of *Listeria* colonies and differentiation of *L. monocytogenes* and *L. ivanovii* from other *Listeria* spp. *L. ivanovii* is considered non-pathogenic to humans but is pathogenic for mice and has been associated with abortions in sheep and cattle (Low and Donachie 1997). In one recent report, abortions were reported in sheep in a mixed sheep and goat flock, but the goats were not affected (Santagada et al. 2004).

Though easily killed by common disinfectants, *L. monocytogenes* can survive in feces, silage, and tissue for five or more years (Dijkstra 1984a). There are now sixteen known serotypes with numerous subtypes. Serotype 4, especially type 4b, and to a lesser extent serotype 1 have been associated with encephalitis and septicemia in goats. Abortion is associated primarily with serotype 1 (Deligaris et al. 1975; Kummeneje 1975; Løken et al. 1982a; Dijkstra 1984b). In one outbreak of listeriosis in goats, the same serotype, 4b, was recovered from goats with encephalitis and from goats with abortion (Wiedmann et al. 1999). It was hypothesized that transmission in this herd outbreak was by the venereal route. Serotypes 1/2a, 1/2b, and 4b are the serotypes most commonly isolated from human cases of listeriosis and from livestock cases.

Because *L. monocytogenes* is widely distributed in nature, characterization of environmental isolates by serotyping or phylogenetic analysis is necessary to confirm their association with disease outbreaks. Techniques such as pulse field gel electrophoresis (PFGE) and ribotyping have become useful tools of molecular epidemiology to improve understanding of the ecology and transmission of *L. monocytogenes* on farms and in food processing facilities and to track the origin of pathogenic strains associated with food-borne outbreaks of listeriosis (Sauders et al. 2003). There is growing evidence that strains of the organism are not host-specific and that food animals and farms may serve as a reservoir for strains of *L. monocytogenes* that can lead to human infections (Nightingale et al. 2004; Okwumabua et al. 2005).

Epidemiology

As many as forty species of birds and mammals, including humans, can be infected with *L. monocytogenes* and the organism has been isolated on six continents. Listeriosis is a well known, sporadic clinical problem in intensively managed dairy goats in North America and Europe. In France, 4.9% of fecal samples from sheep and goats in ninety-eight flocks yielded *L. monocytogenes* (Nicolas et al. 1974). A seroepidemiologic study in Spain identified infection in 5% of goat herds tested (Perea-Remujo et al. 1984). Caprine listeriosis has also been reported from Japan (Asahi et al. 1954), South Africa (Du Toit 1977), Australia (Baxendell 1980), India (Phadke et al. 1979; Chattopadhyay et al. 1985), Brazil (Rissi et al. 2006), and Turkey (Borku et al. 2006). In New Zealand, it was reported as the most common neurologic disease of goats identified at necropsy (Thompson 1985).

Factors predisposing to clinical listeriosis in goats are similar to those reported for other farm animals and include sudden changes in weather, feeding regimens, or general management procedures; confinement in winter, particularly if overcrowded and with poor sanitation; increased stress from poor nutrition, parasitism, or other concurrent disease; advanced pregnancy; and the feeding of silage, particularly poor quality silage. The feeding of silage is often emphasized as a key predisposing factor in ruminant listeriosis (Morin 2004). However, a history of silage feeding is not a prerequisite in outbreaks of caprine listeriosis (Wood 1972; Du Toit 1977). The author has been engaged in several outbreaks of encephalitic listeriosis in goats in which there was no history of silage feeding. Johnson et al. (1996) reported on the occurrence of encephalitic listeriosis in goat herds in Missouri. None of the herds in which the disease was diagnosed had access to silage; all of the affected herds had woody browse as their main source of feed and Angora goats were the most commonly affected breed.

An increased occurrence of listeriosis in fall and winter has also been observed in goats, though cases can occur year-round. The disease is most common in adult goats. Based on experimental challenge studies, goats are more susceptible to *L. monocytogenes* infection than sheep (Gupta et al. 1980). A survey from Greece based on microbial cultures of brains from animals with neurologic signs of disease also found that goat herds were affected with encephalitic listeriosis more frequently than sheep flocks, with serotype 4b being predominant (Giannati-Stefanou et al. 2006).

The source of infection in herds is not always clear. Wild mammals and birds may be original sources of the bacteria, which then persist in soil and on plants. Goats exposed to such soil and crops may become latent carriers. During periods of stress they may become clinically ill, or shed large numbers of organisms in the feces, spreading the infection to other goats, particularly under intensive rearing conditions. Purchase of latent carrier animals may introduce the infection into previously naive herds.

Active proliferation of the bacteria in silage occurs in silage-associated outbreaks, resulting in heavy challenge to animals eating the material. Proliferation of bacteria is enhanced by poor silage quality with pH levels above 5. In one caprine outbreak, pieces of a pheasant were found chopped into the silage and the tissues of the bird were positive for *L. monocytogenes* (Dijkstra 1984b). In addition to the presence of the bacteria, the feeding of silage has been shown to have some intrinsic immunosuppressive effect in sheep, leading to decreased circulating lymphocyte numbers and reduced serum total protein. This may additionally aggravate susceptibility to *Listeria* organisms present in the feed.

Recent studies have identified some differences in the ecology and transmission of *L. monocytogenes* on cattle farms as compared to sheep and goat farms in upstate New York. Cattle farms had a higher level of environmental contamination with *L. monocytogenes* than small ruminant farms whether the cattle had a history of clinical listeriosis (case farms) or not (control farms). When small ruminant case farms were compared with bovine case farms, isolation of *L. monocytogenes* in small ruminant fecal samples was significantly less common than in bovine fecal samples. However, the organism was significantly more common in feed samples from small ruminant case farms than from bovine case farms, indicating that listeriosis on goat and sheep farms is more likely transmitted via feed than feces. On all farms, soil samples were positive more commonly than were feed samples, indicating that soil is an important source of feed contamination with *L. monocytogenes*.

These findings suggest that small ruminants are less likely to appreciably amplify ingested *L. monocytogenes* than cattle (Nightingale et al. 2004). In a related study (Nightingale et al. 2005), it was noted that the prevalence of *L. monocytogenes* on small ruminant farms peaked during the winter and the prevalence of *L. monocytogenes* in all samples collected from small ruminant farms was notably lower during the summer and fall. The number of healthy animals on cattle and small ruminant farms that were shedding *L. monocytogenes* in feces was most affected by season, with the prevalence of fecal shedding peaking in the winter and spring. Confinement housing and the quality of feeds fed in winter were believed to contribute to this pattern.

While direct transmission of *L. monocytogenes* from animals to humans can occur, it is uncommon. In such cases human symptoms are usually limited to localized cutaneous infections. Much more common is the transmission of the infection to humans via foods of animal origin. Zoonotic infection from goat milk and goat milk products is a very real concern. *Listeria monocytogenes* can be shed in the milk of clinically affected goats as well as normal-appearing latent carriers. Shedding is less likely in the encephalitic form of the disease than in the septicemic or abortion forms. In latent carriers, the intensity of shedding is increased toward the end of gestation (Grønstøl 1984). *Listeria monocytogenes* has resisted pasteurization at 143°F (61.7°C) for thirty-five minutes, but is killed by high-temperature short-time pasteurization at 160.9°F (71.6°C) for fifteen seconds. The intraleukocytic location of some of the organisms in milk presumably contributes to this pasteurization resistance (Blenden et al. 1987). Experimentally, the organism has been reisolated from semi-soft, aged, goat milk cheeses made from unpasteurized, *L. monocytogenes*-inoculated goat milk as long as eighteen weeks after preparation (Tham 1988). The organism has been isolated from retailed, pasteurized, fluid goat milk in the UK (Roy 1988). In a study in Sri Lanka, *L. monocytogenes* was recovered from raw goat milk, standard pasteurized milk, and cheese, but not from sterilized milk, ultra-high temperature (UHT) milk, yogurt, or curd (Jayamanne and Samarajeewa 2001).

Not all listerial contamination of processed dairy products has the original milk as its source. Cross-contamination or recontamination after pasteurization can occur in processing plants if the strictest sanitation and hygiene are not observed. It is known that *L. monocytogenes* readily produces biofilms, which are microbial communities that strongly adhere to underlying surfaces. Biofilms can persist on processing equipment that is not scrupulously cleaned and disinfected. This can also occur on the farm, in that biofilms on milking machines can be a recurring source of contamination of bulk tank milk (Zundel et al. 2003). In a survey of 405 goat dairies in Spain, 2.56% of bulk tank samples were positive for *L. monocytogenes*. The isolates were most common in samples taken in the fall and winter and were rare in spring and summer (Gaya et al. 1996).

When goats have the septicemic or abortion form of listeriosis, the organism may be present in large numbers in feces, milk, birth fluids, placenta, fetuses, and newborn kids. Given the zoonotic potential of these materials for veterinarians and animal caretakers, appropriate precautions should be taken against infection when handling such tissues.

Pathogenesis

In the encephalitic form of listeriosis, the organism gains entrance to nerve endings in the oral cavity via breaks in the oral mucosa caused by coarse food, dental abrasions, or the loss of deciduous teeth. It then migrates up the nerves to the brain stem, where it stimulates a localized inflammatory response in the form of microabscesses comprised primarily of neutrophils. It is believed that *L. monocytogenes* primarily induces a cell-mediated immune response in the host and the severity of the resulting lesions may be mediated by the degree of immune recognition of the organism. Microabscesses are most common in the medulla and lead to destruction of cranial nerve nuclei, notably nerves V through IX. The cranial nerve deficits seen clinically reflect this process. Occasionally, generalized meningitis can occur in addition to focal encephalitis. The incubation period in the encephalitic form may be two to three weeks.

In the septicemic form, the incubation period may be as short as one day. The organism is believed to gain entry through the intestinal mucosa. There is an initial bacteremia with fever. This may be followed by recovery, development of a latent carrier state, or progression to more severe clinical disease. Because the morbidity rate is often low in outbreaks of septicemic listeriosis, it is presumed that many animals handle transient bacteremia effectively and are only subclinically infected. When animals do become ill they may die within forty-eight hours or the illness may last for several weeks. Pregnant does abort several days after the initial fever and aborted fetuses also show evidence of septicemia. Septicemic goats may excrete the organism in feces and milk during and after clinical illness. Newborn kids exposed to the colostrum or milk of infected does can show signs of septicemia in the first few days of life. Seroconversion is marked in goats after septicemic listeriosis but mild in goats after encephalitic listeriosis (Løken and Grønstøl 1982).

Ocular forms of listeriosis are also reported in cattle and sheep (Morin 2004). Keratoconjunctivitis and iritis appears to result from direct contact of the eye with *Listeria* present in silage during the act of feeding ("silage eye"). The condition is not well documented in goats. Harwood (2004) reports unilateral or bilateral keratoconjunctivitis occurring in a goat herd concurrently with the encephalitic form of listeriosis, but not specifically in association with silage feeding.

Clinical Findings

The encephalitic form is the most common in goats. Though unusual, septicemic and encephalitic listeriosis have been reported in the same goat herd (Løken and Grønstøl 1982).

The initial signs of the encephalitic form are nonspecific and include depression, decreased appetite, a decrease in milk production, and a transient fever of up to 107.6°F (42°C). These prodromal signs may be followed by incoordination and hemiparesis with a tendency for the goat to lean, stumble, or move in one direction only. This tendency progresses to obvious torticollis and circling in the same direction. In advanced cases, the goat may be recumbent with the head pulled tightly into the flank, unable to straighten the neck voluntarily (Figure 5.4a).

Deficits of the facial nerve are also common and may occur with or without concurrent hemiparesis and circling. The signs are usually unilateral and include ear droop, ptosis, flaccid buccal muscles with accumulation of feed in the buccal pouch, salivation, and a collapsed nostril (Figure 5.4b). Slack jaw, weak tongue, impaired swallowing, and nystagmus may also be seen. When lesions are bilateral, some of these deficits may be paradoxically less obvious since the abnormalities are symmetrical. Keratitis may be observed as a sequela to abnormal eyelid function. Loss of excessive saliva through drooling and the inability to swallow can lead to acid-base imbalance, electrolyte and fluid losses, dehydration, and weakness. The course of encephalitic listeriosis in goats is usually one to four days, which is shorter than that observed in cattle. The morbidity rate is variable, but the mortality rate can be high.

The septicemic form also begins with depression, loss of appetite, decreased milk production, and fever up to 107.6°F (42°C). In these cases, fever may persist and the animal grows progressively weaker over the next several days. Neurologic signs rarely develop, but diarrhea, often bloody, is a common finding in goats. Goats may die within a few days or remain ill for several weeks. Pregnant does abort several days after the onset of septicemia. They may not necessarily show severe signs of septicemia.

Figure 5.4. Clinical presentations of encephalitic listeriosis in goats.

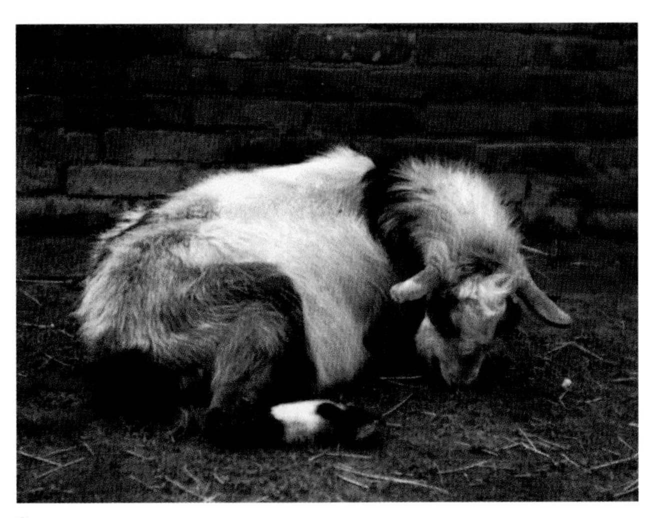

a

Figure 5.4a. An adult buck with listeriosis in recumbency with torso, neck, and head drawn tightly to one side and with profound depression. (Courtesy of Dr. Daan Dercksen.)

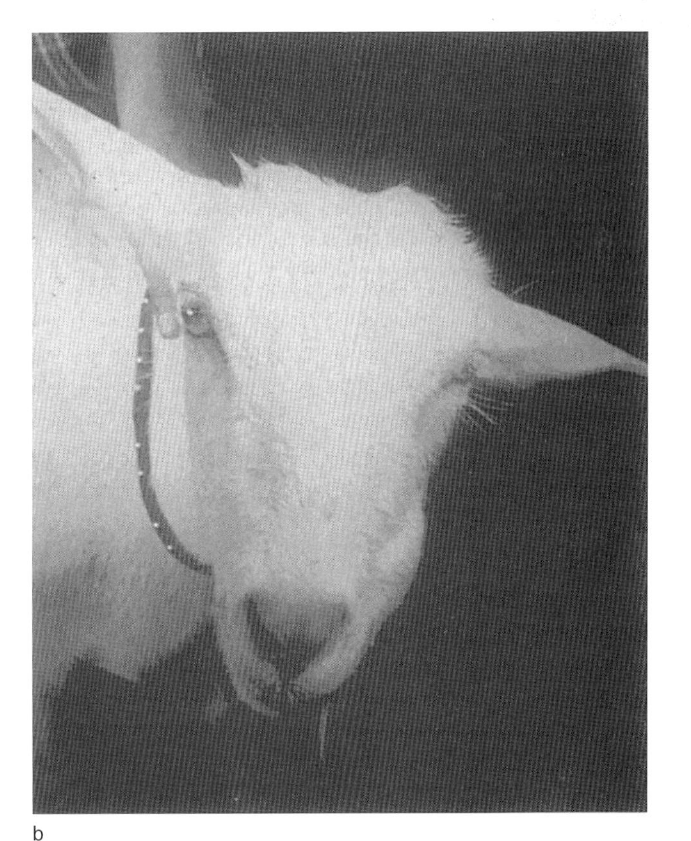

b

Figure. 5.4b. Adult goat with left facial nerve paralysis due to listeriosis. Note drooped left ear and eyelid, swelling of left cheek due to accumulation of food in buccal space, collapsed left nostril, and drooling. (Reproduced by permission of Dr. C.S.F. Williams.)

Clinical Pathology and Necropsy

The hemogram may remain normal, particularly in the encephalitic form of the disease, or show a neutrophilic leukocytosis. The monocytosis seen in laboratory animals does not occur in ruminants. Analysis of the cerebrospinal fluid may be helpful. Protein levels and cell counts are typically moderately elevated. The cells are predominantly monocytes and lymphocytes, with some neutrophils also present. Bacteria are rarely seen in the CSF, and culture from the CSF is almost always unrewarding.

Historically, serology, while useful for epidemiologic studies, has not been widely applied for diagnosis of individual cases (Morin 2004). A number of different serodiagnostic techniques have been employed using crude antigens, but a general limitation for all these techniques was a lack of specificity, with cross reactions to other Gram-positive organisms being common (Low and Donachie 1997). Another practical limitation is that in cases of encephalitic listeriosis, affected animals do not appear to mount a consistent, detectable humoral immune response, in contrast to cases of septicemic listeriosis. An increase in indirect hemagglutination titer is reported after septicemic listeriosis, but not after the encephalitic form (Løken et al. 1982a). Sero-agglutination was found to be unsatisfactory as a screening test for accurately identifying herds with enzootic listeriosis (Nicolas et al. 1974).

ELISA tests have been developed in recent years to detect antibodies against a specific antigen, listeriolysin O, which is an extra-cellular 58 kDa haemolysin, produced by all the pathogenic strains of *L. monocytogenes* (Elezebeth et al. 2007). As with other tests, it does not appear to be a reliable indicator of acute phase disease in cases of encephalitic listeriosis. The kinetics of the antibody response to listeriolysin O in experimentally infected goats has been reported (Rekha et al. 2006).

Culture of *L. monocytogenes* should be attempted for definitive diagnosis, recognizing that the organism may be difficult to isolate without special enrichment methods. In the septicemic and abortion forms of the disease, feces, milk, and aborted fetuses are suitable specimens. Experimentally infected septicemic goats shed *L. monocytogenes* in the feces for twenty-eight days after infection but only two days in milk. Stomach contents, spleen, and liver of the fetus are tissues most likely to be positive on direct culture without enrichment (Gupta et al. 1980). In the encephalitic form, fresh brain should be submitted for culture, especially brain stem. Grinding of brain tissue and refrigeration at 39°F (4°C) before culturing can improve the chance of a positive culture. Occasionally goats with the encephalitic form are fecal culture positive. Culture of silage is also indicated when silage is implicated. However, the distribution of organisms in silage may be uneven and the offending portions may be long gone by the time clinical disease is observed.

Gross post mortem findings are uncommon in the encephalitic form of the disease, though visible, focal gray discoloration and malacia of the brain stem have been observed in affected goats (Wood 1972). The CSF may be cloudy and the meninges congested. In most cases, lesions are identified histologically, and consist of focal microabscesses principally in the medulla but also in the pons and cerebellum. These abscesses are comprised primarily of neutrophils. Perivascular cuffing with mononuclear cells and neutrophils, diffuse microgliosis, and a mononuclear infiltrate of the meninges may also be seen. For definitive diagnosis, a large portion of the brain with brain stem should be submitted fresh for bacterial culture. However, recent reports indicate that immunohistochemistry performed on CNS tissues is much more reliable than bacterial culture for confirming the presence of *L. monocytogenes* in tissues (Ehrensperger et al. 2001; Loeb 2004).

In the septicemic form, multiple foci of necrosis may be seen in liver, spleen, kidney, and heart. Multiple, small yellowish spots on the liver of aborted fetuses are highly suggestive of listeriosis. Placentitis and endometritis may also be observed in does that abort. Successful culture is most likely from the liver, spleen, lung, and uterus of septicemic adults.

Diagnosis

Neurologic diseases that can produce localizing signs consistent with a diagnosis of listeriosis include the neurologic form of CAE, focal brain abscesses, cerebrospinal nematodiasis, coenurosis, middle ear infections, bacterial meningitis, early rabies, and trauma to the facial nerve. Recumbent animals in advanced stage of encephalitic listeriosis may be misdiagnosed. In a survey of sixty-seven encephalitic listeriosis cases in goats and sheep, twelve of the animals were not diagnosed with the disease until necropsy. Six had a working diagnosis of polioencephalomalacia (cerebrocortical necrosis), one was diagnosed with ketosis, one with pulmonary emphysema, and in four no specific diagnosis was made (Braun et al. 2002).

The differential diagnosis for septicemic listeriosis, particularly when diarrhea is present, includes salmonellosis, yersiniosis, and enterotoxemia. When weakness predominates and diarrhea is absent, milk fever, and pregnancy toxemia should be ruled out. Causes of abortion in which the doe shows clinical signs of illness are discussed in Chapter 13.

Treatment

Early intervention improves the prognosis for recovery. Goats already recumbent rarely respond favorably to treatment and a poor prognosis should be given for recumbent animals. Penicillins, tetracyclines, and where permitted, chloramphenicol, are effective antibiotics. Adult goats with the septicemic form of disease responded favorably to intramuscular penicillin administered for three consecutive days at a dose of 2.5 g per day, but shorter courses of therapy were less effective (Løken and Grønstøl 1982). In the encephalitic form, intravenous sodium penicillin at a dose of 40,000 IU/kg every six hours until improvement is noted, followed by a seven-day course of intramuscular procaine penicillin at a dose of 20,000 IU/kg twice a day has been recommended (Brewer 1983). Oxytetracycline should be given intravenously at a dose of 10 mg/kg twice a day for at least three days. These high dosage levels are necessary to promote passage of antibiotic across the blood brain barrier and development of high-tissue concentrations in the CNS.

It has been reported that ampicillin or amoxicillin given in conjunction with gentamicin is the treatment regimen of choice in human listeriosis cases. The use of a combination of gentamicin given at a dose of 3 mg/kg bw IV BID and amoxicillin given at a dose of 7 mg/kg bw IM BID was reported in one retrospective case study in small ruminants (Braun et al. 2002). The outcomes for sheep and goats treated with gentamicin/ampicillin were better than those treated with either penicillin or oxytetracycline. However, more of the animals treated with gentamicin/amoxicillin had a favorable prognosis at the onset of therapy because they were not yet recumbent. The use of gentamicin in goats is problematic due to prolonged antibiotic residues in meat and milk.

Dexamethasone given once a day at a dose of 0.1 mg/kg intravenously has also been used in conjunction with antibiotics in the treatment of encephalitic listeriosis with the rationale that steroids may suppress the infiltration of mononuclear cells that lead to microabscesses in the brain stem. The nonsteroidal anti-inflammatory drug flunixin meglumine has been used at a dose of 2.2 mg/kg bw IV SID in the treatment of goats with encephalitic listeriosis but its contribution to a favorable outcome is not documented.

Supportive therapy in the form of fluid and electrolyte administration, supplemental feeding, and management of exposure keratitis associated with lid paralysis may be necessary in severely affected animals. Large amounts of bicarbonate and fluid may be lost when salivation is prolonged and intense so fluid therapy should be tailored to address these deficiencies.

Control

In outbreaks of disease, aborting does should be isolated from the herd, and kids should be raised separately from adults. Aborted fetuses, placentas, and discharges should be handled wearing gloves and face masks, and disposed of carefully. Kids should not receive unpasteurized colostrum or milk from does involved in the outbreak to avoid neonatal septicemia. Feed samples, particularly silage, should be examined and cultured and infected feeds discarded. Even when culture tests are negative, poor quality silage with a pH more than 5 should be suspect, and not fed. Recently introduced animals also should be considered suspect as carriers. Floors and pens should be thoroughly cleaned and disinfected. After an outbreak, herd-wide fecal cultures with culling of fecal shedders has been used to effectively eliminate infection from goat herds (Dijkstra 1984b). Because of the zoonotic potential, no unpasteurized milk should be consumed from goats in a herd with a history of listeriosis since shedding of the organism in the milk of latent carrier animals does occur.

A vaccine has been in use in central Europe and Norway to protect sheep from listeriosis. While case rates in vaccinated and unvaccinated sheep were similar, the severity of disease was less and the response to treatment better in vaccinated animals (Gudding et al. 1985). A vaccination trial in goats in France produced a sharp reduction in new cases that lasted for at least three months when used in known infected herds. No difference was observed in disease rate or host response to vaccination between a live and killed vaccine except for a rare abortion in does vaccinated with the live vaccine in late gestation (Guerrault et al. 1988).

Goat farmers who produce or market milk, cheese, or other dairy products need to be aware of the zoonotic potential of these products if contaminated with *L. monocytogenes*. There should be no sale of raw milk products from herds where the *Listeria* infection status in not known to be negative. Some of the challenges of keeping cheeses free of listeria contamination in small scale cheese making operations and approaches to reducing the risk of contamination of soft goat cheeses have been reported (Theodoridis et al. 2006).

Tetanus

Tetanus is a well known clostridial disease of humans and animals that produces a characteristic syndrome of muscular rigidity, hyperesthesia, and convulsions. Routine prophylaxis against tetanus in goats is recommended.

Etiology and Pathogenesis

The causative agent is *Clostridium tetani*, an anaerobic, Gram-positive, spore-forming rod found widely in soil and animal feces. Spores are very resistant to destruction and can persist in soil for many years. Proliferation of the organism with release of a potent neurotoxin, tetanospasmin, can occur when spores are subject to a suitable anaerobic environment as can occur in deep puncture wounds or injuries producing necrotic tissue in susceptible hosts. The organism does not disseminate from the site of proliferation, but the neurotoxin ascends the peripheral nerve trunks to the spinal cord where it blocks the inhibitory effect of interneurons on alpha motor neurons. This leads to sustained discharge of motor neurons with resultant signs of tetany. When the toxin reaches the post-synaptic sites where it exerts its effect, it cannot be neutralized by antitoxin and is only removed by gradual degradation. Death is usually caused by respiratory arrest from dysfunction of the tetanic diaphragm. Further explanation of the pathogenesis of tetanus at the cellular and molecular level is available elsewhere (Rings 2004).

Epidemiology

Goats are susceptible to tetanus, and factors that predispose other livestock to the disease also predispose goats. The tetanus organism may be introduced into the goat via puncture wounds; obstetrical interventions; performance of routine procedures such as disbudding, dehorning, tattooing, castration, and hoof trimming; dog bites; fighting by bucks; and penetration of the oral mucosa by fibrous plant awns (King 1980). The use of elastrator bands for castration may be particularly dangerous in establishing conditions for the proliferation of spores. In South Africa, tetanus is frequently encountered in young Angora goats after shearing (Van Tonder 1975). Persistent skin irritation caused by constant rubbing from a metal neck chain (Sinha and Thakur 1978) or a rope tether has been identified as causing tetanus in goats (Figure 5.5).

Spores of *C. tetani* are resident in the intestines of livestock and may be passed in the feces in large numbers, particularly by horses. These spores accumulate in soil, particularly where livestock are kept under intensive management. Goats maintained in barns currently or previously used for horses may be at increased risk of disease.

Clinical Findings

The incubation period varies in tetanus. It can depend in part on the location of the inciting wound or injury and its distance from the CNS as the toxin has to reach the spinal cord before clinical signs are seen. Tetanospasmin moves intra-axonally at a rate of 75 to 250 mm/day (Sanford 1995). Clinical disease has been observed in a one-week-old kid within four days of disbudding and in an adult doe several months after dystocia. In most cases however, the incubation period is ten to twenty days.

Early signs of tetanus include an anxious expression, a stiff gait, and mild bloat. Affected animals adopt a characteristic base-wide, or "sawhorse" stance, and the ears and tail become stiff. There is reluctance to move and difficulty opening the mouth. The animal

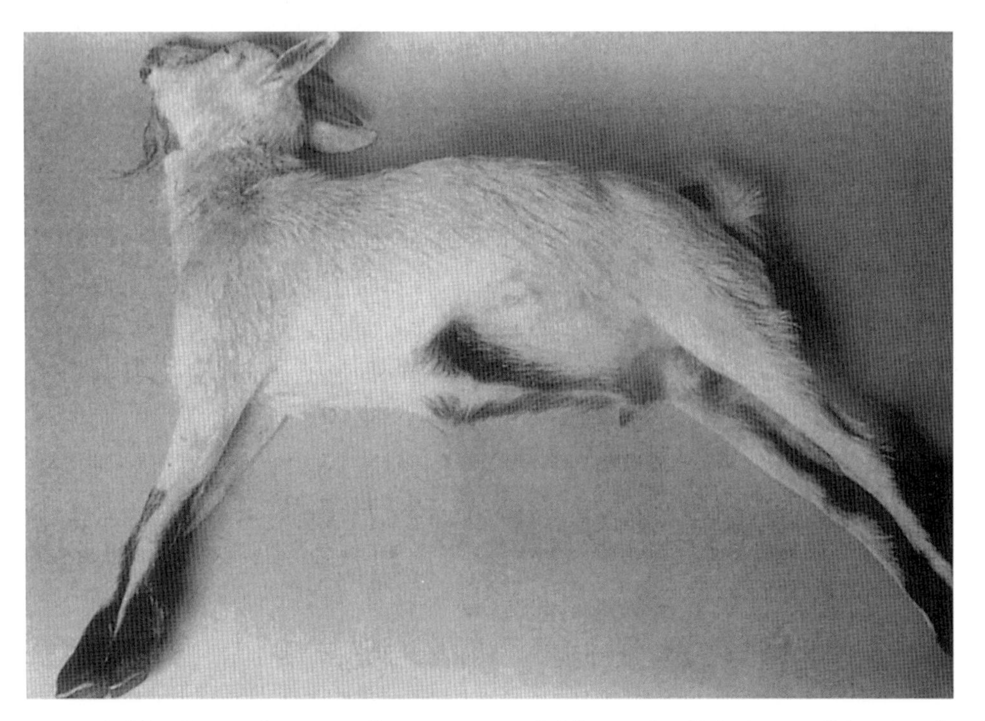

Figure 5.5. Young goat with advanced tetanus. Note extensor rigidity and opisthotonos. This goat developed tetanus secondary to abrasions of the neck associated with prolonged tethering with a tight rope. (Courtesy of Educational Media, Cummings School of Veterinary Medicine at Tufts University, Mr. David Wilman, photographer.)

may become constipated. Food may accumulate in the buccal space and salivation may be observed. Prolapse of the third eyelid may occur. Over time, animals become hyperesthetic and respond dramatically to touch or loud noise by stiffening and collapsing to the ground. This may be followed by seizures. Eventually animals are permanently recumbent, with rigid extension of all limbs and opisthotonos. Rumen tympany may be pronounced. Affected animals convulse periodically at the slightest disturbance. Once recumbent, death usually occurs within twenty-four to thirty-six hours.

Clinical Pathology and Necropsy

There are no characteristic laboratory abnormalities in tetanus and no definitive necropsy findings, as the neurologic lesion is functional rather than physical. A thorough history and careful inspection of the carcass may lead to identification of the wound or infection site of bacterial proliferation where the organism might be cultured. Because the organism may be present in tissues without causing disease, this supports but does not confirm the diagnosis.

Diagnosis

The diagnosis of tetanus is based on the rather characteristic clinical syndrome it produces. However, at different points in the development of full blown tetanus, other differential diagnoses must be considered. Laminitis and nutritional muscular dystrophy can produce a stilted or stiff gait as seen in early tetanus, but not bloat or the other signs. Hyperesthesia and trismus are seen in bacterial meningitis but this condition can be differentiated by CSF analysis. In the terminal stages when recumbency, opisthotonos, and convulsions are present, polioencephalomalacia, which is common in goats, must be differentiated. Strychnine poisoning and hypomagnesemic tetany must also be ruled out, but these are less common in goats. Myotonia congenita, as discussed in Chapter 4, can produce tetanic spasms, but these are intermittent and spontaneously resolve.

Treatment

The prognosis is always guarded, but early identification and intervention improve the recovery rate. Therapeutic goals are to inhibit additional toxin production, neutralize existing unbound toxin, ameliorate the effects of bound toxin, and provide whatever supportive care is necessary. Treatment with systemic penicillin inhibits additional bacterial proliferation and toxin release. Procaine penicillin G at a minimum dose of 25,000 IU/kg bw IM BID for two to three days is recommended with a reduction to once a day treatment after that. Other antibiotics with a Gram-positive spectrum such as ampicillin and amoxicillin may also be used at high, frequent doses.

The drug of choice in human medicine is metronidazole and this is now being used for tetanus cases in small animal practice as well (Linnenbrink and McMichael 2006), but no reports of its use or effectiveness in ruminants were found. The use of metronidazole in food animals (including all goats) is forbidden in the United States (Payne et al. 1999). The site of bacterial proliferation should always be searched for and whenever possible, the wound or infection site should be opened to the air, debrided, flushed with hydrogen peroxide, and infiltrated with penicillin. It is suggested that the area be infiltrated with tetanus antitoxin before the wound cleaning process begins to reduce the chance that more pre-existing toxin will be absorbed during tissue manipulations.

Neutralization of existing unbound toxin is accomplished by parenteral administration of tetanus antitoxin at a dose of 10,000 to 15,000 units intravenously every twelve hours for at least the first twenty-four hours and longer if the proliferation site has not been identified and treated. An alternative approach is the one time administration of antitoxin directly into the CSF via the atlanto-occipital space. In a goat, 5 ml of antitoxin has been introduced into the subarachnoid space after removal of an equivalent amount of CSF (Brewer 1983).

Anticonvulsants, tranquilizers, and muscle relaxants can be administered to reduce the clinical effects of bound toxin. Diazepam can be used at a dose range of 0.5 to 1.5 mg/kg intravenously to effect. Acepromazine works well as a tranquilizer in tetanic animals at a dose of 0.2 mg/kg intramuscularly. Methocarbamol is an effective muscle relaxant at a dose of 22 mg/kg intravenously. Guaifenesin, given intravenously to effect as a 5% solution, may also be used to reduce muscle spasms but care must be taken not to overdose the animal, because it acts by blocking nerve transmission at the level of the interneurons (Rings 2004). Other drugs recommended for use as muscle relaxants but not specifically reported for use in goats are dantrolene sodium, mephenesin, and magnesium sulfate (Rings 2004).

Supportive care includes removing the animal to darkened, quiet surroundings. Intravenous fluids containing dextrose and electrolytes are indicated to counter dehydration and lack of feed intake. An enema may relieve constipation and make the animal more comfortable. The position of the animal should be shifted regularly to avoid decubital ulcers. A nasogastric tube can be passed to relieve bloat and provide fluids and feed per rumen. An egg, honey, milk, glycerine, and oatmeal gruel has been recommended (King 1980). Care must be taken not to traumatize the pharynx and esophagus when the tube is passed repeatedly. When valuable animals are severely affected and the convalescence is expected to be long, surgical creation of a rumen fistula may be indicated to facilitate feeding and bloat control. Any sign of improvement is favorable, but it may take several weeks for complete recovery to occur.

Control

Tetanus can be readily prevented by a combination of improved hygiene and immunoprophylaxis. In general, all wounds should be cleaned promptly and thoroughly. The use of elastrator bands for castration should be avoided. When the immune status of young kids is unknown, routine procedures such as disbudding and castration should be accompanied by injection of 150 to 250 units of antitoxin. When the status of adults is unknown, 500 to 750 units of antitoxin can be administered when treating wounds, dystocias, and other potential sources of tetanus.

It is recommended that routine vaccination for tetanus be incorporated into the herd health program. For small ruminants, tetanus is often included with *Clostridium perfringens* types C and D as a trivalent vaccine which can serve as the foundation for a goat preventive vaccination program. Initially, all goats vaccinated should receive a booster vaccine three to four weeks after their initial vaccination. Then, if pregnant does are vaccinated one month prior to parturition, their kids will be protected by passive colostral antibody for at least several weeks and can be vaccinated for the first time at three to four weeks of age. The kids then should be boostered three to four weeks later, and then revaccinated annually, preferably three to four weeks before kidding. Bucks should also be included in the vaccination protocol.

Botulism

Botulism, a fatal paralysis resulting from the ingestion of the preformed neurotoxin produced by *Clostridium botulinum*, has been reported in goats but is uncommon.

Etiology and Pathogenesis

Clostridium botulinum is an anaerobic, Gram-positive, spore-forming rod found in soil and vegetation and as a normal inhabitant of the intestine of various livestock species including poultry. Seven neurotoxin types (A–G) of *Clostridium botulinum* are known along with different subtypes. As in cattle, botulism in goats is caused principally by types C_β and D. Spores revert to the vegetative state under suitable anaerobic conditions and produce an extremely stable neurotoxin. Bacterial proliferation and toxin production commonly occur in infected, decomposing carcasses and decaying vegetation contaminated with *C. botulinum*. Livestock become ill after consuming preformed toxin. Ingested toxin is absorbed from the intestine and reaches the nervous system via the blood. The toxin acts primarily on lower motor neurons, interfering with the release and function of acetylcholine, the principal neurotransmitter. The result is a general flaccid paralysis that includes the diaphragm and leads to death by asphyxia.

In experimental type C_β botulism in goats, clinical signs usually appeared on day two or three after oral administration of toxin. Doses as small as 0.5 minimum mouse lethal dose (MMLD)/g of bw were fatal and a cumulative toxic effect was observed when small doses were fed over eight days. Goats that grazed pasture or ate silage tolerated higher challenges than goats receiving hay and concentrate, suggesting a protective effect of green forage (Fjølstad 1973). In another experimental study, goats were given type C botulism toxin subcutaneously in doses ranging from 15.6 to 500 LD/kg bw. Goats given doses of 250 or 500 LD/kg bw died at forty-two to forty-six hours post inoculation. Goats given 31.3, 62.5 or 125 LD/kg bw developed subacute disease, while the goat receiving 15.6 LD/kg developed a chronic form of the disease, indicating that clinical response in goats is dose dependent. Toxin was only detectable by the mouse toxicity test in goat serum at the highest dose administered (Santos et al. 1993).

Epidemiology

There is little information on the incidence of botulism in goats throughout the world. In South Africa, where cattle botulism is considered common and is frequently associated with gnawing on the bones of carrion as a result of phosphorus deficiency, botulism in Angora goats is reported, but is comparatively rare. In contrast to cattle, all reported cases in Angora goats were associated with contaminated feed, either milled lucerne containing rodent carcasses or poultry litter containing dead chickens (Van Tonder 1975). In Senegal, a water-borne outbreak of type D botulism killed fifty goats, one hundred sheep, ten cattle, and five horses. The source of toxin was identified as a dead mammal contaminating the well (Thiongane et al. 1984). In a more recent report from South Africa, type D botulism was confirmed in a mixed flock of sheep and Boer goats via the mouse toxicity test using intestinal contents from one of the affected sheep (van der Lugt et al. 1995). Most affected goats and sheep in that outbreak were found dead without first exhibiting clinical signs, or had a short course of disease lasting two to twelve hours.

Clinical Findings

The duration and severity of disease depends on the dose of toxin ingested and can range from peracute to chronic. In experimental caprine botulism (Fjølstad 1973), early signs include a hoarse character of the voice, depression, anorexia, difficulty in chewing, salivation, and a reluctance to stand. When forced to stand, goats show trembling of the limb muscles and stiffness in the hindquarters, and lie down immediately when permitted. Some show an abdominal respiratory effort. Hypersensitivity to light may be seen. As the disease progresses, animals are unable to stand due to flaccid paralysis, but remain sternal. This progresses to lateral recumbency and death, sometimes as early as two days after toxin ingestion. Recoveries are possible after a prolonged illness when low doses of toxin are initially ingested.

In the clinical outbreak reported from South Africa, death without clinical signs was the most common presentation. Goats that did show clinical signs initially showed restlessness, reluctance to move, a stiff gait, muscle tremors, grinding of the teeth, salivation, foaming at the mouth, and pupillary dilatation. They then became recumbent, exhibited paddling of the limbs, and died within minutes to a few hours of lying down (van der Lugt et al. 1995).

Clinical Pathology and Necropsy

There are no characteristic clinicopathological laboratory abnormalities in botulism and no specific necropsy findings because the neurologic lesion is functional rather than physical. Grossly affected animals may show a variety of lesions: congestion of the carcass; some ascites, hydrothorax, and hydropericardium; pulmonary congestion and emphysema; and petechiation of the ruminal, abomasal, and duodenal mucosa (van der Lugt et al. 1995). Stomach contents and suspect feedstuffs may be tested for presence of toxin by toxin neutralization assays in laboratory animals, usually mice. However, distribution of toxin in feeds may be patchy, and ingested toxin may already have been absorbed from the gut, so these tests are often unrewarding in addition to being costly and time-consuming. The blood of goats is unlikely to contain sufficient toxin to be a useful sample for animal challenge studies (Santos et al. 1993). Culture of the organism from feeds or the tissues of affected animals may be misleading, because the organism may be present without participating in disease.

Diagnosis

In most cases, the diagnosis of botulism is presumptive based on identification of a feed source contaminated by likely sources of *C. botulinum*, such as rodent and bird carcasses, in conjunction with a characteristic syndrome of rapidly progressing generalized weakness. Several other conditions should be considered in the differential diagnosis. Enzootic muscular dystrophy should be responsive to vitamin E and selenium therapy in the early stages. Milk fever in lactating does should respond to calcium therapy. Tick paralysis may appear similar, but ticks should be identifiable on the affected goat. The paralytic form of rabies should be considered and can be confirmed at necropsy. Skeletal trauma and spinal cord damage can be ruled out by careful physical examination and supported by radiographs or other imaging techniques.

In the reported South African outbreak, sudden death was the predominant presentation, and the necropsy findings suggested that heart failure was contributory to that outcome. Therefore, the differential diagnosis also included plant poisonings caused by cardiac glycoside- and monofluoroacetate-containing plants, gousiekte-inducing shrubs, and ionophore toxicity (van der Lugt et al. 1995). These cardiotoxic agents are discussed further in Chapter 8.

Treatment

The prognosis is grave in botulism. If type-specific or polyvalent antitoxin were available, it might be useful given early on, but there is little documentation for this in the veterinary literature. Animals with slowly progressive disease may recover gradually over many weeks. Supportive care is necessary and includes maintenance of hydration, tube feeding, slinging or frequent shifting to avoid decubital ulcers, and in extraordinary cases, ventilatory support when the diaphragm is paralyzed.

Control

Because the disease appears to be sporadic in goats, control measures are limited. In cattle, it is recommended that grazing animals be provided adequate protein and phosphorus in the diet to reduce osteophagia. At the least, feed and water supplies should be routinely examined to identify the presence of dead rodents and waterfowl and poultry litter should be fed cautiously. Vaccination can be protective, but is not widely practiced. If goats are vaccinated, a bivalent C and D toxoid should be used.

Clostridium perfringens type D Enterotoxemia

Disease due to *Clostridium perfringens* type D is associated mainly with hemorrhagic enteritis and/or sudden death in goats and is discussed in detail in Chapter 10 in the section on Enterotoxemia.

However, clinical signs of neurologic disease, such as opisthotonos and convulsions, are sometimes observed in cases of enterotoxemia, particularly in calves and lambs (Rings 2004). At necropsy, sheep show a characteristic brain lesion, cerebellar microangiopathy, that is considered pathognomonic for the disease in sheep (Buxton et al. 1978). Until recently, neurologic manifestations of enterotoxemia in goats have been poorly documented. Then, Uzal et al. (1997) reported on the histologic findings of cerebellar microangiopathy with perivascular edema in two goats in Australia which died suddenly and were confirmed with type D enterotoxemia. One goat also demonstrated bilateral symmetrical foci of encephalomalacia in the cerebellar peduncles. Similar histologic findings were subsequently reported from a goat with confirmed enterotoxemia in Brazil (Colodel et al. 2003).

Epsilon toxin of *C. perfringens* type D is not a direct neurotoxin and the pathogenesis of neurologic signs and brain lesions in ruminants with type D enterotoxemia is not fully understood. Experimentally, young goats given high doses of epsilon toxin showed clinical neurologic signs of paddling, opisthotonos, and convulsions, but no brain lesions, while lambs given similar doses showed similar clinical signs and histologic lesions of perivascular edema (Uzal and Kelly 1997). In a related experiment, goat kids were given whole cell cultures of *C. perfringens* type D intraduodenally and these kids did develop characteristic brain lesions, suggesting the possibility that, at least in goats, CNS manifestations of enterotoxemia may be associated with bacterial components other than or in addition to epsilon toxin (Uzal and Kelly 1998).

Meningoencephalitis and Brain Abscesses

Meningoencephalitis in goats can be bacterial or thermal. The latter occurs due to injudicious use of a hot disbudding iron during horn bud removal in the kid. Brain abscesses occur only sporadically in goats.

Etiology and Epidemiology

Bacterial meningoencephalitis is most commonly seen in young kids, occurring as a sequela to neonatal septicemia arising from navel infection. Meningoencephalitis may be the only manifestation of septicemia, or it may be one of a constellation of signs including omphalophlebitis, polyarthritis, pneumonia, diarrhea, and endotoxic shock. Neonatal septicemia is a major cause of kid mortality worldwide but the frequency of CNS involvement is not well established (Sherman 1987). Sporadic cases of meningoencephalitis can also be seen in mature goats.

Multiple factors contribute to the high frequency of bacterial infections in young kids. They include failure of passive transfer of maternal antibodies caused by inadequate colostrum intake by neonates, failure to treat the navel with antiseptics after birth, poor environmental sanitation caused by overcrowding, inadequate drainage or insufficient bedding, and stresses of weather and poor nutrition, among others.

The most commonly involved bacterium in septicemia and subsequent meningoencephalitis is *E. coli*, but other *Enterobacteriaceae* may be isolated as well. In addition, *Streptococcus zooepidemicus* has been identified as the cause of meningoencephalitis in a yearling goat (Gibbs et al. 1981). Cryptococcosis of the CNS has been reported in goats in Brazil (Santa Rosa et al. 1987). *Listeria monocytogenes* may occasionally produce a general meningoencephalitis, but is more commonly associated with focal brain stem lesions. *Corynebacterium pseudotuberculosis* and *Arcanobacterium pyogenes* may occasionally cause meningoencephalitis secondary to extension of infection from superficial lymph node and soft tissue abscesses of the head and neck. There is also a single case report of pyogranulomatous meningoencephalitis in a goat due to *Corynebacterium ulcerans* (Morris et al. 2005). Meningitis also may occur during mycoplasma septicemia in goats (East et al. 1983).

A major noninfectious cause of meningoencephalitis in kid goats is the removal of horn buds with a hot, usually electric, disbudding iron. In contrast to calves, the frontal bone of kids is thin and the frontal sinuses are undeveloped. Excessive heat or prolonged application of the disbudding iron to the skin and horn bud can lead to thermal damage of underlying bone, meninges, and brain. Proper techniques for disbudding are discussed in Chapter 18.

It has been stated that cerebral abscesses caused by *Staphylococcus aureus, Fusobacterium necrophorum*, and *Arcanobacterium pyogenes* are common in both sheep and goats (Brewer 1983). However specific studies on the etiology and pathogenesis of brain abscesses in goats are lacking. As in other ruminant species, goats may be predisposed to pituitary abscesses of hematogenous origin by the presence in ruminants of the rete mirabile, a complex mass of capillaries surrounding the pituitary gland. Five such cases are documented in goats (Lomas and Hazell 1983; Pedrizet and Dinsmore 1986).

Pathogenesis

Bacterial infections are most likely to involve the leptomeninges, choroid plexus, and ventricular walls, and not penetrate into the parenchyma, so that any encephalitis that occurs tends to be superficial. It is speculated that in septicemic animals, bacteria become established on these membranous surfaces via transport within blood monocytes destined to develop into CNS macrophages that normally reside on these membrane surfaces (Cordy 1984). Meningoencephalitis can be focal or diffuse. When the spinal meninges are involved, extension of inflammation to the nerve roots can also occur. In thermal meningoencephalitis caused by disbudding, the lesions are usually focal in the frontal region of the cerebrum. Thermal lesions alone can account for the neurologic dysfunction that occurs, but bacterial invasion also can occur secondary to thermal necrosis of skin and bone overlying the brain (Wright et al. 1983) and infection should be considered as a likely sequela when managing thermal necrosis cases associated with hot iron disbudding (Thompson et al. 2005).

Factors leading to the development of cerebral abscesses in goats are not well defined. The behavioral pattern of frequent head butting with the potential for traumatic injury and the common practice of hot iron disbudding of kids are likely contributors to the potential development of abscesses in young goats. Hematogenous spread from focal or generalized infections is also possible, as in the pituitary abscess syndrome. The clinical signs that develop in cases of brain abscess depend on the size and location of the abscess, and are highly variable. In one instance, a cerebellar abscess in a Nubian doe led to rostral transtentorial herniation of the brain (Kornegay et al. 1983). In another case, a pyogranuloma involving the cerebellum, cerebellar peduncles, and pons in a six-year-old goat appeared to have been an extension of a middle ear infection. In that case, the clinical signs were suggestive of vestibular dysfunction and included circling, vertical nystagmus, and head tilt (Morris et al. 2005).

Clinical Findings

Fever is common in bacterial meningoencephalitis and may also occur in the thermal form. Not all possible signs of meningoencephalitis are seen in all cases. Variability depends on whether the lesions are focal or diffuse, and mild or severe. Possible signs include mania or an anxious expression, trismus, cutaneous hyperesthesia, and hypersensitivity to sound. Muscular spasms or rigidity may also be observed or palpated, especially over the neck and back. Recumbent animals may show extensor rigidity of the limbs, opisthotonos, and convulsions.

In goats, depression occurs more often than mania. Incoordination, paraplegia, and coma are common signs. Blindness is also frequently reported in affected kids, and may be accompanied by hypopyon. When hypopyon is not obvious, fundic examination may reveal papilledema and vascular congestion. While mortality is generally high, spontaneous recoveries from thermal meningoencephalitis have been reported (Sanford 1989).

Kids with signs of meningoencephalitis should be examined for other evidence of septicemia, particularly omphalophlebitis; pneumonia; and hot, swollen joints. Frequently animals with thermal meningoencephalitis may show no prodromal signs and die suddenly hours to weeks after disbudding injury is incurred.

Though variable, signs most often associated with brain abscesses include mental depression, clumsiness, head pressing, blindness, and intermittent attacks of motor irritation, including convulsions (Radostits et al. 2007). In pituitary abscess syndrome, dysphagia, blindness, abnormal pupillary responses, and reduced jaw tone are the most common signs (Pedrizet and Dinsmore 1986).

Clinical Pathology and Necropsy

Characteristic changes in the CSF caused by meningoencephalitis include an increase in white blood cells, particularly neutrophils, and an elevation of the total protein. Bacteria may also be present in the CSF. In severe cases, the CSF may be visibly cloudy on collection. Gram stain of the CSF sediment can be helpful in guiding therapy while cultures are pending.

Brain abscesses that may occur deep in the parenchyma of the brain may not induce inflammatory changes in the CSF. The inflammatory response may be reflected in the hemogram in both meningoencephalitis and brain abscesses. Kids with meningoencephalitis are often hypogammaglobulinemic.

Meningoencephalitis is usually detectable grossly at post mortem as thickening, cloudiness, and hemorrhage of the meninges along with hyperemia and congestion of the adjacent brain tissue. In early cases, histologic examination may be necessary to identify active inflammation. Signs of septicemia may be observed in other tissues, such as hemorrhage of serosal surfaces and cloudy joint fluid. Bacterial culture of liver, heart blood, and CSF should be carried out when there is a potential herd problem. In thermal meningoencephalitis, obvious focal, circular, necrotic, fibrinous lesions of the frontal bones (Figure 5.6) and underlying meninges and cerebrum will be observed, representing

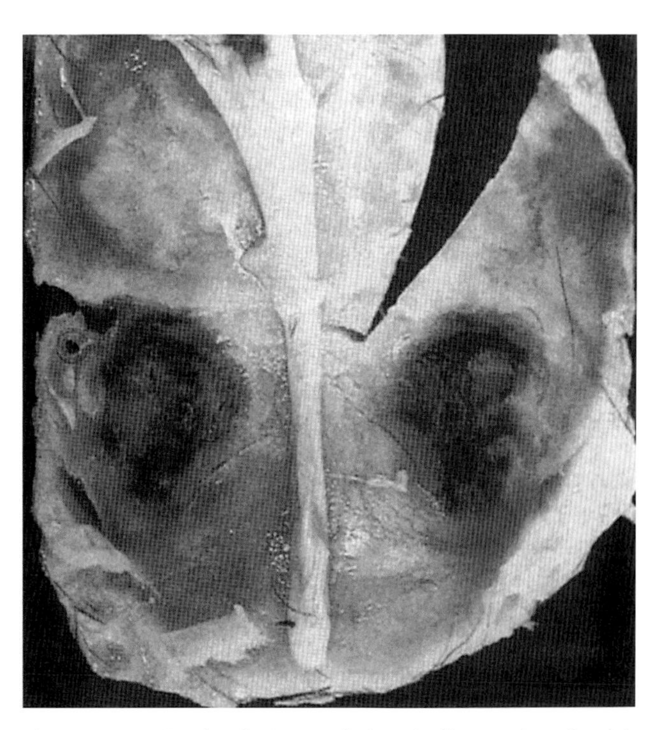

Figure 5.6. Circular lesions of the skull associated with excessive heat applied to the head during a thermal disbudding procedure with a hot iron. (From Wright et al. 1983. Reproduced by permission of Veterinary Medicine Publishing Company.)

the points of application of the disbudding iron. Focal abscesses are revealed by systematic serial section of the brain or inspection of the sella turcica.

Diagnosis

The presumptive diagnosis of meningoencephalitis in young kids is based on typical clinical signs in conjunction with a history of recent hot iron disbudding or identification of management factors that predispose to septicemia. Meningoencephalitis and brain abscesses can virtually always be confirmed by post mortem examination, and this is the most common method of diagnosis for the latter.

Treatment

The prognosis is guarded in meningoencephalitis, but early, aggressive intervention can result in some successful outcomes. Antibiotic therapy is indicated in all cases of meningoencephalitis because there is evidence of secondary bacterial invasion even in cases initiated by thermal injury. Resolution of brain abscesses with antibiotic therapy is rarely achieved.

Treatment should be initiated using broad spectrum, bactericidal antibiotics until culture and sensitivity results are available to guide therapy. Several antibiotics have been recommended for use in ruminants with Gram-negative bacterial meningitis (Jamison and Prescott 1988).

Trimethoprim-sulfonamide combinations are recommended for intravenous use at doses of 16 to 24 mg combined/kg at least every twelve hours. Third generation cephalosporins such as cefotaxime or moxalactam can be used intravenously at 50 mg/kg two to four times a day. Gentamicin can be used at a dose of 3 mg/kg intravenously or intramuscularly three times a day either alone or in conjunction with trimethoprim-sulfonamide combinations, cephalosporins, ampicillin, or penicillin.

The recommended dose for sodium ampicillin is 10 to 50 mg/kg intravenously or intramuscularly given four times a day. The dose for sodium penicillin G is 20,000 to 40,000 IU/kg given intravenously four times a day. Penicillin or ampicillin should not be used alone when there is any likelihood of Gram-negative bacterial involvement, but they are usually effective alone in streptococcal infections. The duration of antibiotic therapy depends to a large extent on the clinical response, but should extend for at least forty-eight hours after the goat appears normal.

Antibiotics should be administered in cases of thermal meningoencephalitis associated with hot iron disbudding. In one report from New Zealand, eighteen of 150 kids showed altered mentation two days after hot iron disbudding and were treated with a single dose of long acting oxytetracycline. On the next day, an additional twelve of the 150 disbudded kids were found dead and five that were necropsied had lesions of cerebral infarction beneath the disbudding sites. It was concluded that the eighteen goats treated the day before also had thermal injury but survived because of the antibiotic therapy which had been given (Thompson et al. 2005).

Nonsteroidal anti-inflammatory drugs are also indicated, including phenylbutazone at a dose of 10 mg/kg given once daily or flunixin meglumine given intravenously or intramuscularly at 1 to 2 mg/kg every twelve hours. Aspirin can be given to goats with a developed rumen at a dose of 100 mg/kg orally every twelve hours.

Affected animals should be kept in quiet, dimly lit, well-bedded surroundings. They should be turned frequently if recumbent to minimize decubital ulcers and hypostatic congestion of the lung. If excitatory signs are present, anticonvulsant therapy or sedation may make the animal more comfortable and manageable as described earlier for tetanus.

Control

When bacterial meningitis is confirmed in kids, a careful review of kid rearing techniques with the owner or herdsperson is necessary to identify deficiencies in management. Special attention must be paid to identifying problems of overcrowding and poor sanitation, inadequate disinfection of navels, and failure of transfer of passive immunity, as discussed in Chapter 7. Serious kid losses caused by septicemia and meningitis have been reported in herds in which kids were deprived of colostrum and instead fed commercial products advertised as colostrum supplements (Scroggs 1989; Custer 1990).

Veterinarians should provide information to clients on the risks of hot iron disbudding and the proper techniques for performing it. If thermal meningoencephalitis does occur in a herd, the veterinarian should ask to be present at subsequent disbudding sessions to identify any problems associated with the disbudding iron or its application. Despite the potential problems of thermal meningoencephalitis, hot iron disbudding still remains the most efficient, reliable way to prevent horn growth when done properly. It has been recommended that a dose of broad spectrum antibiotic be given to kids prophylactically at the time of hot iron disbudding, because some of the losses that occur may be due as much to secondary infection of the meninges and brain entering through devitalized tissue as to the thermal lesion itself (Thompson et al. 2005).

PARASITIC DISEASES

Parelaphostrongylosis and Elaphostrongylosis

Infection with the meningeal worm *Parelaphostrongylus tenuis* is subclinical in its only definitive host, the whitetail deer. In aberrant hosts, including goats, sheep, llamas, and other wild cervids, clinical signs of focal myelitis or encephalomyelitis are produced. The disease is restricted to North America.

In Norway, a similar clinical syndrome of cerebrospinal nematodiasis in goats has been identified. The condition results from infection with *Elaphostrongylus rangiferi*, the elaphostrongyloid nematode of reindeer (Handeland and Sparboe 1991). Though not completely elucidated, the natural history of this disease in goats appears quite similar to parelaphostrongylosis as seen in North America.

More recently, a similar clinical syndrome has been reported in goats in Switzerland associated with *Elaphostrongylus cervi*, the elaphostrongyloid nematode of several species of Eurasian deer, including red deer, roe deer, maral deer, and sika deer.

Etiology and Pathogenesis

Parelaphostrongylus tenuis is a hair-like nematode in the family *Protostrongylidae*. The definitive host is the whitetail deer, *Odocoileus virginianus*. The parasite has an indirect life cycle that involves terrestrial slugs and snails as intermediate hosts. Adult worms reside in the subdural spaces and cranial venous sinuses of the CNS of deer. Eggs laid on the meninges hatch, enter the circulation, and localize in the lungs. Eggs laid in the venous sinuses are carried to the lungs and hatch there. In either case, larvae migrate up the airways, are swallowed, and passed in the deer's feces. They are subsequently ingested by gastropods where they develop into infective larvae over a three- to four-week period. Infective larvae are released from snails and slugs when the gastropods are ingested by grazing mammals. In the deer, larvae penetrate the intestine and migrate to the spinal cord through the peritoneum, reaching the CNS within ten days where they mature in the dorsal horns of spinal gray matter for an additional twenty to thirty days. Adults then travel to the subdural space, migrate to the cranium, and penetrate the dura mater to enter the venous sinuses, thus completing the life cycle.

When infective mollusks are ingested by goats and other aberrant hosts, migration to the spinal cord via the peritoneum also takes place over a ten-day period. However, beyond this point, the normal life cycle goes awry. Maturation of larvae is erratic, and subsequent migrations through the spinal cord are random and unsuccessful in reaching the cranial venous sinuses. Randomly migrating larvae are responsible for the parenchymal destruction and inflammation that leads to clinical neurologic disease in aberrant hosts. The wide variety of neurologic abnormalities observed in clinical cases reflects the frequently multifocal nature and diverse distribution of lesions in the spinal cord or brain. The goat is able to control *P. tenuis* infection in some cases, as recovery has been observed in experimentally challenged animals and in natural outbreaks. In kids experimentally infected orally with 200 or more larvae, severe colitis and peritonitis developed within four to eleven days of infection caused by larval migration through the intestinal wall (Anderson and Strelive 1969). The occurrence of peritonitis in naturally occurring goat cases has not yet been reported.

The life cycles of *E. rangiferi* and *E. cervi* are similar to that of *P. tenuis*, involving gastropods as intermediate hosts. The life cycle of these parasites is completed without damage to the natural hosts, but in goats, as with *P. tenuis*, the life cycle is not completed and aberrant migration through the spinal cord and brain results in clinical disease. Experimental challenges of goats with *E. cervi* did not produce patent infections (Scandrett and Gajadhar 2002)

Epidemiology

Cerebrospinal nematodiasis caused by *P. tenuis* is restricted to North America, reflecting the geographic distribution of the definitive host. The whitetail deer originally was concentrated in the eastern United States and Canada but now has spread throughout much of the two countries and into northern Mexico.

The deer favors forested areas as natural habitat, and commonly grazes pastures and croplands adjacent to woodlands. Goats grazing pastures where deer feed are at increased risk of exposure to *P. tenuis*. Although the intermediate gastropod hosts are terrestrial, there appears to be increased risk of exposure to snails and slugs in low-lying, wet, and poorly drained fields and pastures.

Cool, moist weather is believed to enhance the infectivity of the first stage larvae passed by deer and to promote the activity of intermediate host snails. Pastures in the northern half of North America are most dangerous during late summer to early fall and most cases of clinical disease in goats are seen in fall and early winter. In Texas, clinical disease has been reported in April (Guthery et al. 1979). Additional reports of *P. tenuis* in goats have come from Minnesota, Michigan, and New York (Mayhew et al. 1976; O'Brien et al. 1986; Kopcha et al. 1989). It can be presumed that grazing goats are at risk wherever whitetail deer are found.

In experimental infection of goat kids, clinical signs of neurologic disease appeared between eleven and fifty-two days after introduction of infective larvae into the peritoneum (Anderson and Strelive 1972). In natural infection, onset of clinical signs has been noted as late as nine weeks after removal of goats from pasture. Morbidity rates in affected herds have been reported from 10% to 27%, with mortality rates as high as 65%.

Elaphostrongylus rangiferi is naturally found in reindeer in Scandinavia, and the disease has been well documented in goats in Norway (Handeland and Sparboe 1991). The parasite was introduced into Canada in the early 1900s with the importation of reindeer into Newfoundland. As a result, native caribou herds and moose in Canada became infected (Lankester and Fong 1979). Therefore, the potential for goat cases exists in North America as well. Clinical and pathological findings of experimental infections of goats with *E. rangiferi* have been reported (Handeland and Skorping 1992, 1992a, 1993).

Elaphostrongylus cervi is naturally found in Europe and western Asia in a number of native cervids but was introduced into New Zealand through the importation of red deer (Mason et al. 1976). There are several well documented case reports of cerebrospinal nematodiasis due to *E. cervi* from Switzerland (Pusterla et al. 1997, 1999, 2001).

Aberrant hosts such as the goat are most commonly exposed to these parasites by grazing on pastures that also have been grazed by infected wild ungulate hosts. Goats grazing on these contaminated pastures ingest gastropods that contain infective larvae. As this occurs most commonly in summer and early fall, clinical cases of disease are seen most commonly in late fall and winter.

Clinical Findings

All breeds, sex, and ages of goats can be affected. Animals usually have been on pasture within the past two months. Observation of deer on pasture can often be elicited in the history. Affected animals can have a variable history regarding duration of signs, ranging from a gradual progression of lameness or paresis over several days to a sudden onset of recumbency since the previous day. Angora goats on range have been found dead, entangled in brush, presumably because of limb weakness and locomotor difficulties associated with spinal lesions.

The most common clinical presentations suggest involvement of the spinal cord. Signs include paresis or paralysis of one or more limbs, ataxia, postural reaction deficits, knuckling, toe dragging, abnormal gait, limb weakness, recumbency in a dog-sitting posture, or inability to rise. Any combination of forelimb and hind limb involvement is possible. Reflex responses, muscle tone, and the presence of muscle atrophy are variable, depending on the degree of upper and lower motor neuron involvement. Affected animals may get progressively worse, remain static, or in some cases improve without therapeutic intervention. In most cases they remain mentally alert and continue to eat and drink normally. Pruritus and linear excoriations of the skin may be noted if the larvae migrate through dorsal nerve roots.

Indications of brain involvement in affected goats include circling and blindness, separation from the flock, abnormal posture, and head tilt. Hypopyon has also been noted.

The duration and severity of clinical signs vary. Animals that remain ambulatory should be given at least one month to demonstrate if they will stabilize or recover. Animals unable to rise have a poorer prognosis.

Clinical Pathology and Necropsy

Affected animals frequently have a moderate increase in total protein and white blood cell counts in the CSF with eosinophils frequently noted. In one study of fourteen cases, CSF protein concentration ranged from 29 to 360 mg/dl with a median of 69.5 mg/dl. The white blood cell counts ranged from 0 to 1,000/mm^3 with a median of 54/mm^3. Eosinophils were present in CSF in 57% of cases (Smith 1982). Hemograms are usually normal. The life cycle of *P. tenuis* is not completed in aberrant hosts. Therefore, first stage larvae are not found in the feces of goats.

No serologic tests are currently available commercially, but the potential for serologic diagnosis exists. In experimental infection of two goat kids, antibodies to *P. tenuis* were detectable in the serum and CSF using ELISA. Serum antibodies were detectable before, during, and after the onset of clinical signs and peaked at eight weeks post infection. CSF antibodies peaked at five to eight weeks post infection (Dew et al. 1992).

There are no gross lesions associated with *P. tenuis* infection except perhaps neurogenic muscle atrophy. After preservation of tissue in formalin, however, focal asymmetrical areas of whitish discoloration may be observed in the spinal cord on cut section. Some of these areas may have a greenish tinge and are the most likely areas to find evidence of the parasite itself (Mayhew et al. 1976). Both L4 and L5 stages of *P. tenuis* have been identified in goat tissues, the latter containing reproductive structures.

Microscopically, lesions are usually confined to the spinal cord and brain stem. There are focal areas of malacia and necrosis, especially in white matter, with evidence of degenerating axons. Adjacent to malacic areas there is perivascular cuffing with lymphocytes, sometimes eosinophils, and occasionally plasma cells. The degree of general inflammation is mild, although focal granuloma formation has been reported (Kopcha et al. 1989). Hemorrhage is sometimes observed and a mononuclear or eosinophilic meningitis may occur.

Diagnosis

No definitive antemortem diagnosis is currently possible. Presumptive diagnosis is based on a history of goats grazing where deer are found, a seasonal occurrence of neurologic disease in goats with diverse clinical signs, and the presence of eosinophils in CSF when found. Definitive diagnosis depends on identifying the parasite in nervous tissue at time of necropsy.

Treatment

Currently, there is no proven effective therapy for *P. tenuis* or *Elaphostrongylus* spp. in goats and other aberrant hosts. Reports of successful therapy to date must be viewed cautiously because no controlled studies have been reported and spontaneous recoveries are known to occur in untreated animals.

Diethylcarbamazine has been used at doses ranging from 40 to 100 mg/kg for one to three days, on the basis of its reported efficacy in treatment of cerebrospinal nematodiasis caused by *Setaria digitata* in Asia. However, this filarial worm is not a member of the family *Protostrongylidae* and has a different pattern of anthelmintic susceptibility. More recently, ivermectin has been a focus of therapeutic interest. However, studies in whitetail deer indicate no effect against *P. tenuis* once the larvae have entered the CNS, although larvae are killed during the preceding migration period (Kocan 1985). A newer avermectin, moxidectin, has higher lipid solubility and is more hydrophobic than other avermectins and may therefore be better able to cross the blood-brain barrier to reach nematodes already present in the CNS. Benzimidazoles, notably fenbendazole, also are used empirically, though levamisole has shown no efficacy (Nagy 2004). Steroid therapy may have some value in reducing inflammation in nervous tissue, although its effect on subsequent migratory or developmental activity of larvae is unknown. Nonsteroidal anti-inflammatory drugs such as flunixin meglumine have also been used empirically.

Combination of multiple anthelmintics and anti-inflammatory drugs is commonly reported in the treatment of cerebrospinal nematodiasis, perhaps reflecting the uncertainty of what actually is known to be effective (Nagy 2004). For example, there is a report of treatment of goats for clinical *Elaphostrongylus cervi* infections in seventeen goats using flunixin meglumine at 1.1 mg/kg bw IM and oral administration of fenbendazole at 50 mg/kg and ivermectin at 200 µg/kg SQ for five days (Pusterla et al. 1999). Eleven (64.7%) showed an immediate improvement in neurological signs. Three of them had a complete recovery while eight had some persistent ataxia. Six recumbent goats (35.3%) were killed because of a lack of response. It was concluded that the therapy was effective if neurologic deficits were not already severe when treatment was initiated.

Because goats have been known to recover spontaneously from cerebrospinal nematodiasis, affected animals should be allowed time to show signs of improvement when the situation permits. Supportive care is extremely important during that period. Because animals may be recumbent from paresis or paralysis, ample dry bedding is necessary and periodic lifting or slinging may be appropriate.

Control

Control methods are currently limited to reducing deer access to livestock grazing areas and reducing exposure of goats to gastropods and infective larvae. Practical means of reducing deer access are limited by regulations on hunting and the ability of deer to jump fences. It may be helpful to limit goat pasturing to fields without contiguous woodlands and to pastures that are on high ground and well drained. When feasible, goats should be removed from pasture earlier in the grazing season before weather turns wet and cool. No other practical means of snail and slug control have been reported.

Based on knowledge of the life cycle of the parasite and the effectiveness of ivermectin against migrating larvae, control is theoretically possible by anthelmintic prophylaxis every ten to sixteen days while goats are at pasture; this, however, is costly and may be impractical. It would be useful to have larvicidal anthelmintics that can be administered regularly and inexpensively during grazing periods to prevent entry of ingested larvae into the CNS. Benzimidazoles effective against the larval stages of other *Protostrongylidae* such as *Muellerius* that are available as salt or feed additives are potential candidates in non-lactating goats. Pyrantel tartrate has also been recommended for use in this manner because it is formulated to be fed on a daily basis (Rickard 1994). However, the regular use of anthelmintics to control cerebrospinal nematodiasis could contribute negatively to the growing problem of anthelmintic resistance in gastrointestinal nematodes, a far more common and costly problem.

Setariasis

The filarial worm *Setaria digitata* is nonpathogenic in definitive ungulate hosts, but can produce a cerebrospinal nematodiasis in goats, sheep, and other aberrant hosts in Asia. The disease is commonly referred to as lumbar paralysis or kumri. It is clinically similar to the conditions produced by *Parelaphostrongylus tenuis*, *Elaphostrongylus rangiferi*, and *E. cervi*.

Etiology and Pathogenesis

Setaria digitata is a non-pathogenic parasite of the peritoneal cavity of cattle, buffalo, and zebu. It occurs only in Asia. There was some debate whether *S. labiatopapillosa*, found in the peritoneum of cattle, antelope, deer, and giraffe, was a separate or identical species, but phylogenetic analysis now indicates that the two species are distinct (Jayasinghe and Wijesundera 2003). The life cycle of these filarids is not completely understood, but is known to be indirect. Mosquitoes of various genera, including *Anopheles, Aedes,* and *Armigeres* spp., serve as the intermediate hosts.

In the definitive cattle host, adult worms live in the peritoneal cavity and produce microfilaria that circulate in the blood stream. Mosquitoes ingest the microfilaria along with blood during feeding. Within two weeks these microfilaria mature into infective larvae and enter the salivary glands of the mosquito. During subsequent feedings, they are introduced into the blood stream of new ungulate hosts. In the definitive host these larvae migrate to and mature to adults in the peritoneal cavity to complete the life cycle. In aberrant hosts such as the goat, sheep, and horse, the microfilaria migrate to the CNS, sometimes the eye, and occasionally the fetus of pregnant animals, where they cause mechanical damage and an inflammatory reaction. Clinical signs usually develop one month after infection. The life cycle is rarely completed in aberrant hosts, and microfilaria are not detectable in the blood stream.

Epidemiology

The disease was first suspected in imported goats in Japan in 1927, but the parasitic nature of the disease was not confirmed until much later. It has since been reported in goats in Japan, Korea, and Sri Lanka (Innes et al. 1952); India (Patnaik 1966); China (Wang et al. 1985); Taiwan (Fan et al. 1998); and most recently as a putative outbreak in Saudi Arabia (Mahmoud et al. 2004). The disease occurs as a seasonal epizootic; it is associated with increased numbers of mosquitoes. In Japan, most cases are seen in August and September, in China, June through October, and in India, September through December, after the rains and before winter. Morbidity rates can be high, with as many as 30% to 40% of susceptible animals affected. There appears to be some natural immunity in local animals, with higher morbidity and mortality observed in imported goats. The proximity of large cattle populations infected with *S. digitata* predisposes to infection of aberrant hosts.

The goat is considered an aberrant host for *S. digitata*. Microfilaria are introduced into the goat via the bites of mosquitoes and the parasite generally is considered not to reach maturity in this host. However, patent infections in Saudi goats have now been reported, with adult worms detected in five of forty-eight goats examined at a veterinary diagnostic laboratory. These animals did not show clinical signs of disease, but had male and female *S. digitata* in the abdominal cavities, mostly on the omentum as well as microfilaria in the blood (El-Azazy and Ahmed 1999). It was speculated that the genetic constitution of this local Saudi goat breed may be predisposed to establishment of patent infection.

Clinical Findings

All ages, sex, and breeds of goats may be affected. The appearance of clinical signs may be acute or subacute, and mild to severe. Variable outcomes occur, including acute death, progressive worsening of neurologic signs, stabilization of neurologic deficits, and occasionally spontaneous recovery. Most typically, affected animals show evidence of spinal cord involvement with ataxia, lack of proprioception, paresis, or paralysis. Any or all limbs may be affected, but most often hind limbs are involved. Sensory deficits are minimal. Additional signs suggesting brain involvement include cranial nerve deficits, nystagmus, and circling. In most cases, animals remain mentally alert. Fever is not observed.

Clinical Pathology and Necropsy

As with other parasitic infections of the CNS, eosinophilia of the CSF can occur in caprine setariasis. Gross necropsy lesions are rarely identified and diagnosis depends on thorough microscopic examination of the brain and spinal cord, concentrating especially on those areas that correlate with the clinical neurologic examination. In most cases only a single larva is involved, and rarely more than three. Microscopically, lesions are characterized by a focal malacia that can be identified in serial sections as the migratory tract or channel of the offending parasite. In adjacent areas there may be evidence of axonal degeneration, demyelination, astrocytosis, and perivascular cuffing with mononuclear cells and eosinophils. Hemorrhage is variable. Locating the actual offending larvae in histologic sections is uncommonly achieved.

Diagnosis

Antemortem diagnosis is presumptive based on the seasonal observation of epizootic neurologic disease characterized principally by locomotor dysfunction in countries where setariasis occurs. Definitive diagnosis depends on identification of the parasitic larvae in the CNS of affected animals at time of necropsy.

Treatment

The filaricide diethylcarbamazine can be effective in goats and sheep when animals are treated early in the course of disease. Early signs may represent meningeal irritation or radiculitis caused by the parasite before its entry into the brain or spinal cord and the parasite may still be susceptible to anthelmintic therapy at this stage. Diethylcarbamazine is given orally, suspended in water, once at a dose of 100 mg/kg bw, or at a dose of 40 to 60 mg/kg daily for one to six days (Shoho 1952, 1954). Once the parasite has crossed the meninges, response to therapy is poor. Avermectins may also show efficacy against some species of microfilaria in other livestock species, but reports on use of ivermectins specifically against *S. digitata* in goats are lacking.

Control

To reduce the incidence of setariasis in aberrant hosts such as goats, the parasite should be controlled in the normal host, cattle, particularly at the beginning of the mosquito season. Because the infection is subclinical in cattle, routine treatment of cattle by farmers may be difficult to effect. When possible, goats should be housed separately from cattle. The use of diethylcarbamazine in sheep at an oral dose of 40 mg/kg given one time every three weeks before and during the mosquito season appeared to reduce the number of clinical cases observed in the field compared with untreated controls (Shoho 1954). Reduction of mosquito populations could also reduce the transmission of the parasite from cattle to goats.

Strongyloidosis

Strongyloides papillosus is a nematode parasite of ruminants normally associated with gastrointestinal parasitism. It is discussed in more detail in Chapter 10 in the section on nematode gastroenteritis. However, there were several outbreaks of mortality recorded in young kids and lambs in Namibia in which *S. papillosus* was identified as the cause. Of note in these outbreaks were the signs of neurologic disease in addition to the characteristic signs of gastrointestinal parasitism. Neurologic signs included gnashing of teeth, aimless wandering, and persistent head pressing against objects. The presence of neurologic signs was so unexpected that experimental challenge studies were undertaken to better characterize the clinical syndrome and the underlying pathology seen in the field and to confirm *S. papillosus* as the etiology (Pienaar et al. 1999).

In the experimental studies, some but not all challenged goats showed signs of CNS involvement in their clinical presentation. Signs included gnashing of teeth, wide based stance, ataxia, stupor, nystagmus, and head pressing ("pushing syndrome"). At necropsy, no gross lesions were seen in the CNS, but histopathologic lesions were found in the brain and spinal cord. These lesions were characterized as status spongiosus with marked vacuolation of the white matter but also in the gray matter and in some nuclei. The most common sites for lesions were the roof nuclear area of the cerebellum, corpus striatum, thalamus, and midbrain and medulla; less common sites included the cerebrum, granular layer of the cerebellum, spinal cord, and optic tracts. The severity of lesions was closely correlated with the presence of neurologic signs in challenged goats.

To date, neurologic signs associated with *S. papillosus* have not been reported elsewhere either under field conditions or in experimental challenge studies. It is not clear why neurologic disease was noted in these Boer cross goats in Namibia. Possible explanations include the intensity of the challenge dose; variations in breed susceptibility; or the presence of other toxic, metabolic, or infectious causes that were not recognized in the field outbreaks or the experimental animals. Further documentation of the occurrence of neurologic disease associated with *S. papillosus* infection is needed. When unexplained head pressing, ataxia, or gnashing of teeth is noted in goats, particularly if signs of gastrointestinal parasitism are present as well, then fecal samples should be checked for *S. papillosus* and goats that die should be necropsied with examination of the brain.

Coenurosis

Coenurosis, also known as gid, sturdy, or staggers, is a metacestodal infection of ungulates, especially sheep and goats. It primarily causes a focal encephalopathy.

Etiology and pathogenesis

The metacestode involved in this disease is the intermediate stage of the tapeworm of carnivores, *Taenia multiceps*, formerly known as *Multiceps multiceps*. The metacestode is identified in sheep as *Coenurus cerebralis* and in goats as either *C. cerebralis* or, historically, as *C. gaigeri*. It was thought that a separate species existed because cysts are frequently located outside the CNS in the goat. However, it is now believed that the difference lies with the host, not the parasite (Soulsby 1982).

T. multiceps is a large intestinal tapeworm of dogs, foxes, coyotes, and jackals. Eggs or gravid tapeworm segments are passed in the feces of the host, contaminate herbage, and are ingested by grazing ruminants. Embryos are released after ingestion and penetrate the small intestine, enter portal vessels, and are distributed widely throughout the tissues via the circulation. In sheep, only larvae that reach the CNS develop into metacestodes; all others die.

In goats, metacestode development occurs primarily in the CNS, but frequently in the skeletal musculature and the heart as well. The muscular form of the disease is discussed in Chapter 4. Cysts also have been found in mesenteric lymph nodes and there is a recent report of metacestode cysts within the eye of a goat (Islam et al. 2006). There is a period of migration through nervous tissue that may result in clinical signs of acute meningoencephalitis if large numbers of larvae are present. In most cases, however, this migratory phase is subclinical. After migration, the stationary phase of metacestode maturation lasts from two to seven months. The mature metacestodes are cystic structures up to 7 cm in diameter, transparent, thin-walled, and filled with clear fluid. They contain up to several hundred scolices that are visible as white plaques on the clear cyst wall in excised cysts. The majority of mature cysts are located superficially in the parietal or frontal region of the cerebral cortex, but location is variable throughout the CNS and musculature. The life cycle of the tape worm is completed when carnivores ingest mature cysts while feeding on tissues of infected ruminants.

During early growth of cysts, irritation of adjacent nervous tissue occurs and may be reflected in some cases by early excitatory signs. As the metacestode enlarges, pressure on adjacent tissues increases, and neuronal death occurs, leading to signs of neurologic deficit. The pressure that develops is considerable and is reflected in a high incidence of papilledema and rarefaction of cranial bone adjacent to superficial cysts. Cerebrospinal fluid pressure also can be markedly elevated. The clinical signs that develop reflect the location of the cyst or cysts present.

Epidemiology

T. multiceps is present in carnivores worldwide, but coenurosis is not common in goats in most countries. There are numerous clinical reports originating from the Indian subcontinent. Thirty-two caprine cases were recorded in one year at a single veterinary institution in India (Saikia et al. 1987). A slaughterhouse survey in Bangladesh demonstrated a prevalence range of 1.9% to 13.3% for cerebral coenurosis (Ahamed and Ali 1972). Caprine coenurosis is sporadic in Europe and Africa (Harwood 1986). The disease is rare or absent in goats and sheep in North America, Australia, and New Zealand. The status of coenurosis in Africa and Asia has recently been reviewed (Sharma and Chauhan, 2006).

The disease is most commonly reported in young female goats, but this may reflect their disproportionately large presence in goat herds rather than a predilection to disease. Morbidity rates are low but mortality rates are high in untreated cases. The disease is infrequently reported in humans, with most documented cases reported from Africa. The goat is not directly involved in the zoonotic aspect of the disease.

Clinical Findings

Because of the prolonged development phase for coenurosis, cases may be seen anytime of the year. Affected animals may have a history of ill-defined, low-grade neurologic abnormalities for one month or longer. Animals with the neurologic form of the disease may show a variety of signs.

The clinical presentation is variable, but it has been suggested that there are three phases of development (Saikia et al. 1987). In the first stage, animals may be depressed and show intermittent periods of abnormal head carriage, especially head tilt. There may be short, intermittent convulsions or intermittent circling. This phase lasts four to eight days and may be overlooked. In the second phase, which usually begins eight to sixteen days after onset of signs, signs become more consistent. The most common findings are head tilt, unilateral blindness, circling, and loss of balance with a staggering gait. Some animals may show determined forward walking with the head held high and a hypermetric gait followed by head pressing against obstacles instead of circling. Other signs include grinding of the teeth, salivation, exophthalmos, nystagmus, and irregular rumen contractions. The third or terminal phase usually begins twelve to twenty-five days after onset of signs. Animals become recumbent, exhibit extensor rigidity, and paddle frequently with the hind limbs. These stages overlap considerably and the clinical course is frequently one month or longer.

Papilledema and hemorrhage of the optic papilla are common in coenurosis cases, so a fundic examination should be performed. In addition, firm, digital palpation of the head frequently identifies dissymmetry or softened areas of skull, suggestive of underlying superficial cysts. Digital pressure on such spots may exacerbate clinical signs. Cysts deep in the parenchyma are not associated with bony changes.

Recently a case of coenurosis was reported in a seven-month-old goat in Mongolia which presented with bilateral flaccid paralysis of the hind limbs. The goat had been at pasture and had actually been grazing for some time, dragging its hind limbs behind it. At necropsy, the goat had a metacestode cyst occupying the lumbar vertebral canal, extending along three vertebrae. Impingement of the spinal cord by this space occupying cyst accounted for the clinical signs (Welchman and Bekh-Ochir 2006).

Clinical Pathology and Necropsy

Total protein, cell counts, and pressure are often elevated in the CSF. Mean total protein in affected goats has been reported at 80.3 mg/dl, mean cell counts at 85/mm^3, and mean pressure at 262.4 mm water. Eosinophils and degenerative cells may be common on cytologic examination (Sharma and Tyagi 1975). Allergic skin testing has also been used with positive goats having a reaction of more than 1.2 cm.

Radiographs can reveal metacestode-associated rarefaction of the skull when bone softening has not yet reached the point of detection by digital palpation. Cerebral angiography has been used to identify deep parenchymal cysts in goats. The angiograph reveals stagnation of contrast material around the avascular zone of the cyst surrounded by concentric arches of displaced vessels (Sharma et al. 1974).

At necropsy, cysts ranging in size from 1 to 7 cm in diameter can be identified in predilection sites such as brain, spinal cord, and skeletal muscle.

Diagnosis

Though the clinical course is prolonged, it may not always be recognized as such, and animals may present as acute onset of circling, falling, or head pressing. The differential diagnosis should include listeriosis, CAE, polioencephalomalacia, brain abscesses, sinusitis, cerebral hematomas or tumors, cerebrospinal nematodiasis, and rabies. The nose bot, *Oestrus ovis*, may occasionally penetrate the frontal sinuses and produce a clinical syndrome known as false gid because the signs are similar to those seen in coenurosis.

Treatment

There are no known, consistently effective anthelmintic therapies for elimination of the metacestode in clinically affected animals (Sharma and Chauhan 2006). Praziquantel administered orally at dose of 50 mg/kg bw has given unreliable results in sheep. The drug was more reliably effective at a higher dose of 100 mg/kg given orally (Verster and Tustin 1990).

When bone softening is pronounced so the site of the cyst is obvious, aspiration of cyst contents is accomplished via an aseptic needle passed through the softened or perforated bone. Afterward, a mild antiseptic is introduced, such as 0.1% acriflavine solution. Surgical treatment is possible when bone is still firm but lesions are identifiable by radiography or other imaging techniques. The skull is opened over the area of the cyst and the cyst removed by first bluntly dissecting it from underlying brain tissue and then lifting it out either by application of suction or by a forceps. In two separate studies, 90% of thirty goats and 87.5% of sixteen goats survived and showed good recovery after surgery (Sharma and Tyagi 1975; Ahmed and Haque 1975). Either general or local anesthesia is used.

Control

Control methods involve reducing stray dog populations, restricting the feeding of small ruminant carcasses and offal to dogs, and ensuring strict, regular treatment of dogs kept with livestock for control of mature tapeworms. There are no vaccines commercially available, though research efforts suggest that vaccination could be useful in control of this disease.

Tick Paralysis

Ascending paralysis and death can result from the feeding activity of certain species of ticks on domestic animals including goats. The disease has been reported sporadically in goats in parts of Europe, the Middle East, and South America. It is considered a major constraint on small ruminant production in parts of South Africa where the disease is known as Karoo tick paralysis.

Etiology

At least thirty-one hard ticks in the *Ixodidae* family and six soft ticks of the *Argasidae* family can produce tick paralysis in mammals and birds. In goats, the condition has long been associated primarily with *Ixodes rubicundus* in South Africa, and then later with *Rhipicephalus punctatus* as well (Stampa 1959; Fourie et al. 1991). In Israel, Crete, Turkey, and Bulgaria, *Ixodes ricinus* causes the disease in goats (Hadani et al. 1971; Trifonov 1975). In 1983, tick paralysis was reported for the first time in Brazil, associated with *Amblyomma cajennense* (Serra Freire 1983).

Most reports of tick paralysis involve adult ticks rather than larvae or nymphs and when such ticks have a two- or three-year life cycle, disease outbreaks may be seen only every second or third year. In many cases, the immature tick stages show different host feeding preferences. For example, immature forms of *I. rubicundus* are found primarily on hares and shrews. This is not always the case, however; in Brazil, there is experimental evidence that larval and nymphal stages of *A. cajennense* may also produce the disease. Development of disease appears to be less associated with the number of ticks actually feeding than with the stage of engorgement of the ticks present on the host.

Epidemiology

The incidence of tick paralysis is tied to the life cycle and ecology of the offending ticks and conditioned by livestock management and grazing practices. For example, in Israel, the disease is seen only every third year between December and February when adult ticks are active, and only in the more temperate, inland regions of the country. It usually occurs only in flocks or herds grazing on the more densely vegetated, northern slopes of hills and not the barer, southern slopes (Hadani et al. 1971). In South Africa, Karoo tick paralysis is also seen primarily in the winter months (March to August), on the moister, hillier portions of the Karooveld and tick densities vary with different vegetation types (Stampa 1959). The *Rhipicephalus*-associated disease is seen in September through November and again in February in South Africa. In Brazil, naturally occurring cases were observed between June and December.

Morbidity and mortality can be high in epizootics of tick paralysis. For example, fourteen of fifty-one (27%) South African Angora kids younger than one month of age developed paralysis while grazing over a two-week period in September, and 71% of these died even after ticks were removed (Fourie et al. 1988).

Pathogenesis

Though not proven in all cases, it appears that ticks responsible for paralysis produce a salivary neurotoxin that is introduced into the host animal during active feeding, particularly when the tick reaches a certain stage of engorgement. At least in tick paralysis of dogs infested with *Dermacentor* spp., the toxin is known to interfere with acetylcholine liberation at the neuromuscular junction. In all cases there is a resulting flaccid paralysis that first involves the limbs and may progress to involve the diaphragm with animals dying of respiratory compromise.

The author could not find reports of tick paralysis in goats in North America. However, the disease is reported in cattle, sheep, and New World camelids in western Canada and the western United States, in association with *Dermacentor* and *Argas* spp. ticks, so veterinarians in North America should consider the disease a possibility in goats (Schofield and Saunders 1992; Cebra et al. 1996).

Clinical Findings

The disease is seen most often in grazing animals infested with ticks. Ticks are most common around the head and neck, especially in the ears, and around the tail head, but the entire body should be inspected. Affected goats show evidence of lower motor neuron involvement including muscular weakness of the limbs, unsteady gait, knuckling, ataxia, and hypoesthesia. There is no fever, and animals often remain bright and alert and they continue to eat. Frequently the hind limbs are affected first, but all four limbs may be affected simultaneously, especially in Karoo tick paralysis. As the disease progresses the animal becomes laterally recumbent due to flaccid paralysis. In terminal cases, death is caused by respiratory paralysis or aspiration pneumonia. The clinical course is usually one to three days. If ticks are identified and removed early in the course of disease, before recumbency, many but not all animals recover completely within twenty-four hours.

Clinical Pathology and Necropsy

There are no clinical pathological or necropsy findings that support the diagnosis of tick paralysis, save for the presence of offending species of ticks.

Diagnosis

Diagnosis is presumptive on the basis of identification of ticks known to cause tick paralysis on affected goats under circumstances of likely occurrence. The differential diagnoses for progressive limb paralysis in goats include rabies, enzootic ataxia or swayback, CAE, botulism, cerebrospinal nematodiasis, vertebral trauma or abscesses, and congenital spinal abnormalities. Intramuscular injections affecting the sciatic nerves, nutritional muscular dystrophy, and skeletal trauma must also be considered in sudden loss of mobility in the hind limbs.

Treatment and Control

The only known treatment is removal of feeding ticks and supportive care. Knowledge of the ecology of offending ticks may be used to restrict grazing in high-risk areas during seasons of known adult tick activity. When this is not possible, tick control with the use of topical acaricides is indicated during the high-risk seasons.

NUTRITIONAL AND METABOLIC DISEASES

Polioencephalomalacia

Also known as cerebrocortical necrosis, this nutritional/metabolic disease primarily affects ruminants, including goats. The disease in goats is increasingly recognized under intensive management conditions when goats are fed more grain concentrate feed to encourage accelerated growth or increased production.

Etiology and Pathogenesis

Strictly speaking, polioencephalomalacia (PEM) is a descriptive term for a softening of the gray matter of the cerebral cortex, also referred to as cortical necrosis. The term does not inherently ascribe a particular etiologic basis for the occurrence of such a lesion. Yet, over the years, the term has become closely linked in veterinary medicine to a specific syndrome of ruminants believed to be caused by disturbances of thiamine (vitamin B_1) metabolism and which occurs most commonly in feedlot cattle on high concentrate rations. In recent years, however, there has been a serious movement away from the use of the term to describe a specific disease associated with alterations in thiamine metabolism, largely because other distinct diseases can cause the same lesion of polioencephalomalacia. These include lead poisoning, sulfur toxicity, and salt poisoning/water deprivation.

There are several reasons for the traditional association of PEM with thiamine. In ruminants, thiamine is produced by the activity of rumen bacteria and dietary sources of the vitamin are not required under normal conditions. PEM is most commonly seen in cattle in feedlots on high grain rations. It is documented that when the pH of the rumen is reduced, as occurs with the feeding of grain rations, rumen bacteria that produce thiamine are reduced in numbers while other bacteria which produce thiaminase, an enzyme that degrades thiamine, are increased. It is also documented that in experimental studies and field cases of PEM, there may be markedly decreased concentrations of thiamine in body tissues, decreased activity of a thiamine pyrophosphate-dependent enzyme, transketolase, in blood, and increased levels of thiamine-destroying thiaminases in the gastrointestinal tract (Gould 1998).

But perhaps the most compelling argument for the belief that thiamine plays a central role in the pathogenesis of PEM has been that administration of thiamine to clinical cases, particularly early in the course of disease, frequently results in recovery of affected animals. Nevertheless, current thinking suggests that the positive therapeutic effect of thiamine does not prove that thiamine deficiency or inhibition is the underlying etiologic basis for PEM. Rather, it is now thought that thiamine may improve energy metabolism in the impaired brain regardless of the inciting cause of the polioencephalomalacia (Niles et al. 2002).

Thiamine has important physiologic functions. It is part of the coenzyme thiamine pyrophosphate (TPP), which plays numerous roles in carbohydrate and amino acid metabolism. It participates in the tricarboxylic acid cycle as a cofactor in the oxidative decarboxylation of alpha ketoglutarate to succinate and in the conversion of pyruvate to acetyl CoA. In addition, as a coenzyme of transketolase, it participates in the pentose phosphate pathway to create D-glyceraldehyde-3-phosphate.

The pathophysiology of the polioencephalomalacia lesion is not fully understood. It is believed to result from intracellular edema associated with a dysfunction of the adenosine triphosphate (ATP)-dependent sodium potassium pump (Cebra and Cebra 2004). Failure of the pump results in sodium accumulation within cells and a resulting net influx of water, leading to cell swelling and death. Most neuronal ATP is generated through glycolysis via the pentose phosphate pathway; transketolase is the rate limiting enzyme in the pathway and thiamine pyrophosphate serves as an important cofactor to transketolase. Therefore, the administration of thiamine may help maintain cell function and integrity in nerve cells when energy demands of brain tissue are not being met, regardless of the underlying cause. It is noteworthy that administration of thiamine improves the clinical outcome in cases of ruminant lead poisoning, which are not specifically associated with thiamine deficiency (Coppock et al. 1991). This underscores the point that thiamine therapy in PEM, though effective, may not necessarily be linked to a specific etiology of thiamine deficiency.

Another development that has challenged the central role of thiamine in the pathogenesis of PEM is the emergence of sulfur toxicity as a demonstrable cause of PEM. It has been documented in situations such as cattle feedlots, where cases were historically attributed to thiamine deficiency. Elemental sulfur, as well as inorganic and organic sulfur compounds, may be present in water and a wide range of animal feeds including forages, concentrates, and molasses, and overall dietary intake may present potentially toxic levels of sulfur. The rumen contains a range of bacteria that metabolize sulfur in different ways. So-called assimilatory bacteria reduce sulfate for their own metabolic utilization and to make sulfur-containing amino acids. Dissimilatory bacteria also use sulfur for their own metabolic needs but they produce excess amounts of sulfide, which accumulate in the rumen. A third group of bacteria contain cysteine desulfhydrase and liberate additional sulfide by enzymatic reactions with sulfur-containing proteins (Gould 1998).

It is known that reductions in rumen pH, as occur in feedlots in association with concentrate feeding, favor the accumulation of hydrogen sulfide (H_2S) in the rumen gas cap where it can readily diffuse into the portal bloodstream. If absorbed in excessive amounts, it may override the capacity for hepatic detoxification. In addition, if present in high concentration in the rumen gas cap, eructated H_2S may be inhaled into the lungs and pass directly into the circulation across the pulmonary membranes. Though the pathophysiological effects on nervous tissue are not completely understood, it is known that H_2S and free sulfide radicals are potentially toxic. They can interfere with oxidative processes within mitochondria by blocking cytochrome C, leading to depletion of ATP and resulting in cell anoxia and death.

H_2S has a high affinity for brain tissue because of its high lipid content, and therefore may exert its toxic effects most dramatically in the brain, leading to polioencephalomalacia by mechanisms not yet fully elucidated. The toxic effects of H_2S gas on the respiratory tract are well known, as the inhalation of H_2S from manure pits leads to severe pulmonary edema and has been responsible for the deaths of livestock and humans. While it is known that high sulfur diets can lower ruminal thiamine production, the pathophysiology of sulfur-related PEM does not necessarily involve thiamine deficiency. In reports of clinical cases of PEM in feedlot steers, rumen H_2S levels were elevated while blood thiamine levels remained in the normal range (McAllister et al. 1997). Current perspectives on polioencephalomalacia and its causes, with an emphasis on sulfur toxicity, have been reviewed (Gould 1998, 2000; Niles et al. 2002).

Epidemiology

Information is sparse on the worldwide incidence of caprine polioencephalomalacia. Currently the disease is presumed to occur only sporadically in goats. Nevertheless, it has been reported to be the most commonly seen nervous disease of goats in New Zealand (McSporran 1988).

The pattern of disease in goats is not as well established as in cattle or sheep, but as in those species, dietary and management factors that may alter normal rumen flora appear to play a key role. Sudden changes in diet, excessive feeding of concentrates, use of horse feeds high in molasses, feeding of moldy hay, development of rumen acidosis, dietary stress of weaning, and overdosing of amprolium have all been associated with cases of caprine polioencephalomalacia. Given that it is now well documented in cattle and sheep that excess consumption of sulfur in the water and feed can also produce PEM, it is reasonable to assume that this also can occur in goats. However, at the time of this writing, no field cases have been documented in goats with sulfur toxicity as the confirmed etiology.

In North America, an increased occurrence in winter has been noted, when roughage quality and availability are low and grain feeding is increased (Smith 1979). It is known that sulfur and sulfates can be found in high quantities in drinking water, notably in the Plains and intermountain regions of the United States and Canada, and this could contribute to the development of PEM. In India, cases increased between August and December when lush pasture was available (Tanwar 1987). In South Africa, an outbreak was associated with concentrate supplementation during winter grazing (Newsholme and O'Neill 1985).

Poor growth rate has been associated with subclinical thiamine deficiency in lambs. One study demonstrated that normal goats in herds where clinical polioencephalomalacia occurred had more thiaminase activity in feces than normal goats in herds with no history of the disease. This suggests that subclinical thiamine deficiency may occur in goats as well (Thomas et al. 1987).

Clinical Findings

All goats are susceptible to PEM, but most cases involve weanlings and young adults. The history frequently includes a sudden change in feed, increases in concentrate feeding, difficulties in weaning, or a recent bout of digestive disease. The initial presentation is variable with some animals showing a prodromal period of depression, anorexia, and/or diarrhea with gradual expression of neurologic abnormalities over a period of one to seven days. In most cases, however, the presentation is one of acute neurologic dysfunction. Early neurologic signs include excitability, elevation of the head or opisthotonos while standing, staring off into space (stargazing), aimless wandering, circling, ataxia, muscle tremors, and apparent blindness.

As the disease progresses, dorsomedial strabismus, nystagmus, lack of a menace response, extensor rigidity, odontoprisis, recumbency with opisthotonos, and convulsions are observed. Fever is not seen except in association with convulsions. The pupillary reflexes are variable depending on the degree of cerebral edema. Rumen contractions are present in uncomplicated polioencephalomalacia, but they may be absent if the condition was precipitated by a severe rumen acidosis. If there is no therapeutic intervention, goats usually die between twenty-four and seventy-two hours after onset of clinical signs.

Clinical Pathology and Necropsy

Goats with polioencephalomalacia show little or no change in the CSF except for a slight mononuclear pleocytosis. While CSF pressure would be expected to increase, normal CSF pressures are poorly documented in the goat. In one reported case of polioencephalomalacia, the CSF pressure was 220 mm water (deLahunta 1977).

Measurement of transketolase activity of red blood cells offers an indirect measurement of thiamine levels. In one study, the mean transketolase activity in nine normal goats measured as μmoles pentose/hour/10^9 red blood cells was 0.782 with a range of 0.125 to 2.90 compared with levels of 0.099 and 0.068 in two clinically affected goats (Smith 1979). In another study, mean transketolase activity in normal goats was reported as 35 ± 5 IU/l compared with 18 ± 2 in affected goats (Thomas et al. 1987). To have the transketolase assay performed, heparinized blood should be centrifuged for ten minutes at 3,000 g, the plasma discarded, and the red cells frozen at –4°F (–20°C) for shipment to the laboratory.

Thiaminase activity can be measured in feces of live animals or rumen content at necropsy. Fresh samples should be submitted frozen to the laboratory and at least 60 grams of rumen content provided. In normal goat feces, thiaminase activity has been measured as 0.2 ± 0.1 mU/g and 0.8 ± 0.3 in clinically affected goats. In normal goats, no rumen fluid thiaminase activity was detected while a mean activity of 0.5 ± 0.3 mU/m was measured in clinically affected goats (Thomas et al. 1987).

The calculated normal reference range for blood thiamine levels in goats has been reported as 66 to 178 nmol/l, but the diagnostic value of such measurements in clinically affected goats remains uncertain. At necropsy decreased tissue thiamine levels support the diagnosis of polioencephalomalacia (Rammell and Hill 1988). Liver and brain samples should be submitted frozen. Mean liver thiamine levels in normal goats have been reported as 1.6 ± 0.3 μg/g wet weight and 0.3 ± 0.4 in affected goats. In brain, the mean for normal goats was 0.7 ± 0.1 and 0.3 ± 0.1 in affected goats (Thomas et al. 1987).

Confirming the presence of high concentrations of H_2S in the rumen gas cap can support the diagnosis of sulfate toxicity as the underlying cause of PEM. A technique for sampling the rumen gas cap through the left paralumbar fossa using a commercially available H_2S detection tube has been described (Gould et al. 1997). Normal and diagnostic values for the goat have not been specifically reported, but in cattle, steers on a high carbohydrate diet supplemented with sodium sulfate developed PEM and had rumen H_2S gas concentrations forty to sixty times higher than control steers on the same diet without sodium sulfate supplementation. The H_2S concentration in the supplemented steers was 4,850 ppm by the fifth day of feeding, while the concentration in non-supplemented steers never exceeded 75 ppm during the experimental trial (Gould et al. 1997). It is recommended that in field cases the analysis be performed when possible on healthy herd mates of the clinically affected animals because sick animals that are off feed quickly revert to lowered concentrations of H_2S in the rumen and may therefore give false negative results. If quantitative testing cannot be performed, the breath of affected animals should be checked during eructation for the characteristic "rotten egg" odor of H_2S, which can give a qualitative indication that sulfur toxicity may be involved.

Gross necropsy findings are limited to the brain. In the most severe cases, the cerebrum is soft and edematous with a grayish yellow or yellow discoloration. The cerebral gyri appear flattened from pressure and the cerebellum may be partially herniated through the foramen magnum. In less severe cases, examination of the cerebrum in darkness using an ultraviolet lamp (black light) may demonstrate areas of fluorescence in the cortex associated with cerebrocortical necrosis. Histologically, a laminar necrosis is confirmed in affected gyri with evidence of separation of the gray and white matter, and obvious degeneration of neurons with perineuronal vacuolation.

In cases where grain engorgement is a predisposing factor, evidence of rumenitis and other sequelae of lactic acidosis may be observed.

Diagnosis

Early signs of depression or altered mentation and diarrhea are consistent with enterotoxemia caused by *Clostridium perfringens* or pregnancy toxemia. The former disease might respond favorably to antitoxin administration; the latter occurs in pregnant does usually with positive urine ketones. The combination of blindness, opisthotonos, extensor rigidity, nystagmus, and strabismus is strongly suggestive of polioencephalomalacia in goats. These signs, however, may occur successively, simultaneously, or not at all, and definitive diagnosis is not always easy. The differential diagnosis for acute, central blindness is given in Chapter 6.

Opisthotonos and extensor rigidity are also characteristic of tetanus and goats with advanced polioencephalomalacia can easily be mistaken for tetanus cases. When circling or other unilateral signs are seen, listeriosis, brain abscesses, ear infections, cerebral nematodiasis, and CAE must be considered. Listeriosis is associated with changes in the CSF fluid and the other diseases are more slowly progressive. Terminal cases of polioencephalomalacia are often convulsive and therefore, meningitis, rabies, pseudorabies, and a variety of toxicities must be considered in the differential diagnosis. As discussed above, lead poisoning and salt poisoning can produce the brain lesion of PEM and may therefore also produce similar clinical signs.

While laboratory tests can support the diagnosis of polioencephalomalacia, the critical nature of the disease demands swift intervention by the practitioner, usually before such laboratory results are ever available. In practice, polioencephalomalacia is most often diagnosed by a response to therapy with thiamine. In goats, evidence of therapeutic response may be seen as soon as two hours after treatment.

Treatment

Despite questions concerning the role of thiamine metabolism in the pathogenesis of PEM, administration of thiamine remains the treatment of choice (Niles et al. 2002). Response is variable, depending mostly on the severity of the disease at the time treatment is initiated. The dose is 10 mg/kg bw repeated every six hours for twenty-four hours. The initial dose is usually given intravenously, and subsequent doses can be given intravenously, intramuscularly, or subcutaneously. Thiamine hydrochloride is most frequently used. If only multiple B vitamins are available, be sure that they are dosed according to the thiamine content. In early or mild cases, complete cure frequently occurs. In advanced cases, partial cures may occur with permanent residual blindness or abnormal mentation. Severely affected goats may die despite therapy. In other species, intravenous hyperosmotic mannitol at a dose of 1.5 g/kg bw in a 20% solution and parenteral dexamethasone at 1 to 2 mg/kg bw have been used in severe cases to reduce cerebral edema. The diuretic furosemide has also been used empirically for that purpose at a dose of 1 mg/kg bw IV. Diazepam at 0.5 to 1.5 mg/kg or other anticonvulsants may be required when seizures occur.

In addition to thiamine therapy and the management of cerebral edema, any underlying problems that may have predisposed to polioencephalomalacia, such as grain engorgement, should be identified and treated, as should sequelae such as dehydration and metabolic acidosis.

Control

A careful history is required to identify specific predisposing factors in each affected herd. Common control recommendations include an increase in roughage feeding with a concomitant decrease in concentrate feeding, and avoidance of moldy feeds and those containing large amounts of molasses, such as horse feeds. When weanlings are involved, weaning procedures should be reviewed to ensure that kids obtain adequate roughage before weaning to promote normal rumen development and proper rumen flora. In problem herds, supplementation of the grain ration with thiamine mononitrate or brewer's yeast may be indicated.

New information on sulfur toxicity as a cause of PEM indicates that the total sulfur content of the ration, including the water supply, should be calculated and then reduced if it exceeds requirements. Levels of dietary sulfur able to produce toxicity in goats are not reported. In beef cattle, sulfur content of the total ration is recommended to be between 1,500 to 2,000 ppm (0.15% to 0.20% on a dry matter basis) and to avoid toxicity, should not exceed 4,000 ppm (0.40%) (Niles et al. 2002). The maximum tolerable dietary sulfur level for ruminants is 0.50% when the diet contains at least 40% forage (NRC 2005). Some specific dietary constituents known to have high sulfur content may need to be removed from the ration. These may include cruciferous forages (*Brassica* spp.), molasses, gypsum (calcium sulfate dihydrate), and ammonium sulfate. The latter may be in use in some goat herds as a supplement to acidify urine where urolithiasis is a problem. To avoid the risk of sulfur toxicity, ammonium chloride should be used for that purpose instead of ammonium sulfate.

Enzootic Ataxia and Swayback

Nutritional copper deficiency can lead to neuronal degeneration and secondary demyelination in the CNS and result in progressive paresis of young lambs and kids. The term swayback is applied to the congenital form of this condition, while enzootic ataxia refers to the condition if it develops after birth. Both are discussed here. Some authors consider the terms synonymous.

Etiology

In sheep, nutritional copper deficiency of the ewe during the second half of pregnancy leads to abnormal maturation and subsequent degeneration of neurons and myelin in the developing fetus and the lamb postnatally. The clinical and pathological similarities of enzootic ataxia in kids to the condition in lambs suggests that the cause is similar, if not identical, in both species.

The problem with attributing caprine enzootic ataxia and swayback solely to copper deficiency is that in some reports of naturally occurring disease, serum and tissue copper levels in clinically affected kids and their dams are not always low. In some instances, unaffected control animals have even lower copper levels. Nevertheless, the favorable therapeutic response to copper administration and the cessation of additional cases through copper supplementation in affected goat herds support copper deficiency as playing a central role in the development of the disease in goats. It is very likely that caprine enzootic ataxia and swayback are metabolic diseases of complex origin with conditioned copper deficiency at the core.

Epidemiology

Enzootic ataxia and swayback in goats have been reported from California, New York, Massachusetts, and Louisiana in the United States (Cordy and Knight 1978; Summers et al. 1980; Lofstedt et al. 1988; Banton et al. 1990), Saskatchewan in Canada (Brightling 1983), Argentina (Dubarry et al. 1986; Bedotti and Sanchez Rodriguez 2002), Scotland (Barlow et al. 1962; Owen et al. 1965), the Netherlands (Wouda et al. 1986), Germany (Winter et al. 2002), Switzerland (Beust et al. 1983), Kenya (Hedger et al. 1964), Ethiopia (Roeder 1980), India (Prasad et al. 1982), Australia (O'Sullivan 1977; Seaman and Hartley 1981), and New Zealand (Black 1979).

Copper deficiency in goats can either be primary, caused by low copper levels in soil and forages raised on that soil, or secondary (conditioned), when normal amounts of copper are present in soils and feeds but uptake and absorption are impeded by the presence of copper antagonists such as molybdenum, iron, manganese, cadmium, lead, and sulfates.

A genetic predisposition was postulated in the Netherlands, where dwarf goats were disproportionately represented in a review of twenty-three cases (Wouda et al. 1986). Breed and family line predispositions play a role in the disease in sheep, presumably through differences in intestinal absorption and storage efficiency of copper.

Pathogenesis

Copper plays an essential role in a number of metabolic and developmental functions, serving primarily in tissue oxidation-phosphorylation reactions as part of the cytochrome oxidase system. Copper is specifically involved in myelination, osteogenesis, hematopoiesis, hair pigmentation, and normal growth (Brewer 1987). The role of copper in myelination is believed to involve phospholipid metabolism for production of normal myelin nerve sheaths.

In congenital copper deficiency or swayback, severe, prolonged copper deficiency in the dam affects normal development of myelin throughout the entire CNS of the developing fetus. This form occurs frequently in lambs and is associated with cavitating lesions of the cerebrum. It is rare in kids. Microcytic anemia and fragility of long bones occasionally have been observed in swayback kids, reflecting the roles of copper in hematopoiesis and osteogenesis, respectively. In contrast to swayback, the postnatal disease enzootic ataxia develops when copper deficiency occurs later in gestation, when the deficiency is less severe, or when the deficiency continues in offspring after birth. Neuronal death and myelin degeneration occur, but are more limited to the spinal cord, brain stem, and sometimes the cerebellum (Cordy and Knight 1978; Wouda et al. 1986).

Clinical Findings

Male and female kids of all breeds can be affected. In congenital copper deficiency (swayback), kids are abnormal at birth. They are weak and most are unable to rise unassisted, but may stand unsteadily if helped to their feet. Muscle tremors and persistent nodding or shaking of the head are characteristic signs. Teeth grinding also occurs variably. Affected kids are able to suckle, vocalize, see, and hear. With intensive nursing care, these kids may live from several days to several weeks.

In the delayed form of the disease, enzootic ataxia, kids are born normally and develop a progressive paresis beginning as early as one week or as late as twenty-eight weeks of age. The mean age of onset is thirteen weeks. The clinical course varies from one to fourteen weeks and at least in the early stages, kids remain bright and alert and continue to eat. Early signs include weakness, fatigue, tremors, difficulty in rising, and incoordination. Symmetrical paresis and ataxia are usually observed first in the hind limbs, but sometimes in the forelimbs first. The signs are never unilateral. Periodic spasmodic contractions of the hind limbs and overstretching of the tarsal joints may occur. Hypermetria has been noted when there is cerebellar involvement. Laryngeal stridor was noted in a kid with involvement of the recurrent laryngeal nerve.

Affected kids may adopt a straddle-legged posture and collapse from weakness after standing a few minutes. Kids with forelimb involvement may drop onto their knees, while kids with hind limb involvement adopt a dog-sitting position and pull themselves along with the forelimbs. Rising becomes progressively more difficult as paresis gives way to paralysis. Permanently recumbent kids show flexor contracture of the forelimbs, spastic extension of the hind limbs, decubital ulcers, and muscle wasting. Diarrhea may occur, but affected kids frequently have concurrent coccidiosis or helminthiasis, so attribution of diarrhea to copper deficiency is problematic. Kids with enzootic ataxia are either euthanized or succumb to secondary problems such as pneumonia.

Signs of copper deficiency in adults in affected herds are not usually noted, but may include ill thrift, diarrhea, anemia, and depigmentation of the hair coat.

Clinical Pathology and Necropsy

Normal blood copper levels in goats are reported to be in the range of 9.4 to 23.6 μmol/l (60 to 150 μg/dl or 0.6 to 1.5 ppm) (Underwood 1981). Blood or serum copper levels less than 8 μmol/l (50 μg/dl or 0.5 ppm) and liver copper levels less than 20 ppm dry weight are reported to be diagnostic for enzootic ataxia in kids (Seaman and Hartley 1981). However, these low levels are not consistently recorded in affected goats, and considerable overlap occurs in blood and tissue copper levels among affected goats, nonaffected goats from the same farm, and control goats from premises with no history of the disease (Owen et al. 1965; Cordy and Knight 1978; Wouda et al. 1986; Bedotti and Sanchez Rodriguez 2002). Numerous animals in suspect herds must be tested to assess the overall copper status in the herd.

A microcytic anemia may be seen in affected kids, and hemoglobin values in the range of 5 to 7.7 g/dl have been reported (Hedger et al. 1964). Analysis of CSF has been performed infrequently and most reported cases of enzootic ataxia had concurrent CAE retroviral infections, so the significance of moderate pleocytosis and elevated protein in the CSF is not clear (Summers et al. 1980). In one uncomplicated case of enzootic ataxia, the CSF was normal (Lofstedt et al. 1988).

At necropsy, the cavitation and gelatinization of the cerebral hemispheres common in lambs with swayback are not seen in affected kids. Neither are gross lesions evident in the CNS of kids with enzootic ataxia. These kids are usually emaciated and show evidence of muscle atrophy.

Microscopic lesions are most common in the brain stem and spinal cord. The lesions are bilaterally symmetrical and are particularly obvious in the dorsolateral tracts of the cervical and thoracic spinal cord. Neuronal degeneration and demyelination are characteristic. Swelling of the neuronal cytoplasm with shrunken nuclei and marked chromatolysis is typical. Wallerian degeneration and loss of myelinated axons with gliosis and phagocytosis are evident. Cerebellar atrophy or hypoplasia may also be noted, with degeneration of Purkinje cells and reduced thickness of molecular and granular cell layers (Cordy and Knight 1978; Wouda et al. 1986).

Diagnosis

Definitive diagnosis is based on determination of low tissue copper levels and characteristic lesions at necropsy. A presumptive diagnosis antemortem is based on the typical clinical presentation, evidence of low copper levels or the presence of copper antagonists in the diet, low tissue copper levels, and a therapeutic response to treatment with copper compounds in mildly affected kids.

For congenital copper deficiency, the differential diagnosis includes hydrocephalus, congenital vertebrospinal abnormalities, caprine beta mannosidosis, border disease, hypoglycemia, and hypothermia. There is also a reported case of granulomatous encephalitis in a newborn kid due to congenital infection with *Neospora caninum*, which produced signs similar to those of congenital copper deficiency (Corbellini et al. 2001). This protozoal parasite is more commonly associated with abortion and is discussed further in Chapter 13.

For delayed copper deficiency, the neurologic form of CAE, vertebral trauma, spinal abscesses, cerebrospinal nematodiasis, nutritional muscular dystrophy, floppy kid disease, and listeriosis must be ruled out. In the early stages of disease, ascending paralysis caused by rabies is also a diagnostic consideration. Numerous cases of enzootic ataxia concurrent with CAE have been reported, which complicates the diagnosis (Summers et al. 1980; Lofstedt et al. 1988).

Treatment

Mildly affected congenital cases, and early cases of enzootic ataxia, may respond favorably to treatment with copper compounds, but complete recovery is uncommon. If desired, blood and liver biopsy specimens should be taken before treatment so that interpretation of tissue copper levels is not confused. Copper glycinate has been reported as an effective treatment given parenterally to kids as a single total dose of 60 mg (Seaman and Hartley 1981).

Control

Effective control depends on determining the underlying cause of copper deficiency. It may be necessary to assay feeds, water, and soils to ascertain if there is a primary copper deficiency or a secondary deficiency conditioned by excess molybdenum, sulfates, or other copper antagonists. Copper requirements are not well defined for goats. This is unfortunate because goats appear to metabolize and store copper differently from sheep and extrapolations are probably inaccurate. Nevertheless, for sheep, copper levels in various feeds should be at least 5 ppm and molybdenum levels should not exceed 5 ppm. The copper to molybdenum ratio in the overall diet should be kept between 5:1 and 10:1 (Rankins et al. 2002). The current dietary copper recommendation for goats, as discussed in Chapter 19, is 10 to 20 ppm. Sulfate levels may be high in water and on pastures and may induce conditioned copper deficiency even when Cu:Mo ratios are within acceptable limits. Sulfate levels in feed should not exceed 3,500 ppm (Black 1979). When soils are copper deficient, annual top-dressing of pasture with copper sulfate at a rate of 2 to 3 kg/ha is recommended.

Enzootic ataxia may be prevented by supplementation of copper. In the face of outbreaks of swayback or enzootic ataxia, pregnant does can be given copper glycinate subcutaneously at a total dose of 150 mg at mid gestation to prevent subsequent copper deficiency in kids. Kids can be given 60 mg of copper glycinate subcutaneously at birth if does were not treated earlier in pregnancy. This should protect them at least through weaning. Oral copper sulfate in the drinking water of does at a dose of 1.5 g per head per week during pregnancy has also been used successfully, but may cause corrosion problems in metal pipes and troughs.

The most convenient method of control is to ensure that goats always have adequate copper in the diet. Trace mineralized salts containing copper sulfate in the range of 0.5% to 2% can be made available in blocks free choice or incorporated into the concentrate ration. A number of sustained release copper products for oral administration such as copper oxide needles in gelatin capsules have been used successfully in sheep in copper deficient areas, and there is at least one report of their safe use in goats in a herd with a history of swayback, though at fifteen weeks following administration of 4 g copper oxide needles, copper levels in viscera were no different between treated and untreated goats, suggesting that the intervention may be less effective in goats than in sheep (Inglis et al. 1986).

Hypovitaminosis A

In cattle, vitamin A deficiency is associated with a number of clinical manifestations including lacrimation, nasal discharge, coughing, corneal opacity, abortion, and weak calves. Signs of neurologic dysfunction include night blindness, total blindness, incoordination, and convulsions. The incoordination and convulsions are due to increased intracranial pressure resulting from reduced absorption of CSF caused by biochemical and structural alterations of the arachnoid villi associated with vitamin A deficiency.

It has been demonstrated experimentally in adult goats fed vitamin A-deficient diets that decreased absorption of CSF can result, but CSF pressure does not rise significantly and no papilledema of the optic nerve develops (Frier et al. 1974). Convulsions were not observed in either this study or an earlier one involving both adult and young, growing goats (Schmidt 1941). Signs were limited to a loss of appetite and weight, ropy nasal discharge, corneal opacity, and night blindness. Hypovitaminosis A is not a likely cause of convulsions in goats.

PLANT TOXICITIES

Bitterweed Poisoning

Hymenoxys odorata, an annual of the Texas range, is a major cause of economic loss in sheep and also affects

Angora goats. The plant, known as western bitterweed or bitter rubberweed, is most common in southwest Texas, especially on the Edwards Plateau. It is found between December and May, especially January through March, and may be the only succulent range plant available, particularly during times of drought. Goats are much less inclined to eat this plant than sheep unless forced to do so by a severe lack of forage.

A second plant, *Hymenoxys richardsoni*, known as pingue or Colorado rubberweed, can also produce the disease and is found more extensively in the west from Kansas to Mexico. The major toxin, hymenoxon, a sesquiterpine lactone, is a cumulative toxin that inhibits cellular function by alkylating sulfhydril groups of cellular enzymes. The principal signs are gastrointestinal and neurological. In sheep, the LD_{50} of *H. odorata* is just 1.3% of body weight. Goats are reported to be slightly more resistant, requiring 1.8 times more plant material than sheep to produce death (Rowe et al. 1973).

Acute, subacute, and chronic disease states can occur. The acute form is seen mostly under experimental conditions, after a single large ingestion. The clinical course is one to four days and leads to death. Early signs include bloat, anorexia, arching of the back, teeth grinding, and marked depression. Affected animals become increasingly depressed and may show regurgitation, fine muscle tremors, mucous nasal discharge, mild dyspnea, and head pressing. Terminal animals become recumbent with intermittent paddling, tonic convulsions, opisthotonos, tachycardia, severe dyspnea, and regurgitation.

The subacute and chronic forms are more likely under field conditions, usually after approximately one month of low-level exposure to the plant. In the subacute form, animals show only anorexia, a greenish nasal discharge, and possible regurgitation, and die quietly after one to seven days. Chronically affected animals become anorexic, weak, and thin, and die of starvation or dehydration caused by the inability to gather food. At necropsy, gross findings consist of edema and hemorrhage of lungs and epicardium and congestion and hemorrhage of the abomasum and duodenum.

Though there is no specific therapy, a gradual recovery can occur if affected animals are removed from the plant source and fed fresh feed and water. In severe cases, oral administration of activated charcoal may improve chances of recovery. Control of bitterweed poisoning involves avoidance of overgrazing and reduction of bitterweed or pingue by mowing and burning, fencing, or applying herbicides to reduce plant populations.

Coyotillo Poisoning

Karwinskia humboldtiana, or coyotillo, is a woody shrub indigenous to southern Texas and California and northern Mexico. It grows on gravelly hills and ridges and in canyons, gullies, and river valleys. The leaves and fruit are toxic, and spontaneous poisoning has been reported in goats, sheep, cattle, and humans, especially in winter when the plants are heavy with fruit and other forage is scarce. Losses of more than 1,000 goats caused by coyotillo poisoning have been reported on Texas ranches (Sperry et al. 1962). Consumption of whole fruit in quantities as little as 0.3% of the goat's body weight is lethal. The toxicity is due to polyphenolic compounds in the plant which are not fully characterized. The toxic action is primarily on striated muscle cells and Schwann cells leading to cellular degeneration.

Early signs in goats include increased alertness, hypersensitivity to sound and touch, generalized fine tremors, and a humpbacked posture, soon followed by disturbances of gait. The stride becomes shortened and jerky or hypermetric. These abnormalities are aggravated by forced exercise. The jerkiness of the gait gradually gives way to a marked weakness with hypotonia and loss of stretch reflexes. The goat assumes a crouched posture with marked hock and carpal flexion during standing or ambulation. Stumbling is common. Severely affected goats gradually become recumbent. Patellar and gastrocnemius reflexes are lost. Appetite, urination, and defecation remain normal until close to the time of death. Dyspnea is common in the terminal stages. The course of disease may last from several days to several weeks (Charlton et al. 1971).

Gross lesions in coyotillo poisoning of goats are not described. Histologically, lesions of the nervous system are found in the peripheral nerves and the cerebellum. There is extensive Schwann cell degeneration and demyelination and to a lesser extent Wallerian degeneration of axons. Secondary axonal degeneration is most prominent in distal sections of long motor nerves (Charlton and Pierce 1970). Axonal dystrophy of Purkinje cells is also prominent in the cerebellum of affected goats (Charlton et al. 1970). Myodegeneration of heart and skeletal muscle may also be observed as well as fatty degeneration of the liver (Dewan et al. 1965). The muscle lesions are similar to those seen in nutritional muscular dystrophy.

Treatment is nonspecific and involves removal of affected goats from the plant and providing adequate feed and water. Some recoveries can occur. Goats should not be turned into infested areas for grazing when the plant is in fruit.

Astragalus Poisoning (Alpha mannosidosis; Locoism)

Several distinct disease syndromes of differing pathogenesis are associated with livestock consumption of leguminous weeds of the genera *Astragalus* and

Oxytropis. Three of these syndromes produce signs of nervous disease and have been identified in goats. The first, locoism, is a chronic poisoning that results from prolonged consumption of species containing the indolizidine alkaloid, swainsonine. This alkaloid produces an acquired lysosomal storage disease, alpha mannosidosis, by inhibiting lysosomal alpha mannosidase, which leads to vacuolation and degeneration of the CNS.

Other plants also contain swainsonine and can induce acquired alpha mannosidosis in grazing livestock. These include *Swainsona* spp. and *Sphaerophysa* spp. which are, like *Astragalus* and *Oxytropis*, in the family Fabaceae, *Ipomoea* spp. and *Turbina* spp. in the family Convolvulaceae, and *Sida* spp. in the family Malvaceae. Ingestion of *Ipomoea carnea* (Schumaher-Henrique et al. 2003) and *Turbina cordata* (Dantas et al. 2007) are reported to cause acquired alpha mannosidosis in goats in Brazil and *I. carnea* consumption has been associated with the disease in goats in Mozambique as well (Balogh et al. 1999). Ingestion of *Sida carpinifolia* has caused the disease in Brazilian goats (Colodel et al. 2002). A similar acquired lysosomal storage disease in goats has been reported in association with consumption of *I. hieronymi* in Argentina (Rodriguez Armesto et al. 2004). Several *Oxytropis* spp. in China and *Swainsona* spp. in Australia have also been associated with acquired alpha mannosidosis in grazing livestock, but cases specifically in goats, though possible, have not been reported.

The second syndrome is an acute poisoning resulting from short term consumption of plant species possessing nitro-containing glycosides, notably miserotoxin. The third syndrome is blind staggers, or alkali disease, a condition long thought to be due to chronic selenium poisoning associated with consumption of plant species such as *Astragalus* that act as selenium accumulators. The condition has been known in western rangelands of the United States for more than a century, but in recent years the role of selenium in this disease has been called into question and the theory proposed that this condition is actually a manifestation of polioencephalomalacia resulting from excessive sulfur intake (O'Toole et al. 1996).

Species of *Astragalus* and *Oxytropis* that cause locoism are found in temperate regions worldwide but the disease is of particular concern in grazing stock in the western United States, particularly on open plains in winter. The plants are not palatable and livestock eat them initially only during times of limited forage. They quickly become habituated to locoweeds, however, continuing to eat them even when other feeds become available. The poisoning results from chronic ingestion, with signs appearing six to eight weeks after the onset of grazing locoweed and death four to six weeks later.

While reports of spontaneous locoism in goats in the United States are scarce and the economic impact minor, the clinical effects of two Texas locoweeds, *A. earlei* and *A. wootoni*, have been documented (Mathews 1932). Goats ate 335% of their body weight of *A. earlei* over fifty-four days to produce locoism, but refused to eat *A. wootoni*. Early signs include hind limb weakness characterized by inability to extend the hocks and an intermittent, weaving, rear gait. Startled goats may stumble or suddenly collapse onto their hindquarters but remain supported on the forelimbs. Paresis and ataxia are progressive, eventually involving the forelimbs as well. In advanced stages, goats become sternally recumbent with intermittent opisthotonos, nystagmus, and shaking of the head. There is progressive weight loss. Goats may remain bright and alert until just a few days before death. In comparison, sheep almost always show profound depression in locoism. Documentation of abortion in goats caused by locoism, a common problem in sheep, is lacking. At necropsy, gross lesions are limited to emaciation and possibly abomasal ulceration. Histologically there is vacuolation of neurons in the CNS.

Goats may recover from locoism if they are removed from locoweeds early in the course of the disease and then are well fed and watered. However, they may seek out and resume eating locoweed if allowed subsequent access, due to the habituation that occurs.

The acute neurologic form of *Astragalus* poisoning caused by nitro-containing compounds has been reported in cattle and sheep in Texas and reproduced experimentally in goats by feeding *A. emoryanus*, the red-stemmed peavine (Mathews 1940). Young green plants are most toxic and effects are seen when plants are consumed at a rate of 0.7% to 1.8% of body weight. Goats may show profound depression, anorexia, recumbency, weakness, and death within one to two days of initial consumption. In less severe cases, goats develop pronounced ataxia that is particularly evident in the hind limbs and that can persist for as long as one year after the animals are denied access to the plant. Dyspnea, associated with methemoglobinemia, as observed in sheep poisoned by peavine, was not observed in goats. There are no characteristic gross or microscopic lesions.

"Blind staggers" has been reported in goats and sheep in Iran after prolonged grazing of *Astragalus* spp. (Hosseinion et al. 1972). This form of *Astragalus* toxicity has been ascribed to its role as a selenium accumulator. Emaciation, rough hair coat, anorexia, separation from the flock, impaired vision, circling, and a staggering gait were observed as were foamy salivation, lacrimation, severe constipation, and signs of abdominal pain. The mortality rate was approximately 4%. Selenium concentration of the weeds was 500 ppm.

Guajillo Poisoning

Acacia berlanderi, or guajillo, is a perennial shrub of rangeland in southwest Texas and Mexico. The plant is palatable and routine grazing by goats and sheep is generally permitted. However, it may cause toxicity under drought conditions when the diet is monotonous and consumption extends for six months or longer. The toxic principles are sympathomimetic amines, N-methyl-beta-phenylethylamine (Camp and Lyman 1957) and tyramine. Affected animals retain their appetites and remain bright and alert. The predominant clinical sign is a progressive ataxia that eventually leads to recumbency and death secondary to starvation and thirst. The condition is known locally as limberleg or guajillo wobbles. There are no significant lesions found at necropsy. Recoveries can occur if the condition is identified early and animals removed from the plant.

Carpetweed or Caltrops Poisoning

Kallstroemia hirsutissima, known as carpetweed or caltrops, is a low lying, ground hugging weed of disturbed soils in western North America from Kansas south to northern Mexico. Though not palatable, the plant may be consumed by grazing livestock in summer during periods of drought. Natural cases of poisoning in goats are not documented, but experimental poisoning has been reported (Mathews 1944). The toxic principal is unknown. The susceptibility of goats is variable with clinical disease seen in one goat eating the plant at a rate of 11% of body weight, and no signs seen in another eating 177% of its weight in carpetweed. After three days of consumption, the affected goat showed signs of marked paresis, being unable to stand normally, and walking on the carpi in front with the hocks flexed behind. The animal was killed and no gross lesions were observed. Cattle and sheep also showed marked paresis and walked with prominent knuckling of the fetlocks.

Milkweed Poisoning

There are numerous species of milkweeds in the genus *Asclepias* and many are toxic to livestock. Many are distributed widely throughout the United States. These plants are not normally eaten except in times of drought or limited forage. They also may be baled into hay and retain their toxicity when dry. Goats are poisoned by milkweed (Kingsbury 1964). Consumption of various *Asclepias* species in doses from 0.25% to 2% of body weight can be toxic. Clinical signs appear within a few hours of ingestion of a toxic dose and include profound depression, weakness, and a staggering gait. Bloat and dyspnea may also occur. Severely affected animals go down and exhibit intermittent tetanic convulsions. Pupils become dilated, coma ensues, and death usually occurs between one and two days after the onset of signs. The milkweeds contain toxic resins and steroid glycosides, including cardiac glycosides, but the specific mechanism of neurotoxicity is not known. Nonspecific lesions at necropsy include congestion of liver and kidneys and irritation of intestinal mucosa. There is no known treatment and poisoning is controlled by reducing access to milkweed and by maintaining pastures in good condition.

Cycasin Toxicity or Zamia Staggers

Cycasin is a toxic pseudocyanogenic glycoside found in the nuts, leaves, and young shoots of various tropical cycad palms. Poisoning of cattle has been associated with consumption of leaves or young shoots of four genera: *Cycas, Macrozamia, Zamia,* and *Bowenia* in Puerto Rico, the Dominican Republic, Japan, and Australia. The poisoning of goats with *Cycas media* is a serious problem in parts of Australia, notably Groote Eylandt (Hall 1964). Clinical neurologic disease associated with ingestion of the seeds of the King Sago palm tree, *Cycas revoluta*, has been reported in dogs in the southern United States so the potential for goat exposure exists there (Albretsen et al. 1998).

Chronic consumption leads to incoordination characterized by a lack of proprioception, with abnormal placement of feet, knuckling, and stumbling or falling. Pain responses, motor control, and withdrawal reflexes remain intact. Once signs are observed, the condition is irreversible (Baxendell 1988). Goats experimentally poisoned with cycasin extracts also show marked depression, anorexia, weight loss, and anemia. At necropsy, histologic lesions of the spinal cord include axonal swelling and death with demyelination most prominent in the lateral and ventral funiculi. Hepatic necrosis, biliary hyperplasia, and pancreatic atrophy were additional necropsy findings in experimentally poisoned goats (Shimizu et al. 1986).

Miscellaneous Plant Poisonings

Nervous disease in goats associated with plant ingestions have been reported sporadically from various places in the world. *Solanum* spp. have been reported to produce neurologic dysfunction in goats in Australia (Bourke 1997) and Florida (Porter et al. 2003). In Australia, the implicated plant was *S. cinereum* (Nawarra burr) and in Florida, *S. viarum* (tropical soda apple). The clinical presentation was similar in both instances and strongly suggested involvement of the cerebellum, with grazing goats showing signs of head tremor, wide base stance, hypermetria, incoordination, nystagmus, and proprioceptive deficits. At necropsy, CNS lesions were restricted to the cerebellum and were characterized by cytoplasmic vacuolation, degeneration, and loss of Purkinje fibers. The *Solanum* spp. may contain several toxic principles, including the steroidal glycosides solasonine and solasodine as well as beta-carboline alkaloids. The exact cause of the cerebellar degeneration is not fully clarified.

Albizia is a genus of legumes in the family Mimosaceae. Seed pods of the toxic species in this genus contain 4-methoxy-pyridone, a pyridoxine (vitamin B_6) analog which causes neurologic dysfunction as well as cardiomyopathy and pulmonary edema. An outbreak of *A. versicolor* poisoning of goats and sheep eating ripe, dry, seed pods was reported from Malawi and was confirmed by experimental oral challenge of goats and sheep with dried seed pods (Soldan et al. 1996). Sheep were more susceptible than goats. Signs of intoxication included hyperesthesia, wild running, lateral recumbency with rapid leg movements, nystagmus, and rapid blinking. The condition is reported to be treatable in sheep with 20 to 25 mg/kg pyroxidine hydrochloride/kg bw given twice at an eight-hour interval, even after clinical signs are apparent and well advanced (Gummow et al. 1992).

In Togo, grazing on the shrub *Byrsocarpus coccineus* —especially young shoots—at the beginning of the rainy season in March and April produces toxicity in goats. Clinical signs include anorexia, weight loss, separation from the flock, dizziness, staggering gait, circling, and frantic, aimless flight. In peracute cases, tetanic convulsions are observed. Recovery occurs if goats and sheep are removed to pastures where the shrub is absent (Amégée 1983).

In Tanzania, ingestion of the seeds or leaves of the deciduous shrub *Burttia prunoides* has produced neurologic signs in goats including circling, bleating, lateral recumbency, teeth grinding, convulsions, coma, and death. The disease has been observed naturally and produced experimentally (Msengi et al. 1987). In Sudan, *Azadirachta indica* is reputed to cause toxicity to livestock. Experimentally, continuous feeding of leaves of this plant to goats led to weight loss, weakness, diarrhea, and terminally, ataxia and tremors (Ali 1987).

In Holland, ingestion of fool's parsley *(Aethusa cynapium)* by goats led to signs of ataxia, indigestion, and hyperpnea. Affected goats were treated orally with oak bark, tannalbumin, and purgative salts, and recovered in several days (Swart 1975). This annual weed also occurs in northeastern North America and is found locally in waste places and gardens.

Diplodiosis is a neuromycotoxicosis of cattle and occasionally sheep in South Africa. It occurs when livestock consume maize contaminated with the fungus *Diplodia maydis*. Goats are susceptible based on experimental toxicosis, showing typical signs of ataxia, paresis, and paralysis. The fungus occurs on corn in the United States and Argentina, but poisoning of livestock has not yet been reported from these places (Kellerman et al. 1985).

Larkspurs (*Delphinium* spp.) are an important cause of cattle mortality during spring and early summer grazing in western North America. The plant is readily eaten. Goats are presumed susceptible. Toxic alkaloids in larkspurs block postsynaptic cholinergic receptors. Signs of toxicity include sudden death, or a staggering gait, basewide stance, collapse, difficulty rising, muscle twitching, abdominal pain, constipation, and bloat. Removal from the plant and early treatment with neostigmine at 0.01 to 0.02 mg/kg bw intramuscularly, repeated as needed, may be effective (Knight 1987).

Plant poisonings that produce signs of nervous dysfunction via the mechanism of hepatoencephalopathy secondary to phytogenous hepatosis are discussed in Chapter 11. Plants causing blindness are discussed in Chapter 6.

A number of additional plants have been identified as causing neurologic symptoms in small ruminants (Brewer 1983). While their toxicity in sheep is well established, documentation of goat poisonings is often lacking. These plants include *Solanum esuriale*, the cause of "humpy back" in Australia; *Kochia scoparia*, or Mexican fireweed found in the western United States; and the lupines of the western United States and Australia. In addition, phalaris, paspallum, rye, and dallis grasses have been associated with "grass staggers" in sheep but the condition in goats is not well defined. Periodically, Bermuda grass *(Cynodon dactylon)* has been associated with cattle losses in the southern United States, producing ataxia, tremors, and sometimes death. The toxicity for goats has been demonstrated experimentally (Strain et al. 1982). Convulsive ergotism, well documented in other livestock species, is poorly substantiated in goats.

INORGANIC CHEMICAL NEUROTOXICITIES

Lead Poisoning

Documented cases of naturally occurring lead poisoning in goats are not found in the contemporary veterinary literature. Nevertheless, several reviews of goat diseases identify lead poisoning as a disease of goats producing neurologic signs similar to those seen in affected cattle or sheep. Signs cited include blindness, ataxia, head pressing, circling, hypermetria, grinding of teeth, and diarrhea. However, experimental studies of lead poisoning in goats report either no neurologic dysfunction or nervous signs limited to depression, incoordination, or terminal convulsions. Weight loss, anorexia, abortion, and diarrhea are the more prominent signs in experimental lead poisoning of goats (Dollahite et al. 1975; Davis et al. 1976; Gouda et al. 1985).

Goats are considered resistant to lead poisoning compared to cattle and dogs and have been observed not to become ill under circumstances where companion cattle show signs of disease. Whether this was caused by innate resistance or an unwillingness to consume sources of lead is not clear (Guss 1977). Certainly they are exposed to lead in certain circumstances such as when they graze near lead-zinc smelters, in which case elevated blood lead levels have been documented along with depressed blood copper and cobalt levels (Swarup et al. 2006). At least experimentally, goats refuse to eat lead-based paint or pure lead acetate despite the sweet taste of the latter (Davis et al. 1976). Susceptibility to lead poisoning varies between individual goats and may be increased by pregnancy (Dollahite et al. 1975).

Diagnosis of lead poisoning in goats depends on a strong history of exposure, identification of the source, and confirmation of increased blood or tissue lead levels. Goats appear to accumulate lead less dramatically than other species. Experimentally poisoned, clinically ill goats had whole blood lead levels as low as 0.2 ppm, liver levels as low as 5.5 ppm, and renal cortex levels as low as 26 ppm. Values higher than these should be considered diagnostic for lead poisoning when evaluating field cases. Liver lead levels in aborted fetuses greater than 1.5 ppm are suggestive of lead-induced abortion. It has also been reported that blood porphyrin levels are reliably elevated in lead poisoning in goats. Goats experimentally administered lead acetate for ninety-one days had progressively increasing mean blood porphyrin levels in the range of 31.7 to 56.9 µg/dl, while control goats had levels in the range of 23.5 to 24.6 µg/dl. Most of the lead-exposed goats also showed a so-called lead line in radiographs of forelimbs, with marked radiopaque bands at the distal metaphysis of the radii, indicating incorporation of lead in bone at the growth plates. The goats were eight to nine months old at the onset of the exposure (Swarup et al. 1990).

Because the occurrence of nervous signs in lead poisoning of goats is not firmly established, veterinarians are strongly encouraged to submit whole blood for lead analysis in all suspect cases and to pursue alternate diagnoses while waiting for test results. When blindness is present in conjunction with other neurologic signs, serious consideration must be given to polioencephalomalacia as an alternate diagnosis and intravenous thiamine therapy at 10 mg/kg should be instituted immediately.

When lead poisoning is the working diagnosis, treatment is similar to that of other species and is targeted primarily at chelation of lead for removal from the body. The chelating agent, calcium disodium versanate, remains the standard treatment in ruminants (Cebra and Cebra 2004). The recommended regimen consists of two treatments given intravenously at a dose of 110 mg/kg bw daily at a six-hour interval for up to three to five days (Radostits et al. 2007). Experimentally, meso-2,3-dimercaptosuccinic acid has also shown promise as a chelation treatment for lead removal in ruminants (Meldrum et al. 2003). As an adjunct to chelation therapy, administration of thiamine hydrochloride in cattle with lead poisoning improved the clinical response. It resulted in better remission of nervous signs and also appeared to enhance the reduction of blood lead concentration (Coppock et al. 1991). The dose was 2 mg/kg bw thiamine hydrochloride given intramuscularly once daily.

Treatment efficacy may be monitored by repeated blood lead measurements. High blood levels that persist during a course of therapy suggests the presence of a persistent source of lead in the rumen that may require removal by rumenotomy.

Salt Poisoning

Salt poisoning occurs in livestock when there is excessive salt intake from the feed, inadequate water intake in the face of normal salt intake, or when only saline drinking water is available. The condition is most common in swine, but is also reported in cattle and sheep. Documentation of the condition in goats is rare but it is sometimes included in discussions of diseases showing nervous signs (Guss 1977; Baxendell 1988). In a case report from Italy, one of eight affected goats presented with convulsions, opisthotonos, and respiratory distress while the other seven showed weakness and intense thirst. The severely affected goat died and had cerebral edema at necropsy. The others were successfully rehydrated (Buronfosse 2000).

Signs of acute salt intoxication in other species include tremors, blindness, nystagmus, weakness, incoordination, knuckling of the fetlocks, head pressing, opisthotonos, convulsions, coma, and death associated with cerebral edema. When the disease occurs from a large dose of excess salt, signs of gastrointestinal irritation including vomiting, diarrhea, and abdominal pain may also be seen. When neurologic signs are marked, tranquilization with diazepam and reduction of cerebral edema with diuretics and mannitol solutions may be indicated. The condition and its management in other species is reviewed in detail elsewhere (Cebra and Cebra 2004; Radostits et al. 2007).

Bromide Intoxication

Two separate incidents of bromide poisoning of goats have been reported in the United States. One involved contamination of pastures by sodium bromide from an adjacent chemical dump and the other, contamination of oat hay grown on fields initially treated with methyl bromide as a nematocide (Knight and Costner 1977; Liggett et al. 1985). Although the latter source of bromide is organic, toxicity is believed to be caused by release and uptake by plants of bromide ion from the treated soil. The clinical signs were similar in both cases and developed over a period of days to weeks after exposure. Weakness and locomotor impairment were characteristic, with difficulty standing and turning, stumbling and dragging of the feet while walking. Dribbling of urine; drooping ears, eyelids, and tail; and a progressive somnolence and recumbency were observed. Deaths occurred in both outbreaks.

Measurement of serum bromide can be diagnostic. In the sodium bromide-related outbreak, unexposed, control goats had concentrations less than 0.625 mEq/l, exposed goats with no clinical signs measured 1.6 to 3.2 mEq/l, and clinically affected goats had concentrations more than 21.1 mEq/l. When laboratory measurement of serum chloride is performed using an ion-selective electrode, pseudohyperchloremia may be recorded in animals with bromide poisoning.

There are no definitive necropsy lesions, although necrosis of the ventral horn of the lumbar spinal cord was noted in one goat. There is no specific therapy reported, but some goats did recover after hospitalization with supportive care for four to fifteen days.

Boron or Borax Intoxication

Borax may be found on the farm for use as a soil sterilant or fly control compound. Goats may be accidentally exposed but are unlikely to voluntarily ingest it unless it was accidentally incorporated into the feed. Clinical signs of intoxication may include diarrhea, dehydration, and convulsions before coma and death (Guss 1977).

The toxicity of boron has been demonstrated experimentally in goats (Sisk et al. 1988). A goat given sodium borate fertilizer orally at a dose of 3.6 g/kg bw exhibited signs of weakness and somnolence, with the chin resting on the floor. It developed muscle tremors and pasty feces, and died quietly eight hours after challenge. A second goat given the fertilizer at a dose of 1.8 g/kg did not become ill. Neurotoxicity is presumed to be involved in boron toxicity, but the mechanism is not fully known. A stimulatory effect on serotonergic and dopaminergic neurons has been proposed based on increased metabolites of serotonin and dopamine in CSF fluid of experimentally challenged goats (Sisk et al. 1990). No specific treatment is reported, but efforts to restore hydration may be helpful.

ORGANIC CHEMICAL NEUROTOXICITIES

Organophosphates and Carbamates

Etiology and epidemiology

Organophosphate and carbamate pesticides are commonly found on farms. They are used to treat livestock for internal and external parasites, and to protect soil and crops from insect pests. Toxicities occur when animals are overdosed either by parenteral or topical administration or when livestock gain accidental access to chemicals that are carelessly stored, accidentally spilled, or inadvertently added to feed or water supplies. Toxic doses of various organophosphate and carbamate compounds administered either orally or topically to goats are given in Table 5.5.

Pathogenesis

Organophosphates and carbamates exert their toxic effects by competitive inhibition of acetylcholinesterase, the enzyme ordinarily responsible for the degradation of the neurotransmitter acetylcholine. This inhibition leads to accumulation of acetylcholine at neuromuscular junctions, autonomic ganglia, and effector cells, and causes an increased, prolonged stimulation of skeletal muscle, the entire parasympathetic nervous system, and the post-ganglionic cholinergic nerves of the sympathetic system. These sustained muscarinic and nicotinic effects are responsible for the clinical signs associated with toxicity.

In sheep, a delayed neurotoxicity caused by the organophosphate anthelmintic haloxon is recognized. The pathogenesis of delayed neurotoxicity is believed to involve an inherited esterase deficiency in Suffolk sheep. A distal axonopathy with dying back of neurons, particularly long axons in the spinal cord, develops several weeks after administration of haloxon. The clinical picture is one of progressive, symmetric, spastic paresis of the hind limbs. This syndrome has been suspected in Angora goats, but no additional documentation has emerged (Wilson et al. 1982).

Clinical Findings

The clinical signs of acute toxicity in goats are similar to those seen in other species, and include restlessness, frothing at the mouth, dyspnea, tremors, frequent urination and defecation, bloat, head pressing, teeth grinding, lacrimation, staggering gait, intermittent convulsions, paresis, and finally, recumbency and death (Mohamed et al. 1989, 1990).

Clinical Pathology and Necropsy

Identifying a marked decrease in acetylcholinesterase activity supports the diagnosis of organophosphate and carbamate poisoning. Whole blood is a suitable sample in goats because 89% of acetylcholinesterase activity in blood is in red blood cells (Osweiler et al. 1984). Heparinized blood samples should be submitted refrigerated but not frozen. When carbamates are suspected, blood must be refrigerated immediately and tested as soon as possible because inhibition of acetylcholinesterase by carbamate is reversible. The laboratory should be notified of your suspicion of carbamates so that test methods that require dilution of the sample are not used.

Table 5.5. Toxicity of some organophosphate, carbamate, and chlorinated hydrocarbon insecticides for goats.

Chemical	*Oral dose*		*Dermal dose (%)*	
	Maximum nontoxic dose tested (mg/kg bw)	*Minimum toxic dose found (mg/kg bw)*	*Maximum nontoxic dose tested (% concentration)*	*Minimum toxic dose found (% concentration)*
Organophosphates				
Chlorpyrifos		LD_{50} = 500		
Coumaphos			0.25	0.5
Crufomate		100	2.5	
Crotoxyphos			1	
Demeton		LD_{50} = 8		
Diazinon	20	30		
Dichlofenthion			0.25	0.5
Dioxathion			0.25	
Disulfoton		LD_{50} < 15		
Ethion			0.25	0.5
Fenthion				0.25
Malathion	50	100		
Methyl trithion			0.1	
Monocrotophos		LD_{50} = 20		
Parathion		20		
Phosmet			0.5	
Carbamates				
Carbaryl			1	
Landrin		LD_{50} = 210		
Propoxur		LD_{50} > 800		
Chlorinated hydrocarbons				
Aldrin				4
Chlordane			3	4
DDT	250			8
Dieldrin		LD_{50} = 100		
Endrin		LD_{50} = 25		
Toxaphene	25	LD_{50} > 160		

Traditional test methods determine the change of pH that occurs when acetylcholinesterase hydrolyses acetylcholine or a substitute ester under controlled conditions. The normal range of delta pH for caprine whole blood acetylcholinesterase activity is 0.04 to 0.24, with a mean of 0.14 (Osweiler et al. 1984). In cases of toxicity, delta pH is frequently zero. Titrimetric methods, which do not require sample dilution, report acetylcholinesterase activity as the µmol of substrate hydrolyzed/minute/ml of whole blood or plasma. Normal values in goats using acetylcholine iodide as a substrate have been reported in the range of 4.20 to 5.60 µmol/minute/ml of whole blood and 0.60 to 1 µmol/minute/ml in plasma. Activity was reduced to levels of 20% to 50% of normal after oral administration of toxic doses of diazinon, phosmet, phosphamidon, or trichlorfon, with reported activity ranging from 0.90 to 2.50 µmol/minute/ml in whole blood and 0.27 to 0.32 µmol/minute/ml in plasma (Abdelsalam 1987). Dialkyl phosphates are hydrolytic breakdown products of the phosphate moieties of organophosphate insecticides. Detection of dialkyl phosphates in the urine of goats proved to be a reliable indicator of exposure to diazinon over a range of challenge doses (Mount 1984). The test was more sensitive than measurement of blood cholinesterase activity in goats not showing clinical signs of toxicity.

There are no specific necropsy findings in organophosphate or carbamate poisoning. Chemical analysis of tissues is often unrewarding because organophosphate and carbamate insecticides are rapidly metabolized. Analysis of stomach or rumen content, suspected feeds, or other formulations for insecticide content is preferred.

Diagnosis

Diagnosis is based on the characteristic signs of acute toxicity in conjunction with documentation of decreased or absent acetylcholinesterase activity. In the absence of laboratory support, a favorable clinical response to atropine or oxime therapy supports the diagnosis. Other acute poisonings, such as cyanide, nitrate, and urea toxicity, and anaphylactic reactions must be considered in the differential diagnosis. The pyrethroid insecticide fenvalerate has been shown to produce clinical signs suggestive of organophosphate toxicity when administered orally to Nubian goats at doses more than 112.5 mg/kg (Mohamed and Adam 1990).

Treatment and Control

Treatment can be successful, especially with early intervention. The treatment of choice to counteract signs of toxicity is atropine sulfate given at a dose of 0.6 to 1 mg/kg bw. One-fourth to one-third the total dose should be given intravenously and the remainder subcutaneously or intramuscularly. The higher end of the dose range can be used in severe cases. Repeated dosing may be necessary every four to five hours for as long as two days in severe cases, but dosage should be cut back when possible to avoid serious bloat.

Oximes, such as trimedoxime bromide, 2-pyridine aldoxime methiodide (2-PAM), and pralidoxime chloride, free acetylcholinesterase from organophosphate, but not from carbamate complexes. They are particularly useful in combination with atropine for the treatment of coumaphos, ronnel, dimethoate, and crufomate toxicity, where atropine alone is not always effective (Osweiler et al. 1984). The use of these drugs in goats is not reported. In other ruminants, recommended doses are as follows; 2-PAM, 50 to 100 mg/kg bw; trimedoxime bromide, 10 to 20 mg/kg bw; and pralidoxime chloride, 20 mg/kg bw intravenously.

When poisoning is by the oral route, oral administration of 1 g/kg bw activated charcoal per adult goat by orogastric tube may help to reduce the additional uptake of insecticide. When exposure is dermal, washing animals with soap and water helps to reduce additional absorption. Handlers should wear masks and rubber gloves. Control of these toxicities is difficult because most outbreaks involve accidental exposure. Certainly these chemicals should be treated with respect and used only according to directions. They should be stored securely where animal contact is impossible.

Chlorinated Hydrocarbons

Etiology and Epidemiology

These insecticide compounds, also known as organochlorines, have been used widely in agriculture for treatment of soils, water supplies, crops, seeds, and livestock. Methoxychlor, lindane, DDT, aldrin, dieldrin, chlordane, and toxaphene are common examples. Use of these insecticides directly on livestock is increasingly restricted due to environmental and public health concerns. Nevertheless, accidental exposures or inappropriate use still lead to toxicities in livestock, including goats. Information on toxic doses of various chlorinated hydrocarbons for goats is given in Table 5.5. Because goats are used for both meat and milk production, the potential for relay toxicity to humans from consumption of goat products is similar to cattle. These compounds are noted for persistence in fatty tissues over long periods. Residue levels in goat milk and tissues for various chlorinated hydrocarbons have been reported (Cho et al. 1976).

Pathogenesis

The pathogenesis of toxicity for these compounds is not completely known and may be different for each. At least for chlorophenothane, the compound acts on axonal membranes to prolong the depolarized state by interfering with sodium influx and potassium efflux. Poisoning can occur by single large-dose exposure or chronic lower-dose exposure due to the ability of these insecticides to accumulate in tissues. Absorption of these chemicals can occur through the skin, or by oral ingestion, aspiration, or inhalation. Neurologic signs in all cases are the usual clinical manifestation.

Clinical Findings

Clinical signs are similar in all species. Hypersensitivity, apprehension, and/or aggressiveness are frequent early signs followed by fasciculation of muscles, especially in the head and neck, that extend to muscular spasms over the entire body. Snapping of the eyelids and continuous chewing or teeth grinding are common, sometimes with excessive salivation. Moderate bloating may occur. Loss of coordination with staggering gait, aimless wandering, or circling may be observed. Severe and prolonged convulsions frequently develop. It is not unusual for animals to have a high fever due to seizure activity. Though animals may die during convulsions, death is usually preceded by terminal coma.

The severity of signs is to some extent dose dependent. Experimental poisoning with aldrin at a daily oral dose of 2.5 mg/kg bw led to clinical signs of depression, anorexia, teeth grinding, salivation, staggering gait, and hypersensitivity in one goat after eighteen days of dosing but no signs of toxicity in three others (Singh et al. 1985). Goats given daily aldrin orally at a dose of 20 mg/kg showed signs of hyperexcitability, incoordination of movement, muscle tremors, and convulsions by the ninth day of dosing, and died one to three days later (Omer and Awad Elkarim 1981).

Clinical Pathology and Necropsy

Clinicopathologic data are generally not helpful in the diagnosis before death. There are no specific necropsy findings, although pulmonary congestion and ecchymotic hemorrhages of the heart and other serosal surfaces may be observed. When there have been severe prolonged convulsions with fever, the intestines may have a blanched or cooked appearance.

Diagnosis

Presumptive diagnosis depends on a history of exposure to chlorinated hydrocarbons followed by the development of typical clinical signs. Definitive diagnosis depends on identification of the offending agent by laboratory analysis of hair samples, rumen content, fat biopsies, or milk samples antemortem or in tissue samples post mortem, especially liver, brain, and fat. Concentrations of the various chlorinated hydrocarbons considered diagnostic of toxicity in goat tissue are not well documented. Analyses are complex and costly so there should be some notion of the specific chemical being searched for.

Treatment and Control

Therapy is primarily supportive. When topical poisoning is involved, animals should be washed thoroughly with soap and water. Handlers should wear masks and rubber gloves. In cases of ingestion, gastric lavage may be performed or activated charcoal given at a dose of 1 g/kg bw per adult goat as soon as possible after exposure. Seizures may need to be controlled by use of long-acting barbiturates. Daily oral dosing of recovered animals with small volumes of mineral oil may help to clear chlorinated hydrocarbons from the intestinal tract but will have little or no effect in mobilizing the agents in tissue. Specific guidelines for the safety of meat and milk products from goats recovered from poisoning are not available. Because of the potential harmful effects in humans, the consumption of meat or milk from these recovered animals should be discouraged. Control essentially involves client education concerning the danger, proper usage, and safe storage of chlorinated hydrocarbons.

Miscellaneous Organic Chemical Toxicities

Levamisole, a widely used caprine anthelmintic, is one of the most common potential causes of neurotoxicity in goats. When overdosed, it can produce a clinical syndrome very similar to nicotine poisoning with signs including anxiety, hyperesthesia, increased urination and defecation, muscle tremors, staggering gait, and convulsions. More information on levamisole use and toxicity in goats is given in Chapter 10.

Urea toxicity has been reported in goats. The syndrome is characterized by abdominal pain, bloat, dyspnea, and frothy salivation; neurologic signs include ataxia, tremors, hyperesthesia, and struggling. The condition is discussed in detail in Chapter 19.

Both cyanide and nitrate poisoning can produce signs of nervous dysfunction including excitement, muscle tremors, staggering gait, and dilated pupils secondary to systemic anoxia. These conditions are discussed in detail in Chapter 9.

Diesel fuel poisoning has been reported in goats when the animals drank from a small pond containing fuel from an overturned tank truck (Toofanian et al. 1979). Goats drank the tainted water readily. Clinical signs developed within hours and included anorexia, depression, diarrhea, dyspnea, and a mucopurulent nasal discharge. The breath and the urine smelled strongly of diesel fuel. Affected goats progressively worsened; developed neurologic signs including incoordination, tremors, head pressing, aimless wandering, pica, abnormal vocalization, and recumbency; and died, presumably due to respiratory compromise.

Nitrofurans are a class of antibacterials that were formerly in common use for control of enteric infections in young calves and pigs. Due to public health concerns about their carcinogenicity, the use of nitrofurans in food animals is now severely restricted in many countries, including the United States, where parenteral use was first banned in 1991 and topical use was banned in 2002. The toxicity of furazolidone in Nubian goats has been reported (Ali et al. 1984). At oral daily doses as low as 40 mg/kg for as long as ten days, goats showed signs of anorexia, weight loss, restlessness, incoordination, and hyperexcitability, with constant chewing movements, tail wagging, foot stamping, backward walking, and circling. At daily oral doses of 160 or 320 mg/kg similar signs were more severe and accompanied by frothy salivation, grunting, and bellowing and death within one week of the onset of treatment.

Dinitro compounds such as dinitrophenol and dinitrocresol are used as herbicides and fungicides and are toxic to goats immediately after application to foliage, but not after the residue has dried (Guss 1977). When goats feed on sprayed foliage there may be yellow discoloration of skin and hair around the mouth and nose associated with feeding activity. Clinical signs of toxicity include fever, dyspnea, tachycardia, and convulsions. The clinical course is short and death rapidly ensues. Even with early intervention, the prognosis is guarded. No specific therapies have been reported, but use of antipyretics, anticonvulsants, and supportive care may be of some value.

Pentachlorophenol is commonly used as a wood preservative for lumber. It is toxic to livestock via the mechanism of uncoupling oxidative phosphorylation. It is readily absorbed through the skin, via inhalation, or by ingestion. As a general precaution, pentachlorophenol-treated wood should not be used in goat buildings because of the well known wood chewing and swallowing behavior of goats. Of particular concern is freshly treated wood that has not yet dried or cured. Clinical signs of toxicity can include muscular weakness and lethargy, fever, sweating, dehydration, tachypnea, collapse, and death with rapid onset of rigor mortis. Convulsions have been reported in goats before death (Guss 1977). There is no specific treatment.

Chlorpromazine and piperazine produce a fatal drug interaction when given to goats. The drug combination resulted in immediate, severe, clonic convulsions, and rapid respiratory arrest when chlorpromazine was given intravenously at a dose of 10 mg/kg after oral administration of piperazine at a dose of 220 mg/kg (Boulos and Davis 1969).

CONGENITAL AND INHERITED DISEASES

Beta Mannosidosis

This heritable, lysosomal storage disease in goats is seen only in newborn kids of Nubian breeding and is characterized by intention tremors and an inability to rise. The condition is transmitted as an autosomal recessive trait. There is no treatment and carrier adults can be identified by blood test.

Epidemiology

The condition was first described as a neurovisceral storage disease with dysmyelinogenesis of unknown cause in newborn Anglo Nubian kids in Australia in 1973 (Hartley and Blakemore 1973). It was later characterized as beta mannosidosis in Nubian kids in Michigan in 1981 (Jones and Laine 1981). It was long thought to occur only in the goat, but is now also recognized in humans (Dorland et al. 1988) and the Salers breed of cattle (Abbitt et al. 1991). The specific molecular defect responsible for caprine beta-mannosidosis has been identified and the associated cDNA coding region has been sequenced and characterized (Leipprandt et al. 1996). It involves a single base pair deletion.

Currently the caprine disease is known only in the Nubian breed or Nubian crossbreds (Shapiro et al. 1985). It has been reported in Australia, New Zealand, Fiji, Canada, and the United States. Heterozygous carriers of the trait can be identified by intermediate plasma levels of beta mannosidase. An Australian survey identified 13.7% of 988 Anglo Nubians as carriers (Sewell and Healy 1985). This suggests a significant potential economic loss for Nubian breeders.

Pathogenesis

The lysosomal storage diseases result from an acquired or inherited deficiency of a catabolic lysosomal hydrolase. In cells where the hydrolase is missing, the substrate that is ordinarily catabolized accumulates in lysosomes producing marked vacuolation and destruction of cells. In the case of beta mannosidosis, the condition is inherited as an autosomal recessive trait, transmitted with a frequency of 25% by the mating of two heterozygous parents, and the deficient hydrolase is beta mannosidase. The deficiency results in intracellular accumulation of incompletely catabolized oligosaccharides leading to marked vacuolation of cells, the characteristic histologic lesion. These substances, the disaccharide betamannosyl-(1-4)-*N*-acetylglucosamine and the trisaccharide betamannosyl-(1-4)-*N*-acetylglucosaminyl-(1-4)-*N*-acetylglucosamine, are also excreted in the urine.

While vacuolation occurs in a wide variety of cell types, lesions are most severe in the CNS and clinical manifestations of the disease in neonates are essentially neurologic. Vacuolation of neurons is accompanied by marked dysmyelinogenesis in beta mannosidosis, but the exact relationship of these two findings is unresolved. One study has reported that greater accumulation of oligosaccharide at various locations in the CNS is not directly associated with the severity of myelin deficiency at those sites (Boyer et al. 1990).

Clinical Findings

The clinical presentation is consistent (Kumar et al. 1986). Affected kids of either sex are born alive. They are unable to rise, and lie in lateral recumbency or drag themselves along if placed sternally. They have contracted tendons with carpal flexion, hind limb extension, and hyperextension of the pastern joints. Withdrawal reflexes are intact. There is a varying degree of facial dysmorphism including a domed skull, an elongated and narrow muzzle, small, slit-like palpebral fissures, enophthalmos, and a depressed nasal bridge. Most, if not all, affected kids are deaf, though this may be difficult to establish. Bilateral ptosis as part of Horner's syndrome is present. Pendular nystagmus and intention tremors may be observed. The skin is thickened and the muscle mass may be decreased. Affected kids can see, smell, suckle, defecate, and urinate normally and may survive for several weeks with nursing care.

Clinical Pathology and Necropsy

The hemogram and serum chemistry profile are normal. Despite the facial dysmorphism and locomotor difficulties, radiographs of the skull, vertebrae, and long bones are normal. An abnormal electromyogram, with spontaneous potentials resembling positive sharp waves and fibrillation potentials, occurs in some cases.

Techniques for measuring plasma beta mannosidase activity have been developed and can be used as an aid to distinguish normal goats from affected goats and heterozygous carriers (Healy and McCleary 1982; Cavanagh et al. 1983). Using a fluorometric technique, affected kids have markedly reduced or absent activity, with measurements below 0.2 U/l, while the activity of heterozygous carriers is always below 2.4 U/l and frequently below 1.7 U/l (Healy and McCleary 1982). Most normal, adult, noncarrier goats have activity greater than 2.1 U/l, but some may measure as low as 1.7 U/l, giving false positive results. In screening for heterozygous carriers, false positive identification rates as high as 12% can occur in goat populations when 2.1 U/l is used as the discriminate value and 2% when 1.7 U/l is used (Sewell and Healy 1985). Laboratory values for plasma beta mannosidase activity have also been reported for normal kids in the range of 66 to 222 nmol/hour/ml (Cavanagh et al. 1982). Clinically affected homozygous kids have no beta mannosidase activity in plasma and heterozygous carriers have intermediate activity. In one study, heterozygous carriers had activity measurements that averaged 47% of that of normal goats (Sewell and Healy 1985).

While there is conflicting information on the effect of reproductive status and gender on beta mannosidase activity, the activity is known to decrease with increasing age up to but not after sexual maturity (Dunstan et al. 1983; Sewell and Healy 1985). Severe stresses such as transport and shearing can reduce activity into the heterozygous suspect range, so blood samples should not be taken from goats immediately after obvious stressors (Mason 1986).

Affected kids also have the abnormal oligosaccharides betamannosyl-(1-4)-*N*-acetylglucosamine and betamannosyl-(1-4)-*N*-acetylglucosaminyl-(1-4)-*N*-acetylglucosamine present in the urine (Matsuura et al. 1983). Prenatal testing by ultrasound guided aspiration of fetal fluids has been described (Lovell et al. 1995). Abnormal accumulation of oligosaccharides was confirmed in the allantoic fluid, but not in the amniotic fluid. Diagnosis in live kids may be possible by examination of gingival biopsies for the characteristic lesions of Schwann cell vacuolation and axonal dense bodies in peripheral nerve cells (Malachowski and Jones 1983).

At necropsy, muscles appear pale and small. When the contracted tendons are cut, joint motion is unimpaired. The most prominent gross lesions are in the brain. Ventricular dilation is observed in association with a marked diminution of white matter because of a paucity of myelin, especially in the cerebrum. There is also polypoid hypertrophy of the middle ear mucosa (Jones et al. 1983).

Histologically, the disease is characterized by fine to coarse vacuolation of a wide variety of cell types in all tissues. These are lysosomal storage vacuoles. Fibroblasts, macrophages, and endothelial and perithelial cells are most consistently affected in all tissues. In the CNS there is vacuolation of virtually all cell types. In addition, there is marked demyelination, especially in the brain and to a lesser extent in the spinal cord, and axonal spheroids occur throughout the white matter. Mineralization may be seen, especially in the cerebellum and globus pallidus (Lovell and Jones 1983). Ocular lesions have also been described (Render et al. 1989).

Diagnosis

The diagnosis is based on the characteristic presentation in newborn kids of Nubian descent, confirmation of reduced beta mannosidase activity in plasma or abnormal oligosaccharides in urine, and characteristic histology at necropsy. Differential diagnoses include hydrocephalus, congenital spinal malformations or trauma at birth, Akabane disease, border disease, and swayback.

Treatment and Control

There is no treatment for this condition. Control in individual herds depends on diagnosis of the condition in newborn kids and removal of the parents of affected kids from the breeding program. Goat owners purchasing Nubian goats for breeding purposes may want to screen for heterozygous carriers by assaying plasma beta mannosidase activity. More recently, a genetic test has been developed and is available through the Texas Veterinary Medical Diagnostic Laboratory.

Mucopolysaccharidosis IIID

Mucopolysaccharidosis IIID (MPS IIID) is an inherited lysosomal storage disease first described in human beings and later recognized in the Nubian breed of goats (Thompson et al. 1992). In human medicine the condition is also known as Sanfilippo D syndrome and Nubian goats are now used as a model for studying the human disease.

MPS IIID is caused by a deficiency in N-acetylglucosamine 6-sulfatase (G6S) activity in lysosomes that results from a nonsense mutation in the 5′ region of the gene coding for expression of this enzyme. The result of this enzyme deficiency is that the catabolism of glycosaminoglycans (GAG) is disrupted so that *N*-acetylglucosamine 6-sulfate and heparan sulfate accumulate in the tissues and urine of affected individuals. While multiple tissues are affected, the lysosomal accumulation of these GAG in the central nervous system is mostly responsible for the clinical manifestations seen in humans and Nubian goats. The key lesions seen in the CNS of affected goats are primarily the neuronal accumulation of heparan sulfate and the excess storage of gangliosides in cerebral cortical and spinal cord gray matter as well as dysmyelination (Jones et al. 1998).

The pattern of inheritance for MPS IIID is autosomal recessive with individuals homozygous for the defective gene expressing the disease condition. In a Michigan study of 552 Nubians using a G6S PCR-based mutation test, 25.2% of animals tested were identified as heterozygous carriers and 1.3% were homozygous for the mutation (Hoard et al. 1998).

There is phenotypic variation in MPS IIID disease expression with mild and severe forms recorded in homozygous Nubian goats (Jones et al. 1998). Affected goats may be born with marked neurological deficits. One carefully studied case showed an inability to rise at birth, and a wide based stance and hyperextension of the limbs when lifted to standing. Additional signs included a fine neck tremor and horizontal nystagmus. Though the animal gradually became ambulatory, it remained ataxic and showed delayed and stunted growth. However, six other homozygous individuals in the same study showed no overt clinical signs at birth and continued normally for extended periods of time. One individual, for example, only showed signs beginning at forty-four months of age. These signs included abnormal gait, persistent head tremor, and intermittent hyperextension of the forelimbs. Another homozygous goat began showing aggressive behavior in her second year of life. The one observation common to all six mildly affected goats was growth retardation (Jones et al. 1998). Field reports suggest that mildly affected goats have decreased muscle mass and may be more prone to infection and that overt signs of disease may manifest as animals become older due to progressive accumulation of GAG in CNS and other tissues.

Differential diagnosis for newborn kids should include congenital copper deficiency, congenital skeletal abnormalities such as hemivertebra, hydrocephalus, and beta mannosidosis, the other lysosomal storage disease that occurs only in Nubian goats. Akabane virus infection can also produce kids unable to rise at birth, but these kids have arthrogryposis which is not reported in MPS IIID. When progressive neurological signs appear in adult goats, scrapie must be considered as well as coenurosis where it occurs. The differential diagnosis for animals showing poor growth and decreased muscle mass should include the various nutritional, infectious, and parasitic diseases discussed in Chapter 15 relative to wasting.

Testing for the presence of the G6S mutation can be performed on white blood cells harvested at the laboratory from 1 to 2 ml of blood collected in EDTA. The Texas Veterinary Medical Diagnostic Laboratory currently performs this test in the United States. The condition can be controlled through breeding based on the G6S mutation status of breeding stock determined through testing. There is no treatment for the condition.

Progressive Paresis of Angora Goats

Ataxia, first noted at approximately four months of age, has been seen in Angora goat kids from serial litters of the same parentage in Australia. Kids had normal mental status, cranial nerve function, and reflexes, but exhibited signs of weakness including difficulty in rising, a reluctance to move, and stumbling when forced to do so. Weakness was more apparent in the hind limbs than the forelimbs.

Though clinically similar to enzootic ataxia or caprine arthritis encephalitis, this condition has characteristic pathologic findings. No gross lesions were observed except muscle atrophy. Microscopic lesions were characterized by the occurrence of large cytoplasmic vacuoles in large neurons of the midbrain, brain stem, and ventral horns of the spinal cord. Chromatolysis and pyknosis were also observed. The history of reoccurrence of the condition in kids from serial litters of the same parentage suggested a hereditary basis for the condition, though the pathogenesis of the disease remains unclear (Lancaster et al. 1987).

Spastic Paresis

This condition is well known in cattle and is considered to be inherited in that species. Spastic paresis is characterized by intermittent unilateral or bilateral spastic contracture of the gastrocnemius muscle leading to hyperextension of one or both hind limbs. The hyperextension may be so extreme that the animal is unable to place the foot on the ground and the leg is carried straight behind. The hock is straight and the gastrocnemius muscle is palpably firm or knotted. It has been demonstrated that selective depression of gamma efferent neurons in the spinal cord by epidural administration of dilute procaine alleviates the condition, indicating that the disorder occurs from overstimulation of the myotatic (stretch) reflex (De Ley and De Moor 1980).

Reports of the condition in goats are infrequent. The condition was first reported in Czechoslovakia in 1973 and involved a three-year-old male Saanen (Kral and Hlousek 1973). The goat was reluctant to stand and when forced to do so remained on its carpi with rump in the air, hind limbs overextended with the hocks straight, and the gastrocnemius tendons palpably taut. Though the diagnosis could not be confirmed, tibial neurectomy, as frequently applied in cattle, corrected the condition.

More recently, the condition was reported in two familially related pygmy goats in the United States (Baker et al. 1989). In these cases, the diagnosis was supported by application of a dilute procaine epidural with subsequent alleviation of signs. Despite this evidence of spastic paresis in goats, the diagnosis must be made with caution because of the hereditary implications of the disease, which are not well defined in the caprine species. The author has observed at least two goats with classically described signs of spastic paresis that turned out to be cases of the arthritic form of CAE. The occurrence of joint pain without joint swelling is not uncommon in CAE and could lead to abnormalities of gait and posture that can mimic spastic paresis.

Hydrocephalus and Hydranencephaly

Hydrocephalus occurs sporadically in goats as a developmental anomaly resulting in improper drainage of the CSF. This causes increased intracerebral pressure, with thinning of the cerebral cortices, expansion of the ventricles, and possible distortion of the skull surrounding the brain. Affected kids can be delivered dead or alive. Live kids are usually dull and blind with pronounced muscular weakness; they are unable to stand unassisted or ambulate (Figure 5.7). Obvious doming of the skull is variable and does not have to be present to make a diagnosis of hydrocephalus. Hydranencephaly, which is a normotensive hydrocephalus that results from necrosis or a failure of cell growth, occurs in goats in conjunction with arthrogryposis as a result of fetal Akabane virus infection as discussed in Chapter 4. Kids with hydranencephaly have neurologic deficits similar to those seen in hydrocephalus.

NEOPLASTIC DISEASE

Neoplasms of the CNS in goats are rarely found in large scale surveys of neoplastic disease of livestock. For example, there was one caprine neoplasia, a spongioma, in a report on 400 tumors of the nervous system of domestic animals (Luginbuhl 1963). However, some individual cases have been reported in the literature. In Germany, a fifteen-year-old female goat that suddenly developed a right sided heat tilt that progressed to loss of orientation and ataxia was subsequently euthanized and found to have a choroid plexus carcinoma which manifested as a well circumscribed mass in the left ventricle that compressed the cerebrum and infiltrated the left piriform lobe (Klopfleisch et al. 2006). In a report from North Carolina, glioma was diagnosed in a six-year old castrated male, mixed-breed goat that presented with a one-week history of circling, behavioral change, decreased appetite, and adipsia. A CT scan identified a large cerebral mass which was confirmed at necropsy as a glioma (Marshall et al. 1995). Lymphosarcoma (Craig et al. 1986) and malignant melanoma (Sockett et al. 1984) have also been reported involving the nervous system in goats. A malignant Schwannoma of peripheral nerve sheaths, manifesting as 0.5 to 2 mm nodules, was recently identified in the diaphragm of a two-year-old female goat at slaughter in Spain (Ramírez et al. 2007).

A goat with cerebral gliomatosis was identified in a survey of small ruminant field cases with clinical presentations of neurologic disease carried out in support of Swiss scrapie surveillance activities. The goat also had hair lice and the combination of pruritus from the lice and neurologic signs from the tumor effectively mimicked clinical scrapie (Maurer et al. 2005). Another case report of cerebral gliomatosis from Switzerland involved a three-year old Appenzell goat buck (Braun et al. 2005). The animal showed depression, generalized ataxia, hypermetria of the forelimbs, generalized hypoesthesia, bilateral mydriasis, and a decreased menace response. At necropsy, there were no gross lesions in the brain, but histologically there was extensive diffuse glial cell hyperplasia in the white matter of the cerebral hemispheres and in the brain stem.

NEUROLOGIC DISEASES OF UNKNOWN ETIOLOGY

Polyradiculoneuritis

Polyradiculoneuritis has been reported as a cause of progressive hind limb ataxia, hyporeflexia, and extensor rigidity in a six-week-old male kid in California (MacLachlan et al. 1982). At necropsy, there were no gross lesions but microscopically there was evidence of mononuclear inflammation and demyelination involving the meninges, nerve roots, and peripheral nerves, but not the brain or spinal cord. Similar conditions are known in man and in dogs and are hypothesized to be caused by an auto-immune reaction.

Caprine Encephalomyelomalacia

Caprine encephalomyelomalacia has been reported from California (Cordy et al. 1984). The condition has been described only in kids between three and a half and four months of age of dairy breeds. There is an acute onset of nervous dysfunction characterized by posterior paresis and incoordination progressing rapidly to paralysis. In some cases tetraparesis is observed. All kids were killed after a clinical course of six to ten days.

There are no gross lesions at necropsy. Microscopic lesions are bilaterally symmetrical and are restricted to the gray matter of the spinal cord, particularly in the cervical and lumbosacral enlargements, and certain brain stem nuclei. Necrosis of neurons is observed.

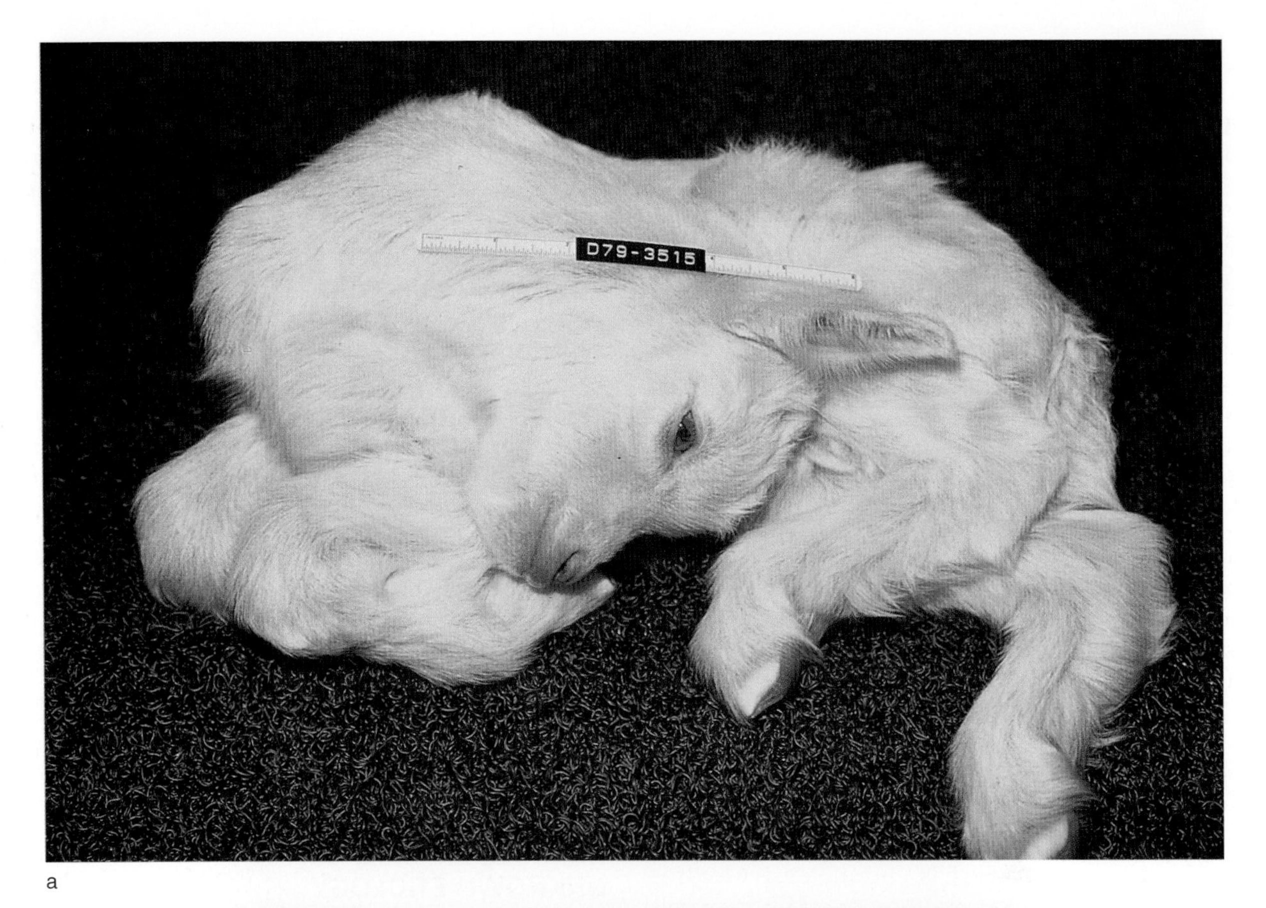

a

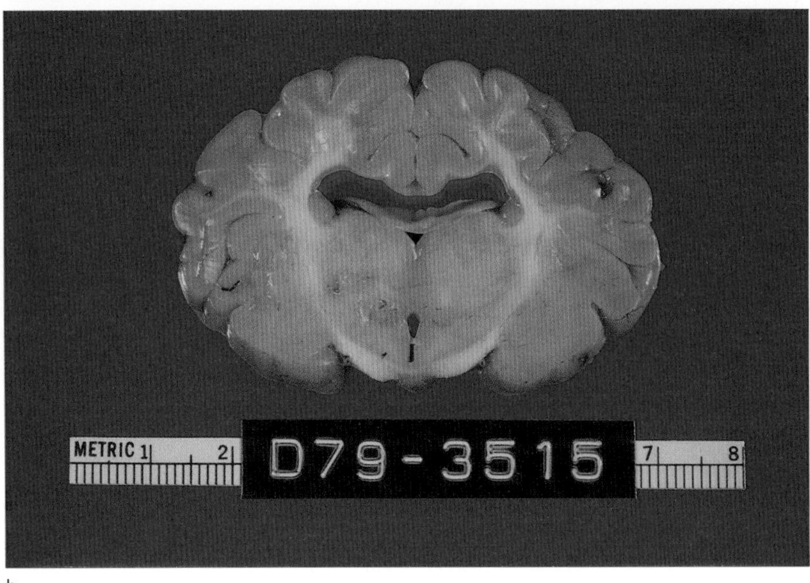

b

Figure 5.7. A two-day-old kid with hydrocephalus. The kid was dull and depressed at birth and could only stand when assisted. It preferred the curled, recumbent position, as shown in Figure 5.7a. Doming of the skull was not prominent, but distension of the ventricular system was evident at time of necropsy (Figure 5.7b). (Courtesy of Dr. T.P. O'Leary.)

REFERENCES

Abbitt, B., et al.: Beta—mannosidosis in twelve Salers calves. J. Am. Vet. Med. Assoc. 198(1):109–113, 1991.

Abdelsalam, E.B.: Comparative effect of certain organophophorous compounds and other chemicals on whole blood, plasma and tissue cholinesterase activity in goats. Vet. Hum. Toxicol., 29:146–148, 1987.

Acutis, P.L., et al.: Identification of prion protein gene polymorphisms in goats from Italian scrapie outbreaks. J. Gen. Virol., 87(4):1029–1033, 2006.

Agrimi, U., et al.: Animal transmissible spongiform encephalopathies and genetics. Vet. Res. Comm., 27(Suppl 1):31–38, 2003.

Agrimi, U., et al.: Epidemic of transmissible spongiform encephalopathy in sheep and goats in Italy. Lancet, 353:560–561, 1999.

Aguzzi A.: Prion diseases of humans and farm animals: epidemiology, genetics, and pathogenesis. J. Neurochem., 97(6):1726–39, 2006.

Aguzzi, A. and Heikenwalder M.: Pathogenesis of prion diseases: current status and future outlook. Nat. Rev. Microbiol., 4(10):765–75, 2006.

Ahamed, S. and Ali, M.I.: Incidence of *Coenurus cerebralis* in goat in Bangladesh. Indian Vet. J., 49:1157–1158, 1972.

Ahmed, J.U. and Haque, M.A.: Surgical treatment of coenurosis in goats. Bangladesh Vet. J., 9:31–34, 1975.

Albretsen, J.C., Khan, S.A. and Richardson, J.A.: Cycad palm toxicosis in dogs: 60 cases (1987–1997). J. Am. Vet. Med. Assoc. 213(1):99–101, 1998.

Alexander, K., Drost, W.T., Mattoon, J.S. and Anderson, D.E.: ^{99m}TC-ciprofloxacin in imaging of clinical infections in camelids and a goat. Vet. Radiol. Ultrasound, 46(4):340–347, 2005.

Ali, B.H., Hassan, T., Wasfi, I.A., and Mustafa, A.I.: Toxicity of furazolidone to Nubian goats. Vet. Hum. Toxicol., 26:197–200, 1984.

Ali, B.H.: The toxicity of *Azadirachta indica* leaves in goats and guinea pigs. Vet. Hum. Toxicol., 29:16–19, 1987.

Amégée, Y.: Le tournis à *Byrsocarpus* des petits ruminants au sud du Togo. Rev. Élev. Méd. Vét. Pays Trop., 36:27–31, 1983.

Amer, A.A. and Misk, N.A.: Rompun in goats with special reference to its effect on the cerebrospinal fluid (CSF). Vet. Med. Rev., 2:168–174, 1980.

Aminlari, M. and Mehran, M.M.: Biochemical properties of cerebrospinal fluid of sheep and goat. Comparison with blood. J. Vet. Med. A, 35:315–319, 1988.

Anderson R.M., et al.: Transmission dynamics and epidemiology of BSE in British cattle. Nature, 382(6594):779–788, 1996.

Anderson, R.C. and Strelive, U.R.: Experimental cerebrospinal nematodiasis in kids. J. Parasitol., 58:816, 1972.

Anderson, R.C. and Strelive, U.R.: The effect of *Pneumostrongylus tenuis* (Nematoda: Metastrongyloidea) on kids. Can. J. Comp. Med., 33:280–286, 1969.

Andréoletti, O., et al.: Bovine spongiform encephalopathy agent in spleen from an ARR/ARR orally exposed sheep. J. Gen. Virol., 87(4):1043–1046, 2006.

Andrésdóttir, V., Torsteinsdóttir, S. and Georgsson, G.: Neurological disease produced by maedi-visna and caprine arthritis-encephalitis viruses, lentiviruses of sheep and goats. In: The Neurology of AIDS. Gendelman, H.E. et al., eds. Oxford University Press USA, New York, pp. 279–287, 2005.

Antognini, J.F., Wang, X.W. and Carstens, E.: Isoflurane anaesthetic depth in goats monitored using the bispectral index of the electroencephalogram. Vet. Res. Commun., 24(6):361–370, 2000.

Arencibia, A., et al.: Anatomy of the cranioencephalic structures of the goat (*Capra hircus* L.) by imaging techniques: a computerized tomographic study. Anat. Histol. Embryol., 26:161–164, 1997.

Arnal, M.C., et al.: A novel pestivirus associated with deaths in Pyrenean chamois (*Rupicapra pyrenaica pyrenaica*). J. Gen. Virol., 85(12):3653–3657, 2004.

Arsac J.N., et al.: Similar biochemical signatures and prion protein genotypes in atypical scrapie and Nor98 cases, France and Norway. Emerg. Infect. Dis. 13(1):58–65, 2007.

Asahi, O., Hosoda, T., Akiyama, Y. and Ebi. Y.: Studies on listeriosis in domestic animals. I. Listeriosis in goats found in Aomori Prefecture. Gov. Exp. Stn. Anim. Hyg. Expt. Rep. 27:289–300, 1954.

Bahmani, M.K., et al.: Varied prevalence of Borna disease virus infection in Arabic, Thoroughbred and their crossbred horses in Iran. Virus Res. 45(1):1–13, 1996.

Baker, J.C., Ciszewski, D., Lowrie, C. and Mullaney, T.: Spastic paresis in pygmy goats. J. Vet. Intern. Med., 3:113, 1989.

Baker, J.C., Esser, M.B. and Larson, V.L.: Pseudorabies in a goat. J. Am. Vet. Med. Assoc., 181:607, 1982.

Balogh, K.K.I.M. de, et al.: A lysosomal storage disease induced by *Ipomoea carnea* in goats in Mozambique. J. Vet. Diagn. Invest., 11(3):266–273, 1999.

Banton, M., et al.: Enzootic ataxia in Louisiana goat kids. J. Vet. Diagn. Invest., 2:70–73, 1990.

Barlow, R.M., et al.: Experiments in border disease. VII. The disease in goats. J. Comp. Pathol., 85:291–297, 1975.

Barlow, R.M., Robertson, J.M., Owen, E.C. and Proudfoot, R.: A condition in the goat resembling swayback in lambs. Vet. Rec., 74:737–739, 1962.

Barnard, B.J.H.: Symptoms of rabies in pets and domestic animals in South Africa and South West Africa J. So. Afr. Vet. Assoc., 50:109–111, 1979.

Bastian, F.O.: Spiroplasma as a candidate agent for the transmissible spongiform encephalopathies. J. Neuropathol. Exp. Neurol., 64(10):833–838, 2005.

Batalla, D., Mendez, J.J. and Garcia, F.: Safety and antigenicity of the rabies vaccine strain acatlan v-319 in goats and sheep. In: Proceedings, 3rd Internat. Conf. Goat Prod. Dis., Scottsdale, Dairy Goat Journal Publ. Co., pp. 297, 1982.

Batcher, J.D. and Potkay, S.: Radial paralysis in a goat: treatment by tendon transplantation. Vet. Med. Small Anim. Clin., 71:1031–1034, 1976.

Baxendell, S.A.: Caprine nervous diseases. In: Proceedings, Refresher Course for Veterinarians, Post-Graduate Committee in Veterinary Science, University of Sydney, 52:333–342, 1980.

Baxendell, S.A.: The Diagnosis of the Diseases of Goats. Sydney South, Post-Graduate Committee in Veterinary Science, 1988.

Baylis, M. and Goldmann, W.: The genetics of scrapie in sheep and goats. Curr. Mol. Med., 4:385–396, 2004.
Becher, P., et al.: Genetic and antigenic characterization of novel pestivirus genotypes: implications for classification. Virol., 311:96–104, 2003.
Becher, P., et al.: Phylogenetic analysis of pestiviruses from domestic and wild ruminants. J. Gen. Virol., 78:1357–1366, 1997.
Bedotti, D.O. and Sanchez Rodriguez, M.: Observations on animal health problems of goats in the west of the province of La Pampa (Argentina). Vet. Argent., 19(182):100–112, 2002.
Bell, F.R. and Itabisashi, T.: The electroencephalogram of sheep and goats with special reference to rumination. Physiol. Behav. 11:503–514, 1973.
Bellworthy, S.J., et al.: Natural transmission of BSE between sheep within an experimental flock. Vet. Rec., 157(7):206, 2005.
Bellworthy, S.J., et al.: Tissue distribution of bovine spongiform encephalopathy infectivity in Romney sheep up to the onset of clinical disease after oral challenge. Vet. Rec., 156:197–202, 2005a.
Bencsik, A. and Baron, T.: Bovine spongiform encephalopathy agent in a prion protein $(PrP)^{ARR/ARR}$ genotype sheep after peripheral challenge: complete immunohistochemical analysis of disease-associated PrP and transmission studies to ovine-transgenic mice. J. Infect. Dis., 195:989–996, 2007.
Benestad, S.L., et al.: Cases of scrapie with unusual features in Norway and designation of a new type, Nor98. Vet. Rec. 153:202–208, 2003.
Bergamasco, L., et al.: Effects of brief maternal separation in kids on neurohormonal and electroencephalographic parameters. Appl. Anim. Behav. Sci., 93(1/2):39–52, 2005.
Bergamasco, L., et al.: Electroencephalographic power spectral analysis of growing goat kids (*Capra hircus*). Small Rumin. Res., 66:265–272, 2006.
Bernkopf H., Levine S. and Nerson R.: Isolation of West Nile virus in Israel. J. Infect. Dis., 93:207–218, 1953.
Bestetti, von G., Fatzer, R., Frese, K. and Fankhauser, R.: Histologische und ultrastrukturelle Untersuchungen zur melanosis thalami beim Tier. Schweiz. Arch. Tierheilk., 122:637–652, 1980.
Beust, B.R. von, Vandevelde, M., Tontis, A. and Spichtig, M.: Enzootische Ataxie beim Zicklein in der Schweiz. Schweiz. Arch. Tierheilk., 125:345–351, 1983.
Biacabe, A.G., Laplanche, J.L., Ryder, S. and Baron, T.: Distinct molecular phenotypes in bovine prion diseases. EMBO Rep., 5:110–114, 2004.
Billinis C., et al.: Prion protein gene polymorphisms in natural goat scrapie. J. Gen. Virol., 83(3):713–721, 2002.
Black, H.: Copper deficiency in Northland. Surveillance, N. Z., 6:2–5, 1979.
Blanton, J.D., Krebs, J.W., Hanlon, C.A. and Rupprecht, C.E.: Rabies surveillance in the United States during 2005. J. Am. Vet. Med. Assoc., 229(12):1897–1911, 2006.
Blenden, D.C., Kampelmacher, E.H. and Torres-Anjel, M.J.: Listeriosis. J. Am. Vet. Med. Assoc., 191:1546–1551, 1987.
Borku, M.K., et al.: Serological detection of listeriosis at a farm. Turkish J. Vet. Anim. Sci., 30(2): 279–282, 2006.
Boulos, B.M. and Davis, L.E.: Hazard of simultaneous administration of phenothiazine and piperazine. New Engl. J. Med., 280:1245–1246, 1969.
Bourke, C.A.: Cerebellar degeneration in goats grazing *Solanum cinereum* (Narrawa burr). Austral. Vet. J., 75(5):363–365, 1997.
Bowen, R.: Personal Communication. Dr. Richard Bowen, Professor, Department of Biomedical Sciences, Animal Reproduction and Biotechnology Laboratory, Colorado State University, Fort Collins, CO, 2007.
Boyer, P.J., Jones, M.Z., Rathke, E.J.S., Truscott, N.K. and Lovell, K.L.: Regional central nervous system oligosaccharide storage in caprine beta-mannosidosis. J. Neurochem., 55(2):660–664, 1990.
Braun, U., Hilbe, M. and Ehrensperger, F.: Clinical and pathological findings in a goat with cerebral gliomatosis. Vet. J., 170(3):381–383, 2005.
Braun, U., Stehle, C. and Ehrensperger, F.: Clinical findings and treatment of listeriosis in 67 sheep and goats. Vet. Rec., 150(2):38–42, 2002.
Brewer, B.D.: Neurologic disease of sheep and goats. Vet. Clin. N. Am., Large Anim. Pract., 5:677–700, 1983.
Brewer, N.R.: Comparative metabolism of copper. J. Am. Vet. Med. Assoc., 190:654–658, 1987.
Brightling, P.: Enzootic ataxia in lambs and kids in Saskatchewan. Can. Vet. J., 24:164–165, 1983.
Brooks, D.L., Tillman, P.C. and Niemi, S.M.: Ungulates as laboratory animals. In: Laboratory Animal Medicine. J.G. Fox, B.J. Cohen, and F.M. Loew. eds. Orlando, Academic Press, 1984.
Brotherston, J.G., et al.: Spread of scrapie by contact to goats and sheep. J. Comp. Pathol., 78:9–17, 1968.
Brown, P., McShane, L.M., Zanusso, G. and Detwiler, L.: On the question of sporadic or atypical bovine spongiform encephalopathy and Creutzfeldt-Jakob disease. Emerg. Infect. Dis., 12(12):1816–1821, 2006.
Buronfosse, F.: Intoxication by sodium chloride in a herd of goats. Summa, 17(1):75–76, 2000.
Buschmann, A., et al.: Atypical scrapie cases in Germany and France are identified by discrepant reaction patterns in BSE rapid tests. J. Virol. Methods, 117:27–36, 2004.
Buxton, D. Linklater, K.A. and Dyson, D.A.: Pulpy kidney disease and its diagnosis by histological examination. Vet. Rec. 102(11):241, 1978.
Callan, R.J. and Van Metre, D.C.: Viral diseases of the ruminant nervous system. Vet. Clin. No. Amer. Food Anim. Pract., 20:327–362, 2004.
Camp, B.J. and Lyman, C.M.: The toxic agent isolated from *Acacia berlandieri*, N-methyl beta-phenylethylamine. Southwest. Vet., 10:133–134, 1957.
Canadian Food Inspection Agency: Accredited Veterinarian's Manual. Chapter 7. Scrapie Flock Certification Program. Appendix 1A. Brain Sampling Procedures. Government of Canada, Ottawa, 2005. http://www.inspection.gc.ca/english/anima/heasan/man/avmmva/avmmva_mod7_a1ae.pdf.
Cantile, C., Del Piero, F., Di Guardo, G. and Arispici, M.: Pathologic and immunohistochemical findings in naturally occurring West Nile virus infection in horses. Vet. Pathol., 38:414–421, 2001.

Caplazi, P., et al.: Die "Bornasche Krankheit" in der Schweiz und im Fürstentum Liechtenstein. Schweiz. Arch. Tierheilk., 141:521–527, 1999.

Capobianco, R., et al.: Conversion of the BASE prion strain into the BSE strain: the origin of BSE?, PloS Pathog 3(3): e31, 2007. http://pathogens.plosjournals.org/perlserv/?request=get-documentanddoi=10.1371%2Fjournal.ppat.0030031

Capucchio, M.T., et al.: Natural occurrence of scrapie in goats in Italy. Vet. Rec., 143(16):452–453, 1998.

Caramelli, M., et al.: Evidence for the transmission of scrapie to sheep and goats from a vaccine against *Mycoplasma agalactiae*. Vet. Rec., 148:531–536, 2001.

Casalone C., et al.: Identification of a second bovine amyloidotic spongiform encephalopathy: molecular similarities with sporadic Creutzfeldt-Jakob disease. Proc. Natl. Acad. Sci. U.S.A., 101:3065–70, 2004.

Cavanagh, K., Dunstan, R.W. and Jones, M.Z.: Measurement of caprine plasma beta-mannosidase with a p-nitrophenyl substrate. Am. J. Vet. Res., 44:681–684, 1983.

Cavanagh, K., Dunstan, R.W. and Jones, M.Z.: Plasma alpha- and beta-mannosidase activities in caprine beta-mannosidosis. Am. J. Vet. Res., 43(6):1058–1059, 1982.

Cebra, C.K. and Cebra, M.L.: Altered mentation caused by polioencephalomalacia, hypernatremia, and lead poisoning. Vet. Clin. N. Am. Food Anim. Pract., 20(2):287–302, 2004.

Cebra, C.K., Garry, F.B. and Cebra, M.L.: Tick paralysis in eight new world camelids. Vet. Med., 91(7):673–676, 1996.

Celedon, M., et al.: Survey for antibodies to pestivirus and herpesvirus in sheep, goats, alpacas (*Lama pacos*), llamas (*Lama glama*), guanacos (*Lama guanicoe*) and vicuna (*Vicugna vicugna*) from Chile. Arch. Med. Vet. 33(2):165–172, 2001.

Chalmers, R.M., Thomas, D.R. and Salmon, R.L.: Borna disease virus and the evidence for human pathogenicity: a systematic review. Q. J. Med., 98(4):255–74, 2005.

Chandna, I.E., Bhargava, A.K. and Tyagi, R.P.S.: Myelographic studies in caprine spinal surgery. Philip. J. Vet. Med., 22:100–109, 1983.

Chandna, I.S., Bhargava, A.K. and Tyagi, R.P.S.: Rupture of dorsal longitudinal ligament in the thoracic region of a goat. Haryana Vet., 17:109–111, 1978.

Charlton, K.M. and Pierce, K.R.: A neuropathy in goats caused by experimental coyotillo *(Karwinskia humboldtiana)* poisoning. III. Distribution of lesions in peripheral nerves. Pathol. Vet., 7:408–419, 1970.

Charlton, K.M., Claborn, L.D. and Pierce, K.R.: A neuropathy in goats caused by experimental coyotillo *(Karwinskia humboldtiana)* poisoning: clinical and neurophysiologic studies. Am. J. Vet. Res., 32:1381–1389, 1971.

Charlton, K.M., Pierce, K.M., Storts, R.W. and Bridges, C.H.: A neuropathy in goats caused by experimental coyotillo *(Karwinskia humboldtiana)* poisoning. V. Lesions in the central nervous system. Pathol. Vet., 7:435–447, 1970.

Chattopadhyay, S.K., Harbola, P.C. and Bhagwan, P.S.K.: Infectious encephalitis in sheep and goats in a farm at arid zone in India. Indian J. Comp. Microbiol. Immunol. Infect. Dis., 6:127–132, 1985.

Chelle, P.L.: A case of scrapie in the goat. Bull. Acad. Vet. Fr., 95:294–295, 1942.

Cho, T.H., Cho, J.H., Whang, D.W. and Lee, M.H.: Studies on organochlorine pesticide residues in livestock products. Organochlorine pesticide residues in milk and tissues of goats fed different pesticide levels. Research Report Office Rural Develop., Korea, 18(12):63–76, 1976.

Cissik, J.H., et al.: Reference standards and the physiologic significance of the pregnant goat *(Capra hircus)* as a human model in obstetrical research. Comp. Biochem. Physiol. A, 88:533–537, 1987.

Clements, J.E. and Zink, M.C.: Molecular biology and pathogenesis of animal lentivirus infections. Clin. Microbiol. Rev., 9(1):100–117, 1996.

Colodel, E.M., et al.: Caprine enterotoxaemia in Rio Grande do Sul, Brazil. Pesq. Vet. Bras., 23(4):173–178, 2003.

Colodel, E.M., et al.: Clinical and pathological aspects of *Sida carpinifolia* poisoning in goats in Rio Grande do Sul, Brazil. Pesq. Vet. Bras., 22(2):51–57, 2002.

Constable, P.D.: Clinical examination of the ruminant nervous system. Vet. Clin. N. Am. Food Anim. 20:185–214, 2004.

Cooley, W.A., Davis, L.A., Keyes, P. and Stack. M.J.: The reproducibility of scrapie-associated fibril and PrP^{Sc} detection methods after long-term cold storage of natural ovine scrapie-affected brain tissue. J. Comp. Pathol. 120(4):357–368, 1999.

Coppock, R.W., et al.: Evaluation of edetate and thiamine for treatment of experimentally induced environmental lead poisoning in cattle. Am. J. Vet. Res. 52(11):1860–1865, 1991.

Corbellini, L.G., Colodel, E.M. and Driemeier, D.: Granulomatous encephalitis in a neurologically impaired goat kid associated with degeneration of *Neospora caninum* tissue cysts. J. Vet. Diagn. Invest., 13:416–419, 2001.

Cordy, D.R. and Knight, H.D.: California goats with a disease resembling enzootic ataxia or swayback. Vet. Pathol., 15:179–185, 1978.

Cordy, D.R., East, N.E. and Lowenstine, L.J.: Caprine encephalomyelomalacia. Vet. Pathol., 21:269–273, 1984.

Cordy, D.R.: Pathomorphology and pathogenesis of bacterial meningoventriculitus of neonatal ungulates. Vet. Pathol. 21:587–591, 1984.

Cork, L.C., et al.: Infectious leukoencephalomyelitis of young goats. J. Infect. Dis., 129:134–141, 1974.

Craig, D.R., Roth, L. and Smith, M.C.: Lymphosarcoma in goats. Comp. Cont. Educ. Pract. Vet., 8:S190–S197, 1986.

Crick, J.: Rabies. In: Virus Diseases of Food Animals, Volume II. E.P.J. Gibbs, ed. London, Academic Press, 1981.

Custer, D.M.: Shortcut to disaster. United Caprine News, 13 (10):6–9, 1990.

Dahme, E., et al.: Clinical and pathological findings in a transmissible granulomatous meningoencephalomyelitis (gMEM) in domestic goats. Acta Neuropathol. (Berl.), 23:59–76, 1973.

Dantas, A.F.M., et al.: Swainsonine-induced lysosomal storage disease in goats caused by ingestion of *Turbina cordata* in northeastern Brazil. Toxicon, 49:111–116, 2007.

Daubney, R.: Viral encephalitis of equines and domestic ruminants in the Near East. Res. Vet. Sci., 8:419–439, 1967.

Dauphin, G., Legay, V., Pitel, P.H. and Zientara, S.: Borna disease: current knowledge and virus detection in France. Vet. Res. 33:127–138, 2002.

Davis, J.W., Libke, K.G., Watson, D.F. and Bibb, T.L.: Experimentally induced lead poisoning in goats: Clinical observations and pathologic changes. Cornell Vet., 66:489–496, 1976.

de la Concha-Bermejillo, et al.: Overview of diseases and drug needs for sheep and goats. Veterinarians' and producers' perspectives. Vet. Hum. Toxicol. 40(Suppl. 1):7–12, 1998.

De Ley, C. and De Moor, A.: Bovine spastic paralysis: results of selective gamma-efferent suppression with dilute procaine. Vet. Sci. Commun., 3(4):289–298, 1980.

De Mia, G.M., et al.: Genetic characterization of a caprine *Pestivirus* as the first member of a putative novel pestivirus subgroup. J. Vet. Med. B., 52:206–210, 2005.

DEFRA: National Scrapie Plan: Atypical Cases of Scrapie. Department for Environment, Food and Rural Affairs, London. UK, 2005. http://www.defra.gov.uk/animalh/bse/othertses/scrapie/nsp/Atypicalcases/index.htm.

DEFRA: Possible BSE in a 1990 UK goat sample. News Release, UK Department for Environment, Food and Rural Affairs, London, February 8, 2005a. http://www.defra.gov.uk/news/2005/050208a.htm.

DEFRA: Incidences of BSE. Department for Environment, Food and Rural Affairs, London. UK, 2007. http://www.defra.gov.uk/animalh/bse/statistics/incidence.html.

deLahunta, A.: Veterinary Neuroanatomy and Clinical Neurology. Philadelphia, W.B. Saunders Co., 1977.

Deligaris, N., Xenos, G. and Doucas, G.: Fréquence de sérotypes de *Listeria monocytogenes* isolés des chèvres. In: Proceedings, Internat. Vet. Cong., 2:1530–1532, 1975.

Dellmann, H.D. and McClure, R.G.: Central nervous system. In: Sisson and Grossman's The Anatomy of the Domestic Animals, 5th Ed., Volume 1. R. Getty, ed. Philadelphia, W.B. Saunders Co., 1975.

Deslys, J.P. and Grassi, J.: Screening tests for animal TSE: present and future. Pathol. Biol. 53(4):221–228, 2005.

Detwiler, L.A. and Baylis, M.: The epidemiology of scrapie. Rev. Sci. Tech. Off. Int. Epiz., 22(1):121–143, 2003.

Dew, T.L., Bowman, D.D. and Grieve, R.B.: Parasite-specific immunoglobulin in the serum and cerebrospinal fluid of white-tailed deer (*Odocoileus virginianus*) and goats (*Capra hircus*) with experimentally induced parelaphostrongylosis. J. Zoo Wildl. Med., 23(3):281–287, 1992.

Dewan, M.L., et al.: Toxic myodegeneration in goats produced by feeding mature fruits from the coyotillo plant *(Karwinskia humboldtiana)*. Am. J. Pathol., 46:215–226, 1965.

Dijkstra, R.G.: Procedure to isolate *Listeria monocytogenes* out of contaminated organic materials (hay, silage, food). In: Les Maladies de la Chèvre, Les Colloques de l'INRA, No. 28. P. Yvore and G. Perrin, eds. Paris, Institut National de la Recherche Agronomique, pp. 183–185, 1984.

Dijkstra, R.G.: Survival of *Listeria* bacteria in suspensions of brain tissue, silage and faeces and in milk. In: Les Maladies de la Chèvre, Les Colloques de l'INRA, No. 28. P. Yvore and G. Perrin, eds. Paris, Institut National de la Recherche Agronomique, pp. 181–182, 1984a.

Dijkstra, R.G.: Aetiological aspects of listeriosis in goats. In: Les Maladies de la Chèvre, Les Colloques de l'INRA, No. 28. P. Yvore and G. Perrin, eds. Paris, Institut National de la Recherche Agronomique, pp. 187–188, 1984b.

Dollahite, J.W., Rowe, L.D. and Reagor, J.C.: Experimental lead poisoning in horses and Spanish goats. Southwest. Vet., 28:40–45, 1975.

Dorland, L., et al.: Beta-mannosidosis in two brothers with hearing loss. J. Inherited Metab. Dis., 11 (Supp. 2):255–258, 1988.

Du Toit, I.F.: An outbreak of caprine listeriosis in the Western Cape. J. S. Afr. Vet. Assoc., 48:39–40, 1977.

Dubarry, J.R., Ganuza, R.O., and Buse, L.G.: Paresia y paralisis enzootica de los cabritos del oeste pampeano. Presuntas causas ecologicas que lo provocan. Vet. Argent. 3(26):560–565, 1986.

Dunstan, R.W., Cavanagh, K. and Jones, M.Z.: Caprine alpha- and beta-mannosidase activities: effects of age, sex and reproductive status and potential use in heterozygote detection of beta-mannosidosis. Am. J. Vet. Res., 44:685–689, 1983.

Dürrwald, R., Kolodziejek, J., Muluneh, A., Herzog, S. and Nowotny, N.: Epidemiological pattern of classical Borna disease and regional genetic clustering of Borna disease viruses point towards the existence of to-date unknown enzootic reservoir host populations. Microbes Infect. 8(3):917–929, 2006.

Dürrwald, R., Kolodziejek, J., Herzog, S. and Nowotny, N.: Meta-analysis of putative human bornavirus sequences fails to provide evidence implicating Borna disease virus in mental illness. Rev. Med. Virol., 17:181–203, 2007.

East, N.E., et al.: Milkborne outbreak of *Mycoplasma mycoides* subspecies *mycoides* infection in a commercial goat dairy. J. Am. Vet. Med. Assoc., 182:1338–1341, 1983.

Ehrensperger, F., et al.: Cerebral listeriosis in sheep and goats: a histopathological and immunohistological study. Wiener Tierärztliche Monatsschrift. 88(8):219–225, 2001.

Ehrensperger, F.: Personal communication. Prof. Dr. Felix Ehrensperger, Department of Veterinary Pathology, University of Zürich, Zürich, Switzerland, 2007.

El-Azazy, O.M.E. and Ahmed, Y.F.: Patent infection with *Setaria digitata* in goats in Saudi Arabia. Vet. Parasitol. 82(2):161–166, 1999.

Elazhary, M.A.S.Y., Silim, A. and Dea, S.: Prevalence of antibodies to bovine respiratory syncytial virus, bovine virus diarrhea virus, bovine herpesvirus-1, and bovine parainfluenza-3 virus in sheep and goats in Quebec. Am. J. Vet. Res., 45:1660–1662, 1984.

Elezebeth, G., Malik, S.V.S., Chaudhari, S.P. and Barbuddhe, S.B.: The occurrence of *Listeria* species and antibodies against listeriolysin-O in naturally infected goats. Small Rumin. Res., 67 173–178, 2007.

Ellis, T.M., Wilcox, G.E. and Robinson, W.F.: Antigenic variation of caprine arthritis-encephalitis virus during persistent infection of goats. J. Gen. Virol., 68:3145–3152, 1987.

Eloit, M., et al.: BSE agent signatures in a goat. Vet. Rec.. 156(16):523–524, 2005.

Espenes, A., et al.: Detection of PrP(Sc) in rectal biopsy and necropsy samples from sheep with experimental scrapie. J. Comp. Pathol., 134(2–3):115–125, 2006.

European Commission: TSE in small ruminants. Directorate General, Health and Consumer Protections, Brussels, 2006. http://ec.europa.eu/food/food/biosafety/bse/mthly_reps_en.htm

European Commission: Commission Regulation EC No. 253/2006 of 14 February 2006 amending Regulation (EC) No. 999/2001 of the European Parliament and of the Council as regards rapid tests and measures for the eradication of TSEs in ovine and caprine animals. Official Journal of the European Union, L44(9):9–12, February 15, 2006a.

European Commission: Commission requests further investigations on three unusual cases of TSE in sheep. Press Release IP/06/288, Brussels, March 9. 2006b. http://europa.eu/rapid/pressReleasesAction.do?reference=IP/06/288andformat=HTMLandaged=0andlanguage=EN.

European Commission: Opinion on the risk of infection of sheep and goats with bovine spongiform encephalopathy agent. Scientific Steering Committee, Directorate General, Health and Consumer Protection, Brussels, Meeting of 24–35 September, 24 pp. 1998. http://ec.europa.eu/food/fs/sc/ssc/out24_en.pdf.

European Commission: Regulation (EC) No. 999/2001 of the European Parliament and of the Council of 22 May 2001 laying down rules for the prevention, control and eradication of certain transmissible spongiform encephalopathies. Official Journal of the European Union, L147:1–40, May 31 2001. http://europa.eu.int/eur-lex/lex/JOHtml.do?uri=OJ:L:2001:147:SOM:EN:HTML.

European Commission: Report on the monitoring and testing of ruminants for the presence of transmissible spongiform encephalopathy (TSE) in the EU in 2002. European Commission, Directorate General, Health and Consumer Protection, Brussels, 2003. http://ec.europa.eu/food/food/biosafety/bse/annual_reps_en.htm.

European Commission: Report on the monitoring and testing of ruminants for the presence of transmissible spongiform encephalopathy (TSE) in the EU in 2003, including the results of the survey of prion protein genotypes in sheep breeds. European Commission, Directorate General, Health and Consumer Protection, Brussels, 2004. http://ec.europa.eu/food/food/biosafety/bse/annual_reps_en.htm.

European Commission: Report on the monitoring and testing of ruminants for the presence of transmissible spongiform encephalopathy (TSE) in the EU in 2004. European Commission, Directorate General, Health and Consumer Protection, Brussels, 2005. http://ec.europa.eu/food/food/biosafety/bse/annual_reps_en.htm.

European Commission: Report on the monitoring and testing of ruminants for the presence of transmissible spongiform encephalopathy (TSE) in the EU in 2005. European Commission, Directorate General, Health and Consumer Protection, Brussels, 2006. http://ec.europa.eu/food/food/biosafety/bse/annual_reps_en.htm.

European Food Safety Authority: Opinion of the scientific panel on biological hazards on classification of atypical transmissible spongiform encephalopathy (TSE) cases in small ruminants. The EFSA Journal, 276:1–30, 2005.

Fan, P.C., Lin, C.Y., Huang, P. and Yen, C.W.: First confirmed case of cerebrospinal setariosis in goat in Taiwan. J. Chinese Soc. Vet. Sci., 24(2):68–72, 1998.

Fankhauser, R., Vandevelde, M. and Zwahlen, R.: Scrapie in Switzerland? Schweiz. Arch. Tierheilk.,124(5): 227–232, 1982.

FAO Animal Health Yearbook, 1988. L. Velloso, ed. Food and Agricultural Organization of the United Nations, Rome, 1989.

Fatzer, R. von: Diffuse Toxoplasmose-encephalitis in der rechten Grosshirnhälfte einer Ziege. Schweiz. Arch. Tierheilk. 116:219–224, 1974.

Fjøelstad, M.: The effects of *Clostridium botulinum* toxin type C_{beta} given orally to goats.; Acta Vet. Scand., 14:69–80, 1973.

Fletcher, W.S., Rogers, A.L. and Donaldson, S.S.: The use of the goat as an experimental animal. Lab. Anim. Care, 14:65–90, 1964.

Flores, E.F., et al.: Bovine virus diarrhea virus (BVDV) infection in Brazil: history, current situation and perspectives. Pesq. Vet. Bras., 25(3):125–134, 2005.

Foster, J., et al.:, Experimentally induced bovine spongiform encephalopathy did not transmit via goat embryos. J. Gen. Virol. 80(2):517–524, 1999.

Foster, J.D., et al.: Clinical signs, histopathology and genetics of experimental transmission of BSE and natural scrapie to sheep and goats. Vet. Rec. 148:165–171, 2001.

Foster, J.D., Hope, J. and Fraser H.: Transmission of bovine spongiform encephalopathy to sheep and goats. Vet. Rec., 133:339–341, 1993.

Fourie, L.J., Horak, I.G. and Marais, L.: An undescribed *Rhipicephalus* species associated with field paralysis of Angora goats. J. S. Afr. Vet. Assoc., 59:47–49, 1988.

Fourie, L.J., Horak, I.G. and Zyl, J.M. van: Sites of attachment and intraspecific infestation densities of the brown paralysis tick (*Rhipicephalus punctatus*) on Angora goats. Exp. Appl. Acarol. 12(3/4): 243–249, 1991.

Franscini, N., et al.: Prion protein in milk. PloS ONE 1(1):e71. doi:10.1371/journal.pone.0000071. 2006. http://www.plosone.org/article/fetchArticle.action?articleURI=info%3Adoi%2F10.1371%2Fjournal.pone.0000071.

Fraser, G.C., Littlejohns, I.R. and Moyle, A.: The isolation of a probable pestivirus from a goat. Aust. Vet. J., 57:197–198, 1981.

Frier, H.I., et al.: Formation and absorption of cerebrospinal fluid in adult goats with hypo- and hypervitaminosis A. Am. J. Vet. Res., 35:45–55, 1974.

Fulton, R.W., Downing, M.M. and Hagstad, H.V.: Prevalence of bovine herpesvirus-1, bovine viral diarrhea, parainfluenza-3, bovine adenoviruses-3 and –7, and goat respiratory syncytial viral antibodies in goats. Am. J. Vet. Res., 43:1454–1457, 1982.

Gao, G.F., et al.: Molecular variation, evolution and geographical distribution of louping-ill virus. Acta Virol. 41(5)259–268, 1997.

Gavier-Widen, D., et al.: Diagnosis of transmissible spongiform encephalopathies in animals: a review. J. Vet. Diagn. Invest. 17(6):509–27, 2005.

Gaya, P., Saralegui, C., Medina, M. and Nunez, M.: Occurrence of *Listeria monocytogenes* and other *Listeria* spp. in raw caprine milk. J. Dairy Sci., 79(11):1936–1941, 1996.

Ghosal, N.G.: Spinal nerves. In: Sisson and Grossman's The Anatomy of the Domestic Animals, 5th Ed., Volume 1. R. Getty, ed. Philadelphia, W.B. Saunders Co., 1975.

Giannati-Stefanou, A., Tsakos, P., Bourtzi-Hatzopoulou, E. and Anatoliotis, K.: Study of microbiological aspects of meningoencephalitis due to *Listeria* spp. in ruminants. J. Hellenic Vet. Med. Soc., 57(4):275–288, 2006.

Gibbs, H.C., McLaughlin, R.W. and Cameron, H.J.: Meningoencephalitis caused by *Streptococcus zooepidemicus* in a goat. J. Am. Vet. Med. Assoc., 178:735, 1981.

Go, T.: Seroepidemiological studies of flavivirus infection among domestic animals in and around Karachi, state of Sind, Pakistan. Japan. J. Vet. Res. 38(2):50, 1990.

Godhinho, H.P., and Getty, R.: Caprine cranial nerves. In: Sisson and Grossman's The Anatomy of the Domestic Animals, 5th Ed., Volume 1. R. Getty, ed. Philadelphia, W.B. Saunders Co., 1975.

Goldmann, W., et al.: The shortest known prion protein gene allele occurs in goats, has only three octapeptide repeats and is non-pathogenic. J. Gen. Virol. 79 (12):3173–3176, 1998.

Goldmann, W., et al.: Novel polymorphisms in the caprine PrP gene: a codon 142 mutation associated with scrapie incubation period. J. Gen. Virol., 77(11):2885–2891, 1996.

Goldmann, W., Perucchini, M., Smith, A. and Hunter, N.: Genetic variability of the PrP gene in a goat herd in the UK. Vet. Rec. 155(6):177–8, 2004.

Gomes, A.A. de B., et al.: Experimental rabies in ovine and caprine inoculated with a Brazilian fox (*Dusicyon vetulus*) isolate virus sample. Sci. Vet. Trop. 8(1/3):29–34, 2005.

Gonzalez, L., et al.: Postmortem diagnosis of preclinical and clinical scrapie in sheep by the detection of disease-associated PrP in their rectal mucosa. Vet. Rec., 158(10):325–331, 2006.

Gouda, I.M., et al.: Changes in some liver functions in experimentally lead-poisoned goats. Arch. Exp. Vet. Med., Leipzig, 39:257–267, 1985.

Gould, D.H., Cummings, B.A. and Hamar, D.W.: *In vivo* indicators of pathologic ruminal sulfide production in steers with diet-induced polioencephalomalacia. J. Vet. Diagn. Invest., 9(1):72–76, 1997.

Gould, D.H.: Update on sulfur-related polioencephalomalacia. Vet. Clin. N. Am. Food Anim. Pract., 16(3):481–496, 2000.

Gould, D.H.: Polioencephalomalacia. J. Anim. Sci., 76:309–314, 1998.

Gould, E.A., Lamballerie, X. de, Zanotto, P.M. and Holmes, E.C.: Origins, evolution, and vector/host coadaptations within the genus *Flavivirus*. In: The Flaviviruses: Current Molecular Aspects of Evolution, Biology and Disease Prevention, Chambers, T.J. and Monath, T.M., eds., Academic Press, London, pp. 277–314, 2003.

Government of Finland: Scrapie found in Finnish goat. MMM Press Release, Ministry of Agriculture and Forestry, Helsinki, November 2, 2002. http://wwwb.mmm.fi/tiedotteet2/tiedote.asp?nro=1029.

Gray, D., Webster, K. and Berry, J.E.: Evidence of louping-ill and tick-borne fever in goats. Vet. Rec., 122:66, 1988.

Griem, W. and Weinhold, E.: Pathology of visna disease in goats. Dtsch. Tierärztl. Wochensch., 82:396–400, 1975.

Grønstøl, H.: Listeriosis in goats. In: Les Maladies de la Chèvre, Les Colloques de l'INRA, No. 28. P. Yvore and G. Perrin, eds. Paris, Institut National de la Recherche Agronomique, pp. 189–192, 195–196, 1984.

Gudding, R., Grønstøl, H. and Larsen, H.J.: Vaccination against listeriosis in sheep. Vet. Rec., 117:89–90, 1985.

Gudmunsdóttir, K.B., et al.: Iron and iron/manganese ratio in forage from Icelandic sheep farms: relation to scrapie. Acta Vet. Scand., 48(1):article 16, 2006. http://www.actavetscand.com/content/48/1/16.

Guerrault, P., Perrin, G. and Fensterbank, R.: Vaccination trial in goats against listeriosis. Bull. Mens. Soc. Vet. Prat. France, 72:223–229, 1988.

Gummow, B., Bastienello, S.S., Labuschagne, L. and Erasmus, G.L.: Experimental *Albizia versicolor* poisoning in sheep and its successful treatment with pyridoxine hydrochloride. Onderstepoort J. Vet. Res., 59(2):111–118, 1992.

Gupta, B.L., Sharma, S.N. and Tanwani, S.K.: Studies on experimental infection of sheep, goats, rabbits, and mice, and serological response with *Listeria monocytogenes* serotype 4. Indian J. Anim. Sci., 50:739–743, 1980.

Guss, S.B.: Management and Diseases of Dairy Goats. Scottsdale, Dairy Goat Journal Publ. Corp., 1977.

Guthery, F.S., Beasom, S.L. and Jones, L.: Cerebrospinal nematodiasis caused by *Parelaphostrongylus tenuis* in Angora goats in Texas. J. Wildlife Dis., 15:37–42, 1979.

Gygi, M., Kathmann, I., Konar, M., Rottenberg, S. and Meylan, M.: Paraparese ber einer Zwergziege: Abklärung mittels Magnetresonanztomographie. Schweiz. Arch. Tierheilk., 146(11):523–528, 2004.

Hadani, A., Tsafrir, N. and Shimshony, A.: Tick paralysis in goats in Israel. Refuah Vet., 28:165–171, 1971.

Hadlow, W.J.: The pathology of experimental scrapie in the dairy goat. Res. Vet. Sci., 2:289–314, 1961.

Hadlow, W.J., et al.: Course of experimental scrapie virus infection in the goat. J. Inf. Dis., 129:559–567, 1974.

Hadlow, W.J., Kennedy, R.C., Race, R.E. and Eklund, C.M.: Virologic and neurohistologic findings in dairy goats affected with natural scrapie. Vet. Pathol., 17:187–199, 1980.

Hall, W.T.K.: Plant toxicoses of tropical Australia. Australian Vet. J., 40:176–182, 1964.

Hamblin, C. and Hedger, R.S.: The prevalence of antibodies to bovine viral diarrhea/mucosal disease virus in African wildlife. Comp. Immunol. Microbiol. Infect. Dis. 2:295–303, 1979.

Handeland, K. and Skorping A.: The early migration of *Elaphostrongylus rangiferi* in goats. J. Vet. Med. Ser. B, 39:263–272, 1992.

Handeland, K. and Skorping A.: Experimental cerebrospinal elaphostrongylosis (*Elaphostrongylus rangiferi*) in goats. II. Pathological findings. J. Vet. Med. Ser. B, 39:713–722, 1992a.

Handeland, K. and Skorping A.: Experimental cerebrospinal elaphostrongylosis (*Elaphostrongylus rangiferi*) in goats. I. Clinical observations. J. Vet. Med. Ser. B, 40:141–147, 1993.

Handeland, K. and Sparboe, O.: Cerebrospinal elaphostrongylosis in dairy goats in northern Norway. J. Vet. Med. B., 38:755–763, 1991.

Harcourt, R.A., and Anderson, M.A.: Naturally-occurring scrapie in goats. Vet. Rec., 94:504, 1974.

Hartley, W.J. and Blakemore, W.F.: Neurovisceral storage and dysmyelinogenesis in neonatal goats. Acta Neuropathol. (Berl.), 25:325–333, 1973.

Harwood, D.G.: Metacestode disease in goats. Goat Vet. Soc. J., 7:35–37, 1986.
Harwood, D.: Diseases of dairy goats. In Practice, 26(5):248–259, 2004.
Healy, P.J. and McCleary, B.V.: Alternative substrates for use in the detection of goats heterozygous for beta-mannosidosis. Res. Vet. Sci., 33:73–75, 1982.
Hedger, R.S., Howard, D.A. and Burdin, M.L.: The occurrence in goats and sheep in Kenya of a disease closely similar to sway-back. Vet. Rec., 76:493–497, 1964.
Heggebø, R., et al.: Distribution of prion protein in the ileal Peyer's patch of scrapie-free lambs and lambs naturally and experimentally exposed to the scrapie agent. J. Gen. Virol., 81:2327–2337, 2000.
Herweijer, C.H. and De Jonge, W.K.: De ziekte van aujeszky bij de geit. Tijdschr. Diergeneesk., 102:425–428, 1977.
Hilbe, M., et al.: Shrews as reservoir hosts of Borna disease virus. Emerg. Infect. Dis., 12(4):675–677, 2006.
Hoard, H.M., et al.: Determination of genotypic frequency of caprine mucopolysaccharidosis IIID. J. Vet. Diagn. Invest., 10(2):181–183, 1998.
Holmala, K. and Kauhala, K.: Ecology of wildlife rabies in Europe. Mammal Rev. 36(1):17–36, 2006.
Hosseinion, M., et al.: Selenium poisoning in a mixed flock of sheep and goats in Iran. Trop. Anim. Health Prod., 4:173–174, 1972.
Hourrigan, J.L., Klingsporn, A.L., McDaniel, H.A. and Riemenschneider, M.N.: Natural scrapie in a goat. J. Am. Vet. Med. Assoc., 154:538–539, 1969.
Houston, F., et al.: Transmission of BSE by blood transfusion in sheep. Lancet, 356:999–1000, 2000.
Huber, R., Deboer, T. and Tobler, I.: Prion protein: a role in sleep regulation? J. Sleep Res. 8(Suppl 1):30–6, 1999.
Huck, R.A.: Transmission of border disease in goats. Vet. Rec., 92:151, 1973.
Ihlenburg, H.: Susceptibility of goats to experimental infection with Borna disease virus. Mh. Vet. Med., 17:337–341, 1962.
Inglis, D.M., Gilmour, D.M. and Murray, I.S.: A farm investigation into swayback in a herd of goats and the results of administration of copper needles. Vet. Rec., 118:657–660, 1986.
Innes, J.R.M., Shoho, C. and Pillai, C.P.: Epizootic cerebrospinal nematodiasis or setariasis. Br. Vet. J., 108:71–88, 1952.
Islam, S., Kalita, D., Bhuyan, D., Rahman, T. and Saleque, A.: Ocular coenurosis in goat. J. Vet. Parasitol. 20(1):53–55, 2006.
Itabisashi, T.: Urea-ammonia poisoning and the electroencephalogram in goats. Natl. Inst. Anim. Health Q., 17:115–123, 1977.
Jackman, R.: Evaluation of a preclinical blood test for scrapie in sheep using immunocapillary electrophoresis. J. AOAC Int. 89(3):720–727, 2006.
Jacobson, E.R., et al.: West Nile virus infection in farmed American alligators (*Alligator mississippiensis*) in Florida. J. Wildl. Dis., 41(1):96–106, 2005.
Jamison, J.M. and Prescott, J.F.: Bacterial meningitis in large animals—part II. Comp. Cont. Educ. Pract. Vet., 10:225–231, 1988.
Jayakumar, R., Thirumurugan, G., Nachimuthu, K. and Padmanaban, V.D.: Detection of rabies virus antigen in animals by avidin-biotin dot ELISA. Zbl. Bakt. 285:82–85, 1995.
Jayamanne, V.S. and Samarajeewa, U.: Incidence and detection of *Listeria monocytogenes* in milk and milk products of Sri Lanka. Trop. Agric. Res. 13: 42–50, 2001.
Jayarao, B.M., et al.: A study of the incidence of rabies in man and animals recorded in King Edward Memorial Hospital and Bai Sakarbai Dinshaw Petit Hospital for animals, Bombay. Indian Vet. Med. J., 9:141–146, 1985.
Jayasinghe, D.R. and Wijesundera, W.S.S.: Differentiation of *Setaria digitata* and *Setaria labiatopapillosa* using molecular markers. Vet. J., 165(2):136–142, 2003.
Jeffrey, M., et al.: Immunohistochemical features of PrP^{d} accumulation in natural and experimental goat transmissible spongiform encephalopathies. J. Comp. Pathol., 134:171–181, 2006.
Jeffrey, M., et al.:, Oral inoculation of sheep with the agent of bovine spongiform encephalopathy (BSE). 1. Onset and distribution of disease-specific PrP accumulation in brain and viscera. J. Comp. Pathol., 124:280–289, 2001.
Johnson, G.C., et al.: Epidemiologic evaluation of encephalitic listeriosis in goats. J. Am. Vet. Med. Assoc., 208(10):1695–1699, 1996.
Jones, M.Z. and Laine, R.A.: Caprine oligosaccharide storage disorder: accumulation of beta-mannosyl(1-4) beta-N-acetylglucosaminyl(1-4) N-acetylglucosamine in brain. J. Biol. Chem., 256:5181–5184, 1981.
Jones, M.Z., et al.: Caprine beta-mannosidosis: clinical and pathological features. J. Neuropathol. Exp. Neurol., 42:268–285, 1983.
Jones, M.Z., et al.: Caprine mucopolysaccharidosis-IIID: clinical, biochemical, morphological and immunohistochemical characteristics. J. Neuropathol. Exp. Neurol., 57(2):148–157, 1998.
Kaneko, J.J.: Clinical Biochemistry of Domestic Animals. 3rd Ed. New York, Academic Press, 1980.
Kellerman, T.S., et al.: Induction of diplodiosis, a neuromycotoxicosis, in domestic ruminants with cultures of indigenous and exotic isolates of *Diplodia maydis*. Onderstepoort J. Vet. Res., 52:35–42, 1985.
Kemp, G.E., et al.: Mokola virus. Further studies on IbAn 27377, a new rabies-related etiologic agent of zoonosis in Nigeria. Am. J. Trop. Med. Hyg., 21:356–359, 1972.
Kim, I.J., et al.: Identification of a bovine viral diarrhea virus type 2 in Korean native goat (*Capra hircus*). Vir. Res., 121:103–106, 2006.
King, N.B.: Clostridial diseases. In: Proceedings, Refresher Course for Veterinarians, Post-Graduate Committee in Veterinary Science, University of Sydney, 52:217–220, 1980.
Kingsbury, J.M.: Poisonous Plants of the United States and Canada. Englewood Cliffs, Prentice-Hall Inc., 1964.
Kleiboeker, S.B., et al.: Diagnosis of West Nile virus infection in horses. J. Vet. Diagn. Invest., 16(1):2–10, 2004.
Klopfleisch, R., Beier, D. and Teifke, J.P.: Choroid plexus carcinoma in a goat. J. Comp. Pathol., 135:12–16, 2006.
Knight, A.P.: Larkspur poisoning. Comp. Cont. Educ. Pract. Vet., 9:F60–F61, 1987.
Knight, H.D. and Costner, G.C.: Bromide intoxication of horses, goats, and cattle. J. Am. Vet. Med. Assoc., 171:446–448, 1977.
Kocan, A.A.: The use of ivermectin in the treatment and prevention of infection with *Parelaphostrongylus tenuis* in white-tailed deer. J. Wildl. Dis., 21:454–455, 1985.

Kopcha, M., et al.: Cerebrospinal nematodiasis in a goat herd. J. Am. Vet. Med. Assoc., 194:1439–1442, 1989.

Koptopoulos, G. and Papadopoulos, O.: A serological survey for tick-borne encephalitis and West Nile viruses in Greece. Arboviruses in the Mediterranean Countries. Gustav Fischer Verlag, Stuttgart, pp. 185–188, 1980.

Kornegay, J.N., Oliver, J.E. and Gorgacz, E.J.: Clinicopathologic features of brain herniation in animals. J. Am. Vet. Med. Assoc., 182:1111–1116, 1983.

Kral, E. and Hlousek, A.: Spasticka parezapanevnichkoncetinukozla. Veterinarstvi, 23:425–426, 1973.

Krametter-Frötscher, R., et al.: Influence of communal alpine pasturing on the spread of pestiviruses among sheep and goats in Austria: first identification of border disease virus in Austria. Zoonoses Public Health, 54(5): 209–213, 2007.

Kumar, K., et al.: Caprine beta mannosidosis: phenotypic features. Vet. Rec., 118:325–327, 1986.

Kummeneje, K.: *Listeria monocytogenes.* Isolation from sheep and goats in northern Norway. Serogrouping and some biochemical reactions. Nord. Vet. Med., 27:140–143, 1975.

Lamontagne, L. and Roy, R.: Presence of antibodies to bovine viral diarrhea-mucosal disease virus (border disease) in sheep and goat flocks in Quebec. Can. J. Comp. Med., 48:225–227, 1984.

Lancaster, M.J., Gill, I.J. and Hooper, P.T.: Progressive paresis in Angora goats. Aust. Vet. J., 64:123–124, 1987.

Lankester, M.W. and Fong, D.: Protostrongylid nematodes in caribou (*Rangifer tarandus caribou*) and moose (*Alces alces*) of Newfoundland. Rangifer. Special Issue 10, 73–83, 1998.

Le Dur, A., et al.: A newly identified type of scrapie agent can naturally infect sheep with resistant PrP genotypes. Proc. Natl. Acad. Sci., 102(44):16031–16036, 2005.

Leipprandt, J.R., et al.: Caprine β-mannosidase: sequencing and characterization of the cDNA and identification of the molecular effect of caprine β-mannosidosis. Genomics, 37:51–56, 1996.

Levine, G.J., et al.: Imaging diagnosis—bacterial diskospondylitis in a goat. Vet. Radiol. Ultrasound, 47(6):585–588, 2006.

Lezmi, S., et al: Comparative molecular analysis of the abnormal prion protein in field scrapie cases and experimental bovine spongiform encephalopathy in sheep by use of western blotting and immunohistochemical methods. J. Virol. 78(7): 3654–3662, 2004.

Liberski, P.P.: Prion protein as a target for therapeutic interventions. Pure and Appl. Chem., 76(5):915–920, 2004.

Liggett, A.D., Jain, A.V. and Blue, J.L.: Pseudohyperchloremia associated with bromide intoxication in a goat herd. J. Am. Vet. Med. Assoc., 187:72–74, 1985.

Ligios, C., et al.: PrP^{Sc} in mammary glands of sheep affected by scrapie and mastitis. Nat. Med., 11(11):1137–1138, 2005.

Lincicome, D.R.: Goat disease: prevalence in the United States and Canada as reflected in autopsy reports for 1977–1979. In: Proceedings, 3rd Internat. Conf. Goat Prod. Dis., Scottsdale, Dairy Goat Publ. Co., pp. 602, 1982.

Linnenbrink, T. and McMichael, M.: Tetanus: pathophysiology, clinical signs, diagnosis, and update on new treatment modalities. J. Vet. Emerg. Crit. Care, 16(3):199–207, 2006.

Loeb, E.: Encephalitic listeriosis in ruminants: immunohistochemistry as a diagnostic tool. J. Vet. Med. Ser. A, 51(9/10):453–455, 2004.

Lofstedt, J., Jakowski, R. and Sharko, P.: Ataxia, arthritis, and encephalitis in a goat herd. J. Am Vet. Med. Assoc., 193(10):1295–1298, 1988.

Løken, T. and Bjerkås, I.: Experimental pestivirus infections in pregnant goats. J. Comp. Pathol., 105:123–140, 1991.

Løken, T., Krogsrud, J. and Bjerkås, I.: Outbreaks of border disease in goats induced by a pestivirus-contaminated orf vaccine with virus transmission to sheep and cattle. J. Comp. Pathol., 104:195–209, 1991.

Løken, T. and Grønstøl, H.: Clinical investigations in a goat herd with outbreaks of listeriosis. Acta Vet. Scand., 23:380–391, 1982.

Løken, T., Aspøy, E. and Grønstøl, H.: *Listeria monocytogenes* excretion and humoral immunity in goats in a herd with outbreaks of listeriosis and in a healthy herd. Acta Vet. Scand., 23:392–399, 1982a.

Løken, T., Bjerkås, I. and Hyllseth, B.: Border disease in goats in Norway, Res. Vet. Sci., 33:130–131, 1982.

Løken, T.: Pestivirus infection in goats. In: Abstracts, 2nd International Colloquium in Niort, Goat Diseases and Production, June 26–29, Niort, France, p. 49, 1989.

Lomas, S.T. and Hazell, S.L.: The isolation of *Mycoplasma arginini* from a pituitary abscess in a goat. Aust. Vet. J., 60:281–282, 1983.

Lovell, K.L. and Jones, M.Z.: Distribution of central nervous system lesions in beta-mannosidosis. Acta Neuropathol., 62:121–126, 1983.

Lovell, K.L., Sprecher, D.J., Ames, N.K. and Jones, M.Z.: Development and efficacy of ultrasound-guided fetal fluid aspiration techniques for prenatal diagnosis of caprine β-mannosidosis. Theriogenology, 44:517–527, 1995.

Low, J.C. and Donachie, W.: A review of *Listeria monocytogenes* and listeriosis. Vet. J. 153(1):9–29, 1997.

Ludwig, H. and Bode, L.: Borna disease virus: new aspects on infection, disease, diagnosis and epidemiology. Rev. Sci. Tech. Off. Int. Epiz., 19(1):259–288, 2000.

Luginbuhl, H.: Comparative aspects of tumors of the nervous system. Ann. N. Y. Acad. Sci., 108:702–721, 1963.

Lundgren, A.L. and Ludwig, H.: Clinically diseased cats with non-suppurative meningoencephalomyelitis have Borna disease virus-specific antibodies. Acta Vet. Scand., 34 (1):101–103, 1993.

Macaldowie, C., et al.: Louping-ill in llamas (*Lama glama*) in the Hebrides. Vet. Rec., 156:420–421, 2005.

MacKay, J.M.K. and Smith, W.: A case of scrapie in an uninoculated goat—a natural occurrence or a contact infection. Vet. Rec., 73:394–396, 1961.

MacLachlan, N.J., Gribble, D.H. and East, N.E.: Polyradiculoneuritis in a goat. J. Am. Vet. Med. Assoc., 180:166–167, 1982.

Mahmoud, O.M., Haroun, E.M. and Omer, O.H.: An outbreak of neurofilariosis in young goats. Vet. Parasitol., 120(1/2):151–156, 2004.

Malachowski, J.A., and Jones, M.Z.: Beta-mannosidosis: lesions of the distal peripheral nervous system. Acta Neuropathol. (Berl), 61:95–100, 1983.

Malkinson, M., et al.: Borna disease in ostriches. Vet. Rec. 133(12):304, 1993.

Mall, M.P., Ashok, K. and Malik, S.V.S.: Sero-positivity of domestic animals against Japanese encephalitis in Bareilly area, U. P. J. Commun. Dis. 27(4):242–246, 1995.
Markotter, W., et al.: Lagos bat virus, South Africa. Emerging Infect. Dis., 104–2(3):504–506, 2006.
Marriott, L., et al.: Detection of louping-ill virus in clinical specimens from mammals and birds using TaqMan RT-PCR. J. Virol. Methods, 137:21–28, 2006.
Marshall, C.L., Weinstock, D., Kramer, R.W. and Bagley R.S.: Glioma in a goat. J. Am. Vet. Med. Assoc., 206(10):1572–1574, 1995.
Mason, P.C., et al.: *Elaphostrongylus cervi* in red deer. N.Z. Vet. J., 24(1/2):22–23, 1976.
Mason, R.W.: Observations on the effects of management stress on beta-mannosidase activity in goats. Aust. Vet. J., 63:339–340, 1986.
Mathews, F.P.: Locoism in domestic animals. Bull. Tex. Agric. Exp. Sta., 456, 1932.
Mathews, F.P.: The toxicity of *Kallstroemia hirsutissima* (carpet weed) for cattle, sheep, and goats. J. Am. Vet. Med. Assoc., 105:152–155, 1944.
Mathews, F.P.: The toxicity of red-stemmed peavine *(Astragalus emoryanus)* for cattle, sheep and goats. J. Am. Vet. Med. Assoc., 97:125–134, 1940.
Matsuura, F., Jones, M.Z. and Frazier, S.E.: Structural analysis of the major caprine beta-mannosidosis urinary oligosaccharides. Biochim. Biophys. Acta, 759:67–73, 1983.
Maurer, E., et al.: Swiss scrapie surveillance. I. Clinical aspects of neurological diseases in sheep and goats. Schweiz. Arch. Tierheilk. 147(10):425–433, 2005.
Mayhew, I.G., de Lahunta, A., Georgi, J.R. and Aspros, D.G.: Naturally occurring cerebrospinal parelaphostrongylosis. Cornell Vet., 66:56–72, 1976.
McAllister, M.M., et al.: Evaluation of ruminal sulfide concentrations and seasonal outbreaks of polioencephalomalacia in beef cattle in a feedlot. J. Am. Vet. Med. Assoc., 211(10):1275–1279, 1997.
McGuire, K., et al.: Tracing the origins of louping-ill virus by molecular phylogenetic analysis. J. Gen. Virol., 79(5):981–988, 1998.
McLean R.G., Ubico, S.R., Bourne, D. and Komar, N: West Nile virus in livestock and wildlife. Cur. Top. Microbiol. Immunol., 267:271–308, 2002.
McSporran, K.D.: Polioencephalomalacia in goats. Surveillance, N.Z., 15:24, 1988.
Meldrum, J.B. and Ko, K.W.: Effects of calcium disodium EDTA and meso-2,3-dimercaptosuccinic acid on tissue concentrations of lead for use in treatment of calves with experimentally induced lead toxicosis. Am. J. Vet. Res. 64(6):672–676, 2003.
Miller D.L., et al.: West Nile virus in farmed alligators. Emerg. Infect. Dis. 9:794–799, 2003.
Mogi, K., et al.: Correlation between spontaneous feeding behavior and neuropeptide Y profile in the third ventricular cerebrospinal fluid of goats. Dom. Anim. Endocrinol., 25:175–182, 2003.
Mohamed, O.S.A., Adam, S.E.I. and El Dirdiri, N.I.: The combined effect of dursban and reldan on Nubian goats. Vet. Hum. Toxicol., 32:47–48, 1990.
Mohamed, O.S.A. and Adam, S.E.I.: Toxicity of sumicidin (fenvalerate) to Nubian goats. J. Comp. Pathol., 102:1–6, 1990.
Mohamed, O.S.A., El Dirdiri, N.I. and Adam, S.E.I.: Toxicity of reldan (chlorpyrifos-methyl) in Nubian goats. Vet. Hum. Toxicol., 31:60–63, 1989.
Monleón, E., et al.: Approaches to scrapie diagnosis by applying immunohistochemistry and rapid tests on central nervous and lymphoreticular systems. J. Virol. Methods, 125:165–171, 2005.
Morin, D.E.: Brainstem and cranial nerve abnormalities: listeriosis, otitis media/interna, and pituitary abscess syndrome. Vet. Clin. N. Am. Food Anim. Pract., 20(2): 243–273, 2004.
Morishima, O.H., et al.: Toxicity of lidocaine in adult, newborn and fetal sheep. Anesthesiology, 55:57–61, 1981.
Morris, W.E., Uzal, F.A. and Cipolla, A.L.: Pyogranulomatous meningoencephalitis in a goat due to *Corynebacterium ulcerans*. Vet. Rec., 156:317–318, 2005.
Mount, M.E.: Diagnostic value of urinary dialkyl phosphate measurement in goats exposed to diazinon. Am. J. Vet. Res., 45:817–824, 1984.
Moynagh, J., Schimmel, H. and Kramer, G.N.: The evaluation of tests for the diagnosis of transmissible spongiform encephalopathy in bovines. Commission of the European Communities, Brussels, 1999. http://ec.europa.eu/food/fs/bse/bse12_en.pdf.
Mravak, S., Bienzle, U., Feldmeier, H., Hampl, H. and Habermehl, K.-O.: Pseudorabies in man. Lancet. 1(8531):501–502, 1987.
Msengi, L.M.K.T., Mosha, R.D., Matovelo, J.A., and Hansen, N.G.: The toxicity of *Burttia prunoides* in rats and goats. Vet. Hum. Toxicol., 29:398–400, 1987.
Nagy, D.W.: *Parelaphostrongylus tenuis* and other parasitic diseases of the ruminant nervous system. Vet. Clin. No. Amer. Food Anim. Pract., 20(2):393–412, 2004.
National Creutzfeldt-Jakob Disease Surveillance Unit, Variant Creutzfeldt-Jakob Disease Current Data (June 2007). University of Edinburgh, Edinburgh, UK., 2007. http://www.cjd.ed.ac.uk/vcjdworld.htm.
NRC: Mineral Tolerance of Animals, 2nd Rev. Ed., National Research Council, Washington D.C., National Academies Press, 2005.
Newsholme, S.J. and O'Neill, T.P.: An outbreak of cerebrocortical necrosis (polioencephalomalacia) in goats. J. So. Afr. Vet. Assoc., 56:37–38, 1985.
Nicolas, M.A., et al.: Enquête epidémiologique de la listeriose des ovins et des caprins. Revue Méd. Vét., 125:1369–1378, 1974.
Nightingale, K.K., et al.: Ecology and transmission of *Listeria monocytogenes* infecting ruminants and in the farm environment. Appl. Environ. Microbiol., 70(8):4458–4467, 2004.
Nightingale, K.K., et al.: Evaluation of farm management practices as risk factors for clinical listeriosis and fecal shedding of *Listeria monocytogenes* in ruminants. J. Am. Vet. Med. Assoc., 227(11):1808–1814, 2005.
Niles, G.A. Morgan, S.E. and Edwards, W.C.: Relationship between sulfur, thiamine and polioencephalomalacia—a review. Bovine Pract. 36(2):93–99, 2002.
Norman, S. and Smith, M.C.: Caprine arthritis-encephalitis: review of the neurologic form in 30 cases. J. Am. Vet. Med. Assoc., 182:1342–1345, 1983.

Nottidge, H.O., Omobowale, T.O., and Oladiran, O.O.: Mokola virus antibodies in humans, dogs, cats, cattle, sheep, and goats in Nigeria. Intern. J. Appl. Res. Vet. Med., 5(3):105–106, 2007.

Nurse, G.H. and Lenghaus, C.: An outbreak of *Toxoplasma gondii* abortion, mummification, and perinatal death in goats. Aust. Vet. J., 63:27–28, 1986.

O'Brien, T.D., et al.: Cerebrospinal parelaphostrongylosis in Minnesota. Minn. Vet., 26:18–22, 1986.

O'Rourke, K.I., et al.: Preclinical diagnosis of scrapie by immunohistochemistry of third eyelid lymphoid tissue. J. Clin. Microbiol., 38(9): 3254–3259, 2000.

O'Sullivan, B.M.: Enzootic ataxia in goat kids. Aust. Vet. J., 53:455–456, 1977.

O'Toole, D., Raisbeck, M., Case, J.C. and Whitson, T.D.: Selenium-induced "blind staggers" and related myths. A commentary on the extent of historical livestock losses attributed to selenosis on western US rangelands. Vet. Pathol., 33:104–116, 1996.

OIE: Manual of Diagnostic Tests and Vaccines for Terrestrial Animals. Chapter 2.3.13., Bovine Spongiform Encephalopathy. Office International des Epizooties, Paris, 2004a. http://www.oie.int/eng/normes/mmanual/A_00064.htm.

OIE: Manual of Diagnostic Techniques and Vaccines for Terrestrial Animals. Chapter 2.2.5 Rabies. Office International des Epizooties, Paris, 2007. http://www.oie.int/eng/normes/mmanual/A_00044.htm.

OIE: Manual of Diagnostic Tests and Vaccines for Terrestrial Animals. Chapter 2.4.8. Scrapie. Office International des Epizooties, Paris, 2004. http://www.oie.int/eng/normes/mmanual/A_00074.htm.

OIE: World Animal Health Situation. Number of cases of bovine spongiform encephalopathy (BSE) reported in the United Kingdom. Office International des Epizooties, Paris, France, 2007a. http://www.oie.int/eng/info/en_esbru.htm.

Okoh, A.E.J.: Rabies in farm livestock in Nigeria. Int. J. Zoon., 8:51–56, 1981.

Okwumabua, O., et al.: Characterization of *Listeria monocytogenes* isolates from food animal clinical cases: PFGE pattern similarity to strains from human listeriosis cases. FEMS Microbiol. Lett. 249(2):275–281, 2005.

Olaleye, O.D., Omilabu, S.A., Ilomechina, E.N. and Fagbami, A.H.: A survey for haemagglutination-inhibiting antibody to West Nile virus in human and animal sera in Nigeria. Comp. Immunol. Microbiol. Infect. Dis. 13(1):35–39, 1990.

Olcott, B.M., Strain, G.M. and Kreeger, J.M.: Diagnosis of partial epilepsy in a goat. J. Am. Vet. Med. Assoc., 191:837–840, 1987.

Omer, O.H. and Awad Elkarim, A.H.: The combined effects of aldrin and sevin insecticides on Nubian goats. Sudan J. Vet. Sci. Anim. Husb., 22:12–18, 1981.

Orr, M.B. and Barlow, R.M.: Experiments in border disease. X. The postnatal skin lesion in sheep and goats. J. Comp. Pathol., 88:295–302, 1978.

Orr, M., Montgomery, H., Gill, J. and Smith, R.: Abortion in goats: a field study. Surveillance, NZ, 14:5–6, 1987.

Orr, M.: Causes of goat abortion: an Otago-Southland study. Surveillance, NZ, 15:19–20, 1988.

Osweiler, G.D., Carson, T.L., Buck, W.B. and Van Gelder, G.A.: Clinical and Diagnostic Veterinary Toxicology, 3rd Ed. Dubuque, Kendall Hunt Publ. Co. 1984.

Owen, E.C., et al.: Pathological and biochemical studies of an outbreak of swayback in goats. J. Comp. Pathol., 75:241–251, 1965.

Papa, A., Pavlidou, V. and Antoniadis, A.: Greek goat encephalitis virus strain isolated from *Ixodes ricinus*, Greece. Emerg. Infect. Dis., 14(2):330–332, 2008.

Pappenheimer, J.R., Heisy, S.R., Jordan, E.F. and Downer, J. deC.: Perfusion of the cerebral ventricular system in unanesthetized goats. Am. J. Physiol., 203:763–774, 1962.

Patnaik, B.: Lumbar paralysis in Beetal goats and their graded progeny in Orissa. 1. A study of the incidence and symptoms of the disease. Indian J. Anim. Health, 5:1–9, 1966.

Pattison, I.H.: Myopathy in sheep. Lancet, I:104–105, 1957.

Pattison, I.H.: The spread of scrapie by contact between affected and healthy sheep, goats, and mice. Vet. Rec., 76:333–336, 1964.

Pattison, I.H., Gordon, W.S. and Millson, G.C.: Experimental production of scrapie in goats. J. Comp. Pathol., 69:300–312, 1959.

Pattison, I.H., Hoare, M.N., Jebbett, J.N. and Watson, W.A.: Spread of scrapie to sheep and goats by oral dosing with foetal membranes from scrapie-affected sheep. Vet. Rec., 90:465–468, 1972.

Payne, M.A., et al.: Drugs prohibited from extralabel use in food animals. J. Am. Vet. Med. Assoc., 215:28–32, 1999.

Pedrizet, J.A. and Dinsmore, P.: Pituitary abscess syndrome. Comp. Cont. Educ. Pract. Vet., 8:S311–S318, 1986.

Pépin, M., et al.: Maedi-visna virus infection in sheep: a review. Vet. Res., 29:341–367, 1998.

Perea-Remujo, A., et al.: Sero-epidemiological survey of listeriosis in cattle, sheep and goats in Cordoba province. Arch. Zootec., 33:265–284, 1984.

Perler, L.: Swollen knees eradicated on Swiss goats. Annual Report 2003. Swiss Federal Veterinary Office. SVFO Magazine, 2:16–17, 2004. http://www.bvet.admin.ch/org/02328/index.html?lan=en.

Petersen, L.R. and Marfin, A.A.: West Nile virus: a primer for the clinician. Ann. Intern. Med., 137(3):173–179, 2002.

Phadke, S.P., Bhagwat, S.V., Kapshikar, R.N. and Ghevari, S..: Listeriosis in sheep and goats in Maharashtra. Indian Vet. J., 56:634–637, 1979.

Pienaar, J.G., et al.: Experimental studies with *Strongyloides papillosus* in goats. Onderstepoort J. Vet. Res., 66:191–235, 1999.

Pisoni, G., Quasso, A. and Moroni, P.: Phylogenetic analysis of small-ruminant lentivirus subtype B1 in mixed flocks: Evidence for natural transmission from goats to sheep. Virology, 339:147–152, 2005.

Porter, M.B., et al.: Neurologic disease putatively associated with ingestion of *Solanum viarum* in goats. J. Am. Vet. Med. Assoc., 223(4):501–504, 2003.

Prasad, T., Arora, S.P. and Behra, G.D.: Note on the dietary investigation of suspected "swayback" in kids. Indian J. Anim. Sci., 52:837–840, 1982.

Pratelli, A., et al.: Genomic characterization of pestiviruses isolated from lambs and kids in southern Italy. J. Virol. Methods. 94:81–85, 2001.

Pratelli, A., et al.: Pestivirus infection in small ruminants: virological and histopathological findings. Microbiologica, 22:351–35, 1999.

Prince, M.J., et al.: Bovine spongiform encephalopathy. In: Risk analysis of prion diseases in animals. C.I. Lasmézas and D.B. Adams, eds. Rev. Sci. Tech. Off. Int. Epiz., Vol. 22, No. 1, pp. 37–60, April 2003.

Prusiner, S.B.: Prions. Proc. Natl. Acad. Sci. U.S.A., 95(23):13363–83, 1998.

Pusterla, N., Caplazi, P. and Braun, U.: Cerebrospinal nematodiasis in seven goats. Schweiz. Arch. Tierheilk. 139(6):282–287, 1997.

Pusterla, N., Caplazi, P., Lutz, H. and Braun, U.: Treatment of cerebrospinal nematodiasis in goats. Deutsche Tierarztliche Wochenschrift, 106(1):22–24, 1999.

Pusterla, N., et al.: *Elaphostrongylus cervi* infection in a Swiss goat. Vet. Rec. 148(12):382–383, 2001.

Quérat, G., et al.: Highly lytic and persistent lentiviruses naturally present in sheep with progressive pneumonia are genetically distinct. J. Virol., 52(2):672–679, 1984.

Race, R., Jenny, A. and Sutton, D.: Scrapie infectivity and proteinase K-resistant prion protein in sheep placenta, brain, spleen, and lymph node: implications for transmission and antemortem diagnosis. J. Infect. Dis., 178(4):949–953, 1998.

Radostits, O.M., Gay, C.C., Hinchcliff, K.W. and Constable, P.D.: Veterinary Medicine. A textbook of the diseases of cattle, horse, sheep, pigs and goats. 10th Edition, Saunders Elsevier, Edinburgh, 2007.

Ramírez, G.A., et al.: Malignant peripheral nerve sheath tumour (Malignant Schwannoma) in the diaphragm of a goat. J. Comp. Pathol., 137:137–141, 2007.

Rammell, C.G., and Hill, J.H.: Blood thiamine levels in clinically normal goats and goats with suspected polioencephalomalacia. N. Z. Vet. J., 36:99–100, 1988.

Rankins, D.L., Ruffin, D.C. and Pugh, D.G.: Feeding and nutrition. In: Sheep and Goat Medicine, D.G. Pugh, ed. W.B. Saunders Co., Philadelphia, pp. 19–60, 2002.

Reid, H.W., Buxton, D., Pow, I. and Finlayson, J.: Transmission of louping-ill virus in goat milk. Vet. Rec., 114:163–165, 1984.

Rekha, V.B., Malik, S.V.S., Chaudhari, S.P. and Barbuddhe, S.B.: Listeriolysin O-based diagnosis of *Listeria monocytogenes* infection in experimentally and naturally infected goats. Small Rumin. Res., 66(1/3):70–75, 2006.

Render, J.A., Lovell, K.L., Jones, M.Z. and Wheeler, C.A.: Ocular pathology of caprine beta-mannosidosis. Vet. Pathol., 26(5):444–446, 1989.

Rickard. L.G.: Parasites. Vet. Clin. N. Am. Food Anim. Pract., 10(2):238–247, 1994.

Rings, D.M.: Clostridial disease associated with neurologic signs: tetanus, botulism and enterotoxemia. Vet. Clin. N. Am. Food Anim. Pract., 20(2):379–391, 2004.

Rissi, D.R., et al.: Meningoencephalitis caused by *Listeria* sp. in goats. Pesq. Vet. Bra., 26(1):14–20, 2006.

Robinson, W.F., Chapman, H.M., Grandage, J. and Bolton, J.R.: Atlanto-axial malarticulation in Angora goats. Austral. Vet. J., 58(3):105–107, 1982.

Rodriguez Armesto, R., et al.: Intoxication in goats due to ingestion of *Ipomoea hieronymi* in Catamarca, Argentina. Vet. Argent. 21(205):332–341, 2004.

Roeder, P.L.: Enzootic ataxia of lambs and kids in the Ethiopian rift valley. Trop. Anim. Health Prod., 12:229–233, 1980.

Ronzon, F., et al.: BSE inoculation to prion diseases-resistant sheep reveals tricky silent carriers. Biochem. Biophys. Res. Commun. 350(4):872–877, 2006.

Rott, R., Herzog, S. and Richt, J.A.: Borna disease. In: Infectious diseases of livestock. Volume Two. Oxford University Press, Oxford, UK, Ed. 2, pp. 1368–1372, 2004.

Rott, R., Herzog, S., Bechter, K. and Frese, K.: Borna disease, a possible hazard for man? Arch. Virol. 118(3–4):143–149, 1991.

Rowe, C.L.: Hemivertebra in a goat. Vet. Med. Sm. Anim. Clin., 74:211–214, 1979.

Rowe, L.D., Dollahite, J.W., Kim, H.L. and Camp, B.J.: *Hymenoxys odorata* (bitterweed) poisoning in sheep. Southwest. Vet., 26:287–293, 1973.

Roy, R.N.: A study of the lipolytic properties of extracellular enzymes from *Listeria monocytogenes* isolated from bulked raw cow milk and pasteurized goat milk. J. Dairy Sci., 71 (Suppl. 1):85, 1988.

Rupprecht, C.E., Hanlon, C.A. and Hemachudha, T.: Rabies re-examined. Lancet Infect. Dis., 2:327–343, 2002.

Saikia, J., Pathak, S.C. and Barman, A.K.: Coenurosis in goats. Indian Vet. Med. J., 11:135–141, 1987.

Sanford, J.P.: Tetanus—forgotten but not gone. N. Engl. J. Med., 332(12):812–3, 1995.

Sanford, S.E.: Meningoencephalitis caused by thermal disbudding in goat kids. Can. Vet. J., 30:832, 1989.

Santa Rosa, J., Berne, M.E.A., Johnson, E.H. and Olander, H.J.: Diseases of goats diagnosed in Sobral, Brazil. In: Proceedings, IV International Conf. Goats, Brasilia, EMBRAPA-DDT, pp. 1360–1361, 1987.

Santagada, G., Latorre, L., Ianuzziello, V. and Petrella, A.: Outbreak of abortion in sheep due to *Listeria ivanovii*: epidemiological considerations. Large Anim. Rev. 10(4):31–35, 2004.

Santos, L.B., et al.: Botulismo experimental em caprinos pela toxina tipo C. Pesq. Vet. Bras., 13(314):73–76, 1993.

Sauders, B.D., et al.: Molecular subtyping to detect human listeriosis clusters. Emerg. Infect. Dis., 9(6):672–680, 2003.

Scandrett, W.B. and Gajadhar, A.A.: Assessment of domestic goats as a patent host of *Elaphostrongylus cervi*. J. Parasitol., 88(1):93–96, 2002.

Schenk, H.C., et al.: Magnetic resonance imaging findings in metabolic and toxic disorders of 3 small ruminants. J. Vet. Intern. Med. 21:865–871, 2007.

Schmidt, H.: Vitamin A deficiencies in ruminants. Am. J. Vet. Res., 2:373–389, 1941.

Schofield, L.N. and Saunders, J.R.: An incidental case of tick paralysis in a Holstein calf exposed to *Dermacentor andersoni*. Can Vet. J., 33:190–191, 1992.

Schreuder, B.E.C. and Somerville, R.A.: Bovine spongiform encephalopathy in sheep? Rev. Sci. Tech. Off. Int. Epiz. 22(1):103–120, 2003.

Schreuder, B.E.C., van Keulen, L.J.M., Vromans, M.E.W., Langeveld, J.P.M. and Smith, M.A.: Tonsillar biopsy and PrP^{Sc} detection in the preclinical diagnosis of scrapie. Vet. Rec., 142:564–568, 1998.

Schuler, L.A., Khaitsa, M.L., Dyer, N.W. and Stoltenow, C. L.: Evaluation of an outbreak of West Nile virus infection in horses: 569 cases (2002). J. Am. Vet. Med. Assoc., 225(7):1084–1089, 2004.

Schumaher-Henrique, B., Gorniak, S.L., Dagli, M.L.Z. and Spinosa, H.S.: The clinical, biochemical, haematological and pathological effects of long-term administration of *Ipomoea carnea* to growing goats. Vet. Res. Commun., 27(4):311–319, 2003.

Scientific Panel on Biological Hazards of the European Food Safety Authority: Opinion on a quantitative assessment of risk posed to humans by tissues of small ruminants in case BSE is present in these animal populations". The EFSA Journal 227:1–11, 2005. http://www.efsa.europa.eu/en/science/biohaz/biohaz_opinions/990.html.

Scientific Panel on Biological Hazards of the European Food Safety Authority: Statement of the EFSA Scientific Expert Working Group on BSE/TSE of the Scientific Panel on Biological Hazards on the health risks of the consumption of milk and milk derived products from goats, EFSA, Brussels, November 26, 2004. http://www.efsa.europa.eu/etc/medialib/efsa/science/biohaz/biohaz_documents/709.Par.0002.File.dat/bdoc_statement_goatsmilk_en1.pdf.

Scroggs, P.: Diary of a tragedy. Dairy Goat J., 67:793–795, 799, 817, 1989.

Seaman, J.T. and Hartley, W.J.: Congenital copper deficiency in goats. Australian Vet. J.: 57:355–356, 1981.

Serra Freire, N.M.: Tick paralysis in Brazil. Trop. Anim. Health Prod., 15:124–126, 1983.

Seuberlich, T., et al.: Atypical scrapie in a Swiss goat and implications for transmissible spongiform encephalopathy surveillance. J. Vet. Diagn. Invest., 19:2–8, 2007.

Sewell, C.A. and Healy, P.J.: The use of plasma beta-mannosidase activity for the detection of goats heterozygous for beta-mannosidosis. Aust. Vet. J., 62:286–288, 1985.

Shah, C., et al.: Phylogenetic analysis and reclassification of caprine and ovine lentiviruses based on 104 new isolates: evidence for regular sheep-to-goat transmission and worldwide propagation through livestock trade. Virology, 319:12–26, 2004.

Shah, C., et al.: Direct evidence for natural transmission of small-ruminant lentiviruses of subtype A4 from goats to sheep and vice versa. J. Virol., 78(14):7518–7522, 2004a.

Shapiro, J.L., et al.: Caprine beta-mannosidosis in kids from an Ontario herd. Can. Vet. J., 26:155–158, 1985.

Sharma, D.K. and Chauhan, P.P.S.: Coenurosis status in Afro-Asian region: a review. Small Rumin. Res., 64(3):197–202, 2006.

Sharma, H.N. and Tyagi, R.P.S.: Diagnosis and surgical treatment of coenurosis in goat. Indian Vet. J., 52:482–488, 1975.

Sharma, H.N., Bhargava, A.K. and Tyagi, R.P.S.: Cerebral angiography for locating the space-occupying lesions in goats. Indian Vet. J., 51:718–721, 1974.

Sherman, D.M.: Causes of kid morbidity and mortality: an overview. In: Proceedings IV International Conf. Goats, Brasilia, EMBRAPA-DDT, pp. 335–354, 1987.

Shimizu, T., et al.: Hepatic and spinal lesions in goats chronically intoxicated with cycasin. Jpn. J. Vet. Sci., 48:1291–1295, 1986.

Shoho, C.: Further observations on epizootic cerebrospinal nematodiasis: I. Chemotherapeutic control of the disease by 1-diethylcarbamyl-4-methyl-piperazine citrate: preliminary field trial. Br. Vet. J., 108:134–141, 1952.

Shoho, C.: Prophylaxis and therapy in epizootic cerebrospinal nematodiasis of animals by 1-diethylcarbamyl-4-methyl-piperazine dihydrogen citrate: report of a second field trial. Vet. Med., 49:459–462, 1954.

Shoji, Y., et al.: Genetic and phylogenetic characterization of rabies virus isolates from wildlife and livestock in Paraiba, Brazil. Acta Virol., 50:33–38, 2006.

Sigurdsson, B., Grimsson, H. and Palsson, P.A.: Maedi, a chronic progressive infection of sheep lungs. J. Infect. Dis., 90:233–241, 1952.

Sigurdsson, B. and Palsson, P.A. Visna of sheep. A slow, demyelinating infection. Br. J. Exp. Pathol., 39: 519–528, 1958.

Sigurdsson, B.: Maedi, a slow progressive pneumonia of sheep: an epizoological and a pathological study. Br. Vet. J., 110: 255–270, 1954.

Sigurdsson, B., Thormar, H. and Palsson, P. A.: Cultivation of Visna virus in tissue culture. Arch. ges. Virusforsch., 10:368–381, 1960.

Sigurdsson, B., Palsson, P.A. and Grimsson, H.: Visna, a demyelinating transmissible disease of sheep. J. Neuropathol. Exp. Neurol., 16:389–403, 1957.

Sigurdsson, B., Palsson, P.A. and Van Bogaert, L.: Pathology of visna. Transmissible demyelinating disease in sheep in Iceland. Acta Neuropathol., 1:343–362, 1962.

Silva, A.E.D.F. and Silva, M.U.D.: Doencas mais frequentes observadas nos caprinos do nordeste. Brasilia, Departamento de Difusao de Technologia, 1987.

Simoens, P., De Vos, N.R., Lauwers, H. and Nicaise, M.: Numerical vertebral variations and transitional vertebrae in the goat. Zbl. Vet. Med. C. Anat. Histol. Embryol., 12:97–103, 1983.

Singh, K.K., Jha, G.J., Chauhan, V.S. and Singh, P.N.: Pathology of chronic aldrin intoxication in goats. Zbl. Vet. Med. A, 32:437–444, 1985.

Sinha, R.P. and Thakur, D.K.: An interesting case of tetanus in a buck. Livestock Adviser, Bangalore. 3:41–43, 1978.

Sisk, D.B., Colvin, B.M. and Bridges, C.R.: Acute, fatal illness in cattle exposed to boron fertilizer. J. Am. Vet. Med. Assoc., 193:943–945, 1988.

Sisk, D.B., et al.: Experimental acute inorganic boron toxicosis in the goat: Effects on serum chemistry and CSF biogenic amines. Vet. Hum. Toxicol., 32(3):205–211, 1990.

Sisó, S., et al.: The neuropathologic phenotype of experimental ovine BSE is maintained after blood transfusion. Blood, 108(2):745–748, 2006.

Smith, M.C.: Polioencephalomalacia in goats. J. Am. Vet. Med. Assoc., 174:1328–1332, 1979.

Smith, M.C.: The diagnostic value of caprine cerebrospinal fluid analysis. In: Proceedings, 3rd Internat. Conf. Goat Prod. Dis., Scottsdale, Dairy Goat Publ. Co., p. 294, 1982.

Sockett, D.C., Knight, A.P. and Johnson, L.W.: Malignant melanoma in a goat. J. Am. Vet. Med. Assoc., 185:907–908, 1984.

Soldan, A.W., Inzen, C. van, and Edelsten, R.M.: *Albizia versicolor* poisoning of sheep and goats. J. S. Afr. Vet. Assoc., 67(4):217–221, 1996.

Soulsby, E.J.L.: Helminths, Arthropods and Protozoa of Domesticated Animals. 7th Ed. Philadelphia, Lea and Febiger, 1982.
Sperry, O.E., Ryerson, D.E. and Pearson, H.A.: Distribution and chemical control of coyotillo, a range shrub poisonous to livestock. Texas Agric. Exp. Sta. Misc. Publ., MP594, 1962.
Staeheli, S., Sauder, C., Hausmann, J., Ehrensperger, F. and Schwemmle1, M.: Epidemiology of Borna disease virus. J. Gen. Virol. 81:2123–2135, 2000.
Stampa, S.: Tick paralysis in the Karoo areas of South Africa. Onderstepoort J. Vet. Res., 28:169–227, 1959.
Stavrou, D., Deutschlander, N., and Dahme, E.: Granulomatous encephalomyelitis in goats. J. Comp. Pathol., 79:393–398, 1969.
Steiner, S., Chvala, S., Krametter-Frotscher, R. and Henninger, W.: Caprine Arthritis-Enzephalitis (CAE) ein Fallbericht: Abklärung mittels Magnetresonanztomographie. Wien. Tierärztl. Mschr., 93:183–188, 2006.
Stemshorn, B.W.: Un cas de tremblante naturelle chez une chèvre. Can. Vet. J., 16:84–86, 1975.
Strain, G.M., Seger, C.L. and Flory, W.: Toxic Bermuda grass tremor in the goat: an electroencephalographic study. Am. J. Vet. Res., 43:158–162, 1982.
Strain, G.M., Claxton, M.S., Olcott, B.M. and Turnquist, S.E.: Visual-evoked brainstem potentials and electroretinograms in ruminants with thiamine-responsive polioencephalomalacia or suspected listeriosis. Am. J. Vet. Res., 51(10):1513–1517, 1990.
Sudarshan, M.K., et al.: Assessing the burden of human rabies in India: results of a national multi-center epidemiological survey. Internat. J. Infect. Dis., 11:29–35, 2007.
Sugawara, H., Katayama, M. and Kimura, T.: Effects of prolonged lighting on the plasma concentration of prolactin and electroencephalogram in goats. Jpn. J. Zootech. Sci., 60(6):567–577, 1989.
Sugawara, H.: Studies on the electroencephalogram in ruminants. I. EEG in goats. Jpn. J. Vet. Sci., 33:25–37, 1971.
Summers, B.A., et al.: Studies on viral leukoencephalomyelitis and swayback in goats. Cornell Vet., 70:372–390, 1980.
Sundquist, B., Jonsson, L., Jacobson, S.O. and Hammarberg, K.E.: Visna virus meningoencephalomyelitis in goats. Acta Vet. Scand., 22:315–333, 1981.
Sundquist, B.: Goat visna virus: isolation of a retrovirus related to visna virus of sheep. Arch. Virol., 68:115–127, 1981.
Swart, F.W.J.: Vergiftiging van geiten door hondspeterselie. Tijdschr. Diergeneesk., 100:989–990, 1975.
Swarup, D., et al.: Lowered blood copper and cobalt contents in goats reared around lead-zinc smelter. Small Rumin. Res., 63: 3, 309–313, 2006.
Swarup, D., Maiti, S.K., and Dwivedi, S.K.: Diagnostic use of blood porphyrin and radiographic changes in lead exposure in goats. Vet. Hum. Toxicol., 32(6):549–551, 1990.
Taniyama, H., et al.: Equine Borna disease in Japan. Vet. Rec. 148(15):480–482, 2001.
Tanwar, R.K.: Polioencephalomalacia, an emerging disease of goats. Indian J. Anim. Sci., 57:1–4, 1987.
Taylor, W.P., Okeke, A.N.C. and Shidali, N.N.: Prevalence of bovine virus diarrhoea and infectious bovine rhinotracheitis antibodies in Nigerian sheep and goats. Trop. Anim. Health Prod., 9:171–175, 1977.
Tham, W.: Survival of *Listeria monocytogenes* in cheese made of unpasteurized goat milk. Acta Vet. Scand., 29:165–172, 1988.
Theodoridis, A.K., Papageorgiou, D.K., Abrahim, A. and Karaioannoglou, P.G.: Fate of *Listeria monocytogenes* during the manufacture and storage of Chevre Metsovo and Pichtogalo Chanion cheeses. Ital. J. Food Sci., 18(1):51–61, 2006.
Thiongane, Y., Leforban, Y., and Doutre, M.P.: Botulism type D in Senegal. A new water-borne outbreak with high mortality. Rev. Élev. Méd. Vet. Pays. Trop., 37:152–154, 1984.
Thomas, K.W., Turner, D.L. and Spicer, E.M.: Thiamine, thiaminase and transketolase levels in goats with and without polioencephalomalacia. Aust. Vet. J., 64:126–127, 1987.
Thompson, J.N., Jones, M.Z., Dawson, G. and Huffman, P.S.: N-acetylglucosamine 6-sulphatase deficiency in a Nubian goat: a model of Sanfilippo syndrome type D (mucopolysaccharidosis IIID). J. Inher. Met. Dis., 15(5):760–768, 1992.
Thompson, K.G.: Nervous diseases of goats. In: Goat Husbandry and Medicine, Publication 106, Massey University, Palmerston North, NZ, pp. 152–161, 1985.
Thompson, K.G., Bateman, R.S. and Morris, P.J.: Cerebral infarction and meningoencephalitis following hot-iron disbudding of goat kids. N.Z. Vet. J., 53(5):368–370, 2005.
Thuring, C.M., et al.: Discrimination between scrapie and bovine spongiform encephalopathy in sheep by molecular size, immunoreactivity and glycoprofile of prion protein. J. Clin. Microbiol. 42(3):972–980, 2004.
Toofanian, F., Aliakabari, S. and Ivoghli, B.: Acute diesel fuel poisoning in goats. Trop. Anim. Health Prod., 11:98–101, 1979.
Topica, V., et al.: Serological survey for group B arbovirus infections among animals in the Banat province of Rumania. Arch. Roumain. Pathol. Exp. Microbiol., 30(2):231–236, 1971.
Toumazos, P. and Alley, M.R.: Scrapie in goats in Cyprus. N.Z. Vet. J., 37:160–162, 1989.
Trifonov, T.: The *Ixodes* fauna along the southern Black Sea littoral. Veterinarnomed. Nauki, 12:70–79, 1975.
Tuo, W., et al.: Prp-c and Prp-Sc at the fetal-maternal interface. J. Biol. Chem., 276(21):18229–34, 2001.
Tyler, J.W., Turnquist, S.E., David, A.T., Kleiboeker, S.B. and Middleton, J.R.: West Nile virus encephalomyelitis in a sheep. J. Vet. Intern. Med., 17:242–244, 2003.
Umoh, J.U.: Post-exposure immunization of ruminants against rabies. Ph.D. Thesis, Graduate School, University of Missouri-Columbia, 1977.
Umoh, J.U. and Blenden, D.C.: Post-exposure immunoprophylaxis of goats against rabies. Int. J. Zoonoses, 8:127–134, 1981.
Umoh, J.U. and Blenden, D.C.: The dissemination of rabies virus into cranial nerves and other tissues of experimentally infected goats and dogs and naturally infected skunks. Int. J. Zoonoses, 9:1–11, 1982.
Underwood, E.J.: The Mineral Nutrition of Livestock. 2nd Ed. Slough, Commonwealth Agricultural Bureaux, 1981.

USDA: Scrapie: Nor98-like Wyoming. Quarterly Report. USDA, APHIS, VS, Centers for Epidemiology and Animal Health. United States Department of Agriculture, p.4, June 2007.

USDA: United States Department of Agriculture. Scrapie Program. FY 2007 Report. USDA, APHIS, VS, National Center for Animal Health Programs, Riverdale, MD, 2007a. http://www.aphis.usda.gov/animal_health/animal_diseases/scrapie/downloads/yearly_report.pps.

USDA: United States Department of Agriculture. Voluntary Scrapie Flock Certification Program Standards. Appendix 1—Specimen Collection and Submission. USDA, APHIS, VS, National Center for Animal Health Programs, Riverdale, MD, pp.28–39, 2007b. http://www.aphis.usda.gov/animal_health/animal_diseases/scrapie/downloads/sfcp.pdf.

USDA: United States Department of Agriculture. SOSS: Phase II: Scrapie: Ovine Slaughter Surveillance Study, 2002–2003. USDA, APHIS, VS, Riverdale, MD, 2004. http://www.aphis.usda.gov/vs/ceah/ncahs/nahms/sheep/SOSSphase2.pdf.

Uzal, F.A. and Kelly, W.R.: Effects of the intravenous administration of *Clostridium perfringens* type D epsilon toxin on young goats and lambs. J. Comp. Pathol., 116(1): 63–71, 1997.

Uzal, F.A. and Kelly, W.R.: Experimental *Clostridium perfringens* type D enterotoxemia in goats. Vet. Pathol., 35(2):132–140, 1998.

Uzal, F.A., Glastonbury, J.R.W., Kelly, W.R. and Thomas, R.: Caprine enterotoxaemia associated with cerebral microangiopathy. Vet. Rec., 141(9):224–226, 1997.

Vaccari, G., et al.: Identification of an allelic variant of the goat PrP gene associated with resistance to scrapie. J. Gen. Virol., 87(5):1395–1402, 2006.

van der Lugt, J.J., et al.: Two outbreaks of type C and type D botulisum in sheep and goats in South Africa. J. S. Afr. Vet. Assoc., 66(2):77–82, 1995.

van Tonder, E.M.: Notes on some disease problems in Angora goats in South Africa. Vet. Med. Rev., 1/2:109–138, 1975.

Verster, A. and Tustin, R.C.: Treatment of cerebral coenuriosis in sheep with praziquantel. J. S. Afr. Vet. Assoc., 61(1):24–26, 1990.

Waggoner, D.J., Bartnikas, T.B. and Gitlin, J.D.: The role of copper in neurodegenerative disease. Neurobiol. Dis. 6(4):221–30, 1999.

Wang, M.Z., Ye, K.X. and Hu, L.S.: Study on etiology of "lumbar paralysis" in horses, sheep, and goats. In: Proceedings, 4th Internat. Sympos. Vet. Epidemiol. Econ., Singapore, November 18–22, pp. 283–284, 1985.

Weinhold, E. and Triemer, B.: Visna in the goat. Zbl. Vet. Med. B, 25:525–538, 1978.

Weissmann, C. and Aguzzi, A.: Approaches to therapy of prion diseases. Annual Rev. Med., 56:321–344, 2005.

Welchman, D. de B. and Bekh-Ochir, G. Spinal coenurosis causing posterior paralysis in a goat in Mongolia. Vet. Rec., 158(7):238–239, 2006.

WHO: Rabies—Epidemiology. World Health Organization, Geneva. 2007. http://www.who.int/rabies/epidemiology/en/.

WHO: Rabies-Bulletin-Europe. Rabies Information System of the WHO Collaboration Centre for Rabies Surveillance and Research. Database queries. World Health Organization, Geneva, 2007a. http://www.who-rabiesbulletin.org/Queries/Trend.aspx.

Wiedmann, M., et al.: Molecular investigation of a listeriosis outbreak in goats caused by an unusual strain of *Listeria monocytogenes*. J. Am. Vet. Med. Assoc., 215(3):369–371, 1999.

Wilesmith, J.W., Ryan, J.B.M., Hueston, W.D. and Hoinville, L.J.: Bovine spongiform encephalopathy: epidemiological features 1985 to 1990. Vet. Rec. 130(5):90–94, 1992.

Wille, H., et al.: Structural studies of the scrapie prion protein by electron crystallography. Proc. Natl. Acad. Sci. U.S.A. 99(6):3563–3568, 2002.

Wilson, J., and Brewer, B.D.: Vestibular disease in a goat. Comp. Cont. Educ. Pract. Vet., 6:S179–S182, 1984.

Wilson, R.D., Witzel, D.A. and Verlander, J.M.: Somatosensory-evoked response of ataxic Angora goats in suspected haloxon-delayed neurotoxicity. Am. J. Vet. Res., 43:2224–2226, 1982.

Winter, P., Hochsteiner, W. and Hogler, S.: Congenital copper deficiency in neonatal German Improved Fawn breed of goats. Tierärztliche Praxis, 30(6):378–384, 2002.

Wood, J.S.: Encephalitic listeriosis in a herd of goats. Can. Vet. J., 13:80–82, 1972.

Wood, J.N.L, Done, S.H., Pritchard, G.C. and Wooldridge, M.J.A.: Natural scrapie in goats: case histories and clinical signs. Vet. Rec., 131:66–68, 1992.

Wouda, W., Borst, G.H.A. and Gruys, E.: Delayed swayback in goat kids, a study of 23 cases. Vet. Q. 8:45–56, 1986.

Wright, H.J., Adams, D.S. and Trigo, F.J.: Meningoencephalitis after hot-iron disbudding of goat kids. Vet. Med. Small Anim. Clin., 78:599–601, 1983.

Yang, W.C., Yeung, E.S. and Schmerr, M.J.: Detection of prion protein using a capillary electrophoresis-based competitive immunoassay with laser-induced fluorescence detection and cyclodextrin-aided separation. Electrophoresis. 26(9):1751–1759, 2005.

Yoshikawa, T.: Atlas of the Brains of Domestic Animals. University Park, The Pennsylvania State University Press, 1968.

Zamir, S.: Personal Communication. Dr. Shmuel Zamir, Chief Sheep and Goat Health Officer, Veterinary Services and Animal Health, Ministry of Agriculture and Rural Development, Government of Israel, 2007.

Zanoni, R.G.: Phylogenetic analysis of small ruminant lentiviruses. J. Gen. Virol., 79:1951–1961, 1998.

Zhang, L., Li, N., Fan, B., Fang, M. and Xu, W.: PRNP polymorphisms in Chinese ovine, caprine and bovine breeds. Anim. Genet., 35:457–461, 2004.

Zhao, L.B., et al.: Detection of Borna disease virus P24 gene in goats in Chongqing. Vet. Sci. Chin., 36(6):460–463, 2006.

Zlotnik, I.: The histopathology of the brain of goats affected with scrapie. J. Comp. Pathol., 71:440–448, 1961.

Zundel, E., et al.: Virulence of *Listeria monocytogenes* as a biofilm: consequences for dairy farming. 10emes Rencontres autour des Recherches sur les Ruminants, Paris, France, 3–4 Decembre 2003. Institut National de la Recherche Agronomique, Paris, France, pp. 211–214, 2003.

6

Ocular System

Although ophthalmologists have in general paid little attention to the goat in their writings, several published reviews are oriented toward caprine ophthalmology (Wyman 1983; Baxendell 1984; Moore and Whitley 1984; Whittaker et al. 1999). Most aspects of anatomy and therapy apply across species lines. Any good ophthalmology text, then, should be useful for the practitioner needing more information than this chapter supplies.

CLINICAL ANATOMY AND EXAMINATION OF THE EYE

The history elicited from the owner may suggest a problem with ocular structures or vision. The goat may have a hesitant gait or refuse to move or pass through a gate. The animal may carry its head abnormally elevated or near the ground. A report of normal vision should be verified by the examiner; visual loss may not be apparent until the goat is placed in unfamiliar surroundings. The eyes should also be examined relative to systemic conditions (i.e., dehydration, anemia, icterus, septicemia, hemorrhagic diseases) and during prepurchase or breeding soundness examinations.

Lids and Lashes

The upper and lower eyelids normally are tightly apposed to the globe. They should neither roll inward (entropion) nor gape outward (ectropion). Lashes should not be in contact with the cornea. The examiner should note the location of any long, tactile hairs before evaluating vision by the menace response. Touching the lids near the medial canthus should evoke the palpebral reflex (blinking and retraction of the globe). This reflex requires function of cranial nerves V (sensory branches of trigeminal nerve) and VII. The third eyelid (nictitating membrane) is normally unobtrusive. It can be seen better if the globe is retropulsed, using digital pressure through the eyelids. Topical anesthesia permits grasping of the third eyelid with smooth forceps so that its posterior surface can be inspected for lesions or foreign bodies. Prolapse of the third eyelid occurs in some cases of tetanus. Passive prolapse of the nictitans occurs in conditions causing enophthalmos, including dehydration or emaciation, as well as in neurologic diseases accompanied by Horner's syndrome (see Chapter 5).

Lacrimal Glands and Ducts

The lacrimal apparatus of the goat has been reviewed by Sinha and Calhoun (1966). Lysozyme has been identified in goat tear samples (Brightman et al. 1991). Plasma cells in the nictitating gland secrete IgA into the tear film (Schlegel et al. 2003). Normally no staining or wetness occurs beneath the goat's eye, neither is there a deep recess filled with exudate near the medial canthus analogous to the infraorbital gland of sheep. The nasolacrimal duct can be catheterized from the ocular puncta (Moore and Whitley 1984).

Ocular Position

The ruminant eye normally maintains a constant position relative to the ground rather than remaining centered between the lids. This can make ocular examination frustrating if the goat's head cannot be restrained in the position required to expose the structures of interest. Abnormal function of the nerves supplying the extraocular muscles (cranial nerves III, IV, VI) affects ocular position. Dorsomedial strabismus, for instance, sometimes occurs in polioencephalomalacia. Mydriasis and strabismus may occur with botulism as a result of paralysis of intrinsic and extrinsic ocular muscles (Wyman 1983). Normal nystagmus (vestibular nystagmus) occurs when the head is slowly turned to one side and has its quick phase in the same direction as the head movement. Normal postrotatory nystagmus (direction opposite the direction of rotation) lasts for less than ten seconds.

Exophthalmos (protrusion of the globe) may be due to a retrobulbar abscess or tumor. Ideally, examination of the orbit by ultrasound or computed tomography, followed by guided aspiration of cells or fluid from the lesion, allows a diagnosis to be made. Enucleation may be required to resolve a retrobulbar abscess. It is unlikely to cure the tumors most likely in this location (lymphosarcoma, enzootic nasal tumor). See Chapter 9 for further discussion of enzootic nasal tumor.

Conjunctiva, Sclera, and Scleral Vessels

Everting the eyelids permits inspection of the conjunctiva (Figure 6.1). Rotating the head upward and to one side exposes bulbar conjunctiva and the deeper sclera and its vessels. A pale white color with almost invisible blood vessels occurs with severe anemia, and yellow sclera is indicative of icterus. A brownish discoloration of this and other mucous membranes occurs with nitrate poisoning, a purplish color with cyanotic conditions, and bright red coloration with cyanide poisoning. Vessels may appear congested with ocular, regional, or systemic inflammatory or toxic diseases.

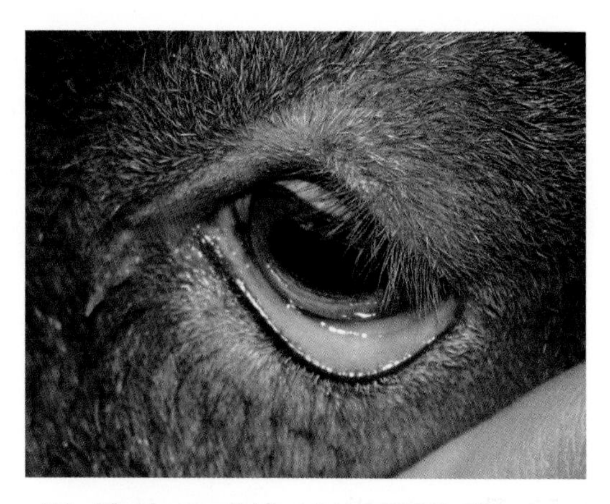

Figure 6.1. The lower lid has been everted to expose the conjunctiva. This goat had a packed cell volume of 21%. (Courtesy Dr. M.C. Smith.)

Cornea

The cornea is normally clear and moist. Oblique lighting and observing the clarity with which the iris can be visualized aid in differentiating cloudiness of the cornea from lens opacity. If the cornea is lightly touched with a finger or a wisp of cotton, the corneal reflex results in the same blinking and globe retraction, via the same pathway, as the palpebral reflex.

Iris, Pupil, and Lens

A strong and well-focused light source should be used to evaluate direct and consensual pupillary response (optic nerve and parasympathetic fibers traveling with the oculomotor nerve, midbrain). Pupillary responses may be intact in a blind animal, and they may be almost impossible to elicit in an apprehensive goat. The pupil is oval, becoming more rectangular in bright light, and has granula iridica (corpora nigra) attached to both its dorsal and its ventral rim. Various toxicities may affect the pupil (e.g., mydriasis with chlorinated hydrocarbons [Choudhury and Robinson 1950] or miosis with organophosphates). The anterior chamber, between cornea and iris, should be examined for hyphema, hypopyon, and aqueous flare (cells and protein, often indicative of anterior uveitis).

If a cataract (opacity of the lens or its capsule) is detected, the density of the cataract should be evaluated. If a portion of the retina is clearly visible in a blind animal, any cataract that may be present is not the cause of blindness.

Retina and Ophthalmoscopic Examination

The goat's fundus can usually be examined without resorting to mydriatics. If a detailed examination is desired, and if the examiner is willing to wait fifteen to thirty minutes for its effect, 1% tropicamide may be used to dilate the pupil (Figure 6.2). This should not be done until after pupillary response has been evaluated and diagnostic cultures or scrapings have been performed.

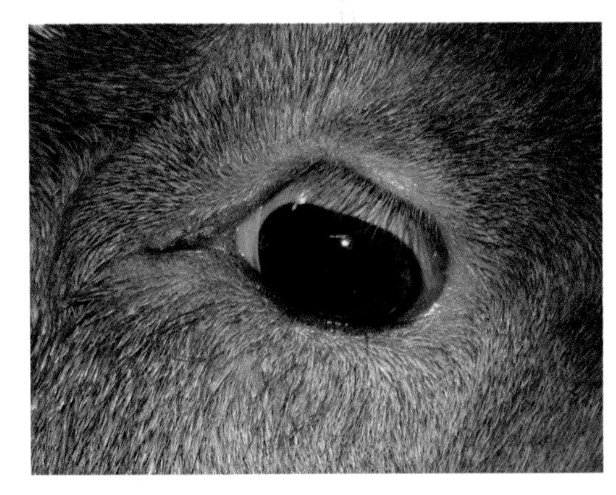

Figure 6.2. The normally rectangular pupil has been dilated with tropicamide to permit a thorough fundus examination. (Courtesy Dr. M.C. Smith)

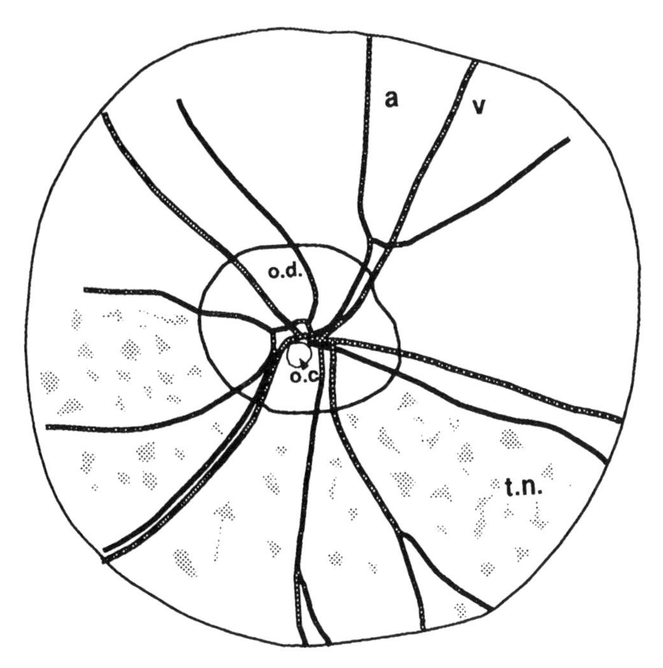

Figure 6.3. The fundus of a Saanen goat. o.d. = optic disc, a = arteriole, t.n. = tapetum nigrum, o.c. = optic cup, v = venule.

Hyaloid remnants on the optic nerve head and continuing into the vitreous body are commonly found in adult ruminants, including four of ten goats in one study (Schebitz and Reiche 1953). Presence of blood within the hyaloid vessel is also considered normal until eight weeks of age in lambs, although this has not been investigated in kids.

Photographs of the fundus of goats have been published (Rubin 1974; Whittaker et al. 1999; Galan et al. 2006b). A diagram of a goat fundus is provided in Figure 6.3 and a normal Boer goat fundus is illustrated in Figure 6.4. The fundus is usually in focus with a direct ophthalmoscopic setting of −1D to −5D. The

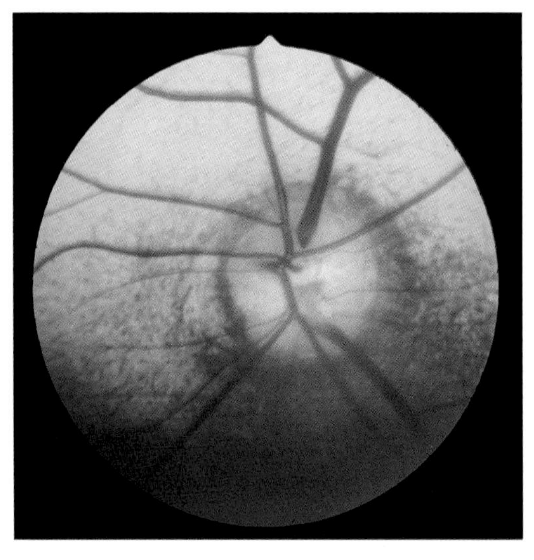

Figure 6.4. The fundus of a normal Boer goat. (Courtesy Dr. M.C. Smith.)

optic disc is rather round or oval, whereas in the sheep it is often more kidney-shaped. The optic disc in goats is frequently located totally within the tapetal fundus (tapetum lucidum, yellow to bluish green). In cattle and sheep it is usually situated in the nontapetal fundus (tapetum nigrum, brownish) just beneath the horizontal junctional area of tapetal and nontapetal fundus. The optic disc is grayish pink and sharply demarcated, and has a small funnel-shaped physiologic cup. The broader veins enter the middle of the disc while the thinner, redder arteries originate like rays from a pericentral location (Schmidt 1973). There are more blood vessels than in sheep or cattle. Galan et al. (2006b) report three to six retinal arteries in the goat, often branching from a common artery that emerges from the dorsotemporal portion of the disc. There are many stars of Winslow which are black dots in the tapetum lucidum where choriocapillaris vessels penetrate the tapetum. Fluorescein angiography of the normal goat fundus has been described (Galan et al. 2006a).

Ultrasonography can be used to evaluate the contents of the globe and the retrobulbar area, as is done routinely in companion animal medicine. Ideally, both a 7.5-MHz probe and an offset pad are used. The globe can be imaged through the upper eyelid or directly through the cornea. Tranquilization is followed by application of a local anesthetic to the cornea, and the probe is placed on lubricating jelly on the lid or on a mound of sterile ocular lubricating gel on the cornea. Normal chamber fluid is hypoechoic, while the posterior lens capsule and retina are hyperechoic. Conditions that might be demonstrated by ultrasound include luxated lens, retinal detachment, or a retrobulbar abscess or tumor (Toal 1996).

Cranial Nerves and Evaluation for Blindness

The optic disc is the optic nerve head. It may be swollen with papilledema or with optic neuritis. Unilateral blindness may be detected by covering one eye and observing the goat's behavior in a strange environment. Young kids often visually follow a bottle of milk when other items fail to attract their interest. The complete visual pathway, including optic nerve and cerebral cortex, is also evaluated by the menace response. Fingers are moved vertically or quickly spread apart (to decrease air currents) in front of each eye in turn. Lashes and tactile hairs must not be touched. The palpebral reflex (cranial nerves V and VII) should be checked if the goat does not blink in response to the menacing gesture.

MALFORMATIONS OF THE GLOBE

Various chemical or viral teratogens may interfere with embryologic development of the eyeball.

Cyclopia

Veratrum californicum, if consumed on approximately day four of pregnancy, can cause cyclopia in kids and lambs (Binns et al. 1972). Deformation of the skull ("monkey face"), absence of the pituitary, and other brain malformations may also occur. This problem can be prevented by not allowing the buck access to the females when grazing on the plant might occur. The author has seen cyclopic kids in New York, where *Veratrum californicum* does not grow, and several case reports from India also did not identify a cause of the malformation (Raju and Rao 2001). It is logical that other toxins or tissue insults occurring at the critical stage of embryologic development, when a single optic field is dividing in two, could also result in cyclopia.

Microphthalmia

Microphthalmia and other congenital deformities including lens luxation or aphakia have been reported in lambs when pregnant ewes have grazed on seleniferous pastures. Anophthalmia has been caused by exposure of a pregnant ewe to apholate, an insect chemosterilant (Younger 1965). The effects on caprine ocular structures of these compounds or of in utero viral infections have not been reported.

LID ABNORMALITIES

Lacerations of the eyelids should be repaired using standard techniques. Skin diseases involving the lids (e.g., contagious ecthyma, mange, staphylococcal dermatitis, zinc deficiency) are described in Chapter 2. When skin lesions are restricted to the eyelids, the possibility that they are caused by ocular discharge or rubbing in response to ocular discomfort should be investigated. Injuries to the face may occur because of blindness. Small palpebral fissures, thickened nonpliable lids, and partial prolapse of the nictitating membrane occur in Nubian kids with inherited beta mannosidosis (Render et al. 1989), which is discussed in Chapter 5.

Entropion

Entropion is the turning inward of the lower lid or both eyelids so that the eyelashes rub on the cornea. The condition is painful and results in tearing and retraction of the eyeball. The lids are partially closed; the lashes may be stuck together with exudate.

Congenital or Primary Entropion

When a kid's eyelids are malformed from birth, the condition is usually recognized within the first few days of life. The longer the entropion remains uncorrected, the more likely that a serious infection or corneal ulceration will result. It is probable, though unproven, that this condition has a hereditary component. Thus, if surgical treatment is required on humane grounds, the identity of the goat should be recorded so that it can be slaughtered for meat or sterilized rather than being permitted to reproduce.

Spastic Entropion

Older animals may develop entropion as the result of prolonged squinting when another painful eye condition is present (Figure 6.5). Typical examples are severe keratoconjunctivitis or the presence of a foreign body in the eye. If one goat continues to suffer from "pinkeye" after the rest of the herd has recovered, a point should be made of examining its eyelids. When the entropion is of spastic origin, surgically altering the eyelids is not always necessary. Instead, the lid position can be corrected by sutures or wound clips long enough for the initial and secondary problems and pain to be resolved.

Other Causes of Secondary Entropion

It is possible for entropion to follow a previous injury to and deformation of the eyelid. A small or collapsed globe also permits the lids to roll inward, as does retraction of a painful eyeball deeper into the orbit. Severe dehydration and emaciation (as from starvation or parasitism) are perhaps the most common causes of secondary entropion.

Corrective Measures

The literature is replete with techniques for correction of entropion in goats and in other species (Rook and Cortese 1981; Wyman 1983; Baxendell 1984; Moore and Whitley 1984; Whittaker et al. 1999). In general, the veterinarian should not rush into a complicated and therefore expensive technique without giving con-

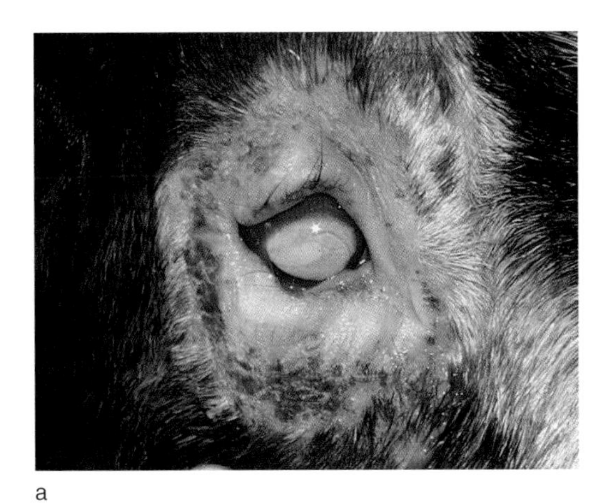

a

Figure 6.5a. Chronic spastic entropion with severe keratitis and hair loss.

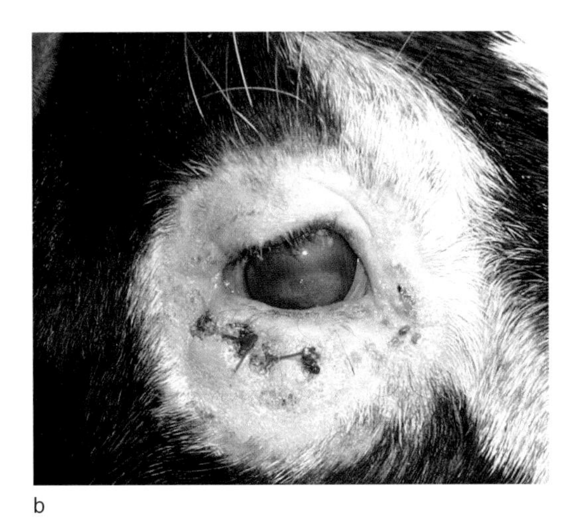

b

Figure 6.5b. Same goat, twelve days after surgical correction of the entropion by removal of an ellipse of skin below the eye. (Courtesy Dr. M.C. Smith.)

sideration to one of the more temporary but often effective methods developed by ingenious shepherds and private practitioners.

One such simple but versatile technique is the use of Michel wound clips (Eales et al. 1984) (Miltex Instrument Co., New York, NY) or metal surgical staples, three or four per affected lid, to pinch up a fold of skin adjacent and parallel to the lid margin. No anesthesia is required; it is simple to remove and replace a clip if the effect of its placement is not immediately satisfying, and the clips fall out on their own over time. The owner of a newborn kid may be able to achieve correction simply by drying the area and manually rolling the lid margin outward as often as possible over the course of one or two days. Another version of this approach is to roll superglue onto the skin below the eyelid with a toothpick (which only serves as the applicator), causing the skin to evert and adhere to itself (Mongini 2007). Tensing of the lid by injection of penicillin in the same site where clips would be placed is also effective. A slightly more traumatic approach is to crush a fold of skin with hemostats; the ensuing swelling everts the lid. Naturally, any additional causes of ocular pain should be identified and treated. An antibiotic ointment is administered for several days, until the eye appears to be comfortable.

Surgical techniques, mostly adapted from canine ophthalmology, include removing an ellipse of skin alone or skin plus orbicularis muscle. Although initially effective, these methods carry the danger of creating an ectropion when the scar contracts. Thus, they should not be used for the treatment of very young kids or of goats with a simple, spastic entropion.

Tumors

A hemangioma of the third eyelid has been reported in a goat in England (Matthews 1992). Tumors of the third eyelid (type not specified) have been observed in Saanen goats in Australia (Baxendell 1984) and other regions where animals are exposed to high intensity sunlight. Conjunctivitis, lacrimation, and even a purulent secretion may result. The tumor is surgically removed with the aid of tranquilization, local anesthesia, and (if available) electrocautery. Eye ointments are used postoperatively. The Angora goat (because of lack of protective pigmentation) is also considered to be predisposed to ocular squamous cell carcinoma.

Warts may involve the eyelids. They are discussed in detail in Chapter 2. Most warts on the face regress spontaneously, but excision may be desirable in select cases. They need to be distinguished from contagious ecthyma lesions, which are also proliferative and self-limiting but have an important zoonotic potential. Almost any lesion on the eyelid, including warts and other tumors, can become secondarily infected with staphylococci.

CONJUNCTIVITIS AND KERATOCONJUNCTIVITIS

Infectious keratoconjunctivitis is known to the layperson as "pinkeye." A number of etiologic agents have been incriminated. When only one or two animals are affected, it becomes more difficult to distinguish between an infectious and an irritant cause. In fact, many sources of irritation, such as bright sunlight, dusty hay, and dust blown into the eyes by wind or transport in an open vehicle, can predispose the goat to development of an infection. Flies and hay or grass contaminated by ocular secretions can spread the agents to other goats. A herd outbreak may follow introduction of a carrier animal or attendance at a show.

Another common source of irritation to conjunctiva and cornea is entropion. Entropion should be suspected in young kids with tearing; its management is discussed above. In an older animal with sudden occurrence of entropion, the possibility that a foreign body remains in the conjunctival sac or beneath the third eyelid must be considered and investigated by thorough examination.

Infectious Keratoconjunctivitis

Etiology

Mycoplasma and *Chlamydophila* are currently believed to be the most common causes of keratoconjunctivitis in goats in the United States. Numerous other agents are rarely involved or are exotic to North America.

Mycoplasma

Mycoplasma conjunctivae has been isolated from naturally occurring cases of pinkeye in goats and in sheep and has induced the disease in experimental studies (Barile et al. 1972; Baas et al. 1977; Trotter et al. 1977). It also can exist in a carrier state in the conjunctival sac of clinically healthy eyes. Mild forms of the disease are self-limiting and last approximately ten days, although clinical signs have been reported as persisting as long as twelve weeks. Other mycoplasma species isolated from goats with keratoconjunctivitis include *Mycoplasma agalactia*, *M. mycoides* subsp. *mycoides*, large colony type (McCauley et al. 1971; Bar-Moshe and Rapapport 1981), *M. capricolum* (Taoudi et al. 1988), and *Acholeplasma oculi* (Al-Aubaidi et al. 1973). Because these agents can be associated with mastitis, pleuropneumonia, or arthritis, it may be easier to demonstrate the organism in other disease processes in the same goat. A report of *M. mycoides* var. *capri* from the United States (Jones and Barber 1969) probably represents a misidentification of *M. mycoides* subsp. *mycoides* (DaMassa et al. 1984). *Chlamydophila* remains an important differential, especially if arthritis or pneumonia is concurrent.

Chlamydophila

Chlamydial conjunctivitis has been recorded as a contagious disease of young goats and adults (Baas 1976; Eugster et al. 1977). In sheep, recurrence of chlamydial keratoconjunctivitis within a few weeks after clinical remission and an outbreak duration of several months have been recorded (Andrews et al. 1987). Lymphoid follicles are reported to develop in the conjunctiva early in the course of the disease. The current name applied to the chlamydial species causing conjunctivitis in small ruminants is *Chlamydophila pecorum* (Nietfeld 2001).

Rickettsia

Colesiota (*Rickettsia*) *conjunctivae* has been proposed as an etiologic agent for pinkeye in goats and sheep (Rizvi 1950). Most reports were based on cytology and predated the knowledge that chlamydia and mycoplasma are commonly involved, and thus rickettsia have fallen out of favor as being involved in the syndrome (Jones et al. 1976). The reported clinical signs, including occasional prolonged outbreaks, are indistinguishable from the disease produced by the other agents. However, experimental subconjunctival injection of the Q fever agent (*Coxiella burnetii*) has produced severe keratoconjunctivitis in goats, with rickettsia demonstrable in scrapings (Caminopetros 1948).

Other Possible Agents

The isolation of a bacterium from the conjunctival sac of a goat with keratoconjunctivitis is not adequate proof of causality. It is possible that *Moraxella (Branhamella) (Neisseria) ovis* is sometimes involved in the pathogenesis (Bulgin and Dubose 1982). Conjunctivitis but not severe keratitis has been reproduced experimentally in goats using a strain of *Moraxella* (*Branhamella*) *ovis* isolated from an outbreak of keratoconjunctivitis (Bankemper et al. 1990), but this same organism appears to be common in normal eyes of goats, at least in some herds (Pitman and Reuter 1988). *Staphylococcus aureus* has also been isolated from ocular swabs of healthy goats (Adegoke and Ojo 1982). In cattle and sheep, *Listeria monocytogenes* has been associated with a keratitis resulting from direct inoculation of contaminated silage into the eye (Evans et al. 2004).

Moraxella bovis, an important cause of pinkeye in cattle, is rarely involved in caprine keratoconjunctivitis. The organism is rod-shaped, whereas *Moraxella* (*Branhamella*) *ovis* is a coccus. Commercial *Moraxella* vaccines have no place in caprine medicine. A very closely related species, *Moraxella caprae*, is also a rod and has been isolated from normal goats (Kodjo et al. 1995). The significance of this organism as a potential cause of keratoconjunctivitis is unknown.

Infectious bovine rhinotracheitis (IBR) virus has been isolated from a goat that developed severe keratoconjunctivitis after five days of treatment with an antibiotic preparation containing corticosteroid for respiratory disease (Mohanty et al. 1972). Most experimental inoculations of goats with the IBR virus have produced seroconversion but only mild clinical signs in addition to fever.

Borna disease is an infectious meningoencephalomyelitis of viral origin that affects horses and sheep in middle and eastern Europe and may be transmitted by ticks. Conjunctivitis and epiphora have been reported as ocular signs. Central nervous system involvement can lead to blindness as well as other neurologic signs. Antibodies have been found in goats, but spontaneous cases of the disease have rarely been reported in this species (see Chapter 5).

The rinderpest and peste des petits ruminants paramyxoviruses cause high fever and erosive lesions in the alimentary tract of ruminants. Ocular signs may include increased lacrimation and a serous conjunctivitis that turns mucopurulent. Gray, elevated fibrinonecrotic lesions in the conjunctiva may eventually slough, leaving an ulcer (Williams and Gelatt 1981).

Goats with capripox infections sometimes develop oculonasal discharge, conjunctivitis, and keratitis, in addition to fever and anorexia (Patnaik 1986). The typical skin lesions caused by the virus are discussed in Chapter 2.

Thelazia spp., the eyeworms, can cause conjunctivitis or keratitis in sheep, and probably in goats. *Thelazia rhodesii* occurs in goats as well as cattle, sheep, and other species, and is cosmopolitan in Europe, Asia, and Africa. *Thelazia californiensis* is widely distributed in the United States, but goats are not mentioned as harboring the parasite (Soulsby 1982). The nematodes are small (7 to 18 mm) and slender. They may be found in the conjunctival cul-de-sacs, behind the third eyelid, or swimming across the surface of the cornea. Sometimes they invade the nasolacrimal duct. A topical anesthetic is applied and the eye is irrigated with sterile saline to remove the worms (Wyman 1983). Alternatively, topical application of an avermectin, such as a drop or two of 1% moxidectin for injection, kills the parasite (Lia et al. 2004). Systemic levamisole or avermectins should also kill the worms (Whittaker et al. 1999). Control of nonbiting flies, which serve as vectors (Otranto and Traversa 2005), is desirable.

A single *Setaria cervi* worm longer than 1 inch was found in the aqueous humor of a goat in India. The goat exhibited continuous unilateral lacrimation. The worm was successfully removed under local anesthesia (Emaduddin 1954).

Migrating larvae of *Gedoelstia hassleri* (nasal botfly) cause keratoconjunctivitis and panophthalmitis in goats and other species in endemic areas of South Africa (Basson 1962). *Trypanosoma brucei* and *T. rhodesiense* cause blepharoconjunctivitis and keratitis in goats (Losos and Ikede 1972). In many tropical and subtropical countries, screwworm larvae may invade fresh wounds on the head or ocular tissues infected with keratoconjunctivitis. A foul odor and brownish exudate are produced. Other opportunistic fly larvae may then infest the lesions.

Besnoitiosis is a parasitic disease of goats as well as cattle and horses in southeastern Europe, Africa, and New Zealand. The causative agent in goats is a *Besnoitia* species, possibly different from *B. besnoiti* of cattle (Njenga et al.1993). Cats that eat cysts in infected tissues develop an intestinal infection and excrete infective forms in their feces. Clinical signs in goats include dermatitis, alopecia, and infertility. Ocular cysts (white, elevated, sand-like foci) on the scleral conjunctiva are useful for field diagnosis of the infection (Bwangamoi et al. 1989).

Mycotic keratitis, although relatively common in horses, seems to be rare in ruminants (Wyman 1983) and specific reports in goats are lacking. Isolation and identification of the fungus are required before the diagnosis can be made. A chronic keratitis, plaque-like growths on the cornea, or severe keratomalacia might prompt attempts to culture a fungus, especially if there is a history of treatment with antibiotics and corticosteroids together. Therapy is difficult and expensive. The practitioner should consult with an ophthalmologist.

Clinical Signs

Early or mild keratoconjunctivitis results in lacrimation; the side of the face is wet below the eye. The conjunctiva is also red and swollen (chemosis) (Figure 6.6). Over several days, hyperemia of the conjunctiva increases, follicle formation occurs, and neovascularization of the cornea may develop. The cornea may be slightly hazy at the limbus or entirely opaque (Baxendell 1984). A few animals develop a corneal ulcer that can be demonstrated with fluorescein stain (Figure 6.7), and that ulcer may perforate. The eye is painful and held partially closed; blinking is frequent. If both eyes are opaque or ulceration occurs, the goat will lose body condition because it does not forage well. Totally blind animals on range may die (Eugster et al. 1977).

Diagnostic Techniques

The various etiologic diagnoses for infectious keratoconjunctivitis cannot be distinguished on the basis of clinical signs; laboratory assistance is required. Mydriatics, topical anesthetics, or vital stains should not be used until after diagnostic samples have been taken.

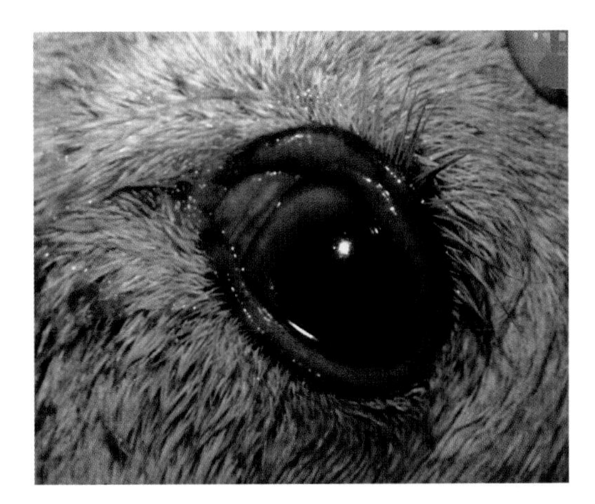

Figure 6.6. Early keratoconjunctivitis with chemosis and slight ocular discharge. (Courtesy Dr. M.C. Smith.)

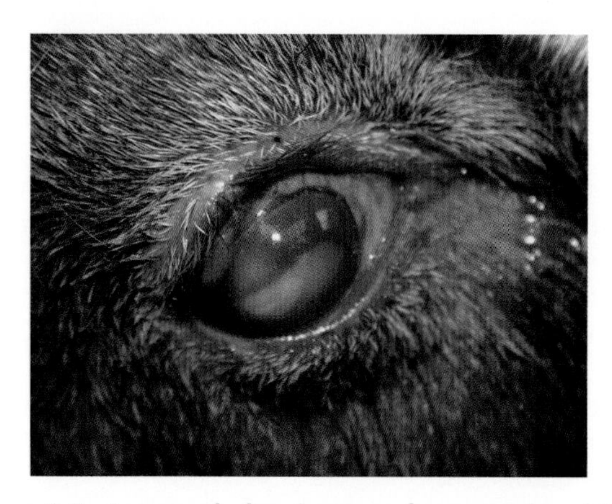

Figure 6.7. A corneal ulcer is green from uptake of fluorescein stain. Marked neovascularization of the cornea indicates chronicity. (Courtesy Dr. M.C. Smith.)

CULTURES. A premoistened sterile polyester or calcium alginate swab is rubbed briskly across the conjunctiva and placed in transport media (such as Amies). If possible, personnel at the diagnostic laboratory should be consulted regarding media, because chlamydia and mycoplasma can be difficult to isolate. If the laboratory does a polymerase chain reaction test for chlamydia, use of transport media may dilute the sample too much for good results. Dry cotton swabs are less desirable for fastidious organisms. It is also important to take samples from early lesions; secondary bacteria, leukocytes, and various products of immune mechanisms interfere with isolation efforts.

SCRAPINGS FOR IMMUNOFLUORESCENCE TESTING. Scrapings from the palpebral conjunctiva (especially lymphoid follicles) can be made with a wooden spatula designed for obtaining Pap smears, the butt end of a disposable scalpel blade, or with the bevel of a sterile, disposable 20-gauge needle. The tissue thus obtained is spread on several microscope slides. Many laboratories consider fluorescent antibody testing for chlamydia to be easier than culturing this agent in embryonated eggs or tissue culture cells.

EXFOLIATIVE CYTOLOGY. Interpretation of cytological preparations from conjunctival scrapings can be very difficult, even for trained people. Practitioners should consider preparing duplicate slides to simplify later consultation with an ophthalmologist or diagnostic laboratory. Superficial cells can be harvested with minimal distortion by rolling a dry swab across the conjunctiva and then across the slide, as is done for canine vaginal smears. Deeper scrapings are obtained with a blade or small spatula. New methylene blue, Wright, Giemsa, Dif-Quik, or Gram stain is typically used. Large basophilic, Gram-negative cytoplasmic inclusion bodies in epithelial cells occur with chlamydial conjunctivitis but are difficult to find after the first week (Wyman 1983). Smaller basophilic coccobacillary (McCauley et al. 1971) and signet-shaped bodies are found attached to or within epithelial cells in mycoplasmal infections. *Moraxella* (*Branhamella*) *ovis* organisms are larger than mycoplasma and more uniform in shape, and stain more intensely (Dagnall 1994). Rickettsia are described as small, Gram-negative, highly pleomorphic bodies that may be both intracytoplasmic and free (Beveridge 1942; Rizvi 1950). Pigment granules or stain precipitates can be confusing, and visible evidence of an etiologic agent may be lacking, even when cultures are positive.

Treatment

The intensity of treatment varies according to the number of infected goats and the concern of the owner. What follows is most appropriate for single pets or valuable animals. The eye should be irrigated with physiologic saline, sterile saline for contact lens wearers, or clean (preferably previously boiled) water to remove exudates and dust or other foreign matter. Although antibiotic drops are theoretically better than ointments, it is inconvenient for the owner to apply drops every two hours. Ointments are generally effective if given at least twice (or better, three to four times) a day. Several antibiotics have been clinically effective, but it must be remembered that many animals heal uneventfully without treatment. Given the spectrum of agents associated with keratoconjunctivitis, a tetracycline eye ointment is a reasonable choice. In countries where its use is permitted, chloramphenicol ointment might be effective, although systemic chloramphenicol was not effective in treating sheep with keratoconjunctivitis (König 1983). It is illegal to administer chloramphenicol to goats in the United States, because all goats are assumed to be food-producing animals despite the owner's plans for the individual.

Powders and aerosols are irritating to the eyes and ideally should not be used, but they have been reported to give good results. When economics become an important consideration, as when many goats are affected or the whole herd is being treated simultaneously to try to end a prolonged epizootic, it may not be possible to use ophthalmic ointments. Experimentation may identify a nonirritant mastitis ointment containing a suitable antibiotic that is better than no treatment at all. Under similar circumstances, intramuscular injections of long-lasting tetracycline have prevented relapses in sheep affected with *Mycoplasma conjunctivae* and other agents (König 1983; Hosie 1988). Intramuscular tylosin (200 mg/goat/day) has afforded good results in goats treated early in the course of chlamydial keratoconjunctivitis (Eugster et al. 1977). Subcutaneous administration of these antibiotics would also be effective and less painful. A newer macrolide antibiotic, tulathromycin, has not yet been evaluated in small ruminants but is effective in treating keratoconjunctivitis in beef cattle (Lane et al. 2006). Milk contamination makes systemic antibiotic treatment unjustifiable in most dairy herds. In fact, the possibility of milk contamination from eye ointments has apparently not been investigated.

Corticosteroids are available in many different topical and injectable preparations of varying anti-inflammatory effect and penetrating ability (Bistner 1986). Corticosteroids are not necessary and are contraindicated if an ulcer is present. A subconjunctival injection of a depot form of corticosteroid may be helpful to control neovascularization after extensive keratitis. The eye must be "quiet" and the cornea free of ulcers, as demonstrated by fluorescein staining, before such a treatment is performed. In general, it is best to dispense an ointment without steroids because the owner is likely to use whatever product is on hand to treat undiagnosed eye problems of goats or other animals at a later date.

Ulcerated eyes should be observed several times a day for descemetocele formation. If perforation of the cornea appears imminent, a conjunctival flap, third eyelid flap, or tarsorrhaphy is indicated to protect and support the cornea. The third eyelid flap is probably easiest. Local anesthesia with an ophthalmic anesthetic, paralysis of the eyelids with 1 or 2 ml of injectable anesthetic (diluted if the goat is small) over the auriculopalpebral nerve (on the lateral surface of the zygomatic arch), and light tranquilization with xylazine are employed. Mattress sutures of 00 chromic gut that pass through the full thickness of the upper lid but do not penetrate the bulbar aspect of the third eyelid pull the cartilaginous portion up to the upper lid (Moore and Whitley 1984); small buttons or pieces of tubing on the outside of the lid prevent pressure necrosis of the skin. Follow-up care includes continued therapy with antibiotic ointment and close observation for loosening of the sutures. Misplaced sutures abrade the cornea. Absorbable sutures dissolve in two to three weeks, and nonabsorbable sutures should be removed at this time.

As a simpler alternative to surgery for severe corneal ulcers, the author has seen excellent response to topical 5% silver nitrate, a few drops applied once a day for five days in conjunction with systemic oxytetracycline. This solution is not available commercially but can be approximated by dissolving the material coated onto one Grafco® silver nitrate applicator stick (Atlanta, GA) in 1 ml of sterile water. The totally opaque soft cornea is firm and shiny again in a few days, although total clearing of the cornea can be expected to require more than a week (Figure 6.8). Because the silver nitrate appears to sting, pretreatment with a topical anesthetic is advised. In human medicine, both 1% silver nitrate solution and 2.5% povidone iodine solution have been effective in killing microorganisms in the eye for prophylaxis of ophthalmia neonatorum (Isenberg et al. 1994).

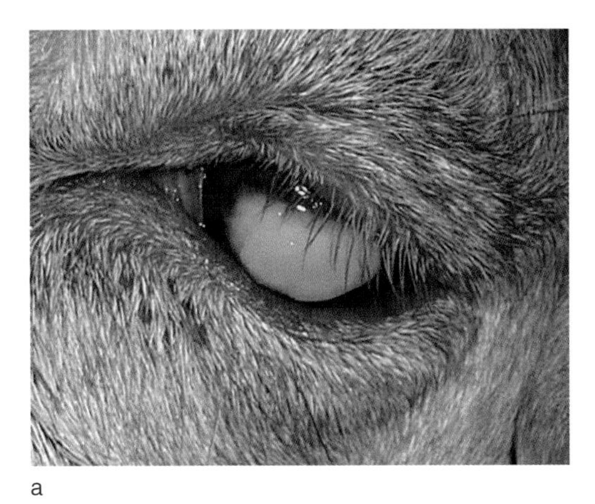

a

Figure 6.8a. A totally opaque and softened cornea from severe bilateral keratoconjunctivitis.

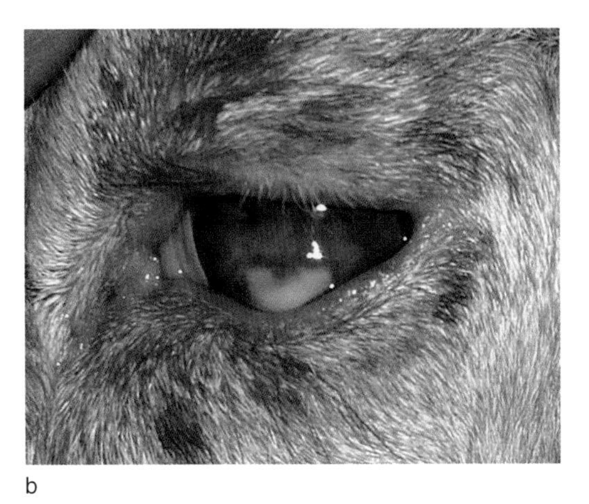

b

Figure 6.8b. The same cornea, five days after initiation of treatment with systemic oxytetracycline and topical 5% silver nitrate. The cornea is firm, shiny, and clearing. (Courtesy Dr. M.C. Smith.)

Noninfectious Keratitis

Not all cases of keratitis begin as infectious conjunctivitis.

Abrasions

Foreign bodies (in addition to eyelashes) may abrade or penetrate the cornea. The eye is painful, and fluorescein staining reveals a defect in the corneal epithelium. Treatment for shallow abrasions is with an antibiotic ointment after careful search for a foreign body in the fornix or behind the third eyelid. If the injury has reached the level of Descemet's membrane, and the inner layer of the cornea bulges outward, a conjunctival or third eyelid flap is indicated. A corneal stromal ulcer with lysis (melting) as a result of collagenase production may appear soft and gelatinous or may resemble a deep abrasion. When any doubt exists as to the origin of the lesion, anticollagenase drugs (Mucomyst® [Bristol-Myers Squibb, Princeton, NJ] topically) and aspirin (100 mg/kg twice daily orally) should accompany placement of a conjunctival flap. If the full thickness of the cornea has been perforated but iris has plugged the hole, consultation with or referral to an ophthalmologist is desirable. A collapsed eyeball is generally best enucleated.

Exposure Secondary to Facial Nerve Deficit

Listeria organisms often enter the brain stem along a cranial nerve. If the facial nerve is thus involved, unilateral paresis or paralysis of the eyelids may occur before any signs of central nervous system disturbance are recognized. The goat that can no longer blink may incur a shallow abrasion to the cornea, which the owner recognizes because of lacrimation, conjunctival injection, corneal clouding, and photophobia. It is very important for the veterinarian to evaluate ipsilateral tonus of lids, ear, and lip. Although it may be impossible to distinguish a facial nerve paralysis of traumatic origin or secondary to otitis media from early listeriosis, treatment with penicillin or tetracycline for one week is justified because the prognosis for an animal with listeriosis is so much worse when the signs are unequivocal.

The cornea dries out and becomes opaque in more advanced listeriosis or other long-standing facial nerve paralysis. A lid-splitting suture pattern to hold the lids in apposition over the cornea prevents additional damage and decreases the frequency with which application of ointments is required during the prolonged recovery period, until nerve function returns. In general, local therapy for exposure keratitis should include antibiotics to prevent secondary infection and atropine for cycloplegia (Rebhun and deLahunta 1982). Uveitis and even hypopyon can be expected in severely affected goats.

Vitamin A Deficiency

Bilateral corneal opacity, lacrimation, and diarrhea were observed in kids born in a goat herd experiencing severe vitamin A deficiency due to six months on dry pasture. All signs disappeared after improvement of the diet (Caldas 1961). Night blindness, lacrimation, and corneal ulceration were reported in adult goats kept on an experimental vitamin A deficient diet for periods as long as two years (Schmidt 1941; Majumdar and Gupta 1960; Dutt and Majumdar 1969).

Toxins

Phenothiazine was once commonly used as an anthelmintic. If metabolism is not complete, phenothiazine sulfoxide reaches the aqueous humor and is a primary photosensitizing agent; it induces uveitis, corneal endothelial damage with subsequent edema, and keratitis (Enzie and Whitmore 1953). Young goats should be kept out of direct sunshine for three days after receiving this drug.

Keratoconjunctivitis sicca, or dry eye, is one of the signs associated with locoweed poisoning (*Astragalus* spp). Drying out of the eyes may be caused by inadequate blinking and failure of neurologic stimulation to the lacrimal glands or by reduced tear production capabilities of the glands.

The imported fire ant (*Solenopsis invicta*) is present in the south central United States. Ants occasionally attack weak or debilitated animals, injecting a necrotoxic venom into the victim. Necrotic ulceration of conjunctiva and cornea has been observed in a goat stung by these ants (Joyce 1983).

Caprine Mucopolysaccharidosis-IIID

A recessive genetic defect (G6S) of Nubian goats which causes a deficiency of *N*-acetylglucosamine-6-sulfatase results in the accumulation of glycosaminoglycans in lysosomes. Growth retardation has been reported clinically. One severely affected kid was ataxic and developed mild, nonprogressive corneal clouding; histologically there was vacuolation of cells in the cornea as well as in the brain (Jones et al. 1998). A survey of 552 purebred Nubian goats in Michigan revealed that 25% of the animals were heterozygous for the mutation and 1.3% were homozygous (Hoard et al. 1998).

ANTERIOR UVEITIS, CATARACTS, AND GLAUCOMA

Anterior uveitis (inflammation of the iris and ciliary body) produces a variety of changes within the eye. These include decreased production of aqueous humor (decreased intraocular pressure), increased protein content of aqueous humor (flare), and accumulation of leukocytes (hypopyon) or erythrocytes (hyphema). Constriction of the pupil is an important diagnostic sign, as is photophobia because of painful inflammation of the ciliary muscle. Organophosphate toxicity, which is also accompanied by miosis, is an important differential. Miosis has also been reported with urea poisoning (Schmidt 1973). Adhesions may form between the swollen iris and the lens or cornea. Retinal detachment and glaucoma are other potential sequelae.

Causes of Anterior Uveitis

Septicemia

Hypopyon, deep neovascularization of the cornea, and other signs of anterior uveitis sometimes accompany neonatal septicemia. The posterior segment of the eye or the brain may also be infected. Appropriate systemic antibiotic therapy is critical to survival of the animal. If the infectious agent is resistant to the antibiotic chosen, the corticosteroids used to treat the secondary anterior uveitis may exacerbate the primary infection.

Toxemia

Constriction of the pupil and anterior uveitis may be noted in goats with severe toxic mastitis or metritis.

Deep Keratitis

Severe keratitis resulting from infectious keratoconjunctivitis or exposure keratitis may extend to or cause reflex inflammation of deeper portions of the globe. *Mycoplasma* spp. infections can also reach the uveal tract by the systemic route during septicemia (Whitley and Albert 1984).

Retroviral Infections

A nonsuppurative chorio-iridocyclitis, sometimes accompanied by granuloma formation, has been documented in the eyes of goats with chronic neurologic disease believed in retrospect to be caused by retroviral infection (Stavrou et al. 1969; Dahme et al. 1973). Clinical signs directly related to the ocular system included corneal opacity, nystagmus, and blindness (usually unilateral). The prevalence of anterior uveitis in goats with caprine arthritis encephalitis or related virus infections (see Chapter 5) is unknown. Clinical blindness could be the result of a brain lesion rather than an eye lesion and few studies have reported histology of the eye. In one group of naturally infected goats where optic nerves and eyes were examined, no histologic lesions were found in these tissues (Sundquist et al. 1981).

Toxoplasmosis

At least in other species, toxoplasmosis can lead to iridocyclitis and necrotizing granulomas on the retina and ciliary body. In one study including sheep (but no goats), granulomatous ocular lesions were demonstrated in eyes from twelve of eighteen sheep with experimental toxoplasmosis (Piper et al. 1970). Systemic therapy with sulfonamides and pyrimethamine and topical treatment with atropine, steroids, and 10% sulfacetamide ophthalmic ointment have been recommended. The possible occurrence of ocular lesions in kids congenitally infected with toxoplasmosis needs to be investigated.

Trauma

Blunt trauma to the head may induce hyphema or an anterior uveitis. This might explain the occasional occurrence of fibrin tags attached to the iris of goats with central blindness because of polioencephalomalacia (Smith 1979). In general, it is wiser to administer thiamine whenever blindness is accompanied by any other neurologic signs rather than to exclude from consideration a common disease based on the presence of an unusual sign.

Treatment of Anterior Uveitis

Even though the exact cause is rarely determined, in the absence of fluorescein uptake by the cornea, treatment of the eyeball showing such signs should include corticosteroids and atropine. The corticosteroids are generally given by bulbar subconjunctival injection with a tuberculin syringe and a 25-gauge needle. The atropine might be given by injection, but more commonly, ointment or drops are instilled every few hours until the pupil dilates, then once or twice a day. Both painful spasm of the ciliary muscle and the danger of adhesion formation are decreased by using atropine. The animal should be allowed access to a darkened stall until the ability to constrict the pupil is regained after discontinuation of therapy. Antiprostaglandin therapy also results in dilation of the pupil.

Cataracts

Cataracts are opacities of the lens or its capsule. Uveal pigment may be deposited on the anterior lens capsule. Fluid accumulation within the lens or denaturation of lens protein may hinder light transmission. A cataract can occur as a sequela to any severe anterior uveitis if not vigorously treated. Congenital cataracts have apparently not been reported in goats (Wyman 1983). Referral to a specialist should precede any surgical attempt at cataract extraction.

Glaucoma

Secondary glaucoma has been reported as occurring after severe anterior uveitis induced by *Mycoplasma agalactia* (Moore and Whitley 1986). The intraocular pressure rises because the iridocorneal angle is closed by the inflammatory process. Both the anterior uveitis and the glaucoma may contribute to corneal edema, as does anterior lens luxation if it occurs. Buphthalmia (enlargement of the globe) may initially protect the retina. When intraocular pressure becomes high enough to damage the retina, permanent blindness occurs. Proper use of mydriatics and corticosteroids to prevent secondary glaucoma is paramount.

Tonometry

The only method available to most large animal practitioners for estimating intraocular pressure is digital tonometry. The index and middle fingers of one hand are used to slightly flatten the globe by applying pressure through the upper lid. The other hand simultaneously evaluates the second eye of the patient. At least until experience is gained, comparison with a normal goat is helpful.

The Schiotz tonometer, although previously available in many small animal practices, is not practical for use in goats. The goat must be in dorsal recumbency for the cornea to be accessible when the tonometer is held vertically. A topical anesthetic is required. Struggling or compression of the jugular veins might artificially elevate the intraocular pressure. By contrast, Tono-Pen tonometers are easy to use on goats. Although a normal range for the goat using this device has not been reported, values from the patient could be compared with intraocular pressure measurements from several normal goats.

Treatment

It is unlikely that glaucoma will be diagnosed in an affected goat until the cornea is "steamy" and the globe is enlarging. In most instances, medical management is impractical. Prompt referral to an ophthalmic surgeon may be appropriate for certain valuable animals. Otherwise, the practitioner should plan to enucleate the glaucomatous eye when the goat appears to be in persistent pain or when the eyelids can no longer cover the enlarged globe well enough to prevent drying of the central cornea. An alternative to enucleation might be an injection of gentamicin plus corticosteroid into the vitreous to destroy the ciliary body.

RETINAL CHANGES

A number of lesions may be recognized in the course of a thorough ophthalmoscopic examination of the retina. Cellular infiltration may appear focal or diffuse or it may follow blood vessels. Infiltrations are white or gray. Edema has a similar appearance but may be better demarcated. Hemorrhages have different shapes depending on the layer of the retina where they are located. Thus, focal or round hemorrhages are deep within the retina, linear lesions (flame hemorrhages) are in the nerve fiber layer, and crescent shaped (keel) hemorrhages are preretinal (beneath the vitreous).

Papilledema

Papilledema is a noninflammatory swelling of the optic disc. It is an important sign of increased intracranial pressure. Causes in ruminants include hypovitaminosis A, acquired and congenital hydrocephalus, space-occupying brain lesions, meningitis, encephalitis, coenurosis, and hexachlorophene toxicity (Whittaker et al. 1999). Papilledema is usually bilateral. The arterioles are more thread-like (and more red) than the congested retinal venules. Hemorrhages may be present on the disc or retina.

Chorioretinitis

Retinitis has been described in association with elaeophorosis in sheep. Trypanosomosis of sheep has caused severe uveitis, chorioretinitis, and optic neuritis. Natural infection with bluetongue or use of an attenuated vaccine in ewes in the first half of pregnancy has caused necrotizing retinopathy in lambs, according to Wyman (1983). Toxoplasmosis, as discussed under anterior uveitis, can cause a granulomatous chorioretinitis in ruminants. These conditions apparently have not been reported in goats.

Chorioretinopathy

This term suggests that active inflammation is not (or is no longer) present. One example would be scars from an earlier septicemia. Retinopathy is manifested by tapetal hyper-reflectivity and pale depigmented areas in the nontapetal fundus. Retinal atrophy has been reported after congenital infection with Akabane virus. A spontaneous retinopathy possibly caused by rod-cone dysplasia has been reported in a young Toggenburg goat (Buyukmihci 1980). Four other closely related Toggenburg kids in Canada were blind from birth and showed a similar tapetal hyperreflectivity and marked retinal vessel attenuation; an inherited disorder was suspected (Wolfer and Grahn 1991). Other causes of retinal degeneration in ruminants, even if unreported in goats, are mentioned below for completeness.

Scrapie

Scrapie, at least in sheep, can cause a central blindness. However, multifocal retinal elevations have also been described. These are blister-like, hyperreflective, with a dark edge, and scattered in the tapetal fundus. They vary from one-fourth to three-fourths the size of the optic disc (Barnett and Palmer 1971).

Border Disease

Because of parallels with lesions identified in cattle affected in utero with bovine virus diarrhea (BVD) virus, border disease might be expected occasionally to be accompanied by retinal changes. Abnormalities reported in cattle include grayness of the optic disc, vascular attenuation, hyperreflective areas of the tapetal fundus, unusual admixtures of tapetal colors, and multifocal depigmentation of the nontapetal fundus. Cataracts may occur and normal pupillary light reflexes may be absent. Such findings have not yet been reported in sheep or goats.

Bright Blindness

Sheep consuming bracken fern (*Pteridium* spp.) (Barnett and Watson 1970) for many months may develop progressive bilateral blindness. The tapetum develops increased reflectivity, and the neuroepithelium degenerates. The pupils become circular and react poorly to light. The arteries and veins of the retina appear narrower than normal. The shepherd notices the blindness when a sheep becomes separated from the flock and runs around with elevated head and a high-stepping gait.

Blind Grass

Stypandra imbricata, or blind grass, is a plant found in western Australia. Goats and sheep that survive acute exposure become permanently blind, with degeneration of photoreceptor cells, optic nerves, and optic tracts. Clinical examination several weeks after blindness develops reveals foci of pigment epithelium hypertrophy, especially prominent in the nontapetal fundus near the optic disc. Pupillary light reflexes are absent (Main et al. 1981). A related Australian plant, *Stypandra glauca* (nodding blue lily), has been associated with blindness in goats consuming the plant during its flowering stage. Acute cerebral edema with subsequent compression of the optic nerve within the optic canal may be important to pathogenesis (Whittington et al. 1988).

Other Plant Toxicities

Helichrysum argyrosphaerum toxicity has caused papilledema and retinal changes in sheep and cattle in Namibia, with spongiform lesions occurring in brain and optic fasciculi as well (Kellerman et al. 2005). Goats appear to be resistant (Basson et al. 1975) but in one blind goat with cerebral and brainstem vacuolation, a slight increase in tapetal reflectivity and pigmented foci in the nontapetal fundus were noted (Van der Lugt et al. 1996).

Some species of *Astragalus* (locoweed) cause a retinal degeneration, at least in cattle and sheep. Many cells in the body are vacuolated, including neurons in the brain and inner ganglionic layer of the retina and secretory cells in the lacrimal gland. The eye appears dull and vision is impaired (Van Kampen and James 1971). *Swainsona* (darling pea) in Australia causes similar signs. Both plants contain substances that inhibit lysosomal mannosidase, thereby producing a storage disease. Similar vacuolation of retinal cells has been seen in goat kids with hereditary beta mannosidosis (Render et al. 1989). *Astragalus* species have also caused blindness, ataxia, and weight loss (blind staggers) caused by high concentrations of selenium (Hosseinion et al. 1972), although it has been speculated that some cases of blind staggers were actually sulfur-related polioencephalomalacia (Whittaker et al. 1999). This condition is discussed in Chapter 5.

Dryopteris filix-mas (male fern) ingestion in cattle causes acute retrobulbar neuropathy that may progress to optic atrophy. Hemorrhages on or around the optic disc and papilledema are noted acutely. Chronic lesions include optic nerve atrophy and reduced retinal vasculature; these animals are blind.

Retinal Detachment

Detachment occurs when transudates or exudates accumulate between the retinal pigment epithelium and the receptor layers. A total detachment results in blindness and is recognized by the presence of a billowing structure containing blood vessels in the vitreous. Case reports in goats are lacking.

AMAUROSIS

Amaurosis is blindness without any externally detectable defect in the visual system. The cornea, lens, and uveal tract appear to be normal. If the lesion is limited to the cerebral cortex and optic nerve and nuclei are intact, the pupillary reflexes are also normal. Blindness becomes apparent because of abnormal behavior or failure to respond to visual stimuli.

Blindness versus Failure to Blink

It is common but inaccurate to equate the ability to blink in response to a menacing hand gesture with the ability to see; this is because the entire visual pathway, from the retina to the cerebral cortex, must be intact for the reflex to function (deLahunta 1983). Because it is a learned response, very young kids may not menace even though they have no trouble seeing and following a moving bottle or other item of interest. A goat with normal vision also fails to blink if facial nerve paralysis is present. This possibility is investigated by actually touching the medial or lateral canthus. Even a blind animal should then blink, unless either sensory or motor function is disturbed.

Blindness versus Severe Depression or Toxemia

Severely obtunded or semi-comatose goats respond minimally to stimuli routinely applied to evaluate cranial nerve function. If the animal is severely depressed, a metabolic disease (hypoglycemia, hypocalcemia, pregnancy toxemia, rumen acidosis), liver disease (see Chapter 11), or terminal septicemic or toxemic (Boermans et al. 1988) condition, rather than a lesion specifically involving visual pathways or cerebral cortex, may be present. It is inappropriate, then, to limit diagnostic consideration to those diseases with blindness as a leading sign.

Polioencephalomalacia

Blindness is almost always present in advanced cases of polioencephalomalacia. Thus, thiamine administration, as discussed in Chapter 5, is indicated (at least initially) for every goat with amaurosis.

Enterotoxemia

Blindness is one sign of focal symmetrical encephalomalacia, an uncommon disease reportedly caused by exotoxins of *Clostridium perfringens*, in sheep. The condition has been reported only rarely in goats (see Chapter 5).

Lead Poisoning

Although blindness is a prominent sign of lead poisoning in cattle, this is not the case in goats. Anorexia and diarrhea, not blindness and convulsions, are reported with experimental lead poisoning in goats (Davis et al. 1976).

Hydrocephalus

A young kid that has a good suckle reflex and a normal gait may become separated from its dam or stuck in corners. Hydrocephalus or other congenital malformation of the brain may be responsible for this abnormal behavior associated with blindness. Sometimes the skull is domed, which increases the suspicion of hydrocephalus. Other kids have no outward conformational changes even though very little brain is in fact present.

Vitamin A Deficiency

Maternal deficiency of vitamin A produces atrophy of the optic nerves in calves. This is because the optic canals have not grown to accommodate the optic nerves, resulting in pressure atrophy and demyelination of the nerves. In the case of acquired avitaminosis A in cattle, there is an initial, often reversible night blindness caused by deficient formation of rhodopsin. If the deficiency continues, the retina degenerates and eventually constriction of the optic nerve can occur in growing calves. Papilledema is an important sign of vitamin A deficiency and is secondary to increased cerebrospinal fluid (CSF) pressure. Vascular congestion and focal superficial hemorrhages also occur. The intraocular pressure is not elevated. Specific reports of this condition in goats are lacking, and in one experimental study adult goats fed a vitamin A depletion ration failed to develop papilledema or increased CSF pressure (Frier et al. 1974).

Severe vitamin A deficiency, as occurs during the dry season or droughts in semiarid regions, causes night blindness that is not always accompanied by corneal opacity and ulceration. These ocular problems are documented in sheep (Eveleth et al. 1949, Ghanem and Farid 1982) and have been reproduced experimentally in goats (Schmidt 1941).

Coenurosis

Coenurus cerebralis is the larval stage of the tapeworm *Taenia multiceps*. It can form a cyst in the cerebral hemispheres or median fissure. A common clinical sign is partial or total blindness in one eye (Sharma 1965; Tirgari et al. 1987; Nooruddin et al. 1996). The head is held in the direction away from the blind eye and the animal circles in that direction, that is, toward the cerebral lesion. Pupillary reflexes generally remain normal, but papilledema may be noted because of increased intracranial pressure (Sharma and Tyagi 1975). In some cases, the skull overlying the cyst is softened and deformed, and pressure on the affected bone elicits signs of pain (loud bleating). Vision usually returns within one day after surgical removal of the cyst. The disease has not been reported in recent years in the United States (Kimberling 1988).

Miscellaneous Causes of Central Blindness

Several other diseases may cause blindness in sheep, and perhaps in goats. Melioidosis is a fatal septicemic disease caused by *Burkholderia* (*Pseudomonas*) *pseudomallei* and occurs mainly in Southeast Asia and Australia. A central blindness can accompany other neurologic signs. Likewise, scrapie can cause blindness but will probably be recognized by other neurologic signs. Caprine arthritis encephalitis can cause a variety of central neurologic signs, including blindness.

Chronic poisoning with some forms of arsenic, in some species, can cause blindness. Acute blindness in cattle and sheep has been associated with consumption of rape (*Brassica napus*), but documentation is meager. In some instances of poisoning with *Brassica* spp., the actual cause of blindness may be polioencephalomalacia (Wikse et al. 1987). Ironwood (*Erythrophloeum chlorostachys*), a tree from tropical Australia, has been reported to poison goats and cause, among other signs, a staring-eyed demeanor with vision apparently affected (Hall 1964). Overdosage with hexachlorophene, rafoxanide, and closantel can cause degeneration of the optic nerve, optic tract, or retina (Button et al. 1987). The pathologic changes (Gill et al. 1999) resemble those caused by *Stypandra* spp, but pigment epithelium hypertrophy has not been described.

Residual Blindness

Blindness may persist for days, weeks, or even the life of a goat that did not receive thiamine early in the course of polioencephalomalacia. Other traumatic or metabolic insults to the cerebral cortex (prolonged application of a disbudding iron, pregnancy toxemia) could also result in amaurosis. Usually there is a history of partial recovery from a previous severe illness.

ENUCLEATION

Enucleation is indicated if the eyeball has collapsed because of trauma or the perforation of an ulcer resulting from infectious keratoconjunctivitis, or whenever a chronic painful eye condition cannot be resolved. Whether local or general anesthesia is used depends on the facilities available to the veterinarian. If necessary, tranquilization with xylazine and infiltration of 1% lidocaine subcutaneously around the eye and in the depth of the orbit can be used. Thus, in a large animal practice, enucleation in a goat can be performed on the farm. The lids are clipped and disinfected; irritating solutions should be kept out of the unaffected eye, and they should not be allowed to pool on the surgery table near the down eye. The lid margins, conjunctival sac, and ocular muscles are dissected free from the orbit with curved scissors. A tight ligature around the optic nerve and accompanying blood vessels should control hemorrhage, although a hematoma may form in the orbit. An everting mattress suture is often chosen to close the skin, and penicillin may be instilled into the cavity created by enucleation.

REFERENCES

Adegoke, G.O. and Ojo, M.O.: Biochemical characterization of staphylococci isolated from goats. Vet. Microbiol., 7:463–470, 1982.

Al-Aubaidi, J.M., Dardiri, A.H., Muscoplatt, C.C. and McCauley, E.H.: Identification and characterization of *Acholeplasma oculusi* spec. nov. from the eyes of goats with keratoconjunctivitis. Cornell Vet., 63:117–129, 1973.

Andrews, A.H., Goodard, P.C., Wilsmore, A.J. and Dagnell, G.J.R.: A chlamydial keratoconjunctivitis in a British sheep flock. Vet. Rec., 120:238–239, 1987.

Baas, E.J.: Infectious keratoconjunctivitis ("pink eye") of goats and sheep. In: Sheep and Goat Practice Symposium, Proceedings. Fort Collins, CO, American Association of Sheep and Goat Practitioners, pp. 58–70, 1976.

Baas, E.J., Trotter, S.L., Franklin, R.M. and Barile, M.F.: Epidemic caprine keratoconjunctivitis: recovery of *Mycoplasma conjunctivae* and its possible role in pathogenesis. Infect. Immun., 18:806–815, 1977.

Bankemper, K.W., Lindley, D.M., Nusbaum, K.E. and Mysinger, R.H.: Keratoconjunctivitis associated with *Neisseria ovis* infection in a herd of goats. J. Vet. Diagn. Invest., 2:76–78, 1990.

Bar-Moshe, B. and Rapapport, E.: Observations on *Mycoplasma mycoides* subsp. *mycoides* infection in Saanen goats. Isr. J. Med. Sci., 17:537–539, 1981.

Barile, M.F., Del Giudice, R.A. and Tully, J.G.: Isolation and characterization of *Mycoplasma conjunctivae* sp. n. from sheep and goats with keratoconjunctivitis. Infect. Immun., 5:70–76, 1972.

Barnett, K.C. and Palmer, A.C.: Retinopathy in sheep affected with natural scrapie. Res. Vet. Sci., 12:383–385, 1971.

Barnett, K.C. and Watson, W.A.: Bright blindness in sheep. A primary retinopathy due to feeding bracken (*Pteris aquilina*). Res. Vet. Sci., 11:289–290, 1970.

Basson, P.A.: Studies on specific oculo-vascular myiasis (uitpeuloog). III. Symptomatology, pathology, aetiology and epizootiology. Onderstepoort J. Vet. Res., 29:211–240, 1962.

Basson, P.A., et al.: Blindness and encephalopathy caused by *Helichrysum argyrosphaerum* D.C. (Compositae) in sheep and cattle. Onderstepoort J. Vet. Res., 42:135–148, 1975.

Baxendell, S.A.: Caprine ophthalmology. In: Refresher Course for Veterinarians, Proceedings No. 73, Goats, The University of Sydney, The Post-Graduate Committee in Veterinary Science, Sydney, N.S.W., Australia, 1984.

Beveridge, W.I.B.: Investigations on contagious ophthalmia of sheep with special attention to the epidemiology of infection by *Rickettsia conjunctivae*. Aust. Vet. J., 18:155–164, 1942.

Binns, W., Keeler, R.F. and Balls, L.D.: Congenital deformities in lambs, calves and goats resulting from maternal ingestion of *Veratrum californicum*: harelip, cleft palate, ataxia and hypoplasia of metacarpal and metatarsal bones. Clin. Toxicol., 5:245–261, 1972.

Bistner, S.: Basic ophthalmic therapeutics. In: Current Veterinary Therapy Food Animal Practice 2. J.L. Howard, ed. Philadelphia, W.B. Saunders Co., 1986.

Boermans, H.J., Ruegg, P.L. and Leach, M.: Ethylene glycol toxicosis in a Pygmy goat. J. Am. Vet. Med. Assoc., 193:694–696, 1988.

Brightman, A.H., Wachsstock, R.S. and Erskine, R.: Lysozyme concentrations in the tears of cattle, goats, and sheep. Am. J. Vet. Res., 52:9–11, 1991.

Bulgin, M.S. and Dubose, D.A.: Pinkeye associated with *Branhamella ovis* infection in dairy goats. Vet. Med. Small Anim. Clin., 77:1791–1793, 1982.

Button, C., Jerrett, I., Alexander, P. and Mizon, W.: Blindness in kids associated with overdosage of closantel. Aust. Vet. J., 64:226, 1987.

Buyukmihci, N.: Retinal degeneration in a goat. J. Am. Vet. Med. Assoc., 177:351–352, 1980.

Bwangamoi, O., Carles, A.B. and Wandera, J.G.: An epidemic of besnoitiosis in goats in Kenya. Vet. Rec., 125:461, 1989.

Caldas, A.D.: Avitaminose A espontânea em caprinos. (Spontaneous avitaminosis A in goats.) O Biologico 27:266–270, 1961.

Caminopetros, J.P.: La "Q" fever en Grèce: le lait source de l'infection pour l'homme et les animaux. Ann. Parasitol. Hum. Comp., 23:107–118, 1948.

Choudhury, B. and Robinson, V.B.: Clinical and pathologic effects produced in goats by the ingestion of toxic amounts of chlordan and toxaphene. Am. J. Vet. Res., 11:50–57, 1950.

Dagnall, G.J.R.: Use of exfoliative cytology in the diagnosis of ovine keratoconjunctivitis. Vet. Rec., 135:127–130, 1994.

Dahme, E., et al.: Klinik und Pathologie einer übertragbaren granulomatösen Meningoencephalomyelitis (gMEM) bei der Hausziege. Acta Neuropathol., 23:59–76, 1973.

DaMassa, A.J., Brooks, D.L., East, N.E. and Moe, A.I.: Brief account of caprine mycoplasmosis in the United States with special reference to *Mycoplasma mycoides* subsp. *mycoides*. In: Proceedings, U.S. Anim. Health Assoc., 88:291–302, 1984.

Davis, J.W., Libke, K.G., Watson, D.F. and Bibb, T.L.: Experimentally induced lead poisoning in goats: Clinical observations and pathologic changes. Cornell Vet., 66:489–496, 1976.

deLahunta, A.: Veterinary Neuroanatomy and Clinical Neurology. 2nd Ed. Philadelphia, W.B. Saunders Co., 1983.

Dutt, B. and Majumdar, B.N.: Epithelial metaplasia in experimental vitamin A deficient goats. Indian Vet. J., 46:789–791, 1969.

Eales, F.A., Small, J., Robinson, J.J. and Gebbie, C.: Correction of entropion in newborn lambs. Vet. Rec., 114:193, 1984.

Emaduddin, M.: *Setaria cervi* in the eye of a goat. Indian Vet. J., 31:111–112, 1954.

Enzie, F.D. and Whitmore, G.E.: Photosensitization keratitis in young goats following treatment with phenothiazine. J. Am. Vet. Med. Assoc., 123:237–238, 1953.

Eugster, A.K., Jones, L.P. and Gayle, L.G.: Epizootics of chlamydial abortions and keratoconjunctivitis in goats. Ann. Proc. Am. Assoc. Vet. Lab. Diagn., 20:69–78, 1977.

Evans, K., et al.: Eye infections due to *Listeria monocytogenes* in three cows and one horse. J. Vet. Diagn. Invest., 16:464–469, 2004.

Eveleth, D.F., Bolin, D.W. and Goldsby, A.I.: Experimental avitaminosis A in sheep. Am. J. Vet. Res., 10:250–255, 1949.

Frier, H.I., et al.: Formation and absorption of cerebrospinal fluid in adult goats with hypo- and hypervitaminosis A. Am. J. Vet. Res., 35:45–55, 1974.

Galan, A., Martin-Suarez, E.M., Granados, M.M. and Molleda, J.M.: Comparative fluorescein angiography of the normal sheep and goat ocular fundi. Vet. Ophthalmol., 9:7–15, 2006a.

Galan, A., Martin-Suarez, E.M. and Molleda, J.M.: Ophthalmoscopic characteristics in sheep and goats: comparative study. J. Vet. Med. A, 53:205–208, 2006b.

Ghanem, Y.S. and Farid, M.F.A.: Vitamin A deficiency and supplementation in desert sheep. 1. Deficiency symptoms, plasma concentrations and body growth. World Rev. Anim. Prod., 18(2):69–74, 1982.

Gill, P.A., et al.: Optic neuropathy and retinopathy in closantel toxicosis of sheep and goats. Aust. Vet. J., 77:259–261, 1999.

Hall, W.T.K.: Plant toxicoses of tropical Australia. Aust. Vet. J., 40:176–182, 1964.

Hoard, H.M., et al.: Determination of genotypic frequency of caprine mucopolysaccharidosis IIID. J. Vet. Diagn. Invest., 10:181–183, 1998.

Hosie, B.D.: Keratoconjunctivitis in a hill sheep flock. Vet. Rec., 122:40–43, 1988.

Hosseinion, M., et al.: Selenium poisoning in a mixed flock of sheep and goats in Iran. Trop. Anim. Health Prod., 4:173–174, 1972.

Isenberg, S.J., et al.: Povidone-iodine for ophthalmia neonatorum prophylaxis. Am. J. Ophthalmol., 118:701–706, 1994.

Jones, A. and Barber, T.L.: *Mycoplasma mycoides* var. *capri* isolated from a goat in Connecticut. J. Infect. Dis., 119:126–131, 1969.

Jones, G.E., Foggie, A., Sutherland, A. and Harker, D.B.: Mycoplasmas and ovine keratoconjunctivitis. Vet. Rec., 99:137–141, 1976.

Jones, M.Z., et al.: Caprine mucopolysaccharidosis-IIID: clinical, biochemical, morphological and immunohistochemical characteristics. J. Neuropathol. Exp. Neurol., 57:148–157, 1998.

Joyce, J.R.: Multifocal ulcerative keratoconjunctivitis as a result of stings by imported fire ants. Vet. Med. Small Anim. Clin., 78:1107–1108, 1983.

Kodjo, A., et al.: *Moraxella caprae* sp. nov., a new member of the classical Moraxellae with very close affinity to *Moraxella bovis*. Int. J. Syst. Bacteriol. 45:467–71, 1995.

Lia, R.P. et al.: Field efficacy of moxidectin 1 per cent against *Thelazia callipaeda* in naturally infected dogs. Vet. Rec., 154:143–145, 2004.

Losos, G.J. and Ikede, B.O.: Review of pathology of diseases in domestic and laboratory animals caused by *Trypanosoma congolense*, *T. vivax*, *T. brucei*, *T. rhodesiense* and *T. gambiense*. Vet. Pathol. Suppl. ad vol 9:1–71, 1972.

Kellerman, T.S., et al.: Plant Poisonings and Mycotoxicoses of Livestock in Southern Africa. 2nd Ed. Oxford, Oxford Univ. Press, 2005.

Kimberling, C.V.: Jensen and Swift's Diseases of Sheep. 3rd Ed. Philadelphia, Lea and Febiger, 1988.

König, C.D.W.: "Pink eye" or "zereoogjes" or keratoconjunctivitis infectiosa ovis (KIO). Clinical efficacy of a number of antimicrobial therapies. Vet. Q., 5:122–127, 1983.

Lane, V.M., George, L.W. and Cleaver, D.M.: Efficacy of tulathromycin for treatment of cattle with acute ocular *Moraxella bovis* infections. J. Am. Vet. Med. Assoc., 229:557–561, 2006.

Main, D.C., et al.: *Stypandra imbricata* ("blindgrass") toxicosis in goats and sheep—clinical and pathologic findings in 4 field cases. Aust. Vet. J., 57:132–135, 1981.

Majumdar, B.N. and Gupta, B.N.: Studies on carotene metabolism in goats. Indian J. Med. Res., 48:388–393, 1960.

Matthews, J.G.: Caprine tumours seen in a mixed practice. Goat Vet. Soc. J., 13:52–54, 1992.

McCauley, E.H., Surman, P.G., and Anderson, D.R.: Isolation of mycoplasma from goats during an epizootic of keratoconjunctivitis. Am. J. Vet. Res., 32:861–870, 1971.

Mohanty, S.B., Lillie, M.G., Corselius, N.P. and Beck, J.D.: Natural infection with infectious bovine rhinotracheitis virus in goats. J. Am. Vet. Med. Assoc., 160:879–880, 1972.

Mongini, A.: Entropion repair with superglue. Wool Wattles, 35(4):10, 2007.

Moore, C.P. and Whitley, R.D.: Ophthalmic diseases of small domestic ruminants. Vet. Clin. N. Am. Large Anim. Pract., 6:641–665, 1984.

Moore, C.P. and Whitley, R.D.: Ocular diseases of sheep and goats. In: Current Veterinary Therapy: Food Animal Practice 2. J.L. Howard, ed. Philadelphia, W.B. Saunders Co., 1986.

Nietfeld, J.C.: Chlamydial infections in small ruminants. Vet. Clin. North Am. Food Anim. Pract. 17:301–314, 2001.

Njenga, J.M., et al.: Preliminary findings from an experimental study of caprine besnoitiosis in Kenya. Vet. Res. Commun., 17:203–208, 1993.

Nooruddin, M., Dey, A.S. and Ali, M.A.: Coenuriasis in Bengal goats of Bangladesh. Small Rumin. Res., 19:77–81, 1996.

Otranto, D., and Traversa, D.: *Thelazia* eyeworm: an original endo- and ecto-parasitic nematode. Trends Parasitol., 21:1–4, 2005.

Patnaik, R.K.: Epidemic of goat dermatitis in India. Trop. Anim. Health Prod., 18:137–138, 1986.

Piper, R.C., Cole, C.R. and Shadduck, J.A.: Natural and experimental ocular toxoplasmosis in animals. Am. J. Ophthalmol., 69:662–668, 1970.

Pitman, D.R. and Reuter, R.: Isolation of *Branhamella ovis* from conjunctivae of Angora goats. Vet. Rec., 65:91, 1988.

Raju, K.G.S. and Rao, K.S.: Cyclopia in a kid. Indian Vet. J., 78:70, 2001.

Rebhun, W.C. and deLahunta, A.: Diagnosis and treatment of bovine listeriosis. J. Am. Vet. Med. Assoc., 180:395–398, 1982.

Render, J.A., Lovell, K.L., Jones, M.Z. and Wheeler, C.A.: Ocular pathology of caprine β-mannosidosis. Vet. Pathol., 26:444–446, 1989.

Rizvi, S.W.H.: Transmission of *Rickettsia conjunctivae* to goats. J. Am. Vet. Med. Assoc., 117:409–411, 1950.

Rook, J.S. and Cortese, V.: Repair of entropion in the lamb. Vet. Med. Small Anim. Clin., 76:571–574, 1981.

Rubin, L.F.: Atlas of Veterinary Ophthalmoscopy. Philadelphia, Lea and Febiger, 1974.

Schebitz, H. and Reiche, F.: Über das Vorkommen der A. hyaloidea persistens bei Rind, Schaf und Ziege. Monatshefte Veterinärmed., 8:181–184, 1953.

Schlegel, T., Brehm, H. and Amselgruber, W.M.: IgA and secretory component (SC) in the third eyelid of domestic animals: a comparative study. Vet. Ophthalmol., 6:157–161, 2003.

Schmidt, H.: Vitamin A deficiencies in ruminants. Am. J. Vet. Res., 2:373–389, 1941.

Schmidt, V.: Augenkrankheiten der Haustiere. Stuttgart, Ferdinand Enke Verlag, 1973.

Sharma, H.N.: *Coenurus cerebralis* in goats. Indian Vet. J., 42:137–139, 1965.

Sharma, H.N. and Tyagi, R.P.S.: Diagnosis and surgical treatment of coenurosis in goat (*Capra hircus*). Indian Vet. J., 52:482–488, 1975.

Smith, M.C.: Polioencephalomalacia in goats. J. Am. Vet. Med. Assoc., 174:1328–1332, 1979.

Sinha, R.D. and Calhoun, M.L.: A gross, histologic, and histochemical study of the lacrimal apparatus of sheep and goats. Am. J. Vet. Res., 27:1633–1640, 1966.

Soulsby, E.J.L.: Helminths, Arthropods and Protozoa of Domesticated Animals. 7th Ed. Philadelphia, Lea and Febiger, 1982.

Stavrou, D., Deutschländer, N., and Dahme, E.: Granulomatous encephalomyelitis in goats. J. Comp. Pathol., 79:393–396 and plates, 1969.

Sundquist, B., Jönsson, L., Jacobsson, S.-O. and Hammarberg, K.E.: Visna virus meningoencephalomyelitis in goats. Acta Vet. Scand., 22:315–330, 1981.

Taoudi, A., Karib, H., Johnson, D.W. and Fassi-Fehri, M.M.: Comparaison du pouvoir pathogène de trois souches de *Mycoplasma capricolum* pour la chèvre et le chevreau nouveau-né. Rev. Elev. Méd. Vét. Pays Trop., 41:353–358, 1988.

Tirgari, M., Howard, B.R. and Boargob, A.: Clinical and radiographical diagnosis of *Coenurosis cerebralis* in sheep and its surgical treatment. Vet. Rec., 120:173–178, 1987.

Toal, R.L.: Ultrasound for the Practitioner. 2nd Ed. Effingham, IL, Professional Veterinary Software and Services, 1996.

Trotter, S.L., Franklin, R.M., Baas, E.J. and Barile, M.F.: Epidemic caprine keratoconjunctivitis: experimentally induced disease with a pure culture of *Mycoplasma conjunctivae*. Infect. Immun., 18:816–822, 1977.

Van der Lugt, J.J., Olivier, J., and Jordaan, P.: Status spongiosus, optic neuropathy and retinal degeneration in *Helichrysum argyrosphaerum* poisoning in sheep and a goat. Vet. Pathol., 33:495–502, 1996.

Van Kampen, K.R. and James, L.F.: Ophthalmic lesions in locoweed poisoning of cattle, sheep, and horses. Am. J. Vet. Res., 32:1293–1295, 1971.

Whitley, R.D. and Albert, R.A.: Clinical uveitis and polyarthritis associated with *Mycoplasma* species in a young goat. Vet. Rec., 115:217–218, 1984.

Whittaker C.J.G, Gelatt, K.N. and Wilkie, D.A.: Food animal ophthalmology. In: Veterinary Ophthalmology, Third Ed. K.N. Gelatt, ed. Philadelphia, Lippincott Williams and Wilkins, pp. 1117–1176, 1999.

Whittington, R.J., Searson, J.E., Whittaker, S.J. and Glastonbury, J.R.W.: Blindness in goats following ingestion of *Stypandra glauca*. Aust. Vet. J., 65:176–181, 1988.

Wikse, S.E., Leathers, C.W. and Parish, S.M.: Diseases of cattle that graze turnips. Comp. Cont. Educ. Pract. Vet., 9: F112-F121, 1987.

Williams, L.W. and Gelatt, K.N.: Ocular manifestations of systemic disease. Part III. Food animals. In: Veterinary Ophthalmology. K.N. Gelatt, ed. Philadelphia, Lea and Febiger, pp. 741–763, 1981.

Wolfer, J. and Grahn, B.: Diagnostic ophthalmology (Retinal degeneration). Can. Vet. J., 32:569–570, 1991.

Wyman, M.: Eye disease of sheep and goats. Vet. Clin. N. Am. Large Anim. Pract., 5:657–675, 1983.

Younger, R.L.: Probable induction of congenital abnormalities in a lamb by apholate. Am. J. Vet. Res., 26:991–995, 1965.

7

Blood, Lymph, and Immune Systems

Caprine hematology has received considerable attention in the past thirty years. A range of discrepant normal values and hematologic responses have been reported. These discrepancies result from variations in age, breed, and health status of the goats evaluated and from differences in environment, climate, methodology, and sample size. Despite inconsistencies, sufficient data exists for reasonable standardization of normal caprine hematologic values and kinetics (Jain 1986; Kramer 2000). In contrast, information on the organization of the caprine immune system and the immune response is limited. Newer information that is available derives from studies of specific diseases. The most notable is caprine arthritis encephalitis (CAE), which emerged as an animal model for study of acquired immunodeficiency syndrome (AIDS) in humans because of the relatedness of the CAE and human immunodeficiency (HIV) lentiviruses (Cheevers et al. 1997; Sharmila et al. 2002; Fluri et al. 2006; Bouzar et al. 2007) as well as paratuberculosis (Storset et al. 2000, 2001) and others.

BASIC CAPRINE HEMATOLOGY

Anatomic Considerations

The principal organ of hematopoiesis in the goat is the bone marrow. The spleen of the goat is located in the left craniodorsal abdomen between the diaphragm and the dorsal sac of the rumen. The anomaly of two distinct spleens in the left abdomen of a goat has been reported (Ramakrishna et al. 1981). As in other ruminants, goats possess a hemal node system. These nodes contain lymphoid tissue and may also participate in blood storage by hemoconcentration. There are five to twelve hemal nodes in a goat, located along the course of the aorta in the abdominal and thoracic cavities (Ezeasor and Singh 1988). The distribution of the lymph nodes is discussed in more detail in Chapter 3.

Bone Marrow

The myeloid to erythroid (M:E) ratio of the bone marrow of the goat has been reported as 0.69, indicating more active erythrocyte than granulocyte production. The proportions of cell types found in normal caprine marrow is reported as follows: myeloblasts, 0.58%; promyelocytes, 0.79%; neutrophilic myelocytes, 2.69%; metamyelocytes, 8.25%; band neutrophils, 8.88%; segmented neutrophils, 9.98%; eosinophils, 1.79%; basophils, 0.06%; monocytes, 0.02%; lymphocytes, 7.49%; and nucleated erythrocytes, 56.33% (Coles 1986). Megakaryocytes were not included in the differential count.

Bone marrow collection procedures should be performed aseptically. Bone marrow biopsies and aspirates can be conveniently obtained from the iliac crest. In addition, an aspirate can be obtained from the dorsal 5 to 10 cm of ribs 10 to 13 using sturdy, 3.8-cm, 16- or 18-gauge styletted needles (Weber 1969). Care must be taken to place the needle on the midline of the narrow goat rib. Marrow aspiration from the third or fourth sternebrae also has been reported (Whitelaw 1985). Because goats are prone to developing chronic abscesses in the sternal region, the sternal site should be used as a last resort.

Blood and Plasma Parameters

Mean blood volume as a percentage of body weight is approximately 7% with a range of 5.7% to 9% (Fletcher et al. 1964; Brooks et al. 1984), or 70 to 85.9 ml/kg of bw (Jain 1986). Blood volume increases in response to increased altitude (Bianca 1969). The mean specific gravity of whole blood is 1.042 with a range of 1.036 to 1.050 (Fletcher et al. 1964; Brooks et al. 1984). The osmotic pressure of serum colloids is 300 mm H_2O.

Mean plasma volumes range from 4.2% to 7.5% of body weight, or 53 to 60.2 ml/kg of bw (Jain 1986). Mean plasma specific gravity is 1.022, with a range of 1.018 to 1.026.

Erythrocyte Parameters

Erythrocyte parameters in the goat are labile, changing markedly over the goat's lifetime (Holman and Dew 1964, 1965; Edjtehadi 1978). So-called normal or average values from the clinical laboratory, then, must be interpreted in the context of the animal's age. The decreases in hemoglobin (Hb) and packed cell volume (PCV) that occur during the first month of life may be due to iron deficiency anemia associated with a milk diet. The decrease can be prevented in kids by administering 150 mg of iron as iron dextran at birth (Holman and Dew 1966). Other age-related variations seen in erythrocyte parameters are shown in Table 7.1.

Seasonal changes are also noted in erythrocyte parameters, with greater red blood cell (RBC), Hb, and PCV values in late summer and fall than in winter and spring. Male goats tend to have higher RBC counts than females. Pregnancy has little effect on erythrocyte parameters, but PCV can decrease during the first five months of lactation.

The goat has the smallest erythrocyte of the domestic mammals, with a diameter of 3.2 to 4.2 microns. As a result, standard methods of determining the PCV may overestimate it by as much as 10% to 15% because of inadequate centrifugation time. For the microhematocrit method, centrifugation for a minimum of ten minutes at 14,000 G is recommended for accurate results. The standard Wintrobe method cannot generate sufficient relative centrifugal force to completely pack goat RBCs, even when centrifugation time is extended. As much as 20% of plasma can be trapped with the erythrocytes (Jain 1986). The standard erythrocyte sedimentation rate (ESR) is not applicable to the goat because there is no settling of goat RBCs within the one-hour interval prescribed for the Wintrobe method. However, a decrease of 2 to 2.5 mm can be observed in normal goat blood held for twenty-four hours.

The small size of the goat RBC is also associated with the highest osmotic fragility among the domestic species. When exposed to hypotonic saline solutions, RBC hemolysis begins at concentrations of 0.62% to 0.74% and complete hemolysis occurs in saline concentrations of 0.48% to 0.60%. Pygmy goat erythrocytes are more fragile than those of Toggenburg goats on the basis of susceptibility to osmotic lysis, possibly because of differences in membrane composition (Fairley et al. 1988).

Goat RBCs have only slight biconcavity. In blood smears, they lack a zone of central pallor and do not exhibit rouleaux formation, except perhaps at the edge of a thick smear. Normal cell shape is quite variable and poikilocytosis is common, with triangular, rod-shaped, pear-shaped, and elliptical cells frequently seen, especially in goats younger than three months of age. Sickle cells can occur in Angora goats similar to those seen in deer (Jain et al. 1980). This morphologic change is associated with filamentous polymerization of hemoglobin and is considered innocuous.

Nucleated RBCs may be seen in newborn goats as old as six weeks of age, but are uncommon afterwards. Reticulocytes are always absent or rare in health. Basophilic stippling of goat erythrocytes has been reported in experimental lead poisoning (Davis et al. 1976). The normal life span of circulating RBCs in the domestic goat, *Capra hircus*, is an average of 125 days, but as long as 165 days in a wild goat, the Himalayan Tahr *(Hemitragus jemlaicus)* (Kaneko and Cornelius 1962).

Hemoglobin

The goat has one embryonic Hb type that occurs very early in fetal development in erythroid precursors. A single distinct fetal Hb (HbF) that comprises alpha and gamma globin chains is present by approxi-

Table 7.1. Erythrocyte parameters in the normal goat from selected reports worldwide.

Country	*Goat description*	*RBC count ($\times 10^6$ ul)*	*PCV (%)*	*Hb (g/dl)*	*MCV (fl)*	*MCH (pg)*	*MCHC (%)*	*References*
India	0–6 months old	16.3	27.9	8.0	17.2	—	28.8	Nangia et al. 1968
	6–12 months old	13.6	24.3	7.0	17.6	—	28.3	"
	1–2 years old	12.8	22.6	7.4	18.0	—	32.6	"
	2–3 years old	12.6	25.5	7.0	20.5	—	27.3	"
	3–4 years old	10.3	21.9	6.5	22.2	—	29.3	"
	4–5 years old	12.2	24.3	7.0	20.0	—	29.0	"
	5 years and older	12.8	26.0	7.2	21.0	—	27.9	"
Nigeria	0–6 months old	13.4 ± 3.3	25.1 ± 3.4	8.4 ± 0.9	19.8 ± 4.8	—	33.9 ± 3.9	Oduye 1976
	6–12 months old	12.9 ± 2.1	27.0 ± 4.6	9.1 ± 1.4	21.2 ± 3.4	—	33.9 ± 3.3	"
	12–24 months old	11.9 ± 1.7	26.9 ± 3.8	8.7 ± 1.3	22.9 ± 3.5	—	32.4 ± 3.2	"
	2 years old	11.8 ± 2.3	25.9 ± 4.4	8.5 ± 1.5	22.4 ± 4.4	—	32.9 ± 3.6	"
	All females	12.2 ± 2.2	26.1 ± 4.5	8.5 ± 1.3	21.8 ± 3.7	—	33.0 ± 4.0	"
	Pregnant females	11.3 ± 2.0	26.9 ± 4.0	8.7 ± 1.6	23.9 ± 3.6	—	32.3 ± 0.9	"
	All males	12.7 ± 2.7	25.9 ± 3.9	8.6 ± 1.3	21.3 ± 4.8	—	33.5 ± 2.9	"
	All goats	12.3 ± 2.4	26.1 ± 4.1	8.6 ± 1.3	21.8 ± 4.4	—	33.1 ± 3.4	"
United Kingdom	Adult males	14.95 ± 2.40	27.2 ± 5.2	10.6 ± 1.6	18.1 ± 1.7	7.2 ± 0.8	39.5 ± 3.6	Wilkins and Hodges 1962
	Adult wethers	16.34 ± 2.10	34.8 ± 3.8	13.1 ± 1.2	21.4 ± 0.8	8.1 ± 0.5	37.7 ± 2.1	"
	Adult females	13.94 ± 2.80	28.9 ± 5.1	11.4 ± 1.6	21.1 ± 3.1	8.4 ± 1.6	39.6 ± 4.4	"
United States	Adults	14.5 ± 2.9	34.0 ± 4.9	12.7 ± 1.5	23.3 ± 2.1	7.9 ± 0.4	34.4 ± 1.5	Lewis 1976

RBC = red blood cell, PCV = packed cell volume, Hb = hemoglobin, MCV = mean corpuscular volume, MCH = mean corpuscular hemoglobin, MCHC = mean corpuscular hemoglobin concentration.

mately forty days of fetal life and persists through birth, diminishing to zero by approximately fifty days of age. Replacing HbF in the young growing goat is HbC, a Hb type peculiar to sheep, goats, and other members of the Caprini family, including the aoudad, Barbary sheep, and the mouflon. In the goat, by fifty days of age, from 80% to 100% of Hb is the HbC type. Hemoglobin C demonstrates decreased oxygen affinity compared with HbF. It is postulated that HbC is a physiologic adaptation that allows the relatively fast-growing kid to satisfactorily oxygenate tissues during rapid growth (Huisman et al. 1969). The marked poikilocytosis commonly observed in kids between one and three months of age may be associated with the switch to HbC during this period.

By 120 days, the final adult types of Hb, comprised of alpha globin chains together with beta globin chains, have largely replaced HbC. However, 5% to 10% of adult Hb may normally persist in the HbC form. In addition to its regular occurrence in growing kids, and its mild persistence in normal adults, Hb switching to HbC also occurs extensively in adult goats during erythropoiesis in response to naturally occurring and experimentally induced anemias and at high altitudes. Erythropoietin is the direct stimulus for Hb switching and the increased production of HbC by developing erythrocytes in the bone marrow (Garrick 1983).

In addition to small amounts of HbC, three adult hemoglobins are commonly recognized and identified as A, B, and D, although a later publication identified the three adult hemoglobins as A, D, and E (Garrick and Garrick 1983). Adult hemoglobins are comprised of both alpha and beta chains and globin chain production is controlled by at least five structural genes. Polymorphism of goat Hb occurs from variation in either beta or alpha chains. Phenotypic variation occurs in the goat with phenotypes AA, AB, BB, and AD previously reported as most common (Huisman 1974). Another Hb type, HbD_{malta} has been identified in high frequency in goats on Malta (Bannister et al. 1979). An association between certain Hb phenotypes and disease resistance has been observed in the goat in relation to helminthiasis (Buvanendran et al. 1981). In a Finnish study of milking goats, increased hemoglobin concentration correlated with increased milk yields and decreased somatic cell counts, though there was no direct explanation for the relationship (Atroshi et al. 1986).

Response to Anemia

The goat demonstrates only a mild to moderate reticulocyte response to anemia. Red cell parameters have been measured after experimental induction of hemorrhagic anemia via controlled venisection that reduced mean RBC counts more than 50% (Dorr et al. 1986). Reticulocyte counts before bleeding were between 0% and 0.5%. Maximum reticulocyte counts occurred six to eight days after bleeding, and ranged from 3.2% to 7.7%. A second reticulocyte peak was seen between eleven and nineteen days with maximum counts between 2.9% and 6.3%. Anisocytosis and persistence of macrocytes for four weeks after bleeding were more dramatic indicators of regeneration than reticulocytosis. The large size of newly released erythrocytes was reflected in a progressive increase in the mean corpuscular volume (MCV), which was highest from twenty-five to twenty-nine days after bleeding, but did not always exceed the normal range of MCV reported for the species. Therefore, the MCV must be interpreted carefully in establishing the presence of regenerative anemia. Hemoglobin and PCV levels returned to before-bleeding levels by five weeks.

Jain et al. (1980) reported a marked poikilocytosis in response to experimentally induced hemorrhagic anemia in normal Angora goats exhibiting increased percentages of erythrocyte sickling. The percentage of fusiform (sickle) cells decreased as new distinct poikilocytic forms developed. Poikilocytosis was maximal between eight and thirteen weeks after bleeding. The change in erythrocyte morphology was attributed to the presence of HbC in regenerative cells.

Blood Types

Currently, most references to the caprine blood grouping system compare it to the sheep system but specific similarities and differences are not always clear. Seven blood groups are known to exist in the sheep, identified as R-O, A, B, C, D, M, and X. The antigens of the R-O group are soluble substances, and naturally occurring anti-R antibodies may be found in R-negative sheep. The M system in the sheep is associated with variation in intracellular RBC potassium concentration, with animals homozygous for the Ma allele having greater intracellular potassium levels. High potassium and low potassium red cell types have also been recorded in goats, but no clear association with the M blood group system has been established despite attempts to do so (Ellory and Tucker 1983). The B system is most complex, with at least fifty-two alleles involved in expression of B-group antigens. Using sheep reagents, at least five of the seven sheep blood groups have been confirmed in goats; B, C, M, R-O, and X. Multiple phenogroups occurred in the B system, similar to sheep (Nguyen 1977).

As with other ruminant species, hemolytic testing is preferred to agglutination testing for blood typing work because of the inherent inagglutinability of erythrocytes in some individuals (Andresen 1984). Neonatal isoerythrolysis is not known in goats. However, hemolytic disease has been reported in one-week-old kids that had received bovine colostrum at birth (Perrin et al. 1988).

In 1992, the American Dairy Goat Association (ADGA) instituted a voluntary blood typing program to assist in indentification and parentage verification of registered goats. In 1998, ADGA replaced identification of individual goats and parentage by blood typing with DNA typing because of the superiority of DNA technology and the limited availability of antisera available for blood typing (Bowen 2007).

Transfusions

In sheep, it has been advised that R-positive blood not be used for transfusion to avoid early donor RBC destruction by isoantibodies (Andresen 1984). In practice, however, cross-matching of goat or sheep blood before single transfusions is not usually performed (Bennett 1983). Nevertheless, naturally occurring antibodies to RBCs can be present in goats and cross matching may be advisable. Transfusion reaction rates of 2% to 3% have been reported (Fletcher et al. 1964). Cross matching is indicated whenever multiple transfusions are anticipated.

Autologously transfused RBCs have a half survival time of eight days while homologously transfused cells have a half survival time of only 2.4 to 5.1 days (Gulliani et al. 1975). Sheep RBCs transfused into goats had a maximum average life span of 4.6 days (Clark and Kiesel 1963). Cross species transfusions in clinical practice are not advised.

Goats are considered to be a "large-spleened" domestic species. As such, the healthy goat can accommodate a blood loss of up to 25% of the red cell mass acutely, and up to a 50% loss over a twenty-four-hour period. In such cases, fluid replacement is of more concern than RBC replacement. In chronic blood loss, as often occurs with parasitic diseases, the PCV may reach levels as low as 9% without overt clinical manifestations of anemia, as long as the animal is not decompensated by stress, activity, or concurrent disease. Treatment of the underlying cause of anemia may be sufficient therapy without the need for blood transfusion. If the anemia is accompanied by profound hypoproteinemia with clinical signs of edema and ascites, plasma transfusions may be indicated.

For transfusions, the safe volume of blood that can be collected from a healthy goat has been reported as low as 6 ml/kg (Mitruka and Rawnsley 1981) to as high as 15 ml/kg bw (Bennett 1983). In practice, 10 ml/kg of bw is a reasonable volume. A 4% solution of sodium citrate is a suitable anticoagulant for blood collection, using 50 to 100 ml per 400 ml of blood collected. Collection bags or bottles should be swirled continuously during blood collection, and blood administered through a filtered system to remove possible clots. Blood can be safely given to recipients in volumes of 10 to 20 ml/kg bw.

Leukocyte Parameters

The mean white blood cell (WBC) count of the goat is generally reported to be 9,000 cells/ul with a range of 4,000 to 14,000. However, total WBC counts and differential cell counts may vary significantly with age as shown in Table 7.2. This is also true of the neutrophil to lymphocyte (N:L) ratio. The following mean N:L ratios have been reported for normal goats at different ages: one day old, 1.6:1; one week old, 0.8:1; one month old, 0.6:1; three months old, 0.3:1; two years of age, 1.1:1; and three years of age and older, 1.0:1 (Holman and Dew 1965a). These changes are partially due to a lower neutrophil count at birth that peaks at one month of age and then returns to and remains at birth levels after three months of age.

More significant is the dramatic two- to three-fold increase in lymphocyte numbers that occurs from birth to three months of age. Lymphocyte numbers begin to decline again and remain roughly equivalent to neutrophil numbers throughout adulthood. Eosinophils, basophils, and monocyte counts did not change notably with age in this study (Holman and Dew 1965a). However, in a field study with samplings of 1,000 goats in Mexico, eosinophil counts in kids younger than seven weeks of age averaged 0.5% of the WBC count, but 4.3% in adults (Earl and Carranza 1980).

Band neutrophils may represent up to 2.5% of the neutrophils in neonates as old as six weeks of age, but are rare or absent in health after this time. Lymphocytes in goats exhibit three distinct sizes: small, medium, and large. Young goats may exhibit two and a half times more small lymphocytes than large. It is postulated that the small lymphocytes represent thymocytes and that small lymphocyte numbers decrease as thymic involution progresses (Earl and Carranza 1980). Morphologically, large lymphocytes may be confused with monocytes. The large lymphocyte is distinguished by a nuclear chromatin that is condensed in large, irregularly shaped clumps, as compared with the looser, stringier chromatin pattern of monocytes.

Interpretation of Leukogram

Guidelines for interpretation of caprine leukograms have been suggested (Coles 1986). A WBC count more

Table 7.2. Total leukocyte numbers and differential counts in normal goats reported worldwide.

Country/reference	*Goat description*	*WBC count* ($\times 10^3$/ul)	*Mature neutrophils* (%)	*Band neutrophils* (%)	*Lymphocytes* (%)	*Monocytes* (%)	*Eosinophils* (%)	*Basophils* (%)	*References*
Mexico	2 days–7 weeks old	—	33.66 ± 12.56	0.90 ± 0.95	64.07 ± 13.00	0.82 ± 0.91	0.52 ± 0.72	0.03 ± 0.18	Earl and Carranza 1980
	Adults	—	50.28 ± 13.73	0.19 ± 0.43	43.43 ± 13.94	1.24 ± 1.11	4.27 ± 2.07	0.60 ± 0.77	"
United Kingdom	First day of life	7.52 ± 2.94	55.2 ± 17.9	—	41.3 ± 14.9	2.0 ± 1.3	0.7	0.2	Holman and Dew 1965
	1 week old	8.90 ± 4.14	42.9 ± 11.8	—	52.4 ± 11.9	2.6 ± 1.2	0.2	0.5	"
	1 month old	9.24 ± 2.42	32.7 ± 10.8	—	62.5 ± 9.4	2.1 ± 1.7	1.0	1.1	"
	3 months old	18.18 ± 3.84	22.5 ± 5.8	—	72.6 ± 11.5	2.0 ± 3.7	1.1	0.4	"
	2 years old	8.08 ± 2.51	49.0 ± 10.7	—	42.3 ± 10.4	3.1 ± 2.5	1.9	0.9	"
	3 years old and older	9.73 ± 2.51	47.7 ± 12.2	—	48.2 ± 12.0	2.2 ± 1.0	1.5	0.2	"
United States	Adults	13.30 ± 2.70	43.0 ± 6.7	—	51.0 ± 11.4	3.0	2.0	1.0	Lewis 1976

WBC = white blood cell.

than 13,000/ul constitutes leukocytosis and a count less than 4,000/ul, leukopenia. A neutrophil count greater than 7,200/ul represents neutrophilia and a count less than 1,200/ul, neutropenia. More than 100 band neutrophils/ul constitutes a left shift. Lymphocytosis is interpreted as a lymphocyte count greater than 9,000/ul and lymphopenia by a count less than 2,000/ul. Monocytosis is represented by a monocyte count more than 550/ul and eosinophilia by an eosinophil count more than 650/ul. Inflammatory responses in the goat often produce a neutrophilia with total WBC counts in the range of 22,000 to 27,000/ul. The maximum WBC count reported in a goat is 36,300/ul observed in association with a kidney abscess (Jain 1986).

A mature neutrophilia is often seen that in association with stress and chronic infections, particularly when abscesses develop as in caseous lymphadenitis or mastitis. Acute bacterial infections can produce a moderate to severe neutrophilia with some degree of left shift. Acute, severe coccidiosis in young kids is a frequent cause of marked neutrophilia and left shift.

Leukopenia is a common finding in infectious conditions of goats associated with the release of endotoxin. Transient leukopenia has been reported with experimental administration of staphylococcal enterotoxin B and *E. coli* endotoxin (Van miert et al. 1986). Leukopenia also occurs in theileriosis and tick-borne fever. Infection of WBCs is a fundamental part of the pathogenesis of these diseases. In theileriosis, lysis of lymphocytes occurs when protozoal merozoites are released into the bloodstream and lymphopenia may be observed. In tick-borne fever, *Ehrlichia phagocytophilia* invade the cytoplasm of granulocytes and monocytes, producing a marked leukopenia. Persistent leukopenia also has been reported in experimental heartwater disease (cowdriosis) (Illemobade and Blotkamp 1978) and as a result of plant poisoning with *Ipomoea carnea* in goats in the Sudan (Tartour et al. 1974).

Neoplastic transformation of lymphocytes may occur in caprine lymphosarcoma. This condition is not common in goats, and leukemia is a rare clinical presentation when the disease does occur. Peripheral lymphadenopathy is the clinical presentation most likely to suggest the diagnosis of lymphosarcoma in goats.

Platelet Parameters

The mean platelet count in the goat is generally considered to be 500,000/ul, with a range of 340,000 to 600,000/ul (Lewis 1976; Mitruka and Rawnsley 1981). One disparate study identified considerably lower counts in goats, with an average count of 116,000/ul during the first two weeks of life, decreasing to 28,000/ul by 1.5 years of age and stabilizing at an average of 62,550/ul by two years of age (Holman and Dew 1965a). These findings have not been duplicated by others. Platelets appear in the peripheral blood, usually in clusters of varying size. The platelets themselves also vary in size and shape, but all contain prominent azurophilic granules that are evenly distributed throughout the cytoplasm.

Coagulation Parameters

Two studies of coagulation parameters in the goat have been reported (Breukink et al. 1972; Lewis 1976). Both general coagulation tests and specific coagulation factor assays were conducted. Reported values are summarized in Table 7.3.

BASIC CAPRINE IMMUNOLOGY

The area of veterinary immunology has made considerable advances in recent years, but specific information on the caprine immune system remains relatively difficult to find in comparison to other domestic animal species. The purpose of this section is to highlight what is specifically known about the caprine immune system. A broader view of veterinary immunology is available from textbooks on the subject (Tizard and Schubot 2004)

There are no reported inherited immunodeficiencies in goats. Acquired immune-mediated diseases are uncommon and those that occur, such as the pemphigus complex, are discussed in the chapters relating to the organ system most affected. The most important immunological disease of goats is that shared with other ruminant species, namely, failure of passive transfer of immunologlobulins to the newborn via the dam's colostrum. Failure of passive transfer (FPT) is discussed in detail later in this chapter.

Immunoglobulins

The structure and function of ruminant immunoglobulins have been reviewed and the categories and distribution of caprine immunoglobulins fit the general ruminant pattern (Butler 1986). The major classes of immunoglobulin identified in the goat are IgG, IgA, and IgM. As in cattle and sheep, there are two distinct IgG subclasses, IgG_1 and IgG_2 (Gray et al. 1969). The major immunoglobulin in goat colostrum is IgG_1, and it is transported preferentially over IgG_2 into the mammary gland from serum (Micusan and Borduas 1976). This is presumably because of a higher affinity of IgG_1 for Fc receptors on mammary epithelial cells. IgG_1 is also the predominant circulating serum antibody produced in response to infection (Micusan and Borduas 1977). Local IgG_1 production has also been

Table 7.3. Coagulation parameters reported from normal goats.

Parameter	*Units*	*Mean*	*Standard deviation*	*Range*	*Reference*
Bleeding time	Minutes	—	—	1–5	Brooks et al. 1984
Clotting time	Minutes	5.5	±0.5	5.0–6.1	Lewis 1976
Lee-White; glass				1.0–5.0	Brooks et al. 1984
Clotting time Lee-White; plastic	Minutes	18.3	±4.5	12.3–23.0	Lewis 1976
Clotting time capillary method	Minutes			1.0–5.0	Brooks et al. 1984
Prothrombin time (PT)	Seconds	11.7	±0.5	9.0–14.0	Brooks et al. 1984
				11.2–12.3	Lewis 1976
		12.6		10.6–14.8	Breukink et al. 1972
Russell viper venom time (RVV)	Seconds	18.5	±1.3	17.2–19.4	Lewis 1976
Activated partial	Seconds	32.4	±7.5	28.4–37.6	Lewis 1976
thromboplastin time (APTT)		41.0		34.0–61.0	Breukink et al. 1972
Thrombin time (TT)	Seconds	27.0	±5.0	20.9–33.4	Lewis 1976
Fibrinogen	mg/dl			100–400	Brooks et al. 1984
		336	±66.1	268–435	Lewis 1976
		462		340–632	Breukink et al. 1972
Platelets/ul	$\times 10^3$	551	±92.9	378–656	Lewis 1976
		483		308–628	Breukink et al. 1972

demonstrated in synovial fluid, specifically in response to caprine arthritis encephalitis (CAE) virus infection (Johnson et al. 1983).

Very little is recorded about caprine IgM, possibly because little difference has been observed in the structure and function of IgM between ruminant species (Aalund 1972; Butler 1986). Caprine IgA has been isolated from serum, colostrum, milk, saliva, and urine. A distinct secretory component occurs in secretions, either in the free state or associated with IgA. The small amount of IgA found in serum is rarely associated with secretory component (Pahud and Mach 1970). IgA is considered the primary immunoglobulin of mucosal surfaces. In all the ruminants, including goats, immunoglobulins with biologic activities typical of IgE have been identified. IgE has become recognized as a useful marker for the development of parasite resistance in ruminant animals and efforts are underway to develop tests for the measurement of IgE to detect resistance. Partial DNA sequencing of caprine IgE has been reported as part of this overall effort (Griot-Wenk et al. 2000). Concentrations of caprine immunoglobulins in serum and various secretions are presented in Table 7.4.

Other Serum Proteins

The range of mean total serum protein concentrations reported in goats is from 6.75 to 7.53 gm/dl with concentrations in individual goats ranging from 5.9 to 8.3 gm/dl (Fletcher et al. 1964; Melby and Altman 1976; Mitruka and Rawnsley 1981). Concentrations for various serum proteins reported in goats are summarized in Table 7.5.

The normal range of plasma fibrinogen levels in goats, 0.1 to 0.4 gm/dl, is less than that of cows. Hyperfibrinogenemia frequently occurs in conjunction with neutrophilia in inflammatory responses. The maximum goat plasma fibrinogen recorded during inflammation is 1.1 gm/dl (Jain 1986).

Reports of complement component concentrations in goats are limited. However, one study demonstrates hemolytic, conglutinating, and bactericidal complement activity and indicates that complement activity is significantly less in kids younger than six months of age than in adults (Bhatnagar et al. 1988).

Cell-mediated Immune System

The induction of the host immune response begins at mucosal surfaces where immune cells in mucosa-associated lymphoid tissue (MALT) come into contact with and process antigens for subsequent transport to regional lymph nodes. The structure, function, and distribution of the caprine MALT system has been reviewed (Liebler-Tenorio and Pabst 2006).

Distinct populations of B and T lymphocytes have been identified in goats (Sulochana et al. 1982) and subpopulations of T lymphocytes also have been identified on the basis of reactivity and nonreactivity to

Table 7.4. Concentrations of immunoglobulin types in various body fluids of normal goats.

Source	*Total IgG (mg/ml ± S.D.)*	*IgG_1 (mg/ml)*	*IgG_2 (mg/ml)*	*IgA (mg/ml)*	*IgM (mg/ml)*	*Reference*
First colostrum	53.27 ± 5.30	50.83 ± 4.95	2.27 ± 1.32			*Micusan and Borduas 1977
	58.0 (50.0–64.0)			1.70 (0.90–2.40)	3.80 (1.60–5.20)	**Pahud and Mach 1970
Mature milk	0.25 (0.10–0.40)			0.06 (0.03–0.09)	0.03 (0.01–0.04)	**Pahud and Mach 1970
Normal adult serum	19.97 ± 1.55	10.92 ± 0.84	9.07 ± 0.78			*Micusan and Borduas 1977
	22.0 (18.0–24.0)			0.32 (0.05–0.90)	1.60 (0.80–2.0)	**Pahud and Mach 1970
Kid serum						
18 hours post suckling	73.59 ± 2.20					***Nandakumar and Rajagopalaraja 1983
1 week old		29.12 ± 4.80	nm			****Micusan et al. 1976
4 weeks old		16.18 ± 1.25	1.71 ± 0.92			**** Micusan et al. 1976
8 weeks old		11.92 ± 0.91	4.56 ± 0.84			****Micusan et al. 1976
12 weeks old		12.08 ± 0.35	8.32 ± 0.94			****Micusan et al. 1976
Adult saliva	0.10 (0.01–0.25)			0.20 (0.03–0.60)	t	**Pahud and Mach 1970

IgG = immunoglobin G, IgA = immunoglobin A, nm = not measurable, t = trace. *standard deviations, **ranges, ***not reported if SE or SD; ****standard errors.

peanut agglutinin (PNA) (Banks and Greenlee 1982). The percentages of B cells and PNA-positive T cells among peripheral blood lymphocytes have been reported, respectively, as 14% and 69% (Banks and Greenlee 1982; Hedden et al. 1986).

There are several reports on optimization, kinetics, and application of the *in vitro* lymphocyte transformation or blastogenesis assay for the measurement of lymphocyte responses using standard mitogens (Staples et al. 1981; Greenlee and Banks 1985), specific antigens, such as CAE virus (DeMartini et al. 1983), steroids (Staples et al. 1983), and allogeneic lymphocytes (van Dam et al. 1978).

Normal caprine neutrophil function has been evaluated in female goats using a variety of indices including migration, chemotaxis, bacterial ingestion, cytochrome C reduction, and antibody-dependent, cell-mediated cytotoxicity (Maddux and Keeton 1987). The effect of dexamethasone and levamisole on neutrophil functions has also been reported (Maddux and Keeton 1987a). Selenium deficiency in goats has been shown to have adverse effects on caprine neutrophil function (Aziz et al. 1984). There is very little information on characterization and function of caprine macrophages and nonneutrophil leukocytes.

Cytokines

Cytokines are proteins that play a central role as immune mediators during host responses against foreign pathogens. The role of cytokines in veterinary medicine has received considerable attention and a recent text on the subject has chapters on cattle, sheep, pigs, horses, dogs, cats, and birds, but alas, not on goats (Schijns and Horzinek 1997). Though knowledge on goat cytokines has not been comprehensively reviewed, information is available in various research reports.

Interleukin 1 (IL-1, endogenous pyrogen) occurs in the plasma of goats during bacterial-induced febrile episodes (Verheijden et al. 1983). Other studies have demonstrated the existence and activity of neutrophil chemotactic factor, leukocyte migration inhibition factor, and interleukin 2 (IL-2) in goats (Aziz and Klesius 1985, 1986). Caprine macrophages stimulated *in vitro* with lipopolysaccharide expressed tumor necrosis factor (TNF) and interleukin 6 (IL-6) (Adeyemo

Table 7.5. Reported concentrations of serum proteins from normal goats.

Protein	*Sex*	*Unit*	*Mean ± SD*	*Range*	*%*	*Reference*
Total protein	Both	gm/dl	6.90 ± 0.48	6.4–7.0	100	Brooks et al. 1984, Kaneko 1980
	Both			5.9–7.8		Mitruka and Rawnsley 1981
	Both		7.53			Hsu 1976
	Male		6.75 ± 0.35			Mitruka and Rawnsley 1981
	Female		6.90 ± 0.38			Mitruka and Rawnsley 1981
Albumin	Both	gm/dl	3.30 ± 0.33	2.7–3.9		Brooks et al. 1984, Kaneko 1980
	Both			2.45–4.35	33.5–66.5	Mitruka and Rawnsley 1981
	Both				44.3	Hsu 1976
	Male		3.46 ± 0.41			Mitruka and Rawnsley 1981
	Female		3.35 ± 0.42			Mitruka and Rawnsley 1981
Total globulin	Both		3.60 ± 0.50	2.7–4.1		Brooks et al. 1984, Kaneko 1980
Total alpha globulin	Both				10.3	Hsu 1976
	Both	gm/dl	0.60 ± 0.06	0.5–0.7		Kaneko 1980
Alpha$_1$ globulin	Both	gm/dl		0.5–0.7	4.2–8.3	Brooks et al. 1984
	Both			0.3–0.6		Mitruka and Rawnsley 1981
	Male		0.45 ± 0.05			Mitruka and Rawnsley 1981
	Female		0.40 ± 0.04			Mitruka and Rawnsley 1981
Alpha$_1$ globulin	Both	gm/dl		0.3–0.9	5.0–12.5	Mitruka and Rawnsley 1981
	Male		0.51 ± 0.06			Mitruka and Rawnsley 1981
	Female		0.68 ± 0.07			Mitruka and Rawnsley 1981
Total beta globulin	Both	gm/dl		1.0–2.0	14.8–28.5	Mitruka and Rawnsley 1981
	Both				14.3	Hsu 1976
	Male		1.33 ± 0.14			Mitruka and Rawnsley 1981
	Female		1.61 ± 0.15			Mitruka and Rawnsley 1981
Beta$_1$ globulin	Both	gm/dl	0.90 ± 0.10	0.7–1.2		Brooks et al. 1984, Kaneko 1980
Beta$_2$ globulin	Both	gm/dl	0.40 ± 0.02	0.3–0.6		Brooks et al. 1984, Kaneko 1980
Total gamma globulin	Both	gm/dl		0.5–1.5	7.0–21.0	Mitruka and Rawnsley 1981
	Both				30.6	Hsu 1976
	Both		1.70 ± 0.44	0.9–3.0		Kaneko 1980
	Male		1.05 ± 0.15			Mitruka and Rawnsley 1981
	Female		0.86 ± 0.14			Mitruka and Rawnsley 1981
A/G ratio	Both	Ratio	0.63 ± 1.26			Brooks et al. 1984, Kaneko 1980
	Both		0.71 ± 1.26			Mitruka and Rawnsley 1981
	Male		1.05 ± 0.11			Mitruka and Rawnsley 1981
	Female		0.95 ± 0.12			Mitruka and Rawnsley 1981
Fibrinogen (plasma)	Both	gm/dl		0.1–0.4		Brooks et al. 1984, Kaneko 1980

et al. 1997). Interleukin 8 (IL-8) and monocyte chemoattractant protein 1 (MCP-1) were expressed by CAE-infected caprine macrophages *in vitro* (Lechner et al. 1997) and interleukin 16 (IL-16) was expressed at higher levels from peripheral blood mononuclear cells and synovial membrane cells of goats infected with CAE than from cells from control goats (Sharmila et al. 2002). Goats with caseous lymphadenitis produced greater interferon gamma (IFN-γ) responses than uninfected goats when cells in whole blood were stimulated *in vitro* with either *Corynebacterium pseudotuberculosis*-secreted antigen alone or with pokeweed mitogen (Meyer et al. 2005).

Major Histocompatibility Complex (MHC)

The MHC of goats is called the goat lymphocyte antigen (GLA) system. Both serologically defined (SD) class I and lymphocyte defined (LD) class II antigens have been identified. Three distinct gene clusters appear to be involved in expression of the GLA: an SD_1, an SD_2, and an LD, producing five, four, and four antigenic specificities respectively (van Dam et al.

1979, 1980, 1981). A more recent report suggests as many as twenty-seven class I antigen specificities (Ruff and Lazary 1987). Cross-matching for GLA antigens prolongs skin graft survival time (van Dam et al. 1978a). Also, the degree of humoral immune response has been associated with GLA type. Increased antibody responses to tetanus toxoid were demonstrated in goats with GLA-SD_{1-2} and SD_{1-4} specificities (van Dam and van Kooten 1980). Additional information on the caprine MHC is available elsewhere (Obexer-Ruff et al. 1996).

DIAGNOSIS OF HEMIC-LYMPHATIC DISEASES BY PRESENTING SIGN

Bleeding Disorders

Indications of bleeding disorders include petechial or ecchymotic hemorrhages of mucous membranes, prolonged bleeding from venipuncture sites or surgical wounds, passage of blood from body orifices, or development of subcutaneous or periarticular swellings. Such signs can result from vasculitis, platelet disorders, or coagulopathies. These categories of disease have received limited attention in goats.

Inherited afibrinogenemia has been reported in a family of Saanen goats (Breukink et al. 1972). The inheritance pattern is incomplete autosomal dominant. There is complete absence of circulating fibrinogen in homozygous individuals, and goats thus affected do not live past the kid stage. Unchecked umbilical hemorrhage at birth is the most common presentation, but recurrent hemarthroses and subcutaneous and mucosal hemorrhage can also be seen. Clotting time, thrombin time, stage 1 prothrombin, and partial thromboplastin times are all prolonged in afibrinogenemia. Fibrinogen concentration, as measured by bioassay of thrombin-clottable protein, is always under 0.15 gm/dl and is usually zero. Acquired coagulation disorders presumably occur in the goat at a rate similar to other species, but the literature on specific causes or cases of coagulopathy in the goat is sparse. Bleeding from the orifices of a dead goat is suggestive of anthrax.

Thrombocytopenia is reported as a consistent finding in African trypanosomosis in all affected species, including goats (Davis 1982). The degree of thrombocytopenia and the development of subsequent hemorrhage are directly correlated to the degree of parasitemia that develops.

Bracken fern *(Pteridium aquilinum)* ingestion by cattle can lead to a syndrome of pancytopenia with leukopenia, thrombocytopenia, and anemia. Melena, epistaxis, and widespread petechial and ecchymotic hemorrhage are major clinical findings. While the morbidity rate may be low, the mortality rate is high. There is one report of naturally occurring bracken fern toxicity in goats, but no signs of hemorrhage were observed (Tomlinson 1983).

Hemorrhagic diathesis is considered to be a clinical manifestation of severe, diffuse liver disease in other farm animal species (Radostits et al. 2007). However, a review of liver diseases of sheep and goats did not identify coagulopathy as a clinical outcome of hepatic disease (Fetcher 1983). The only report documenting decreased clotting activity in goats in association with liver disease involved experimental dosing with carbon tetrachloride (Jones and Shah 1982).

Anemia

Anemia is suggested clinically by pale or white mucous membranes (Figure 7.1), exercise intolerance, tachypnea, tachycardia, possible systolic murmurs, weakness, and (in extreme cases) collapse. When anemia is a result of intravascular hemolysis, then jaundice and hemoglobinuria are also important clinical signs. Signs of anemia are frequently accompanied by signs of hypoproteinemia, particularly intermandibular edema, ascites, and weight loss. Anemia is a common and important clinical presentation in goats.

Causes of Hemolytic Anemia

Important, established causes of hemolytic anemia in goats include the hemoparasitic diseases anaplasmosis, babesiosis, eperythrozoonosis, and theileriosis; nutritional disorders including copper toxicity, kale ingestion, and consumption of other, regional poisonous plants; and an infectious cause, leptospirosis.

Other suspected causes of hemolytic anemia in goats include infections due to *Clostridium novyi* type D *(C. hemolyticum)* and *Clostridium perfringens* type A,

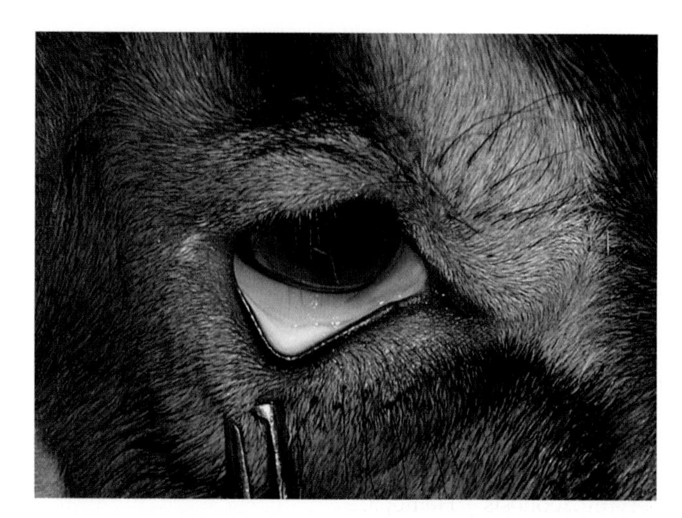

Figure 7.1. White-colored conjunctiva characteristic of a goat with marked anemia. In normal goats, the color is pink to red. (Courtesy of Dr. M.C. Smith.)

as reported in sheep. Experimental poisoning with oak tannins caused marked hemolytic anemia in goats, but naturally occurring oak poisoning is uncommon in this species (Begovic et al. 1978). Experimental infections of sarcocystosis (sarcosporidiosis) produce hemolytic anemia (Dubey et al. 1981), but almost all known naturally occurring infections in goats are subclinical, producing muscle cysts seen at slaughter or necropsy, as discussed further in Chapter 4.

Two reports suggest hypophosphatemia as the cause of hemolytic anemia and hemoglobinuria in female goats, but in two of the three reported cases, serum inorganic phosphorus levels were in the normal range (Setty and Narayana 1975; Samad and Ali 1984). In cattle with post-parturient hemoglobinuria, serum inorganic phosphorus levels are well below the normal range.

Causes of Blood Loss Anemia

Anemia due to loss of blood is of major clinical significance in goats. The condition is most often associated with some form of parasitism. Important causes of blood loss anemia include infestations by *Haemonchus* spp., and liver flukes, especially *Fasciola hepatica*. External parasitic causes include sucking lice, ticks, and fleas (Schillhorn van Veen and Mohammed 1975). Predation may be another important cause of blood loss. While wild predators can be expected to kill goats outright unless interrupted, domesticated dogs often maim goats without killing them. Severe hemorrhagic trauma often results.

Causes of Anemia Due to Impaired Erythropoiesis

Anemias of this type occur infrequently or are overshadowed by other concurrent and more prominent clinical signs. Nutritional causes include cobalt, copper, and iron deficiencies. Toxic causes include fluorosis and possibly bracken fern ingestion. Anemia of chronic infection also occurs in goats (e.g., in paratuberculosis).

Iron deficiency is associated with prolonged feeding of doe's milk to kids without mineral supplementation or access to forage. Copper deficiency manifests primarily as a neurologic disease in young kids. In experimentally induced cobalt deficiency in goats, a macrocytic, normochromic anemia was observed in addition to weight loss (Mgongo et al. 1981). In naturally occurring cases of cobalt deficiency, ill thrift is a consistent finding, but the presence of anemia is variable (Brain 1983; Black et al. 1988). Nonregenerative anemia has been documented in chronic fluorosis of goats grazing near a superphosphate factory in Egypt (Karram et al. 1984). One incident of bracken fern poisoning has been reported goats. Anemia was present, but may have been due to concurrent parasitism (Tomlinson 1983).

Documented causes of anemia in goats are summarized in Table 7.6. The table emphasizes concurrent clinical and laboratory findings, such as hypoproteinemia and hemoglobinuria that can aid in the differential diagnosis of anemia. All of the hemoparasitic diseases, leptospirosis, copper poisoning, phosphorus

Table 7.6. Anemia in goats: Aids for differential diagnosis.

Cause of anemia	*Pathogenesis and morphologic type*	*Role of anemia in disease*	*Total serum protein*	*Icterus*	*Hemoglobinuria*	*Other clinical signs*	*Comments*
Anaplasmosis	Hemoparasitic; extravascular hemolysis; regenerative	Major	Normal	Likely	No	Few; abortions can occur, concurrent disease common	Often subclinical
Babesiosis	Hemoparasitic; intravascular hemolysis	Major	Normal	Likely	Likely	Fever, diarrhea, abortion	Poorly described in goats
Theileriosis	Hemoparasitic; pathogenesis of anemia unclear	Minor	Normal	Variable	Transient	Fever, swollen lymph nodes, lacrimation	Primarily a parasite of white cells
Trypanosomosis	Hemoparasitic; mainly extravascular hemolysis	Major	Normal to low	Unlikely	Unlikely	Fever, edema, lymphadenopathy, weight loss	Seen primarily in Africa
Eperythrozoonosis	Hemoparasitic; mainly extravascular hemolysis	Major	Normal	Likely	No	None, but concurrent disease common	Poorly described in goats

Table 7.6. *Continued*

Cause of anemia	*Pathogenesis and morphologic type*	*Role of anemia in disease*	*Total serum protein*	*Icterus*	*Hemoglobinuria*	*Other clinical signs*	*Comments*
Leptospirosis	Septicemia; intravascular hemolysis	Major	Normal	Yes	Yes	Fever, abortion	Uncommon in goats
Copper poisoning	Nutritional; intravascular hemolysis	Major	Normal	Yes	Yes	Acute death	Goats more resistant than sheep
Haemonchus spp.	Gastric parasite; blood loss anemia	Major	Low	No	No	Weight loss, edema	Major cause of anemia in goats
Coccidiosis	Intestinal parasite; blood loss anemia	Major	Low	No	No	Diarrhea or dysentery; dehydration	Especially young goats affected
Liver flukes	Liver parasite; blood loss anemia	Major	Low	Likely	No	Weight loss, edema, ascites, eosinophilia	
Schistosomosis	Vascular parasite; blood loss anemia	Major	Low	No	No	Weight loss, diarrhea, ascites	Numerous spp. affect the goat
External parasites (ticks, fleas, lice)	Skin parasites; blood loss anemia	Usually minor	Normal to low	No	No	Pruritus, rough hair coat	Sucking lice and fleas may cause severe anemia
Trauma/predation	Blood loss anemia	Minor	Normal to low	No	No	Shock, musculoskeletal	Predation a serious problem
Cobalt deficiency	Nutritional; RBC multiplication reduced; macrocytic anemia	Minor	Normal to low	No	No	Weight loss, diarrhea, lacrimation, weakness	Mimics gastrointestinal parasitism
Copper deficiency	Nutritional; reduced heme synthesis; microcytic anemia	Minor	Normal	No	No	Enzootic ataxia, or "swayback"	Primarily neurologic; mostly in young goats
Iron deficiency	Nutritional; reduced heme synthesis; microcytic anemia	Minor	Normal	No	No	None	Uncommon; seen in milk-fed kids
Phosphorus deficiency	Nutritional; hemolytic anemia	Major	Normal	Yes	Yes	None	Some cases reported from India
Chronic diseases (e.g., paratubercuosis)	Anemia of chronic disease, nonregenerative	Minor	High to low	No	No	Weight loss, possible edema	
Kale poisoning	Plant toxicity; Heinz body anemia; regenerative	Major	Normal	Likely	No	None	Goats more resistant than cattle

RBC = red blood cell.

deficiency, kale ingestion, and other poisonous plants causing anemia are discussed in detail later in this chapter. Other diseases associated with anemia are discussed elsewhere in the text because other clinical signs predominate.

Lymphadenopathy

Transient swelling of select regional lymph nodes can be expected in common, localized infections such as mastitis, or subsequent to vaccinations. Persistent lymphadenopathy, however, is a major clinical finding in many important caprine diseases including caseous lymphadenitis, theileriosis, trypanosomosis, melioidosis, tuberculosis, nocardiosis, and lymphosarcoma. Theileriosis and trypanosomosis are discussed in detail in this chapter because of the significant role of anemia in these diseases. The remainder of the diseases are discussed in Chapter 3.

SPECIFIC DISEASES OF THE HEMIC-LYMPHATIC SYSTEM

RICKETTSIAL DISEASES

Anaplasmosis

Anaplasmosis is an arthropod-borne, rickettsial, hemoparasitic disease of ruminant animals that causes hemolysis. It is usually a subclinical disease in goats and sheep, with goats more likely to manifest clinical signs.

Etiology

In goats, the causative agent is *Anaplasma ovis*. In sheep it is *A. ovis* and a species described in Europe as *A. mesaeterum*, but not listed in the 1980 Approved Lists (Euzéby 2003); in cattle, *A. marginale* and *A. centrale*; and in wild ruminants, *A. marginale* and *A. ovis*. Goats may be transiently infected with *A. marginale* and *A. mesaeterum*, but do not become clinically ill, and are unlikely to be a reservoir of infection for cattle (Maas and Buening 1981). The discussion here is limited to *Anaplasma* organisms that produce erythrocytic anaplasmosis. Some rickettsial organisms that infect white blood cells have been transferred to the genus *Anaplasma* (Dumler et al. 2001) as discussed further in this chapter in the section on tick-borne fever.

Epidemiology

Caprine anaplasmosis has been reported widely in Africa, India, the Mediterranean countries, and the former USSR. In the United States it occurs in sheep but natural infection of goats has not been reported. Because of the largely subclinical nature of the disease in goats, it is often considered to be of minor economic importance (Akerejola et al. 1979). However, clinical disease due to *A. ovis* has been reported sporadically from Nigeria, India, and Iraq (Kuil and Folkers 1966; Mallick et al. 1979; Yousif et al. 1983). More recently, *A. ovis* infection has been implicated in abortion outbreaks in Boer goats in South Africa, and the economic impact of the disease may be more than previously imagined (Barry and van Niekerk 1987).

The disease is spread by a variety of ticks, particularly *Rhipicephalus* and *Dermacentor* spp., while *Haemaphysalis* and *Ornithodoros* spp. have also been incriminated. Ticks become infected by feeding on infected animals; transmission is probably transstadial and intrastadial, as it is in bovine anaplasmosis. The role of other insects, contaminated syringes, and other veterinary equipment in the mechanical transmission of *A. ovis* in goats has not been investigated although such transmission is known in bovine anaplasmosis. *In utero* transmission of *A. ovis* has been established in sheep, and also confirmed in goats (Barry and van Niekerk 1987a).

The severity of clinical disease in cattle increases with advancing age. In experimental infection of goats with *A. ovis*, no correlation of disease severity with age was discernible although older animals did have a greater reduction in red cell mass (Splitter et al. 1956). A carrier state develops with *A. ovis* in goats although sterile protective immunity may occur. Recrudescence of clinical disease is possible when the carrier is sufficiently stressed.

Pathogenesis

The disease produced by *A. ovis* is primarily an anemia. Parasitized RBCs are destroyed in the spleen and bone marrow and the severity of anemia generally correlates with the percentage of parasitized cells. However, immune-mediated destruction of nonparasitized cells may also contribute to the degree of anemia. In experimentally infected goats, the prepatent period was eight to twenty-three days, with parasitized erythrocytes first evident at an average of fifteen days post inoculation. Maximum parasitemia occurred fifteen to thirty days post inoculation and the lowest RBC counts occurred from twenty-three to thirty-four days after inoculation. On average, RBC count, PCV, and Hb decreased more than 50%. Complement fixing antibody began to appear anywhere from eight days before to one week after the appearance of parasitized erythrocytes and remained detectable in carrier animals for as long as one year (Splitter et al. 1956).

Clinical Findings

While *A. ovis* infection is often subclinical in the goat, concurrent disease problems, malnutrition, and other stressors may precipitate clinical anaplasmosis. The most consistent clinical finding may be exercise intolerance, but other signs may be observed including a fever up to 107.5°F (41.9°C), anorexia, depression, weakness, pallor of mucous membranes, dyspnea, and increased heart rate. If anemia is extreme, icterus may be present, but hemoglobinuria is an uncommon event. Subclinically infected animals may show only pallor. Diagnosis of anaplasmosis requires laboratory confirmation.

Clinical Pathology and Necropsy

Unless there is concurrent disease, the leukogram is likely to be unchanged. Erythrocyte parameters are reduced during clinical and, to a lesser extent, subclinical disease. A mean RBC count of 7.45×10^6/ml, mean PCV of 23.4%, and mean Hb of 6.8 gm/dl have been reported in cases with clinical signs of jaundice, weakness, and ill thrift (Yousif et al. 1983). In terminal cases, RBC counts, PCV, and Hb as low as 2.92 10^6/ml, 10%, and 2.8 gm/dl, respectively, have been observed (Mallick et al. 1979). Staining of peripheral blood smears with Wright's or Giemsa stain reveals the organisms in the erythrocytes. Like *A. marginale*, some 60% to 70% of *A. ovis* organisms are found on the periphery of the red blood cell, while as many as 40% of *A. ovis* are submarginal or central in location. The organism is most evident during active parasitemia and may be difficult or impossible to find during the prepatent period or during the carrier state. Even during parasitemia, only a maximum of 6.8% of red cells were observed to be parasitized during experimental subclinical infection, and only 2.7% in naturally occurring clinical disease. Therefore, careful examination of the smear is advisable. Increased MCV, anisocytosis, and polychromasia may be observed during convalescence.

To confirm infection during the carrier state, serologic testing may be necessary. Complement fixing antibody titers are highest during and immediately after active parasitemia but persist with variable intensity during the subsequent carrier state. False-negative tests can occur in some carriers. The most definitive test for establishing the carrier state is the inoculation of a splenectomized goat with blood of the suspected carrier. Other serologic tests include a capillary tube agglutination test, a rapid card agglutination test, a fluorescent antibody test, and an enzyme-linked immunoabsorbent assay test. The capillary tube agglutination test has been reported to be reliable in the diagnosis of caprine anaplasmosis (Mallick et al. 1979).

Necropsy may reveal thin, watery blood, pallor, and jaundice of tissues. The liver may be enlarged and orange in color.

Diagnosis

Anaplasmosis occurs in regions where other caprine hemoparasitic diseases also occur, including babesiosis, eperythrozoonosis, cowdriosis, and theileriosis. In fact, it is not unusual for some of these conditions to occur simultaneously in the same animal, and laboratory confirmation of anaplasmosis is essential to establish infection. Clinically, the absence of hemoglobinuria distinguishes anaplasmosis from babesiosis, leptospirosis, copper toxicity, and other causes of intravascular hemolysis.

Treatment

Treatment is most effective during the parasitemic phase of disease and is directed at reducing the rate of erythrocyte infection. The stress of handling ill animals for repeated therapy may be fatal when anemia is severe. Treatment administered during the prepatent period slows but does not prevent the onset of parasitemia. Oxytetracycline and tetracycline hydrochloride have been used successfully to treat clinically affected goats at an intramuscular dose of 10 mg/kg bw given once a day for one or two days. However, this dose given once a day for three to five days will not eliminate the carrier state. In cattle, the use of long-acting tetracycline preparations at a dose of 20 mg/kg given once a week for two to four weeks has been effective in this regard. Imidocarb diproprionate may be useful in caprine anaplasmosis but information on dosage and treatment schedules for goats is limited.

Control

In general, efforts to control the spread of anaplasmosis by controlling the biologic vectors are not practical except on a local basis through repeated dipping or spraying. There is no evidence that available *A. marginale* bovine vaccines offer any protection against *A. ovis* infection in small ruminants, and no specific vaccine for *A. ovis* is currently available. In lieu of vaccination, prophylactic antibiotic administration might be used to prevent the spread of infection in the case of an outbreak. In exposed cattle, oxytetracycline is administered at a dose of 1 to 2 mg/kg bw daily for ten days to prevent infection. The cost benefit of this program is difficult to evaluate in goats because uncomplicated caprine anaplasmosis is most often a subclinical disease.

Eperythrozoonosis

This hemoparasitic disease of goats is of little clinical and economic significance and is caused by the organism *Eperythrozoon ovis*. This organism, formerly classified in the *Rickettsiales*, is now known to belong to the *Mycoplasmatales* (Neimark et al. 2004), but the differences with classical *Mycoplasma* spp. do not warrant fusion of the two genera (Uilenberg et al. 2006).

Epidemiology

While *E. ovis* infection of sheep is known to occur widely in Europe, Africa, Australia, North America, and the Middle East, reports of infection in goats have come only from Pakistan, South Africa, Australia, and most recently, Cuba (Joa et al. 1987). Transmission is probably by biting insects, contaminated needles, and surgical instruments. In Tasmania, a serologic survey indicated widespread infection in sheep with *E. ovis*, but virtually no infection in goats, suggesting the possibility of different vectors for the two animal species, or a difference in host susceptibility to chronic infection (Mason et al. 1989).

Etiology and Pathogenesis

The same organism, *E. ovis*, is infective for both sheep and goats, though a dimorphism has been noted. On Giemsa-stained smears, the organism on sheep erythrocytes demonstrates a large ring form, while in goats smaller ring and coccoid forms predominate (Daddow 1979, 1979a). In both small ruminant species, subclinical or latent infection is the rule; when clinical disease appears, it is often triggered by concurrent problems such as malnutrition or gastrointestinal parasitism. In experimental infection the prepatent period is six days for both species but the degree and length of parasitemia is shorter in the goat, lasting four weeks compared with six in the sheep. A carrier state developed in goats, with blood infective as long as fourteen months after infection (Daddow 1979).

Clinical Signs

Clinical disease is rarely observed in goats. The disease is characterized in sheep by weakness, unthriftiness, anemia, and mild icterus. Staggering and stiffness of the hindquarters have also been reported in sheep.

Diagnosis

The organism can be found on erythrocytes in Giemsa-stained blood smears during the parasitemia. However, clinical signs of anemia may not be recognizable until the waning stages of parasitemia. Antibody may also be detected with the CF test for up to three weeks after clinical signs are observed. However, false-negative results may occur (Daddow 1977). Low levels of antibody may also be intermittently detectable during subsequent carrier states. It is recommended that the CF test be used on a herd basis rather than for individual diagnosis. Differential diagnoses include other hemoparasites, especially anaplasmosis, malnutrition, gastrointestinal parasitism, and cobalt deficiency.

Treatment and Control

Treatment may alleviate clinical disease, but may not clear the carrier state. Single-dose therapy with either neoarsphenamine at a dose of 30 mg/kg, antimosan at 6 mg/kg, or oxytetracycline at 6.6 mg/kg have been recommended for sheep. No specific therapeutic evaluations have been reported in goats. Control involves good preventive medicine programs to avoid predisposing conditions as well as the single animal use of needles and surgical equipment.

Tick-borne Fever

Tick-borne fever is a tick-transmitted rickettsial disease of goats, sheep, and cattle caused by the organism *Anaplasma phagocytophilum*, formerly classified in the genus *Ehrlichia (E. phagocytophila)*. There are several strains of this organism which differ in host pathogenicity—the zoonotic HGE agent that causes human granulocytic ehrlichiosis (or human anaplasmosis), strains formerly called *E. equi* that cause equine ehrlichiosis (or equine anaplasmosis), and others more adapted to cattle and/or small ruminants that cause pasture fever or tick-borne fever. Dogs can also be infected. The condition is characterized in all ruminant species by fever and leukopenia. Abortions commonly occur in affected sheep and cattle, but not goats. Tick-borne fever in endemic areas causes noticeable losses in goats because of decreased milk production and secondary infections resulting from impaired immune responses.

Epidemiology

The disease occurs in cattle and sheep throughout Europe, wherever its tick vector, *Ixodes ricinus*, occurs. *I. persulcatus* in eastern Europe is also a vector. A similar organism has also been reported from India. Strains causing human and equine ehrlichiosis (or anaplasmosis) in the United States are transmitted by *I. scapularis*. Reports of naturally occurring tick-borne fever in goats have come only from Scotland and Norway (Melby and Grønstøl 1984; Gray et al. 1988). It is reasonable to assume, however, that where the disease occurs in sheep, goats are susceptible. In Europe, the tick vector *Ixodes ricinus* favors wet, cool, woodland pastures, and forest. In Scotland, the infection has been identified in feral goats, which are considered a wildlife reservoir along with the red, roe, and fallow deer (Foster and Greig 1969). The incidence of disease increases in spring and autumn, with increased tick activity.

Etiology and Pathogenesis

The causative agent of tick-borne fever in cattle and small ruminants is *Anaplasma (Ehrlichia) phagocytophilum*, but bovine and ovine strains are recognized. Strains isolated from sheep readily produce the disease experimentally in goats and vice versa. The infectivity of the bovine strains can be less in small ruminants than cattle. Cross immunity between strains is not always complete. Related organisms, with other tick vectors, are *Anaplasma* or *Ehrlichia bovis* in cattle and *Ehrlichia ovina* in sheep.

Infected ticks introduce the organism into host animals in their saliva during blood feeding. Because the organism is passed transstadially and not transovarially in the tick, only nymphal and adult stage ticks can transmit the infection to ruminants. When entering the host's bloodstream, the organism invades neutrophilic granulocytes, and to a lesser extent macrophages, where it replicates. In experimental infection of goats, high fever and granulocyte inclusions are seen by day three after infection. By day seven after infection, the total WBC count may drop to 27% of the level before infection. There is a transient lymphopenia and a persistent neutropenia, with no left shift. A transient eosinophilia is also observed around day five after infection (Van Miert et al. 1984).

It is believed that the invasion of leukocytes stimulates interleukin-1 (endogenous pyrogen) release that accounts for the high fever, rumen stasis, and other signs seen in clinical disease. The transient lymphopenia and neutropenia may impair immune defenses and predispose affected animals to serious secondary infections and increased risk of mortality.

There is limited information on morbidity and mortality rates in goats. In a report from Scotland, twenty-five goats were at risk. Thirteen had detectable antibody responses to tick-borne fever, seven showed clinical signs of disease, and one died (Gray et al. 1988). In a Norwegian report, fifty of 103 goats in a dairy herd were affected by tick-borne fever, including all goats younger than one year of age (Melby and Grønstøl 1984). While a low level of immunity develops after infection, the organism has been reported to persist in the blood stream of infected sheep for as long as two years.

Clinical Signs

Clinical signs reported in goats include a fever often higher than 106°F (41°C) that persists for three to six days accompanied by dullness, anorexia, decreased rumen motility, tachycardia, tachypnea, occasional shivering, and coughing. In lactating does, there is a significant drop in milk production. Animals should be examined for ticks. In contrast to sheep and cattle, abortion and secondary bacterial infections have not played a significant part in reported outbreaks of caprine tick-borne fever. Complete recovery may take several weeks.

Clinical Pathology and Necropsy

By day three of infection, the organism should be readily apparent in neutrophils in peripheral blood smears stained with methylene blue. The organism is located within vacuoles in the cell cytoplasm. Leukopenia is marked, with white blood cell counts commonly less than 3,500 by day seven. Initially there is a reversal of the neutrophil-to-lymphocyte ratio because of a transient lymphopenia. Subsequently, lymphocyte numbers return toward normal and neutrophil numbers continue to decrease. A decrease in serum alkaline phosphatase has been observed in the acute phase of tick-borne fever in goats, but the cause is unclear. There are no remarkable necropsy findings.

Diagnosis

A presentation of high fever in tick-infested goats should suggest tick-borne fever in endemic areas. In the acute phase of disease, identification of the organism in neutrophils in peripheral blood smears is diagnostic. Serologic evidence of infection may be obtained by complement fixation test or counter immunoelectrophoresis (Webster and Mitchell 1988), as well as an indirect immunofluorescent test (Jongejan et al. 1989). Louping-ill, a viral disease, is also transmitted by *Ixodes ricinus* and can produce fever. The two diseases can occur concurrently in endemic areas. Louping-ill produces neurologic signs, and serologic evidence of infection can be obtained.

Treatment and Control

Several drugs have been evaluated for treatment of goats (Anika et al. 1986, 1986a). A single intravenous injection of oxytetracycline at a dose of 10 mg/kg resulted in a return to normal body temperature in six hours and killing of intracellular organisms. A single intravenous dose of trimethoprim (20 mg/kg) in combination with sulphamethylphenazole (50 mg/kg) and sulphadimidine (50 mg/kg) was also effective, as is chloramphenicol in a single intravenous dose of 50 mg/kg, where its use is permitted. Spiramycin and ampicillin were not effective against tick-borne fever.

Control of tick-borne fever involves controlling exposure of goats to ticks. Pasturing young goats in tick-infested areas during seasons of low tick activity may promote immunity and reduce the severity of disease that develops during periods of increased exposure. The use of acaricides during seasons of high tick activity may also be beneficial.

BACTERIAL DISEASES

Leptospirosis

Leptospirosis is a contagious, zoonotic disease caused by various serovars of the spirochete *Leptospira interrogans*. Goats and sheep are less susceptible to leptospirosis than cattle, swine, dogs, and man, and the disease is uncommon in small ruminants. Most leptospiral infections of goats are probably subclinical, although epizootics of abortion have been reported, as have outbreaks of acute septicemia with hemolytic jaundice. The two syndromes can occur simultaneously. Numerous serologic prevalence surveys of caprine leptospirosis have been done, but descriptions of clinical disease are limited.

Etiology

Several serovars of *L. interrogans* have been identified in clinical caprine leptospirosis, most notably *L. pomona, L. grippotyphosa, L. icterohemorrhagiae*, and *L. serjoe*. Additional serovars identified infrequently in apparently healthy goats on serologic survey include *L. autumnalis, L. australis, L. balcanica, L. ballum, L. bataviae, L. bratislava, L. canicola, L. hardjo, L. hyos, L. panama, L. pyrogenes*, and *L. wolfii*.

Epidemiology

Leptospiral infection of goats has been reported from Brazil, Israel, Iran, India, Kenya, Nigeria, Turkey, Spain, Italy, Portugal, the former USSR, Jamaica, Grenada, New Zealand, and the United States. Serious outbreaks of disease with high morbidity and mortality rates in goats have been reported from Iran and Israel. In both countries, *L. grippotyphosa* was involved. In the Iranian epizootic, morbidity was between 90% and 100% for both sheep and goats, but goats showed a mortality rate of 42%, compared with 18% in sheep (Amjadi and Ahourai 1975). In Israel, the morbidity rate was also higher in affected goats than sheep, and goat mortality was also as high as 44% in some herds (Van der Hoeden 1953). In Nigeria, abortions in a university herd of west African dwarf goats were diagnosed as due to leptospirosis. Affected animals also showed diarrhea and jaundice. The predominant serovar was *L. pomona*, but antibodies to *L. grippotyphosa* and *L. icterohemorrhagiae* were also identified in some individuals (Agunloye et al. 1996).

In southern Spain, the seroprevalence was reported as 16.1% in goats and leptospirosis, primarily *L. pomona*, accounted for 2.6% of 262 caprine abortion outbreaks investigated over a fifteen-year period (Leon-Vizcaino et al. 1987). In a Jamaican survey, 35% of 1,545 goats tested were seropositive (Oliveira 1987). In one Brazilian study, the seroprevalence was 0.9% in confined or semiconfined dairy herds, but 6.7% among goats kept under subsistence conditions (Silva et al. 1984). In a more recent study from Brazil, seroprevalence was higher in goats that grazed more than two hours per day as compared to those that grazed less, suggesting a greater risk of exposure to leptospires through grazing. Seroprevalence was also greater in goats in tropical climatic settings than in temperate settings, suggesting that heat stress and rainfall contributed to infection (Lilenbaum et al. 2008). The predominant serovar in the survey was *L. hardjo*

The goat is most likely exposed to infection from wild rodents or other infected livestock shedding the organism in urine, and is not itself considered a persistent reservoir of infection (Schollum and Blackmore 1981). However, goats can shed the organism in urine for at least one month after an acute infection and should be considered as potential sources of new infections during that time.

Leptospires most commonly gain entrance to the host through skin or mucosal abrasions. They are readily killed by drying, but thrive under warm, moist conditions and will persist in contaminated, standing water for long periods. In the Iranian epizootic, the outbreak was attributed to a period of frequent rain, flooding, and warm weather that favored the environmental survival and spread of leptospires. In the Israeli report, the incidence of clinical cases fell off rapidly when the wet winter season ended and dry spring weather began. In Brazil, as well, the occurrence of leptospirosis in goats is associated with increased rainfall (Alves et al. 1996)

Pathogenesis

Infection leads to a septicemic leptospiremia, followed by clearance of the blood as antibody response develops, and subsequent localization of the organism in the kidney with leptospiruria. Death may occur during the septicemic phase. Hemolytic anemia may develop as a result of hemolysin production by certain serovars of *L. interrogans*. In sheep, at least, leptospirosis can also produce immune mediated hemolytic anemia. Abortion results from transplacental passage of leptospires during the septicemic phase with death of the fetus. This is more likely to occur in the second half of pregnancy. In animals that survive acute infection, a strong immunity develops against the inciting serovar, but cross immunity does not occur.

Clinical Signs

In acute leptospirosis goats may show a fever of 104°F to 106.7°F (40°F to 41.5°C), marked depression, and inappetence after an incubation period of four to eight days. Heart rate is elevated and the animals are dyspneic. Icterus of mucous membranes is a prominent finding, and petechial hemorrhages of the conjunctivae may be observed. Reddish brown urine indicative of hemoglobinuria is evident. Pregnant animals often abort. In untreated animals, death can occur within two to three days. Subclinical infections commonly occur in seemingly unaffected herd mates.

Clinical Pathology and Necropsy

A moderate to severe hemolytic anemia develops concurrently with the onset of clinical signs, and hemoglobinuria is present. In animals that do not die, there is soon evidence of a regenerative erythroid response. Leukopenia occurs during the acute phase of disease in cattle, but has not been reported in goats. Thrombocytopenia can occur in all affected species, with or without evidence of concurrent disseminated intravascular coagulation.

At necropsy, icterus is pronounced and extensive in acute leptospirosis (Amjadi and Ahourai 1975). Edema and ecchymosis of the subcutis and serous membranes occur. Lungs may be pale and edematous with widening of the interlobular septa with yellow serous fluid. The liver may be enlarged and friable with extensive subcapsular hemorrhage. The kidneys are swollen, dark brown, and have a rough surface. Grayish streaks may be noted in the renal cortex. Histologic examination indicates renal tubular degeneration and a marked interstitial nephritis. Silver stains reveal spirochetal organisms in the renal tubules.

Diagnosis

Definitive diagnosis depends on isolation of the organism and identification of the serovar. During the leptospiremic phase, the organism may be isolated from blood, but only with difficulty. The potential for isolation from the urine during the leptospiruric phase is somewhat better. It is advised to initiate cultures from fresh specimens right at the farm by inoculating a suitable transport medium, or by injecting urine into guinea pigs or hamsters. In abortion cases, fetal kidney, lung, and pleural fluid should be examined microscopically for leptospires using silver stains or immunofluorescence techniques.

The most practical diagnostic approach is the identification of rising antibody titers in acute and convalescent serum samples taken seven to ten days apart in clinically affected animals. The microscopic agglutination test (MAT) is most commonly used. The MAT measures both IgM and IgG antibody and is more useful in the diagnosis of acute disease than chronic disease. The range of positive titers observed in goats during outbreaks of abortion was 1:200 to 1:12,800 using the MAT (Leon-Vizcaino et al. 1987). In Israel, titers of 1:100 were commonly encountered in animals with no history of clinical leptospirosis. Therefore, titers of 1:300 or more were considered as evidence of active infection. A titer of 1:30,000 was reported as early as day four of illness in a goat (Van der Hoeden 1953). Other serologic tests, including indirect ELISA and antibody-capture ELISA, are also now being used in cattle, but reports of their use in goats are limited.

Where both diseases occur, babesiosis must be ruled out because of the similar presentation of hemolytic anemia, fever, and possible abortion. Identification of characteristic piroplasms in RBCs would confirm babesiosis. Anaplasmosis may also produce fever, anemia, and abortion, but icterus and hemoglobinuria are uncommon. Other differential diagnoses for hemolytic anemia with hemoglobinuria include copper toxicity and plant intoxications, especially kale poisoning.

Treatment

Goats with acute leptospirosis have been reported to respond to a combination of streptomycin and penicillin (Amjadi and Ahourai 1975). In other species, streptomycin used at an intramuscular dose of 12 mg/kg twice a day for three days controls the septicemia. A single intramuscular injection of 25 mg/kg of streptomycin may clear leptospires from the kidney in the subsequent leptospiruric phase. A single intramuscular injection of long acting oxytetracycline at a dose of 20 mg/kg bw may be effective where the use of streptomycin in food animals is prohibited. Tetracyclines administered in the feed at a dose of 3 mg/kg for one week before and two weeks after exposure to leptospirosis has prevented clinical signs in calves, though infection did occur.

Supportive therapy must be considered in acute leptospirosis because anemia can be severe and the potential for renal failure is high due to primary interstitial nephritis and secondary hemoglobinuria with cast formation. Continuous intravenous fluid therapy is indicated to maintain renal output, and blood transfusions may be considered when the degree of anemia appears life-threatening.

Control

Early recognition and initiation of streptomycin or tetracycline therapy may reduce the number of clinical cases. Concurrent use of vaccination with the appropriate serotype vaccine in the face of an outbreak has been shown to reduce the incidence of new cases and abortions in cattle. Active and recovered cases should be isolated because of the possibility of organisms continuing to be shed in the urine. Always remember that leptospirosis is a potential zoonosis.

Prevention is based on environmental hygiene measures such as rodent control, elimination of standing water, and avoidance of damp bedding; screening or prophylactic treatment of newly acquired animals for elimination of the carrier state; and vaccination. Little or no protective cross immunity occurs among the various serovars of *L. interrogans*, so vaccination should be based on serologic evaluation of prevailing serovars. Multivalent vaccines suitable for use in goats are available. All animals older than three months of age should be vaccinated. Kids of vaccinated dams nursing colostrum should be protected by passive antibody up to three months of age. Annual or semi-annual revaccination is practiced in cattle. While the duration of protective immunity in goats has not been reported, semi-annual revaccination of goats has been suggested.

When considering vaccination, bear in mind that leptospirosis in goats is uncommon, and the cost-to-benefit ratio of routine vaccination for leptospirosis in goats is not known. In an American study undertaken to evaluate health status of goats in relation to management practices in forty-three herds, no cases of leptospirosis were reported in any of the herds, regardless of whether they were vaccinated (Hagstad et al. 1984). The prevalence of leptospirosis in the practice area should be assessed in consideration of vaccination programs. Farmers, herders, veterinarians, milkers, and slaughterhouse workers have an increased occupational risk of exposure to this zoonotic disease and should exercise appropriate hygienic precautions to prevent infection.

Anthrax

Anthrax is a well known, infectious disease of livestock with zoonotic potential. The disease in goats is very similar to that in other ruminant species. This septicemic condition is characterized by a failure of the blood to clot. This is commonly noted at death by a bloody discharge from the nose and mouth.

Etiology and epidemiology

Bacillus anthracis is the cause of anthrax in herbivores and humans. The organism is characterized by the ability to produce spores, on exposure to air, that are capable of persisting for longer than fifty years. Anthrax is endemic in many tropical and subtropical regions of the world. The major route of transmission in animals is ingestion of spores residing in soil during periods of grazing. The disease has a seasonal occurrence, and is predisposed by environmental temperatures exceeding 59°F (15°C), periods of drought, or heavy rains. Goats are susceptible to anthrax, but reports of the condition in goats are uncommon, perhaps because they are not ground grazing animals by nature. Outbreaks in goats have been reported from Nigeria (Okoh 1981), Texas (Whitford 1982), China (ProMED-mail 2006), and Ethiopia (Shiferaw, 2004), and are possible wherever anthrax is endemic in other species. Grazing is not an absolute prerequisite for exposure to anthrax. Zero-grazed goats in Texas that were fed hay and a pelleted feed were confirmed with anthrax (ProMED-mail 2008). It is presumed that one or more of the provided feeds was contaminated with anthrax spores. Additional information on the epidemiology of anthrax is available elsewhere (Radostits et al. 2007).

Clinical Findings and Diagnosis

The disease is characterized most commonly by a peracute, fatal course, with most affected animals found dead, the result of bacteremia and toxemia. In acute cases, goats may be noted to be salivating and extremely depressed with the head hanging down. Over a period of one to two days they become recumbent and moribund, and die. Observation of bleeding from the nostrils and mouth of dead animals is characteristic of anthrax. Carcasses of suspect animals should not be opened at the site of death because this will release spores that will contaminate the environment. If movement of the carcass is not possible, then carefully aspirated blood samples and superficial lymph node aspirates can be taken and submitted for bacterial culture. If necropsy is performed, the blood is unclotted and the spleen is dramatically enlarged. Hemorrhages on serosal surfaces suggestive of septicemia are observed. The organism can be cultured from tissue. The differential diagnosis must include all potential causes of sudden death as discussed in Chapter 16.

Treatment and Control

Antiserum and/or antibiotics including tetracyclines, streptomycin, and penicillin may be effective therapies in early cases in the face of an outbreak. In endemic areas, effective vaccines are usually given annually and can be used safely and effectively in goats.

Anthrax is an important zoonotic disease. Transmission is usually by direct handling of hair, wool, skins, or carcasses of infected or contaminated animals. The disease can also be spread by inhalation of spores. A textile mill worker in North Carolina was diagnosed with anthrax that was traced to handling cashmere goat hair imported from endemic regions of western Asia (Briggs et al. 1988). Cases of cutaneous and inhalation anthrax in humans have been reported in the United States in association with the handling of goat skins imported from Africa for drum making (Kaplan 2007). There are numerous reports from developing countries of human cases of anthrax occurring among villagers who eat meat from livestock that have died of anthrax, including goat meat (Boutin et al. 1985; ProMED-mail 2006). Gloves and masks should be worn when handling carcasses or animal products suspected of being contaminated with anthrax. Animals dying of unknown causes or of suspected anthrax should not be eaten. Carcasses should be burned or buried deeply to avoid dissemination and persistence of spores in the environment.

PROTOZOAL DISEASES

Babesiosis

Babesiosis is a tick-borne protozoan hemoparasitic disease of goats. In those regions where it occurs, the economic losses associated with caprine babesiosis may be significant, particularly around the Mediterranean and in the Middle East and India.

Etiology

Two main species of *Babesia* infect sheep, *B. motasi* and *B. ovis*, but in goats *B. motasi* infection predominates. *B. motasi* is classified as a large *Babesia* sp. with a length of 2.5 to 4 microns while *B. ovis* is a small *Babesia* sp. with a length of 1 to 2.5 microns. Another large species, *B. crassa*, has been found in Iran and a few other countries, including Turkey. It is reported to be infective, but probably nonpathogenic, for goats. Another small species, *B. taylori*, infective for goats has been reported from India but the current status of this species is unclear. The agents causing bovine babesiosis are not pathogenic for goats although inapparent infections of goats with *B. bigemina* have been observed. Ticks serve as biological vectors but mechanical transmission is also possible.

Epidemiology

B. motasi infection of small ruminants has been reported from much of Europe, the Middle East, the former USSR, India, southeast Asia, and parts of Africa (Purnell 1981). The primary biological vector for *B. motasi* is the tick *Haemaphysalis punctata*, although it is also likely to be transmitted by other species in the genus *Haemaphysalis*. Reports of transmission by *Dermacentor silvarum* and *Rhipicephalus bursa* are probably erroneous (Uilenberg et al. 1980). Transovarial and transstadial tick transmission occurs.

Several strains of *B. motasi* exist, with variable infectivity and pathogenicity for goats (Purnell 1981a). An outbreak of naturally occurring disease in both sheep and goats caused by *B. motasi* has been reported from India (Jagannath et al. 1974). A strain of *B. motasi* isolated from sheep in Wales produced fever and anemia in a splenectomized goat, but pathogenicity for intact goats was not evaluated (Lewis et al. 1981). Babesiosis was the cause of debilitating disease in sheep and goats in southwest Nigeria but caused death only in goats (Adeoye 1985).

B. ovis is transmitted primarily by *Rhipicephalus bursa*. The geographic distribution of *B. ovis* coincides in part with that of *B. motasi*, but is associated primarily with disease in sheep where it occurs. Natural infection of goats with *B. ovis* has been reported only from Somalia, and the infection was subclinical (Edelsten 1975).

The pathogenicity of *Babesia* spp. in goats and sheep may be intensified by concurrent infections, particularly other hemoparasites. No cross immunity develops after infection with either *B. motasi* or *B. ovis*.

Pathogenesis

Merozoites introduced by feeding ticks invade erythrocytes. Asexual reproduction of the protozoa occurs within the red blood cells to form a pair of trophozoites that are released and re-invade other red blood cells. The release of trophozoites from parasitized red cells results in intravascular hemolysis. The degree of anemia does not always correlate with the degree of parasitemia, and immune-mediated hemolysis may also be occurring. In other species, infection may lead to the development of neurologic signs from cerebral thrombosis, hypotension from activation of plasma kallikrein, and disseminated intravascular coagulation. These syndromes have not yet been reported in the goat. Antibodies are produced in response to infection. A protective immunity develops in nonfatal infections. It does not completely prevent reinfection, but does inhibit recurrence of clinical disease with the same-infecting strain. The development of a carrier state in goats is not addressed in the literature.

Clinical Signs

Affected goats may have fevers as high as 107°F (41.7°C) and show anorexia, weakness, and signs of anemia, including dyspnea and tachycardia. Sheep consistently show icterus and hemoglobinuria, with coffee-colored urine. These signs occur less consistently in goats, but aid in diagnosis when present (Jagannath et al. 1974). Additional signs of coughing and diarrhea have been reported but may be because of other concurrent infections. Affected goats may harbor ticks, though infective ticks may have dropped off before clinical signs develop. Morbidity and mortality rates can be high. Death can occur within forty-eight hours of the onset of signs. Chronic infections may occur, with anemia and ill thrift the prominent findings.

Clinical Pathology and Necropsy

Giemsa-stained blood smears should be examined for evidence of piroplasms. Thin smears are usually adequate at the height of parasitemia, but in chronic cases or when parasitemia is low, thick blood smears prepared from ear vein blood are preferred. Blood from several animals in a suspect group should be examined to avoid missing the diagnosis. *B. motasi* is a large piroplasm and occurs in single and double pear-shaped forms. *B. ovis* is a smaller piroplasm and often assumes a round form near the periphery of the erythrocyte. The *Babesia* piroplasms must be distinguished from *Theileria* piroplasms that can also affect goats and have a similar geographic distribution.

An indirect fluorescent antibody test can be used for the serodiagnosis of *B. motasi* infection, with titers of 1:640 or more considered as evidence of infection (Lewis et al. 1981).

At time of necropsy, the predominant findings are splenomegaly, lymphadenopathy, and enlarged liver. Icterus and hemoglobinuria are variable. Peripheral blood should be examined for piroplasms.

Diagnosis

The diagnosis of caprine babesiosis is suggested by signs of anemia, hemoglobinuria, and acute collapse in animals where babesiosis is known to occur. Definitive diagnosis depends on the identification of the organism in blood smears. Theileriosis can be differentiated by the morphology of piroplasms and a more prominent lymph node enlargement. Anaplasmosis does not normally produce hemoglobinuria. When hemoglobinuria is present, plant poisonings, copper toxicity, anthrax, and leptospirosis must also be considered.

Treatment

A single dose of prescribed treatments is often satisfactory. The diamidine derivatives diminazene and imidocarb diproprionate are effective at doses of 3 mg/kg and 1 to 2 mg/kg, respectively. Diminazene in intramuscular doses as high as 12 mg/kg have been used in goats without adverse effect (Bannerjee et al. 1987). Most of the earlier drugs used for treatment, such as the quinuronium sulfate compounds, are no longer commercially available.

Control

No specific recommendations for control of caprine babesiosis have been made. In cattle and sheep, control efforts are directed at vaccination and reduction of tick infestations using acaricides. Vaccination protocols include vaccination with live protozoa in conjunction with imidocarb chemoprophylaxis, or chemoprophylaxis alone, leading to a controlled natural exposure and self-immunization. Inoculation with indigenous strains of *Babesia* in conjunction with chemoprophylaxis (infection and treatment) may be essential for survival of exotic breeds of goats imported into areas where babesiosis is enzootic.

Theileriosis

Theileriosis is a tick-borne protozoal disease of ruminants affecting primarily the hemic-lymphatic system.

Etiology and Epidemiology

Theileriosis has received little direct attention in goats and much has been inferred from the disease in sheep. As a result, discrepancies occur in the literature concerning pathogenicity for goats. Pathogenic *Theileria* spp. infecting goats and sheep include *T. lestoquardi* (earlier known as *T. hirci*) and two species described recently in China. There is some confusion about the nomenclature of these Chinese species; they have been designated as *Theileria* sp. (China 1) and *Theileria* sp. (China 2) (Ahmed et al. 2006). They have also been named *T. luwenshuni* and *T. uilenbergi* (Yin et al. 2004), but it may not be quite clear to which of the two species each of these names refers.

There are also several nonpathogenic species in small ruminants causing benign theileriosis, which may confuse the picture. *T. ovis* is distributed widely throughout Europe, Asia, and Africa. In Africa, it may be confused with another species, *T. separata*, and in Europe with one or two other species, as yet unnamed.

T. lestoquardi is most often associated with high morbidity and mortality rates and infection with *T. lestoquardi* is known as malignant small ruminant theileriosis. It has produced serious losses in sheep and goats in northern Africa, including the Sudan, Asia, the Middle East, southern Europe, and the southern former USSR. In a report from Iraq, however, a strain of *T. lestoquardi*, responsible for 100% morbidity and 89.7% mortality rates in a flock of sheep, produced no clinical disease when inoculated in a goat (Hooshmand-Rad and Hawa 1973). Similarly, in an Indian study, the infection was transmitted to sheep but not goats (Sisodia and Gautam 1983), and in the Sudan infection of goats with *T. lestoquardi* appears to be rare. Species of *Theileria* highly pathogenic for cattle do not cause disease in small ruminants.

Infections in goats with nonpathogenic small ruminant species of *Theileria* are also much less common than in sheep, and goats may be refractory to some species infective for sheep.

T. lestoquardi is transmitted by *Hyalomma anatolicum* in Asia, while the recently described species in China are transmitted by *Haemaphysalis quinghaiensis*. The tick vectors of *T. ovis* in sub-Saharan Africa are unknown. Transmission of *T. ovis* reported in South Africa by *Rhipicephalus evertsi* in fact involved *T. separata*. *Rhipicephalus bursa* is reported as a vector in the former USSR, north Africa, and Asia. *Haemaphysalis punctata* is the vector in Great Britain of a nonpathogenic species.

Pathogenesis

Sporozoites enter the host by the bite of infected ticks. The parasites are initially located in the spleen and lymph nodes, where they invade lymphocytes and produce schizonts. These schizonts, which early in the infection contain large nuclei, and later small ones, are readily identifiable in Giemsa-stained smears of lymph node aspirates or biopsies, and are referred to as Koch's Blue Bodies. After lysis of lymphocytes, micromerozoites enter the blood stream as piroplasms and invade erythrocytes. The piroplasm is polymorphic in red blood cells, exhibiting ring, oval, comma-shaped, or rod forms. Additional replication occurs in the red blood cells, and the sexual stages of the life cycle occur in the tick. The anemia of theileriosis is less severe than that seen in babesiosis, the other piroplasm of goats.

Clinical Signs

In malignant theileriosis (*T. lestoquardi* infection), clinical signs initially include fever, increased heart and respiratory rates, anorexia, dullness, and depression. Lymph nodes are markedly swollen. Serous nasal discharge and lacrimation develop, and the conjunctivae are congested. The clinical course may last from two to three weeks; during that time, the animal may experience a decrease in milk production, coughing, rough hair coat, emaciation, weakness, recumbency, and death. A mild to moderate anemia may be observed and, in sheep, icterus has been inconsistently reported. In benign theileriosis, transient fever and mild lymph node swelling may occur and be overlooked under field conditions.

Clinical Pathology and Necropsy

Anemia and lymphopenia may be noted in the hemogram. Koch's Blue Bodies may be identified in Giemsa-stained smears of lymph nodes or characteristic piroplasms seen in circulating red blood cells. On examination after death, lymph nodes, spleen, and liver are all enlarged. The liver is yellow and the kidneys may show patchy hemorrhagic infarcts. Necrotizing ulcers ringed by hemorrhage may be seen in the abomasum and intestine.

Diagnosis

Diagnosis is based on identification of Koch's Blue Bodies in lymph nodes or piroplasms in erythrocytes. The piroplasms must be distinguished from those of *Babesia* spp. Molecular methods, comparing selected sequences of nucleotides in DNA, have become important research tools for species identification and phylogenetic studies.

Treatment and Control

Specific information on the treatment of caprine theileriosis is lacking. In cattle, high doses of long-acting oxytetracycline, 20 mg/kg of the 200 mg/ml formulation given intramuscularly, have been therapeutically effective against *T. parva* and *T. annulata*, only when administered very early in the incubation period. A napthoquinone, parvaquone, at 10 mg/kg intramuscularly, given twice to cattle is curative as late as four days into the clinical disease, and a related drug, buparvaquone, is even more effective. An anticoccidial compound, halofuginone, with a single oral dose of 1.2 mg/kg has also been effective against bovine theileriosis. However, even slight overdosing may produce severe adverse effects, so extrapolation to goats is inadvisable without additional evaluation. Control of caprine theileriosis involves control of the tick vectors primarily through dipping programs. Vaccine development is progressing for control of bovine theileriosis, including the use of attenuated schizonts of *T. annulata* in cell culture, but little activity has been reported with small ruminant species of *Theileria*. However, because schizonts of *T. lestoquardi* can be grown in cell culture, attenuation should be attempted.

Trypanosomosis

Trypanosomosis is a major constraint on ruminant livestock production in Africa, including goat production. The impact of South American trypanosomosis on goats is largely unexplored and is only briefly discussed. Salient characteristics of the important animal and human trypanosomes and their pathogenicity for goats are summarized in Table 7.7. Though often referred to as trypanosomosis, the preferred name for disease caused by trypanosome infections is trypanosomosis (Kassai et al. 1988).

Etiology

The trypanosomes are flagellate protozoa characterized by a kinetoplast and an undulating membrane. Most trypanosomes require two hosts to complete their life cycle, a hematogenous insect vector and a vertebrate host. In sub-Saharan Africa, cyclic transmission of the parasite to mammalian hosts occurs via numerous species of tsetse flies (*Glossina* spp.) during feeding by the flies. Elsewhere in the world, mechanical transmission by other species of biting flies is the primary mode of infection. A recent, detailed and informative review of African animal trypanosomes and the diseases they cause is available elsewhere (Connor and van den Bossche 2004).

T. congolense is the most common trypanosome of goats in Africa. *T. vivax* is the second most common. Natural infection of goats with *T. brucei* is also sporadically reported. Goats are susceptible to *T. uniforme*, a trypanosome of the vivax group in Uganda and Zaire, but only mild infections occur. *T. simiae*, a trypanosome of swine and camels, is transmissible to goats by either *Glossina* spp. or biting flies but causes mostly mild or subclinical disease.

Goats and other domestic animals are relatively resistant to *T. gambiense*, the cause of West African human sleeping sickness. When infection does occur, the clinical course is chronic. *T. rhodesiense*, the cause of East African sleeping sickness in humans, is an uncommon cause of caprine disease. A nonpathogenic trypanosome, *T. theodori*, is found incidentally in goats in Israel. It is transmitted by a hippoboscid fly, *Lipoptena caprina*. This organism is morphologically similar to the common, nonpathogenic sheep trypanosome *T. melophagium*.

Information on the pathogenicity of the trypanosomes that occur outside of sub-Saharan Africa, primarily in South and Central America, as well as in Asia, is limited. *T. cruzi* is cyclically transmitted by reduviid bugs in South and Central America, while *T. evansi* and *T. equiperdum* are mechanically or sexually transmitted, respectively, in Africa, South and

Table 7.7. Trypanosomosis in various hosts with the emphasis on goats.

Species	*Morphologic features*	*Major species affected*	*Geographic distribution*	*Vectors involved*	*Natural infection in goats*	*Experimental infection in goats*	*Clinical manifestations in goats*
Cyclically transmitted							
T. vivax	20–27 µm long; monomorphic; short, free flagellum	Domestic ruminants, camels, horses, antelope	Widespread in tropical Africa	*Glossina* spp.	Common	Readily	Acute and chronic forms; usually mild
T. congolense	9–18 µm long; monomorphic; no free flagellum; undulating membrane not seen	All common livestock species and dogs; many wild game species	Widespread in tropical Africa	*Glossina* spp.	Common	Readily	Acute, subacute, and chronic forms; mild to fatal outcome
T. brucei	15–35 µm long; polymorphic; undulating membrane always seen	Domestic ruminants, horses, dogs, and cats	Widespread in tropical Africa	*Glossina* spp.	Common, but with strain variation	Yes, with strain variation	Acute, rapidly fatal outcomes or chronic infections
T. simiae	10–24 µm long; polymorphic; variable undulating membrane	Domestic pigs, camels, wild warthogs	Widespread in tropical Africa	*Glossina* spp. and *Stomoxys*, *Tabanus* flies	Uncommon	Not reported	Mainly subclinical or mild clinical disease
T. gambiense (West African sleeping sickness)	Same as *T. brucei;* slender, intermediate stumpy forms	Humans	Tropical West and Central Africa	*Glossina* spp. and various biting flies	Uncommon; goats very resistant	Very difficult	Noninfective or a chronic form leading to death or spontaneous recovery
T. rhodesiense (East African sleeping sickness)	Same as *T. brucei* and *T. gambiense*	Humans, in addition to species affected by *T. brucei*	East and Southern Africa	*Glossina* spp.	Uncommon	Yes	Experimental infections subacute and fatal
T. cruzi (Chagas disease)	16–20 µm long; in blood forms undulating membrane and free flagellum moderately well developed; tissue forms resemble *Leishmania*	Humans	South and Central America; sporadic in United States	Reduviid blood-sucking bugs	Not reported	Yes	No

Table 7.7. *Continued*

Species	*Morphologic features*	*Major species affected*	*Geographic distribution*	*Vectors involved*	*Natural infection in goats*	*Experimental infection in goats*	*Clinical manifestations in goats*
T. uniforme	12–20 μm long; monomorphic; flagellum is free, shorter than *T. vivax*	Domestic ruminants; antelope	Zaire, Uganda	*Glossina* spp.	Yes	Not reported	Nonpathogenic or subclinical infection
T. theodori	50–60 μm long; well defined undulating membrane and free flagellum	Goats	Israel	*Lipoptena caprina*, a hippoboscid fly	Yes	Not reported	Nonpathogenic
Mechanically transmitted							
T. vivax viennei	15–25 μm long; monomorphic; similar to *T. vivax*	Cattle, water buffalo	North, South, and Central America	Various biting flies	Uncommon but reported	Not reported	Not reported
T. evansi (Surra)	15–34 μm long; usually monomorphic; same as slender form of *T. brucei;* occasional stumpy form	Camels, equines, dogs, water buffalo	India, Far East, Near East, Philippines, North Africa, South and Central America	Various biting flies	Yes	Not reported	Not reported
T. equiperdum (Dourine)	15–34 μm long; same as *T. evansi*	Horses	Northern and South Africa, Central and South America, Mexico, Middle East, Italy, former USSR	Venereal transmission	Not reported	Not reported	Not reported

Central America, and Asia. These trypanosomes cause disease in various species. *T. cruzi* is primarily of importance for humans; *T. evansi* for camels, horses, cattle, and Asian buffalo, and *T. equiperdum* for horses. Their infectivity for goats is presumed to be low. Kids infected experimentally with *T. cruzi* showed no clinical signs of disease and carried the infection for thirty-eight days (Diamond and Rubin 1958).

The goat is a natural host for *T. evansi*, but reports of the disease, surra, in goats are rare. Recently, surra was reported to be occurring in goats in Mindanao in the Philippines, but field confirmation has been difficult. It is believed that the cases may involve a particularly virulent strain of *T. evansi*. Experimental challenge of goats with an equine strain of *T. evansi* from Mindanao produced clinical and pathological changes consistent with surra (Dargantes et al. 2005, 2005a).

Epidemiology

The distribution and intensity of animal trypanosomosis in sub-Saharan Africa follow the distribution and intensity of the various species of the tsetse fly.

Approximately 10 million km^2 or 37% of the African continent is tsetse-infested. This area includes thirty-eight countries. Various estimates suggest that the livestock-carrying capacity of such areas in West and Central Africa could be increased five- to seven-fold by eliminating or controlling animal trypanosomosis (Griffin 1978).

There are more than 200 million goats in Africa with 50 million or more in the tsetse-infested regions of the continent. Natural infections with *T. congolense, T. vivax*, or *T. brucei* resulting in clinical disease have been known in African goats since the early twentieth century. Until recently, however, the perception has persisted that goats are highly resistant to infection, that caprine trypanosomosis is only sporadic, and that the disease in goats is of little economic consequence (Griffin 1978). This opinion is currently undergoing a critical reappraisal. Regional differences do exist in the prevalence of caprine trypanosomosis, but it can be high in some areas (Kramer 1966; Griffin and Allonby 1979). In general, caprine trypanosomosis is more common in East than West Africa. This is attributed to differences in feeding preferences between riverine species of *Glossina* and savannah species; the latter are more inclined to feed on goats. A report from Zambia identified *T. brucei, T. congolense*, and/or *T. vivax* infections in goats naturally transmitted by *Glossina morsitans morsitans* and *G. pallidipes* (Bealby et al. 1996).

Goats may serve as a reservoir of trypanosome infection for other species. In the Sudan, goats infected with *T. congolense* developed a chronic form of disease from which many spontaneously recovered. When the organism was passaged from goats into calves however, acute fatal bovine trypanosomosis occurred (Mahmoud and Elmalik 1977). Goats also have been implicated as a reservoir of *T. rhodesiense*, a nosodeme of *T. brucei* transmissible to man (Robson and Rickman 1973).

The economic impact of trypanosomosis on goat production is beginning to be studied. A Kenyan analysis demonstrated that goats receiving monthly chemoprophylaxis against trypanosomosis had significantly decreased mortality rates, increased weight gains, and improved reproductive performance compared to untreated control goats. Differences in performance were also noted between breeds in the study, with indigenous breeds performing better than nonindigenous breeds or cross breeds (Kanyari et al. 1983).

The existence of inherent trypanotolerance in certain goat breeds has been controversial. It is generally accepted that trypanotolerant breeds of cattle exist, notably the N'dama of West Africa and the West African Shorthorn, and that trypanotolerance is measured by the ability to control trypanosome numbers and resist the effects of the disease, independent of pre-existing immune experience. This inherent ability to control parasitemia and minimize disease is not as great in specific goat breeds, despite the general observation that some breeds of goats readily survive in tsetse infested areas. Dwarf West African goats may, to some extent, be inherently trypanotolerant, yet they can be readily infected experimentally (Murray et al. 1982). While earlier studies suggested that indigenous goat breeds of East Africa may show inherent trypanotolerance, no evidence of genetic resistance was observed in a subsequent study with either natural or experimental challenge in East African, Galla, or East African goats cross bred with Toggenburg, Nubian, or Galla breeds (Whitelaw et al. 1985). One factor contributing to the perceived trypanotolerance of various goat breeds under field conditions may be the feeding preferences of *Glossina* spp. Flies may select other livestock over goats when mixed animal populations are present (Murray et al. 1984). The existence of true trypanotolerance in goats deserves additional careful investigation.

Pathogenesis

Trypanosomes fall into two groups regarding their ability to produce disease. The hematic group, which includes *T. congolense* and *T. vivax*, remains confined to the circulation after introduction into the bloodstream by feeding *Glossina* spp. The disease produced in these infections is characterized by anemia. The humoral group, which includes *T. brucei*, is more invasive, with trypanosomes found in intercellular tissue and body cavity fluids after initial infection. Anemia in these cases is overshadowed by marked inflammatory, degenerative, and necrotic changes.

Anemia in trypanosomosis may be due to extravascular hemolysis and erythrophagocytosis, as well as decreased erythropoiesis in chronic infections (Kaaya et al. 1977). The destruction of red blood cells may result from both non-immune and immune mediated mechanisms. Hemorrhage secondary to disseminated intravascular coagulation (DIC) may also contribute to anemia. Thrombocytopenia, microthrombus formation, and hemorrhage suggestive of DIC have been observed in caprine trypanosomosis due to *T. vivax* (Van den Ingh et al. 1976; Veenendaal et al. 1976). Anemia may be exaggerated by hemodilution because of expansion of blood and plasma volumes, which increased, respectively, 29% and 44% in goats with subacute *T. vivax* infection (Anosa and Isoun 1976).

The pathogenesis of inflammation and tissue damage by humoral trypanosomes such as *T. brucei* is complex and is reviewed elsewhere (Soulsby 1982; Connor and van den Bossche 2004). Immunosuppression can occur in trypanosomosis. *T. vivax* and *T. brucei* infection of goats resulted in depressed responses to mitogen stimulation in lymphocyte transformation tests (van Dam et al. 1981a; Diesing et al. 1983) and goats experimentally infected with *T. congolense* produced a weaker antibody response to vaccination with *Brucella melitensis* vaccine than uninfected controls (Griffin et al. 1980). Impaired immune function may aggravate the severity of concurrent infections. This was suggested by evidence of higher mortality rates and parasite loads in goats concurrently infected with *T. congolense* and *Haemonchus contortus* than in goats infected with only one parasite or the other (Griffin et al. 1981a, 1981b). Under field conditions, goats with chronic trypanosomosis are more susceptible to helminthiasis and carry heavier helminth burdens, probably as a result of immunosuppression.

Trypanosome infection is associated with ovarian dysfunction and irregular estrus cycles (Llewellyn et al. 1987; Mutayoba et al. 1988). Gross testicular atrophy has been reported in bucks with *T. congolense* infection (Kaaya and Odour-Okelo 1980). There is also a variety of endocrine abnormalities reported following inoculation of trypanosomes into the bloodstream of goats, including depression of circulating thyroxine, testosterone, and cortisol levels (Connor and van den Bossche 2004).

One of the most notable features of trypanosomosis is the successive waves of parasitemia that occur every few days in animals that survive initial infection. Each wave of parasitemia is followed by an increase in circulating antibody that temporarily reduces the parasitemia. The effect is only temporary, however, because cyclically transmitted trypanosomes are capable of repeatedly altering their surface antigens and thereby evade the host immune system sufficiently to avoid total elimination of infection. These variant antigens are surface coat glycoproteins. It is the occurrence of variable antigens that has been the major obstacle in the development of effective vaccines.

Clinical Signs

Clinical syndromes produced by the three major tsetse-transmitted trypanosomes are presented separately below. In the early stage of the disease, a prominent skin chancre may be noted at the site of tsetse fly feeding

T. Vivax. Acute, subacute, and chronic forms of disease can occur. Acute disease usually results in recovery or death within four weeks. Subacute disease, with a decreased level of parasitemia, may persist for ten to twelve weeks, and chronic disease for seventeen weeks or longer. The chronic form of the disease is most common. Parasitemia is evident on blood smear within six to seven days after infection and peaks at approximately ten days, but identification of the parasite on blood smears in subacute and chronic cases is less reliable. Successive waves of parasitemia occur at four- to seven-day intervals, accompanied by fluctuating fevers as high as 108°F (42.2°C). Anemia develops rapidly, coinciding with the first wave of parasitemia.

Clinical signs may include depression, anorexia, lack of rumen motility, enlarged lymph nodes, and weight loss. Anemia can become severe with signs including pallor, increased heart rate and respiration, exercise intolerance, and marked listlessness. Jaundice and hemoglobinuria are uncommon findings. Severe emaciation is evident in chronic disease, although surviving animals may begin to gain weight again and the severity of anemia diminish as the level of recurrent parasitemia is brought under control.

T. Congolense. Acute, subacute, and chronic forms of disease also have been described for *T. congolense* infection of goats (Griffin and Allonby 1979a). The acute phase results in death or recovery within six weeks. Fluctuating temperatures up to 106°F (41.1°C) occur and in fatal cases anemia is severe. Weight loss is variable, depending on the duration of disease. In recovered animals, fever and a milder anemia may occur with the initial parasitemia, but PCV returns rapidly to normal. In subacute cases, animals die or recover within six to twelve weeks after infection. In fatal cases, cyclic parasitemia persists and fluctuating fever, progressive emaciation, weakness, lethargy, and pallor are evident clinically. Recovering animals begin to gain weight and strength as fever and anemia subside. Chronic infections, lasting twelve weeks or longer, are almost always fatal. Cyclic fever and parasitemia persist, as does the anemia. Animals become emaciated, hair coat becomes rough, superficial lymph nodes are palpably enlarged, and intermandibular and facial edema develop. Animals become recumbent, then comatose, and die.

T. Brucei. Because *T. brucei* is a humoral trypanosome, clinical signs may be more severe, although pathogenicity varies with the strain. In addition to anemia, fever, and emaciation, keratitis and signs of encephalitis may occur, including head pressing, circling, and opisthotonos. Lymphadenopathy is a consistent finding and may be more pronounced than with *T. vivax* or *T. congolense* infection. The typical course of disease is three to five months, and is usually fatal. Anemia is not as pronounced as it is in infection with the hematic trypanosomes. Parasitemia is also less severe, and detection of trypanosomes on blood smears is more difficult. Examination of lymph node smears may be more rewarding.

Clinical Pathology and Necropsy

In all forms of the disease, the most significant laboratory findings relate to anemia (Edwards et al. 1956). Moderate to severe decreases in PCV, Hb, and RBC numbers can be seen. In the early stages, anemia is macrocytic, while in chronic and terminal cases, a normocytic anemia is more common. This is reflected in the bone marrow, which is often hyperplastic in acute disease and normoplastic or hypoplastic in chronic disease. In experimental infection of goats, all species of trypanosomes produced a significant thrombocytopenia with platelet counts 65% to 82% less than the normal mean (Davis 1982). No consistent changes in the leukogram have been noted in caprine trypanosomosis. In cattle, a transient leukopenia and rebound leukocytosis can occur during the acute phase of disease. Serum chemistry values remain normal. Animals with acute trypanosomosis may show laboratory evidence of DIC.

There are no pathognomonic lesions in trypanosomosis. In acute cases, necropsy findings include an anemic carcass, general lymph node enlargement, marked splenomegaly, serosal and mucosal petechial hemorrhage, and hydropericardium. Microscopically, lymphoid hyperplasia is pronounced and microthrombi may be evident in vessels of numerous organs. In the hematic forms of disease, trypanosomes is present only in vascular spaces, while with *T. brucei* extravascular parasites may be seen in tissues such as the cornea and cerebrospinal fluid. In chronic cases, severe emaciation, with serous atrophy of fat, and muscle degeneration may be observed in addition to petechiation, lymphadenopathy, and splenomegaly (Losos and Ikede 1972).

Diagnosis

Anemia and emaciation in goats from tsetse endemic areas suggest the diagnosis of trypanosomosis. Definitive diagnosis is based on identification of trypanosomes in blood smears or tissues. However, chronic infections in goats are common and trypanosomes may be difficult to find in the blood. In live animals, parasites may be more readily detected in blood samples taken from an ear vein rather than the jugular vein. Thick blood smears examined after lysis of red cells and staining with Romanowsky stain may reveal the presence of parasites, but morphologic identification is better performed on thin smears. Microhematocrital centrifugation of blood and examination of a wet mount of the plasma-buffy coat interface can improve detection. For confirmation of *T. brucei* infection, examination of smears of lymph node aspirates, and mouse inoculation are preferred methods of diagnosis. Because parasitemia is cyclical, examining smears from numerous animals in a suspect group may improve the chances of diagnosis.

Serologic tests employed in the diagnosis of trypanosomosis include an indirect hemagglutination test, a complement fixation test, an indirect fluorescent antibody test, and an enzyme linked immunosorbent assay. Information on interpretation of serologic responses in goats is limited. At present, molecular tools, such as PCR, are commonly employed, but demand well-equipped laboratories and do not replace classical methods in the field.

The differential diagnosis for trypanosomosis should include helminthiasis, malnutrition, and other hemoparasites, notably anaplasmosis, babesiosis, and theilerosis, which occur in trypanosomosis endemic areas.

Treatment

A variety of trypanocidal compounds are available for treatment, but no new drugs have been marketed for quite some time. Subsequently, drug resistance has become a significant problem. Compounds and dosages are formulated for single-dose use and treatment is usually on a herd wide basis because serial treatments on individual animals are difficult to carry out in the semi-nomadic livestock farming systems prevalent in endemic areas. Several of the drugs are locally irritating, so subcutaneous injections should be given in areas of loose skin, and intramuscular injections given deeply, avoiding vessels and nerves. Curative doses used in cattle are also appropriate for goats and sheep on a mg/kg body weight basis (Ilemobade 1986). Treatment is reviewed by Uilenberg (1998).

Diminazene aceturate is given intramuscularly as a 7% cold water solution at a dose of 3.5 mg/kg and is considered effective against the three major trypanosomes. Quinapyramine dimethyl sulfate is little used nowadays, except for treating *T. evansi* in camels and horses, because of toxicity and drug resistance problems. It is given subcutaneously as a 10% cold water solution at a dose of 5 mg/kg. Relapse of infection has been reported in goats treated with diminazene aceturate, presumably because of re-emergence of trypanosomes from the central nervous system where they were inaccessible to the drug during earlier treatment (Whitelaw et al. 1985a).

Homidium chloride (soluble in cold water) or homidium bromide (soluble in hot water) are given in a 2.5% water solution at a dose of 1 mg/kg intramuscularly and are effective against *T. vivax* and *T. congolense.* Isometamidium chloride is currently the most commonly used drug in ruminants. It is effective against the hematic trypanosomes when given at a dose of 0.25 to 0.75 mg/kg intramuscularly as a 1% or 2% solution in water. This drug was shown to produce signs of shock or death in goats if given intravenously at doses greater than or equal to 0.5 mg/kg (Schillinger et al. 1985). All drugs of the phenanthridinium group (homidium and isometamidium compounds) are potentially carcinogenic and should be handled as such.

Control

There are numerous constraints on control, including reservoirs of infection in wild animal populations, the ability of trypanosomes to continuously alter their antigenic character and thus confounding the development of suitable vaccines, a limited availability of effective drugs, the development of resistance to existing trypanocidal drugs, the difficult logistics of widespread tsetse control, lack of economic resources, poorly developed animal disease control programs, limited technical training programs, lack of international cooperation, and political instability (Doyle et al. 1984; Murray and Gray 1984).

Currently, the major fronts in trypanosomosis control in sub-Saharan Africa are reduction or elimination of tsetse populations and chemoprophylaxis of livestock. Tsetse fly control is accomplished by several methods, alone or in combination, including ground or aerial application of insecticides such as chlorinated hydrocarbons and synthetic pyrethroids; tsetse trapping with odor baited, insecticide impregnated traps; and gamma-irradiated sterile fly release. Aerial spraying of insecticides is now less commonly employed for environmental reasons, and trapping has emerged as a viable alternative, albeit for more restricted areas of control.

Isometamidium chloride protects against infection with the three major goat trypanosomes for two to four months. The prophylactic dose of isometamidium is 0.5 to 1 mg/kg bw administered intramuscularly in a 1% or 2% cold water solution. Earlier chemoprophylactic drugs (pyrithidium and quinapyramine chloride) have been discontinued.

Despite intensive research, no effective vaccine is likely in the future because of the continuing problem of antigenic variation in trypanosomes and antigenic strain differences. Given the obstacles to vaccination, there is a keen interest in identifying and promoting trypanotolerant breeds of livestock in endemic areas, as discussed above in the section on epidemiology.

TOXICOLOGICAL DISEASES

Copper Poisoning

Primary copper poisoning has been reported in the goat, but is not common. It can produce a severe hemolytic anemia with hemoglobinuria and death as occurs in the more commonly affected ruminants—sheep and young cattle.

Epidemiology

There is a marked difference in susceptibility between sheep and goats regarding chronic copper poisoning. The condition is harder to produce experimentally in goats than in sheep (Søli and Nafstad 1978; Solaiman et al. 2001), and published reports of naturally occurring caprine copper poisoning are rare. In sheep, several naturally occurring forms of the disease are recognized, including acute copper poisoning, primary chronic copper poisoning, secondary phytogenous copper poisoning, and secondary hepatogenous copper poisoning. Only the acute and primary chronic forms of copper poisoning have been reported to occur naturally in goats. The acute form was reported from Israel (Shlosberg et al. 1978) and involved the oral administration of copper sulfate solution to goats as an anthelmintic. Chronic cases have been reported from New Zealand and the UK, and involved young, hand-reared Angora goats exposed to a variety of copper-containing feeds and supplements (Belford and Raven 1986; Humphries et al. 1987). More recently, primary chronic copper poisoning was reported in dairy goats in the United States (Cornish et al. 2007).

Etiology and Pathogenesis

Acute copper poisoning is sporadic in occurrence and results from an accidental or unintentional ingestion of abnormally high doses of inorganic copper over a short period. Sources of copper include copper sulfate foot baths, improperly mixed feedstuffs or mineral supplements, or inappropriate administration of copper salts for therapeutic purposes. In acute copper ingestions, direct irritation of the gastrointestinal mucosa causes many of the clinical signs observed, including abdominal pain, vomiting, and shock. Death may precede the development of hemolytic anemia. Animals that survive the initial gastrointestinal insult subsequently absorb sufficient copper to initiate hemolysis.

Acute copper poisoning can be induced in sheep and young calves with a single oral dose of copper in the range of 20 to 110 mg/kg bw. The dose is similar in goats, with acute copper toxicity observed after an oral dose of approximately 60 mg/kg of copper sulfate (Shlosberg et al. 1978). Experimentally, acute toxicosis was produced in goats within three to four days by three daily intravenous injections of $CuSO_4 \cdot 5H_2O$ at a total daily dose of 50 mg (Wasfi and Adam 1976).

In all forms of chronic copper toxicity, the ultimate pathway for clinical disease is thought to be the same. Ingested copper accumulates in the liver over time until maximum hepatic levels are reached, at which point there is a sudden release of the accumulated copper into the blood, initiating an acute hemolytic crisis (Radostits et al. 2007). However, this notion may require reconsideration as a recent, well documented herd outbreak of primary chronic copper toxicosis in a dairy goat herd did not involve hemolysis as part of the clinical presentation in affected goats (Cornish et al. 2007).

In primary chronic copper poisoning, copper is ingested continuously as part of the regular ration. The level of copper may be, but need not be, abnormally high, because the uptake of copper from the rumen and subsequent accumulation in the liver are conditioned by the concentrations of other minerals present in the ration. Low dietary levels of molybdenum, zinc, calcium, and sulfates can permit excessive uptake and accumulation of otherwise normal dietary levels of copper.

In secondary phytogenous chronic copper poisoning, grazing of specific pasture plants, notably subterranean clover *(Trifolium subterraneum)*, promotes the accumulation of copper in liver although the plants themselves are relatively low in copper and do not produce any liver damage. The mechanism behind this phenomenon is not known, but British breeds of sheep and Merino crosses seem more susceptible. This syndrome has not been reported in goats. In hepatogenous chronic copper poisoning, hepatotoxic plants are ingested and produce liver damage that increases hepatocyte affinity for copper accumulation. This can accelerate the development of hemolytic crisis even when dietary levels of copper are within normal limits. Plants most often involved are *Heliotropium europaeum* and other pyrrolizidine alkaloid containing species, including *Senecio* spp. and *Echium plantagineum*. This syndrome has not been reported in goats. In fact, goats are relatively resistant to the effects of *Senecio*, and the use of goats has been proposed to clear rangelands of the plant to make them suitable for grazing by cattle (Dollahite 1972).

Primary chronic copper poisoning can be induced in sheep with daily oral doses as low as 3.5 mg/kg bw, but goats require more aggressive challenge. In one study, oral administration of $CuSO_4 \cdot 5H_2O$ twice daily at a dose of 20 mg/kg of bw for fifty-six days produced hemolytic crisis in only one of three Norwegian breed goats. At necropsy, liver copper levels were 1,168 ppm wet weight and kidney levels were 635 ppm wet weight. There were no hemolytic crises in the two other goats killed after seventy-three and 113 days of daily dosing. Liver copper levels of 314 and 384 ppm wet weight and kidney levels of 3 and 4.5 ppm, respectively, were recorded (Søli and Nafstad 1978). In contrast, sheep are reported to experience hemolytic crises when liver copper levels exceed 150 ppm wet weight (Sanders 1983).

In another study with Nubian goats, neither of two goats given $CuSO_4 \cdot 5H_2O$ daily at 20 mg/kg/bw developed hemolytic anemia, while one of two given 40 mg/kg/day and one of two given 80 mg/kg/day did (Adam et al. 1977). In a more recent experimental study, Nubian goats were fed supplemental copper at increasing levels from 100 mg/head/day up to 1,200 mg/head/day for up to thirty-five weeks. Only individuals receiving 600 mg/head/day or higher showed a clinical effect, with signs of thirst, diarrhea, dehydration, lethargy, and weight loss. However, none experienced hemolytic anemia. The authors report that daily doses of copper of 100 mg/head/day are sufficient to produce clinical toxicity in sheep and conclude that goats are more resistant to copper toxicity than sheep (Solaiman et al. 2001). It has been postulated that the difference in susceptibility of sheep and goats to copper poisoning is a function of differences in the distribution of copper- and zinc-binding soluble hepatic proteins (Mjor-Grimsrud et al. 1979).

In goats, as in sheep, development of copper toxicity may be conditioned by influences of other elements. Goats pretreated with vitamin E and selenium injections developed hemolytic crisis after fifty days of oral dosing with 15 mg/kg of copper as copper sulfate, while animals receiving the same copper dose with no vitamin E or selenium pretreatment showed no clinical signs after the same period. Goats with evidence of hemolytic crisis had decreased liver levels of reduced glutathione and higher glutathione disulfide levels (Hussein et al. 1985).

Clinical Signs

Acute copper poisoning in goats resulting from oral ingestion of copper produces signs of gastrointestinal irritation including evidence of abdominal pain, grinding of the teeth, frothing at the mouth, vomiting, and diarrhea. Additional signs include labored breathing, muscle fasciculation, tachycardia, and increased amplitude of heart sounds. Within six hours, severely affected animals may collapse and die. Morbidity and mortality rates are dose-dependent. Mortality rates as high as 53% have been reported in goats given oral copper sulfate at a dose of 60 mg/kg.

In cases of chronic copper toxicity and acute toxicity associated with parenteral administration of copper, dullness, anorexia, thirst, dehydration, and elevated heart and respiratory rates are early signs. Diarrhea may also be present. If hemolytic anemia is part of the clinical syndrome, then icterus will be noted on mucous membranes, serum will be pink, and urine red-brown. Dyspnea may develop as a result of severe anemia, and death may occur in twenty-four to forty-eight hours after the onset of signs. In untreated animals surviving longer, anuria and uremia may develop as a result of hemoglobinuric nephrosis.

However, in the most recent report of chronic copper toxicosis in a dairy goat herd (Cornish et al. 2007), none of the affected animals showed indications of hemolytic anemia. Only lactating does were clinically affected though young goats had laboratory evidence of copper levels consistent with intoxication. Clinical signs in lactating does included anorexia, agalactia, dullness, dehydration, teeth grinding, and drooling. Affected does progressed to recumbency and showed neurologic abnormalities such as paddling and vocalization followed by death. Signs associated with hemolytic anemia such as icterus or hemolyzed plasma were absent (Cornish et al. 2007).

Clinical Pathology and Necropsy

During the acute hemolytic crisis, PCV may fall below 10%, and RBC and Hb levels drop correspondingly. Heinz bodies can be seen in RBCs and there may also be methemoglobinemia. Serum bilirubin is markedly elevated and the urine is strongly positive for hemoglobin. Alterations in clinical chemistry are consistent with liver damage, and elevations of aspartate aminotransferase (AST), gamma glutamyl transferase (GGT), sorbitol dehydrogenase (SDH), and blood ammonia are reported in the goat, though the magnitude of increase is highly variable. Elevation in liver enzymes may precede the acute hemolytic crisis by several weeks and this may be helpful for screening animals in a herd not yet showing clinical disease. None of these changes are diagnostic for copper poisoning and it is important to establish the presence of abnormally elevated copper levels in blood, liver, kidney, or other tissues to confirm the diagnosis.

In a recent report of field cases of primary chronic copper toxicity, it was noted that in clinically affected goats there was no clear association between the magnitude of increase of serum hepatic enzymes and the concentrations of copper in the serum or liver. In clinically unaffected, younger does in the same herd, there was no consistent relationship between serum hepatic enzyme activities, serum copper concentration, and liver copper concentration. It was concluded that serum liver enzymes and serum copper levels are insensitive markers of liver copper concentration and the definitive method for diagnosis antemortem is to measure copper concentrations in liver samples obtained by biopsy (Cornish et al. 2007). Another study confirmed the reliability of liver as the optimal sample for establishing copper toxicosis and pointed out that hair samples did not reflect the copper status of animals (Solaiman et al 2001).

Normal liver copper levels are reported in the range of 0.188 to 1.805 μmol/g (12 to 115 ppm) (Mjor-Grimsrud et al. 1979). The normal kidney copper level in goats has been reported as 0.1 μmol/g (6.4 ppm). Normal serum copper levels in goats are reported to be in the range of 9.4 to 23.6 μmol/L (60 to 150 μg/dl, or 0.6 to 1.5 ppm) (Underwood 1981).

In field cases of chronic copper toxicity in goats in New Zealand, plasma copper levels of 34.6 μmol/l (219.8 μg/dl or 2.2 ppm) and red blood cell copper levels of 95.8 μmol/l (608.6 μg/dl or 6.1 ppm) were observed during acute hemolytic crisis. Liver copper levels were as high as 21.4 μmol/g dry matter (1359 ppm), and kidney levels as high as 6.4 μmol/g dry matter (406 ppm) (Humphries et al. 1987).

In experimental chronic copper intoxication in goats, animals with hemolytic crises had liver copper levels more than 900 ppm and kidney copper levels more than 170 ppm. Goats that were fed excessive copper but did not develop hemoglobinuria had liver copper levels between 300 and 1,100 ppm and kidney levels between 3 and 150 ppm while a control goat not fed copper had liver copper levels of 18.5 ppm and kidney levels of 6.7 ppm (Adam et al. 1977; Søli and Nafstad 1978).

In acute copper toxicity of goats, animals dying shortly after ingestion had normal liver and kidney levels of copper, but the copper contents of rumen ingesta and feces were elevated to 225 ppm and 1,060 ppm, respectively.

Findings at necropsy may include thin, watery blood and general icterus. The liver is enlarged, friable, and yellow. The kidneys are swollen, dark brown to black, metallic, and softened. Hemorrhages on the epicardium and endocardium and congestion of the lungs and spleen may be noted. In acute oral intoxication, marked inflammation of the abomasal and intestinal mucosae is evident. Histologically, the liver lesion is characterized by hemosiderin deposits, centrilobular necrosis and fatty degeneration, and biliary hyperplasia. The kidney exhibits lesions of nephrosis with casts present in tubules. One experimental study of chronic copper poisoning in the goat resulted in liver lesions atypical for the disease and it was suggested that the pathogenesis of chronic copper poisoning in the goat may differ from that in the sheep (Søli and Nafstad 1978). Others have consistently described lesions found in the goat to be similar to those found in sheep.

Diagnosis

When signs of abdominal pain are prominent—as in acute copper toxicosis—intestinal accidents, urethral obstruction, and early infectious enteritis must be considered. When hemolytic anemia is present, the differential diagnosis for chronic copper toxicity in the goat includes the hemoparasites babesiosis and trypanosomosis, where they occur, and several plant poisonings that could lead to hemolytic anemia, particularly kale, which also can produce Heinz bodies. Other intoxications must be ruled out in acute copper toxicity, including arsenic ingestion, organophosphate toxicity, cyanide poisoning, and nitrate poisoning. The recent report of goats with chronic copper toxicosis which had no evidence of hemolytic anemia but did have elevated liver enzymes and neurological signs suggests that various causes of hepatic encephalopathy may have to be considered in the differential diagnosis of chronic copper toxicity.

Treatment

Treatment is directed at the clearance and elimination of copper from the blood and tissues through the use of chelating agents. Until recently, the only treatment reported specifically in goats was ammonium tetrathiomolybdate, administered intravenously at a dose of 1.7 mg/kg for three treatments on alternate days (Humphries et al. 1987). In lambs, a daily oral total dose of 100 mg of ammonium molybdate in combination with 1 g of sodium sulfate given for as long as three weeks has been effective in reducing tissue copper concentrations, and may prevent or ameliorate hemolytic crisis. Other chelating agents also have been used, including oral D-penicillamine at a dose of 52 mg/kg daily for six days. A recent report describes the successful use of penicillamine, ammonium molybdate, and sodium thiosulfate in the treatment of adult goats with primary chronic copper toxicosis (Cornish et al. 2007). Penicillamine was given orally at a dose of 50 mg/kg bw every twenty-four hours for seven days, ammonium molybdenate orally at a total dose of 300 mg every twenty-four hours for three weeks, sodium thiosulfate orally at a total dose of 300 mg every twenty-four hours for three weeks. Vitamin E was also given orally at a total dose of 2,000 U every twenty-four hours for three weeks as an anti-oxidant.

Penicillamine is expensive and, though effective, its use may be limited in commercial herds by cost considerations.

Therapeutic consideration should also be given to management of anemia when present as well as management of potential nephrosis in severely affected individuals. Blood transfusion might be indicated in exceptional cases when PCV is perilously decreased. Continuous intravenous administration of balanced electrolyte solutions helps maintain urine outflow and reduce the potential for irreversible hemoglobinuric nephrosis.

Control

Control of acute copper poisoning in the goat depends on common sense to avoid accidental exposure to and ingestion of high doses of copper. Because chronic copper poisoning in goats is rare, aggressive control methods such as fertilization of crop and grazing lands with molybdenum and molybdenum supplementation of feed are probably unnecessary. However, some caution should be exercised in using feedstuffs formulated for cattle, especially calf milk replacers used in kids. Nutritional requirements for copper in goats are discussed in Chapter 19.

Kale Anemia (*Brassica* Poisoning)

The use of kale *(Brassica oleracea)* as a feedstuff for ruminants may lead to the development of Heinz body anemia with possible mortality. Cattle are most susceptible, and sheep least susceptible. Goats have an intermediate position.

Epidemiology

Clinical outbreaks of Heinz body anemia have occurred in ruminants when kale has a predominant role in feeding programs. This has been a notable problem in Great Britain and Germany. Consumption of large amounts for extended periods increases the likelihood of disease, and anemia rarely develops until animals have been consuming kale for one to three weeks. Mature plants and plants with secondary growth are more toxic. The consumption of plants that have been frosted or frozen also increases the likelihood of disease. Certain varieties of kale are more toxic than others, but heating or ensilage destroys the toxic principle.

The condition is reproducible experimentally in goats (Greenlagh et al. 1969, 1970; Smith 1980). It has been reported as a cause of mortality in Angora goats in New Zealand (Anonymous 1988). Affected goats had been grazing the kale for less than two weeks, while lambs that had preceded kids in grazing were unaffected. It was suspected that kids, already anemic from haemonchosis, were more severely affected by kale toxicity.

Etiology and Pathogenesis

Kale contains high levels of S-methyl cysteine sulfoxide that is converted by rumen bacteria to dimethyl disulfide. This is then absorbed from the rumen and induces Heinz body anemia via the oxidation of hemoglobin in circulating red blood cells. Mature red blood cells are more susceptible to oxidation than young cells so that the anemia may become temporarily self-limiting as the regenerative response increases the relative proportion of young cells to old. As these cells mature, the anemia may worsen again if kale continues to be fed. This phenomenon is associated with higher levels of glutathione reductase in young cells that are protective against oxidation of hemoglobin (Smith 1980).

Clinical Findings

After one to three weeks of kale ingestion, goats develop a marked anemia. Sudden death may be the first reported sign in an affected herd or flock. Closer inspection may identify additional animals that hang back from the flock, appear weak, and have pale mucous membranes. Additional signs include inappetence, tachypnea, and tachycardia. Red-brown urine may be noted because of hemoglobinuria.

Clinical Pathology and Necropsy

Anemia may be pronounced, as hemoglobin levels can decrease below 6 g/dl and sometimes as low as 3 g/dl, with a concomitant decline in RBCs counts and PCV. The appearance of Heinz bodies in RBCs in the peripheral blood may precede the decrease in Hb by as much as a week. Methemoglobinemia, sometimes observed in cattle, is rare in goats. The anemia is regenerative, and reticulocytes and an increase in MCV can be noted.

Necropsy findings specific for the goat have not been reported. In other species, post mortem lesions include pallor, hemoglobinuria, thin, watery blood, dark kidneys, and congestion of the liver with moderate hepatic necrosis. Jaundice, especially of the subcutaneous fat, is pronounced.

Diagnosis

Diagnosis is presumptive based on the presence of Heinz body anemia in conjunction with a history of kale feeding. In other ruminants, rape *(Brassica napus)*, wild onion *(Allium validum)*, cultivated onion, and stubble turnip consumption also produce Heinz body anemia. When widespread jaundice is noted at necropsy, chronic copper toxicity and leptospirosis must be considered in the differential diagnosis.

Treatment and Control

Therapy is limited to supportive care and the possibility of blood transfusion. Removal of kale from the diet results in a return of normal Hb levels within two to three weeks. Affected goats should not be subjected to stress or vigorous exercise during the recovery.

Other Plant-related Anemias

Several reports identify plants toxic to goats with anemia as a clinical manifestation. *Acanthospermum hispidum*, a weed of the Compositae family, has been associated with livestock poisoning in the Sudan, and its toxicity for goats has been confirmed experimentally. Animals fed the plant at a dose of 5 g/kg bw daily showed anorexia, jaundice, and diarrhea within one week, followed by dullness, dyspnea, weakness of the hind end, and terminal neurologic signs, probably because of hepatoencephalopathy. Clinical pathology indicated acute liver dysfunction and development of a marked hemolytic anemia during the course of disease (Ali and Adam 1978).

Ipomoea carnea, in the family Convolvulacae, is a tropical plant with strong drought-resistant properties; it may be an abundant source of browse for goats during adverse climatic periods. Toxicity in goats because of *Ipomoea* spp. has been presumed or documented in India, Brazil, and the Sudan (Tirkey et al. 1987; Dobereiner et al. 1987; Damir et al. 1987). Experimentally, daily repeated doses of fresh leaves of *Ipomoea carnea* as low as 5 g/kg of bw can produce a clinical syndrome of inappetence, depression, pallor, weakness of the hindquarters, dyspnea, weight loss, and death within three weeks, although there is individual variation in response, and some goats survived for longer than three months. A moderate, normocytic, normochromic, occasionally hypochromic anemia is observed in severely affected goats. Packed cell volumes as low as 15% occur, with Hb as low as 5 g/dl. In acute cases, the anemia is nonregenerative, but in animals that survived for longer periods, a macrocytic response was observed. Serum chemistry analysis suggested liver dysfunction with elevated AST and ammonia and hypoproteinemia (Tartour et al. 1974; Damir et al. 1987). Toxicity from *Ipomoea carnea* is dose dependent. In an Indian study, no clinical signs or laboratory abnormalities occurred in goats fed an aqueous extract of the plant at a dose of 160 mg/kg, considered to be one-fifth the LD_{50} dose (Tirkey et al. 1987).

Anemia also has been reported as an incidental finding in several plant poisonings in the Sudan, including *Capparis tomentosa* (Ahmed and Adam 1980), *Tephrosia apollinea* (Suliman et al. 1982), and experimentally, *Solanum dubium*. The latter plant is not routinely eaten by goats but may be consumed during periods of drought (Barri et al. 1983).

Bracken fern *(Pteridium aquilinum)* ingestion has been associated with a number of clinical syndromes in cattle and sheep, including depression of bone marrow activity leading to aplastic anemia, leukopenia with secondary bacterial infections, and ecchymoses secondary to thrombocytopenia, as well as ruminal papillomatosis, progressive retinal degeneration, and enzootic hematuria. There is only one clinical report associating exposure to bracken fern with disease in goats (Tomlinson 1983). Affected goats showed a marked anemia and high fevers that responded to antibiotic therapy, suggestive of secondary bacterial infections. Leukocyte counts and bone marrow evaluations were not performed. The goats concurrently experienced severe gastrointestinal helminthiasis and the contribution of bracken fern ingestion to the anemia and infections was not well established. Currently goats should be considered potentially susceptible to bracken fern toxicity. A report from Venezuela states that bracken fern can cause permanent blindness in goats (Alonso-Amelot 1999).

A number of plants have been associated with hemoglobinuria in sheep, including privet (*Ligustrum* spp.), broom (*Cytisus* spp.), hellebore (*Helleborus* spp.), *Ranunculus* spp., *Colchicum* spp., and frosted turnips (Kimberling and Arnold 1983). Currently, there are no reports of toxicity with these plants in goats, but it is reasonable to assume that a toxic potential exists.

DISEASES OF THE IMMUNE SYSTEM

Thymoma

Neoplasia is comparatively uncommon in goats, but thymoma is one of the two most commonly recognized caprine tumors. It occurs more frequently in goats than in other domestic species. The other common tumor is the adrenal cortical adenoma seen in castrated male goats, as discussed in Chapter 13.

Epidemiology

Thymoma is rarely seen in goats younger than two years of age. There is no sex predilection. Because thymomas rarely produce clinical disease, recognition of thymoma in goats has come mostly from slaughterhouse surveys and as an incidental finding in necropsy studies. The highest prevalence has been reported in a group of Saanen goats used for slow virus research studies. Seventeen of ninety-two goats (18.5%) had thymomas at necropsy, with a prevalence of 25.3% in goats older than two years of age (Hadlow 1978). Slaughterhouse surveys indicate a lesser prevalence in general goat populations, with eight cases per 100,000 goats in one study and fourteen of 2,600 adult Angora goats in another, but this is still more than the prevalence of thymoma in other livestock species (Streett et al. 1968; Migaki 1969).

Clinical Findings

Most occurrences of thymoma are subclinical, but occasionally thymomas have been associated with clinical disease. Congestive heart failure secondary to thymoma was recorded in two aged Nubian goats (Rostkowski et al. 1985). These cases are discussed in more detail in Chapter 8. There is also a case of megaesophagus in an eight-year-old Saanen doe secondary to a thymoma and an associated hematoma which put pressure on the thoracic esophagus. The goat presented with a history of recurrent tympany and regurgitation after eating (Parish et al. 1996).

Occasionally, the thymoma may produce a pronounced subcutaneous swelling visible at the base of the neck. Normal thymic tissue is commonly found near the thyroids and at the base of the neck in healthy goat kids, as discussed in Chapter 3. In other species, notably the dog, thymoma has been associated with myasthenia gravis and polymyositis.

Clinical Pathology and Necropsy

The majority of thymomas occur in the cranial mediastinal cavity and occasionally at the thoracic inlet. Tumor size is variable, with some weighing up to 600 g. The tumors are encapsulated, firm, and grayish-white, and the larger ones tend to be lobulated. On cut surfaces they can contain areas of hemorrhage, cysts, and focal yellow areas of necrosis, sometimes associated with calcification. Metastases are rare, but adhesions to adjacent structures, especially lungs, do occur. In one report, pulmonary metastases from a thymoma were identified in an eight-year-old castrated male French Alpine goat with a history of progressive weight loss, exercise intolerance, and anorexia (Olchowy et al. 1996).

Diagnosis

Lymphosarcoma involving the thymus occurs rarely in goats and must be differentiated from thymoma. In thymoma, the principle neoplastic cell is a polymorphic epithelial cell that is often spindle-shaped, but can be round or ovoid. Lymphocytes are present in thymomas, and may predominate, but they do not exhibit characteristics of neoplastic transformation. The neoplastic cell in lymphosarcoma is the lymphocyte. Because it often produces peripheral lymphadenopathy, lymphosarcoma is discussed in more detail in Chapter 3.

Treatment and Control

Currently there are no methods of control. The reported high incidence of thymoma in Saanen goats used in slow virus research suggests that either genetic or viral factors may play a role in the development of caprine thymoma. This merits additional investigation, particularly because the retroviral disease CAE is now recognized to be widespread in goats.

Failure of Passive Transfer (FPT) of Maternal Immunity

Newborn goats, like the young of other livestock species, depend on the ingestion of antibody-rich colostrum shortly after birth to provide passive immunologic protection until they can actively produce their own array of protective antibodies. The failure to absorb adequate antibodies in the immediate post partum period predisposes young goats to serious infectious disease problems and high mortality rates.

Epidemiology

Unacceptably high levels of death loss in young goats are recognized as a major constraint on goat production wherever goats are raised. The factors contributing to kid death in various goat-producing regions of the world have been reviewed (Sherman 1987; Morand-Fehr 1987). In extensive management systems, kid losses have been reported in the range of 10% to 60% and, in intensive management systems, from 8% to 17%. These deaths most frequently occur in the first few days of life. Numerous factors contribute to this bias toward early death, including low birth weight, premature delivery, large litter size, poor mothering ability, and environmental and weather conditions at the time of kidding. However, the failure to suckle adequate colostrum at birth contributes significantly to the preponderance of early kid deaths, most likely through the mechanism of failure of passive transfer of humoral immunity, as discussed below under pathogenesis. In a French survey, 92% of colostrum-deprived kids that died did so within two days of birth (Morand-Fehr et al. 1984). In an Indian study, serum immunoglobulin (Ig) levels were measured in newborn kids eighteen hours after ingestion of colostrum and the mean serum Ig concentration of these kids was determined to be 735 mg/dl. In the next two months, mortality rates of kids with serum Ig levels less than the mean was 44% but was only 3.8% for those with serum Ig levels more than the mean (Nandakumar and Rajagopalaraja 1983).

In addition to providing immunity against infectious disease and reducing neonatal mortality, there are indications that consumption of adequate colostrum by the neonate is associated with other long term benefits. There are positive correlations between serum IgG concentration at twenty-four hours of age (sIgG-24) and weaning weight in beef calves as well as positive correlations with first lactation milk production and milk fat content in dairy heifers. In goats, a significant correlation is reported between sIgG-24 and average daily weight gain in preweaned dairy goat kids measured up to thirty days of age (Massimini et al. 2007).

Etiology and Pathogenesis

The syndesmochorial (epitheliochorial) placentation of the goat does not permit the transfer of Ig from the maternal circulation to the fetus during gestation. Therefore, the kid is born in an agammaglobulinemic state, and though immunocompetent, is highly susceptible to infection because of the immediate lack of circulating humoral antibody. Passive immunization of the newborn kid depends on early oral ingestion of colostrum containing maternally produced Ig. The doe experiences an increase in antibody production, notably of the IgG_1 class, in the weeks preceding parturition, and IgG_1 antibodies are preferentially transported into the colostrum, aided by the affinity of the Fc fragment of IgG_1 for receptors on mammary epithelial cells. The mean concentrations for IgG_1 and IgG_2 in doe serum are reported as 10.9 and 9.1 mg/ml, respectively, while in colostrum the relative mean concentrations are 50.8 mg/ml for IgG_1 and 2.3 mg/ml for IgG_2 (Micusan and Borduas 1977).

The newborn kid, upon ingesting colostrum, is capable of transporting intact Ig molecules out of the intestinal lumen and into the blood circulation. Survival of intact antibody molecules in the gut lumen probably depends on the presence of trypsin inhibitors present in colostrum. The mechanism of transintestinal transport is pinocytosis through the original neonatal intestinal epithelial cells. It is presumed that as these cells are sloughed and replaced in the normal process by new epithelial cells, the capacity for additional pinocytosis and additional intestinal absorption of Ig is lost. In the calf and lamb, maximal absorptive capacity is believed to persist for six hours after birth, with all absorptive capacity absent by twenty-four hours of age, although this is conditioned to some extent by extrinsic factors such as the time of first suckling. In contrast, the kid may be able to effectively absorb antibody for a longer period, perhaps as long as four days. In one study, kids fed milk only at birth and not given colostrum until seventy-two hours old demonstrated increased serum antibody levels after colostrum administration. The level achieved, however, was not as much as that observed in kids receiving colostrum at birth, and mortality rates were higher (Vihan and Sahni 1982). Therefore, the potentially longer period for intestinal absorption of colostral antibodies in kids is no reason for delaying the ingestion of colostrum. The fact that the concentration of antibody in colostrum decreases rapidly after the first six to twelve hours also underscores the importance of early ingestion.

A number of factors influence the ultimate level of Ig reaching the serum of the kid and the immunity derived from it. Most of these considerations have been elucidated specifically for the lamb but are also considered applicable to the kid (Levieux 1984). These include the ability of the kid to suckle early after birth, volume of colostrum available, absorptive potential of the kid, concentration of antibody in the colostrum, and diversity and activity of the antibody. Small kids, especially if weakened by dystocia, may be unable to rise and therefore experience delayed suckling. Severe weather, disturbance of the doe and kid after birth, and competition by litter mates may also delay suckling or reduce the amount of colostrum available. Normal kids should stand and suckle within approximately one-half hour after birth.

The ability of kids to absorb Ig after ingestion of colostrum depends primarily on the time of colostrum ingestion, with earlier ingestion promoting better absorption. Birth weight and length of gestation are reported to be negatively correlated with absorption of Ig. However, there are apparently other unknown factors that affect the intrinsic ability of individual kids to absorb Ig. When newborn kids were administered colostrum from a common source on a per weight basis at the same time interval after birth, serum antibody levels subsequently varied by as much as a factor of eight. In addition to kid factors, maternal factors affect absorption. The concentration and character of Ig in does can also vary. Older does are likely to have a wider immunologic experience than young does and provide a more diverse spectrum of protective antibodies to kids. Breed variation has been observed in both ewes and does (Nandakumar and Rajagopalaraja 1983a; Levieux 1984). In the dairy breeds, where colostrum is produced well in excess of that required by offspring, IgG concentrations in the colostrum and subsequently in the kids' serum can be present in levels considerably higher than those reported for non-dairy breeds.

The majority of ingested antibody, primarily IgG_1, is absorbed across the intestinal tract to become circulating humoral antibody. Therefore, the key protective role of colostral antibody is prevention of general infection, and the most common cause of death in colostrum-deprived kids is colisepticemia. Doe colostrum also contains small amounts of IgA and IgM, 1.7 mg/ml and 3.8 mg/ml, respectively, but the role of colostral antibody in protecting against local, mucosal infection, particularly in the gut, is rather limited.

While absorbed antibody is clearly beneficial to the kid in terms of immediate disease protection, passive antibody can have a retarding effect on the development of the kid's own active immunity. Experimental evidence demonstrates that in colostrum-deprived kids, circulating IgG_2 appears earlier in the serum than in colostrum-fed kids and that by twelve weeks of age, circulating levels of both IgG_1 and IgG_2 are higher in colostrum-deprived kids than colostrum-fed kids (Micusan et al. 1976).

Based on studies of the disappearance of antibodies specific for *Corynebacterium pseudotuberculosis* from kid serum after colostrum ingestion, the half-life of passively acquired antibody is approximately twelve days, with some antibody still detectable in most kids between five and six weeks of age (Lund et al. 1982). Persistent antibodies may inhibit active immunization with homologous vaccines. When colostrum-fed kids were immunized with human gamma globulin, a protein with which their dams had been previously immunized, they showed no measurable antibody response to immunizations at birth and four weeks of age and responded only at eight weeks of age when passive antibody levels to the protein had diminished (Micusan et al. 1976). These observations are of practical concern when planning vaccination schedules for young goats.

Clinical Findings

There are no specific clinical signs of FPT per se. The condition is suggested by kid deaths occurring within forty-eight hours of birth, in association with clinical signs of septicemia. These include acute collapse, very high or subnormal body temperature, cold extremities, congested mucous membranes, rapid heart rate and thready pulses, and dehydration. Evidence of navel infection, diarrhea, or swollen joints may also be suggestive of septicemia, but many kids die before these signs are observable. Hyperesthesia, seizure activity, or ophistotonos may be observed because of bacterial invasion of the central nervous system or concomitant acidosis. Pneumonia, enteritis, or a pneumoenteritis complex occurring in kids during the first few weeks of life is also suggestive of FPT.

A careful history should be taken to determine if the affected kids were observed to suckle, the time of suckling, whether the caretaker provided colostrum by bottle, and whether navels were disinfected after birth. Examination of the kidding and housing areas for evidence of poor sanitation and lapses in good management technique may suggest that septicemia secondary to FPT is involved.

Clinical Pathology and Necropsy

The most direct method for determining if FPT is involved in death losses is to measure circulating Ig levels in the serum or plasma of kids. The optimal time for obtaining serum samples from kids is between twenty-four and forty-eight hours of life, because maximum antibody absorption from the gut will have occurred during that time. Methods reported specifically for determination of serum Ig in kids are limited compared with other livestock species.

Documented tests include a quantitative zinc sulfate turbidity test and a qualitative glutaraldehyde coagulation test (Vihan 1989; Sherman et al. 1990). Using the zinc sulfate turbidity test, kids receiving 480 ml of heat-treated goat colostrum in the first twenty-four hours of life had mean Ig levels of 1.5 gm/dl when tested twenty-four hours after the last colostrum feeding. Using the glutaraldehyde coagulation test, serum from kids with Ig levels less than 1 gram/dl did not clot after sixty minutes incubation with 10% glutaraldehyde solution. Recently, the use of total protein determination by refractometry and a sodium sulfite precipitation test have been described for deriving reliable estimates of Ig levels in kids under field conditions (O'Brien and Sherman. 1993). When FPT was defined as a serum IgG $< 1{,}200$ mg/dl, all cases of FPT were indirectly identified using total protein determination by refractometry when the cutoff for total protein was set at 5.4 g/dl. Currently, commercial test kits are also available for direct measurement of IgG in goat serum using radial immunodiffusion (Massimini et al. 2007).

Studies correlating antibody level to morbidity and mortality in kids are scarce compared with similar work for calves, lambs, and foals, so minimal acceptable levels of circulating Ig for kids under different systems and conditions of management are not established. In a recent prospective study of kid survival in relation to circulating Ig levels in intensively managed dairy goat kids in New England, in the United States, a serum Ig level of 1,200 mg/dl appeared to be protective (O'Brien and Sherman 1993a).

An indirect method for evaluating Ig absorption by measurement of serum gamma glutamyl transferase

(GGT) levels in kid serum has been reported. The mean serum GGT levels in pre-suckling newborn kids was 19 U/l, with a maximum recorded measurement of 28 U/l. At twenty-four hours after colostrum ingestion, serum GGT levels were on average six and a half times greater than pre-suckle levels, with a mean of 127 U/l and a minimum reported value of 43 U/l. The mean GGT level fell rapidly after twenty-four hours, so timing appeared critical in the evaluation of the test results (Braun et al. 1984).

Goats with septicemia secondary to failure of passive transfer are likely to be severely leukopenic and may show hyperfibrinogenemia. Necropsy results are nonspecific, but bacterial culture results of heart blood and various other organs can establish the presence of septicemia.

Diagnosis

Decreased serum Ig levels in newborn kids twenty-four hours of age or older confirms the presence of FPT. The contribution of this condition to concurrent disease problems can only be inferred. In kids dead before twenty-four hours, FPT may be contributory, but this is more difficult to establish. Hypothermia and hypoglycemia must always be considered in the differential diagnosis of septicemia secondary to FPT. Hypoglycemia may be presumed in the live animal by measurement of blood glucose, although blood glucose is also likely to be decreased in active septicemia. The absence of an inflammatory hemogram supports primary hypoglycemia, as does the absence of a milk clot in the abomasum or ingesta in the small intestine, indicating lack of feed intake. A diagnosis of hypothermia is supported by low body temperature in conjunction with environmental conditions that would promote chilling such as outdoor kidding, cold temperatures, wet weather, and drafts. In individual kids, congenital abnormalities must also be considered as a cause of early death. Under conditions of extremely poor management and with sufficiently virulent organisms, septicemias can occur even when adequate colostrum has been ingested shortly after birth.

Treatment

In most cases, FPT first comes to the veterinarian's attention because of a primary complaint of early deaths or signs of shock suggesting the presence of septicemia. Immediate attention must be given to the management of the infection. Animals should be moved to a warm, dry environment. Intravenous fluid therapy including glucose and sodium bicarbonate should be initiated to counter the hypoglycemia and circulatory effects associated with septic shock. Parenteral nonsteroidal anti-inflammatory drugs such as flunixin meglumine may be helpful. Antibiotic therapy is essential. Choice of drugs ideally should depend on blood culture, but therapy should be initiated immediately with broad spectrum antibiotics, especially those with efficacy against Gram-negative species. Trimethoprim-sulfa combinations or gentamicin combined with ampicillin can be effective. Aminoglycoside drugs must be used cautiously to avoid serious renal damage, particularly if fluid therapy is not used concurrently. Chloramphenicol, where permitted, is also effective in septicemia.

Correction of the hypogammaglobulinemia requires transfusion of plasma or whole blood. The volume required to replace the Ig deficit depends on the known level of circulating Ig in the sick kid and the average or known level of Ig in the blood of the donor goat. The average circulating serum Ig level of does is approximately 20 mg/ml. Although the minimum level of acceptable circulating immunoglobulin required by the kid has not been established, in most cases an initial transfusion of at least 250 ml of plasma is required for an average-sized kid. Repeated evaluation of zinc sulfate turbidity test results after plasma administration can aid in determining the need for additional transfusions.

Prevention

All goat caretakers should be aware of the potential economic losses associated with failure of passive transfer of antibody to newborn kids and educated on aspects of neonatal management related to colostrum administration. Careful observation of goats at kidding time may be necessary to identify individual kids that do not effectively suckle by six hours of age. These kids should be bottle fed or tubed with colostrum at a rate of 50 ml of colostrum per kg bw for each of three feedings over the first twelve to twenty-four hours of life. In intensive management systems, caretakers responsible for kid rearing can be encouraged to electively administer colostrum to all kids routinely within six hours of birth rather than wait for it to occur naturally.

The maintenance of a frozen colostrum bank ensures that all kids have colostrum available regardless of the status of their dams. In preparing frozen colostrum, only that taken from does during the first twelve hours after kidding should be kept for freezing, because the concentration of Ig in colostrum falls off rapidly and dramatically after the first stripping. It is reported that Ig concentration of caprine colostrum shows a strong positive correlation to its specific gravity, so that colostrum quality can be screened using a colostrometer. Colostrum with a specific gravity more than 1.029 is preferred (Ubertalle et al. 1987). Bovine colostrum, either fresh or frozen, has been used successfully as a substitute for ewe colostrum in rearing lambs. This has also gained popularity in goat rearing in an attempt to limit the colostral transmission of CAE virus in kids.

Serum antibody levels achieved in kids suckling bovine colostrum are equivalent to those obtained with caprine colostrum (Sherman et al. 1990). However, this practice must be viewed with caution; in France, a hemolytic syndrome has been reported in some kids at one week of age after consumption of bovine colostrum. It was demonstrated *in vitro* that bovine antibodies were directed against some caprine erythrocytes (Perrin et al. 1988).

Concerns have arisen regarding the impact of heat treatment techniques on immunoglobulin content of goat colostrum used in caprine arthritis encephalitis (CAE) control programs. The original heat treatment protocol of 56°C (132.8°F) for sixty minutes was developed to avoid the denaturing effect on antibody associated with the higher temperatures of pasteurization, while still inactivating the CAE virus (Adams et al. 1983). However, more recent studies demonstrate *in vitro* that heat treatment of colostrum at 56°C for sixty minutes reduces measurable IgG in colostrum by approximately 37% (Argüello et al. 2002). Nevertheless, if the initial concentrations of the colostrum that is heat treated are sufficiently high, successful passive transfer of antibody may still be achieved.

In recent years, a number of commercial products have become available that have been promoted as colostrum supplements for calves, lambs, and kids but have been used by goat owners as colostrum substitutes in part to avoid the need for heat treating colostrum for CAE control, which can be cumbersome and time consuming. These products are usually in the form of soluble powders or boluses. In one study, two of these products were evaluated in kids. There was virtually no detectable increase in circulating serum Ig levels in colostrum-deprived kids receiving these oral products within twelve hours of birth. Therefore, the value of these products as sources of protective Ig must be viewed skeptically (Sherman et al. 1990). Other reports have corroborated the inadequacy of certain colostrum substitutes in achieving adequate immunoglobulin levels in kids receiving the products (Constant et al. 1994).

REFERENCES

Aalund, O.: Immune response of sheep, goats, cattle, and swine. In: Soulsby, E.J.L., ed. Immunity to Animal Parasites. New York, Academic Press, pp. 2–31, 1972.

Adam, S.E.I., Wasfi, I.A. and Magzoub, M.: Chronic copper toxicity in Nubian goats. J. Comp. Pathol., 87:623–627, 1977.

Adams, D.S., et al.: Transmission and control of caprine arthritis-encephalitis virus. Am. J. Vet. Res., 44(9):1670–1675, 1983.

Adeoye, S.A.O.: Disease profiles of sheep and goats in two groups of villages in southwest Nigeria. In: Sheep and Goats in Humid West Africa. J.E. Sumberg and K. Cassaday, eds. Addis Ababa. International Livestock Center for Africa. pp. 13–16, 1985.

Adeyemo, O., Gao, R.J. and Lan H.C.: Cytokine production *in vitro* by macrophages of goats with caprine arthritis-encephalitis. Cel. Mol. Biol. 43(7):1031–1037, 1997.

Agunloye, C.A., et al.: Clinical and serological diagnosis of leptospirosis in aborting West African dwarf goats. Nig. Vet. J. 1(1):9–15, 1996.

Ahmed, J.S., et al.: Phylogenetic position of small-ruminant infecting piroplasms. Ann. N. Y. Acad. Sci., 1081:498–504, 2006.

Ahmed, O.M.M. and Adam, S.E.I.: The toxicity of *Capparis tomentosa* in goats. J. Comp. Pathol., 90:187–195, 1980.

Akerejola, O.O., Schillhorn van Veen, T.W. and Njoku, C.O.: Ovine and caprine diseases in Nigeria: A review of economic losses. Bull. Anim. Health Prod. Afr., 27:65–70, 1979.

Ali, B. and Adam, S.E.I.: Effects of *Acanthospermum hispidum* on goats. J. Comp. Pathol. 88:533–544, 1978.

Alonso-Amelot, M.E.: Bracken fern, animal and human health. Rev. Facult. Agron., Univ. Zulia, 16(5):528–547, 1999.

Alves, C.J., Vasconcellos, S.A., Camargo, C.R.A. and Morais, Z.M.: Influence of regional and climatic factors on the proportion of goats seroreactive for leptospirosis at five breeding centres in the northeastern state of Paraiba, Brazil. Arq. Inst. Biol. (Sao Paulo), 63(2):11–18, 1996.

Amjadi, A.R. and Ahourai, P.: Pathological aspect of leptospirosis in sheep and goats in Iran. Arch. Inst. Razi, 27:71–80, 1975.

Andresen, E.: Blood groups, immunogenetics and biochemical genetics. In: Duke's Physiology of Domestic Animals. 10th edition, M.J. Swenson, ed. Ithaca, Comstock Publishing Assoc., 1984.

Anika, S.M., et al.: Chemotherapy and pharmacokinetics of some antimicrobial agents in healthy dwarf goats and those infected with *Ehrlichia phagocytophilia* (tick-borne fever). Res. Vet. Sci., 41:386–390, 1986.

Anika, S.M., Nouws, J.F.M., Vree, T.B. and Van Miert, A. S.J.P.A.M.: The efficacy and plasma disposition of chloramphenicol and spiramycin in tick-borne fever-infected dwarf goats. J. Vet. Pharmacol. Therap., 9:433–435, 1986a.

Anonymous: Brassica red-water in goats. Goat Health Prod., 2:8, 1988.

Anosa, V.O. and Isoun, T.T.: Serum proteins, blood and plasma volumes in experimental *Trypanosoma vivax* infections of sheep and goats. Trop. Anim. Health Prod., 8:14–19, 1976.

Argüello, A., et al.: Effects of refrigeration, freezing-thawing and pasteurization on IgG goat colostrum preservation. Small Rumin. Res., 48(2):135–139, 2003.

Atroshi, F., Sankari, S., and Lindstrom, U.B.: Somatic cell count and milk yield in relation to haemoglobin concentration in Finnish dairy goats. Vet. Res. Commun., 10:57–63, 1986.

Aziz, E.S. and Klesius, P.H.: Depressed neutrophil chemotactic stimuli in supernatants of ionophore-treated polymorphonuclear leukocytes from selenium-deficient goats. Am. J. Vet. Res., 47:148–151, 1986.

Aziz, E.S. and Klesius, P.H.: The effect of selenium deficiency in goats on lymphocyte production of leukocyte migration inhibitory factor. Vet. Immunol. Immunopathol., 10:381–390, 1985.

Aziz, E.S., Klesius, P.H. and Frandsen, J.C.: Effects of selenium on polymorphonuclear leukocyte function in goats. Am. J. Vet. Res., 45:1715–1718, 1984.

Banerjee, P.K., Guha, C. and Gupta, R.: A note on incidence of *Babesia motasi* infection in a goat in West Bengal. Indian Vet. J., 64:71–73, 1987.

Banks, K.L. and Greenlee, A.: Lymphocyte subpopulations of the goat: Isolation and identification. Am. J. Vet. Res., 43:314–317, 1982.

Bannister, J.V., et al.: The structure of goat hemoglobins. V. A fourth beta chain variant with decreased oxygen affinity and occurring at a high frequency in Malta. Hemoglobin, 3:57–75, 1979.

Barri, M.E.S., et al.: Toxicity of five Sudanese plants to young ruminants. J. Comp. Pathol., 93:559–575, 1983.

Barry, D.M. and van Niekerk, C.M.: *Anaplasma ovis* abortion in Boer goat does: I. Effect on body temperature and haematological picture in infected does. Proc. IV International Conf. Goats, Brasilia, EMBRAPA-DDT, p. 1488, 1987.

Barry, D.M. and van Niekerk, C.M.: *Anaplasma ovis* abortion in Boer goat does: II. Effect on plasma progesterone concentration and transplacental migration of *A. ovis* in infected does. Proc. IV International Conf. Goats, Brasilia, EMBRAPA-DDT, p. 1489, 1987a.

Bealby, K.A., Connor, R.J. and Rowlands, G.J.: Trypanosomosis in goats in Zambia. International Livestock Research. Institute (ILRI), Nairobi, ix + 88 pp., 1996.

Begovic, S., Duaic, E., Sacirbegovic, A. and Tafro, A.: Study of etiology and pathogenesis of function disturbances of haematopoietic system in alimentary intoxications with tannins. Veterinaria, Yugoslavia, 27(4):459–470, 1978.

Belford, C.J. and Raven, C.R.: Chronic copper poisoning in Angora kids. Surveillance, New Zealand, 13:4–5, 1986.

Bennett, D.G.: Anemia and hypoproteinemia. Vet. Clin. N. Am. Large Anim. Pract., 5:511–524, 1983.

Bhatnagar, R.N., Mittal, K.R., Jaiswal, T.N. and Padmanaban, V.D.: Levels of complement activities in the sera of healthy goats. Indian Vet. J., 65:93–97, 1988.

Bianca, W.: Blood volume in young goats at high altitude. Fed. Proc., 28:1220–1222, 1969.

Black, H., Hutton, J.B., Sutherland, R.J. and James, M.P.: White liver disease in goats. N. Z. Vet. J., 36:15–17, 1988.

Boutin, J.P., Debonne, J.M. and Rey, J.L.: Apparition du charbon humain en forêt ivoirienne. Méd. Trop., 45:79–81, 1985.

Bouzar, B.A., et al.: Activation/proliferation and apoptosis of bystander goat lymphocytes induced by a macrophage-tropic chimeric caprine arthritis encephalitis virus expressing SIV Nef. Virol., 364(2):269–280, 2007.

Bowen, J.: DNA Typing. American Dairy Goat Association. Spindale, NC, 2007. http://www.adga.org/dna.htm.

Brain, L.T.A.: Cobalt deficiency in a young goat. Goat Vet. Soc. J., 4:45, 1983.

Braun, J.P., et al.: Transfer of gamma-glutamyltransferase from mother colostrum to newborn goat and foal. Enzyme, 31:193–196, 1984.

Breukink, H.J., et al.: Congenital afibrinogenemia in goats. Zentralbl. Vet. Med. A, 19:661–676, 1972.

Briggs, P.M., et al.: Human cutaneous anthrax—North Carolina, 1987. Morb. Mort. Weekly Report, 37:413–414, 1988.

Brooks, D.L., Tillman, P.C. and Niemi, S.M.: Ungulates as laboratory animals. In: Laboratory Animal Medicine. J.G. Fox, B.J. Cohen, and F.M. Loew, eds. Orlando, Academic Press, 1984.

Butler, J.E.: Biochemistry and biology of ruminant immunoglobulins. Prog. Vet. Microbiol. Immun., 2:1–53, 1986.

Buvanendran, V., Sooriyamoorthy, T., Ogunsusi, R.A. and Adu, I.F.: Haemoglobin polymorphism and resistance to helminths in red Sokoto goats. Trop. Anim. Health Prod., 13:217–221, 1981.

Cheevers, W.P., Beyer, J.C. and Knowles, D.P.: Type 1 and type 2 cytokine gene expression by viral gp135 surface protein-activated T lymphocytes in caprine arthritis-encephalitis lentivirus infection. J. Virol., 71(8):6259–6263, 1997.

Clark, C.H. and Kiesel, G.K.: Longevity of red blood cells in interspecies transfusion. J. Am. Vet. Med. Assoc., 143:400–401, 1963.

Coles, EH.: Veterinary Clinical Pathology, 4th Ed. Philadelphia, W.B. Saunders Co., 1986.

Connor, R.J. and van den Bossche, P.: African animal trypanosomoses. In: Infectious Diseases of Livestock, 2nd Ed. J.A.W. Coetzer and R.C. Tustin, eds., Oxford University Press, Cape Town, pp. 251–296, 2004.

Constant, S.B., et al.: Serum immunoglobulin G concentration in goat kids fed colostrum or a colostrum substitute. J. Am. Vet. Med. Assoc., 205(12):1759–1762, 1994.

Cornish, J., et al.: Copper toxicosis in a dairy goat herd. J. Am. Vet. Med. Assoc. 231(4):586–589, 2007.

Daddow, K.N.: A complement fixation test for the detection of *Eperythrozoon* infection in sheep. Australian Vet. J., 53:139–143, 1977.

Daddow, K.N.: The transmission of a sheep strain of *Eperythrozoon ovis* to goats and the development of a carrier state in the goats. Aust. Vet. J., 55:605, 1979.

Daddow, K.N.: The natural occurrence in a goat of an organism resembling *Eperythrozoon ovis*. Aust. Vet. J., 55:605–606, 1979a.

Damir, H.A., Adam, S.E.I. and Tartour, G.: The effects of *Ipomoea carnea* on goats and sheep. Vet. Hum. Toxicol., 29:316–319, 1987.

Dargantes, A.P., Reid, S.A. and Copeman, D.B.: Experimental *Trypanosoma evansi* infection in the goat. I. Clinical signs and clinical pathology. J. Comp. Pathol., 133(4):261–266, 2005.

Dargantes, A.P., Campbell, R.S.F., Copeman, D.B. and Reid, S.A.: Experimental *Trypanosoma evansi* infection in the goat. II. Pathology. J. Comp. Pathol., 133(4):267–276, 2005a.

Davis, C.E.: Thrombocytopenia a uniform complication of African trypanosomosis. Acta Trop. 39:123–134, 1982.

Davis, J.W., Libke, K.G., Watson, D.F. and Bibb, T.L.: Experimentally induced lead poisoning in goats: Clinical observations and pathologic changes. Cornell Vet. 66:490–497, 1976.

DeMartini, J.C., et al.: Augmented T lymphocyte responses and abnormal B lymphocyte numbers in goats chronically infected with the retrovirus causing caprine arthritis-encephalitis. Am. J. Vet. Res., 44:2064–2069, 1983.

Diamond, L.S. and Rubin, R.: Experimental infection of certain farm animals with a North American strain of *Trypanasoma cruzi* from the raccoon. Exp. Parasitol., 7:383–390, 1958.

Diesing, L., Ahmed, J.S., Zweygarth, E. and Horchner, F.: *Trypanosoma brucei brucei* infection in goats. Response in peripheral blood lymphocytes to mitogen stimulation. Tropenmed. Parasitol., 34:79–83, 1983.

Dobereiner, J., Stolf, L. and Tokarnia, C.H.: Poisonous plants affecting goats. Proc. IV International Conf. Goats, Brasilia, EMBRAPA-DDT, pp. 473–487, 1987.

Dollahite, J.W.: The use of sheep and goats to control *Senecio* poisoning in cattle. Southwest. Vet., 25:223–226, 1972.

Dorr, L., Pearce, P.C., Shine, T. and Hawkey, C.M.: Changes in red cell volume distribution frequency after acute blood loss in goats *(Capra hircus)*. Res. Vet. Sci., 40:322–327, 1986.

Doyle, J.J., Moloo, S.K. and Borowy, N.K.: Development of improved control methods of animal trypanosomiasis: A review. Prev. Vet. Med., 2:43–52, 1984.

Dubey, J.P., Weisbrode, S.E., Speer, C.A. and Sharma, S.P.: Sarcocystosis in goats: Clinical signs and pathologic and hematologic findings. J. Am. Vet. Med. Assoc., 178:683–699, 1981.

Dumler, J.S., et al.: Reorganization of genera in the families *Rickettsiaceae* and *Anaplasmataceae* in the order *Rickettsiales*: unification of some species of *Ehrlichia* with *Anaplasma*, *Cowdria* with *Ehrlichia* and *Ehrlichia* with *Neorickettsia*, descriptions of six new species combinations and designation of *Ehrlichia equi* and "HGE agent" as subjective synonyms of *Ehrlichia phagocytophila*. Int. J. Syst. Evol. Microbiol., 51:2145–2165, 2001.

Earl, P.R. and Carranza, A.B.: Leukocyte differential counts of the Mexican goat. Internat. Goat Sheep Res. 1:6–10, 1980.

Edelsten, R.M.: The distribution and prevalence of Nairobi sheep disease and other tick-borne infections of sheep and goats in northern Somalia. Trop. Anim. Health Prod., 7:29–34, 1975.

Edjtehadi, M.: Age associated changes in the blood picture of the goat. Zentralbl. Vet. Med. A, 25:198–206, 1978.

Edwards, E.E., Judd, J.M. and Squire, F.A.: Observations on trypanosomosis in domestic animals in West Africa. I. The daily index of infection and the weekly haematological values in goats and sheep infected with *Trypanosoma vivax, T. congolense,* and *T. brucei*. Ann. Tropmed. Parasitol. 50:223–241, 1956.

Ellory, J.C. and Tucker, E.M.: Cation transport in red blood cells. In: Red Blood Cells of Domestic Mammals. N.S. Agar and P.G. Board, eds. Amsterdam, Elsevier, 1983.

Euzéby, J.P. Dictionnaire de bactériologie vétérinaire. Approved lists. 2003. http://www.bacterio.cict.fr/bacdico/garde.html.

Ezeasor, D.N. and Singh, A.: Histology of the caprine hemal node. Acta Anat., 133:16–23, 1988.

Fairley, N.M., Price, G.S., and Meuten, D.J.: Evaluation of red blood cell fragility in Pygmy goats. Am. J. Vet. Res., 49:1598–1600, 1988.

Fetcher, A.: Liver diseases of sheep and goats. Vet. Clin. N. Am. Large Anim. Pract., 5:525–538, 1983.

Fletcher, W.S., Rogers, A.L., and Donaldson, S.S.: The use of the goat as an experimental animal. Lab. Anim. Care, 14:65–90, 1964.

Fluri, A., et al.: The MHC-haplotype influences primary, but not memory, immune responses to an immunodominant peptide containing T- and B-cell epitopes of the caprine arthritis encephalitis virus Gag protein. Vaccine, 24(5):597–606, 2006.

Foster, W.N.M. and Greig, J.C.: Isolation of tick-borne fever from feral goats in New Galloway. Vet. Rec., 85:585–586, 1969.

Garrick, M.D. and Garrick, L.M.: Hemoglobin and globin genes. In: Red Blood Cells of Domestic Mammals. N.S. Agar and P.G. Board, eds. Amsterdam, Elsevier, 1983.

Garrick, M.D.: Hemoglobin switching. In: Red Blood Cells of Domestic Mammals. N.S. Agar and P.G. Board, eds. Amsterdam, Elsevier, 1983.

Gray, D., Webster, K. and Berry, J.E.: Evidence of louping ill and tick-borne fever in goats. Vet. Rec., 122:66, 1988.

Gray, G.D., Mickelson, M.M. and Crim, J.A.: The demonstration of two gamma globulin subclasses in the goat. Immunochemistry, 6:641–644, 1969.

Greenlagh, J.F.D., Sharman, G.A.M. and Aitken, J.N.: Kale anemia-I. The toxicity to various species of animal of three types of kale. Res. Vet. Sci., 10:64–72, 1969.

Greenlagh, J.F.D., Sharman, G.A.M. and Aitken, J.N.: Kale anemia-II. Further factors concerned in the occurrence of the disease under experimental conditions. Res. Vet. Sci., 11:232–238, 1970.

Greenlee, A. and Banks, K.L.: Cellular and lipopolysaccharide subunit requirements for the caprine lymphoblastogenic response to endotoxin. Am. J. Vet. Res., 46:75–79, 1985.

Griffin, L.: African trypanosomosis in sheep and goats: a review. Vet. Bull., 48:819–825, 1978.

Griffin, L. and Allonby, E.W.: Studies on the epidemiology of trypanosomiasis in sheep and goats in Kenya. Trop. Anim. Health Prod., 11:133–142, 1979.

Griffin, L. and Allonby, E.W.: Disease syndromes in sheep and goats naturally infected with *Trypanosoma congolense*. J. Comp. Pathol., 89:457–464, 1979a.

Griffin, L., Allonby, E.W., and Preston, J.M.: The interaction of *Trypanosoma congolense* and *Haemonchus contortus* infections in 2 breeds of goat. 1. Parasitology. J. Comp. Pathol., 91:85–95, 1981a.

Griffin, L., Waghela, S. and Allonby, E.W.: The immunosuppressive effects of experimental *T. congolense* infections in goats. Vet. Parasitol., 7(1):11–18, 1980.

Griffin, L., et al.: The interaction of *Trypanosoma congolense* and *Haemonchus contortus* infections in 2 breeds of goat. 2. Haematology. J. Comp. Pathol., 91:97–103, 1981b.

Griot-Wenk, M.E., Obexer-Ruff, G., Fluri, A. and Marti, E.: Partial sequences of feline and caprine immunoglobulin epsilon heavy chain cDNA and comparative binding studies of recombinant IgE fragment-specific antibodies across different species. Vet. Immunol. Immunopathol. 75(1/2):59–69, 2000.

Gulliani, G.L., et al.: Survival of chromium-51-labeled autologous and homologous erythrocytes in goats. Am. J. Vet. Res., 36:1469–1471, 1975.

Hadlow, W.J.: High prevalence of thymoma in the dairy goat: Report of 17 cases. Vet. Pathol. 15:153–169, 1978.

Hagstad, H.V., Hubbert, W.T. and Craig, L.M.: Health status as related to management practices in Louisiana goat herds. Int. Goat Sheep Res., 2:238–242, 1984.

Hedden, J.A., Thomas, C.M., Songer, J.G. and Olson, G.B.: Characterization of lectin-binding lymphocytes in goats with caseous lymphadenitis. Am. J. Vet. Res., 47:1265–1267, 1986.

Holman, H.H., and Dew, S.M.: The blood picture of the goat. II. Changes in erythrocyte shape, size and number associated with age. Res. Vet. Sci. 5:274–285, 1964.

Holman, H.H., and Dew, S.M.: The blood picture of the goat. III. Changes in haemoglobin concentration and physical measurements occurring with age. Res. Vet. Sci. 6:245–253, 1965.

Holman, H.H. and Dew, S.M.: The blood picture of the goat. IV. Changes in coagulation times, platelet counts and leucocyte numbers associated with age. Res. Vet. Sci. 6:510–521, 1965a.

Holman, H.H., and Dew, S.M.: Effect of an injection of iron-dextran complex on blood constituents and bodyweight of young kids. Vet. Rec. 78:772–776, 1966.

Hooshmand-Rad, P. and Hawa, N.J.: Malignant theileriosis of sheep and goats. Trop. Anim. Health Prod., 5:97–102, 1973.

Hsu, C.K.: Immunology. In: Handbook of Laboratory Animal Science, Volume III. E.C. Melby and N.H. Altman, eds. Cleveland, CRC Press Inc. 1976.

Huisman, T.H.J., et al.: Hemoglobin C in newborn sheep and goats: A possible explanation for its function and biosynthesis. Pediat. Res. J., 3:189–198, 1969.

Huisman, T.H.J.: Structural aspects of fetal and adult hemoglobins from nonanemic ruminants. Annals N.Y. Acad. Sci., 241:392–410, 1974.

Humphries, W.R., Morrice, P.C. and Mitchell, A.N.: Copper poisoning in Angora goats. Vet. Rec., 121:231, 1987.

Hussein, K.S.M., Jones, B.-E.V. and Frank, A.: Selenium copper interactions in goats. Zbl. Vet. Med. A, 32:321–330, 1985.

Ilemobade, A.A.: Trypanosomiasis (nagana, samore, tsetse fly disease). In: Current Veterinary Therapy, Food Animal Practice. 2nd Ed. J.L. Howard, ed. Philadelphia, W.B. Saunders Co., pp. 642–645, 1986.

Illemobade, A.A. and Blotkamp, C.: Clinico pathological study of heartwater in goats. Tropenmed. Parasitol. 29:71–76, 1978.

Jagannath, M.S., Hegde, K.S., Shivaram, K. and Nagaraja, K.V.: An outbreak of babesiosis in sheep and goats and its control. Mysore J. Agric. Sci., 8(3):441–443, 1974.

Jain, N.C., Kono, C.S., Myers, A., and Bottomly, K.: Fusiform erythrocytes resembling sickle cells in Angora goats: observations on osmotic and mechanical fragilities and reversal of cell shape during anaemia. Res. Vet. Sci., 28(1):25–35, 1980.

Jain, N.C.: Schalm's Veterinary Hematology, 4th Ed. Philadelphia, Lea and Febiger, pp. 225–239, 1986.

Joa, R., Merino, N., Alonso, M. and Blandino, T.: Eperythrozoonosis *(E. ovis)* in sheep and goats in Cuba. Rev. Salud Anim., 9:85–86, 1987.

Johnson, G.C., Adams, D.S. and McGuire, T.C.: Pronounced production of polyclonal immunoglobulin G1 in the synovial fluid of goats with caprine arthritis-encephalitis virus infection. Infect. Immun., 41:805–815, 1983.

Jones B.E.V. and Shah, M.: Clinico-chemical changes in goats given carbon tetrachloride. Nord. Vet. Med., 34:25–32, 1982.

Jongejan, F., et al.: Serotypes in *Cowdria ruminantium* and their relationship with *Ehrlichia phagocytophila* determined by immunofluorescence. Vet. Microbiol., 21:31–40, 1989.

Kaaya, G.P. and Oduor-Okelo, D.: The effects of *Trypanosoma congolense* infection on the testis and epididymis of the goat. Bull. Anim. Hlth. Prod. Afr., 28(1):1–5, 1980.

Kaaya, G.P., Winqvist, G. and Johnson, L.W.: Clinicopathological aspects of *Trypanosoma congolense* infection in goats. Bull. Anim. Health Prod. Afr., 25:397–408, 1977.

Kaneko, J.J. and Cornelius, C.E.: Erythrocyte survival studies in the Himalayan Tahr and domestic goats. Am. J. Vet. Res. 23:913–915, 1962.

Kaneko, J.J.: Clinical Biochemistry of Domestic Animals. 3rd Ed. Orlando, Academic Press, 1980.

Kanyari, P.W.N., Allonby, E.W., Wilson, A.J. and Munyua, W.K.: Some economic effects of trypanosomiasis in goats. Trop. Anim. Health Prod., 15:153–160, 1983.

Kaplan, T.: Anthrax Is Found in 2 Connecticut Residents, One a Drummer. New York Times, September 6, 2007. http://www.nytimes.com/2007/09/06/hyregion/06anthrax.html

Karram, M.H., Amer, A.A. and Ibrahim, H.A.: Aplastic anaemia in caprine fluorosis. Assiut Vet. Med. J., 12:167–171, 1984.

Kassai, L. et al.: Standardized nomenclature of animal parasitic diseases (SNOAPAD). Vet. Parasitol., 29:299–326, 1988.

Kaaya, G.P. and Oduor-Okelo, D.: The effects of *Trypanosoma congolense* infection on the testis and epididymis of the goat. Bull. Anim. Health Prod. Afr., 28(1):1–5, 1980.

Kimberling, C.V. and Arnold, K.S.: Diseases of the urinary system of sheep and goats. Vet. Clin. N. Am. Large Anim. Pract. 5:637–655, 1983.

Kramer, J.W.: Incidence of trypanosomes in the West African Dwarf sheep and goat in Nsukka, eastern Nigeria. Bull. Epizoot. Dis. Afr., 14:423–428, 1966.

Kramer, J.W.: Normal hematology of cattle, sheep and goats. In: Schalm's Veterinary Hematology, 5th Ed., B.F. Feldman, J.G. Zinkl, and N.C. Jain, eds. Lippincott Williams and Wilkins, Philadelphia, pp. 1075–1084, 2000.

Kuil, H. and Folkers, C.: Een zeer anaemische geit. Tijdschr. Diergeneesk., 91:1247, 1966.

Lechner, F., et al.: Caprine arthritis encephalitis virus dysregulates the expression of cytokines in macrophages. J. Virol., 71:10, 7488–7497, 1997.

Leon-Vizcaino, L., Hermoso de Mendoza, M. and Garrido, F.: Incidence of abortions caused by leptospirosis in sheep and goats in Spain. Comp. Immun. Microbiol. Infect. Dis., 10:149–153, 1987.

Levieux, D.: Transmission de l'immunité passive colostrale chez les petits ruminants. In: Les Maladies de la Chèvre, Les Colloques de l'INRA, No. 28. P. Yvore and G. Perrin, eds. Paris. Institut National de la Recherche Agronomique. pp. 21–30, 1984.

Lewis, D., et al. Investigations on *Babesia motasi* isolated from Wales. Res. Vet. Sci., 31(2):239–243, 1981.

Lewis, J.H.: Comparative hematology: Studies on goats. Am. J. Vet. Res. 37:601–605, 1976.

Liebler-Tenorio, E.M. and Pabst, R.: MALT structure and function in farm animals. Vet. Res., 37(3):257–280, 2006.

Lilenbaum, W., et al.: Risk factors associated with leptospirosis in dairy goats under tropical conditions in Brazil. Res. Vet. Sci., 84(1):14–17, 2008.

Llewelyn, C.A., Luckins, A.G., Munro, C.D. and Perrie, J.: The effect of *Trypanosoma congolense* infection on the oestrous cycle of the goat. Br. Vet. J., 143(5):423–431, 1987.

Losos, G.J. and Ikede, B.O.: Review of pathology of diseases in domestic and laboratory animals caused by *Trypanosoma congolense, T. vivax, T. brucei, T. rhodesiense* and *T. gambiense.* Vet. Pathol. Suppl. 9:1–71, 1972.

Lund, A., Torbjorn, A., Steine, T. and Larsen, H.J.: Colostral transfer in the goat of antibodies against *Corynebacterium pseudotuberculosis* and the antibody status of kids during the first 10 months of life. Acta Vet. Scand., 23:483–489, 1982.

Maas, J. and Buening, G.M.: Characterization of *Anaplasma marginale* infection in splenectomized domestic goats. Am. J. Vet. Res. 42:142–145, 1981.

Maddux, J.M. and Keeton, K.S.: Evaluation of neutrophil function in female goats. Am. J. Vet. Res., 48:1110–1113, 1987.

Maddux, J.M. and Keeton, K.S.: Effects of dexamethasone, levamisole, and dexamethasone-levamisole on neutrophil function in female goats. Am. J. Vet. Res., 48:1114–1119, 1987a.

Mahmoud, M.M. and Elmalik, K.H.: Trypanosomiasis: Goats as a possible reservoir of *Trypanosoma congolense* in the Republic of Sudan. Trop. Anim. Health Prod., 9:167–170, 1977.

Mallick, K.P., Dwivedi, S.K. and Malhotra, M.N.: Anaplasmosis in goats: report of clinical cases. Indian Vet. J. 56(8):693–694, 1979.

Mason, R.W., Corbould, A., and Statham, P.: A serological survey of *Eperythrozoon ovis* in goats and sheep in Tasmania. Aust. Vet. J., 66:122–123, 1989.

Massimini, G., et al.: Effect of passive transfer status on preweaning growth performance in dairy goat kids. J. Am. Vet. Med. Assoc., 231(12):1873–1877, 2007.

Melby, E.C. and Altman, N.H. Handbook of laboratory animal science, Volume III. E.C. Melby and N.H. Altman, eds. Cleveland, CRC Press, 1976.

Melby, H.P. and Grønstøl, H.: Sjodogg (Tick-borne fever) hos geit. Norsk Veterinaertidsskrift, 96:87–90, 1984.

Meyer, R., et al.: In vitro IFN-gamma production by goat blood cells after stimulation with somatic and secreted *Corynebacterium pseudotuberculosis* antigens. Vet. Immunol. Immunopathol., 107(3/4):249–254, 2005.

Mgongo, F.O.K., Gombe, S. and Ogaa, J.S.: Thyroid status in cobalt and vitamin B_{12} deficiency in goats. Vet. Rec., 109:51–53, 1981.

Micusan, V.V. and Borduas, A.G.: Preferential transport into colostrum of Fc fragment derived from serum IgG_1 immunoglobulin in the goat. Res. Vet. Sci., 21:150–154, 1976.

Micusan, V.V. and Borduas, A.G.: Biological properties of goat immunoglobulins G. Immunology, 32:373–381, 1977.

Micusan, V.V., Boulay, G. and Borduas, A.G.: The role of colostrum on the occurrence of immunoglobulin G subclasses and antibody production in neonatal goats. Can. J. Comp. Med., 40:184–189, 1976.

Migaki, G.: Hematopoietic neoplasms of slaughter animals. In: Comparative Morphology of Hematopoietic Neoplasms. National Cancer Inst., Monograph 32, ed. Lingeman and Garner; U.S. Dept. Health Educ. Welfare, Washington D.C., pp. 121–151, 1969.

Mitruka, B.M. and Rawnsley, H.M.: Clinical biochemical and hematological reference values in normal experimental animals and normal humans, 2nd Ed. New York, Masson Publishing Co., 1981.

Mjor-Grimsrud, M., Soli, N.E. and Sivertsen, T.: The distribution of soluble copper- and zinc-binding proteins in goat liver. Acta Pharmacol. Toxicology, 44:319–323, 1979.

Morand-Fehr, P., Villette, Y. and Chemineau, P.: Influence des conditions de milieu sur la mortalité des chevreaux. In: Les Maladies de la Chèvre, Les Colloques de l'INRA, No. 28. P. Yvore and G. Perrin, eds. Paris. Institut National de la Recherche Agronomique. pp. 31–46. 1984.

Morand-Fehr, P.: Management programs for the prevention of kid losses. Proc. IV International Conf. Goats, Brasilia, EMBRAPA-DDT, pp. 405–423, 1987.

Murray, M. and Gray, A.R.: The current situation on animal trypanosomiasis in Africa. Prev. Vet. Med., 2:23–30, 1984.

Murray, M., Morrison, W.I., and Whitelaw, D.D.: Host susceptibility to African trypanosomiasis: trypanotolerance. Adv. Parasitol., 21:1–68, 1982.

Murray, M., Trail, J.C.M., Davis, C.E. and Black, S.J.: Genetic resistance to African trypanosomiasis. J. Infect. Dis., 149:311–319, 1984.

Mutayoba, B.M., Gombe, S., Kaaya, G.P. and Waindi, E.N.: Trypanosome-induced ovarian dysfunction. Evidence of higher residual fertility in trypanotolerant small East African goats. Acta Trop. 45(3):225–237, 1988.

Nandakumar, P. and Rajagopalaraja, C.A.: Growth and mortality in relation to serum immunoglobulin level in neonatal kids. Kerala J. Vet. Sci., 14:49–52, 1983.

Nandakumar, P. and Rajagopalaraja, C.A.: Effect of genetic group, birth weight and type of birth on the post colostral peak of serum immunoglobulin level in kids. Kerala J. Vet. Sci., 14:53–56, 1983a.

Nangia, O.P., Agarwal, V.K., and Singh, A.: Studies on blood cellular constituents of female Beetal goats from birth to over five years of age. Indian J. Anim. Sci., 38:616–625, 1968.

Neimark H., Hoff B. and Ganter M. *Mycoplasma ovis* comb. nov. (formerly *Eperythrozoon ovis*), an epierythrocytic agent of haemolytic anaemia in sheep and goats. Int. J. Syst. Evol. Microbiol., 54:365–371, 2004.

Nguyen, T.C.: Further investigations on the relationships between blood groups of sheep and goats. Anim. Blood Grps. Biochem. Genet. 8(Suppl.):11–12, 1977.

Obexer-Ruff, G., Joosten, I., Schwaiger, F.-W.: The caprine MHC. In: Schook, L., Lamont, S., eds., The Major Histocompatibility Complex Region of Domestic Animal Species. CRC Press, Boca Raton, pp. 99–119, 1996.

O'Brien, J.P. and Sherman, D.M.: Field methods for estimating serum immunoglobulin concentrations in newborn kids. Small Rumin. Res., 11:79–84, 1993.

O'Brien, J.P. and Sherman, D.M.: Serum immunoglobulin concentrations of newborn goat kids and subsequent kid

survival through weaning. Small Rumin. Res. 11:71–77, 1993a.
Oduye, O.O.: Haematological values of Nigerian goats and sheep. Trop. Anim. Health Prod., 8:131–136, 1976.
Okoh, A.E.J.: An epizootic of anthrax in goats and sheep in Danbatta Nigeria. Bull. Anim. Health Prod. Afr., 29:355–359, 1981.
Olchowy, T.W.J., et al.: Metastatic thymoma in a goat. Can. Vet. J., 37(3):165–167, 1996.
Oliveira, D.M.: Profile of caprine disease in Jamaica. In: Proc. IV International Conf. Goats, Brasilia, EMBRAPA-DDT, pp. 1367–1368, 1987.
Pahud, J.J. and Mach, J.P.: Identification of secretory IgA, free secretory piece and serum IgA in the ovine and caprine species. Immunochemistry, 7:679–686, 1970.
Parish, S.M., Middleton, J.R. and Baldwin, T.J.: Clinical megaoesophagus in a goat with thymoma. Vet. Rec., 139(4):94, 1996.
Perrin, G., Polack, B., Gueraud, J.M. and Petat, M.: Anémie hémolytique chez des chevreaux nourris avec du colostrum de vache. Pointe Vét., 20:75–76, 1988.
ProMED-mail: Anthrax, Human, Caprine—China (Shaanxi). International Society for Infectious Diseases. ProMED-mail Post, Vol. 2006, No. 443, Archive No. 20061002.2822, October 2, 2006.
ProMED-mail: Anthrax, Caprine—USA (Texas). International Society for Infectious Diseases. ProMED-mail Post, Vol. 2008, No. 158, Archive No. 20080404.1234, April 4, 2008.
Purnell, R.E.: Tick-borne diseases. Br. Vet. J., 137:221–240, 1981.
Purnell, R.E.: Babesiosis in various hosts. In: Babesiosis. M. Ristic and J.P. Kreier, eds. New York. Academic Press. pp. 25–63, 1981a.
Radostits, O.M., Gay, C.C., Hinchcliff, K.W. and Constable, P.D.: Veterinary Medicine. A textbook of the diseases of cattle, horse, sheep, pigs and goats. 10th Ed. Saunders Elsevier, Edinburgh, 2007.
Ramakrishna, V., Vaish, K.C., and Tiwari, G.P.: Supernumerary spleen in goat *(Capra hircus)*: A case report. Indian Vet. J., 58:685–688, 1981.
Robson, J. and Rickman, L.R.: Blood incubation infectivity test results for *Trypanosoma brucei* subgroup isolates in the Lambwe Valley, South Nyanza, Kenya. Trop. Anim. Health Prod., 5:187–191, 1973.
Rostkowski, C.M., Stirtzinger, T. and Baird, J.D.: Congestive heart failure associated with thymoma in two Nubian goats. Can. Vet. J., 26:267–269, 1985.
Ruff, G. and Lazary, S.: Caprine lymphocyte antigens—serologic and genetic studies. Proc. IV International Conf. Goats. Brasilia, EMBRAPA-DDT, pp. 1317–1318, 1987.
Samad, A. and Ali, M.S.: Non-febrile haemoglobinuria in goats—a record of two cases. Livestock Advisor, 9:53–55, 1984.
Sanders, D.E.: Copper deficiency in food animals. Compend. Cont. Educ. Pract. Vet., 5:S404–S410, 1983.
Schillhorn van Veen, T.W. and Mohammed, A.N.: Louse and flea infestations on small ruminants in the Zaria area. J. Nig. Vet. Med. Assoc., 4:93–96, 1975.
Schillinger, D., Maloo, S.H. and Rottcher, D.: The toxic effect of intravenous application of the trypanocide isometamidium (samorin). Zbl. Vet. Med. A., 32:234–239, 1985.
Schijns, V.E.C.J. and Horzinek, M.C.: Cytokines in veterinary medicine. CAB International, Wallingford, UK: 324 pp, 1997.
Schollum, L.M. and Blackmore, D.K.: The serological and cultural prevalence of leptospirosis in a sample of feral goats. N.Z. Vet. J., 29:104–106, 1981.
Setty, D.R.L. and Narayana, K.: A case of non-febrile haemoglobinuria in a she goat. Indian Vet. J., 52:149, 1975.
Sharmila, C., Williams, J.W. and Reddy, P.G.: Effect of caprine arthritis-encephalitis virus infection on expression of interleukin-16 in goats. Am. J. Vet. Res., 63(10):1418–1422, 2002.
Sherman, D.M., Arendt, T.D., Gay, J.M. and Maefsky, V.: Comparing the effects of four colostral preparations on serum Ig levels in newborn kids. Vet. Med., 85:908–913, 1990.
Sherman, D.M.: Causes of kid morbidity and mortality: An overview. Proc. IV International Conf. Goats, Brasilia, EMBRAPA-DDT, pp. 335–354, 1987.
Shiferaw, G.: Anthrax in Wabessa village in the Dessie Zuria district of Ethiopia, Rev. Sci. Tech. Off. Int. Epiz., 23(3):951–956, 2004.
Shlosberg, A., Egyed, M.N. and Huri, J.: Acute copper poisoning in a herd of goats. Refuah Vet., 35:15, 1978.
Silva, J.A. da, et al.: Aglutinas anti-leptospiras e anti-brucelas em soros de caprinos de diferentes sistemas de produçao do estado de Minas Gerais. Arq. Bras. Med. Vet. Zoot., 36:539–548, 1984.
Sisodia, R.S. and Gautam, O.P.: Experimental cases of *Theileria hirci* infection in sheep and goats. Indian J. Anim. Sci. 53(2):162–166, 1983.
Smith, R.H.: Kale poisoning: The brassica anaemia factor. Vet. Rec., 107:12–15, 1980.
Søli, N.E. and Nafstad, I.: Effects of daily oral administration of copper to goats. Acta Vet. Scand., 19:561–568, 1978.
Solaiman, S.G., et al.: Effects of high copper supplements on performance, health, plasma copper and enzymes in goats. Sm. Rum. Res., 41:2, 127–139, 2001.
Soulsby, E.J.L.: Helminths, Arthropods and Protozoa of Domesticated Animals. 7th Ed. Philadelphia, Lea and Febiger, 1982.
Splitter, E.J., Anthony, H.D. and Twiehaus, M.J.: *Anaplasma ovis* in the United States. Experimental studies with sheep and goats. Am. J. Vet. Res., 17:487–491, 1956.
Staples, L.D., Binns, R.M. and Heap, R.B.: Influence of certain steroids on lymphocyte transformation in sheep and goats studied in vitro. J. Endocr., 98:55–69, 1983.
Staples, L.D., Brown, D. and Binns, R.M.: Mitogen-induced transformation of sheep and goat peripheral blood lymphocytes in vitro: The effects of varying culture conditions and the choice of an optimum technique. Vet. Immunol. Immunopath., 2:411–423, 1981.
Storset, A.K., Berntsen, G. and Larsen, H.J.S.: Kinetics of IL-2 receptor expression on lymphocyte subsets from goats infected with *Mycobacterium avium* subsp. *paratuberculosis* after specific in vitro stimulation. Vet. Immunol. Immunopathol., 77(1/2):43–54, 2000.
Storset, A.K., et al.: Subclinical paratuberculosis in goats following experimental infection: an immunological and microbiological study. Vet. Immunol. Immunopathol., 80(3/4):271–287, 2001.

Streett, C.S., Altman, N.H., Terner, J.Y. and Berjis, C.C.: A series of thymomas in the Angora goat. Edgewood Arsenal Special Publication 100–36, Dept. of the Army, Edgewood Arsenal, Maryland, December 1968.

Suliman, H.B., Wasfi, I.A. and Adam, S.E.I.: The toxic effects of *Tephrosia apollinea* on goats. J. Comp. Pathol., 92:309–315, 1982.

Sulochana, S., Jayaprakasan, V., Pillai, R.M. and Abdulla, P.K.: T and B lymphocytes in the peripheral blood of goats. Kerala J. Vet. Sci., 13:71–78, 1982.

Tartour, G., Adam, S.E.I., Obeid, H.M. and Idris, O.F.: Development of anaemia in goats fed with *Ipomoea carnea*. Br. Vet. J., 130:271–279, 1974.

Tirkey, K., Yadava, K.P. and Mandal, T.K.: Effect of aqueous extract of *Ipomoea carnea* on the haematological and biochemical parameters in goats. Indian J. Anim. Sci., 57(9):1019–1023, 1987.

Tizard, I.R. and Schubot, R.M.: Veterinary Immunology: An Introduction. 7th Ed. Saunders, Philadelphia. 2004.

Tomlinson, C.J.: Bracken poisoning/PGE. Goat Vet. Soc. J., 4:43–44, 1983.

Ubertalle, A., Ladetto, G., Cauvin, E. and Mazzocco, P.: Colostro caprino: caratteristiche del latte ottenuto nelle prime 24 ore post partum. Summa, 4:239–242, 1987.

Uilenberg G., Thiaucourt F. *and* Jongejan F. *Mycoplasma* and *Eperythrozoon* (*Mycoplasmataceae*). Comments on a recent paper. Int. J. Syst. Evol. Microbiol., 56:13–14, 2006.

Uilenberg, G., Rombach, M.C., Perie, N.M. and Zwart, D.: Blood parasites of sheep in the Netherlands. II. *Babesia motasi* (Sporozoa Babesiidae). Vet. Q., 2:3–14, 1980.

Uilenberg, G.: A field guide for the diagnosis, treatment and prevention of African animal trypanosomosis. (Adapted from the original edition by W.P. Boyt.) F.A.O., Rome. 158 pp, 1998.

Underwood, E.J.: The Mineral Nutrition of Livestock. 2nd Ed. Slough, Commonwealth Agricultural Bureaux, 1981.

van Dam, R.H. and van Kooten, P.J.S.: Genetic control of sensitization to defined antigens and its relationship to histocompatibility antigens in goats. Anim. Blood Grps. Biochem. Genet., 11:56, 1980.

van Dam, R.H., Boot, R., van der Donk, J.A. and Goudswaard, J.: Skin grafting and graft rejection in goats. Am. J. Vet. Res., 39:1359–1362, 1978a.

van Dam, R.H., d'Amaro, J. and van Kooten, P.J.S.: The major histocompatibility complex of the goat (GLA). Anim. Blood Grps. Biochem. Genet., 11:55–56, 1980.

van Dam, R.H., et al.: The histocompatibility complex GLA in the goat. Anim. Blood Grps. Biochem. Genet., 10:121–124, 1979.

van Dam, R.H., et al.: Trypanosome mediated suppression of humoral and cell-mediated immunity in goats. Vet. Parasitol., 8:1–11, 1981a.

van Dam, R.H., van Kooten, P.J.S. and van der Donk, J.A.: In vitro stimulation of goat peripheral blood lymphocytes: Optimization and kinetics of the response to mitogens and to allogeneic lymphocytes. J. Immunol. Methods, 21:217–228, 1978.

van Dam, R.H., van Kooten, P.J.S., van der Donk, J.A. and Goudswaard, J.: Phenotyping by the mixed lymphocyte reaction in goats (LD typing). Vet. Immunol. Immunopathol. 2:321–330, 1981.

Van den Ingh, T.S.G.A.M., et al.: The pathology and pathogenesis of *Trypanosoma vivax* infection in the goat. Res. Vet Sci., 21:264–270, 1976.

Van der Hoeden, J.: Leptospirosis among goats in Israel. J. Comp. Pathol., 63:101–111, 1953.

Van Miert, A.S.J.P.A.M., Van Duin, C.T.M., Schotman, A.J.H. and Franssen, F.F.: Clinical, haematological and blood biochemical changes in goats after experimental infection with tick-borne fever. Vet. Parasitol., 16:225–233, 1984.

Van Miert, A.S.J.P.A.M., Van Duin, C.T.M. and Wensing, T.: The effects of ACTH, prednisolone and *Escherichia coli* endotoxin on some clinical hematological and blood biochemical parameters in dwarf goats. Vet. Q. 8:195–203, 1986.

Veenendaal, G.H., et al.: A comparison of the role of kinins and serotonin in endotoxin induced fever and *Trypanosoma vivax* infections in the goat. Res. Vet. Sci., 21:271–279, 1976.

Verheijden, J.H.M., van Miert, A.S.J.P.A.M. and Van Duin, C.T.M.: Demonstration of circulating endogenous pyrogens in *Escherichia coli* endotoxin-induced mastitis. Zentralbl. Veterinaermed. A, 30:342–347, 1983.

Vihan, V.S. and Sahni, K.L.: Role of blood gammaglobulin in relation to the neonatal kid mortality and their subsequent performance. Proc. III International Conf. Goat Prod. Dis., Tuscon, Arizona, pp. 372, 1982.

Vihan, V.S.: Glutaraldehyde coagulation test for detection of hypogammaglobulinaemia in neonatal kids. Indian Vet. J., 66:101–105, 1989.

Wasfi, I.A. and Adam, S.E.I.: The effects of intravenous injection of small amounts of copper sulphate in Nubian goats. J. Comp. Pathol., 86:387–391, 1976.

Weber, W.T.: Evaluation of bone marrow. In: Textbook of Veterinary Clinical Pathology, W. Medway, J.E. Prier, and J.S. Wilkinson, eds. Baltimore, Williams and Wilkins Co., 1969.

Webster, K.A. and Mitchell, G.B.B.: Use of counter immunoelectrophoresis in detection of antibodies to tick-borne fever. Res. Vet. Sci., 45:28–30, 1988.

Whitelaw, D.D., et al: Susceptibility of different breeds of goats in Kenya to experimental infection with *Trypanosoma congolense*. Trop. Anim. Health Prod. 17:155–165, 1985.

Whitelaw, D.D., Moulton, J.E., Morrison, W.I. and Murray, M.: Central nervous system involvement in goats undergoing primary infections with *Trypanosoma brucei* and relapse infections after chemotherapy. Parasitology, 90:255–268, 1985a.

Whitford, H.W.: Anthrax in dairy goats. Southwest. Vet., 35:15, 1982.

Wilkins, J.H. and Hodges, R.R.D.H.: Observations on normal goat blood. J. R. Army Vet. Corps, 33:7–10, 1962.

Yin, H., et al.: Phylogenetic analysis of *Theileria* species transmitted by *Haemaphysalis qinghaiensis*. Parasitol. Res., 92:36–42, 2004.

Yousif, Y.A., Dimitri, R.A., Dwivedi, S.K. and Ahmed, N.J.: Anaemia due to anaplasmosis in Iraqi goats: I. Clinical and haematological features under field conditions. Indian Vet. J., 60:576–578, 1983.

8

Cardiovascular System

The occurrence of clinically recognized cardiovascular disease in goats is very low. As a result, goats have been the least studied of the domestic species regarding normal cardiovascular function and pathophysiology. In recent years, however, goats have received more attention as a suitable animal model for the study of human cardiovascular disease and its management. In particular, goats have been used in studies of the pathophysiology and treatment of atrial fibrillation (Neuberger et al. 2006), chronic heart failure (Tessier et al. 2003), the development of skeletal muscle ventricles (Guldner et al. 2002), the development and testing of artificial heart valves (Björk and Kaminsky 1992), and the use of total artificial hearts (Abe et al. 2007). As reported in 2007, the world record for survival of an animal with a total artificial heart belongs to a goat outfitted with a paracorporeal total artificial heart that survived for 532 days (Abe et al. 2007).

BACKGROUND INFORMATION OF CLINICAL IMPORTANCE

Anatomy and Physiology

Structure of the Heart and Vessels

The heart of the goat extends from the third to the sixth rib and may contact the diaphragm at its caudal edge. The position and orientation within the thorax is similar to that of other ruminants. The adult heart may contain two small cardiac bones, the right and left *os cordis* located around the aortic ring (Aretz 1981). However, a more recent study reported that in a series of fifty goats examined, only a right *os cordis* was present, located beneath the septal cusp of the tricuspid valve near the junction of the interatrial and interventricular septae and that it was only present in 44% of the hearts examined (Mohammadpour and Arabi, 2007). Purkinje fibers extend deep into the myocardium of the goat heart, as in other ruminants, which has clinical implications regarding the diagnostic value of electrocardiography as discussed later in this chapter.

Anomalies of the heart reported in goats include ventricular septal defects (VSD) in the lower, middle, and upper ventricular septum (Parry et al. 1982), and ectopia cordis, with the heart exposed to the outside through a fissured sternum (Narasimha Rao et al. 1980). Kids with ectopia cordis may be born alive and survive for hours or days (Upadhye and Dhoot 2001) or they may be born dead with structural abnormalities of the externalized heart such as a single ventricle (Dadich 2000).

There are no major differences in the structure and distribution of the great vessels of goats compared with other ruminants. Anomalies of the great vessels are uncommon, but persistence of the left cranial vena cava (Waibl 1973), dextroposition of the aorta (Parry et al. 1982), and aortic stenosis (Scarratt et al. 1984) have been reported.

Parameters of Blood Flow

Information on cardiac output, stroke volume, systolic and diastolic arterial pressures, pulmonary arterial pressure, pulmonary arterial flow rates, and central venous pressure has been published, but the numbers of animals involved in the various studies have been limited (Jha et al. 1961; Hoversland et al. 1965; Foex and Prys-Roberts 1972; Ivankovich et al. 1974; Vesal and Karimi 2006).

Mean cardiac outputs in goats of various breeds, age, and sex have been reported in the range of 2.8 ± 0.7 l/minute to 4.8 ± 1.4 l/minute (Hoversland et al. 1965; Foex and Prys-Roberts 1972; Ivankovich et al. 1974; Olsson et al. 2001). More recently, significant differences in cardiac output were confirmed in dairy goats during pregnancy (6.73 ± 0.72) as compared to lactation (6.12 ± 0.52) and the dry period (4.39 ± 0.27) in the same individuals (Olsson et al. 2001).

Mean stroke volumes derived from a measurement of cardiac output and heart rate or measured directly by dye dilution technique have been reported in the range of 20.3 ± 3.1 ml to 46.9 ± 23 ml (Foex and Prys-Roberts 1972; Ivankovich et al. 1974). Mean systolic arterial pressure recorded from goats of varying breeds, age, and sex ranged from 122 to 124.9 mm Hg, while mean diastolic pressures in the same goats ranged from 85 to 97.8 mm Hg (Jha et al. 1961; Hoversland et al. 1965). Mean central venous pressure in goats of both sexes was reported as 1.25 ± 0.14 cm H_2O but there was a statistically significant difference between males (0.80 ± 0.11) and females (1.9 ± 0.26). There was no difference noted, however, between standing goats and those in lateral recumbency (Vesal and Karimi 2006).

Normal Heart Rate and Rhythm

The heart is heard most audibly over the left thoracic wall at the fourth intercostal space. Heart rate varies considerably in goats with age and level of activity. Mean heart rates for small numbers of goats at different ages have been reported from India (Upadhyay and Sud 1977). Barbari goat kids from birth to fifteen days of age had mean heart rates of 255 ± 15 bpm, and 209 ± 6 bpm from sixteen days to one month of age. By one to six months of age, mean heart rates had decreased to 142 ± 6 bpm and to 125 ± 9 bpm between six and twelve months. Goats one to three years of age had heart rates of 126 ± 5 bpm, and goats three to five years of age, 126 ± 7 bpm. In one American study of one hundred male goats one to one and a half years of age, the mean heart rate was 96 bpm with a range of 70 to 120 (Szabuniewicz and Clark 1967). In a second American study of eight adult females of mixed breed, the mean was 105 bpm with a range of 90 to 150 (Jha et al. 1961). While it is generally presumed that fear and distress increase the heart rate in goats, a study involving goat responses to unfamiliar human contact could not demonstrate a significant elevation in heart rate (Lyons and Price 1987).

Using telemetric recording of heart rate, investigators demonstrated a significant increase in heart rate of normal young goats during physical examination (116 ± 11.7 bpm) compared with before (92.2 ± 6.3 bpm) and a significantly higher rate when eating (114.1 ± 2.1 bpm) as compared to standing (84.2 ± 0.9 bpm) or lying down (76.5 ± 1.1 bpm) (Vesal et al. 2000). Other investigators have reported significant differences in heart rates in goats of different breeds kept under similar conditions (Medeiros et al. 2001) and elevated heart rates in pregnant does as compared to the same does when lactating and when non-pregnant and non-lactating (Olsson et al. 2001)

Two heart sounds are normally heard in the goat, S_1 and S_2. A normal respiratory sinus arrhythmia is common, with acceleration occurring in late inspiration. It is more pronounced in younger goats. Second degree A-V block, though uncommon, has been recorded in a normal goat (Szabuniewicz and Clark 1967).

Diagnostic Methods

Electrocardiography

The electrocardiogram (ECG) has been applied relatively infrequently in caprine medicine. Nevertheless, some parameters for the ECG tests in normal goats have been established using standard and augmented limb leads (Szabuniewicz and Clark 1967; Upadhyay and Sud 1977). The goat may be evaluated while standing or in left or right lateral recumbency with little effect on the ECG. Limb leads should be placed on the anteriolateral aspect just above the elbow joint in the forelimb, and just above the stifle joint in the hind limb. Electrocardiography has also been performed with the leads in a sagittal plane between the ears, on the sacrum, and on the sternum (Schultz and Pretorius 1972).

Interval durations, in seconds, have been reported for the P-wave, P-R interval, QRS complex, Q-T interval, and T-wave (Jha et al. 1961; Szabuniewicz and Clark 1967; Schultz and Pretorius 1972; Upadhyay and Sud 1977; Ogburn et al. 1977). Minimal differences occur between various leads (Szabuniewicz and Clark 1967). The amplitudes of ECG deflections are small in the goat. Mean amplitudes for various leads as measured in one hundred goats have been reported (Szabuniewicz and Clark 1967). Duration and amplitude measurements reported for the commonly used lead II are given in Table 8.1.

The P-wave is most often peaked in standard and augmented leads, but is occasionally flat or rounded. Biphasic P-waves are rarely seen. The P-wave is usually positive in the standard leads and the augmented leads, except for aVR. Changes in the shape of P-waves may be observed sometimes in normal goats, representing wandering of the pacemaker in the sinoatrial node.

Table 8.1. Electrocardiographic parameters for lead II reported in normal goats.

Parameter	*P-wave amplitude (mv)*	*P-wave duration (sec)*	*P-R interval duration (sec)*	*QRS complex amplitude (mv)*	*QRS complex duration (sec)*	*Q-T interval duration (sec)*	*T-wave amplitude (mv)*	*T-Wave duration (sec)*
Mean values	0.080	0.04	0.09–0.13	0.258	0.039–0.045	0.295–0.334	0.200	0.07
Range	0.02–0.15	0.02–0.06	0.06–0.16	0.10–0.70	0.03–0.08	0.22–0.38	0.05–0.50	0.04–0.10

QRS = principal deflection in an electrocardiogram.

The shape of the QRS complex is quite variable within and between the different leads. It is usually mono- or diphasic and infrequently triphasic. In lead I, a QS pattern dominates. In lead II, QS or Qr patterns are most often recorded. In lead III, no single pattern is predominant, and the Qr, qR, R, RS, and Rs patterns commonly occur. Q waves are rarely observed in the aVR lead, and the R and Rs patterns predominate. In the aVL lead, the QS pattern is most common, followed in frequency by the rS pattern. In lead aVF, either the Qr or the QS patterns may predominate, with the R, RS, Rs, and rS patterns also common. Because of the variability of the QRS complex in particular, it is generally considered that there is no typical morphologic pattern that is characteristic for the ECG test results of the goat using the common lead systems.

The T-wave occurs most commonly in the peaked form. Flat, round, or diphasic T-waves are uncommon. In most cases, the T-wave is of opposite polarity or deflection to the accompanying QRS deflection, although concurrent positive deflections occur in lead III and concurrent negative deflections in lead aVL.

Vectorcardiography is of limited clinical value in goats. As is the case with other ruminants, Purkinje fibers fully penetrate the ventricular wall with extensive ramification. This permits rapid excitation of both ventricles, resulting in near cancellation of potentials within the wall. As a result, subtle changes in vector orientation or QRS wave structure resulting from cardiac derangements are difficult to distinguish. The occurrence of rapid, simultaneous activation of both ventricles in a period of approximately 10 milliseconds has been well documented in the goat. The pattern of depolarization observed is virtually identical to that of the calf (Hamlin and Scher 1961). In an experimental model of right ventricular hypertrophy, no significant alteration of the QRS complex or vector orientation was identifiable in affected goats. The Q-T interval shortened in goats with right ventricular hypertrophy, but this was attributed to the increased heart rate that occurred (Ogburn et al. 1977). Nevertheless, detailed studies of three goats with naturally occurring ventricular septal defects indicate that prolongation of P-R intervals and P-, QRS, and T-wave intervals and amplitudes may suggest cardiac enlargement (Parry et al. 1982).

Radiography

The radiographic anatomy of the caprine thorax has been described (Singh et al. 1983). In dorsoventral radiographs, the normal heart lies between the second or third intercostal space and the sixth or seventh space, with the base centered over the midline and the apex shifted to the left of midline.

While not universally accepted, measurement of contact area of the heart with the sternum has been used to evaluate cardiac enlargement secondary to ventricular septal defect in the goat. Normal hearts had a mean contact area of 3.3 sternebrae; abnormal hearts had a mean contact area of 6 (Parry et al. 1982).

Echocardiography

While M-mode, two dimensional (B-mode), and Doppler echocardiography are being applied more frequently to the diagnosis of suspected heart disease in goats, published information on normal echocardiographic parameters in the goat remains limited. In one study, mitral, aortic, and tricuspid valves were identified at the right third and fourth intercostal spaces slightly dorsal to the olecranon. The pulmonic valve was identified at the same location on the left (Yamaga and Too 1984). In a more recent study, technical difficulties were noted with regard to echocardiographic examination of the goat. The cranial location of the heart partly covered by the olecranon and the caudal brachial muscles, along with the narrow intercostal spaces, made it difficult to position the ultrasound transducer and limited the acoustic window (Olsson et al. 2001). Nevertheless, echocardiographic and Doppler measurements were obtained in eight normal Swedish domestic goats during pregnancy, lactation, and the dry period. These measurements are presented in Table 8.2. A separate study of eight normal goats in the Philippines also reports normal caprine cardiac parameters measured by B-mode and M-mode ultrasonography (Acorda et al. 2005).

Table 8.2. Echocardiographic and Doppler measurements and calculated stroke volume and cardiac output during pregnancy, lactation, and dry period in the same eight goats (*Capra hircus*).

	Reproductive periods		
Measurements	*Pregnancy*	*Lactation*	*Dry period*
HR (M-mode; beats min^{-1})	148 ± 4***†	123 ± 5	107 ± 9
AO (mm)	23.9 ± 0.7	23.9 ± 0.4	24.3 ± 0.6
LA (mm)	26.2 ± 1.0	27.9 ± 0.6	26.9 ± 0.3
LVEDD (mm)	39.6 ± 1.5	40.5 ± 1.0	40.6 ± 1.0
LVESD (mm)	23.4 ± 1.4	23.8 ± 0.5	24.0 ± 0.8
LVWd (mm)	6.9 ± 0.4	6.5 ± 0.3	6.8 ± 0.3
LVWs (mm)	12.8 ± 0.5	12.3 ± 0.6	12.9 ± 0.6
FS (%)	41.1 ± 2.0	41.1 ± 1.1	40.6 ± 1.2
HR (Doppler; beats min^{-1})	133 ± 3**	114 ± 4	100 ± 6
VTI (cm s^{-1})	10.5 ± 1.1	11.5 ± 0.8	9.5 ± 0.4
V_{max} (m s^{-1})	1.0 ± 0.0	1.1 ± 0.0	0.9 ± 0.0
Stroke volume (ml)	47 ± 5	54 ± 5	45 ± 3
Cardiac output (l min^{-1})	6.73 ± 0.72**	6.12 ± 0.52	4.39 ± 0.27†

HR = heart rate; AO = aortic root; LA = left atrium; LVEDD and LVESD = left ventricular end-diastolic and end-systolic diameter, respectively; LVWd and LVWs = left ventricular wall thickness in diastole and systole, respectively; FS = fractional shortening of the left ventricle; VTI = velocity trace integral; V_{max} = maximal aortic flow. Values are means ± S.E.M. ** $P < 0.01$ and *** $P < 0.001$ vs. dry period; † $P < 0.05$ *vs.* lactation. (From Olsson, K., et al., A serial study of heart function during pregnancy, lactation and the dry period in dairy goats using echocardiography. Experim. Physiol., 86(1):93–99, 2001. Used with permission of Wiley-Blackewll Publishing.)

There is one published case report on the use of echocardiography for the diagnosis of heart disease in a goat (Gardner et al. 1992). In that report, a three-year-old pygmy buck was evaluated for a systolic murmur. Echocardiography revealed an enlarged right atrium and ventricle, an atrial septal defect, and a dysplastic tricuspid valve, while color-flow Doppler echocardiography revealed severe tricuspid regurgitation and a right to left shunt through the atrial septal defect. A diagnosis of Ebstein's anomaly of the tricuspid valve was made, the first such report in goats. Ultrasonography has also been used to identify cardiac and pulmonic abnormalities associated with enzootic calcinosis in goats (Gufler et al. 1999)

Pericardiocentesis

Indications for pericardiocentesis in the goat are limited. Traumatic reticuloperitonitis, which is a well known condition in cattle, is rarely reported in goats in the veterinary literature. Pericardial effusions may occur in caprine heartwater (cowdriosis), but the fluid is not useful for diagnostic purposes. Pericarditis also occurs in conjunction with systemic mycoplasmosis but the organism is more easily isolated from other sites. If attempted, pericardiocentesis is best performed at the right fourth intercostal space low on the chest wall to avoid lung and coronary arteries. The animal can be standing or in lateral recumbency. Chemical restraint such as diazepam is advisable. Surgical access to the pericardium can be accomplished by resection of the left fourth rib.

Computed Tomography

Computed tomography of the caprine thorax has been described (Smallwood and Healey 1982). The heart is visible in cross-section beginning at the caudal aspect of thoracic vertebra T1 and ending at the middle of T5. The right side of the heart is more visible in the anterior cross sections and the left side in the posterior sections. At the level of the caudal aspect of T2, the heart silhouette is in contact with both the right and left thoracic walls.

Angiography

Left ventricular angiocardiograms in goats have been reported for the diagnosis of VSD. Passage of a catheter was performed via the left and right carotid arteries to acquire angiographic and hemodynamic data (Parry et al 1982; Scarratt et al. 1984). Arteriography and ultrasonography also have been applied to studies of the carotid artery diameter and blood flow velocity in goats (Lee et al. 1990).

Clinical Chemistry

The reported use of clinical chemistry in the diagnosis of caprine heart disease is limited. Myocardial damage or necrosis can lead to release of various enzymes into the circulation, including aspartate aminotransferase (AST), lactate dehydrogenase (LDH), and creatine kinase (CK). However, skeletal muscle damage can also result in measurable increases in serum concentrations of these enzymes. In the case of LDH and CK, measurement of cardiac specific isoenzymes might confirm the involvement of heart muscle, but the cardiac specificity and reference values for caprine isoenzymes of LDH and CK are not well documented.

In recent years, measurement of the myofibrillar contractile protein, troponin, in plasma has become the accepted standard biomarker for acute myocardial infarction in human patients and it is also increased in patients with decreased left ventricular function without acute myocardial infarction (Ammann et al. 2003). Reference values for measurement of troponin (cTNI) in plasma of healthy dogs have been recently published, with a median value of 0.03 ng/mL and a range of 0.01 to 0.15 ng/mL (Oyama and Sisson 2004). Goats have intermediate levels of troponin (cTNT) relative to other domestic species and it has been demonstrated that a second generation immunoassay can detect cardiac muscle troponin cTNT in blood (O'Brien et al. 1998).

DIAGNOSIS OF CARDIOVASCULAR DISEASE BY PRESENTING SIGN

Heart disease is not common in goats and the world literature on caprine cardiovascular disease is sparse. One Indian study on the prevalence of gross cardiac abnormalities in slaughtered goats found approximately 3.5% of 2,720 hearts examined to be abnormal (Chattopadhyay and Sharma 1972). A slaughterhouse survey of 29,687 goats in Zimbabwe identified 525 (1.6%) instances of pericarditis (Chambers 1990). Nevertheless, in routine clinical examination, some physical findings may suggest cardiovascular disease in goats, and these findings should be pursued. The differential diagnoses for clinical signs suggesting cardiovascular disease are given below.

Sudden Death

Attribution of sudden death to cardiac disease must be approached cautiously in goats. The presence of gross or microscopic lesions in the heart at necropsy does not always mean that heart disease contributed to the clinical picture. Some changes may be artifactual, related to autolysis, blanching of the heart muscle during rigor mortis, or uneven staining of histologic sections (Newsholme and Coetzer 1984). In addition, a number of abnormalities may be noted in the heart, pericardium, or great vessels that represent subclinical conditions unrelated to the cause of death. These are discussed below in the section on subclinical cardiovascular conditions.

Peripheral evidence of cardiac dysfunction may be a better indicator of heart involvement than abnormalities of the heart itself. These include passive congestion, lung edema, and fluid accumulation in the thorax, pericardium, or abdomen. Histologic evaluation in all cases of the heart should be performed to identify definitive changes when present. The following cardiac causes of sudden death must be considered.

Nutritional Muscular Dystrophy

Nutritional muscular dystrophy or white muscle disease can affect the heart muscle and skeletal muscle and may be responsible for sudden death caused by cardiac failure, particularly in young kids. The disease is discussed in detail in Chapter 4.

Cardiotoxic Plants

A number of plants may cause heart failure and sudden death in goats. In North America, potentially cardiotoxic plants include the ornamental plants oleander *(Nerium oleander)*, foxglove *(Digitalis purpurea)*, lily of the valley *(Convallaria majalis)*, and yew (*Taxus* spp.). Other weeds and shrubs include Indian hemp *(Apocynum cannabinum)*, false hellebore (*Veratrum* spp.), and milkweed (*Asclepias* spp.) (Fowler 1986). Yew and false hellebore contain toxic alkaloids, while the other plants contain cardiac glycosides. In all cases, such poisonings would be sporadic and require careful documentation of exposure. Rumen contents should be examined for identifiable plant parts. The outcomes of these cases often depend on the level of exposure. If nonlethal doses are consumed, clinical signs may persist for several days, because the half-life of most cardiac glycosides is between twenty-four and thirty-six hours.

Successful management of yew toxicity in goats has been reported. Two goats died within twenty-four hours of ingesting the ornamental shrub and three remaining goats showed signs of bradycardia, hypothermia, depression, and weakness. Rumenotomies were performed on these goats to remove ingested plants, and mineral oil, electrolytes, and activated charcoal were added to the rumen. All three survived (Casteel and Cook 1985).

In South Africa, gousiekte, or "quick disease" occurs commonly enough to produce serious economic loss in livestock, including goats. It is caused by six different plants in the family Rubiaceae: *Pachystigma pygmaeum, P. thamnus, P. latifolium, Pavetta schumanniana, P. harborii,* and *Fadogia homblei.* It is a cumulative poisoning and usually requires several weeks of ingestion of these plants before clinical disease occurs. Goats are more susceptible than sheep (Hurter et al. 1972). The toxic principle in these plants has been isolated. It is a water soluble, heat stable, cationic polyamine that has been termed pavetamine (Fourie et al, 1995). The toxin has been shown to inhibit the synthesis of new myosin during the turnover of myocardial proteins (Schultz et al. 2004). Under range conditions, the disease is perceived as one that causes sudden death after a latent period of three to six weeks following ingestion of the offending plants. However, if animals are carefully observed, prodromal signs of lagging behind the flock, lying down with head and neck extended, dyspnea, and coughing may be noted during this latent period (Pretorius and Terblanche 1967). At necropsy, there is gross evidence of heart failure including general congestion, pulmonary edema, ascites, hydrothorax, and hydropericardium. Histologically, the most consistent finding is hypertrophy of myocardial fibers in the subendocardial region (Prozesky et al. 2005).

Other South African plants that can result in sudden death include *Cotyledon orbiculata* and *Dichapetalum cymosum*. The succulent plant *C. orbiculata* contains bufadeniolides, which are cardiac glycosides. When large amounts of the plant are consumed by goats over a short period of time, sudden death from heart failure can occur (Tustin et al. 1984). This may be preceded by signs of weakness, prostration, tachycardia, and pupillary constriction.

The toxic principle in *D. cymosum*, a plant known as gifblaar, is monofluoroacetic acid. Death occurs within a few hours of ingestion. Peritoneal, pericardial, and thoracic effusions may be observed at necropsy, and histological examination of the heart may demonstrate multiple small foci of myocardial necrosis, with lymphocytic infiltration. However, these are not consistent findings (Newsholme and Coetzer 1984). A related species, *D. barteri*, has been identified as a cause of sudden death in goats eating branches of the tree in Nigeria (Adaudi 1975; Nwude et al. 1977).

Sudden death in South African goats has also been reported three days after ingestion of avocado leaves *(Persea americana)*, presumably because of heart failure (Grant et al. 1988). The cardiotoxicity of avocado leaves has since been confirmed experimentally in two goats (Sani et al. 1991). One died suddenly without showing clinical signs while the second developed muffled heart sounds, tachycardia, and tachypnea before dying two days after challenge. At necropsy, there was pleural and pericardial effusion, pulmonary edema, ascites, hepatic congestion, and a pale, flabby heart with widespread degeneration of myocardial fibers seen microscopically. Avocado, oleander, caltrops *(Calotropis procera)*, and red cotton *(Asclepias curassavica)* have also been reported as causes of cardiotoxicity in goats in Australia (Seawright 1984).

In the Sudan, a commonly grazed annual shrub, *Cassia occidentalis*, has been demonstrated to produce a toxic myodegeneration of cardiac muscle in goats (Suliman and Shommein 1986). *C. occidentalis* is also found in the southwestern United States and is known as coffee weed, senna, or coffee senna. It has been associated with death in grazing cattle because of skeletal and cardiac myodegeneration, so goats must be considered at risk.

In all cases of sudden death, when plant toxicity is suspected, additional animals at risk should be removed from the potential source and given activated charcoal orally at a minimum dose of 2 g/kg bw.

Heartwater

Heartwater (cowdriosis), discussed in detail later in this chapter, occurs principally in Africa as well as in some Caribbean islands and can cause peracute death in goats. Lesions observed after death are similar to those described for gousiekte. Where both diseases occur, they must be differentiated by examination of brain tissue for the presence of the rickettsial organisms that cause heartwater.

Foot and Mouth Disease

Foot and mouth disease (FMD) is usually a subclinical infection in goats or it produces mild to moderate signs of lameness in adults. However, very young kids in infected herds may die suddenly of associated viral, lympho-histiocytic myocarditis which can produce a gross lesion of either diffuse gray spots or more organized "tiger" stripes, mainly in the left ventricle and interventricular septum (Kitching and Hughes 2002). FMD is discussed in more detail in Chapter 4.

Other Cardiotoxic Agents

Iatrogenic cardiotoxicity is possible in goats because of overdosage with at least two commonly used substances, calcium salts and ionophore coccidiostats. However, confirmation of sudden death in goats because of these substances is lacking. When treating milk fever (hypocalcemia), it is always advisable to administer intravenous calcium slowly and monitor the heart sounds for arrhythmia, increased rate, or heart block. Goats that are below average weight, have concurrent diseases, or have already been treated by the owner are more likely to experience cardiac irregularities or arrest.

Ionophore toxicity is known to occur in small ruminants. Ionophore antibiotics are used in livestock production as coccidiostats for cattle, sheep, goats, and poultry and the ionophore monensin is also used as a growth promotant that improves feed efficiency and weight gain in beef cattle. Monensin has caused sudden death in sheep fed three or more times the recommended dose of 15 to 22 ppm. The affected sheep readily consumed feed containing this amount, contrary to the general assumption that feed refusal occurs when the level is more than twice the recommended dose. Sudden death occurred in 20% to 40% of affected sheep and microscopic cardiac lesions ranging from focal necrosis with perivascular lymphocytic cuffing to necrotizing myocarditis were present (Bastianello 1988).

Monensin is approved for oral use in confined goats in the United States as a coccidiostat at a dose of 20 g/ton of feed (22 ppm). Goats experimentally given monensin orally at the rate of 55 ppm in feed for three weeks showed anorexia, diarrhea, and an increase in serum sorbitol dehydrogenase, indicating some hepatotoxicity (Dalvi and Sawant 1990). There are no published reports of field cases of monensin toxicity in goats but experimental data indicate that the single dose oral LD_{50} for monensin in goats is 26.4 mg/kg bw (12 mg/lb)(Beasley 1999).

There is however, a report of fatal overdose of goats with the ionophore salinomycin. Angora goats in Turkey were fed salinomycin in their ration at a rate of 680 ppm/kg of feed due to a mechanical mixing malfunction during feed preparation. Thirteen of 70 exposed goats died. Among those for which there was an opportunity for clinical examination before death, signs included listlessness, inappetence, incoordination, dehydration, fluid stool, tachycardia, muscle weakness, salivation, panting, and prostration, and death occurring within fifteen to twenty-four hours. At necropsy there was excessive fluid in the abdomen, thorax, and pericardium. The heart showed petechiation in the ventricles and endocardium and microscopically there was prominent myocardial hemorrhage (Agaoglu et al. 2002). The recommended dose of salinomycin for use in goats as a coccidiostat is 100 ppm of concentrate fed.

Sudden death also has been reported in goats fed excessive amounts of vitamin D. At necropsy, calcification of the coronary arteries and aorta were noted (Neumann et al. 1973).

Trauma

It has been suggested that goats, due to their generally low pain threshold, can die of cardiac failure resulting from neurogenic or catecholamine-induced ventricular dysrhythmias when subjected to painful procedures such as dehorning without appropriate analgesia or anesthesia (Gray and McDonell 1986).

Aortic Rupture

In tropical regions, nematode infections of the aorta with *Spirocerca lupi* and/or *Onchocerca armillata* have been reported in goats (Chowdhury and Chakraborty 1973). These infections may be subclinical or identified at necropsy or slaughter by thickening, nodularity, or calcification of the aorta. However, *S. lupi* in the goat aorta can lead to slow bleeding with anemia and emaciation or to aortic rupture and sudden death (Chhabra and Singh 1972).

Neoplasia

There is one reported case of a three-year-old pregnant female goat that died suddenly when being chased around its pen to be medicated for undiagnosed chronic respiratory disease of about one month duration. On necropsy the goat had ovine pulmonary adenomatosis (jaagsiekte) with tumor in both lungs that had also metastasized to the kidneys and heart. Death was attributed to heart failure secondary to tumor infiltration of the myocardium of the left ventricle (Al-Dubaib 2005). Jaagsiekte is uncommon in goats and is discussed further in Chapter 9.

Abnormal Heart Sounds

Documentation of abnormal heart sounds in goats is limited.

Murmurs

In cases of VSD, grade IV or V out of VI holosystolic murmurs over both the right and left heart base with palpable thrills on both sides have been reported (Scarratt et al. 1984). An audible S4 sound was heard to precede S1 in one case of VSD (Parry et al. 1982). Systolic murmurs can be heard during the prodromal phase of gousiekte (Pretorius and Terblanche 1967).

Reports of abnormal heart sounds associated with valvular abnormalities are rare. A single case of endocarditis has been reported in a Pygmy goat that presented clinically with a continuous rasping cardiac murmur, increased heart rate, dyspnea, inappetence, fever, and depression. It was determined after death to have traumatic peri- and endocarditis because of heart penetration with a sewing needle (Waldman and Woicke 1984). Two additional cases of vegetative endocarditis in goats have been identified only as incidental post mortem findings (Geisel 1973; Krishna et al. 1976). A grade III/V plateau pansystolic murmur was auscultated over the tricuspid valve area and a grade II/V plateau pansystolic murmur was auscultated over the left heart base in a three-year-old male pygmy goat with Ebstein's anomaly of the tricuspid valve (Gardner et al. 1992).

Systolic murmurs of variable character have been reported in cases of enzootic calcinosis in goats in Austria (Gufler et al. 1999) and Switzerland (Braun et al. 2000) in association with the consumption of golden oat grass (*Trisetum flavescens*). Enzootic calcinosis is known to occur in ruminants and horses in various countries around the world where animals consume plants with high concentrations of 1,25 dihdroxycholecalciferol (calcitrol) glycoside or substances that mimic its action. Chronic consumption of such plants leads to excessive absorption of calcium and results in calcification of soft tissues, primarily the cardiovascular system, but also lungs, kidneys, and tendons.

Affected goats show loss of appetite, emaciation, dyspnea, and abnormalities of carriage and gait, including increased recumbency, difficulty rising, kneeling after rising, stilted gait, arched back, shifting weight from leg to leg, and intermittently carrying a limb off the ground. These locomotor signs are associated with calcification of the flexor tendons and blood vessels of the limbs. Calcification of cardiac structures including the heart valves and the great vessels also occurs in enzootic calcinosis. As a result, physical examination and ancillary diagnostic testing may reveal tachycardia, a variety of murmurs, possible arrhythmias, pericardial effusions, pleural effusions, ascites, and abnormalities in the ECG and echocardiogram, including evidence of pericarditis, thickening of the aortic orifice, and calcification of the heart valves. Calcification of the aorta is especially remarkable and may be noted in plain radiographs. There is no treatment for enzootic calcinosis, but the condition can be controlled by eliminating or reducing access to the offending plants in the ration. The calcinogenicity of yellow oat grass is reduced if it is made into hay when mature rather than grazed as fresh young grass.

Muffled Sounds

The principle cause of muffled heart sounds in the goat is hydropericardium resulting from the appropriately named disease heartwater, or cowdriosis. In addition, some of the African poisonous plants cited above may produce pericardial effusions. Lymphosarcoma and traumatic reticulopericarditis, the two most common causes of pericardial effusion in cattle, are rare in goats (Sharma and Ranka 1978; Waldman and Woicke 1984; Craig et al. 1986; Reddi and Surendran 1988). In one reported case of thymoma, the heart was heard over an increased area of the left thorax, and the palpable cardiac impulse was displaced dorsally by the thoracic mass (Rostkowski et al. 1985).

Friction Rubs

Infectious pericarditis, the most likely cause of friction rubs synchronous with the heartbeat, is infrequently reported in goats (Chattopadhyay and Sharma 1972; Hein and Cargill 1981). When it does occur, it is most often associated with general mycoplasmal infections. The pericarditis is often an extension of the pleuropneumonia commonly associated with mycoplasmal infections, notably *M. mycoides* subspecies *mycoides* and *M. ovipneumoniae* (Masiga and Rurangirwa 1979; East et al. 1983; Rodriguez et al. 1995; Williamson et al. 2007). Friction rubs may be heard either in association with the heartbeat or respiration or both. Exudative pericarditis can also occur in caprine tuberculosis (Savey 1984).

Arrhythmias

Arrhythmias are infrequently documented. They have been reported in association with the cardiac form of tuberculosis, in cardiotoxicity resulting from cardiac glycoside-containing plants, and in a case of enzootic calcinosis. Atrial fibrillation has been reported with congestive heart failure and pneumonia (Gay and Richards 1983). Gallop rhythms, tachycardia, splitting of the first heart sound, and arrhythmias occur during the prodromal phase of gousiekte (Pretorius and Terblanche 1967).

Congestive Heart Failure

The clinical signs of congestive heart failure are similar to those seen in other species. They include increased jugular pulse, jugular distension, moist cough, tachycardia, submandibular edema, ascites, exercise intolerance, chronic weight loss, and possibly diarrhea. Not all signs are seen in all cases. Findings in dead goats that are consistent with heart failure include hydrothorax, hydropericardium, hydroperitoneum, pulmonary edema, heart enlargement, and ventricular dilation.

Congestive heart failure in the goat has been attributed to *cor pulmonale* secondary to pneumonia (Gay and Richards 1983), mediastinal thymoma (Rostkowski et al. 1985), and VSD (Parry et al. 1982). Krimpsiekte and gousiekte, usually recognized as sudden death, may show evidence of congestive heart failure at necropsy. Waterpens, another poisonous plant disease of goats and sheep in South Africa caused by *Galenia africana*, produces a marked abdominal ascites and death (van der Lugt et al. 1988). The intoxication results in both hepatic and cardiac lesions. Experimental challenge studies with plant extracts indicate that G. *africana* is primarily hepatotoxic with myocardial involvement occurring only in the terminal stages of the intoxication (van der Lugt et al. 1992). Nutritional muscular dystrophy (white muscle disease) may lead to congestive heart failure when heart muscle damage is not severe enough to produce sudden death.

The differential diagnosis for goats with signs suggesting congestive heart failure should include gastrointestinal helminthiasis and liver fluke disease. These parasitisms can produce edema, ascites, and exercise intolerance secondary to hypoproteinemia and anemia.

Marked jugular distension commonly occurs in goats whose neck chains or collars have been fastened too tightly. This should be differentiated from heart disease.

Reports on therapy for congestive heart failure in goats are limited (Gay and Richards 1983). The principles of therapy and the drugs commonly reported in the dog can be used reasonably as a first approximation in goats. These include reduction of preload with furosemide or other diuretics; reduction of afterload with captopril, hydralazine, or other vasodilators; improvement of contractility with digoxin or dobutamine; and restoration of rate and rhythm with lidocaine, quinidine, procainamide, or other appropriate antiarrhythmic drugs (Kittleson 1985; Wilcke 1985).

SUBCLINICAL CARDIOVASCULAR CONDITIONS

Lesions involving the heart and vasculature are sometimes observed at necropsy in goats when no signs of heart disease have been recognized during the clinical examination. This occurs when other clinical signs overshadow cardiovascular disease, when cardiovascular disease is subclinical, or when lesions observed are non-pathogenic.

Pericardial effusions or pericarditis may be seen in mycoplasmosis, viral goat dermatitis (Patnaik 1986), false blackleg (malignant edema), and enterotoxemia due to *Clostridium perfringens* type D. A nonpathogenic lymphoreticular hyperplasia of the epicardium and pericardium has also been seen histologically from slaughter surveys (Chattopadhyay and Sharma 1972). Hydropericardium has also been reported at necropsy in goats poisoned by consumption of the seed pods of the tree *Albizia versicolor* in Malawi. The predominant clinical picture was one of neurologic disease (Soldan et al. 1996).

Incidental and subclinical myocardial lesions may include gray white foci of necrosis in the ventricles presumed to be caused by earlier plant or bacterial toxic insults, metaplastic cartilage development with or without calcification, focal lymphocytic infiltration of the myocardial interstitium, granulomatous myocarditis, and parasitic myocarditis. Causes of parasitic myocarditis include sarcosporidiosis, hydatid cysts, and metacestodes of other taeniid cestodes including *Cysticercus* and *Coenurus* (Bhalla and Nagi 1962; Chattopadhyay and Sharma 1972; Hein and Cargill 1981).

Aortic abnormalities occur in goats, though in general they contribute little to clinical disease. These include aneurysm, aortitis media, melanosis, intimal fat deposits and intimal fibrosis, cartilaginous and osseous metaplasia, and calcification (Prasad et al. 1972; Geisel 1973). Migratory tracts, nodules, corrugations, aneurysms, and thickening of the aortic wall may be seen in association with onchocerciasis (Kaul and Prasad, 1989). Focal aortic necrosis and calcification in goats is a frequent lesion in caprine paratuberculosis (Majeed and Goudswaard 1971). Calcification of the aorta as well as other great vessels is seen in goats with enzootic calcinosis due to consumption of yellow oat grass (*Trisetum flavescens*), as described above.

SPECIFIC DISEASES OF THE CARDIOVASCULAR SYSTEM

Heartwater

Heartwater, also known as cowdriosis, is an infectious, non-contagious, tick-borne rickettsial disease of domestic ruminants. Historically restricted to sub-Saharan Africa, heartwater has more recently also been identified in the Caribbean. There is considerable concern about the possible spread of heartwater and its vector to tropical and subtropical regions of North, South, and Central America where, moreover, other suitable tick vectors exist.

Etiology

The causative agent is the rickettsia *Ehrlichia* (previously *Cowdria*) *ruminantium*. It is Gram-negative and stains reddish purple to blue in smears with Giemsa stain. Pleomorphism is common. Smaller organisms are usually coccoid while larger ones may be horseshoe, ring, or rod shaped. In mammalian hosts, the organism has a predilection for vascular endothelial cells. In the tick vector, it is found in intestinal epithelial cells and in cells of the salivary glands.

Historically, efforts to perform *in vitro* cultures of *E. ruminantium* have failed, but successful cultivation of several strains of the organism on endothelial cell lines as well as tick cell lines is now possible (Bezuidenhout et al. 1985; Bell-Sakyi et al. 2000). Live organisms in whole blood or tissue homogenates from infected animals may be stored for extended periods by quick freezing in liquid nitrogen using a suitable cryopreservative, for example, dimethyl sulfoxide.

Various strains of the organism exist. Cross-protective immunity may develop after infection with various field strains (Van Winkelhoff and Uilenberg 1981; Uilenberg 1983), but strains are often not or only partially cross-protective when used to challenge ruminants (Uilenberg 1983; Jongejan et al. 1988; Du Plessis et al. 1989), and antigenic diversity is an important feature of *E. ruminantium*. Field isolates often consist of more than one strain. Strains also vary in virulence, and there are isolates, indistinguishable from *E. ruminantium* using molecular methods, that do not cause clinical disease at all (Allsopp et al. 2007), and one of these has even been detected in a goat in the United States (Loftis et al. 2006).

Epidemiology

Heartwater is indigenous to sub-Saharan Africa. It was first recognized in South Africa in 1838 and is still considered a major obstacle to expansion and development of livestock enterprises on the continent. Imported cattle, sheep, and goats in particular are very susceptible to severe infection with high mortality rates.

Heartwater is also found on islands near Africa, including Madagascar, Mauritius, Reunion, the Comoros and São Tome.

The occurrence of heartwater in the Western hemisphere causes concern. The disease was reported on the island of Guadeloupe in 1980. Since that time, its occurrence on other Caribbean islands including Antigua and Marie Galante has been confirmed. The tick vector *Amblyomma variegatum,* originally introduced into the region with an importation of cattle from Senegal in the nineteenth or possibly even in the eighteenth century, has also been found on Puerto Rico, Vieques, St. Croix, St. Martin, Anguilla, St. Kitts, Nevis, La Desirade, Martinique, St. Lucia, St. Vincent, and Barbados, but *E. ruminantium* has not yet been identified on these islands (Camus et al. 1984). An international campaign for the eradication of *A. variegatum* from the Western Hemisphere, operational from 1994 to 2006, has succeeded on some of these islands, but failed in its ultimate objective (ICTTD 2006).

The distribution of heartwater reflects the geographic distribution of the tick vectors of the genus *Amblyomma* that transmit the disease to domestic and wild ruminants. *Amblyomma* spp. are three-host ticks that feed on a wide variety of mammals and birds. The most widespread vector for heartwater in Africa and the Caribbean is *A. variegatum*, also known as the tropical bont tick. Other natural African vectors include *A. hebraeum* in southern Africa, *A. pomposum* in south-central Africa, and *A. gemma* and *A. lepidum* in east and northeastern Africa. Several other African *Amblyomma* spp. may carry the organism but mainly feed on wild animals. At least two ticks found in North and South America, *A. maculatum,* the Gulf Coast tick, and *A. cajennense,* the cayenne tick, are capable of transmitting *E. ruminantium* to domestic ruminants, the former quite effectively (Uilenberg et al. 1984).

In general, *Amblyomma* ticks can passage *E. ruminantium* transstadially but not transovarially, though there is one report of transovarial transfer. Consecutive passage from larval to nymphal stage, nymphal to adult stage, and larval to nymphal to adult stage occurs. Ticks therefore can remain infected for periods as long as several years. The organism resides in the intestinal epithelium of ticks and is thought to be transmitted with the saliva (Kocan and Bezuidenhout 1987).

The hosts for *E. ruminantium* appear to be essentially members of the family Bovidae including both domestic and wild ruminants in Africa. Cervidae are also susceptible. Wild ruminants may serve as a reservoir for infection, but a wildlife reservoir is not necessary to sustain infection. Prolonged survival of *E. ruminantium* in ticks maintains the disease, and the carrier state in ruminants also occurs (Andrew and Norval, 1989).

An age-related resistance to disease occurs in young domestic ruminants, independent of maternally derived passive immunity. The period of resistance in calves and lambs gradually wanes after approximately the first three weeks of life. The period in kids is not well studied but may be even shorter. Young animals exposed during this period are unlikely to develop clinical disease and are resistant to subsequent homologous reinfection. Because the period of host resistance is short and the infection rate and/or number of the tick vectors may be low, the opportunity to develop an immune host population is limited, and serious disease losses can continue to occur in endemic areas.

Goats are the most susceptible natural hosts based on epidemiologic observations and experimental challenge studies. Indigenous goats in endemic areas are more resistant than imported ones, but serious incidents of acute heartwater in local goats do occur in Africa (Aklaku 1980; Gueye et al. 1984). Very young, resistant goats may not be exposed to feeding ticks during their resistant period because of local variations in tick populations, preferential feeding by ticks on cattle over goats, or confinement of kids to villages to avoid theft and predation (Ilemobade 1977). A seroprevalence survey of heartwater in Red Maasai sheep and Small East African goats conducted at three sites in Narok District of Kenya using the MAP1-B ELISA found 62% to 82.5% of sheep and 42.5% to 52% of goats to be seropositive (Wesonga et al. 2006).

Evidence for differences in breed susceptibility is suggested by epidemiologic and experimental observations. In South Africa, Angora goats and Boer goats are quite susceptible to heartwater compared with other indigenous or exotic breeds (Van de Pypekamp and Prozesky 1987). Breed differences in susceptibility have also been reported in Guadeloupe, with native Creole goats showing greater resistance than European breeds of goats. However, differences are also observed between different populations within a given breed based on their history of exposure to cowdriosis. It is presumed that genetic resistance increases over time by natural selection in the face of continued challenge by *E. ruminantium* and that such resistance may be a recessive sex-linked trait (Matheron et al. 1987).

Pathogenesis

E. ruminantium is introduced into the mammalian host by an infected tick while feeding. The early development of infection is not well clarified. It has been suggested that initial replication occurs in regional lymph nodes within macrophages and other reticuloendothelial cells. This is followed by a rickettsemic phase lasting one to four days accompanied by fever. The organism can be demonstrated to occur in the blood plasma as well as in neutrophils (Logan et al. 1987). Subsequently, the organism invades and multiplies in vascular endothelium throughout the body, particularly in the cortex of the brain. The ensuing vasculitis results in fluid and protein loss through capillaries with local edema and hemorrhage that, depending on the location and severity, accounts for the varied clinical and post mortem findings. The incubation period in goats after experimental intravenous inoculation is seven to fourteen days, or even shorter after a massive infective dose.

Clinical Findings

The incubation period to fever after natural tick-transmitted infection is usually from about two to as much as four weeks. There are four clinical forms of heartwater: peracute, acute, subacute, and subclinical. Their development depends on host susceptibility and virulence of the infective strain. Sporadic cases or epizootic outbreaks may occur. Goats most often experience peracute and acute infections.

In peracute disease, affected goats develop a high fever and then suddenly collapse without warning followed by a period of convulsions or paddling lasting from minutes to several hours. The acute form may last from two to five days. The first signs are depression, anorexia, and high fever up to 105.8°F (41°C) accompanied by rapid, labored breathing and cessation of rumination. Auscultation of the chest may suggest pulmonary edema and muffled heart sounds due to hydropericardium. This is followed by nervous signs including bleating, hyperesthesia, muscle twitching, teeth grinding, excessive blinking of the eyelids, nystagmus, frequent urination and defecation, circling, and finally terminal convulsions. Ocular congestion and diarrhea may precede or accompany the nervous signs. Mortality in goats may reach more than 90%.

Signs of subacute disease may be limited to fever, watery eyes, mucous nasal discharge, coughing, dyspnea, and possibly diarrhea and mild nervous signs. Subacute disease is most likely in previously exposed or naturally resistant animals. Subclinical infection, manifested by a transient fever, is uncommonly recognized in goats.

Clinical Pathology and Necropsy

A decrease in packed cell volume, hemoglobin, total plasma protein, and serum albumin are common findings in heartwater. The leukocyte response is variable in goats with either neutropenia and lymphopenia or lymphocytic leukocytosis reported (Ilemobade and Blotkamp 1978; Abdel Rahim and Shommein 1978). Hyperglycemia and lactic acidosis may be recorded terminally. Orange-yellow serum has been reported as a consistent finding in Angora goats affected with heartwater, but the observation has not been repeated in other breeds of goats.

Gross post mortem findings in goats include hydropericardium, variable degrees of hydrothorax, and pulmonary edema. Other possible signs are ascites, edema of lymph nodes, serosal hemorrhage, particularly of the heart, mucosal congestion of the gastrointestinal tract, and swollen kidneys. Splenomegaly, a common sign in other species, was not observed in experimentally infected goats (Ilemobade and Blotkamp 1978). Severe nephrosis is reported in Angora goats (Prozesky and Du Plessis 1985).

Histologically, the disease is characterized by the presence of clusters of *E. ruminantium* in the vascular endothelium of virtually all tissues examined; brain cortex is the most reliable source and liver the least reliable.

For rapid post mortem field diagnosis, squash preparations of Giemsa-stained cerebrocortical gray matter reveal blue- to purple-stained clusters of *E. ruminantium* in vascular endothelium. If removing the entire brain is problematic, cerebellar cortex obtained via the foramen magnum with a spatula or spoon is a suitable sample for examination, or cerebral cortex may be obtained after drilling a hole in the skull, even simply with a good-sized nail and a hammer. Proper precautions in rabies-enzootic countries should of course be taken.

Diagnosis

Diagnosis is presumptive, based on the clinical history and signs, the presence of *Amblyomma* ticks in the region and on the animal, and the demonstration of organisms in vascular endothelium on smears or histologic examinations as described above. Differential diagnosis for the peracute form of disease includes virtually all causes of sudden death in goats, discussed in Chapter 16. The acute or neurologic form of heartwater must be distinguished from tetanus, rabies, pseudorabies, organophosphate toxicity, and various plant poisonings. In particular, one leguminous tree, *Albizia versicolor*, occurs in areas of southern Africa where heartwater is endemic. Consumption of the seed pods by goats can produce both neurologic signs and hydropericardium, which are suggestive of heartwater (Soldan et al. 1996). When diarrhea and fever precede neurologic signs, peste des petits ruminants, rinderpest, and salmonellosis should be ruled out.

Confirmation of heartwater in live animals has long been difficult because the organism cannot be cultured routinely. Intravenous inoculation of 5 to 10 ml of whole blood from suspected cases into known healthy, susceptible goats or sheep with subsequent necropsy of the ill test animal confirms the diagnosis. A technique for cerebral biopsy to examine brain smears from goats for *E. ruminantium* has been described (Synge 1978). It is most diagnostic three to six days after onset of fever (Camus and Barre 1987). At present the infection can be confirmed by molecular methods, specific DNA probes (Waghela et al. 1991), and PCR, which considerably increases sensitivity (Martinez et al. 2004).

There are presently several serological tests for detecting antibodies to *E. ruminantium*, but all suffer to some extent from lack of specificity, as there are cross reactions with some other *Ehrlichia* species or unknown agents. This has partly been overcome by using more specific recombinant antigens instead of crude antigens for enzyme-linked immunosorbent assays (Van Vliet 1995, Katz et al. 1997; Kakono et al. 2003). A direct fluorescent antibody test is capable of detecting E. *ruminantium* in macrophage and buffy coat cultures of infected goats, sheep, and cattle (Sahu 1986). Challenges and advances in the laboratory and field diagnosis of heartwater have been recently reviewed (Mahan 2006).

Treatment

Successful therapy depends on early initiation of antibiotic therapy. Animals treated during the febrile stage of acute heartwater respond favorably to tetracycline, 5 to 10 mg/kg bw intravenously or intramuscularly administered at the first sign of fever and repeated one additional time either one or two days later. Long-acting oxytetracycline given one time intramuscularly at the onset of fever at a dose of 20 mg/kg is also effective. Therapy initiated after the onset of neurologic signs is almost always ineffective. Delaying treatment until after day two may result in poorer success because of development of severe nephrosis secondary to renal ischemia (Prozesky and Du Plessis 1985).

Control

Attempts to control heartwater by controlling tick populations in Africa have been somewhat successful, though eradication of the disease by vector control seems unlikely, and even the attempt at vector eradication from the Caribbean islands has failed

A combination of controlled exposure and treatment has been used to vaccinate exotic livestock in Africa with some success. Infective materials used as vaccines are prepared by snap freezing of blood (or tissue preparations) derived from artificially infected livestock (or ticks). Because these are rather crude preparations, anaphylactic reactions can and do occur in a small percentage of vaccinates, and other pathogens may unintentionally be transmitted. For vaccination these substances are administered by the intravenous route. At the first sign of fever, vaccinated animals are treated with oxytetracycline (10 mg/kg intramuscularly or intravenously) to diminish the signs of disease and impart an immunity to reinfection.

Kids vaccinated during their period of natural resistance may not show a febrile response (Van der Merwe 1987). Because of the logistical difficulty of determining the onset of fever in individual animals, arbitrarily timed treatments after vaccination have been recommended. However, the time of onset of the febrile response depends on the strain and preparation of the vaccine. When Angora goats were monitored after vaccination with a frozen Ball 3 strain vaccine, 97% were in the febrile phase between day ten and day fourteen, while only 76% of goats given a fresh Ball 3 strain vaccine were febrile during that period (Erasmus 1976). Because successful vaccination depends on proper timing of treatment, the mean incubation period for the vaccine to be used should be known in advance if such block treatment is to be used. It may be several days shorter when tick filtrate vaccines are used. Temperatures in goats should reach 103.1°F (39.5°C) before treatment.

The duration of immunity in goats is not well known but may be as short as two months. Field exposure to antigenically different strains may be responsible for a seemingly short duration of immunity, and homologous immunity is likely to be longer. Vaccination should be timed to precede periods of peak tick feeding activity in wet seasons. Vaccination procedures for cowdriosis have been reviewed (Van der Merwe 1987). At present there are ongoing studies on improving and standardizing the classical method of infection and treatment by using infective material obtained in cell culture, which would also largely solve the problem of spreading other pathogens. Other studies concern inactivated as well as attenuated vaccines. Advances in the development of new vaccines and vaccine methodologies for control of heartwater have recently been reviewed (Mahan 2006).

Efforts to control tick populations on goats may help control cowdriosis. However, dipping of Angora goats during pregnancy or cold weather should be avoided because stress-related abortion and hypothermia are common in this breed (Gruss 1987).

Schistosomosis

Schistosomes are trematode parasites of the vascular system. Different species reside in the vasculature of different organs, and can produce a variety of clinical manifestations including rhinitis, enteritis, hepatitis, or pneumonia. All clinical forms occur in goats in endemic regions of the world.

Etiology

In the family Schistosomatidae are two genera that can cause clinical disease in goats: the *Schistosoma* and the *Orientobilharzia*. Numerous species use goats as a definitive host. These are identified in Table 8.3 along with their geographic distribution, intermediate and

Table 8.3. Schistosomes reported to infect goats.

Species	*Geographic distribution*	*Intermediate snail host*	*Definitive hosts*	*Sites of localization*	*Clinical effects*
Schistosoma bovis	Central, East, and West Africa; Mediterranean, Middle East	Various *Bulinus* spp.	Ruminants, equines, camels, rodents, humans	Portal and mesenteric veins	Diarrhea, dysentery, anemia, emaciation, death
S. japonicum	Far East	Various *Oncomeliana* spp.	Ruminants, equines, humans, pigs, dog, cats, rodents	Hepatic, portal, and mesenteric veins	Diarrhea, dysentery, anemia, emaciation, death
S. mattheei	Central, South, and East Africa	Various *Bulinus* spp.	Ruminants, equines, humans, baboons, rodents	Portal, mesenteric, urogenital, and stomach veins	Pneumonia, diarrhea, dysentery, anemia, emaciation, death
S. spindale	Indian subcontinent and Far East	Various *Planorbis*, *Lymnaea*, and *Indoplanorbis* spp.	Ruminants, rodents, and dogs	Mesenteric veins	Diarrhea, dysentery, anemia, emaciation, death
S. indicum	Indian subcontinent	*Indoplanorbis* spp.	Ruminants, equines, camels	Hepatic, portal, mesenteric, pancreatic, and pulmonary veins	Diarrhea, dysentery, anemia, dyspnea, emaciation, death
S. mansoni	Africa, South America, Middle East	Various *Biomphalaria* spp.	Most important in humans; various rodents, wild mammals, including goats	Mesenteric veins	Diarrhea, anemia, dyspnea, emaciation, death
S. nasale	Indian subcontinent	*Indoplanorbis* and *Lymnea* spp.	Goats, cattle, buffalo, sheep, horses	Nasal mucosal veins	Coryza, sneezing, dyspnea
S. incognitum	Indian subcontinent	*Lymnea* spp.	Pigs, dogs, one report in goats	—	Not reported; found at slaughter
S. curassoni	West Africa	Various *Bulinus* spp.	goats, sheep, cattle	Portal and mesenteric veins	Diarrhea, dysentery, anemia, emaciation, death
Orientobilharzia turkestanicum	Mongolia, Iraq, France, Russia	*Lymnaea euphratica*	Ruminants, camels, cats, equines	Mesenteric veins	Chronic debilitation

definitive hosts, and the site of localization within the goat. There is one report of finding *Schistosoma incognitum* in goats in a slaughterhouse survey in Jabalpur, India (Agrawal and Sahasrabudhe 1982), though this species is usually associated with swine. Experimental patent infection of goats with *S. incognitum* was later demonstrated (Gupta and Agrawal 2005). *Schistosoma curassoni,* previously thought to be synonymous with *S. bovis,* is now considered a distinct species infecting goats, sheep, and cattle (Verycruysse et al. 1984), though hybridization is known to occur between the two species (Rollinson et al. 1990). Ongoing phylogenetic studies are helping to clarify the relationships and classification of the pathogenic species of Schistosomatidae (Snyder and Loker 2000; Webster et al. 2006).

The schistosomes are elongated trematodes with distinct male and female forms that are found together in the host as mating pairs. The life cycle of schistosomes is indirect and involves aquatic snails as intermediate hosts. Though there are species variations in life cycle, the general pattern is as follows (Soulsby 1982). Adult schistosomes reside in the vasculature of the target organ of their definitive hosts. These organs are usually the liver, intestine, nasal mucosa, or urinary bladder. Gravid females lay eggs that pass through the vessel walls and gain entrance to the gut lumen, bladder lumen, or nasal passage. These eggs, which may already contain live miracidia, hatch when passed into water. The miracidia are released and infect the appropriate species of aquatic snail, which serves as the intermediate host. Subsequent development in the snail occurs over a variable time period of thirty-eight to 126 days based on environmental factors. Two generations of sporocysts occur in the snail, leading to the formation of cercariae that are released from the snail back into water. When definitive hosts stand in or drink contaminated water, they are infected by the cercariae, either by penetration of the skin or the rumen wall.

After entry into the definitive host, cercariae transform into schistosomula and are carried to the lungs and then the liver via the bloodstream over a period of one week. Schistosomula are usually present in the portal veins by day eight. Mating occurs in the portal vein and adults then migrate to the mesenteric veins where maturation and egg laying occur. When hyperinfection occurs, adult schistosomes may mature in the pulmonary vessels and lay eggs in the lung. Pulmonary schistosomosis due to *S. indicum* has been reported in goats in India (Sharma and Dwivedi 1976). In the case of *S. nasale,* maturation and egg laying occur in the vessels of the nasal mucosa and eggs are passed in nasal discharge. The prepatent period for *S. bovis* infection in goats was recorded as forty-seven to forty-eight days (Massoud 1973).

Epidemiology

Schistosomes infect humans and animals mainly in Asia, Africa, the Middle East, South and Central America, and the Mediterranean region. Schistosomosis, or bilharzia, is an important human disease in Africa, Asia, and South America, caused principally by *S. haematobium, S. japonicum,* or *S. mansoni.* Livestock, including goats, can serve as a reservoir for *Schistosoma* spp. infective for humans (Adam and Magzoub 1977).

The intestinal form of schistosomosis in goats is reported most frequently from Asia and Africa. The nasal form, caused by *S. nasale,* is restricted to the Indian subcontinent. Economic losses because of schistosomosis in goats result from poor growth and performance, treatment costs, mortality, and condemnations, especially of livers, at slaughter (Singh Nara and Nayak 1972; Seydi and Gueye 1982).

The occurrence of schistosomosis is closely tied to the ecology of the intermediate snail hosts. The snails thrive in stagnant or slowly moving water such as is found in irrigation ditches, rice paddies, watering tanks or troughs, shallow ponds or puddles, and ditches during seasons of heavy rain. As such, the occurrence of schistosomosis may be continuous or seasonal depending on the nature of the contaminated water source. Where occurrence is seasonal, snails persist through periods of decreased water habitat, mostly through a strategy of prolificacy. Livestock are infected when they drink from, stand in, or wallow in such water sources. Additional factors contributing to an increased prevalence are poor grazing, limited water supplies, and overcrowding (Hurter and Potgieter 1967).

The prevalence of schistosomosis in various livestock is largely dictated by their behavior relative to water. Pigs and buffalo, the wallowing species, have a high prevalence of infection; cattle, an intermediate prevalence; and sheep and goats, a low prevalence (Agrawal 1981). Goats show a distinct aversion to immersion in water, and even avoid walking through it. This may reduce their potential for exposure (Kassuku 1983). In abattoir surveys, prevalence of schistosomosis in goats is consistently much lower than in buffalo and cattle (Islam 1975; Kassuku et al. 1986). Nevertheless, serious losses of goats can occur, such as reported from China, where summer rains produce marked increases in intermediate host snail populations (Li 1987).

It is fortunate that the goat is less frequently exposed to infection because when cattle, sheep, and goats are experimentally challenged with *S. bovis* or *S. japonicum* cercariae, the intensity and severity of infection is most profound in goats (Massoud 1973; Chiu and Lu 1974).

Pathogenesis

The intestinal form of the disease occurs approximately two months after infection, when adults begin to lay eggs in the mesenteric veins and the spined eggs pass through the intestinal mucosa. This results in injury to all layers of the intestinal wall with hemorrhage and edema, and the formation of microabscesses, granulomas, and progressive fibrosis. These changes lead to diarrhea and dysentery and probably malabsorption, as hypoproteinemia is common. The adult parasites cause phlebitis in the mesenteric vessels and are sometimes also found in vessels of the urinary bladder and the pulmonary arteries. As many as 1,000 pairs of adults have been counted from the mesenteric veins of goats dying with *S. mattheei* infection (Hurter and Potgieter 1967).

The hepatic form of the disease is considered to reflect a severe cell-mediated immune response to *Schistosoma* eggs refluxed back into the portal circulation. Soluble egg antigens induce a marked eosinophilic, granulomatous reaction leading to extensive damage to the portal vasculature and subsequently severe fibrosis of the portal triads (Soulsby 1982). In humans, especially, this results in portal hypertension with development of varices and possibly congestive heart failure. In ruminants, these cardiovascular effects are not expressed clinically and liver involvement is usually detected only at necropsy. It is reported that

O. turkestanicum infection in goats and sheep leads to chronic debility secondary to hepatic cirrhosis and intestinal granuloma formation (Soulsby 1982). Anemia occurs in schistosomosis as a result of hemorrhagic lesions in the intestinal wall from migration of eggs and from blood feeding by adults in the vessels.

The nasal form of the disease represents an inflammatory reaction to the passage of eggs through the nasal mucosa and, to a lesser extent, the presence of adult schistosomes in the nasal vessels. The result is nasal congestion, copious nasal discharge, granuloma formation, and dyspnea.

Pulmonary schistosomosis occurs when the host is challenged with large numbers of cercariae. Maturation of excessive numbers of schistosomes in the liver leads to spread of parasitic emboli back to the lungs. Adult schistosomes lay eggs in the lung vessels and produce multiple, diffuse, nodular granulomata throughout the lung parenchyma. Emaciation and respiratory distress result (Sharma and Dwivedi 1976).

Clinical Findings

All ages, breeds, and sex of goats are affected. Clinical disease occurs in association with the onset of egg excretion. In the intestinal form, diarrhea, anemia, and emaciation are the cardinal signs. The diarrhea is usually watery, but can be mucoid and/or bloody. Anorexia, dehydration, and edema are common accompanying findings. The clinical course is usually weeks to months and can result in death, chronic ill thrift, or sometimes spontaneous recovery. Clinically, the presentation may be indistinguishable from gastrointestinal nematodiasis.

In the nasal form of the disease due to *S. nasale*, there may be weight loss, snoring, sneezing, copious mucoid or foul-smelling purulent nasal discharge, and dyspnea. In pulmonary schistosomosis, emaciation, and dyspnea can occur. The hepatic form of the disease is usually not recognized clinically; it is overshadowed by the enteric or pulmonary forms.

Clinical Pathology and Necropsy

Anemia and sometimes eosinophilia may be noted in the hemogram. Hypoproteinemia, hypoalbuminemia, and hypergammaglobulinemia may also be present (Pandey et al. 1976). In experimental *S. mansoni* infection of goats, there were elevations in serum arginase, AST, and bilirubin, and a depletion of liver glycogen (Adam and Magzoub 1977).

To date, serological tests are generally unreliable for confirmation of individual cases or for prevalence studies, mainly because of cross reactions with other trematodes, notably *Fasciola* spp. and the amphistomes (rumen flukes), which are likely to be present in the same situations as schistosomes. Experimental infections of goats with *S. japonicum* have been confirmed serologically during the prepatent period using ELISA and immunofluorescent antibody techniques (Schumann et al. 1984). A dot ELISA test has recently been evaluated in experimentally and naturally infected goats in India (Vohra et al. 2006). Adjustments necessary to improve specificity of the test resulted in reduced sensitivity, but nevertheless, the test was considered to be potentially useful in the field for conducting prevalence studies in locations where infection status is unknown.

In the field, confirmation requires identification of schistosome eggs in nasal secretions, nasal scrapings, feces, rectal scrapings, or possibly urine. Diagnosis by liver biopsy was also reported to be 100% reliable in goats, whereas fecal examination yielded many false negative results (Agrawal and Sahasrabudhe 1982a). Schistosome eggs are generally larger than nematode eggs. They are elongated and spindle shaped and possess a characteristic terminal spine. Direct smears or sedimentation techniques are preferred to flotation methods for finding these trematode eggs. Microscopic examination of squash preps of rectal mucosa obtained with a bowel forceps was 100% effective in diagnosing schistosomosis in a group of acutely affected sheep and goats (Hurter and Potgieter 1967). In chronic cases, egg shedding may be reduced and diagnosis may depend on identification of adult schistosomes in vessels at necropsy. For the diagnosis of caprine hepatic schistosomosis, it has been reported that egg hatching techniques are more sensitive for detection of eggs in the feces of affected goats than either the formal ether sedimentation technique or the alkaline digestion technique (Vohra and Agrawal 2006a).

At necropsy, the carcass is usually emaciated. Adult schistosomes up to 30 mm in length are most frequently found in mesenteric, portal, intestinal submucosal and subserosal veins. They may also be found in pulmonary veins and veins of the urinary bladder. The liver may have a grayish discoloration and an uneven surface. The lungs may be enlarged, heavy, brown-black, and rubbery with multiple grayish nodular foci on the pleura and on cut surface when pulmonary schistosomosis is present (Sharma and Dwivedi 1984). A catarrhal enteritis is usually present and granulomatous swellings of the mucosa may be noted as well as areas of petechial or ecchymotic hemorrhage with accumulation of blood in the intestinal lumen. In the nasal form, large granulomas protruding from the nasal mucosa may be noted on cut section of the nasal passages.

Histologically, lesions are associated primarily with eggs rather than adult schistosomes. Eggs in the liver, lung, intestinal wall, and nasal mucosa induce a marked inflammatory response with infiltration of eosinophils, lymphocytes, and macrophages.

Granuloma formation around schistosome eggs is common. The liver lesion is characterized by fibrosis in the region of the portal triads in advanced cases.

Diagnosis

The definitive antemortem diagnosis of schistosomosis depends on identification of eggs in excretions or by biopsy. The intestinal form of the disease must be distinguished from other causes of diarrhea in association with anemia and emaciation, notably gastrointestinal nematodiasis, coccidiosis, and fascioliasis. The nasal form of the disease must be differentiated from other causes of rhinitis as presented in Chapter 9. At necropsy, the diagnosis is confirmed by identification of adult schistosomes in the vasculature, or characteristic histologic lesions.

Treatment

In the past, the few drugs available to treat schistosomosis, such as antimony compounds, had narrow margins of safety and frequently produced toxic effects in goats and sheep. Haloxon was also reported to be effective in goats at a dose of 300 mg/kg against the intestinal schistosome *S. mattheei* with no noted side effects (Hurter and Potgieter 1967). Currently, praziquantel is being recommended for ruminants at an oral dose of 25 mg/kg bw repeated one time three to five weeks later. However, a single oral dose of 60 mg/kg was reported to effectively eliminate *S. nasale* infection from a goat with no toxic side effects noted (Anandan and Raja 1987).

Control

Efforts at control are directed at reduction of snail intermediate hosts and exposure of livestock to infective cercariae. When possible, stagnant water sources should be eliminated or fenced off and piped or running water provided instead. Water tanks and troughs should be emptied and cleaned periodically. When ponds or other stagnant water sources must be used, then snail control by application of molluscicides such as copper sulfate or niclosamide have been employed.

To minimize effects on livestock, goats should be treated with praziquantel timed to peaks of likely incidence, such as two months after heavy rains. Currently there are no vaccines against schistosomosis.

REFERENCES

Abdel Rahim, A.I. and Shommein, A.M.: Haematological studies in goats experimentally infected with *Rickettsia ruminantium*. Bull. Anim. Health Prod. Afr., 26:232–235, 1978.

Abe, Y., et al.: Development of mechanical circulatory support devices at the University of Tokyo. J. Artificial Organs, 10(2):60–70, 2007.

Acorda, J.A., Ong, R.A.F. and Maligaya, R.L.: Ultrasonographic features of the heart in Philippine native goats (*Capra hircus*). Philippine J. Vet. Med., 42(2):66–74, 2005.

Adam, S.E.I. and Magzoub, M.: Clinico-pathological changes associated with experimental *Schistosoma mansoni* infection in the goat. Br. Vet. J., 133:201–210, 1977.

Adaudi, A.O.: *Dichapetalum barteri* poisoning in goats. Trop. Anim. Health Prod., 7:56–57, 1975.

Agaoglu, Z.T., et al.: Accidental salinomycin intoxication of Angora goats in Turkey. Small Rumin. Res., 45:159–161, 2002.

Agrawal, M.C.: Some observations on schistosomiasis in Jabalpur area. Livestock Adviser Bangalore. 6:53–55, 1981.

Agrawal, M.C. and Sahasrabudhe, V.K.: A note on natural heterologous schistosome infection in domestic animals. Livestock Advisor, 7(1):58–59, 1982.

Agrawal, M.C. and Sahasrabudhe, V.K.: Evaluation of routine diagnostic methods for detecting hepato-intestinal schistosomiasis in cattle and goats. Indian J. Parasitol., 6:319–320, 1982a.

Aklaku, I.K.: Principal causes of mortality in small ruminants in Ghana. Bull. Off. Int. Epizoot., 92:1227–1231, 1980.

Al-Dubaib, M.A.: Renal and cardiac metastases of Jaagsiekte-like tumour in a goat. Small Rumin. Res., 58(1):75–78, 2005.

Allsopp, M.T., et al.: *Ehrlichia ruminantium* variants which do not cause heartwater found in South Africa. Vet. Microbiol., 120:158–166, 2007.

Ammann, P., et al.: Troponin as a risk factor for mortality in critically ill patients without acute coronary syndromes. J. Am. Coll. Cardiol., 41:2004–2009, 2003.

Anandan, R. and Raja, E.E.: Preliminary trials with praziquantel in *Schistosoma nasale* infection in sheep and goat. Indian Vet. J., 64:108–110, 1987.

Andrew, H.R. and Norval, R.A.I.: The carrier state of sheep, cattle and African buffalo recovered from heartwater. Vet. Parasitol., 34:261–266, 1989.

Aretz, I,: Das Herzskelett von Schaf *(Ovis aries)* und Ziege *(Capra hircus)*. Dissertation, Munich University, 1981.

Bastianello, S.S.: Ionophore toxicity in sheep. J. S. Afr. Vet. Assoc., 59(2):105, 1988.

Beasley, V.: Chapter 45, Organic Compounds that Affect the Heart. In: Veterinary Toxicology, Beasley, V., ed. International Veterinary Information Service, Ithaca NY Document Number A2645.0899. 1999. http://www.ivis.org/advances/Beasley/Cpt14f/chapter_frm.asp?LA=1#Ionophore.

Bell-Sakyi, L., Paxton, E.A., Munderloh, U.G. and Sumption, K.J.: Growth of *Cowdria ruminantium*, the causative agent of heartwater, in a tick cell line. J. Clin. Microbiol., 38:1238–1240, 2000.

Bezuidenhout, J.D., Paterson, C.L. and Barnard, B.J.H.: *In vitro* cultivation of *Cowdria ruminantium*. Onderstepoort J. Vet. Res., 51:113–120, 1985.

Bhalla, N.P. and Nagi, M.S.: Occurrence of larval *Multiceps multiceps* over the heart of a goat. Indian Vet. J., 39:55–56, 1962.

Björk, V.O. and Kaminsky, D.B.: The five-year evaluation of a mechanical heart valve without anticoagulation in goats. J. Thorac. Cardiovasc. Surg. 104:22–5, 1992.

Braun, U., et al.: Enzootic calcinosis in goats caused by golden oat grass (*Trisetum flavescens*). Vet. Rec., 146(6):161–162, 2000.

Camus, E. and Barre, N.: Diagnosis of heartwater in the live animal: Experiences with goats in Guadeloupe. Onderstepoort J. Vet. Res., 54:291–294, 1987.

Camus, E., et al.: Répartition de la Cowdriose (heartwater) aux Antilles. In: Les Maladies de la Chèvre, Les Colloques de l'INRA, No. 28. P. Yvore and G. Perrin, eds. Paris. Institut National de la Recherche Agronomique. pp. 683–688, 1984.

Casteel, S.W. and Cook, W.O.: Japanese yew poisoning in ruminants. Mod. Vet. Pract., 66:875–877, 1985.

Chambers, P.G.: Carcass condemnations of communal goats at meat inspection in Zimbabwe. Zimbabwe Vet. J. 21(1):44–45, 1990.

Chattopadhyay, S.K. and Sharma, R.M.: Macro- and microscopic studies on the lesions encountered in the pericardium and the heart of sheep and goats. Indian J. Anim. Sci., 42:705–710, 1972.

Chhabra, R.C. and Singh, K.S.: Development and pathology of *Spirocerca lupi* in experimentally infected kids and lambs. Indian J. Anim. Sci., 42:232–238, 1972.

Chiu, J.K. and Lu, S.C.: Studies on host-parasite relationships of Ilan strain of *Schistosoma japonicum* in animals. 2. Worm recovery rate. Int. J. Zoonoses, 1:75–81, 1974.

Chowdhury, N. and Chakraborty, R.L.: On concurrent and early aortic onchocerciasis and spirocerciasis in domestic goats *(Capra hircus)*. Z. Parasitenkunde, 42:207–212, 1973.

Craig, D.R., Roth, L. and Smith, M.C.: Lymphosarcoma in goats. Comp. Cont. Educ. Pract. Vet., 8:S190–S197, 1986.

Dadich, G.N.: Ectopia cordis in a goat. Indian Vet. J., 77:898, 2000.

Dalvi, R.R. and Sawant, S.G.: Studies of monensin toxicity in goats. J. Vet. Med. A, 37:352–355, 1990.

Du Plessis, J.L., Van Gas, L., Olivier, J.A. and Bezuidenhout, J.D.: The heterogenicity of *Cowdria ruminantium* stocks: cross-immunity and serology in sheep and pathogenicity to mice. Onderstepoort J. Vet. Res., 56:195–201, 1989.

East, N.E., et al.: Milkborne outbreak of *Mycoplasma mycoides* subspecies *mycoides* infection in a commercial goat dairy. J. Am. Vet. Med. Assoc., 182:1338–1341, 1983.

Erasmus, J.A.: Heartwater: the immunisation of Angora goats. J. S. Afr. Vet. Assoc., 47(2):143, 1976.

Foex, P. and Prys-Roberts, C.: Pulmonary haemodynamics and myocardial effects of althesin (CT 1341) in the goat. Postgrad. Med. J., June Suppl:24–31, 1972.

Fourie, N., Erasmus, G.L., Schultz, R.A. and Prozesky, L.: Isolation of the toxin responsible for gousiekte, a plant-induced cardiomyopathy of ruminants in southern Africa. Onderstepoort J. Vet. Res. 62(2):77–87, 1995.

Fowler, M.E.: Cardiotoxic plants. In: Current Veterinary Therapy, Food Animal Practice, 2nd Ed. J.L. Howard, ed. Philadelphia, W.B. Saunders Co., 1986.

Gardner S.Y., et al.: Echocardiographic diagnosis of an anomaly of the tricuspid valve in a male pygmy goat. J. Am. Vet. Med. Assoc., 200(4):521–523, 1992.

Gay, C.C. and Richards, W.P.C.: Cor pulmonale and atrial fibrillation in goats as a sequel to pneumonia. Aust. Vet. J., 60:274–275, 1983.

Geisel, O.: Zur Pathologie der Ziegenaorta. Vet. Pathol. 10:202–218, 1973.

Grant, R., et al.: Cardiomyopathies caused by januariebos *(Gnidia polycephala)* and avocado *(Persea americana)* leaves. J. S. Afr. Vet. Assoc., 59(2):101, 1988.

Gray, P.R. and McDonell, W.N.: Anesthesia in goats and sheep. Part I. Local anesthesia. Comp. Cont. Educ. Pract. Vet., 8:S33–S38, 1986.

Gruss, B.: Problems encountered in the control of heartwater in Angora goats. Onderstepoort J. Vet. Res., 54:513–515, 1987.

Gueye, A., Mbengue, M.B. and Diouf, A.: Situation épizootiologique actuelle de la cowdriose des petits ruminants dans les Niayes du Senegal. Rev. Élev. Méd. vét. Pays tropic., 37:268–271, 1984.

Gufler, H., Bagó, Z., Speckbacher, G. and Baumgartner, W.: Calcinosis in goats. Dtsch. Tierärztl. Wschr., 106(10):419–424, 1999.

Guldner, N.W., Klapproth, P.. Groβherr, M. and Sievers, H. H.: Development of muscular blood pumps performed in a one-step operation. Artificial Organs. 26(3):238–40, 2002.

Gupta, S. and Agrawal, M.C.: Excretion of eggs and miracidia of schistosomes in experimentally infected goats. J. Parasitic Dis., 29(1):23–28, 2005.

Hamlin, R.L. and Scher, A.M.: Ventricular activation process and genesis of QRS complex in the goat. Am. J. Physiol. 200:223–228, 1961.

Hein, W.R. and Cargill, C.F.: An abattoir survey of diseases of feral goats. Aust. Vet. J., 57:498–503, 1981.

Hoversland, A.S., Parer, J.T. and Metcalfe, J.: The African dwarf goat as a laboratory animal in the study of cardiovascular physiology. Fed. Proc., 24:705, 1965.

Hurter, L.R. and Potgieter, L.N.D.: Schistosomiasis in small stock in the Potgietersrus veterinary area. J. S. Afr. Vet. Med. Assoc., 38:444–446, 1967.

Hurter, L.R., et al.: Ingestion of the plant *Fadogia monticola* as an additional cause of gousiekte in ruminants. Onderstepoort J. Vet. Res., 39:71–82, 1972.

ICTTD: End of the Caribbean *Amblyomma* programme. In: Newsletter on ticks and tick-borne diseases of livestock in the tropics, Integrated Consortium on Ticks and Tick-borne Diseases, no. 30:4–6, 2006.

Ilemobade, A.A.: Heartwater in Nigeria. I. The susceptibility of different local breeds and species of domestic animals to heartwater. Trop. Anim. Health Prod., 29:177–180, 1977.

Ilemobade, A.A. and Blotkamp, C.: Clinico-pathological study of heartwater in goats. Tropenmed. Parasitology, 29:71–76, 1978.

Islam, K.S.: Schistosomiasis in domestic ruminants in Bangladesh. Trop. Anim. Health Prod., 7(4):244, 1975.

Ivankovich, A.D., et al.: Cardiovascular effects of centrally administered ketamine in goats. Anesth. Analg., 53:924–933, 1974.

Jha, S.K., Lumb, W.V. and Johnston, R.F.: Some physiologic data on goats. Am. J. Vet. Res., 22:912–914, 1961.

Jongejan, F., et al.: Antigenic differences between stocks of *Cowdria ruminantium*. Res. Vet. Sci., 44:186–189, 1988.

Kakono, O., Hove, T., Geysen, D. and Mahan, S.: Detection of antibodies to the *Ehrlichia ruminantium* MAP1-B antigen in goat sera from three communal land areas of Zimbabwe by an indirect enzyme-linked immunosorbent assay. Onderstepoort J. Vet. Res., 70:243–249, 2003.

Kassuku, A.A.: Caprine schistosomiasis: infection routes and clinical pathology. Proc. 1st Tanz. Vet. Assoc. Sci. Conf., 1:115–125, 1983.

Kassuku, A., et al.: Epidemiological studies on *Schistosoma bovis* in Iringa region, Tanzania. Acta Trop., 43:153–163, 1986.

Katz, J.B., et al.: Development and evaluation of a recombinant antigen, monoclonal antibody-based competitive ELISA for heartwater serodiagnosis. J. Vet. Diagn. Invest., 9:130–135, 1997.

Kaul, P.L. and Prasad, M.C.: Spontaneous aortic lesions in Indian goats. Indian Vet. J., 66:395–398, 1989.

Kitching, R.P. and Hughes G.J.: Clinical variation in foot and mouth disease: sheep and goats. Rev. Sci. Tech. Off. Int. Epiz., 21(3):505–512, 2002.

Kittleson, M.D.: Cardiovascular diseases. In: Handbook of Small Animal Therapeutics. L.E. Davis, ed. New York, Churchill Livingstone, 1985.

Kocan, K.M. and Bezuidenhout, J.D.: Morphology and development of *Cowdria ruminantium* in *Amblyomma* ticks. Onderstepoort J. Vet. Res., 54:177–182, 1987.

Krishna, L., Kulshrestha, S.B. and Paliwal, O.P.: Vegetative endocarditis in sheep and goat. Indian J. Anim. Health, 15:113–115, 1976.

Lee, S.W., et al.: Comparative study of ultrasonography and arteriography of the carotid artery of xylazine-sedated and halothane-anesthetized goats. Am. J. Vet. Res., 51:109–113, 1990.

Li, Z.D.: Studies on the epidemiology of schistosomiasis and life cycle of *Schistosoma*. Chin. J. Vet. Med., 13:13–15, 1987.

Loftis, D.A., et al.: Infection of a goat with a tick-transmitted *Ehrlichia* from Georgia, U.S.A., that is closely related to *Ehrlichia ruminantium*. J. Vector Ecol., 31:213–223, 2006.

Logan, L.L., Whyard, T.C., Quintero, J.C. and Mebus, C.A.: The development of *Cowdria ruminantium* in neutrophils. Onderstepoort J. Vet. Res., 54:197–204, 1987.

Lyons, D.M. and Price, E.O.: Relationships between heart rates and behavior of goats in encounters with people. App. Anim. Behav. Sci., 18:363–369, 1987.

Mahan, S.M.: Diagnosis and control of heartwater, *Ehrlichia ruminantium* infection: an update. CAB Reviews: Perspectives in Agriculture, Veterinary Science, Nutrition and Natural Resources, 1:055, 2006.

Majeed, S. and Goudswaard, J.: Aortic lesions in goats infected with *Mycobacterium johnei*. J. Comp. Pathol., 81:571–574, 1971.

Martinez D., et al.: Nested PCR for detection and genotyping of *Ehrlichia ruminantium*. Ann. N.Y. Acad. Sci., 1026:106–113, 2004.

Masiga, W.N. and Rurangirwa, F.R.: An outbreak of contagious caprine pleuropneumonia-like disease in Kenya. Bull. Anim. Health Prod. Afr., 27:287–288, 1979.

Massoud, J.: Parasitological and pathological observations on *Schistosoma bovis* Sonsino, 1876, in calves, sheep, and goats in Iran. J. Helminthol., 47:155–164, 1973.

Matheron, G., Barre, N., Camus, E. and Gogue, J.: Genetic resistance of Guadeloupe native goats to heartwater. Onderstepoort J. Vet. Res., 54:337–340, 1987.

Medeiros, L.F.D., Vieira, D.H., Oliveira, C.A. de, and Scherer, P.O.: Cardiac and respiratory frequency in goats from different age and racial groups. Rev. Bra. Med. Vet., 23(5):199–202, 2001.

Mohammadpour, A.A. and Arabi, M.: Morphological study of the heart and os cordis in the sheep and goat. Indian Vet. J., 85:284–287, 2007.

Narasimha Rao, A.V., Suryanarayana Murty, T. and Bucchiah, D.: Ectopia cordis, micromelia and umbilical hernia in a kid. Indian Vet. J., 57:953–954, 1980.

Neuberger, H.R., et al.: Chronic atrial dilation, electrical remodeling, and atrial fibrillation in the goat. J. Am. Col. Cardiol., 47(3):644–53, 2006.

Neumann, F., Nobel, T.A. and Klopfer, U.: Calcinosis in goats. J. Comp. Pathol., 83(3):343–350, 1973.

Newsholme, S.J. and Coetzer, J.A.W.: Myocardial pathology of domestic ruminants in southern Africa. J. S. Afr. Vet. Assoc., 55:89–96, 1984.

Nwude, N., Parsons, L.E. and Adaudi, A.O.: Acute toxicity of the leaves and extracts of *Dichapetalum barteri* in mice, rabbits, and goats. Toxicology, 7:23–29, 1977.

O'Brien, P.J., Dameron, G.W., Beck, M.L. and Brandt, M.: Differential reactivity of cardiac and skeletal muscle from various species in two generations of cardiac troponin-T immunoassays. Res. Vet. Sci., 65(2):135–137, 1998.

Ogburn, P.N., Hamlin, R.L. and Smith, C.R.: Electrocardiographic and vectorcardiographic response to right ventricular hypertrophy in the goat. J. Electrocardiol., 10:215–220, 1977.

Olsson, K., et al.: A serial study of heart function during pregnancy, lactation and the dry period in dairy goats using echocardiography. Exp. Physiol., 86(1):93–99, 2001.

Oyama, M.A. and Sisson, D.D.: Cardiac troponin-I concentration in dogs with cardiac disease. J. Vet. Intern. Med. 18(6):831–839, 2004.

Pandey, G.S., Sharma, R.N. and Iyer, P.K.R.: Serum protein changes in ovine and caprine hepatic schistosomiasis due to *Schistosoma indicum*. Indian J. Vet. Pathol., 1:64–68, 1976.

Parry, B.W., Wrigley, R.H. and Reuter, R.E.: Ventricular septal defects in three familially-related female Saanen goats. Aust. Vet. J., 59:72–76, 1982.

Patnaik, R.K.: Epidemic of goat dermatitis in India. Trop. Anim. Health Prod., 18:137–138, 1986.

Prasad, M.C., Rajya, B.S. and Mohanty, G.C.: Caprine arterial diseases. I. Spontaneous aortic lesions. Exp. Mol. Biol., 17:14–28, 1972.

Pretorius, P.J. and Terblanche, M.: A preliminary study on the symptomatology and cardiodynamics of gousiekte in sheep and goats. J. S. Afr. Vet. Assoc., 38:29–53, 1967.

Prozesky, L. and Du Plessis, J.L.: Heartwater in Angora goats. II. A pathological study of artificially infected, treated and untreated goats. Onderstepoort J. Vet. Res., 52:13–19, 1985.

Prozesky, L., Bastianello, S.S., Fourie, N. and Schultz, R.A.: A study of the pathology and pathogenesis of the myocardial lesions in gousiekte, a plant-induced cardiotoxicosis of ruminants. Onderstepoort J. Vet. Res., 72(3):219–230, 2005.

Reddi, M.V. and Surendran, N.S.: Incidence of traumatic pericarditis in a goat. Indian Vet. J., 65:1131, 1988.

Rodriguez, J.L., et al.: High mortality in goats associated with the isolation of a strain of *Mycoplasma mycoides* subsp. *mycoides* (large colony type). J. Vet. Med. Ser. B, 42(10):587–593, 1995.

Rollinson, D., Southgate, V.R., Vercruysse, J. and Moore, P.J.: Observations on natural and experimental interactions between *Schistosoma bovis* and *S. curassoni* from West Africa. Acta Trop. 47(2):101–114, 1990.

Rostkowski, C.M., Stirtzinger, T. and Baird, J.D.: Congestive heart failure associated with thymoma in two Nubian goats. Can. Vet. J., 26:267–269, 1985.

Sahu, S.P.: Fluorescent antibody technique to detect *Cowdria ruminantium* in *in vitro*-cultured macrophages and buffy coats from cattle, sheep, and goats. Am. J. Vet. Res., 47:1253–1257, 1986.

Sani, Y., Atwell, R.B. and Seawright, A.A.: The cardiotoxicity of avocado leaves. Australian Vet. J., 68(4):150–51, 1991.

Savey, M.: La tuberculose de la chèvre: suspicion clinique et diagnostic différential. L Point Vét., 16(81):60, 1984.

Scarratt, W.K., Lombard, C.W. and Buergelt, C.D.: Ventricular septal defects in two goats. Cornell Vet., 74:136–145, 1984.

Schultz, R.A. and Pretorius, P.J.: An electrocardiographic study of normal goats and cattle using a modified technique. Onderstepoort J. Vet. Res., 39:209–224, 1972.

Schultz, R.A., et al.: Pavetamine: an inhibitor of protein synthesis in the heart. In: Poisonous plants and related toxins. Wallingford, UK, CABI Publishing, pp. 408–411, 2004.

Schumann, N. von, Schmid, K., Boch, J. and Weiland, G.: Antikorpernachweis (IFAT, ELISA) bei experimentell mit *Schistosoma japonicum* infizierten Ziegen. Berl. Münch. Tierärzt. Wochenschr., 97:61–65, 1984.

Seawright, A.A.: Goats and poisonous plants. In: Proceedings, Refresher Course for Veterinarians, Post-Graduate Committee in Veterinary Science, University of Sydney, 73:544–547, 1984.

Seydi, M. and Gueye, K.: Condemnation of meat in the abattoirs of the Cap-Vert district from 1971 to 1980: sanitary aspects and economic and social implications. Med. Afrique Noire, 29:803–816, 1982.

Sharma, D.N. and Dwivedi, J.N.: Pulmonary schistosomiasis in sheep and goats due to *Schistosoma indicum* in India. J. Comp. Pathol., 86:449–454, 1976.

Sharma, K.B. and Ranka, A.K.: Foreign body syndrome in goats—a report of five cases. Indian Vet. J., 55:413–414, 1978.

Singh Nara, R.R. and Nayak, B.C.: Studies on pathology of liver in sheep and goats. J. Remount Vet. Corps, 11:7–15, 1972.

Singh, B., Singh, H., Kumar, A. and Sharma, V.K.: Normal radiographic anatomy of caprine chest. Indian Vet. J., 60:474–479, 1983.

Smallwood, J.E. and Healey, W.V.: Computed tomography of the thorax of the adult Nubian goat. Vet. Radiol., 23:135–143, 1982.

Snyder, S.D. and Loker, E.S.: Evolutionary relationships among the Schistosomatidae (Platyhelminthes: Digenea) and an Asian origin for *Schistosoma*. J. Parasitol., 86(2):283–288, 2000.

Soldan, A.W., van Inzen, C. and Edelsten, R.M.: *Albizia versicolor* poisoning of sheep and goats in Malawi. J. S. Afr. Vet. Assoc., 67(4):217–221, 1996.

Soulsby, E.J.L.: Helminths, Arthropods, and Protozoa of Domestic Animals. 7th Ed. Philadelphia, Lea and Febiger, 1982.

Suliman, H.B. and Shommein, A.M.: Toxic effect of the roasted and unroasted beans of *Cassia occidentalis* in goats. Vet. Hum. Toxicol., 28:6–11, 1986.

Synge, B.A.: Brain biopsy for the diagnosis of heartwater. Trop. Anim. Health Prod., 10:45–48, 1978.

Szabuniewicz, M. and Clark, D.R.: Analysis of the electrocardiograms of 100 normal goats. Am. J. Vet. Res., 28:511–516, 1967.

Tessier, D., et al.: Induction of chronic cardiac insufficiency by arteriovenous fistula and doxorubicin administration. J. Cardiac Surg. 18(4):307–11, 2003.

Tustin, R.C., Thornton, D.J. and Kleu, C.B.: An outbreak of *Cotyledon orbiculata* L. poisoning in a flock of Angora goat rams. J. S. Afr. Vet. Assoc., 55:181–184, 1984.

Uilenberg, G.: Heartwater (*Cowdria ruminantium* infection): current status. Adv. Vet. Sci. Comp. Med., 27:427–480, 1983.

Uilenberg, G. et al.: Heartwater in the Caribbean. Prev. Vet. Med., 2:255–267, 1984.

Upadhyay, R.C. and Sud, S.C.: Electrocardiogram of the goat. Indian J. Exp. Biol., 15:359–362, 1977.

Upadhye S.V. and Dhoot V.M.: A case of ectopia cordis in a goat. Indian Vet. J., 78:1028–1029, 2001.

Van de Pypekamp, H.E. and Prozesky, L.: Heartwater. An overview of the clinical signs, susceptibility and differential diagnoses of the disease in domestic ruminants. Onderstepoort J. Vet. Res., 54:263–266, 1987.

van der Lugt, J.J., Fourie, N. and Schultz, R.A.: *Galenia africana* L. (Aizoaceae) poisoning in sheep. J. S. Afr. Vet. Assoc., 59(2):100, 1988.

van der Lugt J.J., et al.: *Galenia africana* L. Poisoning in sheep and goats: hepatic and cardiac changes. Onderstepoort J. Vet. Res., 59(4):323–333, 1992.

Van der Merwe, L.: The infection and treatment method of vaccination against heartwater. Onderstepoort J. Vet. Res., 54:489–491, 1987.

Van Vliet, A.H., et al.: Use of a specific immunogenic region on the *Cowdria ruminantium* MAP1 protein in a serological assay. J. Clin. Microbiol., 33:2405–2410, 1995.

Van Winkelhoff, A.J. and Uilenberg, G.: Heartwater: cross-immunity studies with strains of *Cowdria ruminantium* isolated in West and South Africa. Trop. Anim. Health Prod., 13:160–164, 1981.

Verycruysse, J., Southgate, V.R. and Rollinson, D.: *Schistosoma curassoni* Brumpt, 1931 in sheep and goats in Senegal. J. Nat. Hist., 18:969–976, 1984.

Vesal, N. and Karimi, A.: Evaluation of central venous pressure in ruminants. Veterinarski Arhiv, 76(1):85–92, 2006.

Vesal, N., Shah-Shahan, S.M. and Rezakhani, A.: The determination of the normal heart rate and the effects of environmental stressors by telemetry in native goats. Iranian J. Vet. Res., 1(1):26–38, 2000.

Vohra, S., Agrawal, M.C. and Malik, Y.P.S.: Dot-ELISA for diagnosis of caprine schistosomosis. Indian J. Anim. Sci., 76(12):988–991, 2006.

Vohra, S. and Agrawal, M.C.: Prevalence of caprine schistosomosis as determined by different coprological methods. Indian Vet. J., 83(11):1160–1163, 2006a.

Waghela S.D., et al.: A cloned DNA probe identifies *Cowdria ruminantium* in *Amblyomma variegatum* ticks. J. Clin. Microbiol., 29:2571–2577, 1991.

Waibl, H.: Left cranial vena cava without corresponding vessel on the right in a domestic goat. Berl. Munch. Tierarztl. Wschr., 86:171–174, 1973.

Waldman, K.H. and Woicke, J.: Traumatic peri- and endocarditis in a male dwarf goat, a case report. Kleintierpraxis, 29:389–390, 1984.

Webster, B.L., Southgate, V.R. and Littlewood, T.J.: A revision of the interrelationships of *Schistosoma* including the recently described *Schistosoma guineensis*. Int. J. Parasitol., 36:947–955, 2006.

Wesonga, F.D., et al.: Seroprevalence of *Ehrlichia ruminantium* (heartwater) in small ruminants in a pastoral production system in Narok district, Kenya. Bull. Anim. Health Prod. Afr., 54:23–33, 2006.

Wilcke, J.R.: Cardiac dysrhythmias. In: Handbook of Small Animal Therapeutics. L.E. Davis, ed. New York, Churchill Livingstone, 1985.

Williamson, M.M., et al.: Pleuropneumonia and pericarditis in a goat with isolation of *Mycoplasma mycoides* subsp. *mycoides* large colony. Aust. Vet. J., 85(4):153–155, 2007.

Yamaga, Y. and Too, K.: Diagnostic ultrasound imaging in domestic animals: two-dimensional and m-mode echocardiography. Jpn. J. Vet. Sci., 46:493–503, 1984.

9

Respiratory System

ANATOMY

The structure of the lungs of the goat is illustrated in Figure 9.1. The lung is divided into bilateral cranial lobes (each with a cranial and a caudal part), a middle (cardiac) lobe on the right side, an accessory lobe of the right lung that extends ventrally on the midline, and bilateral caudal (diaphragmatic) lobes (Constantinescu 2001). The right cranial lobe is supplied by a separate tracheal bronchus which originates before the bifurcation of the trachea. This lobe wraps around anterior to the heart and actually reaches the left side of the thorax. Subpleural lymph nodes 1 to 30 mm in diameter have been reported in the lungs of Angora and feral goats in New Zealand (Valero et al. 1993).

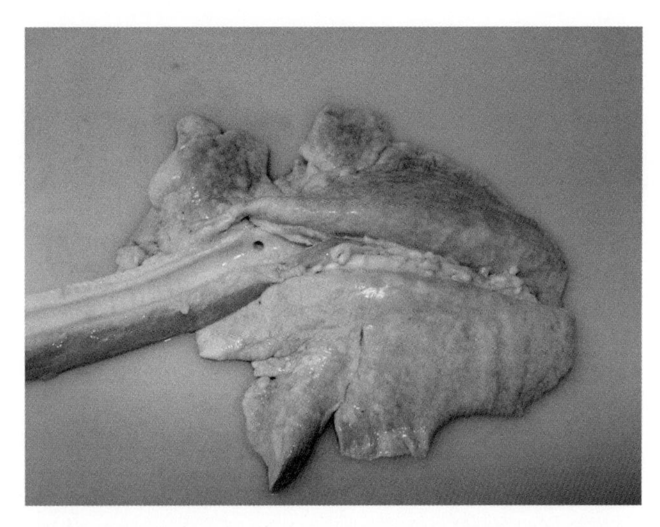

Figure 9.1. Normal goat lung with trachea opened to demonstrate the tracheal bronchus supplying the right cranial lobe. (Courtesy of Dr. M.C. Smith.)

CLINICAL EXAMINATION OF THE RESPIRATORY TRACT

Either a well-taken case history or basic physical exam may suggest the presence of respiratory disease. Signs noted might include increased respiratory rate, labored breathing, rapid tiring (especially with exercise), cyanosis, abnormal sounds associated with breathing, nasal discharge, coughing, or fever. Table 9.1 lists some of these signs and possible etiologies.

If a respiratory disease is suspected, additional herd history is helpful in directing the diagnostic efforts. The owner should always be questioned concerning recent purchase or boarding of animals or attendance at shows, relative to possible introduction of infectious diseases. Do the goats get out of the barn, at least during part of the year? If not, lungworms and nasal bots are less probable. Is the herd known to be infected with or believed to be free of caprine arthritis encephalitis (CAE) virus, caseous lymphadenitis, and mycoplasma mastitis? Are housing and ventilation acceptable? The veterinarian should not accept the owner's answer to this last question without personally inspecting the premises. Is the region selenium-deficient, and is the ration supplemented with vitamin E and selenium? Has the animal been overdosed with injectable selenium, so that it is dyspneic because of heart failure?

It is often impossible to obtain an exact and unquestionable etiologic diagnosis, at least in the living goat. This frustrates recent graduates whose education has suggested that the clever clinician always gets the right answer. On the other hand, more "experienced" practitioners may prescribe their favorite antibiotic for pneumonia rather than determine the cause of the clinical signs observed.

Table 9.1. Some signs suggestive of respiratory disease and possible causes.

Signs	*Possible Causes*
Dyspnea or Tachypnea	Anemia
	Pregnancy toxemia, ketosis
	Rumen acidosis
	Bloat
	Heatstroke
	Urolithiasis
	Nasal obstruction (tumor or foreign body)
	Progressive interstitial retroviral pneumonia (CAEV)
	Peste des petits ruminants
	Contagious caprine pleuropneumonia
	Pasteurellosis
	Septicemia
	Internal caseous lymphadenitis
	Tuberculosis
	Lungworms *(Dictyocaulus)*
	Nutritional muscular dystrophy
	Inhalation pneumonia
	Congenital heart malformation
	Cyanide poisoning
	Nitrate poisoning
	Other assorted toxicities
Cough	Tight collar
	Tracheal stenosis
	Dusty or moldy hay
	Ammonia and other fumes
	Dysphagia (nutritional muscular dystrophy, neurologic disease)
	Contagious caprine pleuropneumonia
	Chronic progressive pneumonia (CAEV)
	Parainfluenza virus (PI3)
	Abscessed retropharyngeal lymph node
	Pasteurellosis
	Cryptococcosis
	Lungworms (*Dictyocaulus*)
	Heart failure
Nasal discharge	Nose bots *(Oestrus ovis)*
	Powdery feeds
	Irritant fumes (ammonia, smoke)
	Cleft palate
	Regurgitation due to nutritional muscular dystrophy
	Atrophic rhinitis (toxigenic stains of *P. multocida*)
	Nasal adenoma
	Paste des petits ruminants, rinderpest
	Parainfluenza virus (PI3)
	Respiratory syncytial virus
	Caprine herpesvirus
	Pulmonary adenomatosis (jaagsiekte)
	Mycoplasma infections
	Pasteurellosis
	Melioidosis
	Cryptococcosis

Not every goat that breathes rapidly or "harshly" has respiratory disease. A complete physical examination always helps avoid embarrassing misdiagnoses. If the mucous membranes are white, think first of anemia, not pneumonia. Do not waste the owner's money on tracheal washes and expensive antibiotics if the kid has an obvious heart murmur, at least not without explaining the seriousness of the underlying heart disease.

Common pulmonary function tests have been adapted to the goat and normal values published (Bakima et al. 1988, 1990). This information should be useful to researchers evaluating respiratory disorders in goats or using goats as models in the study of respiratory physiology.

Respiratory Rate

The normal respiratory rate at rest is approximately ten to thirty breaths per minute (kids twenty to forty per minute). Few goats are "at rest" in the presence of an odoriferous stranger or after a long ride to the clinic in the back of a compact car. In addition, many normal goats pant; a respiratory rate of 270 per minute has been reported for goats held at 104°F (40°C). A goat with a long winter coat will certainly breathe rapidly if brought into a warm and humid room. A curious goat, continually sniffing the examiner, makes just the counting of the respiratory rate frustrating or even meaningless. The movements of the chest and abdominal wall should be observed from a distance, before the patient is disturbed. This is also the best time to note normal costo-abdominal respiration, abdominal pumping, or very shallow and painful chest movements (as with pleuritis).

Many seriously ill goats have an increased respiratory rate because of fever, metabolic disturbances, or pain. Pregnancy toxemia, lactational ketosis, rumen acidosis, or diarrhea can all lead to metabolic acidosis. As part of the respiratory compensation mechanism, goats breathe faster to release carbon dioxide and thereby remove H^+ (along with HCO_3^-) ions from the blood. Goats with listeriosis or other brain stem disease, on the other hand, may have an altered respiratory rate because of acidosis from loss of saliva or lesions in the respiratory centers of the brain. Metabolic alkalosis, which may be accompanied by very slow respiration, is less common in goats than in cattle, because most conditions associated with abomasal stasis (e.g., impaction, displacement, torsion, ulceration) are relatively rare.

Dyspnea

It is helpful to differentiate difficulty in breathing into inspiratory, expiratory, or mixed dyspnea. Strong outward movements of the thorax and longer inspiration are associated with inspiratory dyspnea. Narrowed upper airway passages or bronchopneumonia with reduced respiratory surface in the lungs causes such a pattern. A distended head and neck and dilated nostrils accompany severe inspiratory dyspnea, and audible stenotic sounds may make location of an obstruction possible. With expiratory dyspnea, breathing out is impeded and is accentuated by strong and prolonged expiratory movements of the abdomen. This is less common in goats than in cattle because the caprine lung is not predisposed to interstitial emphysema. Cheek blowing or open mouth breathing with an extended tongue might accompany expiratory dyspnea. Logically, a mixed dyspnea occurs when there is difficulty in both inhaling and exhaling.

Whenever the dyspnea is accompanied by cyanosis, the examiner should proceed cautiously to limit additional stress to the goat. If an upper airway obstruction is suspected, an emergency tracheostomy may become necessary. The heart must also be examined closely, because the cause of dyspnea may reside in the circulatory rather than respiratory system.

Externally Audible Sounds

Sneezing, a brief and powerful expulsion of air through the nose, occurs when the nasal mucosa is irritated by accumulations of secretions, exudates, or foreign matter. Stenotic sounds are caused by constriction in the upper respiratory tract. Snuffling sounds of nasal origin are usually loudest on inspiration. Alternate occlusion of one nostril and then the other helps to determine if the stenosis is unilateral or bilateral. That is, with a unilateral lesion, blocking the nostril on the affected side should decrease the sound while blocking the other nostril should increase the sound by forcing more air through the stenotic nasal passage. Sounds of pharyngeal origin are loudest on expiration, whereas laryngeal stenosis sounds are usually more pronounced on inspiration. Manual compression of the pharynx increases the loudness of pharyngeal sounds while decreasing laryngeal stridor. Sounds originating from a stenotic larynx are accentuated by additional compression of the larynx. If the stenosis is in the trachea, occlusion of one nostril or compression of pharynx or larynx decreases the air flow and the loudness of the stridor. Auscultation along the accessible portion of the trachea may permit localization of the lesion. The character of any stenotic sound (i.e., whistling, hissing, sawing) may be affected by the presence or absence of exudate in the airways.

Coughing

A cough may simply indicate irritation from fumes or dusty feed or compression of the trachea during attempts to reach something theoretically out of reach, such as the neighbor's feed. If irritation lies in the upper respiratory tract, the cough is typically dry and powerful. If the goat has a deep-seated bronchopneumonia, the cough may be moist and feeble. Coughing can be elicited by first briefly preventing respiration. This is done by holding a moist towel or similar object over the nostrils until the goat becomes distressed. When the nose is released, the number and nature of coughs are noted and the lungs are auscultated for abnormal respiratory sounds often accentuated by this procedure.

Nasal Discharge

Possible causes of a nasal discharge are listed in Table 9.1 or discussed under the topic of rhinitis below. Figure 9.2 shows a goat with a mucopurulent nasal discharge during a herd outbreak of infectious keratoconjunctivitis, possibly due to *Mycoplasma conjunctivae* (see Chapter 6). A purulent secretion is more significant than a serous discharge. A clear scanty bilateral nasal discharge is not unusual in adult goats in apparent good health. Clinically normal goats also harbor a wide variety of aerobic bacteria in their nasal passages, including *Pasteurella multocida*, *Mannheimia haemolytica*, and *Streptococcus* spp. (Ngatia et al. 1985).

Closer Examination of the Upper Respiratory Tract

It is useful to smell the breath; rotten odors may suggest the presence of infection or tumor in a sinus or along the airways. Compare with the smell of the open mouth. Some clinicians have the ability to detect ketone bodies on the breath; those who do not should keep a container handy to catch urine because the goat typically urinates on arising or after the stress or insult of close physical examination. If asymmetry in

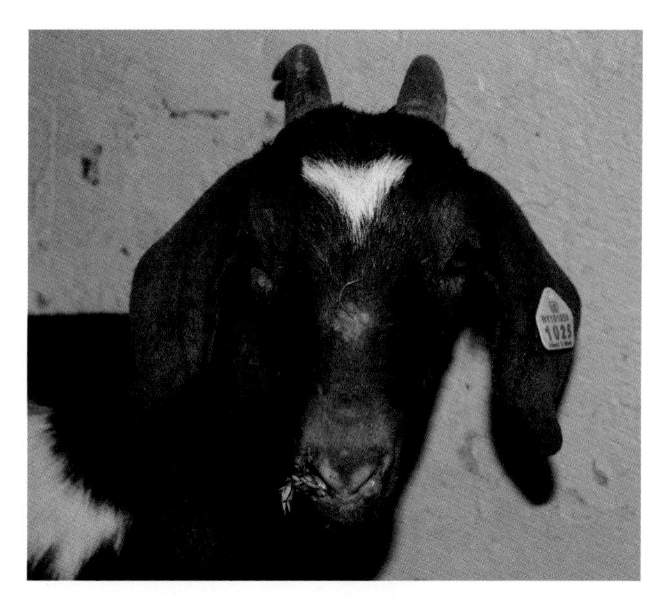

Figure 9.2. Feed particles adhering to a mucopurulent nasal discharge. (Courtesy of Dr. M.C. Smith.)

airflow from the two nostrils is detected while smelling the breath or by holding the palm of the hand before each nostril, a tumor or foreign body may be present.

The frontal and paranasal sinuses should be externally palpated and percussed. If the goat is hornless, the time and method of dehorning should be ascertained. If the goat does not eat hay and chew its cud freely, a tooth root abscess rather than a problem in the respiratory tract may be the source of a bad odor. Radiography may be helpful for diagnosing infections or tumors of the sinuses.

When lesions in the pharynx or larynx are suspected, direct visualization is desirable. Light sedation with xylazine permits a good view of the back of the throat and the teeth. Manual exploration without sedation is hazardous at best. Naturally, in regions where rabies occurs, great care should be taken in all aspects of the physical examination.

Do not neglect to palpate very carefully for the retropharyngeal lymph nodes. Their enlargement may occur with nonspecific local infections, but is more common with caseous lymphadenitis. A progressive dyspnea occurs because of external compression of airway (Jones and Schumacher 1990). Capripox infection can cause a similar obstructive lymph node enlargement in countries where this disease exists (Kitching 2004). Great care should be taken to avoid extending the neck during restraint for physical examination or diagnostic procedures; the increased compromise of the airway may be rapidly fatal.

Endoscopic examination of the nasal passages, pharynx, larynx, and trachea has been performed in awake untranquilized adult goats using a 4-mm flexible endoscope and illustrations of findings in normal animals published (Stierschneider et al. 2007). The normal goat's trachea may be drop shaped, round, or U-shaped in cross section.

The trachea of a goat may be partially obstructed by a mass protruding into the lumen or by tracheal collapse. Coughing, stridor, and exercise intolerance are to be expected. Refrain from diagnosing a hypoplastic trachea without close comparison with healthy goats of the same age and size. That the caprine trachea is relatively small in diameter is well substantiated by the size of endotracheal tube typically required (see Chapter 17). Radiographic evaluation should be helpful in confirming stenotic tracheal lesions or compression from enlarged lymph nodes (Jones and Schumacher 1990). If localization of the problem is possible, excision of a mass or even placement of prosthetic tracheal rings may be attempted (Jackson et al. 1986).

In confined groups of animals, a head tilt, sometimes accompanied by facial nerve paralysis, suggests the possibility of bacterial pneumonia. This is because organisms responsible for pneumonia can also ascend the eustachian tube and cause an otitis media/interna.

Auscultation of the Lungs

Much disagreement exists in the literature regarding terminology for normal and abnormal lung sounds. In addition, harsh inspiratory sounds may be heard over the entire lung field of a goat, especially a thin one, whether the lungs are normal or extensively altered by disease processes. The duration of expiration is also audible in goats, as in sheep. Special efforts should be made to auscultate well forward under the elbow, where cranioventral pneumonias are localized.

Normal breath sounds are loudest on inspiration and are loudest over the trachea and base of the lungs. They are bronchial sounds; the velocity of airflow in alveoli is too low to generate audible sounds, and thus the terms "bronchovesicular" and "alveolar sounds" are inappropriate (Curtis et al. 1986). Increased breath sounds are heard in normal animals with increased rate and depth of respiration (i.e., excitement, exercise, high environmental temperature) or in goats with fever, acidosis, or pulmonary congestion.

"Increased bronchial sounds" are heard on both inspiration and expiration. They occur in disease processes when the bronchial lumen remains open but the surrounding lung tissue transmits sound better because of being consolidated. This is true of most pneumonias of goats. There is no sharp line of demarcation between increased breath sounds and increased bronchial sounds. Crackles are clicking, popping, or bubbling sounds produced by fluid in the airways or by dry airways suddenly popping open. The term "crackles" can be used in preference to "moist rales" because it does not erroneously imply anything about the amount of fluid in the airways. Wheezes (also called rhonchi or dry rales) are whistling or squeaking sounds typically caused by the passage of air through a narrowed airway. Bronchospasm, abscesses, and tenacious exudate are possible causes of wheezes. Both crackles and wheezes may stop or move to another location, as when coughing dislodges fluid or exudate. Stridors (loud wheezing type sounds loudest over the trachea or larynx) may be referred to the lung fields, but they result from stenosis in the upper respiratory tract and are commonly audible without a stethoscope.

Pleuritic friction rubs, described as "sandpaper-like sounds," occur with severe inflammation of the pleura, assuming that adhesion or effusion does not prevent the rubbing.

The absence of breath sounds may be simply because of obesity, as in some Nubians. Pleural effusion, pneumothorax, diaphragmatic hernia, and space occupying thoracic lesions (thymoma) are other possibilities. Breath sounds may be decreased with shallow breathing from pain, weakness, or central nervous disorders (Curtis et al. 1986).

Percussion of the Lung Fields

In the past, the technique of finger-finger percussion or the use of a pleximeter has been more popular in Europe than in America. Thoracic percussion has been reviewed (Roudebush and Sweeney 1990). Veterinarians who expect to obtain useful diagnostic information from the procedure should routinely percuss many goats to become familiar with the normal sounds and lung boundaries. Percussion is usually done on the right side, although the presence of the spleen on the left makes it possible to identify the upper border between lung and rumen. The caudal lung border normally extends in an arc from the dorsal aspect of the eleventh intercostal space to the point of the elbow. A prescapular percussion field is present, and in thin animals the lungs can be percussed through the ventral portions of the scapula. Lifting a flexed forelimb to the side permits clearer percussion of axillary areas (Marek and Mocsy 1960). The full resonance of normal lung is to be contrasted with the more tympanic sound of gas-filled rumen or intestine, the relatively damped or dull sound of ventral abdominal organs, and the absolute dullness of the liver (on the right). A duller than normal sound over the lung fields can occur when large areas of the lung are consolidated by abscess, tumor, or interstitial pneumonia. The dull area is ventrally located and has a horizontal dorsal border if accumulation of fluid in the thorax is responsible. Processes causing increased intra-abdominal pressure (including late pregnancy) can displace the lung borders in a cranial direction.

Blood Gas Measurement

When laboratory testing is accessible, standard blood gas measurements give an indication of pulmonary function, as well as acid-base status of the animal. Venous blood is routinely collected in heparin, avoiding contamination of the sample with room air. Few studies specific to the goat have been published, and ideally each testing laboratory should determine the reference ranges for the apparatus being used, because some variability is to be expected (Kahrer et al. 2006). Time and temperature of blood storage before testing also influence test results. For instance, there is a slight decrease in concentration of HCO_3^- and a marked increase in pO_2 with storage for twenty-four hours at 4°C (39°F), while pH is stable (Piccione et al. 2007). Blood gases determined by Blood Gas Analyzer on twenty-nine adult goats, one each from twenty-nine farms, are presented in Table 9.2 (Stevens et al. 1994). Respiratory acidosis, with increased pCO_2 and HCO_3^-, is expected with impaired pulmonary function.

Table 9.2. Blood gases of adult goats determined on venous blood.

Parameter	*Mean*	*2.5 percentile*	*97.5 percentile*
pH	7.38	7.30	7.50
pCO_2 (mmHg)	40.6	34.6	48.8
HCO_3^- (mmol/L)	25.0	19.6	29.4
TCO_2 (mmol/L) calculated	26.2	20.7	30.7
pO_2 (mmHg)	48.8		

Transtracheal Aspiration

The small diameter of the trachea makes this a more difficult procedure in goats than in cattle.

Indications

Transtracheal aspiration is useful for obtaining samples for cytology and bacteriologic culture in the diagnosis of an etiologic agent. Microbial sensitivity testing aids the choice of antibiotics to be used in treating a particularly valuable goat or one that has failed to respond to previous rational therapy. The frequency of recovery of pathogens from the trachea of goats when pulmonary disease is absent is unknown. Cultures from nasal swabs are of no diagnostic value relative to bacterial pneumonia.

Technique

The hair is clipped midway over the cervical trachea and a small bleb of local anesthetic is injected beneath the disinfected skin. Sterile gloves should be worn. A 14-gauge needle is used to penetrate the trachea and a 3 French polypropylene catheter or a 3 1/2 French tomcat catheter is passed into the trachea. A 16- or 18-gauge intravenous catheter device may be used instead. The needle portion should be withdrawn after placement of the catheter into the trachea to avoid cutting off part of the catheter. Sterile, buffered saline (15 to 20 ml) is injected into the trachea. At once, as much as possible (often only a few milliliters) is aspirated into the syringe and submitted for microscopic examination and culture. The catheter is then removed. No special aftercare is needed.

Bronchoalveolar Lavage

In a hospital or research setting, better samples for cytology are obtained with the goat sedated (acepromazine at 0.3 mg/kg IV) or under general anesthesia and intubated. A tracheal wash catheter is passed through the endotracheal tube to the bronchial bifurcation. In an adult goat, approximately 50 ml of warm sterile saline is flushed into the lungs and then aspirated at once through the same catheter (Berrag et al. 1997). If available, recovery of fluid would probably be improved by use of a pediatric bronchoscope. The authors report that in normal goats the predominant cell type recovered is alveolar macrophage (80% to 95%) with fewer lymphocytes, eosinophils, neutrophils, and epithelial cells.

Radiography of the Lungs

Radiography can document the presence of cranioventral bronchopneumonia, interstitial pneumonia, pleural effusion (often marked in contagious caprine pleuropneumonia), a penetrating metallic foreign body, thymoma, tracheal compression by enlarged mediastinal lymph nodes, or underlying cardiac disease leading to respiratory signs (Ahuja et al. 1985). The value of pulmonary radiographs often comes from confirmation of advanced and extensive changes in the lung fields. Multiple abscesses or massive areas of interstitial pneumonia suggest a very grave prognosis. Sternal and mediastinal lymph nodes should be examined for evidence of enlargement. Sternal abscesses with penetration into the thorax are accompanied by visibly enlarged sternal nodes and often by osteomyelitis of the sternebrae. Both viral and bacterial pneumonias, if chronic, can result in enlargement of mediastinal nodes.

A large thymoma may displace the lungs caudally. Because many thymomas in goats are incidental findings at necropsy (Hadlow 1978), it is conceivable that an asymptomatic tumor might be identified during radiography of a goat with some other thoracic disease. If the lungs are displaced cranially, consideration should be given to a (very rare) diaphragmatic hernia (Tafti 1998).

The radiographic equipment and techniques used for dogs are also appropriate for goats. The forelimbs need to be pulled well forward to expose the cranioventral lung lobes. Light intravenous tranquilization with xylazine (0.05 mg/kg), combined with clever use of tape and sandbags, provides safe restraint.

Ultrasonography of the Thorax

The physical or chemical restraint needed to obtain diagnostic radiographs of the chest may be dangerous to a severely dyspneic animal. Ultrasound examination can be done in a standing animal, usually at less expense than radiography. Scott and Gessert (1998) have described the procedure for sheep, and their findings should be applicable to goats. A sector scanner transducer rather than a linear array transducer is preferred because of the narrow intercostal space, and examination may not be possible in small goats. Hair is clipped from a 7 cm wide strip of skin caudal to the scapula and elbow bilaterally. Starting in the sixth or seventh intercostal space, the thorax is examined in longitudinal and transverse planes. The front limb is adducted and the clipped skin slid forward several spaces to allow access to the ventral aspect of the chest. Examination beginning from the ninth or tenth intercostal space assesses the dorsal lung field. Liberal wetting of the hair with alcohol can be substituted for clipping and application of an ultrasound gel.

Normally aerated lung does not permit penetration of the ultrasound beam, so a bright linear echo and reverberation artifacts are all that are seen during examination of a normal animal. Ultrasound is useful for demonstrating fluid accumulation in the pleural space, abscesses that reach the pleura, tumors, and consolidation by bacterial or interstitial viral pneumonia (Scott and Gessert 1998).

Lung Biopsy and Aspiration of Fluid from the Thorax

If a fluid line is percussed in the thorax or detected by radiography or ultrasonography, thoracocentesis may be indicated. Clipping of hair and thorough disinfection of the skin are mandatory. A site beneath the fluid level but not directly over the heart should be chosen, and the needle should be kept close to the anterior edge of a rib to avoid nerves and blood vessels.

Percutaneous lung biopsy (fine needle aspiration) is rarely performed but can be used to confirm the presence of an extensive interstitial pneumonia or tumor, as is associated with retroviral infections. The technique has been described in small animal medicine textbooks (Johnson 2005) and in sheep (Braun et al. 2000).

EFFECT OF ENVIRONMENT ON RESPIRATORY DISEASE

The veterinarian should not be content with examining only the goat with respiratory disease. The environment should also be analyzed to determine if it is contributing to the pathogenesis of disease. Table 9.3 gives specifications for environmental conditions as recommended for milking goats in temperate climates (Toussaint 1984).

Table 9.3. Optimal housing for goats in temperate climates.

Temperature	Minimal 43°F (6°C) Optimal 50°F to 64°F (10°C to 18°C) Maximal 81°F (27°C)
Relative humidity	Optimal 60% to 80%
Ventilation	Winter 30 m^3/hour/goat Summer 120 to 150 m^3/hour/goat Maximum air speed 0.5 m/s adults, 0.2 m/s kids Air intake at least twice surface area of air exit
Lighting	Window area equal to 1/20 of ground surface area

Temperature

At environmental temperatures above or below the optimal limits given in Table 9.3, the goat has to expend energy specifically to maintain its normal body temperature. As a consequence, production (milk or growth) is adversely affected. In a hot environment, the goat must decrease its heat production (eat less) while losing more heat through evaporation and radiation from lungs and skin. Under cold conditions, the goat must use more energy from feed or body reserves. It will also have increased levels of circulating glucocorticoids. Age and production level both affect the critical temperatures. For instance, the minimum temperature for kids is higher than for adults (Constantinou 1987). Indigenous breeds in many parts of the world are well adapted to more extreme conditions. Moderating the environment for these animals probably causes a loss of some degree of their genetic hardiness after a few generations.

Ventilation

Ventilation affects the purity of the air that the goats breathe. Heat, moisture, and carbon dioxide from the lungs need to be dissipated. Decomposition of feces and urine produces ammonia, hydrogen sulfide, methane gas, and other malodorous substances. A build-up of these chemicals can lead to irritation of the eyes and respiratory tract. Heaters and motorized equipment operating within the barn add to air pollution. Suspensions of dust from feeds and dirt carry with them numerous pathogens and saprophytic organisms. Coughing and sneezing serve to excrete many germs into the air in droplet nuclei (Ojo 1987), while dust helps to keep them airborne. Warm and humid conditions favor the survival of microorganisms in the air.

Animal Density

Overcrowding increases both the temperature and humidity in the barn because more goats generate heat and moisture into the atmosphere. Manure can also significantly increase the temperature. The surface area allotted per goat should be a minimum of 0.5 m^2 per stanchioned animal and 1.5 m^2 per adult in a free stall setting (Toussaint 1984). The minimum per unweaned kid is 0.3 m^2. The minimum feed trough length recommended per goat is 0.4 m. With the inclusion of feed alleys, the typical area per goat in the barn is 2 to 2.4 m^2. The height from the bedding to the ceiling then determines the volume per goat. If the ceiling is too low, temperature and humidity increase. If the air space is too great, the barn may be too cold in the winter.

Building Construction

The building where goats are housed should serve several functions. First, it should shelter the animals from intemperate weather while providing a suitable microclimate for the goats. The comfort of the goat rather than of the owner is paramount. Second, the building should be constructed so that the owner can group animals as necessary and efficiently perform all the tasks required for management of the herd. The building and its equipment must not be so expensive that the owner cannot pay the mortgage.

The barn should be situated where natural ventilation and drainage are good (top of a rise, not the bottom of a slope). In cold climates, exercise lots should have exposure to winter sun and a protective wall relative to prevailing winter winds. The barn should be situated away from wells and streams to avoid contamination of groundwater.

Proper construction of the barn is required to obtain the desired ventilation rate, whether natural or mechanical ventilation is used (Constantinou 1987; Collins 1990). In particular, the placement and size of air inlets and fans are very important. The assistance of an expert in this field should be sought when designing a barn or attempting to correct a preexisting problem (Bates and Anderson 1979). Fans and air intakes must also be cleaned regularly to ensure continuing function of the ventilation system. Plastic netting may be used to temper prevailing winds.

In cold climates, and in kid-raising facilities, insulation of the building avoids the stresses associated with large daily temperature fluctuations. While insulation prevents water condensation on the ceiling it requires more ventilation to remove moisture. A very serious error is the lining of the barn with plastic sheeting with the thought of keeping the goats comfortably warm. High humidity and dripping of condensed water onto the goats predisposes them to pneumonia. Leaky waterers also increase humidity, as does inadequate provision of new bedding.

A last way that building construction can help to limit respiratory disease is in the provision of appropriate isolation facilities. Sick animals should be removed from the main pen, and purchased or boarded animals should be kept isolated from the herd for a minimum of two weeks. If attendance at shows is part of the operation of the herd, the traveling goats should be kept isolated from the stay-at-home animals for an equal time period, though this may in effect mean running two herds during the show season.

UPPER RESPIRATORY TRACT DISEASES

As discussed earlier, clinical signs such as stertor, sneezing, nasal discharge, and cough suggest but are not limited to conditions with upper respiratory tract involvement.

Rhinitis

There are several possible etiologies for inflammation of the nasal passages. Irritation from foreign material or parasites should be ruled out before more esoteric explanations are sought. A single mature goat in Brazil developed *Prototheca*-induced pyogranulomatous lesions of the skin at the nares and extending onto the nasal mucosa, causing inspiratory stertor, dyspnea, and weight loss (Macedo et al. 2008). This report underscores the importance of obtaining a biopsy sample from perplexing cases.

Herpesvirus

Caprine herpesvirus infection (see Chapter 12) has caused severe generalized signs, including bloody diarrhea, fever, dyspnea, and purulent nasal discharge. Fibrinonecrotic ulceration of the nasal septum occurred in one kid experimentally infected (Berrios et al 1975). In other experimental infections, the virus has caused a catarrhal rhinitis and mild tracheitis (Buddle et al. 1990a).

Nasal Bots

Nasal bots (*Oestrus ovis*) cause a chronic catarrhal to purulent discharge (Prein 1938) that may contain many eosinophils. This parasite is less common (larval burdens are smaller) in goats than in sheep (Dorchies et al. 1998). The adult fly deposits larvae around the nostrils of animals on pasture. First instars enter the nasal cavity and develop into second instars, which invade the sinuses of the head. Mature larvae return to the nostrils (if they have not grown too large to escape from the sinuses) after two to ten months and are expelled by sneezing (Kimberling 1988). Pupation occurs in the ground. Adult flies emerge after four weeks or longer, or possibly the next spring. Occasionally larvae are deposited about the eyes of humans, causing painful conjunctival ophthalmomyiasis (Cameron et al. 1991).

Nose bots in goats can be suspected if nasal discharge is profuse and contains eosinophils. Frequent violent sneezing and avoidance behavior in late summer are typical. Caked-on dust leads to mouth breathing and interference with feeding, while inhaled bacteria and eosinophils may induce lung damage. Repeated infections induce a hypersensitivity and immunity in goats (Dorchies et al. 1998). Sometimes the bots are just an incidental finding in the sinus upon dehorning of adult goats.

The condition can usually be ignored if it does not interfere with feed consumption. Various questionable products have been sprayed into the nasal passages in late fall and winter to kill larvae, including ruelene aerosol and concentrated lysol diluted 1:5 with water. Ivermectin (even at 0.2 mg/kg level) is highly effective against all stages of nose bots. A prolonged milk withdrawal of nine days is suggested if ivermectin is administered orally to goats producing milk for human consumption, and forty days if given subcutaneously (Baynes et al. 2000). Eprinomectin pour-on at 0.5 mg/kg has been shown to be effective against *Oestrus ovis* in sheep (Hoste et al. 2004) and does not contaminate milk.

Nasal Leech

The nasal leech (*Dinobdella ferox*) infests ruminants grazing at altitudes of 900 to 1,800 m in the foothills of the Himalayas. The leeches live in permanent pools and springs; young leeches attach themselves to the nostrils of animals that drink there during the dry season. Leeches migrate to the nasal passages to feed but drop back into the water at the onset of the monsoon season (mid-June). Clinical signs include sneezing, blood-tinged mucoid nasal exudate, intermittent epistaxis, and anemia (Mahato et al. 1993). When leeches become large enough to protrude through the nostrils (fifteen days after infection) and restrict breathing, goats become restless and anorectic. Treatment is achieved by wetting the goat's nostrils with water to encourage leeches to protrude, then permitting the leeches to dip their bodies in a (reusable) solution of 10 mcg/ml ivermectin. Leeches are expelled within a few hours after this therapy. Systemic ivermectin is not effective (Mahato 1989).

Nasal Schistosomosis

The blood fluke *Schistosoma nasale* has caused nasal obstruction in goats in India. This parasite is discussed in Chapter 8.

Foreign Matter

Foreign body rhinitis is often caused by powdery feeds. Regurgitation is a more serious possible cause. Assuming the absence of a cleft palate, nutritional muscular dystrophy (white muscle disease) should be considered whenever milk runs out a kid's nose. This is discussed under inhalation pneumonia. Vagal nerve irritation in the abdomen or thorax or poisoning by plants of the Ericaceae (rhododendron) family may cause regurgitation through the nose and mouth, but the distinctive smell and green color of rumen contents on the muzzle make the identification of the irritating substance simple.

Bacterial Rhinitis

Atrophic rhinitis associated with toxigenic strains of *Pasteurella multocida* has been recognized in goats in Norway (Baalsrud 1987). Signs observed in affected herds include purulent nasal discharge, nose bleeding, sneezing, and occasionally tender or distorted noses. Turbinate atrophy can be recognized when heads are sectioned at the level of the first premolar teeth. In tropical countries, purulent rhinitis with raised coalescing nodules on the nasal septum and turbinates has been observed in goats with melioidosis (Omar 1963).

Neoplasia

An enzootic nasal tumor of young adult goats has been reported from France and Spain and recognized in individual animals elsewhere in the world (Fontaine et al. 1983; Pringle et al. 1989; De las Heras et al. 1991a, 2003b). The lesion is unilateral or bilateral and papillary and results in lysis of the turbinates. Histologically, the tumor is benign. Retroviral-like particles have been demonstrated in the tumors of several goats that had negative agar gel immunodiffusion tests for maedi-visna (and therefore CAE) virus (De las Heras et al. 1988, 1991a). Nasal secretions and the associated type D retroviral particles have transmitted the tumor experimentally (De las Heras et al. 1991b, 1995). Affected animals show profuse seromucous nasal exudate, coughing, dyspnea, and stertor. One or both eyes may protrude and pressure on softened cranial bones causes expulsion of mucous nasal exudate. The outcome is eventually fatal, the result of emaciation and asphyxiation (De las Heras et al. 1991a). Presumably, select cases might be amenable to surgical extirpation, as has been performed for nasal tumors of sheep (Rings and Rojko 1985, Trent et al. 1988). Lymphosarcoma can also invade the nasal sinuses of goats (Craig et al. 1986). A fungal granuloma caused by *Cryptococcus neoformans* has been reported to obstruct the nasal cavity of a goat in Australia (Chapman et al. 1990) and could be easily mistaken for a tumor.

Pharyngitis

Balling gun injuries can cause severe cellulitis in the region of the pharynx. Small plastic balling guns are particularly dangerous because the goats soon make them very rough by chewing on the plastic when bolus administration is attempted. Common clinical signs include cough, nasal discharge, and secondary inhalation pneumonia. The breath may have a foul odor, and the region of the pharynx is swollen and sensitive to palpation. Examination is simplified by tranquilization. Broad-spectrum antibiotics are given for treatment. Prevention typically involves using an alternative to anthelmintic or sulfonamide boluses.

Abscessation of Retropharyngeal Lymph Nodes

An enlarged retropharyngeal lymph node (Figure 9.3) may cause stertor, dyspnea, and coughing because of pressure on the pharynx or trachea. The mass can be detected by careful palpation and by radiography. The abscess is often caused by *Corynebacterium*

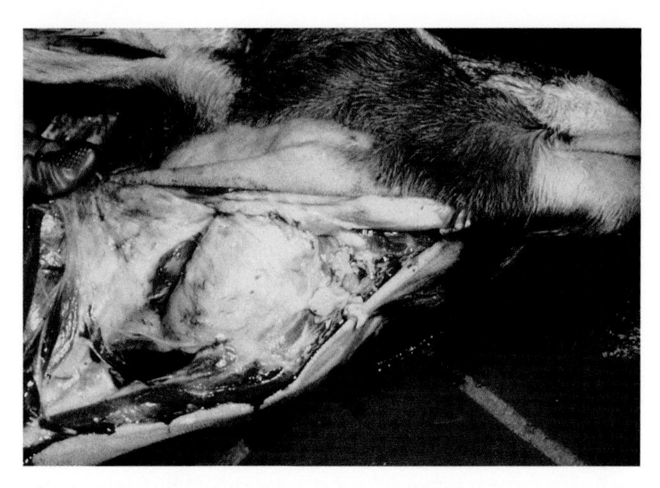

Figure 9.3. Abscessation of the retropharyngeal lymph node caused marked dyspnea in this goat. (Courtesy of Dr. J.M. King.)

pseudotuberculosis. A brave and careful surgeon is required to marsupialize the abscess without severing carotid artery, vagus nerve, or other important structures. Placement of a cuffed tracheostomy tube under local anesthesia has been recommended before induction of general anesthesia (Benson 1986). Caseous lymphadenitis is discussed in detail in Chapter 3.

Laryngitis or Tracheitis

These conditions are suspected when stridors are audible and can be localized to the corresponding portions of the upper respiratory tract. As discussed earlier, the trachea of a normal goat feels quite small.

Common Causes

Collars that press on the trachea may induce coughing in a tethered goat or one that is led by a collar. The cough is far less important than the danger of leg injury from the tether. Tracheitis because of irritants such as smoke, dust, whitewash, and ammonia in urine-soaked bedding has already been alluded to in the discussion of coughing. The diagnostician should get down to goat level and inhale deeply. If hay is dusty, the owner should try shaking it out while the goats are out of stall. If a goat is eating well and maintaining normal production and body condition, occasional coughing when fed or aroused is of no real concern.

The possible role of *Mycoplasma ovipneumoniae* (see below) in chronic cough of otherwise healthy kids on certain farms remains to be studied. This cough is usually outgrown by about eight months of age.

A single case of laryngeal hemiplegia has been reported in an adult Alpine goat (Tschuor et al. 2007). No etiology was determined, even with full necropsy and evaluation of the (normal) laryngeal nerve and musculature.

Necrotic Laryngitis

Fusobacterium necrophorum is a sporadic cause of laryngitis and of necrotic stomatitis in goats. The condition is discussed in Chapter 10.

Cilia-associated Respiratory Bacillus

Recently, a Gram-negative filamentous bacterium called cilia-associated respiratory bacillus, or CAR, has been associated with respiratory tract disease in laboratory rodents and cattle. This organism has also been found by histological examination (Warthin Starry stain and immunohistochemistry) and electron microscopy in the trachea of kids and adult goats with chronic tracheitis (Fernández et al. 1996; Orós et al.1997a) and in the lungs of slaughtered goats with enzootic pneumonia (Orós et al. 1997b). The bacteria are interspersed with cilia and oriented perpendicular to the surface of the tracheal and bronchial epithelium. The significance of CAR in goats remains to be determined.

Infectious Bovine Rhinotracheitis

Infectious bovine rhinotracheitis (IBR) virus (bovine herpesvirus type I) is rarely isolated from goats, but experimentally causes pyrexia and mild clinical signs. Cough and nasal discharge would be expected if any signs at all occurred, although there is one report of severe respiratory disease (Mohanty 1972). The use of IBR vaccination is not recommended for goats. In fact, several caprine isolates have been indistinguishable from bovine vaccine strains (Whetstone and Evermann 1988). Goats may be latent carriers of the virulent bovine virus, potentially interfering with eradication attempts in cattle herds (Six et al. 2001).

LOWER RESPIRATORY TRACT DISEASES

A clinician can only rarely be sure of the etiology of lung disease in a particular live goat. To make a more specific diagnosis than "pneumonia," it is necessary to rely on the history of this or nearby herds or to await the proclamations of a microbiologist or pathologist (Ojo 1977). The etiology of pneumonia is usually multifactorial, and treatment often precedes diagnosis. A general discussion of therapy and prophylaxis for pneumonia, then, can be found following the discussion of etiologic agents.

VIRAL CAUSES OF PNEUMONIA

Viral pneumonias in goats can be chronic or acute. Secondary bacterial infections are often superimposed.

Respiratory Syncytial Virus

A single caprine isolate of respiratory syncytial virus (RSV, a single stranded RNA pneumovirus of the family *Paramyxoviridae*, subfamily *Pneumovirinae*) has been characterized in the United States (Lehmkuhl et al. 1980). This isolate is very closely related to strains of bovine respiratory syncytial virus (BRSV) (Trudel et al. 1989). An RSV similar to BRSV has been isolated from goat kids with respiratory disease in Spain (Redondo et al. 1994). Clinical signs reported in this outbreak included fever, loss of appetite, conjunctivitis, nasal discharge, cough, and tachypnea. Animals with a simultaneous fibrinous *Mannheimia haemolytica* bronchopneumonia had higher fevers and more labored breathing. Crackles were heard over the lungs of all affected animals.

Several surveys have documented antibodies against this virus or the closely related bovine RSV in healthy goats. This includes 36% of 112 adult goats from forty herds studied in Quebec (Lamontagne et al., 1985), 31% of 318 goats in twenty-two herds in another Quebec study (Elazhary et al. 1984), 50% of 332 goats in Louisiana (Fulton et al. 1982) and eleven of forty goats from farms in the Netherlands that also harbored cattle (Van der Pool et al. 1995). Goats in England were found to have antibodies against BRSV without ever having shown respiratory signs (Morgan et al. 1985), whereas goats seroconverted during a pneumonia outbreak in Zaire (Jetteur et al. 1989). The importance of RSV as a respiratory pathogen in goats remains unclear. There are no publications available concerning possible benefits of vaccination, although some veterinarians have used BRSV vaccines to prevent respiratory disease in show goats.

Progressive Interstitial Retroviral Pneumonia

Retroviruses (lentiviruses) are believed to cause both subclinical and fatal pneumonia in goats.

Etiology

The caprine arthritis encephalitis virus (CAEV, viral leukoencephalomyelitis) has been reported to cause subclinical interstitial pneumonia (Cork et al. 1974). Occasional kids with neurologic lesions also have diffuse involvement of one or more lung lobes.

A clinical syndrome indistinguishable from ovine progressive pneumonia and maedi-visna has been identified in CAEV-infected adult goats (Robinson 1981; Oliver et al. 1982). The sheep and goat viruses are still considered to be distinct by most researchers, but serologic tests cross react and both viruses are spread through milk, as discussed in Chapter 4.

To date it has not been possible to reproduce this condition experimentally. Therefore there is a suspicion that an additional agent, such as a helper virus, may be involved. There is currently no evidence that the production of interstitial pneumonia depends on the strain of CAEV with which the goat is infected (Ellis et al. 1988b). Inoculation of CAEV into Merino lambs has failed to produce clinical disease in the sheep (Dickson and Ellis 1989). Natural transmission of small ruminant lentiviruses between sheep and goats has been documented in mixed herds (Shah et al. 2004).

Clinical Signs

The first signs of dyspnea usually occur after a stress such as kidding or mastitis. The clinical course may be several weeks in advanced pregnancy or many months in the doe first affected after kidding. Exercise intolerance, dyspnea, and wasting often accompanied by a cough are prominent. Some but not all affected goats have enlarged carpi. Secondary bacterial pneumonias may be superimposed, and antibiotics often appear to give temporary relief. The pulmonary form of caseous lymphadenitis has a similar clinical appearance.

Diagnosis

Radiographs show small patches of interstitial pneumonia early in the course. A more advanced case is depicted in Figure 9.4 and elsewhere (Koenig et al. 1990). As debilitation progresses, large areas of lung are consolidated and bullous emphysema may damage the remaining lung parenchyma. Either caudal lung lobes or cranioventral lung lobes may be involved (Ellis at al. 1988a). At necropsy, the affected areas are swollen, grey-pink, and firm (Figure 9.5); numerous 1- to 2-mm whitish gray foci are visible on cut section as shown in Figure 9.6 (Robinson and Ellis 1984). Mediastinal lymph nodes are enlarged. Lung biopsies might confirm the diagnosis before death. Serologic testing is of no diagnostic value, but should identify an infected herd.

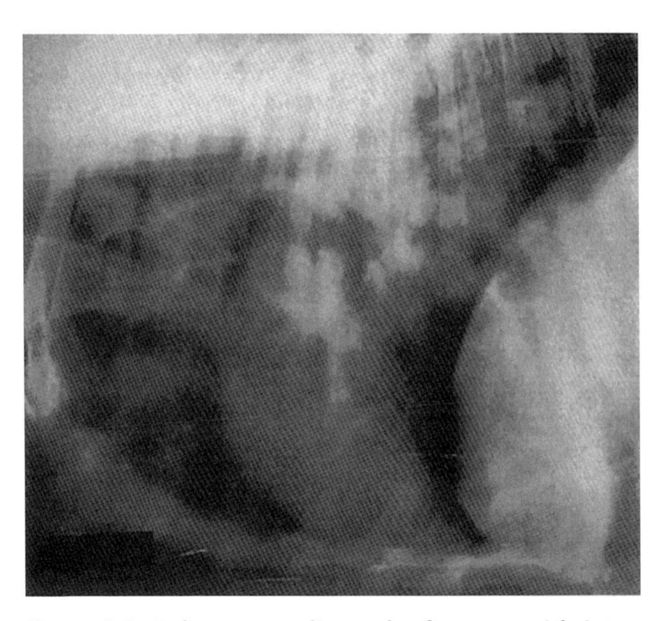

Figure 9.4. Pulmonary radiograph of a goat with interstitial pneumonia (Courtesy of Dr. M.C. Smith.)

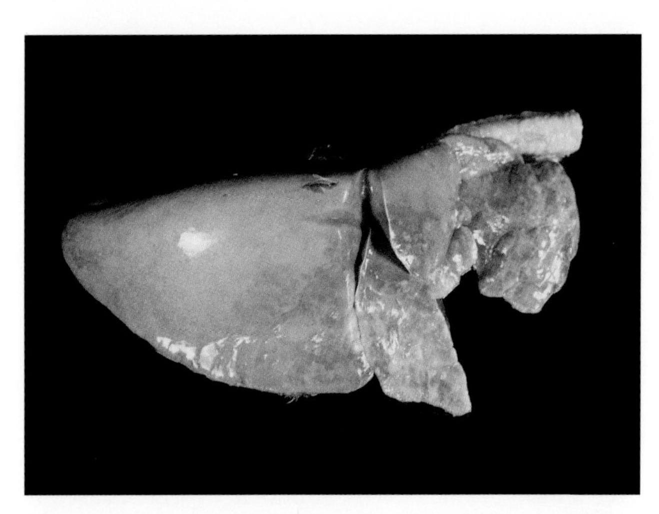

Figure 9.5. Goat lung with CAE interstitial pneumonia distending the diaphragmatic lobe. (Courtesy of Dr. M.C. Smith.)

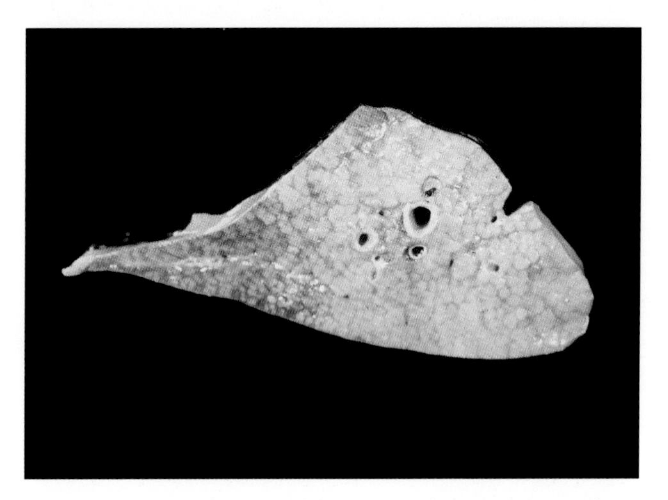

Figure 9.6. Cross section of an affected lung lobe, showing infiltration of the pulmonary parenchyma. (Courtesy of Dr. M.C. Smith.)

Histological study of caprine progressive pneumonia reveals interstitial (peribronchiolar) accumulation of mononuclear cells and proliferation of type II pneumocytes. Alveoli are filled with an eosinophilic material that resembles surfactant when examined with the electron microscope (Robinson and Ellis 1984; Robinson and Ellis 1986).

Discussions of the other CAEV-associated syndromes (i.e., arthritis, neurologic disease, mastitis) can be found elsewhere in this text. Control procedures are discussed in detail in Chapter 4.

Ovine Pulmonary Adenocarcinoma, Sheep Pulmonary Adenomatosis, Jaagsiekte

This contagious lung tumor of sheep has been reported infrequently in goats (Rajya and Singh 1964; Stefanou et al. 1975). The disease has been reported in sheep on all continents except Australia. The cause is an oncogenic beta-retrovirus (De las Heras et al. 2003a). Transmission appears to be via respiratory secretions. Experimental infection is much more difficult to produce in goats than in sheep (Sharp et al. 1986; Tustin et al. 1988).

Clinically affected animals are mature and afebrile (in the absence of secondary bacterial infections) and show prolonged weight loss and dyspnea. Fluid accumulates in the lungs, which results in auscultable crackles or rales. A simple test used to differentiate the condition from chronic progressive pneumonia is to elevate the animal's hindquarters. Fluid is expected to run out the nose if the animal is severely affected with adenomatosis. The disease is considered to be invariably progressive and fatal. There is no known treatment and no serologic test. Control is usually limited to culling goats that are wasting, although recently a PCR test for proviral DNA in leukocytes has permitted identification of subclinically infected sheep (Gonzalez et al. 2001). Removal at birth and artificial rearing on colostrum substitutes and milk replacer (essentially a CAE eradication program) has also been successful in creating a disease-free sheep flock (Voigt et al. 2007).

At necropsy, many grayish nodules or extensive solid tumors are found in the lungs. The respiratory passages are filled with white froth. Histologically, there are alveolar and intrabronchiolar growths composed of masses of cuboidal and columnar cells. Metastases to regional lymph nodes have not been reported in goats (Sharma et al. 1975).

Peste des Petits Ruminants

This important infectious disease of sheep and goats is also called PPR, stomatitis pneumoenteritis complex, and Kata (Hamdy et al. 1976).

Etiology and Pathogenesis

The etiologic agent is a paramyxovirus of the *Morbillivirus* genus that is not pathogenic for cattle. The closely related rinderpest virus of cattle causes similar signs in goats. The two viruses seriously limit goat production in West Africa, the Middle East, India, and Southeast Asia.

The virus is shed in secretions to infect other animals by direct contact. It can persist in the environment for as long as thirty-six hours, and thus holding pens can be a source of infection. The disease is discussed in detail in Chapter 10.

Clinical Signs

The disease is characterized by fever persisting five to seven days and a profuse, even bloody diarrhea. Necrotic stomatitis, foaming at the mouth, and an ocular discharge are also noted. Pregnant animals may abort (Abu Elzein et al. 1990). Respiratory signs occur during the acute stages; these include malodorous, mucopurulent nasal discharge, frequent sneezing, increased respiratory rate, extended head, and mouth breathing. Severe leukopenia persists for ten days in animals that recover (Scott 1990). Some goats die two to three weeks later of a secondary bronchopneumonia (Whitney et al. 1967). The highest incidence of disease occurs during the rainy season, and goats most commonly affected are six to twelve months of age. Kids younger than three months of age usually have colostral immunity.

Diagnosis

Fluorescent antibody testing is useful for identifying the virus in nasal discharges and intestinal scrapings. Ocular or nasal discharges collected after two to three drops of phosphate buffered saline are placed in the eye or nostril can be used as the antigen in a hemagglutination test using 0.6% piglet red blood cell suspension (Wosu 1991). This test permits differentiation of peste des petits ruminants from simple bacterial pneumonia in live goats in situations where sophisticated laboratory facilities are not available. When available, a reverse transcriptase polymerase chain reaction test can be used to identify the virus in oculonasal swabs, oral lesions, or blood (Çam et al. 2005). Serological testing using a competitive ELISA also permits monitoring of the infection in endemic regions (Singh et al. 2004, 2006).

The necropsy findings relative to the gastrointestinal tract are described in Chapter 10. There may be consolidation of cranioventral lung lobes. Histologic lesions reported in the lung include a giant cell pneumonia with eosinophilic intracytoplasmic inclusions in epithelial cells in perhaps half of the goats dying because of peste des petits ruminants. Less commonly there is necrosis of the tracheal epithelium. Diagnosis is complicated by secondary *Pasteurella, Mannheimia,* or *Mycoplasma* pneumonia.

Prophylaxis

Vaccination against this disease in endemic areas is both feasible (Gibbs et al. 1979) and economically sound (Opasina and Putt 1985). Prophylaxis is covered in Chapter 10.

Hyperimmune serum (5 ml intravenously) reverses the signs of peste des petits ruminants if given during the febrile stage of the disease, when the temperature is 104.9°F (40.5°C) or higher. However, reinfection or relapse occurs after ten days and even those goats that develop labial scabs and appear to recover are susceptible to later challenge (Ihemelandu et al. 1985). Thus, goats treated with hyperimmune serum should still be vaccinated.

Goat Pox

The capripox virus, discussed in detail in Chapter 2, causes systemic signs that include pyrexia, anorexia, and an arched back. Case fatality rates are increased when the respiratory tract is involved. At necropsy, multiple foci of consolidation (0.5 to 2 cm diameter) are commonly found beneath the pleura. These lesions may be hemorrhagic (Kitching 2004). Similar lesions may be seen in other organs such as liver, kidney, and abomasum. Secondary bacterial pneumonia is commonly the cause of death (Davies 1981).

MYCOPLASMA, CHLAMYDIA, AND RICKETTSIA PNEUMONIAS

Of these organisms, mycoplasma are most frequently isolated and of the greatest economic importance.

Several species of mycoplasma have been shown to cause pneumonia in goats (Hudson et al. 1967; Ojo 1987; Nicholas 2002). Some of these (belonging to the *Mycoplasma mycoides* cluster) cause specific syndromes known as contagious caprine pleuropneumonia and pleuropneumonia and are discussed separately. Because of changes in classification schemes, it is very difficult to interpret the older literature and to know exactly which organism was involved in a given report (Moulton 1980).

Mycoplasma are generally fragile outside the host animal. They are easily inactivated by heat, sunlight, and disinfectants. Mycoplasma have been isolated from the external ear canal of goats (Ribeiro et al. 1997). Ear mites have been proposed as possibly disseminating the infection (Cottew and Yeats 1982; DaMassa 1983; DaMassa and Brooks 1991).

Nonspecific Mycoplasma Pneumonia

Several species are isolated sporadically from goats, either alone or in conjunction with other causes of pneumonia.

Etiology and Pathogenesis

Mycoplasma ovipneumoniae can be isolated from the trachea and lungs of healthy goats. When found in pneumonic lungs, the numbers of organisms present do not correlate with the severity of the lesion (Bolske et al. 1989). Fever and subacute fibrinous pleuritis have been produced experimentally with *M. ovipneumoniae* (Goltz et al. 1986), and natural cases also have been reported in goats (Livingston and Gauer 1979; Jones and Wood 1988). Production of a capsule may contribute to this organism's pathogenicity (Niang et al. 1998). It lacks the "fried egg" colony appearance typical of other mycoplasmas when grown on solid medium (DaMassa et al. 1992). Note that *M. ovipneumoniae* may accompany other mycoplasma species that are more pathogenic but also more difficult to isolate.

Oral administration of *M. capricolum* (*M. capricolum* subsp. *capricolum*) causes acute pneumonia and polyarthritis in kids via the septicemic route (DaMassa et al. 1983b, 1992; Bölske et al. 1988; Taoudi et al. 1988). The pneumonia is only rarely accompanied by pleurisy. The organism can then spread to contact kids, probably via respiratory secretions. *Mycoplasma agalactiae*, which typically causes mastitis in sheep and goats, has been shown capable of causing pneumonia in kids (Guha and Verma 1987). *Mycoplasma arginini* is isolated occasionally but is of doubtful pathogenicity (DaMassa et al. 1992). *Mycoplasma bovis* has been isolated from the lungs of goats, and could potentially have been acquired by consumption of milk from infected cows (DaMassa et al. 1992).

Associated Clinical Syndromes

In addition to respiratory disease, other conditions associated with mycoplasma include polyarthritis, mastitis, conjunctivitis, and keratitis (see Table 4.3). This combination of clinical signs has been termed the MAKePS syndrome, standing for mastitis, arthritis, keratitis, pneumonia, and septicemia (Thiaucourt and Bölske 1996). The differential diagnoses of these syndromes are considered elsewhere in this text.

Diagnosis

Thoracocentesis has been suggested for the diagnosis of mycoplasmal pneumonia in living goats. Pleomorphic coccoid, ring, and filamentous organisms can be seen with the dark field microscope or, alternatively, after staining with a 5% nigrosin solution (Ojo 1987). Although special media are required, the MAKePS mycoplasmas (including those that cause pleuropneumonia, see below) grow on modified Hayflick's mycoplasma medium (Rosendal 1994). It is relatively easy to isolate mycoplasma from acute cases, but difficult or impossible to culture the organism from chronically infected goats. Swabs should be shipped in transport media (without charcoal), refrigerated but not frozen. Tissue samples from the interface between consolidated and unconsolidated areas are chopped or pulverized in culture medium.

Peribronchiolar lymphocytic infiltrations and diffuse nonsuppurative pleuritis at necropsy are suggestive of mycoplasma, but secondary pasteurellosis complicates the diagnosis. Serologic tests are not available for many mycoplasmal species, and in fact few laboratories are capable of typing mycoplasma isolates to determine if a known pathogenic species is present.

Therapy

Penicillin and related drugs are ineffective because mycoplasma lack a cell wall. Tylosin (10 to 20 mg/kg once daily) and tiamulin (Ojo et al. 1984) (20 mg/kg once daily) are considered to be superior to tetracycline in the treatment of pulmonary mycoplasmosis. Adverse reactions associated with intramuscular injection of these drugs include lameness and collapse. Side effects may be reduced by diluting the drug with an equal quantity of sterile saline solution just before injection or administering the drug subcutaneously. The newer macrolide drug tulathromycin, which has a prolonged pulmonary half-life and activity against bovine mycoplasma, has not yet been evaluated in small ruminants. Isolation of infected animals is desirable, but very difficult in free-ranging systems, especially where communal water holes are used. Control measures used for pleuropneumonia are applicable if herd outbreaks occur.

Contagious Caprine Pleuropneumonia

Contagious caprine pleuropneumonia (CCPP) is a disease that naturally infects only goats, not sheep. Lesions are confined to the respiratory tract (Harbi et al. 1983). The disease is notifiable to the OIE (Office International des Epizooties).

Etiology and Pathogenesis

Mycoplasmologists have reclassified the etiologic agent several times (Martin 1983). In the 1980s the organism was specified as the highly fastidious F38 biotype *Mycoplasma* (McMartin et al. 1980), but currently it is named *Mycoplasma capricolum* subsp. *capripneumoniae* (Thiaucourt and Bölske 1996). Previously, *M. mycoides* subsp. *capri* was cited as the cause of CCPP, but now the disease associated with the latter organism is designated as pleuropneumonia, as discussed below. Although not identified in the Western Hemisphere, CCPP is prevalent in Africa, Turkey, the Middle East, and Asia (Thiaucourt and Bölske 1996). The organism is transmitted by aerosol during cohabitation and is highly contagious. The incubation period is typically six to ten days or longer. All ages are affected.

Clinical Signs and Diagnosis

In countries where this infection occurs, the signs are considered to be specific enough to permit an easy clinical diagnosis (Ojo 1987). These signs include fever, cough, and a painful respiration with grunting and the forelimbs held widely separated. The head is held low, there may be a frothy nasal discharge and salivation, and the goat is unwilling to move. Death occurs within two to ten days after onset of clinical signs. Typically there is a 100% morbidity rate and as much as 50% to 100% mortality rates in a susceptible flock (Ojo 1977).

Necropsy Findings and Diagnosis

Serofibrinous pleuritis results in accumulation of straw colored pleural fluid. Pneumonia usually causes hepatization of entire lobes and is often unilateral. The lung appears granular or variegated, with red, yellow, white, and gray foci. Several reports include color photographs (Kaliner and MacOwan 1976; Thiaucourt et al. 1996; Nicholas 2002). There is extensive bronchoalveolar cellular exudate. In contrast to the findings in goats with pleuropneumonia caused by other organisms, there is no thickening of the interlobular septa (Thiaucourt et al. 1996; Nicholas 2002).

The isolation of the CCPP mycoplasma is difficult and requires special media. Techniques have been described elsewhere (Rosendal 1994; OIE 2004). The agent can be identified by immunofluorescence, growth inhibition, or metabolism inhibition tests (U.S. Animal Health Association 1998). Serologic cross-reactions and similarity in biochemical tests can cause confusion in distinguishing *M. capricolum*. subsp. *capripneumoniae* from *M. capricolum* subsp. *capricolum* (Jones 1989). Paired serology with samples taken three to eight weeks apart is useful for diagnosing the disease in animals that recover, but in acute cases death typically occurs before seroconversion (OIE 2004). A latex agglutination test for field detection of antibodies to *M. c.* subsp. *capripneumoniae* polysaccharide antigen has been reported to be specific for CCPP in goats (Rurangirwa et al. 1990). A PCR testing scheme, when available, is considered conclusive (Hotzel et al. 1996) unless the disease has not been diagnosed in the country before. A very important advantage of the PCR testing is that a sample of pleural fluid from an untreated sacrificed animal can be allowed to dry on filter paper and then transported to a reference laboratory without having to maintain a constant "cool chain."

In countries where CCPP exists, the disease must be differentiated from other or coexisting infections such as pleuropneumonia caused by other mycoplasma infections, peste des petits ruminants, pasteurellosis, heartwater, and goat pox.

Treatment and Control

As with other mycoplasma, treatment with tylosin, tetracycline (El Hassan et al. 1984), tiamulin, or streptomycin (30 mg/kg) (Rurangirwa et al. 1981) is recommended. When tylosin (11 mg/kg), oxytetracycline (15 mg/kg), chloramphenicol (22 mg/kg), and penicillin plus streptomycin (dose per kg not indicated) were compared experimentally, tylosin caused more rapid recovery than oxytetracycline, while fevers were more persistent and some deaths occurred with the other two treatments (Onoviran 1984). More recently, fluoroquinolones have also been found to be effective against caprine mycoplasmas (Al-Momani et al. 2006) but their veterinary use is discouraged or forbidden in food animals because of importance of the antibiotic class in human medicine.

Treatment should be continued for five days or provided with a long duration product (Thiaucourt et al. 1996). The prognosis for recovery with prompt treatment is approximately 87% (Rurangirwa et al. 1981; El Hassan et al. 1984). Animals recovered from clinical disease may remain carriers (El Hassan et al. 1984) and spread the disease to other herds. One study found dihydrostreptomycin-treated goats did not remain carriers (Rurangirwa et al. 1981) but use of this antibiotic is discouraged because of rapid development of resistance (Lefèvre and Thiaucourt 2004). Farmers usually retain animals that survive the infection.

An experimental vaccine has shown good protection for as long as one year after a single immunization (Rurangirwa et al. 1987). Vaccination of 10,000 goats in Kenya with an inactivated F38 vaccine was followed by cessation of reported losses to CCPP after three weeks. None of 400 closely monitored goats showed any evidence of clinical CCPP during the six-month period after vaccination (Litamoi et al. 1989). A commercial vaccine is currently available in Kenya (OIE 2004).

Pleuropneumonia

Etiology

Currently two different species of mycoplasma (*M. mycoides* subsp. *capri* and *M. mycoides* subsp. *mycoides* Large Colony [LC] or caprine type) are believed to cause very similar syndromes known as pleuropneumonia (Pearson et al. 1972). Earlier reports of *M. mycoides* subsp. *capri* from the United States probably reflect a misidentification of *M. mycoides* subsp. *mycoides* LC (DaMassa et al. 1984). *Mycoplasma mycoides* subsp. *capri* has been isolated from a high mortality respiratory outbreak in goats in Mexico (Hernandez 2006).

A closely related species, *Mycoplasma mycoides* subsp. *mycoides* Small Colony type (the cause of contagious bovine pleuropneumonia), has been isolated from pneumonic lungs of goats in Africa (Kusiluka et al. 2000).

Clinical Signs

Incubation is from two to twenty-eight days, depending on virulence. Clinical signs include high fever, cough, painful dyspnea, increased nasal secretion, ear droop, and anorexia. Morbidity rates are near 100%, but mortality rates vary with the organism, less than 40% for the large colony type and close to 100% for the *M. m. capri* subspecies. Since the discovery of *Mycoplasma capricolum* subsp. *capripneumoniae* (F38 biotype), mortality rates attributed to *M. m. capri* have been questioned (Jones 1989).

Diagnosis

In the pleuropneumonia caused by *M. mycoides* subsp. *mycoides* LC, which is common in California, the organism is easily isolated from many internal organs and from joints and milk. The lungs of fatal cases are enlarged and firm. There is hepatization of cardiac and diaphragmatic lobes and marked pleural effusion and fibrinous pleuritis (Thigpen et al. 1981; DaMassa et al. 1986, 1992; Rodriguez et al. 1995). Both subspecies cause similar histopathologic changes; pulmonary edema is extensive and interlobular septa are distended and pale. Arterial and arteriolar vasculitis with necrosis of vessel walls and thrombi formation are seen (Jones 1989).

Mycoplasma mycoides subsp. *mycoides* LC is less fastidious in its growth requirements than many mycoplasma and can be isolated on blood agar. Growth is slow, beta hemolysis appears by day six or seven, and colonies have a "fried egg" appearance (DaMassa et al. 1983a). Biochemical characteristics and antisera can be used to differentiate the various mycoplasma causing pleuropneumonia and contagious caprine pleuropneumonia, but a polymerase chain reaction scheme has also been devised for differentiating these organisms (Hotzel et al. 1996).

Treatment and Prevention

Kids are often infected by ingestion of milk, and the entire kid crop may be infected by pooled colostrum or milk (DaMassa et al. 1983a). Pasteurization of milk is routinely suggested to control an outbreak. Kids should be raised isolated from adults. Burning or deep burial of placentas and stillborn kids is also important. Tylosin (11 mg/kg intramuscularly for five days to two weeks) has been reported to be more rapidly effective for treatment than oxytetracycline at 15 mg/kg.

Ear mites, which may spread mycoplasma to additional animals or herds, can be controlled with ivermectin (see Chapter 2).

Chlamydiosis

The role of chlamydia in caprine pneumonia is very unclear. A serious outbreak of pneumonia in goats in Japan seemed to originate with goats imported from the United States after World War 2 (Omori et al. 1953; Saito 1954). Elementary bodies of various sizes were seen in bronchial epithelial cells and stained by the Machiavello stain. An agent was isolated in embryonated eggs that caused mild chronic respiratory signs such as slight cough, nasal discharge, and fever after intratracheal inoculation, although secondary bacterial infections were often fatal. Experimentally infected goats were successfully treated with tetracycline (7 mg/kg intramuscularly for eleven days) (Ishii et al. 1954). A cough without dyspnea or nasal discharge developed in two of eleven goats experimentally inoculated with an abortion strain of *Chlamydophila abortus* (*C. psittaci*) and persisted one to two months in another study (Rodolakis et al. 1984).

Texas researchers have proposed that chlamydia are usually primary, with *Pasteurella* and mycoplasma causing a secondary pneumonia (Sharp et al. 1982). This theory does not seem to be commonly espoused, except perhaps in India. Fluorescent antibody tests, as have been used for diagnosis of abortion caused by chlamydiosis, would be a useful tool for additional study of the importance of the organism in pneumonia outbreaks. In a slaughterhouse study in India involving 3,799 apparently healthy goats, chlamydia were identified from fourteen of 218 (6.4%) pneumonic lungs by fluorescent antibody tests (Rahman and Singh 1990). Special stains identified elementary bodies in only eight of these cases. Gross lung lesions were mostly cranioventral. Histologically, there was an interstitial pneumonia and macrophages filled alveoli. Additional slaughterhouse studies have identified chlamydia in lung lesions of unknown clinical relevance by special stains or fluorescent antibody tests (Chauhan and Singh 1971; Patnaik and Nayak 1984; Kumar et al. 2004).

Too little is known about the condition to formulate control programs. Different chlamydia serotypes are incriminated from those included in anti-abortion vaccines. Long-lasting oxytetracycline would be appropriate for therapy if involvement of this agent were suspected in field cases of pneumonia.

Q Fever

Q fever, caused by *Coxiella burnetti*, is occasionally associated with abortion in sheep and goats but is otherwise considered to be nonpathogenic for livestock. Its importance is as a zoonosis. However, experimental intrapulmonary or intranasal inoculation has produced febrile bronchopneumonia in goats (Caminopetros 1948). Kids from an abortion outbreak have also shown nonsuppurative interstitial pneumonia (Moore et al. 1991).

BACTERIAL PNEUMONIA

Pasteurella and Mannheimia Pneumonia

Pneumonic pasteurellosis is a cranioventral fibrinous bronchopneumonia. The disease occurs in goats throughout the world.

Etiology

Both *Pasteurella multocida* and *Mannheimia* (previously *Pasteurella*) (Angen et al. 1999) *haemolytica* cause pneumonia in goats (Ojo 1977). Both species are Gram-negative, tiny, ovoid rods that do not form spores. They grow well on blood agar, where only *P. haemolytica* causes hemolysis. Colonies are 1 to 2 mm in diameter. *Pasteurella multocida* but not *M. haemolytica* produces indole.

Mannheimia (Pasteurella) haemolytica was previous divided into two biovars: biovar A, which ferments arabinose, and bivoar T, which ferments trehalose (Bingham et al. 1990). Subsequently, the T biovar was designated as *Pasteurella trehalosi*, and then the organism was assigned to a new genus, becoming *Bibersteinia trehalosi* (Blackall et al. 2007). How this might clarify the epidemiology of pasteurellosis in goats remains to be determined. The *trehalosi* organism has been cultured from the pharynx of healthy pack goats (Ward et al. 2002). A biotype T isolate obtained from an acute fatal case of caprine pneumonia has been used to experimentally produce a proliferative and exudative pneumonia (Ngatia et al. 1986). Biotype T *Mannheimia haemolytica* has also been cultured in association with an outbreak of contagious caprine pleuropneumonia in Ethiopia (Shiferaw et al. 2002). When typing has been performed of *Mannheimia* isolates from goats with pneumonia, *M. haemolytica* type A2 has been reported most frequently (Fodor et al. 1984; Midwinter et al. 1986; Hayashidani et al. 1988).

Epidemiology and Pathogenesis

Both of these organisms commonly reside in the upper respiratory tract of normal goats. While a previous viral infection would increase the probability of lung invasion by *Pasteurella* or *Mannheimia*, field conditions often provide enough stress for the organism to be a primary pathogen. Poor ventilation is a major factor permitting invasion of the lungs, but crowding, parasitism, and malnutrition all contribute to development of disease (Brogden et al. 1998). Some affected goats have been recently stressed by transport (Mugera and Kramer 1967), and steroid administration appears to increase the proliferation of *M. haemolytica* in the nasal passages of transport-stressed goats (Jasni et al. 1991).

The virulence of the *Pasteurella* organism is either very high or increases during an outbreak, so that the disease may spread to unstressed herd members (Pande 1943). In other instances, pneumonia is recognized only in animals exposed to newly introduced goats (Hayashidani 1988; Buddle et al. 1990).

A ruminant-specific leukotoxin produced by *M. haemolytica* is believed to be very important in the pathogenesis of pasteurellosis (Shewen and Wilkie 1985; Zecchinon et al. 2005). This toxin impairs and lyses alveolar macrophages and neutrophils that arrive in the lung to fight the infection. Enzymes released by the dying neutrophils cause additional injury to lung tissue. The deleterious effects of other toxins and cell-associated products of *M. haemolytica* have been reviewed (Brogden et al. 1998).

Clinical Signs

In the acute case, there is typically a fever of 104°F to 106°F (40°C to 41.1°C) and also mucopurulent nasal and ocular discharge. Lethargy, anorexia, dyspnea, and a moist, painful cough are noted. Auscultation may reveal crackles, areas of consolidation (increased bronchial tones), or pleuritis (friction rub early, muffled sounds later). Mortality rates may be 10% or more. Commonly, one goat is found suddenly dead before any are noticed to be ill (Borgman and Wilson 1955; Mugera and Kramer 1967).

Diagnosis and Post Mortem Lesions

Diagnostic cultures may be obtained from tracheal washes or from necropsy specimens. Cultures taken from the nasal passages are not acceptable substitutes. Kids with acute pasteurellosis often have a septicemia, and bipolar organisms may be visible in stained blood smears (Ojo 1987). A radiographic examination documents the cranioventral distribution and rules out the presence of a penetrating metallic foreign body from the reticulum, which rarely acts to introduce infection into the thoracic cavity (see Chapter 10).

At necropsy, the cranioventral lung lobes are usually affected bilaterally. There is a red to purple consolidation of these lobes, sometimes accompanied by a fibrinous pleuritis (Figure 9.7). Histologic changes are typical of pasteurellosis in other species and include hemorrhage, necrosis, and exudation of fibrin, edema fluid, and neutrophils or macrophages into airways.

A *Pasteurella* or *Mannheimia* infection may be secondary to an interstitial pneumonia or possibly may upregulate the CAE virus when macrophages are activated in the lung. If poor body condition suggests that a dead goat has been ill for weeks or months, the dorsal lung lobes should be palpated very carefully. If they seem firmer than normal, histological examination to detect concurrent interstitial pneumonia should be requested.

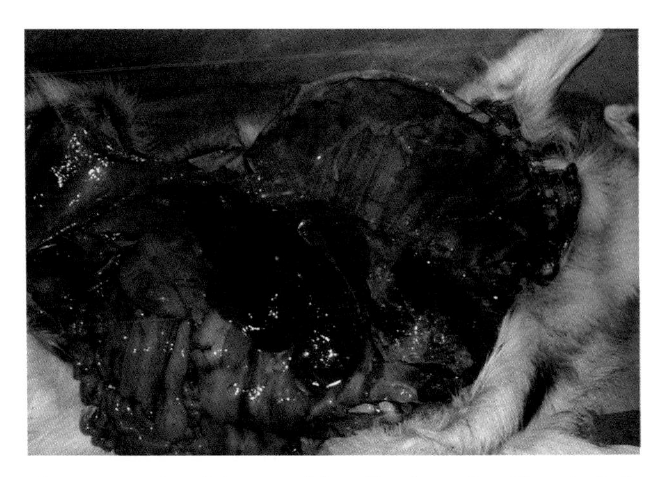

Figure 9.7. Cranial ventral localization of a *Mannheimia* pneumonia with marked fibrinous pleuritis. (Courtesy of Dr. M.C. Smith.)

Treatment and Prevention

Antibiotics commonly used for parenteral treatment include penicillin (20,000 to 40,000 IU/kg once daily), ampicillin (5 to 10 mg/kg twice daily), tetracycline (5 mg/kg once or twice daily), tylosin (10 to 20 mg/kg once or twice daily), ceftiofur (1.1 to 2.2 mg/kg daily), and florfenicol (40 mg/kg every one to two days SC). A sample for culture obtained by tracheal wash or at necropsy should be submitted for sensitivity testing when dealing with herd outbreaks, chronic cases, or very valuable goats. However, caprine isolates of *Mannheimia* and *Pasteurella* are not often resistant to antibiotics routinely used for respiratory disease, as determined by the disk diffusion assay method (Berge et al. 2006). Ventilation should be corrected to decrease humidity in the barn, so that there is no condensation on windows and walls. Nutrition, including vitamin E and selenium, should be optimized. Newly introduced goats should be kept isolated from the herd for at least two weeks.

In some outbreaks, young kids appear to be especially susceptible to pasteurellosis in a septicemic or pneumonic form. Colostral transfer of antibodies may be very important in preventing these infections of the neonate (Gourlay and Barber 1960).

No bacterin has been proven effective against pasteurellosis in goats. This is partly because of a multitude of serotypes possible (Ward et al. 2002) and partly because the antibodies produced in response to vaccination may contribute to damage of pulmonary tissue when infection occurs. A commercial vaccine containing multiple sheep isolates decreased lung lesions in goats in one small trial (Zamri-Saad et al. 1999). A toxoid vaccine directed against the leukotoxin produced by *M. haemolytica*, as developed for cattle (Bechtol et al. 1991), may prove more useful but needs further evaluation in goats (du Preez et al. 2000). Recently, *M. haemolytica* A1 organisms embedded in microagar beads and deposited in lung tissue by the transthoracic (Purdy et al. 1990, 1993) or subcutaneous (Purdy 1996) route have induced significant immunity to challenge exposure in goats. If goats become more popular models for bovine respiratory disease, an effective vaccine may eventually be developed.

Caseous Lymphadenitis Abscesses in the Lungs

Corynebacterium pseudotuberculosis abscesses are most commonly found in the head and neck lymph nodes (see Chapter 3), but abscesses may form in the lung parenchyma or mediastinal lymph nodes. In one slaughterhouse study of 25,467 goats in India, pseudotuberculosis lesions were seen primarily in the lungs of eighty-nine (0.349%) goats, and thirty of these animals had similar lesions in bronchial or mediastinal lymph nodes (Sharma and Dwivedi 1976b).

Clinical and Necropsy Signs and Diagnosis

Because the incubation period is long, this is a chronic pneumonia in adult goats and sheep. Clinical signs of dyspnea, exercise intolerance, and weight loss resemble the signs of progressive interstitial retroviral pneumonia. One to many abscesses may be present in any part of the lung. The abscesses are round, greenish-yellow, encapsulated, and caseo-purulent or caseo-calcified. Radiographic studies help distinguish the pneumonia from the cranioventral, lobar distribution of pasteurellosis. Pleuritis may occur when abscesses rupture into the pleural cavity, but crackles from exudate moving in airways are not routinely auscultated. Histologic examination reveals concentric zones of necrotic neutrophils, round cells (i.e., macrophages, lymphocytes, and occasional giant cells), and fibrosis. Presence of Gram-positive diphtheroid bacteria and absence of acid-fast bacteria help to rule out tuberculosis (Sharma and Dwivedi 1976b).

Diagnosis

In the absence of external abscesses, diagnosis is difficult without a tracheal wash or necropsy examination. If the goat is in a closed herd that has never experienced contagious abscesses, the probability of caseous lymphadenitis is minimal. Serological test results for the organism (see Chapter 3) in affected goats are usually positive, but this cannot be used to confirm a diagnosis of the pneumonic form of caseous lymphadenitis in a herd in which goats are frequently affected with external abscesses. Positive serologic test results also occur during the incubation period of an external abscess and after its resolution by drainage.

Treatment

Long-term antibiotic treatment has little effect on the abscesses. A possible exception might be the combination of penicillin or oxytetracycline and rifampin (Chapter 3). Because the condition is most readily confused with the equally untreatable retroviral pneumonia, euthanasia is warranted when other conditions amenable to therapy have been excluded from the differential diagnosis.

Prevention

The pulmonary form of caseous lymphadenitis is reportedly common in infected flocks of sheep that are driven through a dipping vat immediately after shearing. The dipping solution becomes contaminated with pus from open abscesses and is then swallowed or inhaled by other animals in the flock. Angora and Cashmere goats should be at similar risk. Dipping should be postponed until at least two weeks after shearing if the disease is present in the flock. Another mode by which infection reaches the lungs is by drainage of the thoracic duct into the systemic circulation. Finally, aerosol transmission from another animal with pulmonary abscesses is possible, although intranasal inoculation failed to produce abscesses in experimental goats (Brown et al. 1985). Thus, culling all goats with external abscesses or chronic wasting is important to preventing pulmonic caseous lymphadenitis.

Tuberculosis

Contrary to the fervent belief of many hobbyists, goats are susceptible to tuberculosis (Ramirez et al. 2003). Goats may serve as a reservoir of infection for cattle or they may directly infect humans. On the other hand, humans with tuberculosis (especially if immunocompromised by concurrent human immunodeficiency virus infection) are a potential source of tuberculosis infection for goats.

Etiology

Mycobacterium bovis typically causes pulmonary lesions in goats, whereas *M. avium* is generally associated with intestinal involvement. Infection of goats seems to occur infrequently, even in regions where cattle and swine tuberculosis is prevalent (Nanda and Singh 1943; Thorel 1984). *Mycobacterium tuberculosis* (human type) is a rare cause of generalized caprine tuberculosis (Sharma et al. 1985). Recently, some strains of *M. tuberculosis* isolated from goats, cattle, wildlife, and humans in Europe and having multiple IS*6110* insertion sequences have been classified as a new species, *M. capra*e (Prodinger et al. 2005). These include strains previously identified as *M. bovis* subsp. *caprae* or *M. tuberculosis* subsp. *caprae,* calling into question the species identification in the earlier literature. *Mycobacterium kansasii* has been cultured from the mediastinal lymph nodes of one tuberculin positive goat during a tuberculosis eradication effort in the Canary Islands (Acosta et al. 1998).

Tubercle bacilli are Gram-positive, acid-fast, and aerobic. Culture is easily done in Dorset or Stonebrinks medium. Primary cultures require three to four weeks before colonies are visible. The organisms are killed by pasteurization but may survive for a long time in moist soil or organic matter.

Clinical Signs

In countries where tuberculosis still occurs in livestock, pulmonary tuberculosis caused by *Mycobacterium caprae* and possibly other species may cause severe respiratory signs in goats or remain in a subclinical stage. Weight loss, poor milk production, anemia, and moderate coughing are possible clinical signs (Bernabé et al. 1991) but are nonspecific. Some goats also have firm nodular lesions in the udder.

Diagnosis

Diagnosis in living goats is ordinarily made by an intradermal tuberculin test, performed as for cattle. In the United States, only federal, state, and accredited veterinarians may perform a tuberculin test. A 26-gauge, 1-cm needle is used to inject 0.1 ml of PPD Bovis tuberculin intradermally in one tail fold. The test result is determined by observation and palpation at seventy-two (±6) hours (USDA 2006). Other countries may require injection of the tuberculin in the cervical skin, and this site is used in the United States for a comparative cervical test where the reaction to *M. bovis* antigen is compared to the reaction to *M. avium* antigen. False-positive skin tests may be seen in herds infected with or practicing vaccination against paratuberculosis, because of a potential for mycobacterial cross reactions. Numerous dual infections with the two mycobacterial species have been observed, however, in goats in Spain (Bernabé et al. 1991).

An appropriate serologic test may be helpful in confirming a diagnosis of tuberculosis in animals from herds that are also infected with paratuberculosis (Acosta et al. 2000). A bovine gamma interferon test for cell mediated response using bovine PPD was positive in one tuberculin skin test positive goat from which *M. bovis* was isolated but was also positive in twelve other skin test negative goats which were negative on culture (Cousins et al. 1993). Thus, the gamma interferon test may have poor specificity in exposed but apparently uninfected goats.

Various authors report caseation, calcification, and encapsulation of lesions in lymph nodes; in the parenchyma of the lung, liver, and spleen; and in the peritoneal and pleural cavities (Murray et al. 1921; Carmichael 1938; Bernabé et al. 1991). When caseous granulomas are found in the lungs at slaughter or at necropsy, histology (including acid fast stains) and culture are necessary to confirm the diagnosis. Other agents that might cause a similar pneumonia include *Yersinia pseudotuberculosis* (Rajagopalan and Sankaranarayanan 1944), *Burkholderia (Pseudomonas) pseudomallei, Rhodococcus equi* (Carrigan et al. 1988), and *Corynebacterium pseudotuberculosis.* Granulomatous pneumonia caused by the opportunist *Cryptococcus neoformans* together with *M. bovis* has been reported in a goat that was negative on intradermal and serologic tests for tuberculosis, suggesting an underlying immunodeficiency (Gutiérrez and García Marin 1999).

Control

Government regulations concerning herd quarantine and removal of infected animals must be followed. Cleaning and disinfection with Virkon® (Antech International) or a cresol product such as 5% phenol solution should be stressed, with special attention to feed troughs and water containers. Other livestock species on the premises and the human caretakers should be tested for tuberculosis. Milk fed to goats and humans should be pasteurized.

Melioidosis and Rhodococcal Pneumonia

Melioidosis is a disease in tropical regions caused by *Burkholderia (Pseudomonas) pseudomallei.* Infected goats may develop respiratory signs including coughing and dyspnea on exercise. Abscesses often form in external lymph nodes and lungs. Abscesses are frequently 2 to 5 mm in diameter (but may be larger) and may coalesce in the lungs. Abscess contents are white, cream colored, or greenish, and are viscous, caseous, or dry (Thomas et al. 1988). Affected animals are culled because of the danger of human infection. This condition is discussed in Chapter 3.

Disseminated *Rhodococcus equi* infection was identified in two goats, one of which had raised nodules in the lungs containing off-white caseous material arranged in concentric layers. An enteric route of entry was suspected because of extensive abscessation of the liver. The organism isolated appeared to lack virulence antigens normally present in strains pathogenic for foals (Davis et al. 1999). Similarly, rhodococcal pneumonia in a yearling Angora was confirmed by culture of *R. equi* from pulmonary abscesses that ranged from 0.5 to 4 cm in diameter and resembled the lesions of caseous lymphadenitis (Fitzgerald et al. 1994).

FUNGAL PNEUMONIA

Fungi rarely cause primary pneumonia in goats.

Cryptococcosis

Cryptococcus neoformans is a saprophytic fungus common in soil and in bird droppings. It is yeast-like when grown on Sabouraud's glucose agar. A halo-like capsule surrounds the single cell, which may be budding; this morphology is distinctive (Gillespie and Timoney 1988). Focal lesions have been found in the lungs of goats slaughtered in the West Indies (Sutmoller and Poelma 1957). The major loss seems to be associated with carcass condemnation. In Western Australia, cryptococcal pneumonia is reported to be associated with clinical signs that include nasal discharge, coughing, dyspnea and ill thrift (Baxendell 1988; Chapman et al. 1990). In Spain, affected goats had wasting and respiratory signs, but sometimes liver or brain was also involved (Baro et al. 1998). No effective, economical treatment has been developed.

Other Fungi

Although reports are few, other fungi can contribute to pneumonia in a goat that is immunosuppressed or that experiences inhalation of rumen contents. Animals that receive corticosteroids simultaneously with antibiotics may be at special risk.

Mycotic organisms isolated from goat lungs in slaughterhouse or necropsy studies include *Aspergillus fumigatus*, *A. flavus*, *Nocardia* spp., *Penicillium* spp., and *Candida* spp. (Ikede 1977; Pal and Dahiya 1987; Chattopadhyay et al. 1992). Grayish nodules in the lungs may be seen and observation of organisms in histologic sections of lung and lymph node confirms the nature of the lesion, but clinical significance is unknown.

ENZOOTIC PNEUMONIA

Enzootic pneumonia is an ill-defined term that has been applied to both acute exudative bronchopneumonia and to chronic, nonprogressive, pneumonic lesions found at slaughter or necropsy. Cranioventral lobes are typically affected; they are a darker red than the rest of the lung and are consolidated. It is often assumed that viruses or mycoplasma initiated the pneumonia but that only secondary bacteria such as *Pasteurella* and *Mannheimia* spp. and *Arcanobacterium* (previously *Actinomyces) pyogenes* can still be isolated from the lungs.

Enzootic pneumonia is also a term used to encompass a variety of lung infections occurring in stressed animals. The stress may be provided by malnutrition, shearing, a change in the weather (cold or rain), or the presence of other diseases. Coccidiosis, because of the malnutrition produced by this very common intestinal disease, could be a major predisposing factor for enzootic pneumonia. Increased levels of glucocorticoids then lower the animal's resistance to infection by adversely affecting both cellular and humoral immunity.

In a scenario similar to the shipping fever complex of cattle, it has been proposed that viruses interfere with macrophage function and with the ability of cilia in the tracheal mucosa to transport inhaled bacteria away from the lungs (i.e., mucociliary clearance) (Brogden et al. 1998). A variety of viruses have been incriminated in the process (Daft and Weidenbach 1987); in general, documentation of pathogenicity to goats is scanty. Research conducted with lambs, however, is assumed to be applicable to both species. Parainfluenza virus 3 (Obi and Ibu 1990) and several serotypes of adenovirus (Woods et al. 1991; Lehmkuhl et al. 1997) may participate in multifactorial pneumonic processes.

Some sheep flocks in the United States have used a half dose of PI3 or IBR-PI3 vaccine intranasally because parainfluenza 3 predisposes the sheep to pneumonia. All adults are vaccinated, and then lambs are vaccinated as soon after birth as possible (Lehmkuhl and Cutlip 1985; Rodger 1989). There has been apparent efficacy in some flocks, but a practitioner should certainly not recommend such a program in goats without first documenting the activity of the PI3 virus in the disease process to be combated, either by viral isolation or paired serology. It is also undesirable to inoculate goats or sheep with a live IBR vaccine because of the possibility that they will shed the virus later and thereby infect cattle or even become sick themselves with the bovine vaccine strain.

A respiratory syncytial virus distinct from bovine RSV also has been isolated from goats with severe coughing, oculonasal discharge, and fever (Lehmkuhl et al. 1980; Martin 1983), as discussed above.

Caprine herpesvirus (bovid herpesvirus type 6) has been isolated from the lungs and from nasal swabs of goats dying of *M. haemolytica* pneumonia (Buddle et al. 1990b). Experimental inoculation of the virus followed six days later by *M. haemolytica* resulted in pneumonia in five of six goats (Buddle et al. 1990a). *Mannheimia* alone also caused pneumonia (three of six), but the virus alone caused only catarrhal rhinitis and mild tracheitis. Thus, the role of this virus in producing pneumonia remains uncertain.

PARASITIC PNEUMONIA

Verminous pneumonia resulting from one or more species of lungworms occurs in most parts of the world. Liver flukes and tapeworm cysts have more restricted ranges.

Dictyocaulus Pneumonia

Etiology and Epidemiology

Although *Dictyocaulus filaria* is cosmopolitan, in many parts of the world this lungworm is not very common in goats. This may be caused in part by the tendency to keep young goats off pasture under intensive management systems. In India, sheep and goats graze the same infested pastures, and goats are believed to be more susceptible to the parasite (Dhar and Sharma 1978a).

Pathogenesis

Dictyocaulus filaria lungworms have a direct life cycle (Bowman et al. 2003; Panusaka 2006). Adults live in bronchi and are approximately 30 to 80 mm long. First-stage larvae approximately 550 µm long are coughed up and eliminated in the feces. Development to an infective stage takes one to two weeks. These third-stage larvae are long-lived in damp, cool surroundings. After ingestion, there is a one-month prepatent period and three months patency. Signs can occur as early as three weeks after the goats are put on pasture in the spring, but usually occur in autumn. Kids are most severely affected during their first season on pasture; age resistance is via prior exposure (Wilson 1970). The L4 can last the winter in lungs, but freezing kills larvae on pasture, as does a hot, dry summer.

Clinical Signs

The main sign during the prepatent period is polypnea; dyspnea develops later in the course of infection. The worms cause bronchial irritation, resulting in cough, moderate dyspnea, and loss of condition. Pathologic findings include bronchitis, bronchiolitis, atelectasis, and emphysema. Auscultable crackles and wheezes, fever, and toxemia occur if there is a secondary bacterial infection. Eosinophilia is marked in reexposed animals. An acute shock syndrome is seen when a significant reinfestation occurs after immunity has weakened.

Diagnosis

The diagnosis of verminous pneumonia is best done by the Baerman technique. Feces are collected fresh from the rectum to avoid confusion with *Strongyloides* larvae. Fecal pellets are put in a tea strainer or wrapped in gauze and half submerged in a funnel of warm 77.7°F (25°C) water; larvae fall to the neck of the funnel. A conical flask may provide a better yield than the traditional funnel system (McKenna 1999). The larvae are harvested after four to twenty hours and compared with photos in a parasitology text. The posterior is blunt in *Dictyocaulus*, whereas it is slender and pointed in *Protostrongylus* and has a definite dorsal spur in *Muellerius* (Bowman et al. 2003). Fecal exams for *Dictyocaulus* are positive during the patent period of the first infestation only.

Treatment and Control

Anthelmintics effective against *Dictyocaulus* are routinely used in goats, which probably decreases the prevalence of the disease. Treatments include tetramisole (15 mg/kg) (Kadhim et al. 1972) or levamisole (7.5 mg/kg) orally or subcutaneously. The drug is eliminated by the respiratory tract. Also reported to be effective are mebendazole (15 to 20 mg/kg), fenbendazole (5 to 10 mg/kg), febantel (5 mg/kg), and ivermectin (0.2 mg/kg). Owners should be advised not to sell milk or make it into cheese for at least four days after unapproved drugs are used. The milk withdrawal period for ivermectin should probably last at least nine days after oral use and forty days after subcutaneous injection (Baynes et al. 2000).

Treatment does not allow establishment of immunity, so goats should not be returned to infected pastures. Frequent pasture rotation is often an impractical means of control because moving the goats every four days would be required. Putting the goats out on pasture early in the season allows progressively increasing exposure and immunity. New goats should be separated from yearlings, and kids should not be placed on pastures inhabited by yearlings within the last year. The goats are treated after stabling in the fall (a warm, humid barn allows the cycle to continue) to limit pasture contamination next spring. Other suggestions include avoiding overpopulation, draining wet pastures, and replacing ponds with watering devices on concrete slabs. An irradiated *Dictyocaulus* larvae vaccine has protected goats against experimental challenge (Dhar and Sharma 1978b; Sharma 1994).

Protostrongylids

Etiology

Protostrongylid lungworms include at least five genera. Two are well recognized in the United States; *Muellerius capillaris* is diagnosed more frequently than *Protostrongylus rufescens*. Two more (*Cystocaulus ocreatus* and *Neostrongylus linearis*) are recognized in Europe and northern Africa (Genchi et al. 1984; Perreau and Cabaret 1984; Berrag and Urquhart 1996), while *Varestrongylus pneumonicus* (*Bicaulus schulzi*) is found in eastern Europe and India.

Epidemiology and Pathogenesis

All types have an indirect life cycle and use a variety of snails and slugs as intermediate hosts. The mollusks remain infective for at least one year. Goats and sheep become infected by eating mollusks or third-stage larvae liberated on foliage by death of the intermediate host.

Protostrongylus rufescens adults live in bronchi and are approximately 16 to 35 mm long. The first stage larvae are 370 to 400 μm long and have a pointed tail (Gerichter 1951). Massive infections are unlikely, and only kids show any clinical involvement.

Muellerius lungworms usually cause clinically insignificant focal lesions in the lung parenchyma. Adults are present twenty-five to thirty-eight days after infection (Panuska 2006). They are 12 to 23 mm long and located in subpleural alveoli, never in the bronchi. First stage larvae approximately 300 to 320 μm long (Gerichter 1951) with a distinctive dorsal spur on the tail (Figure 9.8) are passed in the feces if both sexes are present in the same nodule. The infestation is carried over from one year to the next in the goat. Fewer adult worms are established following reinfection but the inflammatory response in the lungs is much more severe (Berrag et al. 1997). Goats do not develop a marked age resistance, and in fact older animals often have heavier infections than those on pasture for only one season. This is in contrast to sheep, which tend to clear the infection.

At least forty species of snails and slugs serve as intermediate hosts for *Muellerius*. A French study found abundant *Helix aspersa* in spring and *Deroceras reticulatum* in autumn to be associated with an increased risk of infection in grazing goats (Cabaret et al. 1986). Almost any goat that has been on pasture in temperate regions of the United States has *Muellerius* larvae on Baerman examination (see above). In a Norwegian study, larvae were found in the feces of 447 out of 457 goats from seven flocks (Helle 1976).

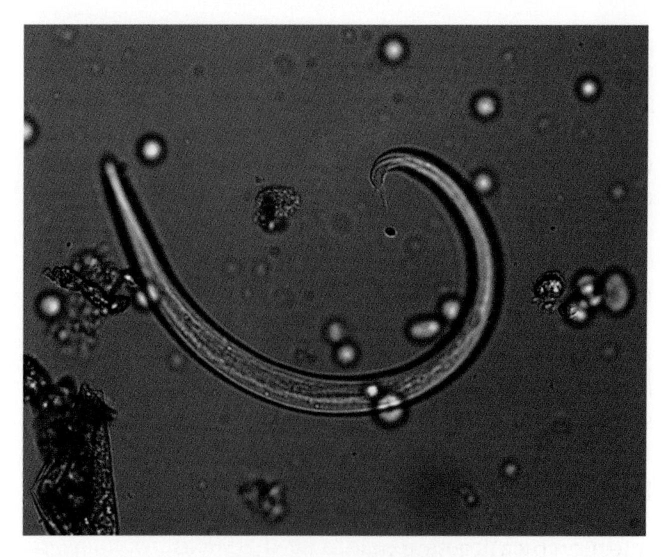

Figure 9.8. Larva of *Muellerius capillaris*, showing dorsal spur on tail. (Courtesy of A. Lucia-Forster.)

Cystocaulus ocreatus has a very similar life cycle to *Muellerius*. It also forms nodules in the lung parenchyma, and uses many of the same mollusks as intermediate hosts. The first stage larvae are 390 to 420 μm long. The larvae are identified by a distinctive tail tip with two appendages (Gerichter 1951). The two species may be found simultaneously in the same goat.

Clinical Signs and Necropsy Findings

Muellerius infestations are usually subclinical. However, there are scattered reports of serious, even fatal pneumonia resulting from heavy *Muellerius* infestations. For instance, Lloyd and Soulsby (1978) found twenty of twenty-four herds infected with *Muellerius*. Eighty-three percent of 169 goats in these herds were passing larvae, including 100% of goats three years of age or older. Dyspnea and a persistent cough were noticed in four adult goats with higher than average larval counts, suggesting that the parasite may be pathogenic in heavily infested goats. In a Swiss herd of CAE-free Saanen goats, all nine adults displayed coughing that abated only temporarily with anthelmintic treatment. Many *Muellerius* larvae were present in the feces of all and in several goats first stage larvae and neutrophils were demonstrated in an increased amount of viscid bronchial secretion by endoscopy (Braun et al. 2000). Hematology and serum biochemistry test results were unremarkable in these goats. A possible association of *Muellerius* with decreased body weight has been reported in New Zealand (Valero et al. 1992).

Lesions (firm tan nodules) are most common in the caudal dorsal lung lobes and are less well localized in goats than in sheep. A frequently cited report (Nimmo 1979) ascribed a diffuse thickening of alveolar septa with mononuclear cell infiltrates to *Muellerius*. That paper suggested that diffuse (non-nodular) lesions occurred in cases of reduced host resistance, because eosinophils were more prominent in focal nodular lesions. Because L1 larvae, eggs, and adult worms in "brood nodules" are readily identified in histologic preparations of the lung (Gregory et al. 1985), it must be remembered that other conditions (such as progressive retroviral pneumonia) must be excluded before ascribing a clinically important pneumonia to these parasites. Also worth considering is the possibility that *Muellerius* lungworms contribute to clinical retroviral infection by attracting many macrophages to the lungs (Ellis et al. 1988a).

Treatment

Recommended treatments for *Protostrongylus* include levamisole and fenbendazole at dosages used for *Dictyocaulus*.

Levamisole is not effective against *Muellerius*. When considering drugs and dosages for *Muellerius* given in the literature, it is not always evident if efficacy was determined by death of the protostrongylids or a temporary infertility of the worms (Cremers 1983). Two treatments with fenbendazole at 15 mg/kg, three weeks apart, relieved clinical signs and completely eliminated shedding of larvae two weeks later (Kazacos et al. 1981). Extended studies revealed that larval shedding resumed in most goats by seven weeks after 30 mg/kg fenbendazole (Bliss and Greiner 1985). Another study found that shedding of larvae resumed many weeks after treatment with either fenbendazole or ivermectin; 25% of ivermectin-treated animals resumed shedding from four to more than nine weeks later. The authors assumed that immature *Muellerius* in the lungs resumed development after death of adult worms (McCraw and Menzies 1986, 1988). Treatment at approximately thirty-five-day intervals has been suggested. Topical eprinomectin at 0.5 mg/kg has been shown to prevent larval shedding for six weeks or maybe more (Geurden and Vercruysse 2007). Netobimin at 20 mg/kg (once orally or divided into two or three doses) failed to completely eliminate shedding or kill all adult *Muellerius* at day eighteen (Cabaret 1991). For other drugs such as mebendazole (20 to 40 mg/kg) and oxyfendazole (7.5 to 10 mg/kg) (Cabaret et al. 1984), the dose suggested is typically double that used for digestive strongyles.

Control

In Scandinavia, a protocol has been developed to specifically control *Muellerius* in goats. During the period when the goats are stabled and not lactating, fenbendazole is fed at 2 mg/kg/day for fourteen days. Prolonged low-level treatment reduces larval shedding for five to seven months (Helle 1986). This treatment is believed to decrease the prevalence of coughing and increase subsequent milk production and bodyweight gains (Hammarberg 1992). The possible teratogenic effects of anthelmintics have not been well studied in goats, and it is prudent to avoid treatment during the first thirty-five days of pregnancy. Also, such a treatment program should not be undertaken when the goats are on pasture, because it might select for resistant gastrointestinal parasites.

Wet, undrained pastures should be avoided. It may be helpful to prevent grazing in early morning or evening when the herbage is damp and snails are up and about. It is best to treat before pasture season in the spring, to prevent contamination of mollusks. A second treatment in early fall is used in heavily contaminated environments.

Eimeria and Other Protozoa

A persistent cough is often associated with severe coccidial infection in young kids, though no adequate explanation has been advanced. The connection may be only that kids stressed by the poor nutritional state that accompanies coccidiosis are more prone to bacterial pneumonia. Prophylaxis includes keeping kids out of feeders, separate from adults, and in a dry environment. A systemically absorbed sulfonamide would be reasonable treatment for such kids.

There is a single case report of the presence of cysts and trophozoites of *Balantidium coli* in the lungs of a goat with interstitial pneumonia and *Dictyocaulus filaria* larvae (Parodi et al. 1985). Because this ciliated protozoon normally inhabits the large intestine, it might have been carried to the lungs by lungworm larvae.

Pneumocystis carinii was found filling the alveolar air spaces of a four-month-old Boer goat with severe diffuse interstitial pneumonia (McConnell et al. 1971). In other species, at least, this organism is usually associated with immunosuppressive conditions.

Besnoitia cysts (diameter 60 to 280 μ) were reported in the alveolar septa of the lungs of two adult goats from Kenya with purulent necrotizing bacterial pneumonia (Kaliner 1973). It has been proposed that the species of *Besnoitia* infecting goats, *B. caprae*, is distinct from that infecting cattle, at least in Kenya (Njenga et al. 1993).

Echinococcosis, Hydatidosis

Echinococcus granulosus hydatid cysts occur in goats in many parts of the world, especially Mediterranean countries, India (Upadhyaya 1983), and Africa. Dogs are the definitive host and herbivores or humans are intermediate hosts. Goats appear to be less susceptible to infection than sheep in a given area, possibly because browsing causes less exposure to dog feces than does grazing (Rausch 1995). Cysts are most often observed in liver and lungs in goats (Pandey 1971; Perreau and Cabaret 1984), and the condition is discussed in greater detail in Chapter 11. Transplacental infection is possible. The cysts can be as large as a fist but are typically pea- to plum-size. The surface of the lung is distorted by focal collapse and emphysema. Older goats have more and larger cysts. They rarely cause specific clinical signs. No practical treatment has been found effective against the parasite in goats (Thompson and Allsopp 1988).

Prevention of zoonotic infection requires breaking the cycle between definitive and intermediate hosts (Gemmell 1979). All dogs should be treated (preferably with praziquantel) and feces passed after treatment should be destroyed. Eggs excreted in feces of dogs remain infective for at least one year. Wild dogs must be controlled. Access by dogs to carcasses of ruminants that die or are slaughtered on the farm or at the local slaughterhouse must be prevented. These measures are very difficult to enforce. More recently, vaccination of ruminants using a recombinant oncosphere peptide combined with twice-a-year dog dosing has shown promise (Craig and Larrieu 2006). Lambs and sheep are vaccinated twice at a one month interval, with a booster six to twelve months later. Reports of the use of this vaccine in goats are not yet available.

The dog tapeworm *Taenia multiceps* (*Multiceps gaigeri*) has also caused cysts within the thoracic and abdominal cavities and in muscles of goats in the Sudan (Hago and Abu-Samra 1980).

Liver Flukes

Both *Fasciola hepatica* and *Fascioloides magna* occasionally invade the lung. Their large size and the dark pigment that often accompanies them make the diagnosis at necropsy simple. Accompanying liver disease would be expected to overshadow any clinical signs originating from the lungs.

Schistosomosis

Pulmonary schistosomosis (*Schistosoma indicum*) has been reported in goats in India (Sharma and Dwivedi 1976a; Dadhich and Sharma 1996). Granulomas occur diffusely throughout the lung where adult parasites have laid eggs in pulmonary vessels. Emaciation and dyspnea may occur. The lesions grossly resemble retroviral interstitial pneumonia. Schistosomosis is discussed in Chapter 8.

INHALATION PNEUMONIA

Inhalation or aspiration of feed, saliva, or medication causes a cough and a nonspecific pneumonia from which a mixture of organisms can often be isolated. Unless foreign material such as a plant awn (King 1989), feed particles, or mineral oil is found in the affected lung at necropsy, the true etiology of the pneumonia may be overlooked.

Nutritional Muscular Dystrophy

Aspiration is a common sequela to nutritional muscular dystrophy (white muscle disease) in rapidly growing, well-fed kids. These kids cough after drinking and milk may appear at the nostrils because of weakness of the muscles of deglutition in the pharynx and tongue. Other animals in the herd may show stiffness, heart failure, dandruff, or off-flavored milk. A subcutaneous injection of vitamin E and selenium is reasonable adjunctive therapy for any kid with pneumonia. The diagnosis and prevention of nutritional muscular dystrophy are discussed in detail in Chapters 4 and 19.

Iatrogenic Inhalation Pneumonia

Although cleft palate and inadequate function of pharyngeal and laryngeal muscles due to nutritional muscular dystrophy can occur in very young kids, improper force feeding is a common cause of inhalation in this age group. It is far better for a kid to be tube-fed (see Chapter 19) than for milk to be dripped or squirted into the mouth of a kid that is unable to swallow.

Errors in administration of medication (e.g., anthelmintic drench, propylene glycol, mineral oil) can cause inhalation pneumonia. Dyspnea, cyanosis, mild fever or subnormal temperature, nasal discharge, mild coughing, crackles, and wheezes are often noted within a few hours after improper drenching. A radiograph reveals a ground glass appearance of involved areas of the lung (Ahuja et al. 1985).

When eliciting a complete history, it is prudent to ask if anything has been given orally before questioning the carefulness of administration. If surgery has been recently performed by another veterinarian, that veterinarian rather than the owner should be asked if a cuffed endotracheal tube was used. Proper positioning of the anesthetized goat so that the thorax is above the abdomen and the head hangs lower than the neck usually avoids inhalation problems when use of an endotracheal tube is not possible.

Neurologic Causes of Dysphagia

Any neurologic disease that interferes with the goat's ability to swallow can cause secondary pneumonia. The most common of these are listeriosis and caprine arthritis encephalitis, but pituitary abscess, cerebrospinal nematodiasis, and botulism are other possibilities.

Plant Poisoning

Plant poisoning with members of the heath family (*Ericaceae*), including rhododendrons, laurels, and Japanese pieris, produces a syndrome of abdominal discomfort that normally includes vomiting as a prominent sign (Knight and Walker 2001). Goats that have received a sublethal dose of the toxic principles, grayanotoxins, may develop inhalation pneumonia subsequent to vomiting. Therefore, prophylactic antibiotics are indicated when poisoning with these plants occurs. Consumption of sneezeweeds (*Helenium* and *Dugaldia* spp.), bitterweed (*Hymenoxys* spp.), and desert baileya (*Baileya multiradiata*) on ranges in the western United States has also produced inhalation pneumonia in sheep and goats (Knight and Walker 2001).

GENERAL CONSIDERATIONS REGARDING TREATMENT AND PROPHYLAXIS OF PNEUMONIA

Antibiotic therapy should be begun with a drug that is normally effective against the organisms suspected to be present in the pneumonic process. Anthelmintics should also be given if verminous pneumonia is suspected.

Choice of Antibiotic and Duration of Therapy

Initial treatment is usually determined by the practitioner's previous experiences. If a culture and sensitivity report is available from a tracheal aspirate or a necropsy, the choice of the antibiotic should be guided by that report. Commonly, however, additional or different organisms are involved in the pneumonia. The practitioner should re-evaluate the patient after forty-eight hours. If a definite response to therapy has not occurred (i.e., decreased fever, improved appetite and demeanor), another antibiotic should be chosen and administered for forty-eight hours. When a response is obtained, the effective drug should be continued until at least forty-eight hours after the goat is clinically normal. This means a minimum of four to five days of therapy for any goat with pneumonia. On the other hand, weeks of treatment are generally not possible because of the pain and mental anguish most goats suffer during a prolonged series of injections. Mycotic pneumonia is also a possible sequela to prolonged antibiotic use.

Ideally, any sick animal receiving treatment should be removed from the herd and kept in isolation facilities. This often is not possible, or the owner refuses to put forth the required effort. In such herds it is important to mark the sick animal so that it can be relocated after it is clinically healthy; otherwise, an adequate duration of therapy will rarely be achieved.

Drug Dosage and Extralabel Use

The dosage rate should be enough to achieve the tissue levels in the lungs that are necessary for the desired antimicrobial effect. When this dose is increased or is given more frequently than labeled dosage rates, or when the drug is not approved for goats, the practitioner must deal with government regulations regarding extralabel drug use. The animal to be treated must be carefully examined by the veterinarian, and provision must be made for prolonged withdrawal periods to prevent contamination of milk or meat for human consumption. In the United States, all goats of all breeds are defined by the Food and Drug Administration as food animals, which limits the choice of legal antibiotics (fluoroquinolones are forbidden). Routine milk and urine antibiotic residue tests after treatment are recommended because pharmacokinetic data for goats to establish withholding times is rarely available (Lofstedt 1987).

Routes of Administration

Except for sulfonamides and lesser doses of tetracyclines, oral use of antimicrobial drugs generally leads to severe systemic illness by interfering with rumen flora. In addition, sick animals usually do not eat or drink well enough to dependably consume medication in feed or water. It is the personal preference of the author to give most antibiotics by subcutaneous injection. Painful muscle necrosis is thereby avoided, as is paralysis from accidental injection into the sciatic nerve. There are several caveats with subcutaneous injections. First, sterile abscesses sometimes occur and can be confused with caseous lymphadenitis. Therefore, injection ahead of the shoulder should be avoided in show goats. Second, the pharmacokinetic disposition of most drugs in goats has not been studied after subcutaneous administration and residue persistence is apt to be erratic. Third, subcutaneous injection of a drug labeled only for intramuscular use is an extralabel use of that drug, even if the government-approved dosage is used.

Supportive Therapy

Many supportive drugs have been used to treat pneumonia. Naturally, a drug effective against lungworms should be administered if historical or laboratory findings suggest parasite involvement. In general, vitamins (including vitamin E and selenium) are part of the routine regimen. Bronchodilators and nonsteroidal anti-inflammatory drugs probably have a place in select cases, but proper dosages have not been determined scientifically. Corticosteroids are best avoided because they increase the frequency of relapse when treatment is discontinued. If an antipyretic agent has been administered (such as acetylsalicylic acid

100 mg/kg orally twice daily or flunixin intravenously, intramuscularly, or orally at 2.2 mg/kg, Königsson et al. 2003), body temperature cannot be used as an indicator of response to antimicrobial therapy. Exudates should not be allowed to obstruct the nares, and aromatic oils can be tried if rapid production of mucus is adding to the distress of the goat. The goat should be kept comfortable with a coat in cold weather, fan under very hot conditions, dry bedding, and good food and water within easy reach.

Pneumonia Prophylaxis

Prophylaxis of pneumonia, except of contagious mycoplasma pneumonia, is almost never through vaccination. Instead, careful attention must be paid to proper ventilation, housing, and nutrition. An increased colostrum intake should be encouraged and dry bedding provided for kids. In cold climates, supplying newborn kids with wool body socks prevents chilling without interfering with barn ventilation. Angora and Cashmere kids should not be shorn during inclement weather and supplemental feed may be required after shearing. When animals must be worked in a dry and dusty corral, wetting down the area with a 5% formalin solution has been proposed to decrease the quantities of both irritant dust and infectious microorganisms inhaled by the goats. Crowding must be avoided.

Strict isolation of purchased animals or those stressed by traveling and showing is also important. The etiology of the febrile illness accompanied by coughing that frequently sweeps through a goat herd after a show is rarely identified. Viruses, mycoplasmas, chlamydia, and pasteurellosis are possible suspects. One approach to handling the herd is to administer tetracycline or tylosin to goats that are off feed or febrile. Close observation, good feed, and good ventilation suffice if the animals are eating well.

In some instances, specific infectious diseases are controlled by separating kids from adults and feeding heat-treated colostrum and pasteurized milk. Pooled milk from other goats at a show should not be fed to members of one's own herd.

PULMONARY EDEMA AND PLEURITIS

The signs associated with pulmonary edema include dyspnea, increased bronchial sounds, crackles, and cough. Thus, it may be difficult to distinguish the condition from a pleuritis or pneumonia of infectious origin. In severe cases of edema, froth may appear at the mouth and nares. Various gastrointestinal diseases discussed in Chapter 10 can cause severe hypoproteinemia and subsequent hydrothorax and pulmonary edema.

Anaphylaxis and Fluid Therapy

Acute lung edema may be caused by an anaphylactic reaction to, for example, a serum or vaccine product. Emergency treatment measures for such an animal include epinephrine (1 ml of 1:1,000 strength per 50 kg), the diuretic furosemide (5 mg/kg), and possibly atropine (100 µg/kg) (Black 1986). If the edema occurs during the course of intravenous fluid therapy, the fluids should be temporarily discontinued and furosemide administered.

Cardiac Disease

Pulmonary edema may occur with severe exertion (as when chased by dogs), heart failure (i.e., because of white muscle disease, ionophore coccidiostats, or toxic plants), or a congenital heart defect. Vitamin E and selenium and symptomatic therapy such as diuretics are indicated.

Pulmonary Disease

Edema may occur in pneumonias caused by many of the infectious and parasitic agents already discussed. It is quite pronounced in certain other conditions affecting the lungs.

Toxic Gases and 3-methylindole

Toxic gases, particularly hydrogen sulfide, can cause pulmonary edema, but goats are rarely exposed to high levels of gases under normal housing conditions. Ruminal administration of 3-methylindole, a metabolite of L-tryptophan, causes severe pulmonary edema and respiratory distress and moderate emphysema in goats (Carlson et al 1972; Dickinson et al. 1976; Huang et al. 1977; Mesina et al. 1984). It is uncertain if this toxin causes naturally occurring disease in goats.

Cor Pulmonale

Chronic edema occasionally occurs along with cor pulmonale in severe long-term lung diseases such as progressive pneumonia and adenomatosis (Gay and Richards 1983). Goats thus affected also have ascites. Treatment is unrewarding.

Heartwater

In endemic areas (sub-Saharan Africa, Caribbean), infection with the tick-borne rickettsia *Ehrlichia (Cowdria) ruminantium* (heartwater) may cause hydrothorax and pulmonary edema because of increased capillary permeability. In addition to dyspnea, clinical signs may include fever, central nervous system dysfunction, and death (Brown and Skowronek 1990). Edema of other organs such as lymph nodes and brain also occurs (Mebus and Logan 1988). Organisms may be demonstrated in endothelial scrapings of the aorta and jugular vein or in capillaries in histologic sections or smears of the brain, as discussed in Chapter 8.

Pleuritis

Mannheimiosis, pasteurellosis, and mycoplasmosis are the most common causes of pleuritis in goats. Infections resulting in abscessation, such as caseous lymphadenitis, can also result in pleuritis if an abscess ruptures into the pleural cavity.

Of special note is the condition of sternal abscess or osteomyelitis. Goats that spend much time recumbent, as with arthritis, may develop a chronic draining tract over the sternum. Radiography is important in offering a prognosis, because if the infection extends between ribs or through sternebrae into the chest (Figure 4.8), neither antibiotic nor surgical treatment is likely to be effective. Such animals have enlargement of sternal lymph nodes and, commonly, pleuritis.

PULMONARY AND THYMIC NEOPLASIA

The most commonly reported neoplasm in the chest of the adult goat is the thymoma (Figure 9.9). Clinical signs of thymoma may include dyspnea and muffled lung sounds, often unilaterally. However, some animals develop congestive heart failure (Rostkowski et al. 1985; Hanselaer 1988) or rumen tympany and megaesophagus (Parish et al. 1996). Either radiographic or ultrasonographic findings of a mediastinal mass, which may be cystic, support the diagnosis, although an abscess could have a similar appearance (Hanselaer 1988). Some affected animals have copious thoracic fluid, which obscures the mass and contains normal lymphocytes. Either epithelial or lymphocytic cells may predominate in the tumor, but the neoplastic cell population is the epithelial cell. Asymptomatic thymomas have been reported in both female and castrated male Saanen goats (Hadlow 1978).

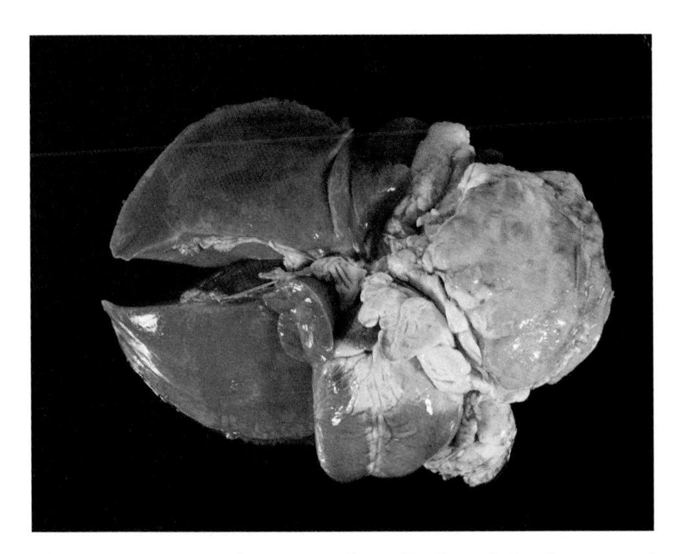

Figure 9.9. Large thymoma that displaced the heart and lungs caudally. (Courtesy Dr. M.C. Smith.)

Lymphosarcoma produced nodular lesions in the lung parenchyma of six of eleven goats in one necropsy study. Only two of these six animals had been reported to by dyspneic antemortem (Craig et al. 1986). Another goat with pulmonary lymphosarcoma detected radiographically was initially believed to have pulmonary nocardiosis originating from a chronic mastitis (Rozear et al. 1998). A viral-induced neoplasm of the lung has been discussed under the topic of jaagsiekte (see above). Although rarely reported, other primary or metastatic lung tumors might be found occasionally in older goats. In one eight-year-old Alpine wether, a thymoma metastasized to the lungs and spleen (Olchowy et al. 1996).

PLANT POISONINGS CAUSING ACUTE RESPIRATORY SIGNS

Perilla frutescens (perilla mint) and moldy sweet potatoes can be expected to produce severe pulmonary edema, emphysema, and adenomatosis in goats, as in other ruminants (Linnabary et al. 1978; Belknap 2002). There is no specific therapy, and exertion by affected animals may precipitate death. Dyspnea may be a prominent sign associated with cardiotoxic effects of avocado (*Persea*) (Sani et al. 1991) or other plants discussed in Chapter 8. *Acacia nilotica* subsp. *kraussiana* causes methemoglobinemia, hemolysis, anoxia, and dyspnea that may be severe enough to cause abortion or death (Terblance et al. 1967).

Even though cyanide and nitrate toxicities are conditions that interfere with cellular respiration rather than affecting the respiratory tract per se, the severe dyspnea associated with these poisonings suggests respiratory tract disease.

Cyanide Poisoning

Hydrocyanic acid (HCN), or prussic acid, is present as a glycoside in certain plants. Hydrolysis in the course of wilting, frosting, or digestion within the rumen releases free HCN. A plant enzyme, glycosidase, hydrolyzes the terminal glucose on a cyanogenic glycoside such as amygdalin, producing the aglycone compound hydroxynitrile. Another enzyme catalyzes a further breakdown into HCN and benzaldehyde (Conn 1978). The cyanide is absorbed directly from the rumen.

Etiology and Epidemiology

A variety of plants are potentially cyanogenic; the level of HCN can be affected by genetic selection. Immature or rapidly growing plants, and plants heavily fertilized with nitrogen, tend to have higher concentrations of cyanogenic glycosides. Damage to the plants by drought, wilting, frosting, or chewing increases toxicity because glycoside and enzyme combine more rapidly. Other ingesta in the rumen may react with cyanide and prevent absorption.

There are few reports of cyanide poisoning in goats (Webber et al. 1985; Shaw 1986; van der Westhuysen et al. 1988; Gough 1995; Tegzes et al. 2003; Radi et al. 2004), but toxicity levels should be comparable with those reported in other ruminants. The goat's propensity for browsing and for escaping from enclosures increases the potential hazard of cyanogenic shrubs and trees. A list of some potentially toxic plants follows.

- *Cynodon* spp. (quick grass, star grass)
- *Eucalyptus cladocalyx* (sugar gum)
- *Heteromeles arbutifolia* (toyon, California holly)
- *Linum* (flax)
- *Lotus corniculatus* (birdsfoot trefoil)
- *Manihot esculenta* (cassava)
- *Phaseolus lunatus* (lima bean [tropical varieties])
- *Prunus* spp. (cherries, apricots, peaches)
- *Pyrus malus* (apple)
- *Sambucus canadensis* (elderberry)
- *Sorghum* spp. (Sudan grass, Johnson grass)
- *Suckleya suckleyana* (poison suckleya)
- *Triglochin maritima* (arrow grass)
- *Trifolium repens* (white clover)
- *Zea mays* (corn)

Pathogenesis and Clinical Signs

The cyanide ion binds to the ferric ion in cytochrome oxidase, yielding a stable complex that cannot transport electrons in the process whereby O_2 is used in metabolic respiration. Oxygen is not released from hemoglobin in the blood and thus is not available within cells; cellular asphyxiation occurs. The oxygen-laden blood is bright red but the animal rapidly becomes severely dyspneic. Cerebral anoxia leads to the clinical signs; initial excitement and muscle tremors are followed by gasping and convulsions. Pupils are dilated. Signs are generally peracute, with death occurring within fifteen minutes to a few hours after plant consumption.

Diagnosis

Venous blood is bright red in peracute cases but cyanosis of mucous membranes supervenes if death is delayed. There may be an odor of "bitter almond" because of benzaldehyde in the rumen contents. Feed, blood, rumen contents, liver, or muscle tissue may be analyzed. Quick freezing or immersing in 1% to 3% mercuric chloride prevents additional release and loss of HCN from the sample. Levels in plants of 200 mg/kg HCN or more are considered potentially toxic, and with cyanide, toxic usually means lethal. A field test using picrate paper has been described (Kingsbury 1964; Radostits et al. 2007), but this detects cyanide at less than the toxic level. Other causes of sudden death (see Chapter 16) must be considered.

Treatment

Because death occurs so rapidly (often in two to three minutes), treatment is rarely possible. However, prompt intravenous injection of sodium nitrite (22 mg/kg) converts some hemoglobin to methemoglobin, which preferentially picks up CN ions from the cytochrome oxidase enzymes. Simultaneous sodium thiosulfate (67 mg/kg) converts cyanide to stable, less toxic thiocyanate. More recently, an increased intravenous dosage of sodium thiosulfate (660 mg/kg) has been proposed (Burrows and Way 1979). Oral or intraruminal sodium thiosulfate (perhaps 6 g to a large goat) at hourly intervals is recommended to fix free HCN in the rumen of affected or exposed animals.

Nitrate Poisoning

Ruminant digestion converts ingested nitrates to nitrites and then reduces the nitrites to ammonia. Nitrite is considered to be ten times more toxic than nitrate (Kingsbury 1964; El Bahri et al. 1997).

Etiology and Epidemiology

Atmospheric nitrogen is converted to nitrate (NO_3^-) by nitrogen fixing bacteria, including those associated with the roots of certain plants such as legumes. The plants can then reduce nitrates to nitrites and eventually convert the nitrogen into plant protein. Animal wastes (urea and ammonia) can also enter into the nitrogen cycle.

Animals most often consume excess nitrates by eating plants containing increased nitrate concentrations. Water contaminated with animal wastes or runoff from fertilized fields and direct consumption of fertilizers are other possible sources. Sources of nitrate are cumulative. Some plants that may accumulate toxic levels of nitrates are listed below.

- *Amaranthus* (pigweed [Agouroudis et al. 1985])
- *Avena sativa* (oats)
- *Beta vulgaris* (beet)
- *Chenopodium* spp. (lambsquarters, goosefoot)
- *Medicago sativa* (alfalfa)
- *Sorghum* spp. (Sudan grass, Johnson grass)
- *Zea mays* (corn)

Heavily fertilized soils make more nitrates available for plant uptake. Uptake is also favored by acid and moist soils, soils deficient in certain minerals (molybdenum, phosphorus, or sulfur), and low temperatures. Rapidly growing plants after drought or hormonal herbicide application accumulate increased nitrates. Finally, decreased light results in accumulation of nitrates within plants because nitrate reductase enzyme requires light for normal activity. Nitrates accumulate in vegetative tissue rather than fruits or grains, and nitrate levels in the whole plant decrease rapidly after flowering and setting of fruit. Corn, for instance, is not dangerous after tasseling out.

Pathogenesis and Clinical Signs

Nitrate toxicity is caused by nitrite formation within the rumen or, occasionally, in ensiled forages. Starved animals are at greatest risk because they are less selective grazers. Also, active rumen microorganisms supplied with rapidly digestible carbohydrates (the well-fed animal) can convert nitrates to microbial protein and thereby escape toxicity.

Nitrite is absorbed from the rumen. The nitrite causes oxidation of ferrous hemoglobin to ferric hemoglobin (methemoglobin) that cannot transport oxygen. The blood turns a dark, chocolate brown color. In addition to cyanosis, clinical signs include weakness, trembling, severe dyspnea, and frothing at the mouth.

Clinical signs are visible when 30% to 40% of the hemoglobin is converted to methemoglobin. Death occurs at 80% to 90% conversion, although this is influenced by stress and exertion. Death usually occurs within twelve to twenty-four hours after ingestion.

Plants containing more than 1% nitrates (as KNO_3) on a dry weight basis and water with more than 1,500 ppm nitrates may cause acute toxicity (Osweiler et al. 1985). Toxicity to goats caused by low-level nitrate exposure has not been described (Mondal et al. 1999).

Diagnosis

Unless there is a history of direct nitrate consumption (e.g., with fertilizer), diagnosis usually requires laboratory confirmation. Dark brown blood and cyanotic membranes indicate the need for methemoglobin determination. Use of a phosphate buffer as a preservative is recommended if testing of heparinized blood will be delayed longer than a few hours (Osweiler et al. 1985). Nitrate levels may be determined in feed, water, rumen contents, or body fluids (including aqueous humor). Nitrite is converted to nitrate very rapidly after death and is often undetectable in field specimens (Boermans 1990). Samples should be preserved by freezing.

Treatment

If nitrate toxicity is likely and respiratory signs are present, the clinician should not delay therapy while awaiting laboratory confirmation. Affected animals are treated intravenously with 4 to 15 mg/kg of methylene blue as a 1% solution in distilled water (Burrows 1984; Mondal and Pandey 2000); this is repeated if necessary. The methylene blue is reduced in blood and body tissues to leucomethylene blue, which in turn rapidly reduces methemoglobin to hemoglobin. When methylene blue is given intravenously to goats, it passes readily into the milk (Ziv and Heavner 1984). Another injectable dye, tolonium chloride, has also been used successfully to treat goats with experimental nitrate toxicity (Mondal and Pandey 2000).

Ruminal lavage with cold water or administration of oral antibiotics or a laxative may decrease additional ruminal reduction of nitrate to nitrite.

DEVOCALIZATION

Certain goats bleat almost continuously when separated from something they want, such as human companionship, or during estrus. Providing the goat with a pen mate (another goat or sheep, a cat, or even a pony) may alleviate the problem. Ovariectomy (see Chapter 13) may solve the problem of vocalization during estrus. In other cases the goat persists in its vocalizations, and the family, the neighbors, or the research group threatens mayhem. Displeased neighbors are especially dangerous to suburban goats because most zoning laws classify the pet wether as livestock. Under these circumstances, surgical removal of the vocal cords is justified.

Two techniques of devocalization are described in the literature and summarized here. Anesthetic agents that might be used include xylazine/ketamine and barbiturates. These are discussed in detail in Chapter 17. Atropine (0.08 mg/kg) administered intramuscularly twenty minutes before induction of anesthesia is recommended to decrease salivation (Tillman and Brooks 1983).

Traditional Surgical Technique

For the older surgical approach (Durant 1974), the goat is positioned in dorsal recumbency with the head lower than the neck. This is achieved by placing a sand bag beneath the neck. Food should be withheld for twenty-four hours and water for six hours before surgery; it is not possible to use a cuffed endotracheal tube to prevent regurgitation and aspiration during the surgery. Skin over the larynx is prepared as for an equine roarer operation. A midline skin incision 35 to 40 mm long is made, with careful attention to hemostasis. The first tracheal ring is incised and that incision is carried forward on the midline through the cricoid cartilage and crico-thyroid ligament to but not through the anterior border of the larynx (see Figure 9.10a). A small divider is used to spread the larynx and expose the vocal cords. Each cord (about 6 mm long) is clamped and removed down to the surface of the cartilage with curved scissors. After hemostasis is achieved the divider is removed and the skin incision closed.

Electrosurgical Technique

The second technique involves electrosurgical destruction of the vocal cords via the oral cavity (Tillman and Brooks 1983). The anesthetized

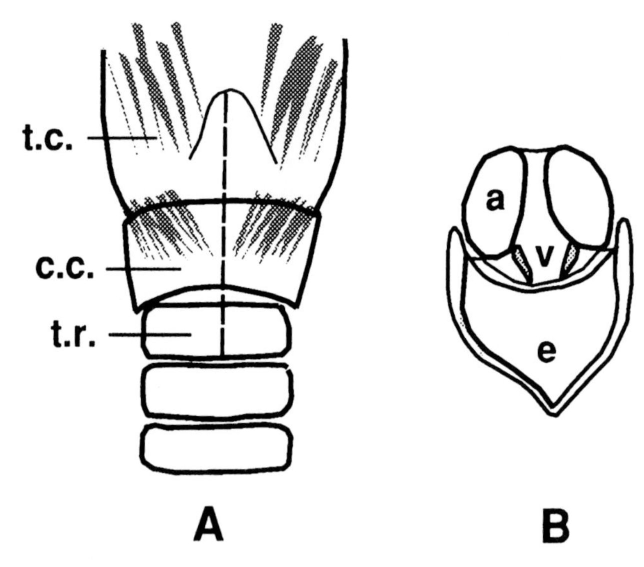

Figure 9.10. Removal of the vocal folds for devocalization. (a) Ventral view of larynx showing initial incision through cartilages of larynx. (b) Larynx as viewed from oral cavity.
a = arytenoid cartilage, v = vocal folds, e = epiglottis, t.r. = first tracheal ring, c.c. = cricoid cartilage, t.c. = thyroid cartilage.

(ketamine/xylazine) goat is placed in sternal recumbency with its chest on the ground plate of an electrocautery unit. A 38-cm tonsil snare arm (without the snare wires) is allowed to protrude 2 to 3 mm from its insulating sheath and is used as a long electrode. A long laryngoscope blade for ruminants (Soper laryngoscope blade 257 or 385 mm, Penlon Ltd., Abingdon, England) is also needed. The goat's head and neck are fully extended by an assistant and the tip of the laryngoscope blade is used to depress the epiglottis. The vocal cords are positioned just posterior to the arytenoid cartilage. They are much smaller than the arytenoids and almost meet ventrally, forming a "V" (Figure 9.10b). Using a coagulation setting, each vocal fold is pressed against the wall of the larynx (5 o'clock and 7 o'clock positions). The energized cautery tip is drawn forward over the vocal fold for a distance of about 1 cm, although closure of the larynx usually prevents visualization while this is being done. The aim is to create scar tissue to prevent elevation of the vocal fold; cautery is repeated if the first attempt has not cauterized an adequate area to ensure this result. Recovery from the adverse effects of surgery takes only a few days, and voice loss is permanent. Devocalization by carbon dioxide laser surgery, as done in dogs, has apparently not been described in goats.

REFERENCES

Abu Elzein, E.M.E., et al.: Isolation of peste des petits ruminants from goats in Saudi Arabia. Vet. Rec., 127:309–310, 1990.

Acosta, B., et al.: Isolation of *Mycobacterium kansasii* from a tuberculin-positive goat. Vet. Rec., 142:195–196, 1998.

Acosta, B., et al.: ELISA for anti-MPB70: an option for the diagnosis of goat tuberculosis caused by *Mycobacterium bovis*. Aust. Vet. J., 78:423–424, 2000.

Ahuja, A., Mathur, P.D. and Sharma, S.N.: Clinical and roentgenological diagnosis of caprine respiratory disease. Indian J. Vet. Med., 5(2):84–87, 1985.

Al-Momani, W., et al.: The in vitro effect of six antimicrobials against *Mycoplasma putrefaciens*, *Mycoplasma mycoides* subsp. *mycoides* LC and *Mycoplasma capricolum* subsp. *capricolum* isolated from sheep and goats in Jordan. Trop. Anim. Health Prod., 38:1–7, 2006.

Angen, O., et al.: Taxonomic relationships of the (*Pasteurella*) *haemolytica* complex as evaluated by DNA-DNA hybridizations and 16S rRNA sequencing with proposal of *Mannheimia haemolytica* gen. nov., comb. nov., *Mannheimia granulomatis* comb. nov., *Mannheimia glucosida* sp. nov., *Mannheimia ruminalis* sp. nov. and *Mannheimia varigena* sp. nov. Int. J. Syst. Bacteriol., 49:67–86, 1999.

Arguroudis, S., Spais, A.G. and Emmanouilidis, I.: (Poisoning in goats by *Amaranthus* plants rich in nitrates.) Ellenike Kteniatrike 28:1–7, 1985. Abstract 7361 in Vet. Bull., 55:904, 1985.

Baalsrud, K.J.: Atrophic rhinitis in goats in Norway. Vet. Rec., 121:350–353, 1987.

Bakima, M., Gustin, P., Lekeux, P. and Lomba, F.: Mechanics of breathing in goats. Res. Vet. Sci., 45:332–336, 1988.

Bakima, M., Lomba, F. and Lekeux, P.: Growth-related changes in the pulmonary function of goats. Vet. Res. Commun., 14:141–146, 1990.

Baro, T., et al.: First identification of autochthonous *Cryptococcus neoformans* var. *gattii* isolated from goats with predominantly severe pulmonary disease in Spain. J. Clin. Microbiol., 36:458–461, 1998.

Bates, D.W. and Anderson, J.F.: Calculation of ventilation needs for confined cattle. J. Am. Vet. Med. Assoc., 174:581–589, 1979.

Baxendell, S.A.: The Diagnosis of the Diseases of Goats. Vade Mecum Series for Domestic Animals Series B, No. 9, Univ. of Sydney Post-Grad. Foundation in Vet. Sci., Sydney, Australia, 1988.

Baynes, R.E. et al.: Extralabel use of ivermectin and moxidectin in food animals. J. Am. Vet. Med. Assoc., 217:668–671, 2000.

Bechtol, D.T., Ballinger, R.T. and Sharp, A.J.: Field trial of a *Pasteurella haemolytica* toxoid administered at spring branding and in the feedlot. Agri-Practice, 12(2):6–7, 10–12, 14, 1991.

Belknap, E.B.: Diseases of the respiratory system. In: Sheep and Goat Medicine. D.G. Pugh, ed. Philadelphia, W.B. Saunders, pp. 107–128, 2002.

Benson, G.J.: Anesthetic management of ruminants and swine with selected pathophysiologic alterations. Vet. Clin. N. Am. Food Anim. Pract., 2(3):677–691, 1986.

Berge, A.C.B., Sischo, W.M. and Craigmill, A.L.: Antimicrobial susceptibility patterns of respiratory tract pathogens from sheep and goats. J. Am. Vet. Med. Assoc., 229:1279–1281, 2006.

Bernabé, A., et al.: Pathological changes of spontaneous dual infection of tuberculosis and paratuberculosis in goats. Small Rumin. Res., 5:377–390, 1991.

Berrag, B. and Urquhart, G.M.: Epidemiological aspects of lungworm infections of goats in Morocco. Vet. Parasitol., 61:81–95, 1996.

Berrag, B., et al.: Bronchoalveolar cellular responses of goats following infections with *Muellerius capillaris* (Protostrongylidae, Nematoda). Vet. Immun. Immunopathol., 58:77–88, 1997.

Berrios, P.E., McKercher, D.G. and Knight, H.D.: Pathogenicity of a caprine herpesvirus. Am. J. Vet. Res., 36:1763–1769, 1975.

Bingham, D.P., Moore, R. and Richards, A.B.: Comparison of DNA: DNA homology and enzymatic activity between *Pasteurella haemolytica* and related species. Am. J. Vet. Res., 51:1161–1166, 1990.

Black, L.: Hypersensitivity. In: Current Veterinary Therapy Food Animal Practice 2. J.L. Howard, ed. Philadelphia, W.B. Saunders Co., 1986.

Blackall, P.J., et al.: Reclassification of [*Pasteurella*] *trehalosi* as *Bibersteinia trehalosi* gen. nov., comb. nov.. Int. J. Syst. Evol. Microbiol., 57:666–674, 2007.

Bliss, E.L. and Greiner, E.C.: Efficacy of fenbendazole and cambendazole against *Muellerius capillaris* in dairy goats. Am. J. Vet. Res., 46:1923–1925, 1985.

Boermans, H.J.: Diagnosis of nitrate toxicosis in cattle, using biological fluids and a rapid ion chromatographic method. Am. J. Vet. Res., 51:491–495, 1990.

Bölske, G., et al.: *Mycoplasma capricolum* in an outbreak of polyarthritis and pneumonia in goats. Acta Vet. Scand., 29:331–338, 1988.

Bölske, G., et al.: Experimental infections of goats with *Mycoplasma mycoides* subspecies *mycoides*, LC type. Res. Vet. Sci., 46:247–252, 1989.

Borgman, R.F. and Wilson, C.E.: Pasteurellosis and enzootic pneumonia in goats. J. Am. Vet. Med. Assoc., 126:198–204, 1955.

Bowman, D.D., et al.: Georgis' Parasitology for Veterinarians. 8th Ed. Philadelphia, W.B. Saunders Co., 2003.

Braun, U., et al.: Protostrongyliden-Pneumonien bei Saanen-Ziegen. Tierärztl. Umschau, 55:338–345, 2000.

Braun, U., et al.: Ultrasound-guided percutaneous lung biopsy in sheep. Vet. Rec., 146:525–528, 2000.

Brogden, K.A., Lehmkuhl, H.D. and Cutlip, R.C.: *Pasteurella haemolytica* complicated respiratory infections in sheep and goats. Vet. Res., 29:233–254, 1998.

Brown, C.C., Olander, H.J., Biberstein, E.L. and Moreno, D.: Serologic response and lesions in goats experimentally infected with *Corynebacterium pseudotuberculosis* of caprine and equine origins. Am. J. Vet. Res., 46:2322–2326, 1985.

Brown, C.C. and Skowronek, A.J.: Histologic and immunochemical study of the pathogenesis of heartwater (*Cowdria ruminantium* infestation) in goats and mice. Am. J. Vet. Res., 51:1476–1480, 1990.

Buddle, B.M., et al.: Experimental respiratory infection of goats with caprine herpesvirus and *Pasteurella haemolytica*. N. Z. Vet. J., 38:22–27, 1990a.

Buddle, B.M., et al.: A caprine pneumonia outbreak associated with caprine herpesvirus and *Pasteurella haemolytica* respiratory infections. N. Z. Vet. J., 38:28–31, 1990b.

Burrows, G.E.: Methylene blue: Effects and disposition in sheep. J. Vet. Pharmacol. Therap., 7:225–231, 1984.

Burrows, G.E. and Way, J.L.: Cyanide intoxication in sheep: Enhancement of efficacy of sodium nitrite, sodium thiosulfate, and cobaltous chloride. Am. J. Vet. Res., 40:613–617, 1979.

Cabaret, J.: Efficacy of netobimin against *Muellerius capillaris* and resistant strain of digestive tract strongyles in dairy goats. Am. J. Vet. Res., 52:1313–1315, 1991.

Cabaret, J., Anjorand, N., Leclerc, C. and Mangeon, N.: Le traitement de la muelleriose caprine: Efficacité comparée de l'oxfendazole. In: Les Maladies de la Chèvre, (Les Colloques de l'INRA, no. 28) Niort, France, pp. 357–366, 1984.

Cabaret, J., Mangeon, N. and Anjorand, N.: Relationship between the prevalence of *Muellerius capillaris* infection in the molluscan intermediate hosts and that in goats in Touraine. Ann. Parasitol. Hum. Comp., 61:651–658, 1986.

Çam, Y., et al.: Peste des petits ruminants in a sheep and goat flock in Kayseri province, Turkey. Vet Rec., 157:523–524, 2005.

Cameron, J.A., Shoukrey, N.M. and Al-Garni, A.A.: Conjunctival ophthalmomyiasis caused by the sheep nasal botfly (*Oestrus ovis*). Am. J. Ophthalmol., 112:331–334, 1991.

Caminopetros, J.P.: La "Q" fever en Grèce: le lait source de l'infection pour l'homme et les animaux. Ann. Parasitol. Hum. Comp., 23:107–118, 1948.

Carlson, J.R., Yokoyama, M.T., and Dickinson, E.O.: Induction of pulmonary edema and emphysema in cattle and goats with 3-methylindole. Science, 176:298–299, 1972.

Carmichael, J.: Tuberculosis of goats in Uganda. Vet. Rec., 50:1147–1154, 1938.

Carrigan, M.J., Links, I.J. and Morton, A.G.: *Rhodococcus equi* infection in goats. Aust. Vet. J., 65:331–332, 1988.

Chapman, H.M., et al.: *Cryptococcus neoformans* infection in goats. Aust. Vet. J., 67:263–265, 1990.

Chattopadhyay, S.K., Parihar, N.S. and Sikdar, A.: Caprine pulmonary mycosis in India: spontaneous and experimental studies. Fifth International Conference on Goats, New Delhi, India. Abstracts of Contributory Papers, Volume I, p. 457, March 1992.

Chauhan, H.V.S. and Singh, C.M.: Studies on the pathology of pulmonary adenomatosis complex of sheep and goats. II: Viral pneumonitis (atypical pneumonia). Indian J. Anim. Sci., 41:272–276, 1971.

Collins, E.R., Jr.: Ventilation of sheep and goats barns. Vet. Clin. North Am. Food Anim. Pract., 6(3):635–654, 1990.

Conn, E.E.: Cyanogenesis, the production of hydrogen cyanide, by plants. In: Effects of Poisonous Plants on Livestock. R.F. Keeler et al., eds. New York, Academic Press, 1978.

Constantinescu, G.M.: Guide to Regional Ruminant Anatomy Based on the Dissection of the Goat. Ames, IA, Iowa State Univ. Press, 2001.

Constantinou, A.: Goat housing for different environments and production systems. In: Proceedings, Fourth International Conference on Goats, Brasilia, Brazil, EMBRAPA, Volume 1, pp. 241–268, 1987.

Cork, L.C., et al.: Infectious leukoencephalomyelitis of young goats. J. Infect. Dis., 129:134–141, 1974.

Cottew, G.S. and Yeats, F.R.: Mycoplasmas and mites in the ears of clinically normal goats. Aust. Vet. J., 59:77–81, 1982.

Cousins, D.V., et al.: *Mycobacterium bovis* infection in a goat. Aust. Vet. J., 70:262–263, 1993.

Craig, D.R., Roth, L. and Smith, M.C.: Lymphosarcoma in goats. Compend. Cont. Educ. Pract. Vet., 8:S190-S197, 1986.

Craig, P.S. and Larrieu, E.: Control of cystic echinococcosis/hydatidosis: 1863–2002. Ad. Parasitol., 61:443–508, 2006.

Cremers, H.J.W.M.: Effectiveness of oxfendazole against *Muellerius capillaris* (Nematoda: Proto-strongylidae) in goats. Tijdschr. Diergeneeskd., 108:863–867, 1983.

Curtis, R.A., et al.: Lung sounds in cattle, horses, sheep and goats. Can. Vet. J., 27:170–172, 1986.

Dadhich, H. and Sharma, G.D.: Pulmonary schistosomiasis in goats in Rajasthan. Indian Vet. J., 73:677–678, 1996.

Daft, B.M. and Weidenbach, S.: Isolation of parainfluenza type 3 virus associated with a respiratory epizootic in goats in California. Agri-Practice 8:35–36, 1987.

DaMassa, A.J.: Prevalence of mycoplasmas and mites in the external auditory meatus of goats. Calif. Vet., 37(12):10–13, 17, 1983.

DaMassa, A.J. and Brooks, D.L.: The external ear canal of goats and other animals as a mycoplasma habitat. Small Rumin. Res., 4:85–93, 1991.

DaMassa, A.J., Brooks, D.L. and Adler, H.E.: Caprine mycoplasmosis: widespread infection in goats with *Mycoplasma mycoides* subsp *mycoides* (large-colony type). Am. J. Vet. Res., 44:322–325, 1983a.

DaMassa, A.J., et al.: Caprine mycoplasmosis: acute pulmonary disease in newborn kids given *Mycoplasma capricolum* orally. Aust. Vet. J., 60:125–126, 1983b.

DaMassa, A.J., et al.: Brief account of caprine mycoplasmosis in the United States with special reference to *Mycoplasma mycoides* subsp. *mycoides*. In: Proceedings, Ann. Meeting U.S. Anim. Health Assoc., 88:291–302, 1984.

DaMassa, A.J., Brooks, D.L. and Holmberg, C.A.: Induction of mycoplasmosis in goat kids by oral inoculation with *Mycoplasma mycoides* subspecies *mycoides*. Am. J. Vet. Res., 47:2084–2089, 1986.

DaMassa, A.J., et al.: Mycoplasmas of goats and sheep. J. Vet. Diagn. Invest., 4:101–113, 1992.

Davies, F.G.: Sheep and goat pox. In: Virus Diseases of Food Animals. Vol. II. Disease Monographs. E.P.J. Gibbs, ed. New York, Academic Press, 1981.

De las Heras, M., Garcia de Jalon, J.A. and Sharp, J.M.: Pathology of enzootic intranasal tumor in thirty-eight goats. Vet. Pathol., 28:474–481, 1991a.

De las Heras, M., González, L. and Sharp, J.M.: Pathology of ovine pulmonary adenocarcinoma. In: Jaagsiekte Sheep Retrovirus and Lung Cancer. H. Fan. ed. Cur. Top. Microbiol. Immunol., 275:25–54, 2003a.

De las Heras, M., et al.: Retrovirus-like particles in enzootic intranasal tumours in Spanish goats. Vet. Rec., 123:135, 1988.

De las Heras, M., et al.: Enzootic nasal tumor of goats: Demonstration of a type D-related retrovirus in nasal fluids and tumours. J. Gen Virol., 72:2533–2535, 1991b.

De las Heras, M., et al.: Experimental transmission of enzootic intranasal tumors of goats. Vet. Pathol., 32:19–23, 1995.

De las Heras, M., et al.: Enzootic nasal adenocarcinoma of sheep and goats. In: Jaagsiekte Sheep Retrovirus and Lung Cancer. H. Fan, ed. Cur. Top. Microbiol. Immunol., 275:201–223, 2003b.

Dhar, D.N. and Sharma, R.L.: Studies on the comparative susceptibility of sheep and goats to infection with *Dictyocaulus filaria*. Indian J. Anim. Sci., 48(1):29–31, 1978a.

Dhar, D.N. and Sharma, R.L.: A note on the immunological response of goats to vaccination with the radiation-attenuated *Dictyocaulus filaria* vaccine. Indian J. Anim. Sci., 48:762–764, 1978b.

Dickinson, E.O., Yokoyama, M.T., Carlson, J.R. and Bradley, B.J.: Induction of pulmonary edema and emphysema in goats by intraruminal administration of 3-methylindole. Am. J. Vet. Res., 37:667–672, 1976.

Dickson, J. and Ellis, T.: Experimental retrovirus infection in sheep. Vet. Rec., 125:649, 1989.

Dorchies, P., Duranton, C., and Jacquiet, P.: Pathophysiology of *Oestrus ovis* infection in sheep and goats: a review. Vet. Rec., 142:487–489, 1998.

Du Preez, E.R., Odendaal, M.W. and Morris, S.D.: Protection of vaccinated goats against experimental challenge with *Mannheimia haemolytica* α1 leukotoxin. In: 7th International Conference on Goats, Tours, France. Proceedings Vol. 1, p. 297, 2000.

Durant, A.J.: Removing the vocal folds of dairy goats. Dairy Goat J., 52(9):30–31, 1974.

El Bahri, L., Belguith, J. and Blouin, A.: Toxicology of nitrates and nitrites in livestock. Compend. Contin. Educ. Pract. Vet., 19:643–648, 1997.

El Hassan, S.M., Harbi, M.S.M.A. and Abu Bakr, M.I.: Treatment of contagious caprine pleuropneumonia. Vet. Res. Commun., 8:65–67, 1984.

Elazhary, M.A.S.Y., et al.: Prevalence of antibodies to bovine respiratory syncytial virus, bovine viral diarrhea virus, bovine herpesvirus-1, and bovine parainfluenza-3 virus in sheep and goats in Quebec. Am. J. Vet. Res., 45:1660–1662, 1984.

Ellis, T.M., Robinson, W.F. and Wilcox, G.E.: The pathology and aetiology of lung lesions in goats infected with caprine arthritis-encephalitis virus. Aust. Vet. J., 65:69–73, 1988a.

Ellis, T.M., Robinson, W.F. and Wilcox, G.E.: Comparison of caprine arthritis-encephalitis viruses from goats with arthritis and goats with chronic interstitial pneumonia. Aust. Vet. J., 65:254–257, 1988b.

Fernández, A., et al.: Morphological evidence of a filamentous cilia-associated respiratory (CAR) bacillus in goats. Vet. Pathol., 33:445–447, 1996.

Fitzgerald, S.D., Walker, R.D. and Parlor, K.W.: Fatal *Rhodococcus equi* infection in an Angora goat. J. Vet. Diagn. Invest., 6:105–107, 1994.

Fodor, L., Varga, J., Hajtos, I. and Szemerédi, G.: Serotypes of *Pasteurella haemolytica* isolated from sheep, goats and calves. Zbl. Vet. Med. B., 31:466–469, 1984.

Fontaine, J.J., Crespeau, F., Guerau, J.M. and Parodi, A.L.: Observation d'une enzootie d'adenome pituitaire de la chèvre. Recueil Méd. Vét. École Alf., 159(4):383–388, 1983.

Fulton, R.W., Downing, M.M. and Hagstad, H.V.: Prevalence of bovine herpesvirus-1, bovine viral diarrhea, parainfluenza-3, bovine adenoviruses-3 and -7, and goat respiratory syncytial viral antibodies in goats. Am. J. Vet. Res., 43:1454–1457, 1982.

Gay, C.C. and Richards, W.P.C.: Cor pulmonale and atrial fibrillation in goats as a sequel to pneumonia. Aust. Vet. J., 60:274–275, 1983.

Gemmell, M.A.: Hydatidosis control—a global view. Aust. Vet. J., 55:118–125, 1979.

Genchi, C., Manfredi, M.T. and Sioli, C.: Les infestations naturelles des chèvres par les strongles pulmonaires en milieu alpin. (The natural infection by lungworms of goats grazing on alpine pastures.) In: Les Maladies de la Chèvre, (Les Colloques de l'INRA, no. 28) Niort, France, pp. 347–352, 1984.

Gerichter, C.B.: Studies on the lung nematodes of sheep and goats in the Levant. Parasitol., 41:166–183, 1951.

Geurden, T. and Vercruysse, J.: Field efficacy of eprinomectin against a natural *Muellerius capillaris* infection in dairy goats. Vet. Parasitol., 147:190–193, 2007.

Gibbs, E.P.J., Taylor, W.P., Lawman, M.J.P. and Bryant, J.: Classification of peste des petits ruminants virus as the fourth member of the genus Morbillivirus. Intervirology, 11:268–274, 1979.

Gillespie, J.H. and Timoney, J.F.: Hagan and Bruner's Microbiology and Infectious Diseases of Domestic Animals. 8th Ed. Ithaca, N.Y., Cornell Univ. Press, 1988.

Goltz, J.P., Rosendal, S., McCraw, B.M. and Ruhnke, H.L.: Experimental studies on the pathogenicity of *Mycoplasma ovipneumoniae* and *Mycoplasma arginini* for the respiratory tract of goats. Can. J. Vet. Res., 50:59–67, 1986.

Gonzalez, L., et al.: Jaagsiekte sheep retrovirus can be detected in the peripheral blood during the pre-clinical period of sheep pulmonary adenomatosis. J. Gen. Virol., 82:1355–1358, 2001.

Gough, J.F.: Black cherry poisoning in an Angora goat. Can. Vet. J., 36:45, 1995.

Gourlay, R.N. and Barber, L.: A strain of *Pasteurella haemolytica* isolated from goats in Uganda. J. Comp. Pathol., 70:211–216, 1960.

Gregory, E., Foreyt, W.J. and Breeze, R.: Efficacy of ivermectin and fenbendazole against lungworms. Vet. Med., 80(2):114–117, 1985.

Guha, C. and Verma, B.B.: Contagious caprine pleuropneumonia: experimental infection of kids with local strain of *Mycoplasma agalactiae*. Indian J. Vet. Med., 7(1):10–13, 1987.

Gutiérrez, M. and García Marin, J.F.: *Cryptococcus neoformans* and *Mycobacterium bovis* causing granulomatous pneumonia in a goat. Vet. Pathol., 36:445–448, 1999.

Hadlow, W.J.: High prevalence of thymoma in the dairy goat. Vet. Pathol., 15:153–169, 1978.

Hago, B.E.D. and Abu-Samra, M.T.: A case of *Multiceps gaigeri* coenurosis in goat. Vet. Parasitol., 7:191–194, 1980.

Hamdy, F.M., et al.: Etiology of the stomatitis pneumoenteritis complex in Nigerian dwarf goats. Can. J. Comp. Med., 40:276–284, 1976.

Hammarberg, K.E. Hudiksvall, Sweden. Personal communication, 1992.

Hanselaer, J.R.: A thymoma in a Nubian goat. Vlaams Diergeneeskundig Tijdschr., 57:113–117, 1988.

Harbi, M.S.M.A., et al.: Experimental contagious caprine pleuropneumonia. Trop. Anim. Health Prod., 15:51–52, 1983.

Hayashidani, H., et al.: Outbreak of pneumonia caused by *Pasteurella haemolytica* infection in Shiba goats in Japan. Jpn. J. Vet. Sci., 50:960–962, 1988.

Helle, O.: Lungworms in goats in Norway. Nor. J. Zool., 24:463, 1976.

Helle, O.: The efficacy of fenbendazole and albendazole against the lungworm *Muellerius capillaris* in goats. Vet. Parasitol., 22:293–301, 1986.

Hernandez, L., et al.: *Mycoplasma mycoides* subsp. *capri* associated with goat respiratory disease and high flock mortality. Can. Vet. J., 47:366–369, 2006.

Hoste, H., et al.: Efficacy of eprinomectin pour-on against gastrointestinal nematodes and the nasal bot fly (*Oestrus ovis*) in sheep. Vet. Rec., 154:782–785, 2004.

Hotzel, H., Sachse, K. and Pfützner, H.: A PCR scheme for differentiation of organisms belonging to the *Mycoplasma mycoides* cluster. Vet. Microbiol., 49:31–43, 1996.

Huang, T.W., Carlson, J.R., Bray, T.M. and Bradley, B.J.: 3-methylindole-induced pulmonary injury in goats. Am. J. Pathol., 87:647–666, 1977.

Hudson, J.R., Cottew, G.S. and Adler, H.E.: Diseases of goats caused by mycoplasma: a review of the subject with some new findings. Ann. N.Y. Acad. Sci., 143:287–297, 1967.

Ihemelandu, E.C., Nduaka, O., and Ojukwu, E.M.: Hyperimmune serum in the control of peste des petits ruminants. Trop. Anim. Health Prod., 17:83–88, 1985.

Ikede, B.O.: The pattern of respiratory lesions in goats and sheep in Nigeria. I. Lesions in goats. Bull. Anim. Health Prod. Afr., 25:49–59, 1977.

Ishii, S., et al.: Study on an infectious pneumonia of goat caused by a virus, IV: Tetracycline treatment of experimental pneumonia in goats caused by the goat pneumonia virus. Jpn. J. Exp. Med., 24:377–383, 1954.

Jackson, P.G.G., White, R.A.S., Dennis, R. and Gordon, D.F.: Tracheal collapse in a goat. Vet. Rec., 119:160, 1986.

Jasni, S., Zamri-Saad, M., Mutalib, A.R. and Sheik-Omar, A. R.: Isolation of *Pasteurella haemolytica* from the nasal cavity of goats. Br. Vet. J., 147:352–355, 1991.

Jetteur, P., Lefèbvre, P. and Schandevyl, P.: Séroconversion envers le virus respiratoire syncytial bovin dans on élevage caprin atteint de pneumonie au Zaire. Rev. Élev. Méd. Vét. Pays Trop., 42:493–494, 1989.

Johnson, L.R.: Fine needle aspiration and lung biopsy. In: Textbook of Veterinary Internal Medicine, Vol. 1. 6th Ed. S.J. Ettinger and E.C. Feldman, eds. St. Louis, Elsevier Saunders, pp. 344–345, 2005.

Jones, G.E.: Contagious Caprine Pleuropneumonia. Paris, Office International des Epizooties. Technical Series No. 9, 1989.

Jones, G.E. and Wood, A.R.: Microbiological and serological studies on caprine pneumonias in Oman. Res. Vet. Sci., 44:125–131, 1988.

Jones, S.L. and Schumacher, J.: What is your diagnosis? Case 1. J. Am. Vet. Med. Assoc., 197:395–396, 1990.

Kadhim, J.K., Jabbir, M.H. and Altaif, K.I.: A comparison between the efficacy of tetramisole and morantel/diethylcarbamazine in experimentally induced *Dictyocaulus filaria* infection in goats. Res. Vet. Sci., 13:597–599, 1972.

Kahrer, E., Lang, C. and Sommerfeld-Stur, I.: [Comparison of two blood gas analysers for measuring blood gases and electrolytes in accord with defined reference values of different ruminants.] Tierärztl. Umschau, 61:575–581, 2006.

Kaliner, G.: Vorkommen von Besnoitienzysten in der Ziegenlunge. Berl. Münch. Tierärztl. Wochenschr., 86:229–230, 1973.

Kaliner, G. and MacOwan, K.J.: The pathology of experimental and natural contagious caprine pleuropneumonia in Kenya. Zbl. Vet. Med. B., 23:652–661, 1976.

Kazacos, K.R., et al.: Fenbendazole for the treatment of pulmonary and gastrointestinal helminths in pygmy goats. J. Am. Vet. Med. Assoc., 179:1255–1258, 1981.

Kimberling, C.V.: Jensen and Swift's Diseases of Sheep. 3rd Ed. Philadelphia, Lea and Febiger, 1988.

King, J.M.: Pneumonia from inhaling a grass awn. Vet. Med., 84:261, 1989.

Kingsbury, J.M.: Poisonous Plants of the United States and Canada. Englewood Cliffs, NJ, Prentice-Hall, Inc., 1964.

Kitching, R.P.: Sheeppox and goatpox. In: Infectious Diseases of Livestock, Volume Two, 2nd Ed. J.A.W. Coetzer and R.C. Tustin, eds. Oxford Univ. Press, Oxford, pp. 1277–1281, 2004.

Knight A.P. and Walter, R.G.: A Guide to Plant Poisoning of Animals in North America. Jackson, Wyoming, Teton NewMedia, 2001.

Koenig, G.J., Partington, B.P., Hull, B.L. and Haibel, G.K.: What is your diagnosis? Case 2. J. Am. Vet. Med. Assoc., 197:396–397, 1990.

Königsson, K., et al.: Pharmacokinetics and pharmacodynamic effects of flunixin after intravenous, intramuscular and oral administration in dairy goats. Acta Vet. Scand., 44:153–159, 2003.

Kumar, R., et al.: Pathoetiology of pneumonic Gaddi goats in Himachal Pradesh. Ind. J. Anim Sci., 74:569–571, 2004.

Kusiluka, L.J., et al.: Demonstration of *Mycoplasma capricolum* subsp. *capripneumoniae* and *Mycoplasma mycoides* subsp. *mycoides*, Small Colony type in outbreaks of caprine pleuropneumonia in Eastern Tanzania. Acta Vet. Scand., 41:311–319, 2000.

Lamontagne, L., Descôteaux, J.-P. and Roy, R.: Epizootiological survey of parainfluenza-3, reovirus-3, respiratory syncytial and infectious bovine rhinotracheitis viral antibodies in sheep and goat flocks in Quebec. Can. J. Comp. Med., 49:424–428, 1985.

Lefèvre, P.-C. and Thiaucourt, F.: Contagious caprine pleuropneumonia. In: Infectious Diseases of Livestock, Volume Three, 2nd Ed. J.A.W. Coetzer and R.C. Tustin, eds. Oxford Univ. Press, Oxford, pp. 2060–2065, 2004.

Lehmkuhl, H.D. and Cutlip, R.C.: Protection from parainfluenza-3 virus and persistence of infectious bovine rhinotracheitis virus in sheep vaccinated with a modified live IBR-PI-3 vaccine. Can. J. Comp. Med., 49:58–62, 1985.

Lehmkuhl, H.D., Smith, M.H. and Cutlip, R.C.: Morphogenesis and structure of caprine respiratory syncytial virus. Arch. Virol., 65:269–276, 1980.

Lehmkuhl, H.D., et al.: Pathogenesis of infection induced by an adenovirus isolated from a goat. Am. J. Vet. Res., 58:608–611, 1997.

Linnabary, R.D., et al.: Acute bovine pulmonary emphysema (ABPE): perilla ketone as another cause. Vet. Human Toxicol., 20:325–326, 1978.

Litamoi, J.K., Lijodi, F.K. and Nandokha, E.: Contagious caprine pleuropneumonia: some observations in a field vaccination trial using inactivated *Mycoplasma* strain F38. Trop. Anim. Health Prod., 21:146–150, 1989.

Livingston, C.W., Jr. and Gauer, B.B.: Isolation of *Mycoplasma ovipneumoniae* from Spanish and Angora goats. Am. J. Vet. Res., 40:407–408, 1979.

Lloyd, S. and Soulsby, E.J.L.: Survey of parasites in dairy goats. Am. J. Vet. Res., 39:1057–1059, 1978.

Lofstedt, J.: Antimicrobial therapy in sheep and goats. In: The Bristol Veterinary Handbook of Antimicrobial Therapy 2nd Ed. D.E. Johnston, ed. Evansville, IN, Bristol-Myers Animal Health, 1987.

Macedo, J.T.S.A., et al.: Cutaneous and nasal protothecosis in a goat. Vet. Pathol., 45:352–354, 2008.

Mahato, S.N.: Leech infestation of livestock. Vet. Rec., 124:641–642, 1989.

Mahato, S.N., Thakuri, K.C. and Gatenby, R.M.: Nasal leeches in goats in the hills of Nepal. Pathologie Caprine et Productions, 2e Colloque International de Niort, 26–29 juin, 1989. CIRAD, pp 342–345, 1993.

Marek, J. and Mocsy, J.: Lehrbuch der Klinischen Diagnostik der Inneren Krankheiten der Haustiere. Jena, Gustav Fischer Verlag, 1960.

Martin, W.B.: Respiratory diseases induced in small ruminants by viruses and mycoplasma. Rev. Sci. Tech. Off. Int. Epiz., 2:311–334, 1983.

McConnell, E.E., Basson, P.A., and Pienaar, J.G.: Pneumocystosis in a domestic goat. Onderstepoort J. Vet. Res., 38:117–126, 1971.

McCraw, B.M. and Menzies, P.I.: Treatment of goats infected with the lungworm *Muellerius capillaris*. Can. Vet. J., 27:287–290, 1986.

McCraw, B.M. and Menzies, P.I.: *Muellerius capillaris*: resumption of shedding larvae in feces following anthelmintic treatment and prevalence in housed goats. Can. Vet. J., 29:453–454, 1988.

McKenna, P.B.: Comparative evaluation of two emigration/sedimentation techniques for the recovery of dictyocaulid and protostrongylid larvae from faeces. Vet. Parasitol., 80:345–351, 1999.

McMartin, D.A., MacOwan, K.J. and Swift, L.L.: A century of classical contagious caprine pleuropneumonia: from original description to aetiology. Br. Vet. J., 136:507–515, 1980.

Mebus, C.A. and Logan, L.L.: Heartwater disease of domestic and wild ruminants. J. Am. Vet. Med. Assoc., 192:950–952, 1988.

Mesina, J.E., Jr., Bisgard, G.E. and Robinson, G.M.: Pulmonary function changes in goats given 3-methylindole orally. Am. J. Vet. Res., 45:1526–1531, 1984.

Midwinter, A.C., Clarke, J.K. and Alley, M.R.: *Pasteurella haemolytica* serotypes from pneumonic goat lungs. N. Z. Vet. J., 34:35–36, 1986.

Mohanty, S.B.: Natural infection with infectious bovine rhinotracheitis virus in goats. J. Am. Vet. Med. Assoc., 160:879–880, 1972.
Mondal, D.B., Pandey, N.N. and Charan, K.: Effects of prolonged low nitrate intoxication in goats. Indian Vet. J., 76:800–803, 1999.
Mondal, D.B. and Pandey, N.N.: Dosage regimen of methylene blue and its comparative therapeutic efficacy with tolonium chloride and ascorbic acid in induced acute nitrate toxicity in goats. Indian J. Anim. Sci., 70:572–575, 2000.
Moore, J.D., Barr, B.C., Daft, B.M. and O'Connor, M.T.: Pathology and diagnosis of *Coxiella burnetii* infection in a goat herd. Vet. Pathol., 28:81–84, 1991.
Morgan, K.L., et al.: Serum antibody to respiratory syncytial virus in goats in the UK. Vet. Rec., 116:239–240, 1985.
Moulton, W.M.: Contagious caprine pleuropneumonia in the United States? J. Am. Vet. Med. Assoc., 176:354–355, 1980.
Mugera, G.M. and Kramer, T.T.: Pasteurellosis in Kenya goats due to *Pasteurella haemolytica*. Bull. Epizoot. Dis. Afr., 15:125–131, 1967.
Murray, C., McNutt, S.H. and Purwin, P.: Tuberculosis of goats. J. Am. Vet. Med. Assoc., 59:82–84, 1921.
Nanda, P.N. and Singh, G.: Tuberculosis amongst goats at the government cattle farm, Hissar. Indian J. Vet. Sci. Anim. Husb., 13:70–74, 1943.
Ngatia, T.A., et al.: Nasal bacterial flora of clinically normal goats. J. Comp. Pathol., 95:465–468, 1985.
Ngatia, T.A., et al.: Pneumonia in goats following administration of live and heat-killed *Pasteurella haemolytica*. J. Comp. Pathol., 96:557–564, 1986.
Niang, M., Rosenbusch, R.F., Andrews, J.J. and Kaeberle, M.L.: Demonstration of a capsule on *Mycoplasma ovipneumoniae*. Am. J. Vet. Res., 59:557–562, 1998.
Nicholas, R.A.J.: Contagious caprine pleuropneumonia. In: Recent Advances in Goat Diseases. M. Tempesta, ed. International Veterinary Information Service, Ithaca NY (www.ivis.org). 2002.
Nimmo, J.S.: Six cases of verminous pneumonia (*Muellerius* sp) in goats. Can. Vet. J., 20:49–52, 1979.
Njenga, J.M., et al.: Preliminary findings from an experimental study of caprine besnoitiosis in Kenya. Vet. Res. Commun., 17:203–208, 1993.
Obi, T.U. and Ibu, J.: Parainfluenza type 3 (PI-3) virus infection in goats in Nigeria. Small Rumin. Res., 3:517–523, 1990.
OIE: Manual of Diagnostic Tests and Vaccines for Terrestrial Animals, Vol. 2, 5th Ed. Office International des Épizooties (OIE), Paris, 2004.
Ojo, M.O.: Caprine pneumonia. Vet. Bull., 47:573–578, 1977.
Ojo, M.O.: Pathology of young goats—respiratory diseases. In: Proceedings, Fourth International Conference on Goats, Brasilia, Brazil, 1987, EMBRAPA, Volume 1, pp. 389–403, 1987.
Ojo, M.O., Kasali, O.B. and Bamgboye, D.A.: In vitro and in vivo activities of tiamulin against caprine mycoplasmas. In: Les Maladies de la Chèvre, (Les Colloques de l'INRA, no. 28) Niort, France, pp. 287–293, 1984.
Olchowy, T.W.J., et al.: Metastatic thymoma in a goat. Can. Vet. J., 37:165–167, 1996.
Oliver, R.E., et al.: Isolation of caprine arthritis-encephalitis virus from a goat. N. Z. Vet. J., 30:147–149, 1982.
Omar, A.R.: Pathology of melioidosis in pigs, goats and a horse. J. Comp. Pathol., 73:359–372, 1963.
Omori, T., et al.: Study on an infectious pneumonia of goat caused by a virus. I. Isolation of the causative agent and its characteristics. Jpn. Govt. Expt. Sta. Anim. Hygiene, Report, pp. 109–117, 1953.
Onoviran, O.: The comparative efficacy of some antibiotics used to treat experimentally induced mycoplasma infection in goats. Vet. Rec., 94:418–420, 1974.
Opasina, B.A. and Putt, S.N.H.: Outbreaks of peste des petits ruminants in village goat flocks in Nigeria. Trop. Anim. Health Prod., 17:219–224, 1985.
Orós, J., et al.: Association of cilia-associated respiratory (CAR) bacillus with natural chronic tracheitis in goats. J. Comp. Pathol., 1997; 117:289–294, 1997a.
Orós, J., et al.: Bacteria associated with enzootic pneumonia in goats. J. Vet. Med. Series B, 1997; 44:99–104, 1997b.
Osweiler, G.D., Carson, T.L., Buck, W.B. and Van Gelder, G.A.: Clinical and Diagnostic Veterinary Toxicology. 3rd Ed. Dubuque, Iowa, Kendall/Hunt Publ. Co., 1985.
Pal, M. and Dahiya, S.M.: Fungi in pneumonic lungs of goats. In: Proceedings, Fourth International Conference on Goats, Brasilia, Brazil, EMBRAPA, Volume II, p. 1363. (Abstract), 1987.
Pande, P.G.: Pleuropneumonia in goats with special reference to *Pasteurella* infection. Indian J. Vet. Sci. Anim. Husb., 13:44–58, 1943.
Pandey, V.S.: Observations pathologiques sur l'échinococcose à *Echinococcus granulosus* chez la chèvre et le chien. Ann. Med. Vet., 115:519–527, 1971.
Panuska, C.: Lungworms of ruminants. Vet. Clin. Food Anim., 22:583–593, 2006.
Parish, S.M., Middleton, J.R. and Baldwin, T.J.: Clinical megaoesophagus in a goat with thymoma. Vet. Rec., 1996; 139:94, 1996.
Parodi, A.L., Samaille, J.P., Guérard, J.M. and Fiocre, B.: Observation d'un cas de pneumonie associée à *Balantidium coli* chez la chèvre. Bull. Acad. Vét. Fr. 58:47–51, 1985.
Patnaik, R.K. and Nayak, B.C.: Studies on pathology of chlamydial pneumonia in goats. Indian Vet. J., 61:821–824, 1984.
Pearson, J.E., et al.: Contagious caprine pleuropneumonia in Arizona. J. Am. Vet. Med. Assoc., 161:1536–1538, 1972.
Perreau, P. and Cabaret, J.: Les affections parasitaires et bactériennes de l'appareil respiratoire de la chèvre. In: Les Maladies de la Chèvre, (Les Colloques de l'INRA, no. 28) Niort, France, pp. 297–308, 1984.
Piccione, G., et al.: Changes in gas composition and acid-base values of venous blood samples stored under different conditions in 4 domestic species. Vet. Clin. Pathol., 36:358–360, 2007.
Prein, W.: *Hypoderma bovis* und *Oestrus ovis* bei Ziegen. Dtsch. Tierärztl. Wochenschr., 46:33–35, 1938.
Pringle, J.K., Wojcinski, Z.W. and Staempfli, H.R.: Nasal papillary adenoma in a goat. Can. Vet. J., 30:964–966, 1989.
Prodinger, W.M., et al.: Characterization of *Mycobacterium caprae* isolates from Europe by mycobacterial interspersed repetitive unit genotyping. J. Clin. Microbiol. 43:4984–4992, 2005.

Purdy, C.W., Straus, D.C., Livingston, C.W. and Foster, G.S.: Immune response to pulmonary injection of *Pasteurella haemolytica*-impregnated agar beads followed by transthoracic challenge exposure in goats. Am. J. Vet. Res. 51:1629–1634, 1990.

Purdy, C.W., Straus, D.C., Struck, D. and Foster, G.S.: Efficacy of *Pasteurella haemolytica* subunit antigens in a goat model of pasteurellosis. Am. J. Vet. Res., 54:1637–1647, 1993.

Purdy, C.W., Straus, D.C., Sutherland, R.J. and Ayres, J.R.: Efficacy of a subcutaneously administered, ultraviolet light-killed *Pasteurella haemolytica* A1-containing vaccine against transthoracic challenge exposure in goats. Am. J. Vet. Res., 57:1168–1174, 1996.

Radi, Z.A., Styer, E.L. and Thompson, L.J.: *Prunus* spp. intoxication in ruminants: a case in a goat and diagnosis by identification of leaf fragments in rumen contents. J. Vet. Diagn. Invest., 16:593–599, 2004.

Radostits, O.M., et al.: Veterinary Medicine. A Textbook of the Diseases of Cattle, Horses, Sheep, Pigs, and Goats. 10th Ed. Edinburgh, Saunders Elsevier, 2007.

Rahman, T. and Singh, B.: Chlamydial pneumonia in goats. Indian J. Anim. Health, 29:65–67, 1990.

Rajagopalan, V.R. and Sankaranarayanan, N.S.: A case of pseudotuberculosis (*Pasteurella pseudotuberculosis* infection) in the goat. Indian J. Vet. Sci. Anim. Husb., 14:34–36, 1944.

Rajya, B.S. and Singh, C.M.: The pathology of pneumonia and associated respiratory disease of sheep and goats, 1: Occurrence of jagziekte and maedi in sheep and goats in India. Am. J. Vet. Res., 25:61–67, 1964.

Ramirez, I.C., Santillan, M.A. and Dante, V.: The goat as an experimental ruminant model for tuberculosis infection. Small Rumin. Res., 47:113–116, 2003.

Rausch, R.L.: Life cycle patterns and geographic distribution of *Echinococcus* species. In: *Echinococcus* and Hydatid Disease. R.C.A. Thompson and A.J. Lymbery, eds. CAB International, Oxon, U.K., 1995.

Ribeiro, V.R., et al.: An improved method for the recovery of mycoplasmas from the external ear canal of goats. J. Vet. Diagn. Invest., 9:156–158, 1997.

Rings, D.M. and Rojko, J.: Naturally occurring nasal obstructions in 11 sheep. Cornell Vet., 75:269–276, 1985.

Robinson, W.F.: Chronic interstitial pneumonia in association with a granulomatous encephalitis in a goat. Aust. Vet. J., 57:127–131, 1981.

Robinson, W.F. and Ellis, T.M.: The pathological features of an interstitial pneumonia of goats. J. Comp. Pathol., 94:55–64, 1984.

Robinson, W.F. and Ellis, T.M.: Caprine arthritis-encephalitis virus infection: From recognition to eradication. Aust. Vet. J., 63:237–241, 1986.

Rodger, J.L.: Parainfluenza 3 vaccination of sheep. Vet. Rec., 125:453–456, 1989.

Rodolakis, A., Boullet, C. and Souriau, A.: *Chlamydia psittaci* experimental abortion in goats. Am. J. Vet. Res., 45:2086–2089, 1984.

Rodondo, E., et al.: Spontaneous bovine respiratory syncytial virus infection in goats: pathological findings. J. Vet. Med. B, 41:27–34, 1994.

Rodriguez, J.L., et al.: High mortality in goats associated with the isolation of a strain of *Mycoplasma mycoides* subsp. *mycoides* (Large Colony Type). J. Vet. Med. Ser. B, 42:587–593, 1995.

Rosendal, S.: Ovine and caprine mycoplasmas. In: Mycoplasmosis in Animals: Laboratory Diagnosis. H.W. Whitford et al., eds. Iowa State Univ. Press, Ames, pp. 84–96, 1994.

Rostkowski, C.M., Stirtzinger, T. and Baird, J.D.: Congestive heart failure associated with thymoma in two Nubian goats. Can. Vet. J., 26:267–269, 1985.

Roudebush, P. and Sweeney, C.R.: Thoracic percussion. J. Am. Vet. Med. Assoc., 197:714–718, 1990.

Rozear, L., Love, N.E. and van Camp, S.L.: Radiographic diagnosis: pulmonary lymphosarcoma in a goat. Vet. Radiol. Ultrasound, 39:528–531, 1998.

Rurangirwa, F.R., Kouyate, B., Niang, M. and McGuire, T.C.: CCPP: antibodies to F38 polysaccharide in Mali goats. Vet. Rec., 127:353, 1990.

Rurangirwa, F.R., McGuire, T.C., Kibor, A. and Chema, S.: An inactivated vaccine for contagious caprine pleuropneumonia. Vet. Rec., 121:397–402, 1987.

Rurangirwa, F.W., et al.: Treatment of contagious caprine pleuropneumonia. Trop. Anim. Health Prod., 13:177–182, 1981.

Saito, K.: Pneumonie contagieuse de la chèvre. Bull. Off. Int. Epiz., 42:676–691, 1954.

Sani, Y., Atwell, R.B. and Seawright, A.A.: The cardiotoxicity of avocado leaves. Aust. Vet. J., 68:150–151, 1991.

Scott, G.R.: Peste-des-petits-ruminants (goat plague) virus. In: Virus Infections of Vertebrates. Vol. 3. Virus Infections of Ruminants. Z. Dinter and B. Morein, eds. New York, Elsevier Science Publ., pp. 355–361, 1990.

Scott, P.R. and Gessert, M.E.: Ultrasonographic examination of the ovine thorax. Vet. J., 155:305–310, 1998.

Shah, C., et al.: Direct evidence for natural transmission of small-ruminant lentiviruses of subtype A4 from goats to sheep and vice versa. J. Virol., 78:7518–7522, 2004.

Sharma, D.N. and Dwivedi, J.N.: Pulmonary schistosomiasis in sheep and goats due to *Schistosoma indicum* in India. J. Comp. Pathol., 86:449–454, 1976a.

Sharma, D.N. and Dwivedi, J.N.: Pseudotuberculosis lesions in lungs of sheep and goats. Indian J. Anim. Sci., 46:663–665, 1976b.

Sharma, D.N., Rajya, B.S. and Dwivedi, J.N.: Metastasizing pulmonary adenomatosis (Jaagziekte) in sheep and goats. Patho-anatomical studies. Indian J. Anim. Sci., 45:363–370, 1975.

Sharma, R.L.: Parasitic bronchitis in goats and the possible use of *Dictyocaulus filaria* vaccine for its control. Vet. Parasitol., 51:255–262, 1994.

Sharma, R.N., Francis, B.K.T., Pandey, G.S. and Chizyuka, H.G.B.: Goat tuberculosis in Zambia. Indian J. Vet. Pathol., 9:29–32, 1985.

Sharp, C.L., Livingston, C.W. and Renshaw, H.W.: Etiologic agents of caprine pneumonia. In: Proceedings, Third Internl. Conf. on Goat Production and Disease. Scottsdale, Arizona, Dairy Goat Journal Publ. Corp., p. 501, 1982.

Sharp, J.M., Angus, K.W., Jassim, F.A. and Scott, F.M.M.: Experimental transmission of sheep pulmonary adenomatosis to a goat. Vet. Rec., 119:245, 1986.

Shaw, J.M.: Suspected cyanide poisoning in two goats caused by ingestion of crab apple leaves and fruits. Vet. Rec., 119:242–243, 1986.

Shewen, P.E. and Wilkie, B.N.: Evidence for the *Pasteurella haemolytica* cytotoxin as a product of actively growing bacteria. Am. J. Vet. Res., 46:1212–1214, 1985.

Shiferaw, G., et al.: Contagious caprine pleuropneumonia and *Mannheimia haemolytica*-associated acute respiratory disease of goats and sheep in Afar Region, Ethiopia. Rev. Sci. Tech. Off. Int. Epiz., 25:1153–1163, 2006.

Singh, R.P., et al.: Prevalence and distribution of peste des petits ruminants virus infection in small ruminants in India. Rev. Sci. Tech., 23:807–819, 2004.

Singh, R.P., et al.: Comparison of diagnostic efficacy of a monoclonal antibody-based competitive ELISA test with a similar commercial test for the detection of antibodies to peste des petits ruminants (PPR) virus. Vet. Res. Commun., 30:325–330, 2006.

Six, A., et al.: Latency and reactivation of bovine herpesvirus 1 (BHV-1) in goats and of caprine herpesvirus 1 (CapHV-1) in calves. Arch. Virol., 146:1325–1335, 2001.

Stefanou, D., Tsangaris, T. and Lekkas, S.: Pulmonary adenomatosis in the goats in the district of Pieria (Greece). In: Proceedings, Twentieth World Vet. Congress, Thessalonika, Greece, pp. 1204–1208, 1975.

Stevens, J.B., et al.: Hematologic, blood gas, blood chemistry, and serum mineral values for a sample of clinically healthy adult goats. Vet. Clin. Pathol., 23:19–24, 1994.

Stierschneider, M., Franz, S. and Baumgartner, W.: Endoscopic examination of the upper respiratory tract and oesophagus in small ruminants: Technique and normal appearance. Vet. J., 173:101–108, 2007.

Sutmoller, P. and Poelma, F.G.: *Cryptococcus neoformans* infection (torulosis) of goats in the Leeward Islands regions. W. Indian Med. J., 6:225–228, 1957; Abstract 571, Rev. Med. Vet. Mycol., 3(1958–60):121.

Tafti, A.K.: Diaphragmatic hernia in a goat. Aust. Vet. J., 76:166, 1998.

Taoudi, A., Karib, H., Johnson, D.W. and Fassi-Fehri, M.M.: Comparaison du pouvoir pathogène de trois souches de *Mycoplasma capricolum* pour la chèvre et le chevreau nouveau-né. Rev. Élev. Méd Vét. Pays Trop., 41:353–358, 1988.

Tegzes, J., et al.: Cyanide toxicosis in goats after ingestion of California holly (*Heteromeles arbutifolia*). J. Vet. Diagn. Invest., 15:478–480, 2003.

Terblance, M., Pienaar, J.G., Bigalke, R. and Vahrmeyer, J.: *Acacia nilotica* (L.) Del. subsp. *kraussiana* (Benth.) Brenan. as a poisonous plant in South Africa. J. S. Afr. Vet. Med. Assoc., 38(1):57–63, 1967.

Thiaucourt, F. and Bölkse, G.: Contagious caprine pleuropneumonia and other pulmonary mycoplasmoses of sheep and goats. Rev. Sci. Tech. Off. Int. Epiz., 15:1397–1414, 1996.

Thiaucourt, F., et al.: Diagnosis and control of contagious caprine pleuropneumonia. Rev. Sci. Tech. Off. Int. Epiz., 15:1415–1429, 1996.

Thigpen, J.E., et al.: Pneumonia in goats caused by *Mycoplasma mycoides* subspecies *mycoides*. J. Am. Vet. Med. Assoc., 178:711–712, 1981.

Thomas, A.D., Forbes-Faulkner, J.C., Norton, J.H. and Trueman, K.F.: Clinical and pathological observations on goats experimentally infected with *Pseudomonas pseudomallei*. Aust. Vet. J., 65:43–46, 1988.

Thompson, R.C.A. and Allsopp, C.E.: Hydatidosis: Veterinary Perspectives and Annotated Bibliography. Wallingford, U.K., CAB International, 1988.

Thorel, M.F.: Tuberculose de la chèvre. Mise au point et synthèse. In: Les Maladies de la Chèvre, (Les Colloques del'INRA, no. 28) Niort, France, pp. 551–557, 1984.

Tillman, P.C. and Brooks, D.L.: A rapid method for devocalizing goats. Lab. Anim. Sci., 33:98–100, 1983.

Toussaint, G.: Importance des conditions d'ambiance dans la propagation des maladies respiratoires en production caprine. In: Les Maladies de la Chèvre, (Les Colloques de l'INRA, no. 28) Niort (France), pp. 309–324, 1984.

Trent, A.M., Smart, M.E. and Fretz, P.B.: Surgical management of nasal adenocarcinoma in sheep. J. Am. Vet. Med. Assoc., 193:227–229, 1988.

Trudel, M., et al.: Comparison of caprine, human, and bovine strains of respiratory syncytial virus. Arch. Virol., 107:141–149, 1989.

Tschuor, A.C., et al.: [Clinical and laryngoscopic findings in a Swiss Alpine goat with left grade 4 laryngeal hemiplegia.] Schweiz. Arch. Tierheilkd., 149:548–552, 2007.

Tustin, R.C., Williamson, A.-L, York, D.F. and Verwoerd, D. W.: Experimental transmission of jaagsiekte (ovine pulmonary adenomatosis) to goats. Onderstepoort J. Vet. Res., 55:27–32, 1988.

United States Animal Health Assoc., Committee on Foreign Animal Diseases: Foreign Animal Diseases. Richmond, VA, U.S.A.H.A., revised 1998.

Upadhyaya, T.N., Datta, B.M. and Rahman, T.: Studies on the pathology of caprine pneumonia. Verminous pneumonia and hydatidosis. Indian Vet. J., 60:787–790, 1983.

USDA: Veterinary Services Memorandum no. 552.15: Instructions and recommended procedures for conducting tuberculosis tests in cattle and bison. Animal and Plant Health Inspection Service, Washington D.C., August 2, 2006.

Valero, G., Alley, M.R. and Manktelow, B.W.: A slaughterhouse survey of lung lesions in goats. New Z. Vet. J., 40:45–51, 1992.

Valero, G., Alley, M.R. and Manktelow, B.W.: Subpleural lymph nodes in goat lungs. N. Z. Vet. J., 40:45–51, 1992.

Van der Pool, W.H.M., et al.: Bovine respiratory syncytial virus antibodies in non-bovine species. Arch. Virol., 140:1549–1555, 1995.

van der Westhuysen, J.M., Wentzel, D. and Grobler, M.C.: Angora Goats and Mohair in South Africa. 3rd Ed. Port Elizabeth, South Africa, NMB Printers, 1988.

Voigt, K., et al.: Eradication of ovine pulmonary adenocarcinoma by motherless rearing of lambs. Vet. Rec., 161:129–132, 2007.

Ward, A.C.S., et al.: Characterization of *Pasteurella* spp. isolated from healthy domestic pack goats and evaluation of the effects of a commercial *Pasteurella* vaccine. Am. J. Vet. Res., 63:119–123, 2002.

Webber, J.J., Roycroft, C.R. and Callinan, J.D.: Cyanide poisoning of goats from sugar gums (*Eucalyptus cladocalyx*). Aust. Vet. J., 62:28, 1985.

Whetstone, C.A. and Evermann, J.F.: Characterization of bovine herpesvirus isolated from six sheep and four goats by restriction endonuclease analysis and radioimmunoprecipitation. Am. J. Vet. Res., 49:781–785, 1988.

Whitney, J.C., Scott, G.R. and Hill, D.H.: Preliminary observations on a stomatitis and enteritis of goats in southern Nigeria. Bull. Epizoot. Dis. Afr., 15:31–41, 1967.

Wilson, G.I.: The strength and duration of immunity to *Dictyocaulus filaria* infection in sheep and goats. Res. Vet. Sci., 11:7–17, 1970.

Woods, L.W., Walters, N.G. and Johnson, B.: Cholangiohepatitis associated with adenovirus-like particles in a pygmy goat kid. J. Vet. Diagn. Invest., 3:89–92, 1991.

Wosu, L.O.: Haemagglutination test for diagnosis of peste des petits ruminants disease in goats with samples from live animals. Small Rumin. Res., 5:169–172, 1991.

Zamri-Saad, M., Sharif, H. and Basri, K.: Microbiological and pathological evaluation of vaccination against naturally occurring caprine pasteurellosis. Vet. Rec., 124:171–172, 1989.

Zecchinon, L., Fett, T. and Desmecht, D.: How *Mannheimia haemolytica* defeats host defence through a kiss of death mechanism. Vet. Res., 36:133–156, 2005.

Ziv, G. and Heavner, J.E.: Permeability of the blood-milk barrier to methylene blue in cows and goats. J. Vet. Pharmacol. Ther., 7:55–59, 1984.

10

Digestive System

The structure and function of the caprine digestive system are typical of the basic ruminant design and closely resemble that of sheep. The goat does exhibit some known anatomic and physiologic characteristics, however, that distinguish it from the sheep and reflect both its specialized feeding behavior and adaptability to environments hostile to other domesticated ruminants.

The spectrum of diseases that affect the caprine digestive system is similar to that seen in sheep and cattle. Infectious and metabolic conditions predominate, and many of the same diseases occur. However the frequency of occurrence may differ significantly in goats for certain conditions. For example, abomasal displacement and traumatic reticulitis are commonly encountered in dairy cattle, but rarely diagnosed in the goat.

A discussion of differential diagnosis of caprine digestive diseases is provided in this chapter, organized on the basis of presenting clinical signs. The major diseases that affect primarily the digestive system are discussed in detail in the last section of the chapter.

BASIC CAPRINE GASTROENTEROLOGY

Several atlases of topographic anatomy and dissection guides of the goat are available (Chatelain 1987; Constantinescu 2001; Popesko 2008), but most anatomic texts focus on cattle or sheep with goats mentioned comparatively, if at all. The situation is very similar for caprine digestive physiology. The following discussion serves to identify known differences in the structure and function of the caprine digestive system that are anatomically distinctive, functionally adaptive, or clinically relevant. Readers requiring a more general review of ruminant anatomy and physiology are referred to comprehensive texts in these areas (Habel 1975; Church 1993; Cronje 2000; Reece 2004).

Clinical Anatomy

Oral Cavity

The upper lip of the goat is complete and muscular and lacks the dividing philtrum of the sheep. This favors the grasping and tearing of browse while the philtrum in the sheep favors consumption of grasses close to the ground. The tongue of the goat is not used for prehension of feed, as it is in cattle. It is shorter and smoother and not as easily extracted or displaced from the oral cavity during oral examination. Taste buds on the tongue can discriminate bitter, sweet, salty, and sour tastes and the tolerance for bitter taste exceeds that of cattle and sheep. This favors the browsing of a wider range of plant species.

There are four main pairs of salivary glands: the parotids, mandibulars, sublinguals, and buccals. The latter are divided into dorsal, middle, and ventral portions. The histology of these glands has been described (Nawar 1980). The parotid and ventral buccal glands are serous, the dorsal and middle buccal glands are mucous, and the mandibular and sublingual glands are mixed. In addition, numerous mucus-secreting labial glands occur in the lips, particularly near the commissures of the mouth. Lingual and palatine glands are minor. Parotid salivary glands must be distinguished from adjacent lymph nodes, especially when diseases such as caseous lymphadenitis cause lymph node enlargement.

The dental formula of the goat is 0033/4033. The upper incisors are replaced by a dental pad that facilitates the tearing of forage. The lower incisors must properly appose the dental pad for efficient acquisition of feed during grazing or browsing. Brachygnathism and prognathism both occur in goats and adversely affect feeding behavior under range conditions. Deciduous lower incisors, or milk teeth, occur in young goats. The central pair may be present at birth or appear within the first week of life. The second pair generally appears at one to two weeks, the third pair at two to three weeks, and the lateral pair at three to four weeks of age.

Permanent incisors generally appear according to the following schedule: central incisors usually are present by one year of age but appear as late as one and a half years of age; second pair, one and a half to two years of age; third pair, two and a half to three years of age; and lateral or fourth pair, three and a half to four years of age. Occasionally, there is a failure of eruption of the permanent incisors. Aged goats with persistent deciduous central incisors have been observed. Aging of older goats using teeth is difficult. Incisors continue to wear over time and the teeth become rounded rather than rectangular. The speed of this process varies considerably with type of feed and management.

Anodontia, or absence of the mandibular incisor teeth, has been reported in a West African Dwarf goat (Emele-Nwaubani and Ihemelandu 1984). Congenital absence of the first cheek tooth (P2) has been noted in feral goats (Rudge 1970).

Molars are present at birth and elongate throughout life, but are continuously worn down by the grinding action of mastication. Shortened molars may be expelled altogether in older goats, leading to accumulation of feed in empty sockets and excessive growth of the unopposed molar.

The lower dental arcades are closer together than the upper arcades. Because the goat chews with a strong lateral grinding motion, extremely sharp dental points may develop on the lateral aspect of the upper molars and the medial aspect of the lower molars, and care must be taken in carrying out an oral examination so that fingers are not injured.

Cleft palate occurs in goats as a congenital malformation. Usually the cause is unknown. However, plants containing piperidine alkaloids, notably *Lupinus formosus*, can produce teratogenic effects, including cleft palate and multiple tendon contractures, when consumed by dams between thirty and sixty days of gestation (Panter et al. 1990, 1994). Cleft palate has also been reported in fetal monsters, associated with duplication of the pelvis and hind limbs (monocephalus dipygus) in one case (Corbera et al. 2005), and with two faces (diprosopus) in another (Mukaratirwa and Sayi 2006).

Esophagus

The embryonic development of the caprine esophagus has been described (Jung et al. 1994). In adult dairy goats of the European breeds, the esophagus is approximately 1 m in length, so at least that length of tube should be used to reach the rumen for relief of bloat or administration of medications. A speculum should be used to avoid the goat chewing the tube. The movement of swallowed boluses, eructated gas and cud, and correctly placed stomach tubes may be seen in the esophagus along the left jugular furrow.

An esophageal or reticular groove is present in the goat and reflexively closes in response to suckling in the neonate, allowing milk to bypass the rumenoreticulum and directly enter the abomasum via the omasal groove. This reflex wanes after weaning and is vestigial in adults, although it can be stimulated by drinking after severe, prolonged water deprivation. There are practical advantages to inducing the reflex in adult animals, particularly for the purpose of administering oral medications directly into the abomasum that otherwise would be deactivated or diluted if introduced into the rumen. The esophageal groove in the goat can be closed reliably by the intravenous administration of lysine-vasopressin at a dose of 0.25 IU/kg. Administration of vasopressin (antidiuretic hormone) is presumed to mimic the natural physiologic response occasioned by prolonged water deprivation (Mikhail et al. 1988). Copper sulfate solution (1 tablespoon $CuSO_4$ in a liter of water) is also thought to reliably close the groove when 5 cc is given orally.

The surgical establishment and maintenance of esophageal fistulae for collection of dietary samples in goats have been described (Pfister et al. 1990). An apparatus for the remote control collection of esophageal fistulae samples and its long-term performance have also been reported (Raats and Clarke 1992; Raats et al. 1996)

Forestomachs and Abomasum

The structure of the forestomachs is quite similar in goats and sheep (Gueltekin 1953; Horowitz and Venzke 1966; Bhattacharya 1980; Chungath et al. 1985). The reticulorumen occupies most of the left half of the abdomen, and extends cranially to the eighth intercostal space and caudally to the tuber coxae, in contact with the left body wall. The cardia occurs at the eighth intercostal space.

The omasum of the goat is much smaller than the reticulum. In small ruminants, the omasum is proportionately smaller and lighter than in the cow. Internally, the longitudinal folds, or leaves of the omasum, produce *laminae omasi* of four different lengths in sheep, but only three in goats; the fourth or shortest lamina is absent. The average number of laminae in the goat is around thirty-five, compared with 169 in cattle (McSweeney 1988). The omasum is situated deep to the eighth and ninth intercostal spaces on the right-hand side of the abdomen, and does not contact the body wall. It sits on the dorsal aspect of the abomasum. In the cow, the heavier larger omasum drops to the abdominal floor and displaces the abomasum more to the left in the abdominal cavity. This anatomic difference may be a factor in explaining why cattle are more likely to develop clinical disorders associated with abomasal displacement than are goats.

The abomasum in small ruminants is proportionately larger and longer than in the cow. The abomasum of the goat is situated on the abdominal floor in the right anterior abdomen and runs caudally along the costal arch.

A wide variety of stomach volumes have been reported for mature goats. Much of the variation is probably caused by breed differences, rations fed, and the method of measurement. The range for rumen volume is 12 to 28 liters, although in most cases, the upper limit is around 20 liters. For the reticulum, the range is 1.6 to 2.3 liters; for the omasum, 0.75 to 1.2 liters; and the abomasum, 2.1 to 4 liters.

The goat is born with an undeveloped rumen and a proportionately larger abomasum (Tamate 1956; Benzie and Phillipson 1957). During the first three weeks of life, the body of the abomasum is located mainly on the left side of the abdomen, adjacent to the diaphragm with the pyloric antrum to the right of the midline. It gradually moves to its adult position in the right abdomen as the forestomachs enlarge on the left. At birth, the ratio of reticulorumen capacity to abomasal capacity is 1:4, with a reticulorumen volume of 70 ml and an abomasal volume of 290 ml. Omasal volume is negligible. In kids given access to roughage, the ratio at six weeks has become 5.7:1. Full rumen capacity is usually reached by twelve weeks of age. Acceleration of rumen development can be achieved by early introduction of roughage and concentrate into the diet of the suckling kid (Tamate 1957).

Small Intestine and Cecum

The small intestine accounts for approximately 77% of the length of the alimentary tract distal to the forestomachs, and the cecum an additional 2%. The measured mean length of the small intestine is 18 meters (and the cecum 0.3 meters) in Barbari goats, a relatively small breed (Rai and Pandey 1978), and up to 25 meters in larger breeds. The common bile duct enters the duodenum approximately 25 to 40 cm distal to the pylorus in the goat. The small intestines and cecum are located for the most part on the right side of the abdomen due to dislocation by the large reticulorumen on the left. Except for the duodenum, the remainder of the small intestine is enclosed within the supraomental recess or omental sling. The blind end of the cecum usually points caudally, but the orientation is variable.

Colon and Rectum

The structure of the caprine colon is typical of the ruminants in that there is a proportionately elongated ascending colon that is spirally coiled, followed by shorter transverse and descending colon segments leading to the rectum and anus. In the goat and sheep, there are usually three centripetal and three centrifugal turns in the spiral segment. The colon and rectum account for approximately 21% of the length of the alimentary canal distal to the forestomachs, and the mean length is 5 meters in most breeds. The diameter is approximately 8 cm at the cecum and 2 cm at the rectum. The colon also is largely displaced to the right abdomen by the reticulorumen. The spiral colon lies medial to the small intestine and cecum.

Omentum and Mesentery

The goat shows a marked predilection for the deposition of fat in omentum and mesentery compared with cattle and sheep. This undoubtedly has adaptive value when goats inhabit environments with scarce feed supplies. It also may be significant in the pathogenesis of pregnancy toxemia because overfeeding in early pregnancy can result in considerable deposition of intra-abdominal fat. This space-occupying fat can reduce feed capacity throughout the digestive tract, leading to decreased feed intake, negative energy balance, and ketosis. Intra-abdominal fat can also be misleading when assessing body condition. Goats that appear underconditioned, with little palpable subcutaneous fat, may have considerable intra-abdominal fat stores. Goats with little mesenteric fat at necropsy have been severely malnourished for an extended period of time.

Digestive Physiology

Feeding Behavior

With regard to diet selection, the goat has been characterized as intermediate between the true grazers, such as the domesticated cow and buffalo, and the true browsers or concentrate selectors, exemplified by wild ruminants such as the moose and whitetail deer (Demment and Longhurst 1987; Hofmann 1988). This means that the goat can exploit a range of plant materials to meet nutrient requirements. This diversity accounts in large part for the growing interest in goats as a desirable livestock species where intensive cropping or maintenance of abundant grassland is not possible. The goat is also being exploited in mixed farming systems, where stocking of goats along with sheep and cattle reduces weeds and shrubs. This improves grass quality and availability for the grazing species, and increases overall yields of animal products per acre.

The typical feeding behavior of goats also has a negative side. They are so successful at exploiting limited feed resources that when overstocking occurs in environments with marginal plant growth, permanent destruction of the flora with desertification of the environment can occur. Traditionally, the goat has been blamed for instances of desertification that are as much a result of failure of livestock population management by stock owners as the goat's superior foraging ability (Dunbar 1984; El Aich and Waterhouse 1999). The ecology of feeding behavior and its impact on animal productivity and environmental quality have been reviewed (Merrill and Taylor 1981; Owen-Smith and Cooper 1987; Van Soest 1987; Devendra 1987).

Nutrient Use

It has long been suggested that the goat has more digestive efficiency than cattle or sheep. Many studies have been carried out regarding comparative digestive efficiency and the results have not been consistent in identifying a distinct advantage for the goat. In general, goats and sheep show equal efficiency on high-quality, low-fiber diets. When fed low-quality, high-fiber diets, however, the two species show different compensatory advantages. Sheep digest fiber more completely than goats, but have a decreased rate of intake, while goats have a greater rate of intake and a faster rate of removal of nondigested fiber from the rumen (i.e., shorter rumen retention time) (Brown and Johnson 1984). The subject of comparative digestive efficiency in domestic ruminants with emphasis on the goat has been reviewed (Morand-Fehr 1981; Devendra 1983; Brown and Johnson 1984).

Digestive Activities

Goats eat more frequently and rapidly than sheep (Geoffroy 1974). In the process, they produce more abundant saliva. Goats produced parotid saliva at the rate of 110 ml/hour compared with 40 ml/hour in sheep when eating the same diet of fresh cut Egyptian clover (Seth et al. 1976). In addition to the known functions of bolus lubrication, urea recycling, and rumen buffering, copious saliva may have adaptive significance for goats regarding diversity of diet. Goat saliva may contain proportionately higher levels of mucin or proline than that of grazing ruminants, enabling binding of potentially toxic tannins found in many of the tree and shrub species browsed by goats (Van Soest 1987, 1994). The rumen flora of feral goats may also contain streptococcal bacteria that can degrade tannins (Brooker et al. 1994; Sly et al. 1997).

The rumination cycle of goats averages sixty-three seconds, or once per minute. The cycle is fairly constant, but may be slightly shorter on silage rather than hay diets. The motility pattern of rumenoreticular contraction of the goat is similar to that of sheep and differs in similar ways from the bovine pattern (Dziuk and McCauley 1965). Involuntary rumen contraction in goats is under vagal control (Iggo 1956). In confinement, on a hay and concentrate ration, goats were observed to actively ruminate approximately 7.75 hours per day, with 75% of cud chewing activity occurring at night (Bell and Lawn 1957).

Descriptions of normal caprine rumen fluid composition are limited, but it is known that certain properties of rumen fluid can vary markedly with changes in water intake. In desert breeds that may have access to drinking water only every three to four days, the rumen plays a vital role as a fluid reservoir. Desert goats are able to maintain a constant serum osmolarity in the face of severe dehydration and subsequent overhydration by pooling fluid in the rumen. After four days without water, the average rumen osmotic concentration in black Bedouin goats is 360 mOsm/kg, but only 82 mOsm/kg immediately after drinking as much as 32% of their original bodyweight. The sudden hypo-osmotic effect reduces rumen protozoa numbers presumably by rupture, but causes no decrease in bacterial numbers or fermentation activity (Brosh et al. 1983).

An interesting aspect of the caprine rumen microflora has to do with the ability to detoxify the feedstuff *Leucaena leucocephala.* This leguminous shrub or low tree is widely distributed throughout the tropics and subtropics. It can contribute considerably to improved animal nutrition and productivity when used as a protein-rich feed for ruminants (Jones 1979). However, when the plant comprises more than 30% of the diet, cattle, sheep, and goats in certain countries develop a variety of clinical abnormalities including alopecia, wool loss, excessive salivation, poor appetite, hypothyroidism, cataracts, poor reproductive performance, weight loss, and death. Goats are reported to show hypothyroidism and erosions of the esophageal mucosa and rumen papillae (Jones and Megarrity 1983).

Some of these toxic effects are directly caused by the amino acid mimosine, which is present in the leaves of *Leucaena leucocephala*, at levels of 2% to 5%. The thyroid effects are caused by a breakdown product of mimosine, 3,4-dihydroxypyridine (DHP), a potent goitrogen. The DHP is produced during mastication and subsequent rumen bacterial degradation. In animals not suffering ill effects from *Leucaena* consumption, DHP is additionally degraded in the rumen to harmless breakdown products by specific anaerobic rumen bacteria (Allison et al. 1990). It has been demonstrated that cultures of rumen bacteria from goats in Hawaii, where clinical *Leucaena* toxicity is not observed, can prevent clinical signs when inoculated into the rumens of goats and cattle in Australia, where *Leucaena* toxicity is widespread (Jones and Megarrity 1986).

Studies on the rate of passage of foodstuffs through the gastrointestinal tract of goats have been carried out using stained markers (Castle 1956, 1956a, 1956b). Stained particles first appear in goat feces from eleven to fifteen hours after ingestion, and have disappeared by six to seven days. The maximum appearance of stained particles is at approximately thirty hours after ingestion. The majority of the time spent by ingesta traversing the alimentary canal occurs in the forestomachs. Passage of ingesta through the entire small intestine takes an average of three hours.

Approximately 58% of the total dry matter digested by the goat is digested in the forestomachs, as is 93% of the crude fiber, 11% of the crude protein, and 80% of the soluble carbohydrate (Ridges and Singleton 1962). Most of the soluble carbohydrate digested in the forestomachs is absorbed from the rumen after fermentation as volatile fatty acids. Some carbohydrate absorption and most protein absorption occurs in the intestine.

Extensive removal of water from intestinal contents occurs in the large intestine of goats and sheep. This serves as an adaptation for water conservation. The average time for passage of ingesta through the large intestine is eighteen hours, compared with three hours in the small intestine, despite the fact that the small intestine is at least three times as long. This delayed transit accounts for the dry consistency of goat and sheep feces. The dry matter content of normal goat feces is usually between 50% and 60%, compared with 15% to 30% for cattle.

Clinical Pathology and Diagnostic Aids

Clinical Chemistry

Normal values for clinical chemistry parameters associated with the organs of digestion are given in Table 10.1

Serum electrolyte levels may change dramatically in digestive disease. Hypokalemia and especially hypochloremia are associated with gastrointestinal stasis. In obstructive diseases such as intussusception and blockage by phytobezoars or foreign bodies, hypochloremia and hypokalemia may be marked (Sherman 1981). Metabolic alkalosis may also occur in these conditions, but if surgical obstructions are severe enough to cause shock, acidosis may prevail. Displacements of the abomasum, the most common cause of hypochloremic, hypokalemic, metabolic alkalosis in dairy cattle, rarely occur in goats. Experimental goats with surgically induced right abomasal displacement, left abomasal displacement, or abomasal torsion were hypochloremic, hyponatremic, and hypokalemic following induction of these abnormalities and also had increased chloride ion levels in rumen fluid (Kwon et al. 1997).

The major chemical abnormalities associated with diarrhea are metabolic acidosis, with decreased serum bicarbonate, and hyponatremia, caused by sodium and bicarbonate loss in the diarrheic feces. Marked acidosis is also commonly seen in d-lactic acidosis due to grain overload or engorgement toxemia. In this condition, serum lactate levels are also markedly increased.

Abdominocentesis

The examination of peritoneal fluid may help in the diagnosis of digestive disease, particularly when lack of forestomach motility and abdominal distension are prominent clinical signs. The most common use of abdominocentesis in goats is to differentiate gastrointestinal causes of abdominal distension from nonalimentary causes. In male goats, ruptured bladder secondary to obstructive urolithiasis is common and leads to accumulation of urine in the abdomen. Hydrops conditions associated with abnormal pregnancy in the female must also be ruled out.

In cattle, abdominocentesis is most often performed immediately behind the xiphoid cartilage to confirm the presence of localized peritonitis in the anterior abdomen from traumatic reticulitis or perforated abomasal ulcers. Because goats rarely experience these conditions, and the main intent is generally to rule out genito-urinary conditions, abdominocentesis is better performed at the lowest point of the ventral abdomen, 2 to 4 cm to the right of the midline to avoid penetrating the rumen. Care must be taken to avoid mammary

Table 10.1. Normal values for blood constituents used in the assessment of diarrheal and other gastrointestinal diseases.

Parameter	*Sample Type*	*Units*	*Range*	*Mean*	*Reference*
Anion gap	S	mmol/l	8–20		Sherman and Robinson 1983
Bicarbonate	VB	mmol/l		24.2 ± 1.52	Cao et al. 1987
Chloride	S, HP	mmol/l	99–110.3	105.1 ± 2.85	Kaneko 1980
Cholesterol, total	S, P, HP	mg/dl	80–130		Kaneko 1980
CO_2, total	S, P	mmol/l	25.6–29.6	27.4 ± 1.4	Kaneko 1980
CO_2, pressure	VB	mm Hg		36.7 ± 4.81	Cao et al. 1987
Glucose	S, P, HP	mg/dl	50–75	62.8 ± 7.1	Kaneko 1980
Lactic acid	S	mg/dl	8.25–10.40	9.53 ± 0.45	Verma et al. 1975
Lipids, total	S	mg/dl		298.6 ± 84.8	Castro et al. 1977
Total Cholesterol	P	mg/ml		0.77 ± 0.01	Bassissi et al. 2004
VLDL		%		3.16 ± 1.06	
LDL		%		22.09 ± 1.42	
HDL		%		72.79 ± 1.82	
LPDF		%		1.96 ± 0.52	
Pepsinogen	P	mU tyrosine	<800		Kerbouf and Godu 1981
pH	VB			7.35 ± 0.30	Cao et al. 1987
Potassium	S, HP	mmol/l	3.5–6.7	5.6 ± 1	Kaneko 1980, Castro et al. 1977a
Sodium	S, HP	mmol/l	142–155	150.4 ± 3.14	Kaneko 1980

CO_2 = carbon dioxide, mmol/l = millimoles per liter, S = serum, VB = venous blood, P = plasma, HP = heparinized plasma, VLDL = very-low-density lipoproteins, LDL = low-density lipoproteins, HDL = high-density lipoproteins, LPDF = lipoprotein deficient fraction.

veins in does or the penis and prepuce in males. The sampling site should be aseptically prepared and a local anesthetic administered. If the animal is nervous, tranquilization should be considered before proceeding, but the animal should remain standing. Penetration of the ventral abdominal wall and peritoneum usually can be accomplished with a standard disposable 18- or 20-gauge needle. If fluid does not flow freely when the peritoneum is traversed, the needle should be rotated gently and a mild suction applied with an attached syringe.

Rumen Fluid Evaluation

Rumen fluid evaluation has not received much attention in goats as a diagnostic aid, but it may be helpful in the diagnosis of intoxications, high intestinal obstruction, indigestion, and grain overload. Rumen fluid analysis has been reported several times in control animals before the experimental induction of d-lactic acidosis (Tanwar and Mathur 1983; Cao et al. 1987) or water loading (Brosh et al. 1983). These reported values are summarized in Table 10.2. Changes observed in rumen fluid during experimental grain overload included decreased pH, decreased protozoal counts, increased lactic acid concentration, and increased bacterial counts. In experimental rumen acidosis, the normal olive green color of rumen fluid changed first to milky gray at twelve hours post induction and then to cream colored from twenty-four hours onward (Shihabudheen et al. 2006).

At necropsy, examination of rumen content is essential for the detection of toxic plants and their subsequent identification. In lead poisoning, lead levels in rumen fluid may be diagnostic because most cases of lead intoxication involve ingestion.

Obtaining a usable sample of rumen fluid by stomach tube can be difficult in goats. Passage of the tube orally with a speculum can cause excessive saliva contamination of the fluid sample, which can erroneously elevate the sample pH. A smaller diameter tube can be passed nasally into the esophagus and rumen, but aspiration of viscous rumen fluid can be difficult with a small diameter tube. A specially designed device for obtaining rumen fluid is illustrated in Figure 19.7. Alternatively, a transabdominal sample can be collected. The fluid/gas interface of the rumen content can be estimated by ballotment or percussion of the left flank and a point selected below the fluid line. After aseptic preparation, a 3-inch (7.6-cm) 18-gauge needle can be passed through the abdominal and adjacent rumen wall and a fluid sample aspirated by syringe. This procedure presents no more risk of inducing peritonitis than routine abdominocentesis. In outbreaks of accidental grain overload involving numerous animals, this method allows for rapid determinations of rumen pH in affected goats to establish treatment priorities.

Table 10.2. Normal values reported for rumen fluid constituents.

Constituent	*Unit*	*Reported range*	*Reported mean*	*Comments/reference*
pH			7.35 ± 0.3	Re-domesticated feral goats with rumen fistulae. Lucerne chaff and water diet fed free choice (Cao et al. 1987).
Osmolarity	mOsmol/kg		248 ± 14.2	"
Lactate	mmol/l		0.0	"
Sodium	mmol/l		115 ± 27	"
Potassium	mmol/l		40 ± 18.2	"
Chloride	mmol/l		21 ± 2.2	"
pH		6.9 (pre-drinking)—6 (post-drinking)		Black Bedouin goats with rumen fistulae. Lucerne hay free choice. Water once a day (Brosh et al. 1983).
Osmolarity	mOsmol/kg	330 (pre-drinking)—178 (post-drinking)		"
Bacterial count	$\times 10^9$/ml	24–26 (no change with drinking)		"
Protozoal count	$\times 10^4$/ml	43–60 (no change with drinking)		"
pH			7.40	Marwari goats with rumen cannulae. No feed for 24 hours before sampling. Water free choice (Tanwar and Mathur 1983).
Lactate	mg/dl		0.0	"
Bacterial count	$\times 10^9$/ml	100–160		"
Protozoal count	$\times 10^4$/ml	20–30		"
Protozoal count	$\times 10^6$/ml	0.25–2.83	0.96	150 Black Bengal goats at slaughter (Mukherjee and Sinha 1990).

mOsmol/kg = milliosmoles per kilogram, mmol/L = millimoles per liter.

Fecal Examination

The gross and microscopic examinations of feces are indispensable aids to the diagnosis of diseases of the digestive system. Normal goat feces is usually voided in piles of individual pellets 0.5 to 1.5 cm in diameter, although it is not necessarily abnormal if the pellets are sometimes caked together. Feces less well formed may be seen from animals grazing lush pasture. Feces similar to that normally produced by the dog, with poorly discernible pellets, should be considered abnormal. It is most often seen associated with gastrointestinal parasitism and sometimes paratuberculosis.

Whole kernels or identifiable portions of grain are rarely observed in goat feces unless the goat is on a very high level of grain feeding because the goat normally produces a consistently fine particle size of ingesta during mastication and regurgitation. Grain in the feces on a low-grain diet suggests dental disease or rumen disease.

Small, stony, darker pellets suggest constipation, most commonly caused by dehydration, and the cause should be pursued. Mucus coating the feces suggests prolonged transit through the alimentary tract and possible dehydration.

Fresh blood is uncommon in normal-appearing goat feces, but may be seen mixed in diarrheic feces in a number of conditions, including Nairobi sheep disease, rinderpest, enterotoxemia, coccidiosis, nodular worm infection, chabertiosis, and Japanese pieris toxicity. Dark, tarry stools (melena) can be seen in coccidiosis. Diarrhea is discussed in detail below.

Microscopic examination of goat feces, using direct smear or fecal flotation techniques, is valuable in the diagnosis and monitoring of most gastrointestinal parasitic infections. Samples for analysis should be fresh because ova will hatch rapidly and larvae will be undetectable using fecal flotation methods. Interpretation of results is discussed under the various specific parasitic diseases.

Imaging Techniques

Because of the goat's small size, radiographic studies can be readily performed and can be helpful in diagnosing intestinal obstruction, congenital atresia, foreign body penetrations, and mass lesions. The radiographic anatomy of the caprine digestive tract and contrast studies have been described (Cegarra and Lewis 1977; Chhadha and Gahlot 2006). Adult goats are fasted for forty-eight hours and given 600 ml of barium sulfate via stomach tube. The first film should be taken within one hour because in some cases the media may rapidly leave the rumen and already be in the abomasum. If the media is still in the rumen, the next film can be taken six to eight hours later and then at four-hour intervals until twenty-four hours, when most of the gastrointestinal tract will have been visualized.

DIAGNOSIS OF GASTROINTESTINAL DISEASE BY PRESENTING SIGN

The purpose of this section is to assist in the differential diagnosis of gastrointestinal diseases on the basis of common presenting signs. The possibilities offered are not geographically restricted, so some of the diseases listed for a given presenting sign may not apply to the sick goat at hand.

The major infectious, parasitic, and metabolic diseases of the digestive system are mentioned when appropriate for a given presenting sign, but are discussed in detail later in the chapter. Other diseases that occur infrequently or sporadically, that are very localized geographically, or that are not well described in goats are discussed fully in this section and are not addressed again later in the chapter. For conditions discussed elsewhere in the text outside of this chapter, the reader is referred to the appropriate chapter number.

Inappetence

A history of inappetence often tempts the clinician into presuming a primary digestive disorder. However, many multisystemic diseases, particularly if they produce fever, reduce appetite. The likelihood that inappetence reflects a digestive dysfunction increases if it is accompanied by changes in rumen motility, vomiting, the development of abnormal feces, tenesmus, or distortions of the abdominal contour.

Frothing at the Mouth

Frothing at the mouth may be seen independently of excessive salivation, slobbering, and drooling as discussed below. In all species, frothing is commonly associated with uncontrolled chewing or lip smacking during convulsive activity. In goats, frothing is probably seen most commonly as a mild adverse reaction to administration of the anthelmintic levamisole. Frothing or excessive salivation, depression, and hyperesthesia may occur in some goats shortly after administration of the drug, even at the suboptimal dose of 8 mg/kg orally or parenterally. Frothing, along with dyspnea, frequent urination and defecation, and clonic convulsions may occur when levamisole is overdosed, particularly by parenteral administration.

Idiopathic frothing at the commissures of the lips associated with cud chewing has been observed by the author in several individual French Alpine and Nubian does in different herds. The animals were normal in all other respects and were not receiving medications of any kind. Owners reported the condition occurred intermittently in individuals over periods of months to years.

Frothing at the mouth in conjunction with dyspnea, diarrhea, and ataxia was reported in goats from the Sudan poisoned by the plant *Cadaba rotundifolia* (El Dirdiri et al. 1987). In Kenya, frothing at the mouth in conjunction with bloat, incoordination, and death was caused by ingestion of *Cestrum aurantiacum*, a shrub used for hedges and windbreaks (Mugera and Nderito 1968). At necropsy, there was severe hemorrhagic gastroenteritis.

Excessive Salivation, Slobbering, or Drooling

Stomatitis, or inflammation of the mucosa of the oral cavity, is most often responsible for excess salivation, slobbering, or drooling in the goat. A foul odor to the breath may accompany salivation if necrosis of the oral mucosa has occurred. If pain is severe, dysphagia may also occur.

Infectious causes of stomatitis include contagious ecthyma, goat pox, unclassified viral dermatitis, foot and mouth disease, bluetongue, vesicular stomatitis, rinderpest, peste des petits ruminants, caprine herpesvirus, necrotic or ulcerative stomatitis caused by *Fusobacterium necrophorum* infection, and alveolar periostitis.

Contagious ecthyma (soremouth, orf) is the most common cause of stomatitis in goats worldwide. The virus produces papular eruptions mainly at the commissures of the lips that may become secondarily infected with bacteria. The lesions heal spontaneously within six weeks, but excess salivation, reluctance to eat, and mild dysphagia leading to weight loss can precede resolution.

Goat pox may produce ulcerative lesions on the lips and in the mouth in addition to the characteristic skin nodules, pyrexia, and conjunctivitis. The disease is absent from the Americas and Australia and has been largely eliminated from Europe. A highly fatal, unclassified viral dermatitis has been observed in India since 1946 (Haddow and Idnani 1948). The condition is distinct from goat pox clinically and pathologically, although a pox virus has been isolated from clinical cases (Patnaik 1986). Widespread cutaneous eruptions may include the lips, gums, and tongue. Rubbery, nonexudative nodules and papules develop on the oral surfaces and lead to necrotic ulcers in seven to ten days.

Foot and mouth disease may have drooling or lip smacking as presenting signs resulting from vesicles in the oral cavity. In goats and sheep, as compared with cattle, however, foot lesions are more common than oral lesions. The disease is endemic in much of Asia, Africa, and South America.

Bluetongue rarely causes clinical disease in goats, although serologic evidence of exposure occurs extensively. When clinical signs do occur, they include stomatitis associated with edema and congestion of the oral mucosa and ulceration of the lips and dental pad. These signs are accompanied by high fever, nasal discharge, diarrhea, and lameness caused by coronitis.

Vesicular stomatitis, caused by a rhabdovirus, occurs only in the Americas. Goats are less susceptible than cattle, horses, and swine. In goats, the only sign may be salivation with vesicles at the commissure of the lips, and the condition should be differentiated from contagious ecthyma by virus isolation.

Rinderpest produces a necrotic stomatitis involving the gums, cheeks, and tongue. However, salivation is not a dominant sign; it can be overshadowed by profuse, mucopurulent, oculonasal discharge, and later, diarrhea. Until recently, rinderpest was endemic in Africa, the Middle East, and south Asia, but the disease is close to being eradicated worldwide as a result of internationally coordinated control efforts. Goats are less severely affected than cattle.

Peste des petits ruminants is similar to rinderpest in clinical presentation, causing necrotic stomatitis, diarrhea, and bronchopneumonia. It affects goats severely. It occurs in much of Africa the Middle East and South Asia.

Caprine herpesvirus has been reported as a cause of severe illness and fatality in kids in Switzerland. Marked oral erosions were observed in conjunction with nasal discharge and conjunctivitis, and at necropsy, erosions of the cecum, colon, and urinary bladder (Mettler et al. 1979).

Necrotic stomatitis, caused by *Fusobacterium necrophorum* and other secondarily invasive bacteria, has been reported in four- to six-week-old Boer goat kids in South Africa (van Tonder et al. 1976). Clinical signs included fever, salivation, frothing, lip smacking and chewing movements, mucopurulent nasal discharge, anorexia, weight loss, and a mortality rate of 21%. Lesions were confined to the mouth, tongue, and throat and consisted of well circumscribed necrotic ulcers up to 4 cm in length. Treatment with parenteral chloramphenicol twice daily for five days was effective. Sodium sulfadimidine, penicillin, streptomycin, and tetracycline are all effective treatments for this condition in calves. A similar outbreak in India involved adult goats and kids. Pregnant does aborted and there was evidence of *F. necrophorum* septicemia (Nayak and Bhowmik 1988).

Dental disease, particularly alveolar periostitis, can produce pain in the mouth and inflammation of the gums leading to dysphagia and salivation. Oral examination should include careful inspection of the molars. Radiographs of the dental arcades may be helpful, because thorough visual examination of the teeth is awkward.

Noninfectious causes of stomatitis include chemical irritants, traumatic injuries, plant and chemical poisonings, and possibly neoplasia. If caustic dehorning pastes are used to remove horn buds on young kids, their licking the paste from each other's polls leads to chemical stomatitis. Caustic soda used to clear drains on farms may also cause stomatitis if the drains are backed up and goats drink the standing water. Battery acid from automotive storage batteries carelessly discarded can taste salty and has been consumed by curious goats, leading to chemical stomatitis (King 1980).

Giant hogweed *(Heracleum mantegazzianum)* has caused ulcerative stomatitis with anorexia and profuse salivation in a goat in Britain (Andrews et al. 1985). Other specific references to plant or chemically induced stomatitis in goats are rare. Agents known to cause stomatitis in other species can presumably affect the goat. These include mercurial and arsenical compounds and plants containing ranunculin, such as buttercup and crocuses.

Traumatic stomatitis with salivation can result from sharp dental points on the buccal aspect of the upper molars and lingual aspect of the lower molars. Abrasion and ulceration of the mucosa can lead to secondary bacterial infections and abscesses, particularly in the cheek. Certain plant awns, such as barley, foxtail, and thistle, can also traumatize the oral mucosa.

Rough or careless administration of medications using dose syringes and balling guns is a common cause of traumatic stomatitis of the hard palate and pharynx. Resulting injuries can produce salivation, dysphagia, regurgitation of feed, and possibly aspiration pneumonia.

Neoplasia of the oral cavity is rare in goats but three cases of lymphosarcoma or adenocarcinoma have been reported to involve oral structures, leading to loosening and displacement of molar teeth (Baker and Sherman 1982; Lane and Anderson 1983; Craig et al. 1986). A rare, primary parotid salivary gland tumor of mixed epithelial and mesenchymal elements has been reported in a two-month-old Jamnapuri crossbred female goat (Omar and Fatimah 1981).

Salivation may occur independent of stomatitis, usually caused by neurologic disease, systemic poisonings, or obstructions of the digestive tract distal to the oral cavity. Neurologic diseases associated with salivation or drooling in the goat are listeriosis, caprine arthritis encephalitis virus infection, migrations of the nematode parasite *Parelaphostrongylus tenuis*, and trauma to the facial nerve. Rabies and polioencephalomalacia may also produce excessive salivation, but usually in conjunction with other neurologic signs that are more general or progressive than those seen with the focal conditions just mentioned. Botulism produces a general weakness of the muscles including the tongue and muscles of mastication. Therefore, dysphagia and drooling can be seen along with recumbency. Neurologic diseases are discussed in detail in Chapter 5. Nutritional muscular dystrophy, or white muscle disease, can produce necrosis of the muscles of the tongue and pharynx, leading to dysphagia and drooling. The condition is discussed in detail in Chapter 4.

Profuse salivation may be one of the first recognized signs of organophosphate and carbamate poisoning. Additional signs include muscle stiffness and fasciculation, frequent urination and diarrhea, pupillary constriction, colic, dyspnea, nervousness, and sudden death. Some of these same signs, including salivation, may be seen in urea toxicity as discussed in Chapter 19. Acute chlorinated hydrocarbon poisoning also produces an abundant flow of ropy saliva in conjunction with signs suggesting neurologic dysfunction, such as belligerence, muscle twitching, clonic and tonic convulsions, and death. Xylazine produces excessive salivation at doses used for tranquilization.

Some plant poisonings produce salivation without stomatitis in goats. Plants of the family Ericaceae produce salivation and vomiting as discussed later in the section on regurgitation. *Cotyledon orbiculata* is common in South Africa. The plant is cardiotoxic, but excessive salivation is an important presenting sign after ingestion (Tustin et al. 1984).

Consumption of *Prosopis juliflora* (mesquite) and *Prosopis glandulosa* (honey mesquite) can be toxic to goats. When ingested in sufficient quantities, the unknown plant toxin can produce signs of salivation, dysphagia, protrusion of the tongue, and tremors of the mandible (Washburn et al. 2002; Misri et al. 2003). Vacuolation of neurons in the trigeminal motor nucleus and neuronal necrosis and loss in the trigeminal ganglia are associated with these clinical signs (Washburn et al. 2002).

"Slobbers" is caused by the fungus *Rhizoctonia leguminicola*, or "black patch," that grows on legume forages, particularly red clover, during wet weather and high humidity. It can persist on stored forages. The fungus produces an alkaloid, slaframine, which produces copious salivation within one hour of ingestion and may last for twenty-four hours after a single exposure. The condition is seen primarily in the United States and Japan and is reported in goats (Isawa et al. 1971). Slobbering may be the only clinical sign, but lacrimation, frequent urination, diarrhea, dyspnea, abortion, and even death may be seen with prolonged exposure. There is no specific treatment except for rapid diagnosis of the problem and removal of goats from the offending feed.

Cyanide poisoning, associated with ingestion of numerous plant species, can have salivation as the initial sign. The disease is discussed in Chapter 9.

Physical obstruction of the esophagus or pharynx can prevent the normal swallowing of saliva and lead to excess salivation. Bloat accompanies salivation when obstruction of the pharynx or esophagus is complete. Foreign bodies likely to produce obstruction are fruits, tubers, and roots.

No specific treatment for excessive salivation is recommended. Atropine may reduce saliva flow, but the additional effects of reduced gastric motility argue against its use. The major goal is to identify and treat the underlying cause of salivation. It should be remembered, however, that saliva is produced in very large amounts and contains many electrolytes, including bicarbonate. Prolonged loss of saliva may lead to dehydration, electrolyte imbalance, and acidosis. These sequelae should be managed with fluid and electrolyte therapy.

Dysphagia

Dysphagia may be manifested by prolonged chewing, retaining feed in the mouth, dropping feed from the mouth (quidding), and as just discussed, drooling or slobbering. Many of the causes of stomatitis also can produce dysphagia depending on the extent and severity of the oral lesions present.

Focal neurologic diseases such as listeriosis, brain abscess, parasitic larval migration, and CAE can produce dysphagia when damage to the cranial nerve roots VII, IX, X, or XII occurs. Nutritional muscular dystrophy affecting the tongue and pharyngeal muscles can mimic these neurologic deficits. Accumulation of feed in the buccal space can be associated with the loss of one or more molars secondary to aging or alveolar periostitis. This can also occur with facial nerve paralysis resulting in flaccidity of the cheek muscles. Holding feed for prolonged periods in the mouth without chewing may be observed in rabies, tetanus, botulism, and polioencephalomalacia.

Developing teeth are subject to structural modification by chronic exposure to fluoride. Fluorosis can produce pitting, a rough, chalky enamel, discoloration, and accelerated wearing of teeth (Milhaud et al. 1980). The excessive tooth wear and associated pain can produce signs of dysphagia. The third and fourth pairs of incisors are most often affected. Exostoses of the mandible and maxilla may also occur. Fluorosis is discussed in detail in Chapter 4. Excessive tooth wear is also associated with grazing of sandy soils by goats.

Additional dental problems that may lead to dysphagia include over-eruption of teeth; broken teeth; vestigial teeth; and displaced, rotated, or migrated teeth (Rudge 1970). Fibrous osteodystrophy, discussed in Chapter 4, can lead to severe inward rotation of the dental arcades.

In recent years, there have been unsubstantiated reports from Kenya that goats grazing on the seed pods of *Prosopis juliflora* (mesquite) are losing their teeth as a result of the seeds sticking between the teeth and gums, leading to gingivitis, alveolitis, disfigured jaws, impaired ability to eat, and inanition (Mwangi and Swallow 2005). While tooth loss is unsubstantiated, *Prosopis* spp. can produce salivation and dysphagia without a direct effect on teeth, as discussed above in the section on salivation.

Presence of milk or chewed feed at the nares and coughing in kids may result from cleft palate. Retropharyngeal abscess caused by *Corynebacterium pseudotuberculosis* in older goats may block normal swallowing by compression of the soft palate leading to coughing and nasal expulsion of feed. Balling gun or dose syringe injuries may initiate these abscesses. Attempts at surgical drainage carry a guarded prognosis. There is a reported case of a goat whose tongue was encircled by the neck of a broken bottle, leading to trauma to the tongue and dysphagia. To correct the condition, the glass ring was snapped with a bone forceps and with supportive treatment the goat recovered (Alhendi et al. 1999).

Treatment of animals with dysphagia should include broad-spectrum parenteral antibiotics until normal swallowing resumes because the risk of aspiration pneumonia in association with dysphagia is high. Correction of dehydration and nutritional supplementation through a stomach tube must also be considered during prolonged disease.

Regurgitation, Retching, or Projectile Vomiting

Partial or complete obstructions of the pharynx or esophagus can lead to regurgitation of feed in goats (Fleming et al. 1989). Acute copper toxicity in a herd of goats given an overdose of oral copper sulfate resulted in repeated attempts to vomit, as well as abdominal pain, muscle fasciculations, labored breathing, tachycardia, and frothing at the mouth before death (Shlosberg 1978).

In other species, notably dogs, megaesophagus is associated with vomiting. However, in the one reported case of megaesophagus in a four-year old Nubian doe there was no history of vomiting. The only clinical signs were an obvious swelling of the dilated esophagus in the ventral portion of the neck and gurgling sounds audible from a few meters. Contrast radiography indicated that the esophageal dilation extended through the thorax to the cardia (Ramadan 1993).

The toxic plants most often associated with vomiting in goats are members of the heath family (Ericaceae) and include rhododendrons, laurels, azaleas, lily of the valley tree (*Clethra arborea*), and Japanese pieris. They contain the toxic principle grayanotoxin (also referred to as andromedotoxin), which acts primarily on the autonomic nervous system, stimulating the vomiting center via the vagus nerve and producing hypotension (Smith 1978; Knight 1987; Gibb 1987). Clinical signs can occur when as little as 0.1% of the animal's bodyweight is ingested as fresh leaves.

Within six hours of ingestion of Ericaceae, goats may show signs of depression, weakness, anorexia, salivation, abdominal pain, vomiting, and possibly bloat and diarrhea. Tenesmus and blood in the feces were reported in a goat consuming *Pieris formosanum* (Hollands and Hughes 1986). While the condition may be self-limiting within days if only small amounts of the plants are eaten, ingestion of large quantities may cause death (Visser et al. 1988). Exposure of eighteen goats to clippings of *Rhododendron macrophyllum* resulted in convulsions and death in two, weight loss in all, and agalactia in seven (Casteel and Wagstaff 1989). Sublethal ingestion of Japanese pieris has been associated with fetal mummification in a goat (Smith 1979).

If known exposure has occurred, rumenotomy before the onset of signs is recommended. After onset of signs, treatment should include intravenous fluid therapy to counter hypotension, relief of bloat by stomach tube if necessary, oral magnesium hydroxide and activated charcoal, and parenteral calcium gluconate, as well as parenteral antibiotic to minimize the risk of aspiration pneumonia associated with vomiting. The antispasmodic hyoscine-*n*-butylbromide has also been used to control vomiting.

Prevention involves educating goat owners regarding the potential danger of these plants to livestock. Members of the heath family are widely used as ornamental plantings, and goats should be kept away from plantings and not fed prunings because these will be readily eaten.

Other plants may cause vomiting in goats. A spontaneous case of vomiting in conjunction with constant bellowing, rumen atony, and depression was reported in a goat ingesting *Raphanus sativus*, a member of the Cruciferae, or mustard, family (Drahn 1951). Vomiting, depression, and a staggering gait were observed in a goat in England after ingestion of *Solanum nigrum*, or black nightshade (Gunning 1949). Gladiolus corms eaten by goats produced bleating or moaning, vomiting, staggering, and depression within hours.

Exposure was fatal in some cases. The prominent finding at necropsy was watery-brown rumen content (Anonymous 1988).

Rumen Atony

Normal rumen mixing contractions may be reduced in frequency when goats are fed rations low in coarse roughage and high in finely ground concentrate. Contractions may disappear when goats are excited or fearful, when parasympathomimetic drugs such as atropine are administered, or when central nervous system anesthetics and depressants such as barbiturates have been given.

Pathologic processes occurring outside the digestive system can inhibit rumen motility. These include pain from any source, severe dehydration, electrolyte or acid-base imbalances, hypocalcemia, high fever, and toxemias. Peritonitis as a cause of rumen atony is uncommon in goats as compared with cattle, mainly because of the infrequent occurrence of traumatic reticuloperitonitis in goats. There are few references to this condition in the goat (Maddy 1954; Sharma and Ranka 1978; Tanwar and Saxena 1984). It is presumed that the more selective, discriminating food prehension behavior of goats limits the ingestion of foreign bodies capable of penetrating the reticulum. When traumatic reticulitis does occur in goats, signs are similar to those in cattle. There is a report of experimentally induced traumatic reticuloperitonitis in seventeen goats fed wires, nails, and/or needles (Roztocil et al. 1968). The clinical presentation reflected what is seen in naturally occurring bovine cases, namely fever, anorexia, depression, cessation of rumen motility, elicitation of pain with application of pressure in the region of the xiphoid cartilage, and neutrophilia with a left shift. Some individuals also developed traumatic pericarditis, pneumonia, and/or hepatitis, depending on the ultimate locations of the metal foreign bodies.

Pathologic processes within the digestive system leading to rumen atony include simple indigestion, bloat, rumen acidosis caused by acute carbohydrate engorgement, and rumen alkalosis associated with urea poisoning. In general, plant and chemical poisonings frequently include rumen atony as one of the presenting signs.

Abdominal Distension

There is considerable variation in the normal abdominal silhouette. Pygmy goats are achondroplastic dwarfs, and as such, their abdominal girth is proportionately greater for their height and weight compared with other breeds. As young pygmy goats develop full rumen capacity, they sometimes appear to inexperienced owners to be abnormally distended in the abdomen. An inherited condition identified as "dropped stomach" has been reported in Toggenburg does. It involved permanent stretching of the ventral abdominal musculature in late pregnancy. After parturition, the ventral abdomen remains pendulous but affected animals are otherwise normal (Wirth 1980). The condition has also been observed in other breeds (Figure 10.1).

Ruminal tympany, or bloat, is not uncommon in goats, and both the frothy (nutritional) and free gas forms can occur. In all types, abdominal distension is initially most prominent in the left paralumbar fossa, and may also involve the entire left side of the abdomen and the right ventral abdomen if severe.

The single case of left displaced abomasum reported in the goat was associated with intermittent bloat (West et al. 1983). Acute carbohydrate engorgement can also produce a similar pattern of abdominal distension due both to gas accumulation and fluid pooling in the rumen. The presence of fluid can be established by ballotment of the ventral rumen and by reflux through a stomach tube.

Rumen impaction produces a distended rumen palpable as a firm mass low on the left side of the abdomen behind the ribs. The causes and management of rumen impaction are discussed later in this chapter. Abdominal distension predominantly in the lower right quadrant is most commonly associated with late pregnancy as the rumen displaces the expanding uterus to the

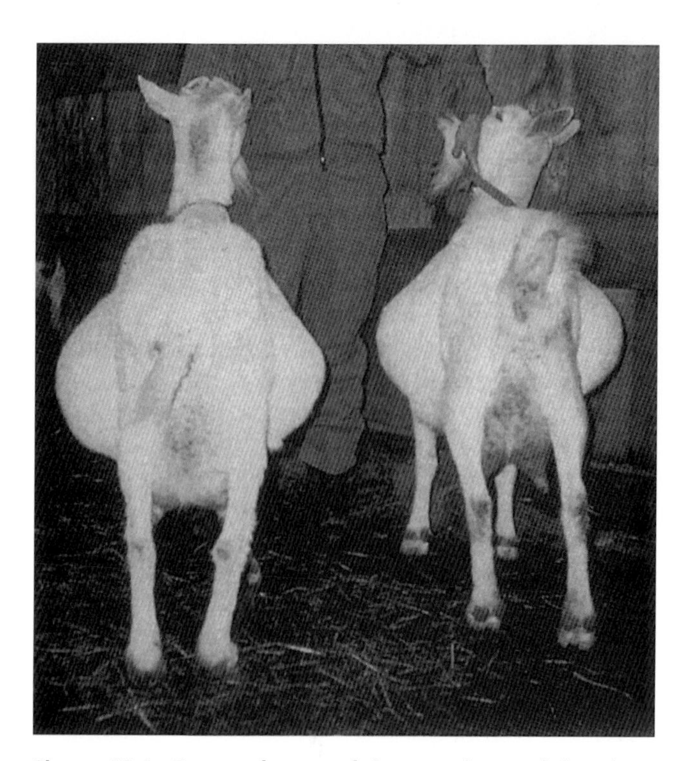

Figure 10.1. Dropped stomach in a mother and daughter pair of Saanen goats. Note prominent abdominal distension. Neither goat is pregnant. (Courtesy of Dr. David M. Sherman.)

right. Herniation of the gravid uterus through the right abdominal floor causing prominent right ventral abdominal distension occasionally occurs (Horenstein and Elias 1987).

Abnormal distension of the right ventral abdomen also can be associated with abomasal disorders. Abomasal impaction with metal shavings has been reported in an adult goat from India (Purohit et al. 1986). Numerous abomasal impactions with phytobezoars have been reported from South Africa. The concretions are composed of the pappus hairs of the seeds of Karoo bushes. Goats are more often affected than sheep and Boer goats more often than Angora goats (Bath 1978). The clinical syndrome is one of progressive abdominal distension and weight loss. Occasionally animals are found dead due to rupture of the stomach. The phytobezoars, which are multiple and round, may be felt in the abomasum by deep palpation behind the xiphoid cartilage. Early recognition and quick slaughter for salvage are recommended because no satisfactory treatment has been identified (Bath and Bergh 1979).

The feeding of high-fiber roughages of low digestibility mentioned as a cause of rumen impaction can also produce abomasal impaction, particularly in pregnant does. In these cases, the lower right abdomen is distended, or a doughy abomasal content can be palpated. Animals are thin and feces are soft, fibrous, and malodorous. Treatment includes dietary improvement and the use of laxatives such as mineral oil. The value of abomasotomy has not been reported. Pregnancy toxemia is a possible sequela, and the prognosis is guarded.

Abrupt changes in feeding, from milk to milk replacer or milk pellets, are associated with abomasal bloat. The pathogenesis of abomasal bloat may involve the rapid fermentation of sugars by gas-producing, anaerobic bacteria present in the abomasum, such as *Sarcina* spp., which were identified during an epidemic of abomasal bloat in kids six to ten weeks of age that occurred in a large goat dairy in California (DeBey et al. 1996). Abomasal bloat is also seen predictably in young kids in artificial rearing systems, particularly when milk is fed directly from a trough or bucket without a nipple (Thompson 1987). This is presumed to be caused by too rapid ingestion followed by excessive fermentation of milk. Because the abomasum in the suckling goat is the largest stomach, gas distension may occur on the left and right sides of the abdomen. The condition can be fatal. Alternative methods of feeding using nipple feeders or feeding *ad libitum* should be considered (Morand-Fehr et al. 1982; Thompson 1987). Successful treatment of a series of abomasal bloat cases in kids one to two weeks of age has been reported using a single intramuscular injection of hyoscine at 0.3 mg/kg bw plus metaclopramide at 0.5 mg/kg bw and a vitamin E/selenium compound at 0.1 mg/kg bw (Kojouri 2004).

Overfeeding of milk can also lead to ruminal bloat when excessive volumes of milk reflux into the developing rumen (Chennells 1981). Overfeeding may also predispose to acute enterotoxemia with signs of hemorrhagic enteritis, nervous dysfunction, or death.

Bilateral ventral distension of the abdomen due to chronic indigestion secondary to abomasal impaction, as described above, may be seen in goats. It also has been observed in a goat with acute duodenal obstruction caused by a phytobezoar (Sherman 1981). Accumulation of ascites fluid secondary to conditions causing hypoproteinemia or cardiac insufficiency also may produce such bilateral distension. There is a report of marked fluid distension of the abdomen of an eleven-year-old pygmy goat secondary to extensive abdominal fat necrosis attributed to tall fescue toxicity in North Carolina (Smith et al. 2004). In young goats, gastrointestinal nematodiasis and tapeworm infestations can lead to a marked "pot-bellied" appearance.

In female goats of breeding age, pseudopregnancy or hydrometra is a common cause of bilateral ventral abdominal distension. In male goats, the most common cause is urine accumulation in the abdomen after ruptured bladder caused by obstructive urolithiasis. This condition is discussed in detail in Chapter 12.

Intestinal and ovarian adenocarcinomas have been associated with accumulations of as much as 30 liters of intra-abdominal fluid in aged, female goats with progressive abdominal distension and discomfort (Haibel 1990; Memon et al. 1995). There is also a single case report of abdominal mesothelioma involving the peritoneum in an eight-year-old female Toggenburg goat in Austria that presented with marked ascites and a distended, pear-shaped abdomen (Krametter et al. 2004). Peritoneal mesothelioma was also diagnosed in a goat in South Africa (Bastianello 1983).

Generalized distension of the abdomen may occur secondary to conditions causing generalized ileus such as severe peritonitis and sporadic intestinal accidents. General abdominal distension in young kids may occur before the onset of diarrhea in the early stages of infectious bacterial enteritis, when the causative organisms are potent gas producers. Congenital atresia ani and atresia coli or recti occur in newborn kids. Atresia can usually be diagnosed by a history of progressive abdominal distension, straining to defecate with no fecal output, depression, and waning appetite in kids from one to four days old. However, kids as old as fourteen days of age have been presented for veterinary attention with a history of no defecation. Atresia ani has been successfully corrected surgically in goats by creation of anal patency (Ali et al. 1976). Atresia coli or recti may require a colostomy to salvage the affected animal (Philip 1973). In the goat, atresia ani also can occur associated with rectovaginal fistula, which allows for fecal voiding and may not be recognized until doelings approach breeding age or vaginitis occurs (Johnson et al. 1980). Animals with congenital anomalies of the anus, rectum, and colon should not be used for breeding if salvaged by surgical repair. A high incidence of atresia ani has been reported in the Shami breed of goat in Jordan (Al-Ani et al. 1998).

Focal distortions of the abdominal silhouette can be seen. Causes include umbilical hernia and spontaneous or traumatic ruptures of the abdominal wall, sometimes associated with fighting between horned goats (Figure 10.2). Ventral abdominal herniation in the doe has been associated with stretching of the ventral musculature during pregnancy and the subsequent increased weight of the enlarging udder (Misk et al. 1986). In Saudi Arabia, 193 goats with hernial swellings were presented to a veterinary teaching hospital over a five-year period. Umbilical, ventral abdominal, inguinal, scrotal, and perineal hernias were all diagnosed, some with the assistance of contrast radiography (Abdin-Bey and Ramadan 2001).

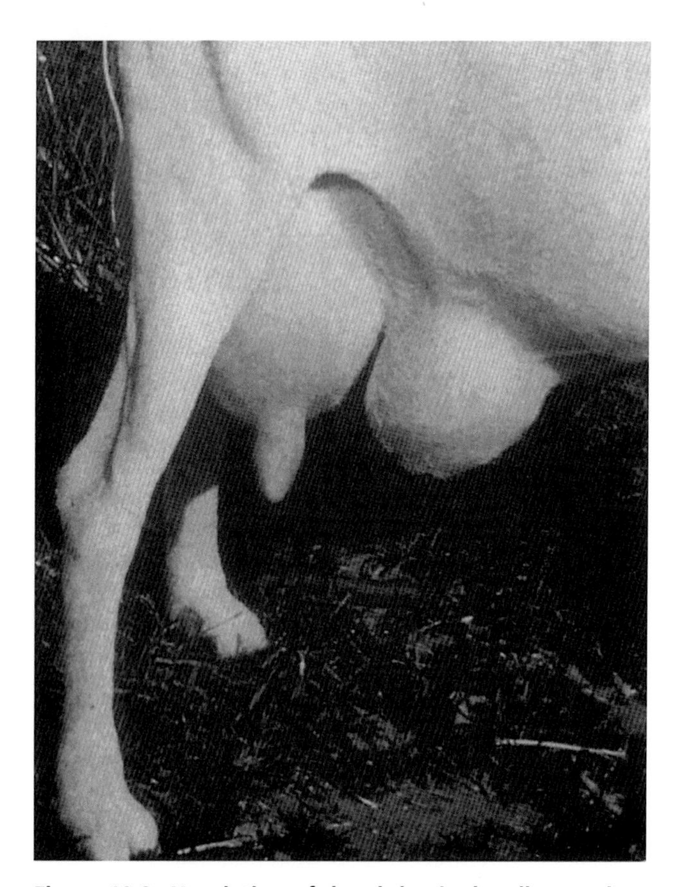

Figure 10.2. Herniation of the abdominal wall secondary to fighting with a horned goat. (Reproduced by permission of Dr. C.S.F. Williams.)

Abdominal Pain or Colic

Abdominal pain in goats may be manifested by depression, restlessness, bleating, teeth grinding, reluctance to move, increased shallow respiration, increased heart rate, tenesmus, or an abnormal posture with an arched back and tucked-up abdomen. Overt colic signs such as kicking at the belly or rolling are less common.

Mechanical Causes

In young kids, abdominal pain may be caused by feeding very cold milk or too much milk. Cecal torsion, intussusception (Mitchell 1983), and torsion of the root of the mesentery are sporadically occurring intestinal accidents more common in young goats than mature goats and are associated with pain. Torsion of the root of the mesentery is most common in unweaned kids fed by bottle or in *ad libitum* systems (Thompson 1985). In pregnant does, uterine torsion can produce abdominal pain. There is a report of rumen impaction in a goat in which extension and stretching of the fore and hind limbs and muscular rigidity, typical of a colicky horse, were presenting signs (Otesile and Akpokodje 1991).

Infectious Causes

Signs of severe abdominal pain may occur in conjunction with diarrhea, screaming, and convulsions before death from acute *Clostridium perfringens* type D enterotoxemia. Episodes of abdominal discomfort or pain may be observed during or immediately after eating in young goats with acute coccidiosis, before the onset of diarrhea. In young kids, enterotoxemia and coccidiosis must be differentiated from intestinal accidents such as torsion of the root of the mesentery at necropsy.

Peritonitis

Peritonitis can produce abdominal pain in addition to ileus, abdominal distension, and fever. Causes of infectious peritonitis in goats include rumen trocharization, uterine tears associated with dystocia, and extension of metritis from the uterus to the abdominal cavity. It can also occur as a sequela to rumenitis after acute carbohydrate engorgement. Organisms commonly associated with infectious peritonitis are *E. coli*, streptococci, staphylococci, *Fusobacterium necrophorum*, and *Clostridium* spp. Systemic mycoplasmosis in goats can produce a serositis-arthritis disease complex that includes peritonitis (DaMassa et al. 1983). Filarial worms of the genus *Setaria* may be found in the peritoneal cavity of goats, but are considered nonpathogenic (Subramanian and Srivastava 1973).

Noninfectious causes of peritonitis in goats include chemical irritation caused by intraperitoneal injections of sulfa drugs or calcium solutions, talc from surgical gloves (Hall 1983), and bile.

Toxicities

Several ingested plants and chemical toxins can produce abdominal pain. The Ericaceae can produce signs of colic, as can acute oral copper poisoning, acute carbohydrate engorgement, and organophosphate insecticide toxicity.

Urolithiasis

Perhaps the most common cause of abdominal pain in goats is obstructive urolithiasis seen in male goats. The appearance of pain is characterized by frequent and strained attempts to urinate. This is often misinterpreted by owners as straining to defecate caused by constipation.

Absence of Feces or Constipation

A history of no fecal output in association with tenesmus, abdominal pain, or abdominal distension strongly suggests an intestinal blockage caused by volvulus, intussusception, incarceration, or luminal obstruction by foreign body. Digital palpation of the rectum may reveal feces that arrived at the rectum before the obstruction occurred. The fecal matter should be removed and the animal rechecked later. If the rectum contains mucus only or mucus mixed with blood, this is strong evidence of intestinal obstruction. In neonates, atresia ani and atresia coli must be considered when there is no feces.

Constipation may be observed as a side effect of normal pregnancy or as a sign of pregnancy toxemia during late gestation (Pinsent and Cottom 1987). It may also be seen when access to water is limited or when diets are fibrous and of poor quality.

Extraluminal compression of the intestine by intra-abdominal abscesses due to *Corynebacterium pseudotuberculosis* may impede fecal output in goats. While clinical coccidiosis is noted for producing diarrhea, subclinical coccidiosis, which is common in young goats, produces constipation in conjunction with anorexia and reduced growth rate (Aumont et al. 1984).

Diarrhea

There are numerous known infectious and parasitic causes of diarrhea and their frequency of occurrence varies to a large extent with the age of goats affected, as presented in Table 10.3. Diarrhea in young goats results from a complex interaction of etiologic, immunologic, and husbandry factors. The topic is discussed separately at the end of this chapter under the heading Neonatal Diarrhea Complex.

Noninfectious causes of diarrhea include overfeeding in kids, simple indigestion, acute carbohydrate engorgement (lactic acidosis), copper deficiency, and

Table 10.3. Reported infectious causes of diarrhea in young kids.

1 day to 4 weeks of age	*4 weeks to 12 weeks of age*	*Over 12 weeks of age*
Viruses	**Viruses**	**Viruses**
Rotavirus	Rotavirus**	Peste des petits ruminants
Coronavirus	Peste des petits ruminants	Rinderpest
Adenovirus	Rinderpest	**Bacteria**
Herpesvirus	**Bacteria**	*Salmonella* spp.
Peste des petits ruminants*	*Salmonella* spp.	*Yersinia* spp.
Rinderpest*	*Yersinia* spp.	*Clostridium perfringens*
Bacteria	*Clostridium perfringens*	**Protozoa**
Escherichia coli	**Protozoa**	*Eimeria* spp.
Salmonella spp.	*Eimeria* spp.	**Nematodes**
*Clostridium perfringens**	*Cryptosporidium***	*Trichostrongylus* spp.
Yersinia spp.*	**Nematodes**	*Ostertagia* spp.
Protozoa	*Trichostrongylus* spp.	*Cooperia* spp.
Cryptosporidium	*Ostertagia* spp.	*Nematodirus* spp.
Eimeria spp.*	*Cooperia* spp.	*Strongyloides papillosus*
Giardia	*Nematodirus* spp.	**Trematodes**
Nematodes	*Strongyloides papillosus*	Paramphistomes
Strongyloides papillosus	**Trematodes**	
	Paramphistomes	

*Reported, but more common in kids older than 4 weeks of age.
**Reported, but more common in kids younger than 4 weeks of age.

intoxications. Though not as well documented, it is reasonable to assume that toxic agents known to produce diarrhea in other species, such as arsenic and organophosphates, would also do so in goats.

A number of plant intoxications have been documented as causing diarrhea in goats. These include *Parthenium hysterophorus, Nerium* spp. (oleanders), *Euphorbium* spp. (spurge), members of the Ericaceae family, *Aristolochia bracteata, Ipomoea sericophylla, Citrullus colocynthis, Lagneria siceraria, Jatropha* spp., *Sesbania vesicaria, Tephrosia apollinea, Malus sylvestris* (crab apple), *Abrus precatorius, Brachiaria mutica* (para grass), *Cassia senna* (coffee senna), and *C. italica* (Prasad et al. 1981; El Sayed et al. 1983; Galal et al. 1985; Shaw 1986; Dobereiner et al. 1987; Barri et al. 1990).

Goats are considered resistant to the toxic effects of oak ingestion and are often used to clear oak from pastures to allow grazing by cattle and sheep. Nevertheless, hemorrhagic gastroenteritis with bloody diarrhea caused by oak ingestion *(Quercus floribunda)* has been reported in goats in India and resistance of goats to oak toxicity cannot be considered absolute (Katiyar 1981).

Selenium toxicosis related to the ingestion of selenium-concentrating plants can also produce diarrhea. Experimental daily dosing of goats with sodium selenite at 6 mg/kg produced constipation followed by diarrhea with blood and mucus, as well as polydipsia, polyuria, lacrimation, coughing, and nasal discharge (Pathak and Datta 1984).

Oral ochratoxin administration produced diarrhea and death in a doe fed 3 mg/kg for five days (Ribelin et al. 1978). This is less than one-fourth the lethal dose rate in cattle.

Weight Loss

The major causes of weight loss associated with the alimentary tract are inadequate nutrition, gastrointestinal nematodiasis, and paratuberculosis. In addition, numerous diarrheal diseases such as enterotoxemia, salmonellosis, rinderpest, and peste des petits ruminants have chronic forms that lead to weight loss. However, there are numerous causes not associated with the alimentary tract. Progressive weight loss is a clinical presentation so common in goats that the differential diagnosis of this condition is discussed in detail in Chapter 15.

SPECIFIC DISEASES OF THE DIGESTIVE SYSTEM

VIRAL DISEASES

Peste des Petits Ruminants

This virus disease of goats and sheep in Africa and Asia is clinically similar to rinderpest in cattle in that animals are affected by fever, stomatitis, and diarrhea, but in contrast to cattle, respiratory signs and pneumonia are prominent features. The comparative aspects of the two diseases in small ruminants have been reviewed (Lefèvre 1982; Roeder and Obi, 1999).

Etiology

Peste des petits ruminants (PPR) is caused by a morbillivirus in the family Paramyxoviridae. The morbillivirus genus also includes the canine distemper, measles, and rinderpest viruses and the related viruses of cetacean and phocine marine mammals. These RNA viruses are enveloped, contain RNA in tightly coiled, helical nucleocapsids, and are structurally, physicochemically, and antigenically similar.

Serologic cross-reactions between PPR and rinderpest virus are observed in immunodiffusion and complement fixation reactions. The shared antigens occur in the nucleocapsid and envelope. Cross-reactive serum neutralizing antibodies also occur, but the reaction to the two viruses can be distinguished based on quantitative antibody assays. There is no evidence of antigenic differences among various field isolates of PPR virus; all belong to one serotype. However, phylogenetic analysis based on amplification and sequencing of a fragment of the viral fusion (F) protein indicates that there are four distinct lineages for the PPR virus (Shaila et al. 1996). Lineages 1 and 2 are found exclusively in West Africa. Lineage 3 has been found in eastern Africa, the Arabian peninsula and southern India, while lineage 4 is found from Turkey eastward through the Middle East and the Indian sub-continent (Dhar et al. 2002).

Peste des petits ruminants virus can be cultivated in sheep or goat kidney cell, Vero cell, and embryonal or neonatal testicular cell cultures. A cytopathic effect with formation of syncytia and clock-faced giant cells is observed. Intracytoplasmic and intranuclear inclusions occur.

Epidemiology

Peste des petits ruminants was first described as a disease mimicking rinderpest in sheep and goats in the Ivory Coast in 1942 (Gargadennec and Lalanne 1942). Serologic cross-reactions with rinderpest virus confused early recognition of the disease as a distinct entity of separate etiology. By the late 1970s, experimental infections, virological studies, and serologic studies established that PPR was a disease distinct from rinderpest and that the small ruminant disease syndromes of West Africa known as Kata and stomatitis pneumoenteritis complex were in fact PPR (Rowland et al. 1971; Hamdy et al. 1976; Gibbs et al. 1979).

From the 1970s PPR has been identified progressively further eastward in sub-Saharan Africa (Roeder et al. 1994), in the Middle East and South Asia. It is now becoming apparent that PPR is in fact caused by an Asian virus which was introduced to West Africa in the early part of the twentieth century (Taylor and Barrett 2007). Much of what was earlier reported to be rinderpest in small ruminants in South Asia is now considered to have been PPR.

An epizootic of highly virulent PPR appears to have developed in South Asia in the early 1990s and to have spread widely between Bangladesh, Turkey, and the Middle East. It is still gaining ground as evidenced by widespread infection in the Central Asian countries in recent years (Roeder, personal communication 2007). The People's Republic of China reported PPR to the World Organization for Animal Health (OIE) for the first time in July 2007. The outbreak occurred in Tibet.

The principal hosts of PPR are sheep and goats, with goats more susceptible to development of disease. Breed variation in susceptibility among goats has been suggested. However, some studies suggest that management and climatic factors may be confounders in this analysis (Ezeokoli et al. 1986). For example, different rates of breeding may affect population susceptibility, as the more prolific breeds may have a higher proportion of younger, more susceptible animals in the population. The disease is considered to be a major constraint in the development of small ruminant productivity among small-holders, mainly by causing high mortality in young stock (Sumberg and Mack 1985).

Virus replication occurs in cattle and pigs, and serum neutralizing antibodies may occur. Neither species, however, is considered to play an active role in disease transmission. Rats can be subclinically infected but do not appear to transmit the virus to other rats or goats (Komolafe et al. 1987).

There is evidence that some wild ruminants can be infected with PPR and experience clinical disease, but the role of wild ruminant populations in the epidemiology of the disease remains unclear. The white tail deer of North America is readily infected experimentally (Hamdy and Dardiri 1976). An outbreak of PPR in a zoological park in the United Arab Emirates resulted in peracute deaths in gazelles, ibex, and gemsbok. Goats grazing on the zoo perimeter were believed to be the source of infection (Furley et al. 1987). In 2002, a PPR outbreak was confirmed in semi-free ranging Dorcas gazelles and Thomson's gazelles in Saudi Arabia with case fatality rates of 100% (Abu Elzein et al. 2004). The source of the infection was not confirmed.

When populations of naive, susceptible goats are suddenly exposed to infected animals, morbidity and mortality from PPR can approach 100%. In outbreaks of PPR in endemic areas, it is young goats between three and twelve months of age that are most often and most seriously affected. Concurrent diseases, such as parasitism or goat pox, can increase mortality. Older animals are protected by antibody derived from previous natural exposure or by vaccination, while newborn animals up to three or four months of age have maternally derived immunity from colostrum. In places where kidding occurs year-round, the continuous supply of susceptible young kids with waning maternal antibody facilitates maintenance of endemic PPR infection.

Seasonal peaks of disease may be observed during the heavy rains of summer or the dry cold winds of winter in some endemic countries. These increases may simply reflect peaks in susceptible young kid populations, but the pattern of disease may also be conditioned by variations in climate, geography, and differences in livestock management practices (Obi et al. 1983; Ezeokoli et al. 1986). Pastoralism and/or transhumance which leads to high densities of susceptible animals on seasonal pastures is often associated with increases in disease.

Goats and sheep that recover from infection do not shed the virus, and no carrier state has been identified for PPR. Recovered animals develop a strong immunity of at least several years' duration. Slaughterhouse surveys of apparently healthy goats in northern Nigeria indicated a seroprevalence of PPR antibody in 44% of goats tested, with goats older than three years of age having the highest rates of prevalence (Taylor 1979).

Pathogenesis

Infected animals shed the virus in oculonasal discharges, saliva, and feces during the clinical stages of disease. The disease is transmitted by direct contact or by aerosol via the coughing and sneezing that occur. After entry into the respiratory tract, virus localizes in the tonsils and in mandibular and pharyngeal lymph nodes during an incubation period of four to six days. Viremia follows with subsequent localization of virus in the visceral lymph nodes, spleen, bone marrow, and mucosae of the respiratory and digestive systems. Virus replication in the mucosal epithelium of the digestive tract produces mucosal erosions resulting in stomatitis and diarrhea. Diarrhea can be severe, with many deaths resulting from dehydration and electrolyte imbalances. Virus replication in the lymphoid tissue produces a marked loss of lymphocytes. Immunity is impaired and secondary infections contribute to the severity of clinical disease and increased mortality, most notably in association with bacterial pneumonias.

Clinical Findings

Exposure to newly introduced goats or sheep during the preceding few days to weeks is a common history in explosive outbreaks of PPR. After an incubation period of four to six days, a fever of 104°F to 106°F

(40°C to 41.1°C) or higher develops, and the animals become depressed, with a rough hair coat and dry muzzle. Within a few hours of the onset of fever, a serous nasal or oculonasal discharge is observed. Superficial necrosis of the lips may also be seen at this time.

The next day, affected animals become anorexic and the nasal and ocular discharges become mucopurulent. Ocular discharges are sometimes accompanied by conjunctivitis but keratitis is not seen. Erosive lesions may be found inside the mouth on the cheeks, lips, gums, and tongue (Figure 10.3). These lesions may be covered with necrotic tissue and inflammatory debris and there is a fetid odor to the breath. Similar erosive lesions sometimes occur on the vaginal mucosa or within the prepuce. A profuse, watery, brown diarrhea may begin one or two days after the onset of fever. Coughing and sneezing are prominent signs at this time.

Fever usually persists for five to eight days; during that time, the animals grow progressively weaker and lose weight. Pregnant does may abort. The eyes, muzzle, and lips are increasingly crusted and matted and animals sneeze in attempts to clear the nares. Diarrhea persists, and marked dehydration ensues. Signs of secondary bacterial pneumonia may also develop. Although fever eventually subsides and erosive lesions in the oral cavity may heal, many animals grow steadily worse due to the persistent anorexia, severe dehydration, and complications of pneumonia. Prostration and death usually occur seven to twelve days after the onset of fever.

Subclinical infections are common, especially in arid regions. In these cases, PPR may go unrecognized, but affected animals are likely to develop fevers and respiratory signs caused by secondary bacterial pneumonia.

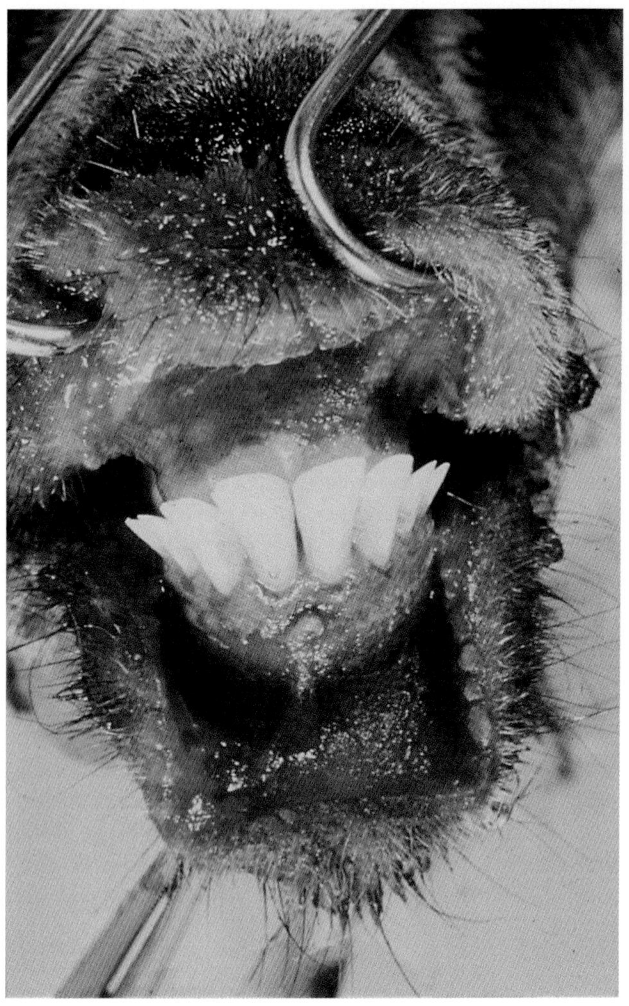

a

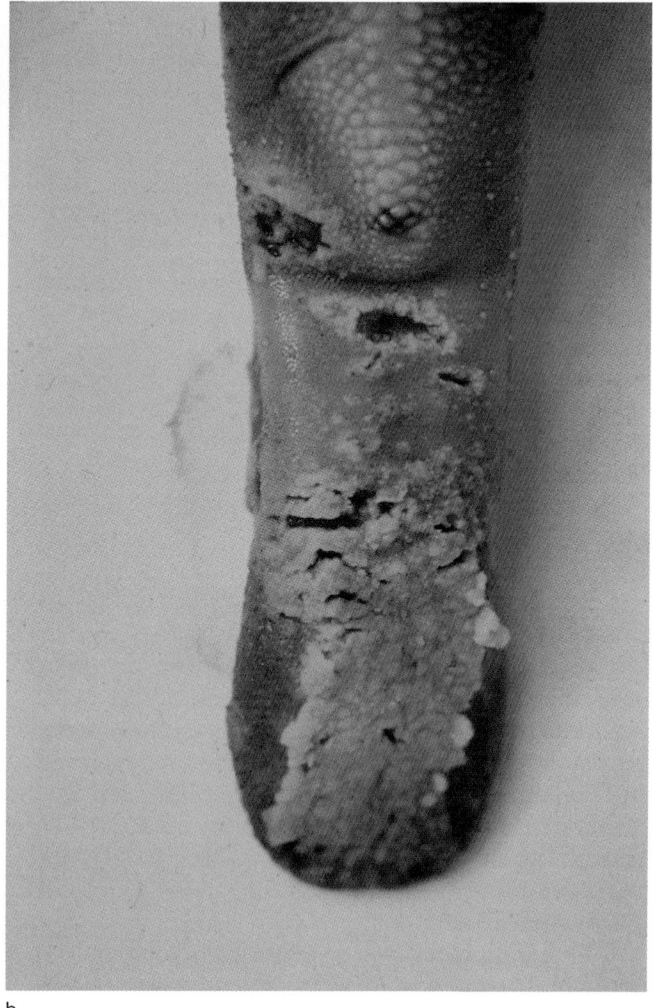

b

Figure 10.3. Ulceration of the gums (Figure 10.3a) and tongue (Figure 10.3b) of a goat with acute peste des petits ruminants. (From the collection of the Institute d'Élevage et de Médecine Vétérinaire des Pays Tropicaux [IEMVT].)

Clinical Pathology and Necropsy

The hemogram demonstrates leukocytosis during the incubation period, and leukopenia during the acute phase of clinical disease. The leukopenia is predominantly a lymphopenia. Neutrophil responses are variable depending on the development of secondary bacterial infections.

During the early febrile stage of the disease, which coincides with viremia, the virus can be isolated from the buffy coat of whole blood. Circulating antibody is not detectable during the febrile stage of the disease, but an increase in convalescent titer can be observed in recovering animals. The virus neutralization test (VNT) and the competitive ELISA are the tests of choice for identifying antibody to PPR. The VNT is the prescribed test for international trade. In areas where rinderpest and PPR both occur, the quantitative serum cross-neutralization test is useful because it does not only quantify the increase in titer, but it discriminates between PPR and rinderpest by demonstrating higher neutralizing antibody titers to PPR (OIE 2004). Convalescent antibody is detectable for at least one year after recovery.

At necropsy, the carcass is emaciated, dehydrated, and soiled around the hindquarters. The eyes, muzzle, and mouth are heavily crusted. Red, raw, shallow mucosal erosions are most common on the lips, tongue, and cheeks near the commissures, and in severe cases, on the soft and hard palate. The pharynx, esophagus, ruminal pillars, and abomasal leaves may also demonstrate mucosal erosions. Intestinal erosions are less common, but congestion is a consistent finding, with a streaky "zebra stripe" pattern of congestion or hemorrhage common in the large bowel near the ileocecal valve, cecocolic junction, and rectum. Peyer's patches may slough from the intestinal wall. Catarrhal inflammation of the upper respiratory tract with occasional petechiation and a necrotic tracheitis may be observed. The lungs may be dark red, congested, and firm. Lobular lung consolidation and airway exudate caused by secondary bacterial pneumonia are common. Lymph nodes and spleen are enlarged, congested, edematous, and possibly hemorrhagic.

Histologically, the mucosal lesions show marked epithelial necrosis with hydropic degeneration of epithelial cells at the edge of erosions. Intranuclear and intracytoplasmic inclusion bodies are common in areas of alimentary and respiratory epithelial necrosis. Syncytial cells in the oral epithelium and giant cells in lung alveoli may be observed. In the small intestine, villous atrophy and cellular casts in the crypts are seen. Lymph nodes and Peyer's patches show a dramatic depletion of lymphocytes and collapse of germinal centers. Lymphocyte necrosis is evident and macrophage numbers are increased. Multinucleated giant cells with eosinophilic intracytoplasmic inclusions are seen. Hemorrhagic necrosis occurs in the spleen.

Virus isolation should be attempted in cell culture from nasal, conjunctival, or buccal mucosal swabs in live animals or from tissues derived at post mortem, especially lymph nodes, spleen, tonsils, and lung. For detection of viral antigen in samples, the agar gel immunodiffusion test is the preferred assay. The immunocapture ELISA can be used when it is necessary to differentiate the PPR and RP viruses. Other assays which can be used to identify the PPR virus or its antigens include counter immunoelectrophoresis, polymerase chain reaction, immunofluorescence, and immunoperoxidase (OIE 2004).

Diagnosis

Peste des petits ruminants is easily confused with rinderpest, which produces a very similar spectrum of clinical signs. However, rinderpest is currently uncommon in places where PPR is endemic as a result of effective international control efforts. If characteristic clinical signs are seen in cattle, buffalo, or yaks, as well as in goats and/or sheep, then rinderpest becomes the more likely diagnosis. Goats and sheep are less severely affected by rinderpest and have morbidity and mortality rates that are lower than those usually seen with PPR. During the early febrile stage, heartwater (cowdriosis) should be considered in the differential diagnosis. In heartwater, however, neurologic signs develop as the disease progresses.

When oral lesions without diarrhea are observed, contagious ecthyma, bluetongue, and goat pox must be considered. While goats are more severely affected by PPR than sheep, the opposite is true in bluetongue, and goats rarely show clinical disease in endemic regions. Goat pox may present as fever followed by oculonasal discharges, but subsequent skin changes are widespread over the body. When diarrhea predominates, salmonellosis, Nairobi sheep disease, and coccidiosis must be ruled out. In recent years, there has been an increasing overlap in the endemic ranges of PPR and Nairobi sheep disease. Coccidiosis is particularly common in the age group most often affected with PPR but can be readily identified by examination of intestinal smears or feces. When pneumonic signs predominate, pasteurellosis and contagious caprine pleuropneumonia need to be considered. In areas where PPR has not occurred previously, the disease is commonly misdiagnosed as pneumonic pasteurellosis. A thorough physical examination that includes inspection of the oral cavity for erosive or ulcerative lesions should help to avoid such misdiagnosis.

Treatment

There is no specific treatment for PPR, although hyperimmune serum temporarily reverses clinical signs if given early, as discussed in Chapter 9. Affected animals should be placed on parenteral broad-spectrum antibiotics early in the disease to reduce the risk of likely secondary bacterial infections. Long-acting oxytetracycline, requiring an injection only every third day, is useful when repeated daily injections are impractical. The dose is 20 mg/kg given intramuscularly. Oral or parenteral fluid and electrolyte therapy may reduce mortality associated with diarrhea and dehydration.

Control

Because control of livestock movement through markets and between villages is so difficult, the main thrust of PPR control in endemic regions currently is vaccination using homologous tissue culture vaccines. The most common of these is derived from a West African strain, Nigeria 75/1, but there are other attenuated vaccines produced with strains from India, Bangladesh, and Kazakhstan. In the past, rinderpest vaccine was used to control PPR. While it offered good cross protection, its use is now contraindicated because it prevents countries from entering on the OIE pathway for accreditation of rinderpest freedom. PPR vaccine produced according to OIE guidelines provides protection against PPR for at least three years (OIE 2004).

In endemic areas, vaccination efficiency can be increased by targeting young animals in the first year of life after the loss of colostral immunity at three to four months of age. This is the group most at risk of infection. In the face of outbreaks, the spread of PPR is limited by ring vaccination of herds surrounding the index herd. When PPR occurs in nonendemic areas, total eradication is advised by slaughter and proper disposal of all sick and exposed sheep and goats.

Efforts are currently being made to develop effective PPR marker vaccines to enable differentiation between infected and vaccinated animals which would allow countries to implement both vaccination and disease surveillance programs at the same time (Diallo et al. 2007). A heat stable PPR vaccine has also been developed that would obviate the need for maintenance of cold chain in the field and thereby facilitate vaccination in remote areas to improve PPR control efforts (Worrall et al. 2001).

Rinderpest

Rinderpest, or cattle plague, is best known as a devastating disease of cattle. At the time of this writing, there is growing confidence that rinderpest has now been eradicated from the world. Formerly a disease widespread in Africa and Asia, the disease and its causative virus were last seen in eastern Africa in Cape buffaloes in 2001 (Roeder et al. 2005). Global accreditation of freedom from rinderpest is expected to be achieved by 2010 by following guidelines in a process overseen by OIE.

Goats are a mildly susceptible host. Frank clinical disease in goats is rarely observed and is associated with spill-over of infection from cattle or buffaloes. Neither goats nor sheep display any ability to maintain virus transmission in the absence of large ruminant infection. Diagnosis of rinderpest in goats can be complicated by the more common occurrence of peste des petits ruminants (PPR), a disease of similar geographic distribution, clinical presentation, and related etiology.

Etiology

Rinderpest virus, like PPR virus, is a morbillivirus in the family Paramyxoviridae. The virus does not survive well away from its mammalian hosts, which include all domestic and wild ruminants and swine. It has been identified in insects feeding on infected cattle, but it does not replicate in insects. In the field, it is readily killed by desiccation, heat, and common disinfectants. In the laboratory, it can remain infective for as long as one year or more in the frozen or lyophilized state. Numerous strains of the virus exist. They are all antigenically similar and immunologically cross-reactive. However, there is a great variation in their infectivity and virulence for different ruminant hosts, including goats (Lefèvre 1982).

Epidemiology

Waves of panzootic rinderpest spread around Africa and Asia throughout history. These epizootics almost always have been associated with the introduction of infected domestic or wild ruminants, frequently following in the wake of military campaigns as last observed in Iraq, Turkey, and Iran in the early 1990s. The introduction of infected goats has been documented as the cause of several major epidemics: in the Himalayas in 1900, Malaya in 1935, and Ceylon in 1943 (Scott 1957).

Reports of clinical caprine rinderpest are uncommon compared with the body of documented work in cattle. The disease has never been reported as a major cause of illness of sheep and goats in Africa, even during the massive rinderpest epizootics that swept the continent in the 1890s; from then until 1955, only two more epizootics involving small ruminants were reported (Scott 1955). Over the next thirty years, reports of caprine rinderpest were limited to the isolation of the virus from a kid in Uganda in 1958 (Libeau and Scott 1960) and to a putative epidemic in the eastern Sudan in 1971 that may actually have been PPR (Ali 1973; Scott 1985). A laboratory confirmed case of rinderpest was identified in a goat in northern Pakistan in association with a severe epizootic in cattle and yaks during 1994 to 1995 in which more than 40,000 large ruminants died (Rossiter et al. 1998).

In contrast with the lack of clinical reports, serologic surveys indicate that exposure of goats to rinderpest was previously common in endemic areas of Africa (Rossiter et al. 1982; Obi et al. 1984). Antibodies were also found in a number of wild ruminant species (Rossiter et al. 1983, 1983a). Wildlife play a minimal role as a disease reservoir for perpetuation of the disease in cattle and are more appropriately considered as victims of epizootics involving domestic ruminants (Karstad et al. 1981). The maximum period for independent maintenance of rinderpest in wildlife appears to be three years (Kock et al. 2006).

Unlike in Africa, outbreaks of clinical rinderpest in goats and sheep in India have been reported more commonly. In the southern states of Karnataka, Andhra Pradesh, and Tamil Nadu, between 1981 and 1986 there were 984 documented outbreaks of rinderpest and 374 (38%) occurred in sheep and goats only, with mortality rates between 44.5% and 67.8% (Ramesh Babu and Rajesekhar 1988). Mortality rates as high as 80% have been reported in Indian goat flocks (Mohan Kumar and Christopher 1985). Subclinical infections are also common and the maintenance of virus in small ruminant populations is considered to encumber control of the disease in cattle. Until recently it was unclear why clinical disease is more common in small ruminants in India compared with Africa. Current understanding indicates that most, but not all, of what was described as rinderpest in small ruminants was in fact PPR (Taylor et al. 2001). Rinderpest in small ruminants is now essentially seen as being acquired from infected cattle with which they are in contact and they do not sustain infection independently (Taylor and Barrett 2007).

Transmission of rinderpest is by direct contact with infected animals shedding virus in nasal, oral, ocular, or other secretions and excretions. The virus can be shed during the early, subclinical, febrile stage of the disease, making it difficult to detect inapparent shedders at markets or during livestock drives. In addition, cross-species transmission occurs among domestic ruminants and between domestic and wild ruminants and these animals may commonly share watering holes and grazing grounds in endemic regions. Contact transmission from cattle to goats and goats to cattle has been confirmed under experimental conditions (Zwart and Macadam 1967, 1967a; Macadam 1968) but appears not to be of major significance in the maintenance of rinderpest transmission chains. Prolonged carrier states are not known to exist in any susceptible species. Infected animals either die or eventually recover with a lifelong immunity.

The endemic nature of rinderpest may be sustained by year-round calving. Newborn cattle are protected from infection by maternal antibody while adults are protected by antibody from past exposure or vaccination. Young stock with waning maternal antibody act as the bridge for maintaining infection in livestock populations throughout the year.

Pathogenesis

There are few studies or reports on the pathogenesis of rinderpest specifically in goats (Wafula and Wamwayi 1988; Brown et al. 1991; Bidjeh et al. 1997). In cattle, animals are exposed by inhalation of infective aerosols. The virus penetrates the epithelium of the upper respiratory tract and primary growth occurs in the tonsils and lymph nodes of the nasopharynx. From there, the virus enters the blood in mononuclear cells and is disseminated to other lymphoid organs, lungs, and epithelial cells of mucous membranes, with a high affinity for alimentary tract mucosa. The lesions which develop are a direct result of the replication of virus in the mucosal cells with cytopathic effect. Stomatitis and diarrhea result from inflammation and disruption of normal mucosal integrity and function. The virus also has a predilection for lymphocytes and the destruction of lymphocytes underlies the leukopenia which develops. The virus induces a strong host antibody response and in cases that are not fatal, the affected animal clears the virus and develops a strong immunity (Radostits et al. 2007).

Clinical Findings

Goats exposed to rinderpest virus may experience either subclinical or clinical infections. The clinical course of acute rinderpest is very similar to PPR, although the progression may be slower. The early phase of disease after incubation is one of fever (104°F to 105.8°F; 40°C to 41°C), rough hair coat, anorexia, and depression. This is accompanied by, or followed within one to two days by, oculonasal discharge that is initially serous but soon becomes mucopurulent. By the second or third day of fever, small epithelial erosions may be seen in the oral cavity, particularly on the inside of the lower lip and on the gums around the incisors. During the next few days, these can spread to the cheeks, commissures, tongue, soft and hard palate, and pharynx. The necrotic epithelium produces a cheesy looking cover to the erosions, which are shallow and red underneath. Around day four or five after the onset of fever, affected animals can develop a profuse watery diarrhea that may be bloody.

Animals with severe diarrhea may die of dehydration, electrolyte imbalance, and general weakness. In animals that survive, a convalescence phase begins around day nine after the onset of fever. Diarrhea may begin to slow and oculonasal discharges abate, and there may be evidence of healing of oral erosions. Animals may still die, however, because of extensive debilitation or the development of severe secondary infections. Bacterial pneumonia, often a fatal sequel of PPR in goats, is less common in goats with rinderpest; this may help to discriminate the two conditions clinically.

Clinical Pathology and Necropsy

Leukocytosis occurs during the incubation period and a leukopenia characterized by lymphopenia develops concurrently with the onset of fever. Dehydration can cause increases in packed cell volume and total protein, and persistent diarrhea may cause electrolyte and acid-base imbalances.

With regard to serologic diagnosis, detectable serum-neutralizing antibodies may take longer to develop in goats than cattle, perhaps as long as twenty-eight days after infection (Afshar and Myers 1986; Wafula and Wamwayi 1988). In general, serum neutralization titers less than 0.3 log10 VN_{50} are considered negative for rinderpest, 0.3 to 0.6 are trace-positive, and more than 0.6 are considered positive. However, evidence of rising titers in convalescent goats should be evaluated.

The virus neutralization test (VNT) and the competitive ELISA are the tests of choice for identifying antibody to rinderpest. The VNT is the prescribed test for international trade (OIE 2004). Antibodies to rinderpest can be discriminated from antibodies to PPR by the quantitative serum cross-neutralization test.

Tests for the detection of rinderpest virus or viral antigen include virus isolation in cell culture; the agar gel immunodiffusion test; immunohistochemistry; and reverse transcription polymerase chain reaction. The differential immunocapture ELISA test can be used to discriminate between PPR and rinderpest viral antigens in tissue samples (OIE 2004).

Studies in goats indicate that, unlike cattle, ocular and nasal secretions are less reliable sources of antigen than prescapular lymph node aspirates for performing these tests in live animals (Wafula and Wamwayi 1988). Samples should be maintained at 39°F (4°C).

Goats dying of clinical rinderpest are emaciated, dehydrated, soiled on the hind end from diarrhea, and have prominent crusting of exudate on the face. Extensive mucosal erosions are present in the oral cavity and possibly also in the pharynx. The abomasum will also demonstrate mucosal erosion, but forestomach lesions are minimal. Ulcerations and hemorrhage of the colonic and cecal mucosa are common. Small intestinal lesions are less prominent and may be limited to congestion and swollen or necrotic Peyer's patches. Lung involvement is less common in rinderpest than in PPR. Histologically, lesions are similar to those described earlier for PPR.

Tissues to be submitted for virus isolation and virus neutralization studies include noncoagulated whole blood, lymph nodes, spleen, and gut lesions. They should be shipped on ice at 39°F (4°C) but not frozen. Where maintenance of cold chain for samples is not possible, formalin fixed third eyelid or mucosal tissue can be submitted for immunohistochemical confirmation of rinderpest viral antigen.

Diagnosis

In countries where both diseases occur, the primary differential for rinderpest in goats is PPR. Definitive diagnosis depends on performance of serum neutralization tests specific for one virus or the other, or on the post mortem isolation of virus from tissues. In the field, concurrent disease in large ruminants points toward rinderpest. There are a number of other diseases that could be mistaken for rinderpest or PPR at different times during the disease. These are presented earlier in the chapter in the diagnosis of PPR.

The differential diagnosis of rinderpest in cattle must include bovine virus diarrhea-mucosal disease, infectious bovine rhinotracheitis, and malignant catarrhal fever. These diseases have never been reported in goats.

Treatment

There is no specific treatment for caprine rinderpest. As rinderpest is now a highly regulated disease on the verge of eradication, suspect cases are likely to be destroyed for diagnostic and control purposes rather than treated.

Control

Rinderpest control is usually carried out by national and international authorities and the approach is two-pronged: control of animal movements and vaccination. Rinderpest-free countries distant from endemic regions simply do not allow the importation of stock from endemic regions. When rinderpest does enter a disease-free country, rapid destruction of all sick and exposed livestock with appropriate disposal by burial or burning can bring the epidemic under control and eliminate the disease (Scott 1981). Countries bordering rinderpest-endemic areas may be obliged to permit livestock movements because of local political and social considerations, but three-week segregation periods are required. In practice, these segregation periods are difficult to monitor and enforce.

In endemic areas, vaccination is the most important means of rinderpest control. This is particularly true in Africa, where migrating herds of wild ungulates exist. Internationally orchestrated rinderpest control campaigns, including Joint Project 15, the Pan-African Rinderpest Campaign, and most recently the Pan-African Control of Epizootics program, were mounted under African Union coordination over the last fifty years. These contributed to the Global Rinderpest Eradication Program (GREP), hosted by FAO, which has the goal of eliminating rinderpest from the world by 2010 (Food and Agriculture Organization 1985; Roeder et al. 2005). The last time rinderpest virus was encountered in the field was in 2001 when African buffaloes were found infected in Kenya. There is now growing confidence that rinderpest has been eradicated and the focus of GREP attention is now on proving freedom from rinderpest by an OIE country accreditation process (Roeder 2005).

The Plowright tissue culture-derived vaccine was used widely in vaccination programs (Plowright and Ferris 1962; Plowright 1984) but is now rarely used, even for protection of small ruminants against PPR, because it can interfere with rinderpest serosurveillance programs and because attenuated homologous PPR vaccines are now widely available. The most common is based on the Nigeria 75/1 isolate.

Modified lyophilization techniques have been applied to enhance and prolong the thermostability of the rinderpest tissue culture vaccine while maintaining antigenicity (Mariner et al. 1990, 1990a). This has allowed the vaccine to be carried into more remote endemic regions without the need for a costly, supportive cold chain to maintain vaccine viability. This innovation has been an important factor in achieving control of rinderpest through vaccination. As global rinderpest eradication efforts have advanced, emphasis has moved from control by vaccination to surveillance for confirmation of rinderpest free status.

Bluetongue

Bluetongue is an infectious, non-contagious, arthropod-borne, viral disease of ruminants. While goats are frequently infected, clinical disease is uncommon or mild in this species, even during epizootics severely affecting sheep. Direct economic losses caused by bluetongue disease in goats are minimal, although historically, importation restrictions existed in bluetongue-free countries resulting in limitations on trade of live goats, semen, and embryos. These restrictions are now becoming less stringent as scientific understanding of the disease ecology of bluetongue has improved (MacLachlan and Osburn 2006).

Etiology

Bluetongue is caused by a non-enveloped, RNA orbivirus in the Reoviridae family. It has a genome of ten segments of double-stranded RNA that produce seven structural and four non-structural proteins. There are currently twenty-four different known serotypes of the bluetongue virus that are distinguished by epitopes on the outer capsid protein VP2 which is encoded by the L2 gene. Individual serotypes are identified in the laboratory by serum neutralization tests. Various serotypes may share common complement fixing and precipitating antigens but cross-protective immunity against heterologous serotypes is poor. Virulence between serotypes varies.

Bluetongue virus (BTV) can be grown in embryonating chicken eggs as well as mouse L, baby hamster kidney-21, African green monkey kidney (Vero), or *Aedes albopictus* cells in culture (OIE 2004a). The virus is very resistant to environmental degradation. It remains infective in citrated blood held at 39°F (4°C) or room temperature for years. Three percent sodium hydroxide (lye) is an effective disinfectant (Kohler 1989).

Epizootic Hemorrhagic Disease (EHD) virus is a closely related Orbivirus infecting primarily wild ruminants. It has caused disease outbreaks in whitetail deer (*Odocoileus virginianus*) in North America. Goats challenged intravenously with EHD virus produce low levels of neutralizing antibodies but show no evidence of viremia or clinical disease (Gibbs and Lawman 1977). Another mosquito-transmitted Orbivirus, Orungo virus, causes febrile disease in humans in Africa. There is serologic evidence of infection in goats, but clinical disease is not reported (Ezeifeka et al. 1984).

The principal insect vectors responsible for transmission of BTV are members of the genus *Culicoides*, variously referred to as biting midges, sandflies, no-seeums, or gnats.

Epidemiology

Bluetongue disease was first recognized in European sheep imported into South Africa in 1870 and the disease was originally thought to be restricted to Africa. The first major epizootic confirmed outside of Africa occurred in Cyprus in 1943. The disease was identified in sheep in Texas in 1948 and the BTV-10 serotype isolated from sheep in California in 1952.

Bluetongue was first confirmed in the laboratory in Israel in 1950, but it is suspected that the disease was occurring in the Middle East since the 1920s (Shimshony 2004). Major epizootics occurred in Spain and Portugal in 1956 and 1957 and over the past fifty years there have been several incursions of bluetongue into the Mediterranean region. There have been large, notable outbreaks in Europe in recent years and the epidemiology of these European outbreaks has recently been reviewed (Saegerman et al. 2008). The first was in southern Europe beginning in 1998 (Gomez-Tejedor 2004), involving the Greek mainland and islands, Bulgaria, Turkey, Serbia and Montenegro, Macedonia, Croatia, and Italy. BTV-9 was mainly reported but also serotypes 1, 4, and 16. A second wave of outbreaks occurred in 1999 in Tunisia, Algeria, and various island groups in the Mediterranean. This outbreak involved BTV-2 but serotypes 4 and 9 were also reported. Successive Mediterranean outbreaks occurred through 2004.

The most recent outbreak began in northern and western Europe in 2006 due to BTV-8 (Elliott 2007). It continued well into 2007. The most recent information at the time of this writing is that vector activity persisted over the winter of 2007–2008 with new cases occurring in 2008. The main countries involved include Belgium, Luxembourg, the Netherlands, Germany, France, and the UK, with Denmark, Switzerland, and the Czech Republic also reporting small numbers of cases in 2007. These European epizootics may be facilitated by climate change as discussed further below.

The global distribution of BTV reflects the distribution of competent *Culicoides* spp. vectors. The virus is found on all continents except Antarctica. Within those continents, it is found mainly in tropical and subtropical regions. Historically the global distribution of bluetongue virus was considered to be between 40°N latitude and 34°S latitude, except in western North America and eastern Asia where the northern demarcation may extend as far as 50°N. The recent European outbreaks are noteworthy because the 1998 outbreak extended northward to 44°N latitude in Serbia and the current 2006–2008 outbreak extends above 51°N latitude in the U.K. In light of these new realities, OIE puts the global distribution of BTV between 53°N and 34°S latitudes (OIE 2007).

From an epidemiological standpoint, the geographic distribution of BTV can be categorized into three ecological zones: enzootic, epizootic, and incursive. Enzootic zones are mainly tropical regions where BTV transmission occurs throughout the year and subclinical infection is common. Clinical disease usually occurs only when immunologically naïve ruminants are introduced to the zone. Epizootic zones include temperate areas where outbreaks occur seasonally, generally in late summer when vector populations are at their highest. Incursive zones are areas that experience sporadic outbreaks when climatic conditions favor disease transmission by vectors (Gibbs and Greiner 1994).

In any given country there may be areas where infection is enzootic and areas free of infection. This is because local climate and geography, host populations, patterns of animal movements, and presence of competent vector species can all influence the presence of infection. For example, BTV was first isolated from a pool of trapped *Culicoides* in northern Australia in 1975, but to date, except for one case in a sentinel flock maintained in the north, there are no reports of disease in sheep, which are raised mainly in the southern portion of the country (Kirkland 2004). Similarly, in the United States, the northeast remains free of bluetongue, while it is enzootic in much of the west and south, with seasonal outbreaks occurring in the northwest.

More than 1,400 *Culicoides* spp. exist worldwide but only seventeen to twenty of these species have been identified as capable of BTV transmission, and the competent *Culicoides* spp. vectors vary regionally. Vector competency appears to be linked to BTV serotype so that distinct regional disease ecologies or episystems exist involving particular *Culicoides* spp. and particular BTV serotypes (Tabachnick 2004). The current, regional distribution of these vectors and serotypes is given in Table 10.4. In addition to *Culicoides*, the sheep ked, *Melophagus ovinus*, certain ticks, and biting flies have been implicated as mechanical vectors for transmission of BTV, but these are of minor importance in the dissemination of BTV. Because the virus is associated with blood cells, iatrogenic transmission by repeated use of needles when administering injections is possible.

All domestic ruminants are susceptible to BTV infection. Among sheep, European fine wool and mutton breeds, are more susceptible to bluetongue than tropical and subtropical breeds. Goats and cattle most often have subclinical infections and are generally considered as reservoir hosts. However, in the recent outbreaks of bluetongue in Europe, disease in cattle and to a lesser extent in goats has occurred. Even when goats are present with severely affected sheep during major epizootics, they usually have lower morbidity and mortality, exhibit milder clinical signs, or most likely, remain clinically normal. The reasons for these differences in ruminant species susceptibility are not well understood.

In tropical and subtropical regions, where *Culicoides* are active year-round, there may be a continuous cycle of new infection in animals and the infection becomes enzootic. In temperate regions, disease is more likely to be seasonal, occurring in the summer and fall when populations of infected *Culicoides* have rebounded from die-offs in winter associated with cold or freezing temperatures. Vector, host, and environmental factors can influence overwintering of BTV. *Culicoides* do not pass BTV virus transovarially so immature stages of the insect are not infective. Therefore, overwintering of the virus in the vector depends on the survival of at least some adult *Culicoides*, which can have life spans as long as three months. The other major factor is the presence of virus in host animals on which *Culicoides* feed. The viremic period in sheep and goats is shorter than that of cattle. Most small ruminants are no longer viremic thirty to forty days post infection and cattle after fifty to sixty days.

In recent years, global warming appears to be altering arthropod-borne disease ecology in Europe. Increases in nighttime temperature and winter temperature along with increases in precipitation in summer and autumn have led to an increased geographical and seasonal incidence of BTV transmission by increasing the range, abundance, and seasonal activity of vectors, by increasing the proportion of the vector species that are competent, and by increasing

Table 10.4. Global distribution of bluetongue virus serotypes and the associated *Culicoides* vector species.

Region	*Bluetongue virus serotypes*	*Major Culicoides vector(s)*	*Other secondary or possible Culicoides vectors*	*Comments*	*Reference*
North America	2, 10, 11, 13, 17	*C. sonorensis, C. insignis* (serotype 2 only)	*C. variipennis*	Serotype 2 restricted to Florida	Walton 2004
Central America and the Caribbean	1, 3, 4, 6, 8, 12, 14, 17	*C. insignis*	*C. pusillus, C. furens, C. filarifer, C. trilineatus*		Walton 2004
South America	4, 6, 12, 14, 17, 19, 20	*C. insignis*	*C. pusillus*		Lager 2004
Europe	1, 2, 4, 8, 9, 16	*C. imicola*	*C. obsoletus, C. pulicaris*		Saegerman et al. 2008
Africa	1–15, 18–20, 22, 24, 25	*C. imicola*	*C. bolitinos* and possibly others		Walton 2004
South Asia	1–9, 11–20, 23	?	*C. imicola, C. oxystoma,*	Details on competent vector species lacking	Sreenivasulu, et al. 2004
Southeast Asia	1–3, 9, 12, 14–21, 23	*C. brevitarsis*	*C wadai, C. actoni, C. fulvus,* and possibly others.		Walton 2004
Australia and Oceania	1, 3, 9, 15, 16, 20, 21, 23	*C. brevitarsis, C. wadai*	*C. actoni, C. fulvus, C. oxystoma, C. peregrinus*		Australian Veterinary Emergency Plan (1996)

the development rates of the virus within vectors, thereby extending transmission ability to other *Culicoides* species. For example, *C. imicola*, the widely distributed midge of Africa and Asia, has been the primary vector in outbreaks of bluetongue in southern Europe. The vector competence of the more temperate palearctic groups of midges, *C. pulicaris* and *C. obseletus*, were known from laboratory studies but only suspected in the absence of *C. imicola* in outbreaks of bluetongue in Greece and southern Bulgaria in 1999 and in the Balkans in 2000–2001 (Purse et al. 2005). However, in 2006 in northwest Europe, these midges clearly established themselves as competent vectors for BTV (Elliott 2007; Saegerman et al. 2008).

Historically, it was considered that the movement of infected livestock was a key element in the global dissemination of bluetongue and this had a significant impact on international trade in live animals, semen, and embryos, with disease-free countries prohibiting the importation of these products from countries where the disease was present. However, it is now understood that trade plays a comparatively minor role in the dissemination of bluetongue. There are two main reasons for this. First, is the recognition that viremia in ruminants has a limited duration and that persistent carriers do not occur. Some early studies, on which trade regulations were based, suggested that bovine fetuses exposed to BTV *in utero* become immunotolerant, persistent carriers (Luedke et al. 1977, 1977a). The existence of persistent carriers has since been disproven (Roeder et al. 1991; MacLachlan et al. 1994; Bonneau et al. 2002).

Second is the recognition that the regional occurrence of bluetongue depends on the particular disease ecology of that region with regard to the specific *Culicoides* vectors and associated BTV serotypes that occur there. There is little evidence that alien serotypes become established or persist if accidentally introduced into a region. The introduction of a new serotype to a region, such as the recent finding of BTV-8 in northern Europe, had more to do with the dissemination of competent *Culicoides* vectors than the movement of animals. Issues of trade policy relative to bluetongue have been reviewed (MacLachlan and Osburn 2006).

Recognition of goats as a host species for bluetongue virus was established experimentally in 1905 (Spruell 1905). The susceptibility of goats to clinical bluetongue, however, remained obscure for years as sick goats were not observed in mixed flocks with sick sheep during outbreaks (Hardy and Price 1952).

Reports of clinical bluetongue in goats are infrequent, as the infection in goats is generally subclinical. The first reported epidemic involving goats occurred in Israel in 1950. Cattle and sheep were the principal species affected. Prevalence was less in goats and signs less severe (Komarov and Goldsmit 1951). The second reported epidemic of bluetongue affecting goats occurred in southern Spain in 1956. While losses in sheep were extreme, with more than 100,000 animals dead, cases in goats were infrequent and mild, with limited mortality (Lopez and Botija 1958). A more severe involvement of goats in a bluetongue epidemic occurred in India in 1961 (Sapre 1964). The clinical disease appeared with equal severity in sheep and goats, though variation in breed susceptibility was noted. Clinical bluetongue associated with BTV-4 occurred in goats in Portugal in December of 2004 with twenty-three cases and two deaths reported to the OIE. In the epizootic in Northern Europe which began in 2006, clinical cases in goats due to BTV-8 were seen in the Netherlands (Dercksen et al. 2007; Backx et al. 2007).

The epidemiology of caprine bluetongue has been studied in the northwestern United States (Osburn 1981; Stott 1985). As in sheep and cattle, there is a seasonal variation in both virus isolation and serologic evidence of infection. The season of maximal infection, June through December, correlates with increases in insect vector populations. Goats are an unlikely reservoir of bluetongue infection, as no virus isolations from goats were made in California from January and June, indicating that the virus does not persist. The prevalence of infection in goats was half that recorded in cattle and sheep. All four of the major American serotypes were found in goats and multiple serotype infections occurred. However, no clinical disease was associated with infection in goats during a three-and-a-half-year period of study.

The epidemiology of caprine bluetongue has received considerable attention in Africa. In Zimbabwe, bluetongue antibody was present in 71% of goats tested, but no evidence of clinical disease has been observed (Jorgensen et al. 1989). Serologic surveys in goats in North African countries in the intertropical zone show a range of seroprevalence from 5% to 54%, with distinct differences in seroprevalence rates between different climatic regions. Low-lying and humid regions tend toward a greater prevalence rate than drier and higher regions (Lefèvre and Calvez 1986). Seroprevalence in goats increases with advancing age (Obi et al. 1983a).

Pathogenesis

There are few if any studies on the pathogenesis of bluetongue specifically in the goat. Therefore, most available information is extrapolated from sheep or cattle. Infection results from cutaneous inoculation of the host with virus during feeding by infected insects. Initial viral replication takes place in the lymph nodes draining the feeding site and dissemination in mononuclear cells to secondary sites of replication. Viremia is usually detectable by day three and peak viremia along with fever and leukopenia usually occurs six to seven days post infection. With viremia, there is localization of the virus in vascular endothelium leading to cell damage and necrosis, with thrombosis, hemorrhage, and edema in affected organs, most notably in the tongue, mouth, esophagus, rumen, and skin, causing hyperemia, erosions, or ulcers. The virus may cross the placenta. It can also be found in semen. The clinical signs of stomatitis, glossitis, rhinitis, enteritis, and coronitis are attributable to the primary endothelial necrosis and loss of capillary integrity. In sheep, disseminated intravascular coagulation may occur, exacerbating the severity of clinical signs. In cattle, endothelial cell damage is minimal and the cell-associated viremia involves mainly erythrocytes and platelets (Radostits et al. 2007).

Recent research on the *in vitro* response of ovine and bovine endothelial cells to BTV suggests that inherent species-specific differences in the production and activities of endothelial cell-derived inflammatory and vasoactive mediators contribute to the greater sensitivity of sheep to BTV-induced microvascular injury. No such comparison has been carried out yet with goat cells (DeMaula et al. 2002).

Experimental challenge studies indicate that viremia in goats can last as long as twenty-one days after challenge and that measurable antibody responses occur during viremia (Barzilai and Tadmor, 1971; Luedke and Anakwenze 1972).

Clinical Findings

In the majority of cases, bluetongue infection in goats is subclinical. When clinical illness does occur, it is often limited to mild depression, temporary loss of appetite, fever, and hyperemia of the oral and nasal mucosa.

Occasionally, more severe cases are seen. The initial signs are fever and anorexia lasting for three to four days. This is followed by hyperemia of the oral mucosa with excoriations of the tongue, lips, and gums that become ulcerative and necrotic. Affected goats salivate excessively. Edema of the face ensues (Figure 10.4) and a watery to mucoid nasal discharge develops.

This is sometimes followed by diarrhea. Coronitis also develops, with hyperemia and swelling around the coronet leading to obvious lameness in one or more legs. In affected goats in India, walnut-sized skin eruptions appeared and were distributed all over the body (Sapre 1964). This presentation appears unique to goats and perhaps to the outbreak in India because it has not been reported again elsewhere. The clinical course is eight to twelve days.

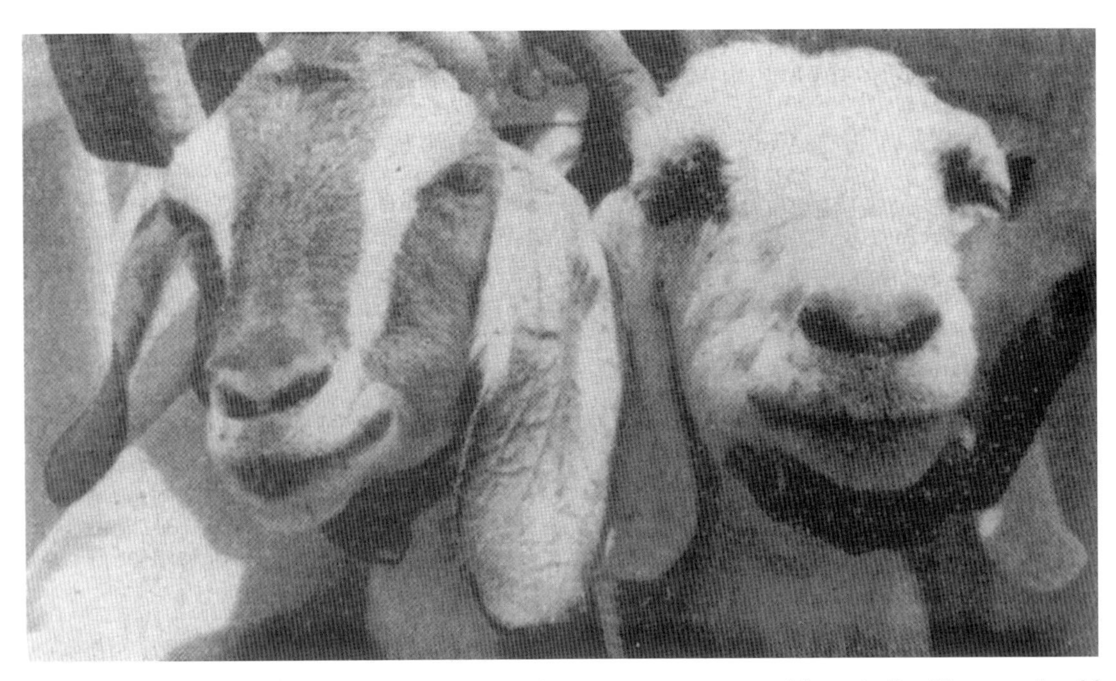

Figure 10.4. Edema of the face in goats affected with bluetongue, as reported from India. Most caprine bluetongue infections are subclinical. (From Sapre 1964.)

Clinical cases were seen in goats in the Netherlands in August, 2006, during the BTV-8 outbreak in northern Europe (Dercksen et al. 2007). The most obvious clinical signs were an acute drop in milk production and a high fever, up to 107.6°F (42°C). Other clinical signs were less obvious than usually seen in sheep, but a few goats had edema of the lips and head, some nasal discharge, scabs on the nose and lips, erythema on the skin of the udder, and some small subcutaneous hemorrhages. When the field strain of BTV-8 was administered intravenously to two experimental goats, both developed viremia and antibody responses, but one remained clinically normal while the second developed fever and became depressed, standing apart with head hanging down. It also showed dysphagia, diarrhea, and lameness. Sheep inoculated in the same experiment showed more severe clinical signs (Backx et al. 2007).

In sheep, the convalescent phase is prolonged and is characterized by emaciation and weakness secondary to active myositis. This has not yet been described in goats. Abortions have been ascribed to bluetongue virus infection in goats, but the causal role is poorly documented (East 1983).

Clinical Pathology and Necropsy

Clinicopathologic changes have not been reported in field cases of caprine bluetongue. In experimental infections, leukopenia occurs and is most pronounced five to ten days after inoculation (Luedke and Anakwenze 1972).

Several serologic tests are available for identifying antibody to bluetongue virus. These include complement fixation, agar gel precipitation, and more recently, the competitive enzyme-linked immunosorbent assay (ELISA). The latter two are considered prescribed tests for international trade (OIE 2004a). In experimentally infected goats, antibody was first detectable at day thirteen post inoculation using a blocking ELISA (Backx et al. 2007).

Virus isolation from blood and tissues is best carried out in embryonated eggs or in cell culture. However, where bluetongue is enzootic, the presence of the virus in individual animals does not establish causality when clinical signs are nonspecific (Inverso et al. 1980).

The development and application of the reverse transcriptase polymerase chain reaction has allowed for the detection of bluetongue viral nucleic acids in blood. This has revolutionized the laboratory diagnosis of bluetongue. Using this tool, antibody positive animals can be confirmed negative for the presence of virus, allowing them to enter international trade when, in earlier times, without PCR this would not have been possible (OIE 2004a).

Identification of bluetongue serogroup can be done using a number of techniques, including immunofluorescence, antigen capture ELISA, and the immunospot test using serogroup-specific reagents. For serotyping of BTV, virus neutralization tests are conducted in tissue culture systems using BTV serotype-specific antisera. Techniques employed include plaque reduction, plaque inhibition, microtiter neutralization, and fluorescence inhibition (OIE 2004a)

Gross necropsy lesions in goats with full-blown clinical bluetongue are similar to those observed in sheep (Sapre 1964). There is hyperemia and edema of the buccal mucosa and ulceration of the palate. Lung congestion and secondary pneumonia may be present. Severe hemorrhagic gastroenteritis may be seen in the abomasum, small and large intestines, and rectum. Pinpoint hemorrhages and congestion occur in the spleen and on the epicardium. Hydropericardium is variable. The mesenteric lymph nodes are enlarged and edematous. Hyperemia and hemorrhage may be noted on the skin of the limbs above the coronets.

Diagnosis

Definitive diagnosis of clinical bluetongue depends on isolation of the virus from animals showing typical clinical signs during seasons of insect activity. Historically, bluetongue has been recognized in goats only when clinical disease occurs simultaneously in sheep or cattle. Subclinical bluetongue in goats may be identified by changes in antibody titers in paired serum samples.

The differential diagnosis for caprine bluetongue includes foot and mouth disease, contagious ecthyma, goat pox, and photosensitization. Stomatitis and enteritis can occur in rinderpest and peste des petits ruminants, but coronitis, lameness, and edema are not prominent findings.

Treatment

There are no specific treatments for bluetongue. In sheep, prophylactic antibiotics are used to prevent secondary bacterial infections. Clinically ill animals should be kept out of direct sunlight, because sunlight appears to aggravate skin lesions. Affected animals should be fed separately so they do not need to compete for food.

Control

Control methods are not routinely directed toward goats because the infection is generally subclinical. In general, recommendations for sheep apply. Animals should not graze in low-lying, wet areas during seasons of insect activity so as to avoid spread of infection, and paddocks and flooring of animal houses should be kept dry. *Culicoides* feed mostly at dusk and early evening so animals should be removed from pastures at these times. Use of chemical insect repellants can be considered if approved for use in food animals.

In areas where seasonal occurrence of bluetongue is a known problem, vaccination is the major means of control, and vaccine should be administered prior to the onset of *Culicoides* feeding. Because the various serotypes offer little cross-immunity, to be effective, vaccines must contain the serotypes known to be problematic in the area. In the United States, only a monovalent vaccine employing serotype 10 is commercially available. Multivalent vaccines against twenty-one serotypes are produced in South Africa. Vaccination against the full complement of serotypes requires three separate injections at three-week intervals.

In 2007, the UK tendered for the development of a serotype 8 vaccine for use in controlling the newly emergent BTV-8 serotype in northern Europe. The vaccine became available in May of 2008 and vaccination began in Protected Zones in the UK in the same month. The vaccine is approved only for use in sheep and cattle, but under the European cascade system, it can be administered to goats by veterinarians, with no withdrawal times necessary.

There are some problems with modified-live, tissue culture virus vaccines. Passively acquired maternal antibody can impair the vaccinal response, so kids and lambs younger than three months of age may not be effectively vaccinated. Vaccination of ewes in the first five to ten weeks of pregnancy can lead to fetal malformations or early embryonic death. This has not been reported in goats, but vaccination before breeding or after kidding is recommended. Vaccination should be timed to precede the insect season to promote maximum protection during high-risk periods.

In the past, bluetongue-free countries had strict prohibitions on the importation of livestock, embryos, and semen, but as of 2005, OIE revised and adopted new, less stringent international trade provisions to reflect improved understanding of the transmission of bluetongue infection as described above. The new regulations set the infective period for bluetongue in animals at sixty days and establish protocols by which livestock, semen, and embryos can be imported into bluetongue free countries from known positive bluetongue countries and zones through the use of quarantines and testing for antibody and virus. The availability of highly sensitive PCR tests to detect the presence or absence of virus in animals independent of their antibody status has helped to facilitate these new protocols. The current OIE provisions for bluetongue are available at http://www.oie.int/eng/normes/mcode/en_chapitre_1.8.3.htm.

Nairobi Sheep Disease

Nairobi sheep disease is an infectious, noncontagious, zoonotic, viral disease transmitted by ticks. Goats, sheep, and humans are affected. The disease occurs in Africa and is characterized by fever and gastroenteritis.

Etiology

The causative virus, Nairobi sheep disease virus (NSDV), is a single-stranded RNA virus in the genus

Nairovirus of the family *Bunyaviridae*. There are thirty-four tick-borne viruses in the Nairovirus genus, classified into seven serogroups. NSDV is the prototype virus of the Nairobi sheep disease serogroup. This serogroup also includes the Dugbe virus and the Ganjam virus. Earlier serologic analysis suggested that NSDV and Ganjam virus were closely related. More recently, sequence analysis of the S RNA genome segment and encoded proteins of both viruses indicate that they are in fact the same virus (Marczinke and Nichol 2002).

Cultivation of NSDV can be accomplished in lamb kidney, baby hamster kidney, or Vero cell culture. Intracerebral inoculation of infant mice is also used. The virus is moderately resistant to environmental degradation and can persist in blood at room temperature for as long as forty-five days (Liebermann 1989).

Epidemiology

Nairobi sheep disease was first described in Africa in 1910. A major epizootic occurred when large numbers of sheep and goats were brought into Kenya in 1915 to feed troops in World War I. The close relationship of Ganjam virus in India to NSDV has led to speculation that NSDV is a variant of Ganjam virus introduced by livestock trading between India and East Africa. Nairobi sheep disease now occurs in Kenya, Uganda, Tanzania, Somalia, Ethiopia, Rwanda, Burundi, Botswana, Mozambique, and the Democratic Republic of Congo. In 1996, it was reported that NSDV was isolated from *Haemaphysalis intermedia* ticks collected on goats in the North Western Province of Sri Lanka (Perera et al. 1996). This same tick is responsible for transmission of Ganjam virus in India, where clinical disease has been reported in sheep and serologic evidence of infection documented in sheep and goats. The full extent of Ganjam virus as a cause of disease in small ruminants in South Asia remains largely undetermined.

Transmission of NSDV is principally by the brown ear tick, *Rhipicephalus appendiculatus*, in which it can be transmitted transovarially and transtadially. The distribution of the disease closely follows the geographic range of this tick and the disease is unlikely to occur in parts of Africa where *R. appendiculatus* has a seasonal rather than a continuous breeding cycle (Davies 1997). In Somalia, it is reported that the main vector is *R. pulchellus*, a tick that can transovarially transmit the virus (Groocock 1998). *Amblyomma variegatum* also transmits NSDV but plays a minor role. *A. variegatum* is a less effective vector because transovarial transmission of the virus does not occur in this tick.

Infected ticks are rendered non-infectious by feeding on immune or resistant hosts. Ticks and subclinically infected sheep and goats are considered the agent reservoir. Wild ruminants and cattle are not implicated.

A seasonal occurrence of clinical disease is observed during rainy periods when tick activity increases. Sheep and goats born in enzootic regions generally are subclinically infected. Clinical disease is seen in imported stock or stock transported from non-enzootic areas. Goats in general are less severely affected than sheep. Goat mortality may be high, but is usually less than the 50% to 90% mortality that occurs in sheep. Experimental inoculation of goats and sheep with blood from infected sheep resulted in lower morbidity, milder clinical signs, and lower mortality in goats (Montgomery 1917).

Human infection is acquired by tick bites. Though seroprevalence in endemic human populations is high, clinical disease is rare. In the case of Ganjam virus in India, human disease was reported in seven laboratory personnel in association with laboratory exposure (Banerjee et al. 1979).

Pathogenesis

The pathogenesis is not completely known. The virus is introduced into goats and sheep by feeding ticks. The incubation period is four to fifteen days under natural conditions and one to three days with experimental inoculation (Groocock 1998). Incubation is followed by viremia and localization of virus in tissues. There is an apparent predilection for epithelial cells of the gut. Bone marrow suppression also occurs. Necrosis of the mucosal epithelium of the intestines and rupture of capillaries leads to a hemorrhagic enteritis. Fluid and electrolyte loss in diarrhea is considerable and may result in death (Kimberling 1988). Recovered animals develop lifelong immunity. Kids and lambs of immune dams are probably protected by maternal antibody during the first few months of life.

Clinical Findings

The disease begins with a fever of 104°F to 106.7°F (40°C to 41.5°C) accompanied by anorexia, pronounced depression, and a variable mucous nasal discharge that may become blood-tinged. This is followed by profuse, watery, diarrhea that may progress to a bloody dysentery with straining or even some colicky signs. Fever usually subsides at the time of onset of diarrhea. Depending on the severity of the disease, affected animals may die during the febrile stage before the onset of diarrhea or after one to six days of diarrhea, or they may gradually recover. Pregnant animals may abort. Swelling of the external genitalia is reported in ewes, but not in goats. Animals that recover maintain a lifelong immunity against reinfection.

Clinical Pathology and Necropsy

Affected sheep and goats have a marked leukopenia during the febrile period. Serum antibody is detectable using the hemagglutination inhibition test, enzyme-linked immunoabsorbent assay, complement fixation, or indirect immunofluorescent antibody test. Paired acute and convalescent serum samples should be evaluated for changes in titer. The virus may be isolated from plasma of the live animal during the febrile stage of disease. Cytopathic effect (CPE) in cell culture may vary with strain of NSDV and cell type used. When CPE is absent, direct immunofluorescence staining or the indirect fluoroscein antibody test confirms presence of virus. At necropsy, virus is best isolated from spleen and mesenteric lymph nodes. In the absence of cell culture, agar gel immunodiffusion, complement fixation, or ELISA can be used to detect NSDV antigen in tissues (OIE 2004b).

Animals that die in the acute, febrile phase of the disease before onset of diarrhea may not have obvious or specific gross lesions at necropsy and this may mistakenly lead the investigator away from a diagnosis of Nairobi sheep disease. In more advanced cases, lesions are found mainly in the gastrointestinal tract, lymph nodes, and spleen. The abomasal mucosa is hyperemic and may contain petechial hemorrhage. The gut lumen content may be bloodstained and there are numerous hemorrhages in the gut mucosa, especially in the cecum and anterior portion of the colon. These hemorrhages may have a linear or streaked appearance along the crest of mucosal folds. The spleen is considerably enlarged and blood-engorged. The mesenteric lymph nodes are also enlarged and edematous. Petechial hemorrhage may also be seen in the epicardium and endocardium and other serosal surfaces. Hyperemia of the genital tract may be noted and when fetuses are present, their tissues may show focal hemorrhages. Histologically, there is a characteristic nephritis with hyaline, epithelial casts, myocardial necrosis, and hemorrhagic gastroenteritis.

Diagnosis

Nairobi sheep disease occurs only in areas where the known tick vectors occur. Disease is most likely to affect recently introduced sheep and goats. The disease should be suspected when high mortality occurs in sheep and goats with vector tick infestations, especially if the animals have been recently moved into an enzootic area or when tick populations have increased due to heavy rainfall. The definitive diagnosis is based on isolation of the virus or detection of viral antigen from clinically affected animals or documentation of seroconversion after clinical disease.

The differential diagnosis includes rinderpest, peste des petits ruminants, Rift Valley fever, heartwater, salmonellosis, anthrax, and bluetongue. Because fever may have subsided when diarrhea begins, coccidiosis and helminthiasis must also be considered.

Treatment

There is no specific treatment for this viral disease. Therapy should be directed at managing the effects of diarrhea and should include fluid and electrolyte therapy and adequate nutrition. Affected animals become leukopenic, so broad-spectrum antibiotics are indicated to reduce the risk of secondary bacterial infections.

Control

Use of acaricides may reduce the risk of exposure for sheep and goats moving into enzootic areas, particularly following rainy seasons when tick numbers and activity increase. Vaccination of susceptible sheep and goats prior to moving them into enzootic areas has been recommended but no vaccines are commercially available. Both an attenuated live vaccine and a killed vaccine have been developed, but there has been little demand for their use from the field (OIE 2004b).

BACTERIAL DISEASES

Enterotoxemia

Enterotoxemia, caused by *Clostridium perfringens*, is recognized worldwide as a common, frequently fatal disease of goats. The disease also occurs in sheep and cattle, but species differences occur in the epidemiology, pathogenesis, clinical presentation, and management of enterotoxemia. Distinctive characteristics of enterotoxemia in goats include the clinical prominence of diarrhea, the presence of severe enterocolitis at necropsy, and the frequent failure of vaccination to protect from clinical disease.

Etiology

Clostridium perfringens causes enteric disease in a wide range of species including domesticated mammals, poultry, and humans. There are five main types of *C. perfringens* based on the lethal exotoxins that they produce, as presented in Table 10.5. This discussion focuses on the disease in goats. Broader discussions of *C. perfringens* and the enteric diseases it produces in other species are available elsewhere (Songer 1996, Radostits et al. 2007).

The principal cause of caprine enterotoxemia worldwide is *C. perfringens* type D. This Gram-positive, nonmotile, spore-forming, toxin-producing, anaerobic, rod-shaped bacterium is resident in the ruminant digestive tract, generally in low numbers. It is passed in feces and may persist in soil, though it dies out more quickly in soil than other *Clostridium* spp. The organism has a quick generation time, as short as eight minutes, allowing for rapid proliferation in the intestine under favorable conditions. It is the rapid proliferation of this resident organism and the associated release of toxins that causes disease in the host.

Table 10.5. ***Clostridium perfringens*** **types and the toxins produced.**

C. perfringens type	*Toxins produced (Gene expressing the toxin)*						*Occurrence in goats*
	Alpha (cpa)	*Beta (cpb)*	*Beta-2 (cpb-2)*	*Epsilon (etx)*	*Iota (iA)*	*Enterotoxin*** (cpe)*	
A	+		+*			±	Infrequently reported
B	+	+		+		±	Rarely reported
C	+	+	+**			?	Infrequently reported
D	+			+		±	Most common cause
E	+				+	±	Not reported

*There is one reported case of caprine enterotoxemia involving a *C. perfringens* expressing alpha toxin and beta-2 toxin (Dray 2004). Similar findings were reported from cases of enterocolitis in horses (Herholz et al. 1999).

**The original identification of beta 2 toxin involved a *C. perfringens* type C associated with necrotic enterocolitis in a pig. The organism expressed alpha, beta, and beta-2 toxins.

***Expression of enterotoxin is not consistent within types. It is most often associated with type A isolates but may be associated with other *C. perfringens* types as well.

C. perfringens type D produces two main toxins: alpha and epsilon. While both toxins are important for typing the organism, epsilon toxin is considered to be the principal virulence factor as discussed later under pathogenesis.

C. perfringens type C has also been cited as a cause of caprine enterotoxemia in the United States and Britain, though definitive confirmation of its role is scarce (Barron 1942; Guss 1977). There is also a report of type C enterotoxemia in goats and sheep in Greece (Tarlatzis et al. 1963). The major toxins of type C are alpha and beta. Because beta toxin is degraded by trypsin, type C enterotoxemia is most common in very young animals with low concentrations of intestinal trypsin, usually under ten days of age.

Enterotoxemia due to *C. perfringens* type B, which causes lamb dysentery, is also uncommon in goats. Type B contains alpha, beta, and epsilon toxins. In Iran, anomalous *C. perfringens* type B strains (lacking hyaluronidase) were isolated from goats in two different but nearby outbreaks of clinical enterotoxemia (Brooks and Entessar 1957). In Germany, type B enterotoxemia was confirmed in a dairy goat herd and a herd of dwarf goats. Mortality of kids up to twelve days of age was reported following bouts of watery, yellow, blood-stained diarrhea (Scharfe and Elze 1995).

In Greece, *C. perfringens* type A was cited as the most common cause of enterotoxemia in sheep and goats (Deligaris 1978). However, ascribing pathogenicity in goats to type A remains controversial because it is considered to be the *C. perfringens* type most widespread in the intestines of warm-blooded animals and the environment and can rapidly overgrow in organs following death (Songer 1996). Another early report of type A enterotoxemia involved captive Siberian ibex (*Capra sibirica*) at a zoo (Russell 1970). Experimental challenge of domestic goats by intraduodenal administration of type A in broth culture produced only a transient diarrhea at twelve hours post inoculation which resolved twelve hours later with no other clinical signs or deaths. In contrast, a second group of goats given type D in the same manner all developed diarrhea and convulsions and died within thirty-six hours (Phukan et al. 1997.)

More recently, a fatal case of enterotoxemia in a five-week-old Boer goat kid in Canada was reported as due to type A (Dray 2004). This was an unusual case in that the *C. perfringens* isolated from the gut at necropsy was found to have genes which expressed alpha toxin and beta-2 toxin, making it an atypical type A isolate. Pathogenicity of type A is usually associated with alpha toxin alone. Beta-2 toxin has been characterized only relatively recently, originally in association with a *C. perfringens* type C organism (Gilbert et al. 1997). *C. perfringens* organisms that produce beta-2 toxin have now been associated with necrotic enterocolitis in piglets (Waters et al. 2003) and horses (Herholz et al. 1999) as well as this single reported case of caprine enterotoxemia (Dray 2004).

C. perfringens can also produce an enterotoxin (Songer 1996). Though most commonly associated with *C. perfringens* type A, it has been found in some isolates of types B and D as well. The gene for enterotoxin expression has been identified in type E isolates but the toxin is not produced (Billington et al. 1998). The role of enterotoxin in the pathogenesis of enterotoxemia in goats has not been studied and its importance, if any, remains unknown.

Epidemiology

Enterotoxemia is frequently cited by producers, veterinarians, and extension personnel around the world as a common and important disease of goats. Paradoxically, there is little documentation of caprine enterotoxemia in the veterinary literature and comparatively little research that relates specifically to the disease in goats.

Descriptions of caprine enterotoxemia have come from Australia (Oxer 1956), Britain (Shanks 1949), Canada (Blackwell and Butler 1992), France (Delahaye 1975), South Africa (van Tonder 1975), Sri Lanka (Wanasinghe 1973), Switzerland (von Rotz et al. 1984) and the United States (Boughton and Hardy 1941; Guss 1977). Most outbreaks of caprine enterotoxemia involve dairy goats raised under intensive or semi-intensive management conditions. When fiber goats have been affected, as in South African or Texas Angoras, the disease is far more likely to occur during periods of corralling or restricted grazing in grain fields than during normal free-range grazing and browsing (van Tonder 1975; Ross 1981). The greatest losses caused by enterotoxemia in sheep occur in growing lambs on concentrate rations in feedlots, but this management situation is rarely encountered in goat practice.

Sudden changes in feedstuffs or feeding practices have been associated with triggering outbreaks of enterotoxemia in all affected species. Specific situations that make goats predisposed to this disease have included turnout to lush pasture, feeding of bread or other bakery goods, feeding of a bran/molasses mash to recently fresh does, excessive grain consumption after accidental access to feed storage sheds, and feeding of garden greens to goats unaccustomed to green feed (King 1980a). Feed changes, however, are not a prerequisite for enterotoxemia to occur. The author has observed an explosive outbreak of enterotoxemia in a herd of commercial antibody-producing goats that were fed an unchanging diet of hay and concentrate for many months before the outbreak.

Abrupt changes in weather have also been associated with onset of enterotoxemia in other species but this has not been well documented in goats. Nor has a strong seasonal pattern been identified. Intestinal tapeworm infections are believed to predispose feedlot lambs to enterotoxemia by slowing transit time of grain rations through the gut, allowing for more extensive proliferation of clostridia, but this association has not been reported in goats either.

While sporadic cases of caprine enterotoxemia are common, outbreaks of enterotoxemia in goat herds with high morbidity rates also occur. On some premises, the outbreak of enterotoxemia can become well established, with new cases occurring over several weeks or months. The epidemiologic factors contributing to this disease pattern are unknown. A buildup of *C. perfringens* type D in the environment from earlier diarrheic cases is probably contributory.

Pathogenesis

Specific studies on the pathogenesis of enterotoxemia in goats are limited. In other ruminant species it is believed that commensal *C. perfringens* type D organisms reside in the gut without producing much damage, because bacterial numbers are low and any toxins that are produced are moved quickly through the gut by normal peristalsis. Sudden ingestion of readily fermentable, carbohydrate-rich feeds permits more undigested starch to pass through the rumen to the abomasum and intestine where it serves as a nutrient substrate for rapid proliferation of the organism. Excess carbohydrate intake may also predispose to reduced motility. This proliferation of *C. perfringens* type D in conjunction with reduced peristalsis enhances the concentration and pathogenic potential of the epsilon toxin produced by the organism. Epsilon toxin, after being converted from the prototoxin by intestinal trypsin, increases vascular permeability in the gut, thereby facilitating its own absorption into the bloodstream. A generalized toxemia ensues. The toxin is necrotizing, and specifically neurotoxic. Death is attributable to damage of vital neurons, generalized toxemia, and shock (Kimberling 1988).

There is evidence that the pathogenesis of enterotoxemia in goats is different in terms of the intestinal effects. In field cases, diarrhea is a predominant clinical finding in goats relative to other species, and at necropsy, marked enterocolitis is often present (Blackwell and Butler 1992). This enterocolitis is an infrequent finding in lambs and calves.

The predilection of the gut as a target organ in caprine enterotoxemia has been demonstrated experimentally. Lambs and kids given broth infusions of *C. perfringens* type D intraduodenally via a cannula showed markedly different clinical and pathologic responses (Blackwell et al. 1991). In general, lambs showed lethargy, overt neurologic signs, minimal diarrhea, and death. Kids showed more prominent diarrhea and abdominal discomfort with fewer neurologic signs preceding death. At necropsy, intestinal lesions in lambs were limited to a moderate edema of the colon and watery gut content, while in kids, a severe necrotizing colitis was seen grossly and confirmed histologically.

More recent experiments involving introduction of epsilon toxin into ligated gut loops of lambs and kids has suggested a possible mechanism for the different clinical responses in sheep and goats. At two hours post inoculation, kids had accumulated much larger volumes of fluid and sodium in the small intestinal lumen than lambs. It was hypothesized that the more rapid endotoxin-induced accumulation of fluid in the small intestine of goats could more quickly flush away bacteria and toxin, moderating the intestinal toxin absorption. In contrast, the delayed physiological response in the small intestine in sheep might result in greater absorption of epsilon toxin from the small intestine of this species, leading to the neurologic signs, brain lesions, and lung edema that is more commonly observed in naturally occurring cases of enterotoxemia in sheep as compared to goats (Fernandez Miyakawa and Uzal, 2003).

Clinical Findings

Three distinct clinical forms of enterotoxemia are recognized in goats, namely peracute, acute, and chronic. The peracute form occurs more frequently in young goats than adults. The clinical course is usually less than twenty-four hours and may go unnoticed. Finding one or more dead animals is often the first indication of peracute enterotoxemia in a herd. In milk-fed kids, it is frequently the larger, more robust, aggressively feeding individuals that are affected. In weaned kids, the history may reflect some recent change in feeding practices or an opportunity to overeat. Clinical signs include a sudden loss of appetite, profound depression, marked abdominal discomfort manifested by arching of the back and kicking at the belly, loud and painful screaming, and profuse watery diarrhea containing blood and shreds of mucus. Fevers of 105°F (40.5°C) are recorded. Affected goats quickly become weak and recumbent. They may show paddling or convulsions, but frequently they just lapse into a coma without excitatory signs. Death ensues within hours. Recoveries are rare, even with treatment. When the peracute form occurs in milking goats, the onset of signs may be foreshadowed by a sudden drop in milk production.

In the acute form, similar clinical signs are seen but with less severity. Abdominal pain and screaming may be absent or reduced. Feces may first turn pasty or soft, but then become watery. The clinical course lasts from three to four days. Severe dehydration and acidosis, caused by the profuse diarrhea, become complicating factors in these cases. Spontaneous recoveries may occur, but most animals die if not treated. The acute form more often affects mature goats. It can occur in herds with a solid history of vaccination against *C. perfringens* type D, so enterotoxemia should not be ruled out on the basis of previous vaccination. A history of recent feed changes may or may not be elicited.

In the chronic form, intermittent, recurring bouts of illness are observed over several weeks. Mature animals are usually affected. These goats are dull and listless with reduced appetite and milk production if lactating. There is progressive weight loss with intermittent episodes of pasty or loose feces. It has been emphasized that the chronic form is extremely difficult to recognize as enterotoxemia unless there is prior knowledge of acute or peracute cases in the herd (Shanks 1949).

Clinical Pathology and Necropsy

Reports on hematologic and clinical chemistry changes during caprine enterotoxemia are limited. The author has recorded complete blood counts on goats with the acute form of the disease. There is a distinct trend toward neutrophilic leukocytosis. In thirty-nine affected goats, the mean white blood cell count was 16,200/mm^3 with individual counts as high as 47,700/mm^3 recorded. Packed cell volumes as high as 57% were noted in cases with severe dehydration. Hyperglycemia, azotemia, and increased serum osmolarity may occur in the later stages of enterotoxemia (Blackwell et al. 1991) but they are not specific to this disease.

Reports on necropsy findings in caprine enterotoxemia also are limited. In a series of ten goat necropsies, enterocolitis was the most consistent finding in enterotoxemia (Blackwell and Butler 1992). The gut lesions were hemorrhagic, fibrinous, or necrotic in character. Enterocolitis was followed in frequency by pulmonary edema, renal tubular necrosis, and edema of mesenteric lymph nodes. Hydropericardium, a common finding in sheep, was seen in only one goat. Glucose may be detected in bladder urine of affected goats. If necropsy is performed shortly after death, the detection of soft or pulpy kidneys supports the diagnosis of enterotoxemia. However, if necropsy is delayed, the pulpy kidney loses its diagnostic significance, because kidney autolysis eventually occurs post mortem regardless of the cause of death. Gross lesions may be entirely absent in some cases of enterotoxemia (Blackwell 1983).

Cerebral microangiopathy has been rarely reported in caprine enterotoxemia, though it is a prevalent finding in sheep with the disease. This may reflect a failure to examine the brains of affected goats histologically since neurologic signs are not prominent clinically in caprine enterotoxemia. When tissues from two goats in Australia diagnosed with enterotoxemia where examined retrospectively, cerebral microangiopathy was noted in both goats (Uzal et al. 1997).

In experimentally induced type D enterotoxemia in goats, produced by administration of starch into the abomasum along with duodenal instillation of either whole cultures, culture supernatant, or washed cells, goats developed diarrhea and a necrotizing colitis, as is typical of the species. They also developed lesions similar to those found more often in ovine enterotoxemia, including lung edema and cerebral vasogenic edema (Uzal and Kelly 1998).

Abnormal appearing areas of bowel mucosa can be used to support the diagnosis of enterotoxemia. Impression smears of affected mucosa reveal a predominant population of large Gram-positive rods typical of *C. perfringens* (Figure 10.5). A similar

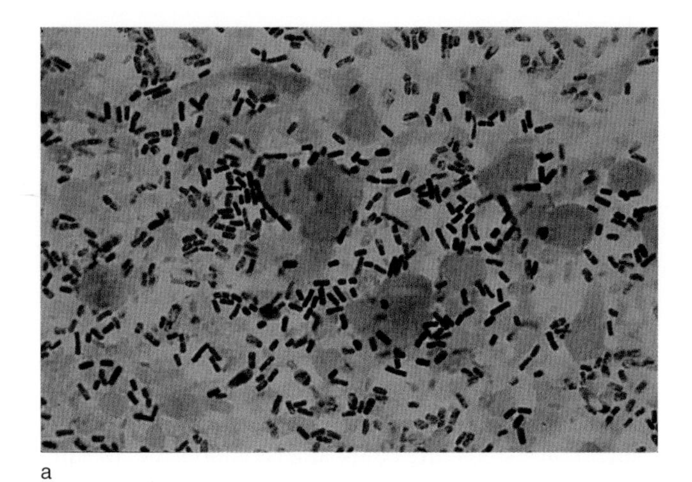
a

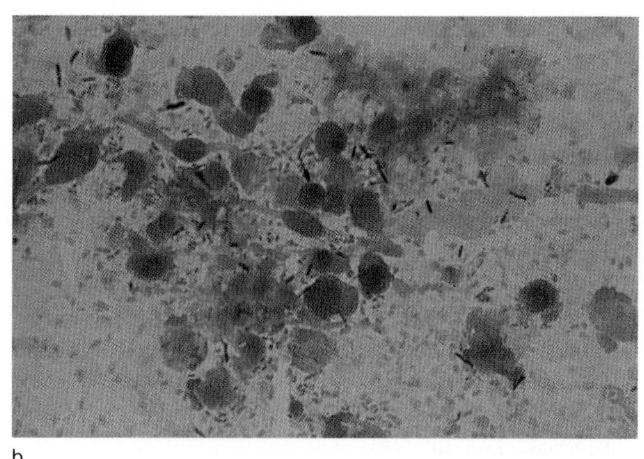
b

Figure 10.5. Gram-stained impression smear of intestinal mucosa of goat with enterotoxemia (Figure 10.5a). Note abundance of large Gram-positive rods compared to intestinal smear taken from a normal goat at necropsy (Figure 10.5b). (Courtesy of Dr. David M. Sherman.)

preponderance of large Gram-positive rods plus spores may be seen in smears made from diarrheic feces *ante mortem*.

Swabs from intestinal lesions can be submitted for anaerobic culture. Because *C. perfringens* type D may be isolated from the gut of normal goats, culturing the organism from the gut has been considered by some to have little diagnostic significance. However, survey studies of abomasal and intestinal culture from normal, healthy goats indicate that only 61% of goats sampled carried any type of enteric clostridial organism, and only 3% carried *C. perfringens* type D (Sinha 1970). Therefore, the isolation of the organism from swabs of necrotic intestine in animals dying of signs typical of enterotoxemia may have more diagnostic significance than is usually ascribed to it.

The most convincing indication of enterotoxemia, however, is the presence of epsilon toxin in diarrheic feces or intestinal content. At least 10 ml of intestinal content should be submitted, taken from the areas of the bowel exhibiting lesions. The toxin is fragile, so gut content should be sent to the lab refrigerated or frozen. When type D enterotoxemia is suspected, intestinal content should be collected as soon as possible after death and frozen for shipment because the epsilon toxin is especially labile.

Traditionally, toxin types have been identified by *in vivo* toxin neutralization assays using mouse lethality and guinea pig or rabbit dermonecrosis as endpoints. More recently, both ELISA and counter immunoelectrophoresis (CIEP) procedures have been described that eliminate the need for lab animals and have improved the availability of confirmatory testing. Both methods have been reported as comparable to mouse lethality tests (Naylor et al. 1987; Hornitzky et al. 1989). However, another study indicated considerable variability in sensitivity of a polyclonal ELISA, monoclonal ELISA, and CIEP when compared to the mouse neutralization test for detection of epsilon toxin in intestinal content and other body fluids. The study also urged that a final diagnosis be based not only on toxin testing but also clinical signs and post mortem findings (Uzal et al. 2003).

Beginning in the 1990s, polymerase chain reaction (PCR) tests have been developed that identify the presence of the bacterial genes responsible for the production of the various *C. perfringens* toxins, thus obviating the need for direct identification of toxin for typing the organism (Daube et al. 1994; Meer and Songer 1997). Multiplex PCR genotyping is now routinely available in some diagnostic laboratories and can be applied to identify and type *C. perfringens* strains present in the gastrointestinal content or feces of goats (Uzal et al. 1996) or from paraffin-embedded tissues of goats (Warren et al. 1999).

Diagnosis

Diagnosis is based on a combination of characteristic clinical history and signs, evidence of enterocolitis at necropsy, isolation of *C. perfringens* from the feces or gut lumen, and identification of epsilon toxin or the gene expressing epsilon toxin in *C. perfringens* cultures from feces or gut lumen content. It has been suggested that a presumptive antemortem diagnosis of enterotoxemia can be made by observation of clinical improvement in response to administration of *C. perfringens* type D-specific antitoxins (Guss 1977). However, this has been reported as unreliable by others (Blackwell and Butler 1992).

Differential diagnosis of the peracute form must include all causes of sudden death, with particular emphasis on plant and chemical toxicities. Peracute deaths in kids younger than three weeks of age are not likely to be due to type D enterotoxemia because normal gut trypsin levels may be inadequate to activate the epsilon prototoxin. Type C enterotoxemia, however, can cause death in these young kids.

When diarrhea is present in peracute or acute disease, the differential diagnosis should include coccidiosis, salmonellosis, yersiniosis, and in younger animals cryptosporidiosis and colibacillosis.

In milking does, the early stages of the acute form of the disease may mimic milk fever or hypocalcemia, but favorable response to administration of parenteral calcium salts in cases of milk fever should clarify the diagnosis. The chronic form of enterotoxemia and chronic salmonellosis may be clinically undifferentiable and diagnosis depends on bacteriologic methods.

Treatment

The prognosis for recovery is guarded in caprine enterotoxemia, even with treatment. Aggressive intervention is required. Affected animals should be managed in a warm and dry hospital pen. Intravenous fluid therapy providing mixed electrolyte solutions with bicarbonate is indicated in peracute and acute cases to counter shock, dehydration, and acidosis. Nonsteroidal anti-inflammatory drugs such as flunixin meglumine (1 mg/kg intravenously every twelve hours) may be helpful in stabilizing animals in toxemic shock and will alleviate pain.

Commercially available type C and D antitoxins should be administered parenterally, preferably intravenously, in severe cases. Though recommended prophylactic doses are usually around 5 ml, therapeutic doses up to 100 ml have been administered. Because the antitoxin products are relatively expensive, a minimum effective dose is desirable. Fifteen to 20 ml has been effective in Australian practices (King 1980a). In those cases responsive to antitoxin, a rapid though sometimes temporary improvement may be noted within one to two hours. Equal or decreased doses can be repeated every three to four hours until the animal's condition has obviously stabilized. In the chronic form of the disease, 2 doses of 20 ml of antitoxin given four days apart was reported to be a reasonably effective treatment (Quarmby 1946). Diarrhea ceased in affected does and their milk production and body condition improved.

Decades ago, there were reports of allergic protein sensitivities to antitoxin observed in Saanen goats after repeated administration (Quarmby 1947). Though this may reflect impurities in older serum products, the potential for anaphylaxis, particularly in the Saanen breed, should be anticipated, and epinephrine (0.03 mg/kg intravenously) kept close at hand.

Antibiotic therapy may be helpful in reducing bacterial proliferation. Oral sulfas have been used successfully. To ensure that the drugs reach the abomasum and intestine, pretreatment with 5 cc of copper sulfate solutions (1 tablespoon $CuSO_4$/liter of water) to close the esophageal groove followed rapidly by antibiotic administration has been recommended (King 1980a). Parenteral antibiotics including penicillin, tetracyclines, or trimethoprim-sulfa combinations may also be useful. *C. perfringens* isolates are often resistant to aminoglycosides (Songer 1996).

To limit the uptake and promote elimination of intestinal epsilon toxin, various cathartics and adsorbents have been given orally, including activated charcoal, magnesium sulfate, magnesium hydroxide, caffeine, and kaolin/pectin. Though the rationale for use is valid, therapeutic efficacy has not been proven.

In the face of outbreaks of enterotoxemia, all animals on the premises should be considered to be at risk. Previously vaccinated goats should be boostered, and unvaccinated goats should receive a prophylactic dose of antitoxin in conjunction with an initial vaccination to be boostered two to three weeks later. Any excessive feeding of carbohydrate should be curtailed immediately.

Control

Goats are considered highly susceptible to enterotoxemia and it is universally recommended that all goats be vaccinated against the disease as part of any basic caprine herd health program. At the same time, it is recognized that vaccination does not afford the same level of protection to goats that occurs in sheep, and that the persistence of serum antibodies against toxin at protective levels in goats is limited (Shanks 1949; Blackwell et al. 1983).

This species difference has been experimentally demonstrated. When sheep and goats were given equivalent doses of three different multivalent clostridial vaccines that included *C. perfringens* type D, levels of serum anti-epsilon toxin antibodies increased significantly in sheep and remained significantly higher than prevaccination levels at twenty-eight days after vaccination. In goats, only one of the same products produced a significant increase in serum anti-epsilon toxin antibody titers, and titers returned to prevaccination levels for all products by twenty-eight days (Green et al. 1987).

The required level of anti-epsilon toxin antibody in serum that protects goats from clinical enterotoxemia is not fully established, but recent research suggests that it is likely 0.25 IU/ml (Uzal and Kelly 1998; Uzal et al. 1998). In one study, goats vaccinated with an incomplete Freund's adjuvanted vaccine had high anti-epsilon antibody titers between 2.45 IU/ml and 230 IU/ml. They showed no clinical signs or post mortem lesions after intraduodenal administration of *C. perfringens* type D culture supernatant. In contrast, goats receiving a commercially available aluminum hydroxide adjuvanted vaccine only produced antibody levels in the range of 0.22 to 1.52 IU/ml and four of five goats developed diarrhea and some evidence of colitis at necropsy, while unvaccinated control goats all developed severe enterocolitis (Uzal and Kelly 1998). It seems, therefore, that the occurrence of enteritis in vaccinated goats derives from the fact that conventional, commercial vaccines, which are generally approved for sheep, may not produce sufficiently high antibody responses in goats to effect protection against the enterocolitic form of the disease common in goats (Uzal and Kelly 1998).

In a second study, antibody levels were measured after vaccination with a standard commercial vaccine following a single injection alone or after booster injections given either twenty-eight days later or forty-two days later. In all three protocols, antibody levels had dropped below the putative protective threshold of 0.25 IU/ml in most of the goats by ninety-eight days after the initial vaccination (Uzal et al. 1998).

These findings support the recommendation that goats should be vaccinated at intervals of three to four months to maintain adequate protection against enterotoxemia using currently available vaccines, especially in herds where there is a history of enterotoxemia. At the least, goats should be vaccinated semi-annually. Initial vaccinations should be followed by a booster vaccination three to six weeks later and semi- or tri-annual vaccinations should be timed so that the last vaccination occurs two to three weeks before parturition in pregnant does. This enhances the protective effect of colostrum for suckling kids. Kids should be vaccinated initially at four to six weeks of age and certainly before weaning. They should also be boostered three to six weeks later, depending on product recommendation.

Vaccines limited to *C. perfringens* types C and D with or without tetanus may be preferable to the use of more complex, polyvalent clostridial vaccines commonly approved for sheep and cattle. These polyvalent vaccines may be more expensive and provide unneeded protection against clostridial diseases that occur uncommonly in goats. Furthermore, in at least one study, anti-epsilon toxin antibody titers were sometimes significantly lower in goats in response to a multivalent vaccine than to a bivalent *C. perfringens* types C and D vaccine (Blackwell et al. 1983). Few products are approved specifically for goats, and in general, sheep dosages are used.

There is a marked tendency for goats to develop local tissue reactions at the vaccine injection site. This is quite troublesome in show goats, and also complicates caseous lymphadenitis control because owners may have trouble differentiating between lymph node abscesses and injection site reactions. The occurrence of sterile abscesses of 2 to 5 cm in diameter after clostridial vaccination is well documented and does not necessarily result from careless injection technique, but rather is intrinsic to some vaccine preparations (Smith and Klose 1980; Blackwell et al. 1983; Green et al. 1987).

Scrupulous vaccination technique should be observed when vaccinating show goats to avoid any implication that technique was at fault, should abscesses develop. Use a new needle for each vaccination. Subcutaneous vaccination in the loose skin on the chest wall behind the elbow is recommended as a site where reactions will be less visible in show goats. However, if reactions occur at this site and become secondarily infected, they may grow quite large before they are noticed. In commercial goats, therefore, vaccination on the neck is recommended. Practitioners should sample several vaccine products to determine which produces the least tissue reaction. No correlation between tissue reaction and immunogenicity has been demonstrated (Green et al. 1987).

In addition to vaccination, control of enterotoxemia depends on avoidance of sudden feed changes, vigilance against overeating, and guarding against accidental access to grains and other stored feeds.

Salmonellosis

Salmonellosis continues to be an important infectious disease for several reasons: changing patterns of infection and morbidity rates in virtually all domestic species of livestock and poultry, public health concerns regarding human illness from animal sources, increased occurrence of multiple drug resistance, and economic losses to producers and food processors caused by condemnations and adverse publicity relating to the zoonotic potential of the infection. These issues are all relevant to the goat industry.

Etiology

Salmonella are Gram-negative, nonspore-forming, rod-shaped bacteria in the family Enterobacteriaceae. There are more than 2,400 serotypes, also known as serovars. On a worldwide basis, the serovar S. Typhimurium is the most common cause of the diarrheal and septicemic forms of clinical salmonellosis in cattle, sheep, horses, and swine. This serovar has been associated with clinical salmonellosis in goats in the United States (Bulgin and Anderson 1981). In two British reports, however, S. Dublin was isolated from sick goats (Levi 1949; Gibson 1957), while in a Nigerian investigation of diarrheic kids, S. Poona was the sole isolate identified (Falade 1976). In an Australian outbreak, four serovars were isolated from goats dying with severe diarrhea: S. Adelaide, S. Typhimurium, S. Muenchen, and S. Singapore (McOrist and Miller 1981). Isolates from cases of gastroenteritis and septicemia in goats in India include *S.* Typhimurium, *S.* Bere, *S.* Colombo, *S.* Newport, *S.* Tennessee, and *S.* Worthington (Janakiraman and Rajendran 1973). *S.* Enteriditis, *S.* Abony, and *S.* Cerro were cultured from cases of kid diarrhea in Greece (Zdragas et al. 2000).

Salmonella can also cause caprine abortion. Abortions may occur as a sequela to septicemia with any *Salmonella* serovar, but a specific epizootic abortion syndrome of goats and sheep caused by *S.* Abortusovis occurs in Mediterranean and Middle Eastern countries (Leondidis et al. 1984). S. Abortusovis may also cause enteric salmonellosis (Sanchis and Cornille 1980). *Salmonella* are an infrequent cause of mastitis in goats, gaining entry to the mammary gland through the teat canal from a contaminated environment.

Numerous *Salmonella* serovars have been isolated from the feces of healthy goats (Kapur et al. 1973; Abdel-Ghani et al. 1987) and more than forty serovars from the viscera of healthy goats at slaughterhouses around the world (Nagaratnam and Ratatunga 1971; Kumar et al. 1973; Gupta et al. 1974; Arora 1978; Nabbut and Al-Nakhli 1982; Subasinghe and Ramakrishnaswamy 1983; Faraj et al. 1983; Diaz-Aparicio et al. 1987; Woldemariam et al. 2005; Chandra et al. 2006). *S.* Paratyphi, the cause of paratyphoid in humans, has been isolated from mesenteric lymph nodes of slaughtered goats in the Middle East and Asia, suggesting that the goat can act as a source of infection for humans. In slaughterhouse surveys of viscera, *Salmonella* are most often isolated from mesenteric lymph nodes and gall bladders.

Epidemiology

The occurrence and outcome of salmonellosis in livestock can be influenced by a number of factors. These include the existence of host-adapted *Salmonella* serovars, the development of a carrier state, impaired immunity of the host, the occurrence of severe stress including prolonged transport or deprivation of food and water, intensive management practices, and exposure to contaminated feeds or infected animals. The role of all these various factors in caprine salmonellosis is not fully described.

There are no known host-adapted *Salmonella* serovars in goats. *S.* Dublin, which is considered to be host-adapted to cattle in Britain, caused clinical disease in goats but there was no indication that a carrier state or persistent shedding occurred in exposed or recovered goats based on repeated fecal cultures or tissue cultures at necropsy (Levi 1949; Gibson 1957).

Reports of naturally occurring salmonellosis indicate that latent carrier states occur in goats and that latent infections can progress to active fecal shedding of *Salmonella* or to overt clinical disease in response to stress of transport, excessive handling, feed or water deprivation, sudden feed changes, or parturition. The frequent isolation of *Salmonella* from the organs of healthy goats at slaughter, as cited above, also indicates the existence of a carrier state.

A latent carrier state in goats has been demonstrated experimentally with *S.* Typhimurium (Arora 1983). Goats challenged orally showed peak fecal shedding at three days after challenge but all shedding ceased by two weeks. During the three subsequent weeks, no organisms were recovered from feces. However, when these goats were later stressed by transport, 60% resumed fecal shedding of S. Typhimurium. The organism was isolated from mesenteric lymph nodes, livers, and spleens at necropsy. In contrast, attempts to confirm the existence of a nasal carrier state in kids from premises with a history of salmonellosis were unsuccessful, though calves and piglets on the same premises yielded the organism (Garg and Sharma 1979).

Transmission is most commonly by the fecal-oral route. The introduction of unrecognized carrier animals into susceptible populations is of major importance in the spread of salmonellosis. Cross species infection can also occur as reported in the transmission of *S.* Dublin from calves to goats via fecal contaminated pens and bedding, and of *S.* Typhimurium from ducks to goats via consumption of contaminated water (King 1980). Other potential sources of infection for goats include raw sewage, contaminated feedstuffs, rodents, birds, and other livestock species, although documentation of such transmissions to the goat is rare.

Other factors that may predispose to clinical salmonellosis in goats include close contact with active shedders, excessive buildup of organisms in the environment caused by poor hygiene or poorly constructed feeders and waterers, concurrent disease, particularly severe gastrointestinal parasitism, stress of capture in feral goats, and in neonates, failure of passive transfer of antibody from the does' colostrum. There is little documentation that intensive management with many goats maintained in confinement housing increases the risk or spread of salmonellosis, although this is considered to be a major factor in regard to dairy cattle.

Human infections with *Salmonella* from goat products have been documented. Raw or undercooked goat meat can pose the risk of salmonellosis, but so can goat milk or goat milk cheese, especially if unpasteurized. Severe gastroenteritis and even fatalities can occur. In France in 1993, a commercial goat cheese made from unpasteurized goat milk led to 273 human cases of salmonellosis with one death. Though the processing plant derived milk from forty goat herds, the offending organism, *S.* Paratyphi B, was traced back to a single goat farm. Thirty-three tons (30 tonnes) of cheese stored at the plant had to be destroyed (Desenclos, et al. 1996). More recently, three brands of unpasteurized goat cheese derived from a single herd of 260 goats in

France were associated with fifty-two cases of human disease in seven European countries: France, Switzerland, Sweden, Austria, Germany, the UK, and the Netherlands. The causative agent was a relatively rare serovar, *S.* Stourbridge (Espié and Vaillant 2005). Milk samples from all goats in the source herd were cultured in the ensuing epidemiologic investigation and the organism was found in the milk of only one asymptomatic carrier. This outbreak underscores, among other things, how widely zoonotic disease can be disseminated under modern systems of marketing and trade.

Pathogenesis

The pathogenesis of enteric and septicemic salmonellosis has not been specifically studied in goats and is presumed to be similar to that described in other species (Radostits et al. 2007). After ingestion, the organism becomes established in the intestines, most commonly in the ileum. A marked enteritis develops, most likely as a result of release of endotoxin from dying organisms. Diarrhea results at least in part from the inflammatory enteritis, but the organisms may also elaborate enterotoxins that have a hypersecretory effect on villous epithelial cells leading to accelerated fluid and electrolyte loss from the gut.

Salmonella are invasive bacteria and can penetrate the mucosa, gaining entry to the lymphatics. Several outcomes are possible. In individuals with decreased disease resistance or severely impaired immunity, the organism can then gain entrance to the blood, producing a generalized septicemia with marked endotoxemia and usually death, while animals with a strong immune system may clear the infection entirely. In animals with moderate disease resistance, a transient bacteremia may occur with subsequent localization of the organism in liver, gall bladder, spleen, and mesenteric lymph nodes. These animals become latent carriers, and in the face of subsequent stresses they may develop clinical septicemia or enteritis, or they may remain subclinical but initiate fecal shedding of the organism, usually as a result of re-inoculation of the gut via the infection in the gall bladder. In carrier does that are pregnant, the stress of parturition may induce bacteremia and result in exposure of the kid either *in utero* or via the milk or by fecal contamination of the udder.

Animals experiencing infection may produce detectable antibodies against flagellar (H) and somatic (O) antigens of *Salmonella*. In goats experimentally infected with S. Typhimurium, antibodies to O and H antigens were detectable by five days post infection in one study (Sharma et al. 2001) and not until after seven days in another (Otesile et al. 1990). The flagellar antibodies appear to be more persistent in goats. The role of antibody in subsequent immunity is not clear. Immunity to the same strains of *Salmonella* may develop after initial exposures, but cross immunity is limited. This fact has impeded the development of broadly efficacious vaccines.

Clinical Findings

Three age patterns of salmonellosis have been identified in goats, namely neonatal septicemia during the first week of life, preweaning enteritis in kids two to eight weeks of age, and enteritis/septicemia of mature goats. The prognosis is grave in the first, poor in the second, and guarded in the third.

In neonatal septicemia, kids usually appear normal at birth and may die acutely by thirty-six hours with no signs other than depression. Occasionally, signs of gaseous abdominal distension with pain or diarrhea may be seen.

In enteritis of older kids, there is an acute onset of depression and anorexia. A profuse, watery, foul-smelling, yellow to greenish-brown diarrhea develops, accompanied by fever up to 107°F (41.7°C). Affected kids rapidly become severely dehydrated, weak, and recumbent. Some may die within eight hours of the onset of diarrhea, with most dying within twenty-four to forty-eight hours. Fever may subside after twenty-four hours and temperature can become subnormal as animals develop shock. Morbidity and mortality rates can be high, particularly as kid births are often concentrated into a short period and numerous kids on the premises may be at risk.

The adult form of the disease tends to be more sporadic, with lower morbidity and mortality rates. Affected goats become acutely depressed, anorexic, and febrile, and develop a watery, foul smelling diarrhea that can be yellow, gray, or greenish-brown. Dehydration and weakness rapidly ensue and death can occur within twenty-four to forty-eight hours of the onset of signs. A chronic form of adult disease can also occur in which similar but milder signs are seen with subsequent recovery, followed by intermittent, recurring bouts of diarrhea. These animals tend to become progressively emaciated and may develop anemia.

In published cases of caprine salmonellosis, bloody diarrhea or fibrinous casts are rarely reported. This is in marked contrast to the disease as described in cattle or sheep.

Clinical Pathology and Necropsy

Goats with salmonellosis may have a marked leukopenia early in the course of disease followed by a rebound leukocytosis, with neutrophilia and a left shift in animals that do not die acutely. Severe metabolic acidosis can be expected along with losses of sodium and potassium caused by diarrhea. Liver-specific enzymes may be elevated in septicemic salmonellosis due to foci of infection in the liver. In chronic salmonellosis, anemia and hypoproteinemia may be observed. In neonates, serum immunoglobulin levels may be low if failure of passive transfer of antibody from the dam has predisposed to clinical salmonellosis. Bacterial culture of the doe's milk and feces is also indicated to identify the dam as the possible source of infection.

For a definitive antemortem diagnosis in enteritis cases, repeated attempts at fecal culture should be made. Appropriate enrichment media should be used. In some cases, attempts to culture the organism from diarrhea are unsuccessful, but positive culture results may be obtained from formed feces after the diarrhea has resolved. Subsequent biochemical characterization and serotyping of isolates at a reference laboratory are recommended because of the different zoonotic implications of various *Salmonella* serovars. Blood cultures may be attempted on septicemic cases before antibiotic therapy, and antibiotic susceptibility testing of isolates should be requested because the occurrence of antibiotic resistance in *Salmonella* is increasing.

Serology may be of some value in the diagnosis of acute salmonellosis, particularly in evaluating a herd outbreak. In outbreaks of S. Dublin infection, goats had strong persistent antibody responses to flagellar H antigens of homologous S. Dublin for several months after exposure. Nonexposed control goats had background agglutination titers up to 1:80, whereas exposed goats had titers as high as 1:20,480.

At necropsy, kids dying acutely of septicemia may show minimal gross lesions consisting of some hemorrhage on serosal surfaces, increased pericardial and peritoneal fluid, and gas distended bowel. Histologically, edema of the abomasum and dilation of the tips of the intestinal villi have been observed. Culture should be attempted from multiple organs.

In older kids and adults with enteritis, gross lesions can be more apparent and include petechial hemorrhage of serosal surfaces, pericardial and peritoneal effusions, enlarged and edematous mesenteric lymph nodes, congestion of the lungs and liver, edematous thickening of the gall bladder, and marked, diffuse inflammation of the intestinal mucosa. The small and large intestines can be involved and the inflammation can range from catarrhal, to hemorrhagic, to necrotic, with diphtheritic membranes present in more prolonged cases. In chronic cases, lack of abdominal fat, miliary nodules in the liver, and hepatic lipidosis may also be seen.

Histologically, the intestinal inflammation is confirmed. The small intestine may show dilated mucosal crypts containing cellular debris and neutrophils, submucosal infiltrates of neutrophils and lymphocytes, and edema of the lamina propria. There may be small foci of hepatic necrosis containing aggregates of mononuclear cells. It is reported from experimental infection in goats with S. Typhimurium that histological lesions in mesenteric lymph nodes may be severe, even when enteric lesions are not conspicuous (Sharma et al. 2001). In goats, the mesenteric lymph nodes are the most promising source for bacterial isolation. Intestinal content, spleen, liver, and bile may also be cultured successfully.

Diagnosis

In newborn kids, starvation, hypothermia, lethal congenital defects, and colisepticemia must be considered in the differential diagnosis. In older kids with acute enteritis, the major differential diagnoses are coccidiosis, cryptosporidiosis yersiniosis, enterotoxemia caused by *Clostridium perfringens* type D, and, if pastured, gastrointestinal nematodiasis. In adult animals, enterotoxemia and gastrointestinal nematodiasis should be ruled out. Peste des petits ruminants and rinderpest must be considered in countries where they occur.

Treatment

Treatment should be directed at rehydration and maintenance of circulatory volume, correction of acid-base and electrolyte imbalances, amelioration of endotoxic effects, and the control of bacteremia when present. Intensive fluid therapy is indicated, and it is unlikely that any route other than intravenous will be of value. Balanced electrolyte solutions supplemented with sodium bicarbonate and potassium are indicated. In septicemic neonates, glucose supplementation is also advisable. If neonates are hypogammaglobulinemic, whole blood or preferably plasma transfusions are desirable. Nonsteroidal anti-inflammatory drugs such as flunixin meglumine administered parentally can be helpful.

The use of antibiotics in the treatment of salmonellosis is controversial because in other species it is associated with prolonged fecal excretion of bacteria, increased likelihood of developing a carrier state, and the promotion of drug resistance in the organism. These associations have had limited investigation in the goat. Two goat isolates made in India, S. Typhimurium and S. Weltevreden, were shown to possess R-factor that imparted multiple drug resistance to tetracycline, oxytetracycline, and chlortetracycline (Kumar and Misra 1983). An abattoir survey of 204 slaughtered goats in India yielded sixty *Salmonella* isolates with forty patterns of antibiotic resistance. All isolates were susceptible to chloramphenicol and imipenem, while 70% were resistant to nitrofurantoin and 52% to amikacin. Multiple resistance to three or more drugs occurred in 52% of the isolates while only 8% of isolates were sensitive to all drugs tested. Thirteen percent were resistant to gentamicin and 18% to tetracycline (Chandra et al. 2006).

It is unlikely that septicemic kids have any chance of survival without the use of antibiotics. In addition, it is extremely difficult to establish clinically if there is a component of septicemia in advanced cases of enteritis where severe dehydration and electrolyte imbalance lead to weakness and recumbency, suggestive of endotoxic shock. The use of antibiotics in these cases is justified. The major concern is that antibiotic-treated animals should not be subsequently introduced into naïve herds because it is impossible to be sure that the carrier state has not developed.

Where its use is permitted, chloramphenicol, at a dose of 10 mg/kg intravenously every twelve hours, has proven to be a drug to which most caprine isolates of *Salmonella* are susceptible. Caprine isolates are also frequently susceptible to cephalothin, the aminoglycosides gentamicin and kanamycin, and trimethoprim-sulfonamide combinations. The aminoglycosides must be used cautiously in these cases because the severe dehydration that is often present can aggravate the inherent renal toxicity of these drugs.

Gentamicin is given intramuscularly or subcutaneously at a dose of 1 mg/kg every eight hours, and kanamycin at 5 mg/kg every eight hours. Trimethoprim is rendered inactive by rumen degradation and therefore trimethoprim-sulfa combination drugs must be given intravenously or subcutaneously to adults. They should also be given intravenously to septicemic neonates to provide rapid plasma concentrations. They may be given orally to young preruminant kids with enteritis. The dose is 30 mg/kg orally once a day or 15 mg/kg intravenously every twelve hours. Sensitivities to tetracyclines, nitrofurantoin, sulfonamides, neomycin, streptomycin erythromycin, and ampicillin are more variable. Resistance to penicillin is typical (Nabbut et al. 1981; Mago et al. 1982; Kumar and Misra 1983). In outbreaks, mass medication with sulfonamides or tetracyclines can be helpful if the isolate is susceptible to these drugs. Drugs should be added to the water rather than the feed, because many affected animals will not eat but may continue to drink.

Control

To prevent introduction of *Salmonella* into a naïve herd, purchase of outside animals should be discouraged. If purchases are made, they should be directly from healthy source herds and not through sales barns or markets. Because the stress of transport and introduction to new surroundings may trigger fecal shedding or overt clinical disease, newly purchased animals should be isolated from the herd for at least three weeks after purchase and, if practical, bacterial cultures of feces should be performed, particularly if the animal develops diarrhea during isolation.

In the face of an outbreak, it is important to identify the source of infection. Because the source of *Salmonella* can be contaminated feed or water, subclinical carrier animals, newly introduced livestock, or other animals on the premises, including rodents and birds, extensive animal and environmental sampling may be necessary to identify and remove the offending source.

Affected animals and their cohorts should be isolated away from the rest of the herd and rigorous hygienic measures should be practiced when dealing with these animals. If affected animals have been moved from the original site of the outbreak, those premises should be thoroughly cleaned, repeatedly disinfected, and allowed to remain unused for several weeks. Common household bleach is an inexpensive and effective disinfectant as long as organic material has been removed from floors, pens, feeders, and waterers.

When sporadic cases or recurrent outbreaks of salmonellosis continue to occur in a herd, the presence of carrier animals must be considered. Repeated herd-wide fecal culture testing with culling of shedders may be costly but effective. Strict attention must be paid to ensuring that kids receive adequate colostrum and that kidding facilities and feeding equipment are kept clean. Kids should be reared in a separate facility away from adults and preferably in individual pens or hutches rather than in groups.

Vaccination can play an important role in the control of *Salmonella* infection in ruminant livestock, but at present the options are limited for goats, because there are no vaccines approved specifically for use in this species. A bivalent killed bacterin containing *S.* Typhimurium and *S.* Dublin is available for use in cattle in many countries, including the United States, but the effectiveness of whole cell killed *Salmonella* bacterins is limited. Vaccines based on the core lipopolysaccharide (LPS) common to Gram-negative bacterial cell walls are also commercially available for cattle and may offer better cross protection between serovars, because the repeat polysaccharide units of the LPS which confer serotype specificity are not present in the vaccine.

There is active research on the development of new vaccine technologies to improve cellular and humoral responses and especially to overcome the general lack of cross protection provided by monovalent vaccines against heterologous *Salmonella* serovars. One promising advance has been the development of a vaccine that produces antibodies against siderophore receptor sites and porin proteins found on the outer cell membrane of Enterobacteriaceae, including *Salmonella*. The receptor sites and proteins are necessary for the transfer of iron into the bacterial cell, a requisite for bacterial multiplication and survival. The receptor site structures are conserved across various *Salmonella* serovars, so cross protection against multiple serovars by using this approach can be significant. A commercial vaccine based on this technology is now available in the United States but is limited to use in cattle (Stevens and Thomson 2005). At present, the use of autogenous bacterins made from *Salmonella* isolated on the premises can be considered for control of infection in known infected herds of goats.

Yersiniosis

Yersiniosis has emerged as a common cause of enteritis and death in goats in New Zealand, where it appears to have become enzootic. It is also sporadically associated with enteritis, abortion, mastitis, internal abscesses, and mortality caused by septicemia in goats throughout the world. Yersiniosis is a zoonotic disease.

Etiology

Yersinia spp. are Gram-negative, aerobic and facultatively anaerobic, nonlactose-fermenting coccobacilli of the family *Enterobacteriaceae*. They grow readily on blood agar and MacConkey's agar, but may be quickly overgrown, particularly when isolating from fecal specimens.

There are three pathogenic species in the genus *Yersinia*. *Y. pestis* causes plague in humans and rodents and will not be considered further except to note that there are recorded cases of human plague traced to the slaughter, skinning, and butchering of sick goats. The goat is considered a sentinel animal in plague epidemics (Christie et al. 1980).

Y. enterocolitica and *Y. pseudotuberculosis* are pathogenic for humans and a range of animal species including goats. *Y. enterocolitica* is ubiquitous in the environment. *Y. pseudotuberculosis* is a common inhabitant of the gut of many domestic and wild animals. The conditions caused by either of these two species are known collectively as yersiniosis.

Different serotypes are recognized, based primarily on somatic O antigens. There are six main serotypes (I to VI) of *Y. pseudotuberculosis*. Serotypes I and especially III are most often associated with disease in goats (Hubbert 1972; Jones 1982; Hodges et al. 1984; Slee and Button 1990; Seimiya et al. 2005). Serotype III produces an exotoxin that may be a virulence factor.

Yersinia enterocolitica isolates are classified according to biotype, which refers to their biochemical characteristics, and serotype, which refers to their antigenic characteristics, mainly associated with somatic O antigens. Because some antigens are common to both pathogenic and nonpathogenic isolates, ideally, organisms should be described by first their biotype and then serotype, though these full descriptions are not always included in the earlier literature. There are five main biotypes or biovars of *Y. enterocolitica*, and many serotypes or serovars. Biotype 5 serotype O:2,3 has been associated with caprine enteritis in Norway (Krogstad et al. 1972) and was also associated with enteric disease of goats and sheep in Australia and New Zealand (Slee and Button 1990a).

In standard serological tests, such as the microagglutination test, *Y. enterocolitica* serotype O:9 is cross-reactive with *Brucella abortus* and can confound surveillance in brucellosis control programs. It was demonstrated in Canada that normal goats may be infected with serotype O:9 and possess antibody that leads to false positive brucellosis test results when using *B. abortus* antigen (Mittal and Tizzard 1980). More recently, an ELISA technique using refined antigens from *B. abortus* has been reported to serologically differentiate *Brucella* infected animals from those with *Yersinia enterocolitica* O:9 (Erdenebaatar et al. 2003).

Epidemiology

Many sporadic episodes of yersiniosis have been reported in animals and humans throughout the world for most of the twentieth century. In recent years, gastrointestinal illness in humans caused by *Y. enterocolitica* is increasing and links to animal contact and animal food sources are often suspected or confirmed (Nesbakken 2006). *Y. enterocolitica* has been isolated from raw goat milk offered for sale in Northern Ireland and Australia (Hughes and Jensen 1981; Walker and Gilmour 1986), and yersiniosis in a goat keeper was recorded in Norway during an epizootic of diarrhea in goats with *Y. enterocolitica* biotype 5 serotype O:2,3, possibly as a result of animal or fecal contact (Krogstad et al. 1972).

Nevertheless, goats are not considered to be significant carriers of human pathogens (Nesbakken 2006). A recent sampling survey of 575 goats in twenty-four goat herds in northern Germany yielded seventeen *Y. enterocolitica*-positive fecal samples from five herds. All isolates were biovar 1A, which is considered to be nonpathogenic, and it was concluded that milk, cheese, or meat from these goats did not represent a risk of human yersiniosis (Arnold et al. 2006). However, a serosurvey in the same region of Germany during the same time frame indicated that sera from 66% of 681 goats from twenty-eight farms had antibodies to *Yersinia* outer proteins (Yop) generally associated with pathogenicity (Nikolaou et al. 2005). One possible explanation is that goats are indeed often exposed to subclinical infections with pathogenic *Yersinia* but mount effective immune responses which eliminate these infections. This explanation is supported by the findings of a longitudinal study in New Zealand wherein pathogenic *Yersinia* cultured from the feces of young goats could not be identified again on subsequent monthly samplings from those same goats (Lãnada et al. 2005).

Epizootics in lab animal colonies and aviaries due to *Y. pseudotuberculosis* have been the most common form of the disease in animals, but livestock epizootics also occur (Obwolo 1976). Stress, overcrowding, and sudden cold weather can be predisposing factors. Birds and rodents are considered reservoirs of infection and may introduce virulent strains into susceptible herds by contaminating feedstuffs. Swine are a carrier source of *Y. enterocolitica* and may infect ruminant species when commingled. Because *Yersinia* organisms are often present in the gut of normal animals, factors that compromise gut mucosal integrity, such as concurrent parasitism, or coarse feed-related abrasions or ulcerations can predispose to septicemic yersiniosis.

Yersiniosis has been increasingly recognized as a cause of various disease problems in goats in the past two decades. Abortion and post-parturient deaths in goats because of *Y. pseudotuberculosis* have been reported from Germany (Albert 1988), India (Sulochana and Sudharma 1985), Japan (Morita et al. 1973), and the United States (Witte et al. 1985). Liver abscesses and granuloma formation in goats because of *Y. pseudotuberculosis* have been documented in the United States, Japan, and Australia (Hubbert 1972; Morita et al. 1973; Slee and Button 1990). Chronic mastitis in does caused by *Y. pseudotuberculosis* has been reported from California (Cappucci 1978) and the UK (Jones 1982). Clinical mastitis caused by *Y. enterocolitica* has not been reported in goats, and efforts to induce it experimentally were unsuccessful (Adesiyun and Lombin 1989).

Yersiniosis has become enzootic in goats in New Zealand. In a large study of goat mortality on the North Island, yersiniosis, mainly due to *Y. enterocolitica* biotype 5, was the fourth most common documented cause of death, and the most prevalent infectious cause (Buddle et al. 1988). It was also the most common bacterial cause of caprine enteritis identified in diagnostic laboratories (Vickers 1986). The disease occurs mostly in late autumn or winter and has been linked to the stress of transport, excessive handling of feral goats, nutritional deprivation, winter shearing, cold and wet weather, inadequate shelter, and, in one outbreak, contact with pigs (Orr et al. 1987). Young goats are more often affected but all ages are at risk. *Y. enterocolitica* is more frequently identified than *Y. pseudotuberculosis* (Thompson 1985). Enteric yersiniosis also has been reported in goats in Norway (Krogstad et al. 1972) due to *Y. enterocolitica*, in Australia due to *Y. enterocolitica* and *Y. pseudotuberculosis* (Slee and Button 1990, 1990a), and most recently in Japan due to *Y. pseudotuberculosis* (Seimiya et al. 2005).

A cohort study of *Yersinia* infection in goats in New Zealand indicated a clear seasonal and age related pattern of infection in goats, with most fecal excretion of pathogenic biotypes of *Y. enterocolitica* and *Y. pseudotuberculosis* occurring in the colder winter months and dropping off in summer, while excretion of non-pathogenic or environmental *Yersinia* spp. (e.g., *Y. frederiksenii*) showed a more persistent temporal pattern. The shedding of pathogenic *Yersinia* was highest in goats less than one year of age, with pathogenic strains rarely isolated from adults (Lãnada et al. 2005). It is likely that young goats normally experience subclinical infections due to environmental exposures and develop immunity, but if they are stressed during those infections, they may manifest clinical disease (Orr et al. 1990)

Pathogenesis

Infection is usually via the oral route, though in the case of mastitis, entry via the teat canal is more likely. The two *Yersinia* spp. causing yersiniosis are known to contain two plasmid-mediated virulence factors, the V and W antigens, similar to those of *Y. pestis.* In addition, some *Y. pseudotuberculosis* serotype III organisms produce an exotoxin that may enhance virulence (Obwolo 1976). *Yersinia* organisms multiply in the intestine, producing enteritis, but the organisms also produce bacteremia via the portal circulation and lymphatics, leading to internal abscesses, abortions, and acute deaths.

Clinical Findings

The enteric form of yersiniosis occurs most often in kids between one and six months of age, but all ages and breeds can be affected. In an outbreak in Japan, for instance, twenty-nine of one hundred adult lactating does developed diarrhea, but no kids, males, or dry does on the premises became ill (Seimiya et al. 2005). The initial signs were anorexia and a significant drop in milk production followed by depression and a watery diarrhea containing mucus one or two days later that lasted for four to six days. The case fatality rate was 13.7% (four of twenty-nine). There was no fever recorded in any affected animals but fever has been associated with enteric yersiniosis in other reports. In young animals, cases of sudden death without diarrhea may occur along with cases of diarrhea. The diarrhea is watery and not bloody. The course of diarrhea may be short, up to several days, and is often fatal. A more prolonged illness with dehydration and weight loss also may be seen.

In the abortion form, spontaneous abortions may occur in a herd in conjunction with the birth of weak, term kids that die shortly after birth. The cotyledons on placentas from affected does may be entirely white or have focal white spots on their surfaces (Witte et al. 1985). An abortion rate of 24% was recorded in one affected herd over a period of ten days and affected does died (Albert 1988).

Both acute and chronic forms of mastitis occur. There is udder swelling and clots in the milk in the acute form and there may be blood in the milk in the chronic form. Induration of the udder may persist for weeks after infection is cleared.

Clinical Pathology and Necropsy

Goats with enteritis may show a pronounced leukocytosis with neutrophilia and a marked left shift (Seimiya et al. 2005). There may also be laboratory evidence of hemoconcentration due to dehydration from diarrhea. The causative organism can be isolated from diarrheic feces, mastitic milk, and uterine discharges. Because the organism may be present in feces as a normal gut inhabitant, serotyping is necessary to confirm the isolate as a likely pathogen. Serologic testing can be used to support a diagnosis of yersiniosis. Goats with diarrhea caused by *Y. enterocolitica* may show marked increases in agglutination titers between sera taken at the time of diarrhea and two to three weeks later (Krogstad 1974).

At necropsy, goats with the enteric form of yersiniosis are thin and often emaciated. The large, multiple, internal abscesses (pseudotuberculosis) characteristic of the disease in laboratory animals are not reported in goats, though occasional, single, abscesses have yielded *Y. pseudotuberculosis.* The most consistent gross finding is enlargement and edema of the mesenteric lymph nodes. Gross lesions in the intestines may be limited to hyperemia or edema of the mucosa or a catarrhal enteritis, but careful inspection of the mucosal surface frequently reveals small focal areas of necrosis visible as small, whitish, circular lesions 1 to 2 mm in diameter. Histologically, there are microabscesses in the superficial mucosa or lamina propria of the intestine that contain colonies of Gram-negative bacteria surrounded by neutrophils (Vickers 1986). Gross thickening of the cecum and proximal colon and mucosal ulceration and fibrin plaque formation have also been observed in at least one goat with intestinal yersiniosis (Slee and Button 1990). Microabscesses in the small and large intestines are strongly suggestive of *Y. enterocolitica* infection (Slee and Button 1990a).

In the abortion form of the disease, the uterus may be hemorrhagic or filled with pus. Goats that die with the abortion form of the disease may also have swollen, edematous mesenteric lymph nodes. Splenomegaly, renal infarcts, and swelling of the intestinal mucosa with edema also have been noted. *Yersinia* organisms can be cultured from mesenteric nodes and uterine content.

Diagnosis

Because of the zoonotic potential of yersiniosis, definitive diagnosis by bacteriological or serologic methods should be attempted whenever human exposure is a concern. In the enteric form of the disease, all potential causes of diarrhea must be considered. In the age group most often affected, kids one and six months of age, coccidiosis and nematode parasitism are the most likely causes of diarrhea and must be ruled out. Salmonellosis and enterotoxemia are also likely to produce diarrhea in conjunction with sudden deaths. The differential diagnosis for abortion is discussed in Chapter 13, and for mastitis, in Chapter 14. Internal abscesses in goats are most likely caused by *Corynebacterium pseudotuberculosis*, but yersiniosis, tuberculosis, and melioidosis must also be considered as potential causes.

Treatment

Yersinia are generally susceptible to a wide range of broad-spectrum antibiotics. Most reports of successful treatment, however, have involved use of tetracyclines. Tetracycline was effective in halting outbreaks of both the enteric and abortion forms of the disease (Orr et al. 1987; Albert 1988;). Antibiotic therapy is most successful when initiated early in the course of disease. In severe diarrhea cases, supportive fluid therapy may improve outcome. Antibiotic sensitivities were conducted on the *Y. pseudotuberculosis* serotype III isolates associated with diarrhea in lactating goats in Japan. All were sensitive to enrofloxacin, ceftiofur, gentamicin, tetracycline, oxytetracycline, colisitin, and fosfomycin (Seimiya et al. 2005).

Control

Because the epidemiology of caprine yersiniosis is incompletely understood, control recommendations are largely empirical. In New Zealand, it is suggested that to minimize stress, hair goats normally sheared in winter be well fed before shearing and have good shelter available immediately afterwards. It is also recommended that newly captive feral goats not be sheared at all their first winter to avoid compounding their stress (Thompson 1985). Other general recommendations include avoidance of overcrowding and other stressors, provision of adequate nutrition and feeder space, separation of goats from swine, good nematode parasite control, and good rodent and bird control in intensive housing and feeding arrangements. Water supplies should be tested for the presence of pathogenic *Yersinia*. There are no commercial vaccines available for *Y. enterocolitica* or *Y. pseudotuberculosis* in livestock.

Paratuberculosis

Paratuberculosis, also known as Johne's disease, is an economically important infectious disease of domestic and wild ruminant animals primarily affecting the digestive tract. Infection leads to gradual debilitation and death through a mechanism of digestive dysfunction that is not completely understood.

Because the disease has been studied most intensively in cattle, many aspects of the bovine disease traditionally have been assumed to hold true for goats. However, this is not the case. Diarrhea, which is the cardinal sign in cattle, is an uncommon clinical sign in goats. Caprine paratuberculosis is characterized mainly by chronic, progressive weight loss in adults.

Etiology

Paratuberculosis is caused by the bacterium formerly known as *Mycobacterium paratuberculosis* (also previously called *M. johnei*). Based on advances in the molecular characterization of the organism that occurred in the 1990s, the organism has since been reclassified as a subspecies of *Mycobacterium avium* and is referred to as *M. avium* subsp. *paratuberculosis (Map)*. The characterization and molecular epidemiology of *Map* have been reviewed (Harris and Barletta 2001). Analysis of *Map* strains from different geographic locations and different host species using various molecular techniques indicates that there are two main groups of strains. The C, or cattle, strains occur mainly in cattle but are also the predominant strains in goats. The C strains also occur in deer and, rarely, sheep. The S, or sheep, strains occur mainly in sheep but also in farmed deer and sometimes goats. The presence of S strains in goats, though less frequent than the C strains, occurs mainly when goats are commingled with infected sheep. Restriction endonuclease analysis and DNA hybridization studies indicate that there may be a unique *Map* strain that is isolated from Norwegian goats that falls neither in the C nor S strain groups (Collins et al. 1990), but other studies could not distinguish Norwegian goat strains from cattle strains (Thoresen and Olsaker 1994). Previous experimental challenge studies indicated that the Norwegian goat strain has little or no pathogenicity for cattle (Saxegaard 1990). However, further evaluation of goat strain pathogenicity for cattle is ongoing, and there are indications that infection and shedding in cattle may in fact occur (Holstad et al. 2003).

Map is a small mycobacterium (0.5 × 1 microns) compared with other pathogenic mycobacteria. It demonstrates typical acid fastness with Ziehl-Neelsen stain. In tissues, the organism tends to be found in clumps inside macrophages rather than as individual bacteria. The bacterium is very resistant to environmental degradation and can persist in barnyards and in manure spread on pastures for longer than one year. Shade on pastures prolongs the survival time and there are indications that *Map* may be genetically capable of dormancy, i.e., being able to enter a viable but noncultivable state and later reverting to a vegetative form (Whittington et al. 2004). Disinfectants capable of eliminating the organism from the environment include cresylic compounds diluted 1:64 and sodium orthophenylphenate diluted 1:200.

The C strain of *Map* is a fastidious, slow-growing organism *in vitro*. Positive cultures are rarely identifiable before six weeks and should be held at least twelve weeks for confirmation of negative cultures. The cultivation of field isolates of *Map* requires supplementation of the culture media with mycobactin, an iron-chelating substance found in other *Mycobacterium* spp. Mycobactin dependence has long been considered a distinguishing culture characteristic of the paratuberculosis organism. However, it is now known that certain strains of *M. avium* subsp. *avium* and *M. avium* subsp. *sylvaticum* (formerly known as the wood pigeon mycobacterium) also demonstrate mycobactin dependence and may sometimes infect ruminants. These other mycobactin-dependent species can be distinguished from *Map* by molecular techniques based on the fact that *Map* contains multiple copies of the genetic insertional sequence IS900 while the other species contain the genetic insertional sequences IS901 (*M. avium* subsp. *avium*) or IS902 (*M. avium* subsp. *sylvaticum*).

Until recently, the S strains of *Map* could not be grown using the standard culture techniques successfully employed for cultivation of the C strains. Reliable growth is now possible by use of liquid modified BACTEC 12B medium. Solid media (modified Middlebrook 7H10 and 7H11 agars) can also support growth but may be less sensitive (Whittington et al. 1999).

The interspecies infectivity of *M. paratuberculosis* was established in 1913 when clinical paratuberculosis was produced in a goat with a bovine-derived inoculum (Twort and Ingram 1913). In general, when different ruminant species are managed together on a single farm premises and one species is infected, the risk of cross-infectivity is considerable. The development of paratuberculosis in feral goats in New Zealand after introduction into paddocks with known paratuberculous cattle has been documented (Ris et al. 1988).

Epidemiology

Paratuberculosis was first definitively described in cattle in 1895 (Johne and Frothingham 1895) and in goats in 1916 (McFadyean and Sheather 1916). It has traditionally been considered a disease of temperate regions with sporadic occurrence in tropical environments, primarily as a result of importation of infected livestock from endemic areas. Today, paratuberculosis is generally considered a disease of worldwide distribution. However, accurate details on the geographic distribution of caprine paratuberculosis are difficult to ascertain, because statistics on goat disease are often reported together with sheep by governments and international agencies.

Caprine paratuberculosis has been specifically described in numerous countries representing all continents but Antarctica. These countries include the Sudan (Chaudhari et al. 1964) in Africa; India (Rajan et al. 1976), Nepal (Singh et al. 2007), and Korea (Lee et al. 2006) in Asia; Turkey (Alibasoglu et al. 1973), and Israel (Shimshony and Bar Moshe 1972) in the Middle East; Cyprus (Polydorou 1984), France (Yalcin and Des Francs 1970), Greece (Xenos et al. 1984), Norway (Government of Norway 1985), Spain (Leon Vizcaino et al. 1984), and Switzerland (Tontis and König 1978) in Europe; Canada (Morin 1982; Moser 1982), the United States (West 1979; Sherman and Gezon, 1980; Ullrich et al. 1982), and Mexico (Ramirez et al. 1983; Estevez-Denaives et al. 2007) in North America; Chile (Kruze et al. 2007) in South America; and Australia (Lenghaus et al. 1977; Straube and McGregor 1982) and New Zealand (Thompson 1986).

The prevalence of caprine paratuberculosis is not well documented and presumably it may vary widely between countries because of local management conditions, infectivity of *Map*, and other factors. The prevalence is likely to be higher in intensively managed goats than in extensively managed goats. For example, in Norway, where goats are kept intensively for dairying and a goat-specific strain of the organism is recognized, nationwide prevalence was as high as 53% before the introduction of a vaccination program. In India, with generally smaller herds and more extensive management, a thirteen-year necropsy study indicated a prevalence of only 5.2% (Kumar et al. 1988).

A significant development in the epidemiology of paratuberculosis over the past twenty years has been the suggestion of a putative association between *Mycobacterium avium* subsp. *paratuberculosis* and Crohn's disease, a granulomatous enteritis of humans. Paratuberculosis was proposed as a possible model for the study of Crohn's disease in 1972 because of the clinical and histopathologic similarities of the two conditions, but at that time there was no suggestion that the *Map* organism itself might be involved in the pathogenesis of the human disease (Patterson and Allen 1972). However, in 1984 the *Map* organism was identified in tissues of four Crohn's disease patients (Chiodini et al. 1984), suggesting an etiologic role for the organism. This also suggested that paratuberculosis might be a zoonotic disease, potentially transferable by contact with infected livestock or by consumption of food products from those animals.

Since then considerable research has been carried out on the possible role of *Map* in the pathogenesis of Crohn's disease and that literature has been reviewed (Hermon-Taylor et al. 2000; National Research Council 2003). A body of research has also evolved relative to the potential for zoonotic transmission from infected animals, meat, milk, or milk products, and this also has been reviewed (Grant et al. 2001; Grant 2006). Concerns about the risk of dairy products were heightened when it was demonstrated in the UK that *Map* in milk can survive standard high temperature—short time pasteurization of 161.6°F (72°C) for fifteen seconds (Grant et al. 1999). This prompted regulators and processors to extend the pasteurization time to twenty-five seconds. Still, *Map* could be identified in containers of pasteurized milk offered for sale at the retail level (Grant et al. 2001; O'Reilly et al. 2004).

A comprehensive study by the National Research Council published in 2003 concluded that "there remains insufficient evidence to prove or disprove that *Mycobacterium avium* subsp. *paratuberculosis* is a cause of some or all cases of Crohn's disease in humans" (National Research Council 2003). However, it was also concluded that a causal link between paratuberculosis and Crohn's is plausible and a new research approach is needed to definitively establish or disprove that relationship. Nevertheless, there are members of the human medical community who believe quite strongly that sufficient evidence exists to make that link and they call for a strong and immediate public health response (Hermon-Taylor and Bull 2002). Others believe that the evidence for involvement of *Map* in Crohn's disease remains unconvincing (Eckburg and Relman 2007). In the meantime, public perceptions have spurred regulators and producers to take the control of paratuberculosis in cattle, sheep, and goats far more seriously than in decades past.

Pathogenesis

The primary mode of transmission of paratuberculosis is fecal-oral, with the organism shed in the manure of infected adults and ingested by susceptible young stock, particularly when animals are overcrowded and sanitation is poor. An age-related resistance to infection is well known to exist in cattle, and this appears to hold true for goats as well (Levi 1948). Neonates are considered most susceptible to new infections, particularly when their own dam is an active fecal shedder and the kid is allowed to remain with the doe. However, age-related resistance is not absolute, and it is probable that adult animals may remain at risk for new infection if kept in overcrowded, heavily contaminated environments.

In utero infection of the fetus is considered a less common form of transmission, but is documented in cattle (McQueen and Russell 1979) and sheep (Tamarin and Landau 1961). The role of *in utero* transmission in the goat remains unknown, although the organism has been recovered from the uterus and fetal organs of some experimentally infected goats (Goudswaard 1971). If fetal infections were shown to occur naturally in goats, then currently accepted disease control practices would require modification.

As with cattle and sheep, goats are most likely infected at an early age by ingestion of the organism.

Following ingestion, the organism localizes in the mucosa of the small intestine and associated lymph nodes. The organism is transported across the intestinal mucosa by M cells associated with the Peyer's patches or by enterocytes (Sigurdðardóttir et al. 2005). While some exposed individuals may develop resistance to chronic infection, many infected goats subsequently carry the infection in a dormant state in the Peyer's patches of the intestine and the mesenteric lymph nodes for a variable period into adulthood. At some point, triggered by stress or other ill-defined factors, some infected animals begin to shed the organism in the feces. They may begin to show clinical signs concurrently or at a later time. These signs include diarrhea and weight loss in cattle, and progressive weight loss without diarrhea in sheep and goats.

It is not known why diarrhea is the distinguishing characteristic in bovine paratuberculosis but an infrequent finding in the caprine and ovine forms of the disease. Because small ruminants normally produce a drier feces than the cow, it may require a more severe derangement of colonic water resorption capacity in the goat or sheep to produce evidence of clinical diarrhea than in the cow.

In general, small ruminants with paratuberculosis tend to have less severe lesions of granulomatous enteritis than affected cattle. There have been a number of recent studies of experimental paratuberculosis infection in goats aimed at gaining a better understanding of the pathogenesis of the disease at a cellular level and the associated cell mediated and humoral immune responses (Storset et al. 2001; Valheim et al. 2002, 2004; Sigurdðardóttir et al. 2005; Munjal et al. 2005; Stewart et al. 2006). A standard experimental challenge model for caprine paratuberculosis has been proposed (Hines et al. 2007).

There is experimental evidence that bacteremia occurs in goats with clinical paratuberculosis based on isolation of the organism in blood cultures and numerous tissues at necropsy, including the udder and uterus (Goudswaard 1971). This suggests that offspring born to clinically infected does have a very high likelihood of infection through the birth process or when suckling, if not already infected as fetuses.

Because of the prolonged dormancy of infection, the persistence of the organism in the environment, and the endemic nature of the disease, all goats in a known-infected herd must be considered at risk of infection. Goats in an infected herd may fall into one of four categories: resistant or non-infected individuals; infected, non-shedders; subclinically infected, inapparent-shedders; and clinically affected, apparent-shedders. Only individuals in the last group can be identified as abnormal on physical examination, although a definitive diagnosis can never be made on physical examination alone. The subclinical infection rate in an infected herd is likely to be much higher than the rate of clinically apparent cases.

Clinical Findings

Overt clinical disease rarely occurs before one year of age and is most common in goats two and three years of age. Clinical disease is often triggered by some episode of stress, such as parturition or recent introduction into a new herd. Affected individuals begin a course of progressive weight loss, which may extend from weeks to months and can lead to dramatic emaciation (Figure 10.6). Appetite may remain intact initially, but decrease later on, and the animal becomes increasingly lethargic and depressed. A rough hair coat and flaky skin are common. Animals in the advanced state of disease may become immunologically anergic. Advanced cases eventually succumb to debilitation, inanition, exposure, or secondary infections.

Unlike cattle, goats rarely show persistent watery diarrhea, except possibly in the terminal stages of disease. When it occurs, diarrhea may actually be due to concurrent parasitism, although sometimes it may be directly because of paratuberculosis. Soft stool, like dog feces in appearance, may occur intermittently through the course of disease, but normal pelleted feces are the rule.

As the disease progresses a moderate anemia of chronic infection may develop and clinical evidence of hypoalbuminemia such as intermandibular edema may be seen. The nonspecific nature of these clinical signs makes a definitive diagnosis of paratuberculosis by clinical examination impossible.

Clinical Pathology and Necropsy

Anemia and hypoalbuminemia are likely to be present in advanced clinical cases, but are not specific for paratuberculosis. Hypergammaglobulinemia and hypocalcemia have also been reported in affected goats (Schroeder et al. 2001). Definitive diagnosis of paratuberculosis requires bacteriologic or serologic testing and/or histopathologic examination of tissues.

Infection with paratuberculosis slowly evolves in such a way that no single diagnostic test can possibly detect all infected animals at any given time in the course of the disease. The earliest detectable reactions to develop involve the cell mediated immune (CMI) response. Humoral immune response, with the production of circulating antibodies, occurs after the CMI response, later in the course of subclinical infection. The detection of infection by culture of organisms from the feces can only occur in animals that are actively shedding the bacteria. This usually occurs after or concurrent with the development of the antibody response, though some subclinically infected animals with a detectable antibody response may remain non-shedders for a significant period of their infection. One

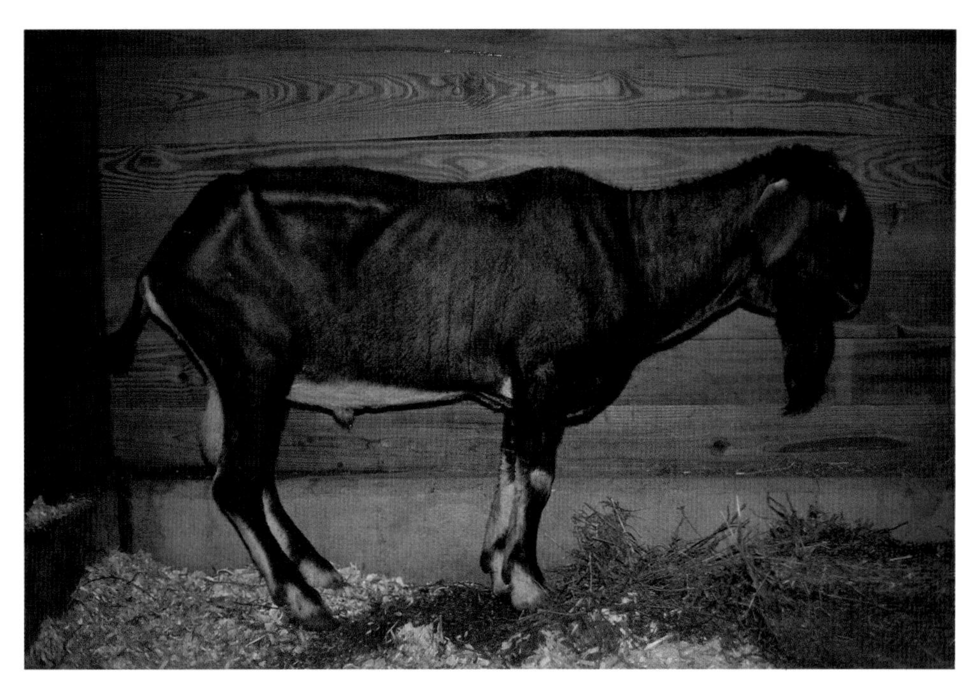

Figure 10.6. Adult Nubian buck with advanced clinical paratuberculosis. Note severe emaciation. (Courtesy of Dr. David M. Sherman.)

recent experimental study illustrates the progression of the goat host response to *Map* infection. The CMI response, as measured by the lymphocyte proliferation test, was detectable at sixty days post infection (dpi); fecal shedding of *Map* began between 150 and 180 dpi; and antibody response, measured by ELISA and AGID, became detectable at 180 dpi (Munjal et al. 2005).

During clinical disease, tests of cell mediated and humoral immunity as well as fecal culture can be employed for diagnosis but in the advanced stages of clinical disease, anergy may occur in some individuals and cell mediated and humoral immune responses may be lost, yielding false-negative results. Furthermore, even when tests are applied at the appropriate times, there is no single bacteriological or serologic test with sufficient sensitivity to identify all clinical and subclinical cases of caprine paratuberculosis or with sufficient specificity to avoid some false-positive results. For these reasons, more than one type of test needs to be applied for implementation of herd control programs that are based on testing and culling of infected animals.

Traditionally, the CMI response has been assessed by *in vivo* intradermal skin test using johnin purified protein derivative (PPD-J) or the intravenous johnin test. These *in vivo* assays have largely been replaced by newer techniques involving the identification of cytokines released by immune cells, such as the production of gamma interferon (IFNγ) produced *in vitro* by stimulation of peripheral blood mononuclear cells with mycobacterial antigens, and then measured using a sandwich enzyme immunoassay (Rothel et al. 1990). The IFNγ assay was used to monitor the progression of paratuberculosis in a naturally infected herd of pygmy goats along with fecal culture, ELISA, and AGID. The IFNγ assay produced both false positive (one of three) and false negative (three of ten) results in live animals based on the true infection status determined subsequently by necropsy and culture of *Map* from tissues (Manning et al. 2003). In experimentally challenged goats, CMI was measured by IFNγ assay, but also by interleukin 2 receptor expression and by lymphocyte proliferation test (Storset et al. 2001). CMI responses were detectable by nine weeks post inoculation and persisted with variation through the two years of the study, though responses were stronger in the first year.

The tests currently in use for identification of antibody responses in goats are the complement fixation (CF) test, the agar gel immunodiffusion (AGID) test, and the ELISA test. In general, when applied to goats, these tests have a sensitivity in the range of 85% to 100% when applied to clinical cases but only 20% to 50% when applied to subclinical cases (Stehman 2000).

The CF test is probably the least commonly employed but remains in use because a number of countries require a negative CF test for importation of ruminant livestock. One problem with the CF test is that anticomplementary activity with goat serum may confound interpretation of the test, yielding neither clear positive nor negative results (Stehman 1996).

Specificity may also be reduced in the CF test due to cross reactions with other mycobacteria or *Corynebacterium pseudotuberculosis* as discussed further below in relation to the ELISA test.

The AGID test is very effective in confirming suspect clinical cases of caprine Johne's disease, with a sensitivity of 86% or greater, and it provides results within twenty-four to forty-eight hours. It can also identify subclinical shedders with moderate reliability, but sensitivity falls dramatically when the test is applied to subclinically infected non-shedders. Agar gel immunodiffusion tests performed as well as fecal culture when both tests were used for several years in a large, naturally infected goat herd (Sherman and Gezon 1980). Precipitating antibody was detectable in infected goats at approximately the same time that the animals began to shed the organism in their feces. Similar results were reported independently in a large goat herd studied for three years in England, where fecal culture and the AGID test proved more useful than intradermal and complement fixation tests for detecting infected individuals (Thomas 1983). Nevertheless, false-negative AGID test results do occur in subclinically infected goats and a single negative test should not be presumed to indicate non-infected status (Ramirez Casillas et al. 1984).

The application of ELISA tests for the diagnosis of paratuberculosis emerged in the 1990s and since then a number of studies have reported its use specifically in goats (Milner et al. 1989; Molina et al. 1991; Molina Caballero et al. 1993; Burnside and Rowley 1994; Rajukumar et al. 2001; Whittington et al. 2003; Dimareli-Malli et al. 2004; Munjal et al. 2004; Gumber et al. 2006). Differences in performance are noted, often as a result of the type of antigens that are employed in the assay. In general, these ELISA tests have sensitivity in the range of 54% to 88%; they are more reliable for confirmation of clinical cases than detection of subclinical cases. In experimentally infected goats, enzyme-linked immunosorbent assay and agar gel immunodiffusion test were found to be 100% sensitive from 180 and 210 dpi onward, respectively (Munjal et al. 2005).

The specificity of ELISA tests may suffer because of the occurrence of cross reactions. *Map* is known to share common antigens with other *Mycobacterium* spp., *Nocardia* spp., and *Corynebacterium* spp. Corynebacterial infections may produce cross reactivity in serologic tests used to diagnose *Map* infection (Ridell 1977). This is of particular concern in goats because caseous lymphadenitis caused by *C. pseudotuberculosis* is a common disease in the species. The problem of cross reaction occurs mainly with ELISA and CF tests, while the AGID test is not influenced by antibodies to *C. pseudotuberculosis* (Van Metre et al. 2000). In one study comparing specificity of two paratuberculosis ELISA kits and the AGID test, 344 goats with known exposure to *C. pseudotuberculosis* but with negative fecal cultures for *Map* were tested. The AGID gave no false-positive results. One ELISA kit gave five false-positive results (1.5%), while the second kit gave eighty-nine false positive results (25.9%)(Manning et al. 2007). Clearly, if the infection status of a herd is not known relative to paratuberculosis and caseous lymphadenitis, the ELISA test would not be a wise choice for screening the herd to determine the prevalence of paratuberculosis.

Commercial test kits for performance of the ELISA are available. Until recently, the kits available in the United States were approved only for use in cattle to test serum and plasma. In Europe, and more recently in the United States, an ELISA (Paracheck®) is marketed that is approved for serologic diagnosis of paratuberculosis from cattle, sheep, and goat serum or plasma as well as from bovine milk. The comparative performance of a commercial ELISA has recently has been evaluated for goat milk and serum from the same animals. Sensitivity of the milk ELISA was lower than for the serum ELISA, but the specificity was higher than that of the serum ELISA (Salgado et al. 2005, 2007).

There have been some notable advancements in techniques for identification of the organism in the feces or tissues of infected animals. Conventional fecal cultures on solid media grow slowly. Positive cultures can take six weeks or more to develop and culture tubes have to be held for a minimum of twelve weeks to ensure that they are negative. The use of liquid media has allowed for faster cultivation. Radiometric techniques for culture of mycobacteria on liquid media have been adapted for growth of *Map* and provide more rapid results with equal or greater sensitivity than conventional culture on solid media (Collins et al. 1990a; Sockett et al. 1992; Eamens et al. 2000). The use of radiometric liquid medium has also enabled laboratories to culture the S strain of *Map* from sheep (Whittington et al. 1999). Because goats can be infected with either the C or S strain of *Map*, use of radiometric culture should be considered, especially when there is clinical or serologic evidence of paratuberculosis, and fecal cultures on conventional solid media are negative.

Molecular probes and PCR techniques have also been developed to confirm the presence of *Map*-specific genetic material in feces or tissue samples, in an effort to bypass the need for culture. However, inhibitors in feces and inefficient DNA release from clinical samples have hampered the general application of these techniques, particularly with regard to fecal samples.

Most laboratories with the capacity to culture *Map* still offer the conventional solid media technique as the main or sole method for detection of *Map* in feces. Radiometric culture is increasingly available but can be more expensive. Expense is an issue in herd-wide testing for paratuberculosis and may be an obstacle in getting herd owners to undertake testing either to establish herd prevalence or to follow through with test and cull programs for control. One approach to reducing costs has been the use of pooled fecal cultures to determine a herd's infection status. This is done by combining samples from groups of animals of the same age for testing. The sensitivity of this method depends on the prevalence of infection in the herd and the intensity of shedding among herd members. There is one report from Australia on the use of pooled samples for culture of *Map* in goats. Based on the conditions prevailing in that study, pools of twenty-five samples were considered to be suitable for producing meaningful test results (Eamens et al. 2007).

Because clinical caprine paratuberculosis is invariably a terminal disease, necropsy provides the opportunity for definitive diagnosis. Gross lesions are more variable in occurrence in the goat as compared with cattle. Therefore, histologic examination of tissues and bacterial culture of selected organs also should be performed.

The gross and microscopic lesions of caprine paratuberculosis are well described (Levi 1948; Harding 1957; Nakamatsu et al. 1968; Fodstad and Gunnarsson 1979). The prominent, accordion-like, corrugated thickening of the intestinal wall and mucosa commonly seen in cattle is not often observed in goats. When gross lesions are present in small ruminants, they usually present as focal or diffuse thickening or edema of the ileum, cecum, or spiral colon. Adjacent lymph nodes may be enlarged and edematous, and caseation of nodes with focal calcification occurs more often in goats than cattle. Emaciation is a constant finding, although persistence of abundant mesenteric fat deposits is not unusual in goats, even when the general body condition is one of emaciation. Calcification of the aorta often occurs in goats with prolonged paratuberculosis, though the pathogenesis is unknown.

Histologically, paratuberculosis produces characteristic granulomatous lesions in the intestinal tract, lymph nodes, and possibly liver. At a minimum, tissues submitted for microscopic examination should include a section of the ileocecal junction and adjacent ileocecal lymph node, ileum, spiral colon, and another mesenteric node. Where available, PCR can be applied to paraffin embedded tissues to detect the IS900 insertional sequence characteristic of *Map*. Otherwise, acid-fast Ziehl-Neelsen or immunohistochemical staining should be requested on these samples when paratuberculosis is suspected. Bacterial culture of fresh or frozen tissues is also possible. In areas where both tuberculosis and paratuberculosis occur in goats, microbiological diagnosis is imperative because necropsy lesions may be similar.

Diagnosis

The differential diagnosis of paratuberculosis in goats is essentially the differential diagnosis of chronic weight loss. The causes of this common presenting sign in goats are covered in detail in Chapter 15.

Treatment

There are no known effective treatments for the elimination of *Map* infection and none are specifically approved for the treatment of paratuberculosis. Various antimycobacterial drugs have been used with limited effect in goats. Attempted unsuccessful therapies have included isoniazid, isoniazid plus rifampin, isoniazid plus ethambutol, or all three drugs together (Gezon et al. 1988). However, some treatment regimens have alleviated clinical signs in individual cases as long as therapy is continued. Nevertheless, the organism can still be isolated from cultures prepared from tissues at necropsy. One such regimen is daily streptomycin sulfate (0.5 g intramuscularly) plus isoniazid (25 mg by mouth) plus sodium aminosalicylate (850 mg by mouth) for six months (Zahinuddin and Sinha 1984). A second regimen is daily dihydrostreptomycin (0.5 g intramuscularly) plus rifampin (300 mg by mouth) and isoniazid (300 mg by mouth) twice daily (Slocombe 1982). Long-term administration of monensin has been reported to have some therapeutic effect in cattle, reducing the severity of paratuberculous lesions in the digestive tract (Brumbaugh et al. 2000) and reducing fecal shedding of *Map* in calves (Whitlock et al. 2005), but no trials in goats have been reported. Treatment has little economic application in goats except for the possibility of keeping known infected, high-quality, breeding does in good health long enough to achieve embryo transfers or to prolong the life of pet goats. However, in light of the putative connection between paratuberculosis and Crohn's disease, owners of pet goats should be made aware of that link before deciding to treat and maintain a known infected goat as a pet.

Control

Interest in the control of paratuberculosis has increased in recent years, mainly for two reasons. The first is increased understanding of the economic losses associated with the disease, particularly in dairy herds. In dairy cattle, losses are associated with decreased milk production, decreased milk fat and protein, premature culling, reduced slaughter weight at culling, decreased fertility, reduced feed efficiency, and increased incidence of mastitis (Radostits et al. 2007). Losses have been estimated to be as high as $200/cow/year in high prevalence herds. While similar types of loss could be expected in goat dairies, no specific findings on the economic impact have been reported.

The second major stimulus for control of paratuberculosis is the much publicized zoonotic potential of the disease relative to Crohn's disease in humans, which has caused concern among public health officials, regulatory veterinary agencies, and livestock producers about public perception of milk and meat as wholesome foods. As a result, numerous countries have initiated or expanded their paratuberculosis control programs in recent years. Most programs focus on cattle, but some may include sheep and goats. Readers should contact their own regulatory veterinary authorities to determine the status of goats in existing paratuberculosis control programs. In the United States, for example, there is now a national Voluntary Bovine Johne's Disease Control Program that focuses on control of the disease in cattle. Johne's programs for sheep and goats are administered through the individual states rather than at the national level. In 2006, six states responded to a survey indicating that they have some activity, albeit limited in some cases, related to control of goat paratuberculosis. The states were Illinois, Nebraska, New York, Ohio, Wisconsin, and Wyoming.

Paratuberculosis is almost always a herd problem rather than an individual animal problem, unless the individual goat diagnosed with paratuberculosis was recently introduced into the herd. When a clinical case is diagnosed from within a long established herd, the herd almost inevitably includes additional subclinical shedders and infected, non-shedding goats. These subclinical infections are likely to be present in far greater numbers than the clinical cases, often in the range of one to five subclinical cases for each clinical case, depending on herd size, how long the herd has been in existence, and various management factors that affect the level of bacterial contamination on the farm.

There are three basic elements to consider in developing a strategy for eliminating paratuberculosis from infected herds: identifying and removing infected individuals from the herd; reducing the rate of new infections in susceptible kids through improved sanitation and modified kid-rearing techniques; and vaccinating to increase host resistance to new infections. It is unlikely that any one of these components of the control program taken alone will effectively eliminate paratuberculosis, but the emphasis on each component in the overall control program will vary with local conditions. On the national level, paratuberculosis has been controlled in Norway largely through vaccination (Saxegaard and Fodstad 1985). At the local level, elimination of paratuberculosis in a large commercial herd in the United States was achieved without vaccination by testing and culling in conjunction with altering management procedures (Gezon et al. 1988). In another dairy goat herd, infection in adult goats was significantly reduced over a two-year period by serological testing with ELISA and AGID, culling of positive animals, and improving herd management practices (Hutchinson et al. 2004).

The best techniques currently available for identifying infected goats are the bacterial culture of feces and the AGID or ELISA tests. Because these tests do not reliably identify all infected non-shedders, testing must be carried out at frequent intervals to assure that infected non-shedders are rapidly identified as they convert to subclinical, inapparent-shedder status. Testing at intervals of at most six months is recommended. In aggressive eradication programs, all offspring of positive test animals are culled in addition to the positive animal itself. This reflects the belief that kids of infected dams are also very likely to be infected.

Improved management and sanitation help reduce the incidence of new infections in young stock. In intensive dairy operations, kidding pens should be cleaned or rebedded between kiddings. Kids should be taken immediately from the does and raised in separate facilities on heat-treated colostrum and pasteurized milk or milk replacer. Kids should not commingle again with adult animals until they themselves have kidded. Adult animals should not be overcrowded, manure should be removed frequently from the pens, and feed and water should be provided in a manner that does not allow for fecal contamination. If manure is spread on pastures, goats should not be allowed to graze those pastures for at least one year. The use of pastures in general may be problematic as it has become clear that wildlife reservoirs exist for *Map* which may contaminate pastures, even when paratuberculous livestock have been kept off those pastures. An association between *Map*-infected wild rabbits on farms in Scotland and paratuberculosis in cattle on those farms has been reported (Greig et al. 1999). Wild ruminants are often seen in pastures in North America, and *Map* has been isolated from a number of species, including whitetail deer, mule deer, bison, and elk (Harris and Barletta 2001).

Management recommendations for extensively managed goat herds are more difficult to make. At the least, does should be turned out on clean, uncontaminated pastures before kidding so they can spread out to kid and minimize cross contamination. Herd-wide testing by culture of feces or AGID tests to identify infected dams should be performed before the

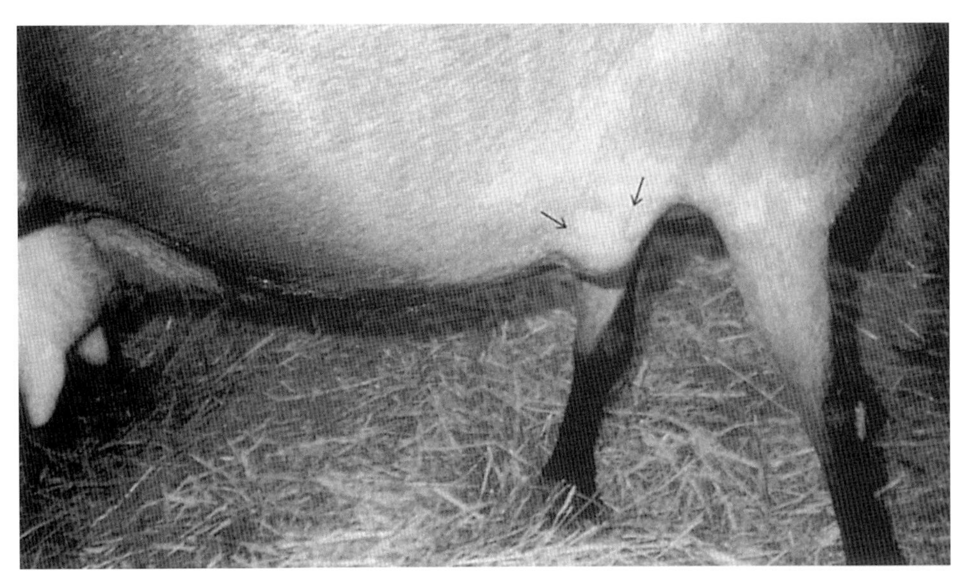

Figure 10.7. Persistent granulomatous reaction (arrows) at site of vaccination for paratuberculosis with live vaccine. (Courtesy of Dr. David M. Sherman.)

kidding season begins. Infected dams should either be culled or segregated from the non-infected animals before kidding.

Vaccination of goats for paratuberculosis in Norway has been extremely effective in reducing the national prevalence of caprine paratuberculosis (Saxegaard and Fodstad 1985). The vaccine employed is a live, attenuated, adjuvanted vaccine containing two strains of *Map* and is given to goat kids between two and four weeks of age. Post mortem evaluation of vaccinated and unvaccinated goats over a fifteen-year period indicated that the infection prevalence was reduced from 53% in 1966 to 1% in 1982, primarily through the use of vaccination. The majority of infected goats identified in 1982 were not vaccinated. Because caprine paratuberculosis in Norway may involve a unique caprine-specific strain of *Map*, this success with vaccination may not be transferable to all situations worldwide.

Currently, data on extensive field experience from other nations is lacking. More recently, it was reported that a killed vaccine administered to adult goats in a known infected herd was very useful in the control of paratuberculosis. Half the goats were vaccinated and the other half left unvaccinated and all goats culled for any cause were necropsied to determine the presence of paratuberculosis. By the end of two years, three times as many goats had been culled from the unvaccinated group as the vaccinated group, and three times as many of the cases culled in the unvaccinated group were cases of paratuberculosis (Corpa et al. 2000). This killed vaccine is now registered in or available for use by special permit in Australia, Cyprus, Germany, Greece, India, the Netherlands, New Zealand, Norway, Spain, South Africa, the United Arab Emirates, and the UK (Colmeiro, 2008).

Two potential drawbacks to the use of all vaccines containing *Map* are the appearance of a granulomatous nodule at the site of vaccination (Figure 10.7) and the fact that animals vaccinated against *Map* may develop cross-reactivity to standard tuberculosis tests, thus complicating the testing procedures for regulatory programs designed to control tuberculosis. Implementation of paratuberculosis vaccination, then, may be restricted by regulatory agencies in countries where tuberculosis is monitored or still endemic. Under the new Voluntary Bovine Johne's Disease Control Program in the United States, some vaccination may be permitted with regulatory approval and supervision in herds actively involved in Johne's control that have been shown to be free of tuberculosis. Vaccination is limited to cattle and not all states allow vaccination. An additional caution involves accidental injection of live vaccines into the vaccinator. A serious, persistent granuloma can result at the accidental injection site in people.

PROTOZOAL DISEASES

Coccidiosis

Coccidiosis is the most likely cause of diarrhea in young goats between three weeks and five months of age, particularly when young goats are group-housed in confinement.

Etiology

Coccidiosis is caused by protozoal parasites of the genus *Eimeria*. In the past, the *Eimeria* species infecting goats and sheep were presumed to be the same. In 1979, however, well-controlled experiments using *E. ninakohlyakimovae* and *E. christenseni* demonstrated that each small ruminant host has its own host specific *Eimeria* species that are not readily cross-infective (McDougald 1979). This led to a reexamination of *Eimeria* morphology and a renaming of species thought to be cross-infective. The current nomenclature for the recognized *Eimeria* of goats is given in Table 10.6, with information on comparable sheep species, oocyst morphology, pathogenicity, geographic distribution, and prevalence in goats (Norton 1986; Soe and Pomroy 1992).

Historically, the *Eimeria* have been classified based on phenotypic characteristics such as morphology, ultrastructure, life cycles, and host specificity. However, more recent molecular phylogenetic studies of *Eimeria* spp. have called into question the accuracy of some of these classifications. Readers should be aware that as a result, names of *Eimeria* spp. affecting goats may be subject to change (Tenter et al. 2002). Furthermore, additional new species of *Eimeria* are being identified in goats such as *E. minasensis* reported from Brazil (Silva and Lima 1998) and *E. sundarbanensis* reported from India (Bandyopadhyay 2004).

The typical life cycle of the various *Eimeria* spp. is as follows. Oocysts passed in the feces sporulate in the goats' environment to produce infective sporocysts containing sporozoites. These sporocysts are ingested

Table 10.6. The *Eimeria* species infecting goats (*Capra hircus*).

Current name	*Comparable Eimeria species in sheep*	*Morphologic characteristics of oocysts (length × width in µm)*	*Prepatent period (days)*	*Pathogenicity*	*Distribution; occurrence*
E. alijevi	*E. parva*	Spherical to subspherical; 16 × 14 µm; no micropyle, no cap; yellow to yellow-green wall	16–17	Mild	Worldwide; very common
E. apsheronica	*E. faurei*	Ovoid; 29 × 21 µm; distinct micropyle, no cap; brownish yellow to pink wall	20	Mild	Worldwide; very common
E. arloingi	*E. bakuensis (E. ovina)*	Ellipsoidal to ovoid; 27 × 18 µm; distinct micropyle and cap	?	moderate to severe	Worldwide; most common
E. capralis	Unknown	Ellipsoidal; 29 × 20 µm micropyle and cap; smooth wall	?	?	New Zealand only
E. caprina	None	Ellipsoidal; 32 × 23 µm; distinct micropyle, no cap; yellow brown outer wall, inner wall clear	?	Moderate to severe	Known in US, UK, Brazil; common
E. caprovina	Same species infects sheep	Ellipsoidal to ovoid; 30 × 24 µm; distinct micropyle, no cap; yellow-brown inner wall, outer wall clear	14–20	Moderate	Known in US, UK; uncommon
E. charlestoni	Unknown	Ellipsoidal; 23 × 17 µm; indistinct micropyle; no cap	?	?	New Zealand only
E. christenseni	*E. ahsata*	Ovoid; 38 × 25 µm; distinct micropyle, dome-shaped cap	17	Moderate to severe	Worldwide; very common

Table 10.6. *Continued*

Current name	*Comparable Eimeria species in sheep*	*Morphologic characteristics of oocysts (length × width in μm)*	*Prepatent period (days)*	*Pathogenicity*	*Distribution; occurrence*
E. hirci	*E. crandallis*	Spherical to ellipsoidal; 23 × 19 μm; flat, saucer-shaped micropylar cap	?	Nonpathogenic	Worldwide likely; common
E. jolchijevi	*E. granulosa*	Ellipsoidal to urn-shaped; 29 × 21 μm; distinct micropyle and cap; brownish-yellow wall	?	?	Known in US, UK, Australia; uncommon
E. kocharli	*E. intricata*	Ellipsoidal; 47 × 32 μm; distinct micropyle and light-colored cap; very thick wall	20–27	Mild	Known in India, Africa, Russia; uncommon
E. marisca	Same species may also occur in sheep	Ellipsoidal; 19 × 13 μm; faint micropyle, shallow, domed cap; polar granule, colorless to pale yellow	14–16	Mild	Reported in Spain only
E. masseyensis	Unknown	Ellipsoidal to ovoid; 22 × 17 μm; micropyle and cap	?	?	New Zealand only
E. minasensis	Unknown	Ellipsoidal; 35 × 24.5 μm; micropyle and cap; two-layered wall; inner brown, outer colorless	19–20	?	Recently reported from Brazil
E. ninakohlyakimovae	*E. ovinoidalis*	Ellipsoidal to ovoid; 23 × 18 μm; no micropyle or cap; faint brownish-yellow wall	15–17	Most severe	Worldwide; very common
E. pallida	Same species may also occur in sheep	Ellipsoidal; 14 × 10 μm; micropyle indistinct, no cap; yellowish green wall	?	Nonpathogenic	Known in U.S., Turkey, India, Sri Lanka; uncommon
E. punctata	Questionable status in sheep and goats	Subspherical to spherical, 21 × 17 μm; micropyle and small cap; obvious pitting in wall and greenish tint	?	Nonpathogenic	Reported in Germany and Zimbabwe
E. sundarbanensis	Unknown	Pyriform, 28 × 20 μm, micropyle and cap; yellowish, two-layered wall	?	?	Newly reported from India

by other goats. Ingested sporocysts release their sporozoites which then enter host cells to form schizonts. Schizonts undergo asexual reproduction to produce a first generation of daughter merozoites. Depending on the species of *Eimeria*, anywhere from a few dozen to one hundred thousand merozoites may be formed by each schizont. The merozoites then break from the disrupted host cell and each is capable of invading a new host cell to form a second generation of schizonts. The number of cycles of schizogony varies among *Eimeria* spp. The final cycle of schizogony leads to the differentiation of merozoites into male and female gametes. Male gametes (microgametes) then are released from host cells to fertilize female gametes (macrogametes) within their host cells. Zygote formation results in oocyst formation with release of oocysts from disrupted host cells and subsequent passage in the feces.

Epidemiology

Eimeria spp. have been isolated from goats on all continents. Prevalence studies throughout the world demonstrate that *Eimeria* oocysts are widely present in the feces of both normal and diseased goats, with a reported range of 38% to 100% of all goats infected (Lima 1980). Concurrent infection with multiple *Eimeria* spp. is the rule. For example, in a survey from Iran of 150 goats, 110 animals were infected with at least one species, but ninety-three of these (84.5%) were infected with multiple species (Razavi and Hassanvand 2007). Similarly, in Zimbabwe, in a survey involving more than 1,000 goats, 89.9% of adults and 94% of kids were found to be infected. All had multiple infections, with the number of species ranging from two to eleven. Just over 75% were infected with six to eight different *Eimeria* spp. (Chhabra and Pandey 1991). It is reasonable to assume that where there are goats, there are coccidia; however, it is important to discriminate between infection with coccidia and disease caused by coccidiosis.

All ages of goats may be infected with *Eimeria*, but numerous factors contribute to the highest incidence of clinical disease occurring in young goats between three weeks and five months of age. These include host, parasite, management, and environmental factors.

Host Factors. Age-related resistance to clinical coccidiosis is reported in all ruminant species. The resistance is immunologic in nature and is maintained by continuous exposure to coccidial infection. Immunity is relative and not absolute because it does not eliminate infection, but effectively checks the rate of coccidial reproduction in the host intestinal tract. This is reflected in a good correlation of oocysts shed in feces with age of infected goats. There is a steady decline in oocyst numbers from six months through six years of age, followed by an increase in goats seven years and older as immunity begins to wane in older goats (Kanyari 1988).

Complete elimination of coccidial infection may lead to a failure of immunity and the development of clinical disease on reexposure to pathogenic *Eimeria*. The immunity that develops is specific for a given *Eimeria* species and animals of any age may develop clinical disease if exposed to a population of *Eimeria* spp. not previously encountered. In most management situations, goats become resistant to clinical disease at approximately five months of age. Resistance may be impaired, however, by stresses such as concurrent illness, lactation, transport, feed changes, weather changes, increased levels of exposure, or exposure to new species of *Eimeria*. Therefore, sporadic outbreaks of clinical coccidiosis may occur in a variety of unexpected settings besides the predictable occurrence in confined weanlings. Breed variation may exist in resistance to coccidia. In Australia, Angora goats and feral goats are considered more susceptible to clinical coccidiosis than dairy breeds (Howe 1984). However, a study of fecal oocyst counts in three Australian breeds showed approximately equal counts for Angoras and Anglo-Nubians, and significantly lower counts for Saanens (Kanyari 1988).

Parasite Factors. Oocysts are quite resistant to environmental degradation, and are even more resistant when sporulation occurs. Overwintering of sporocysts is not uncommon, and many disinfectants, including 5% formalin, do not destroy them. Sporulation depends on a combination of oxygen availability, temperature, and moisture conditions. In general, with adequate moisture and oxygen, sporulation of oocysts occurs optimally within two to five days at temperatures between 75°F and 90°F (24°C to 32°C) and readily at temperatures down to 53.6°F (12°C). Synchronous sporulation can occur among oocysts accumulating in a contaminated environment when optimal conditions prevail. This means that susceptible goats may be challenged by massive numbers of infective sporocysts under appropriate conditions of warmth and humidity.

Some of the more pathogenic *Eimeria* spp. such as *E. ninakohlyakimovae* produce thousands of merozoites per schizont during asexual reproduction inside the goat intestine. The various species may also differ in the number of cycles of schizogony involved in reproduction. The more merozoites produced, the more intestinal epithelial cells are disrupted because every merozoite potentially can invade a target host cell. Prepatent periods also vary among goat *Eimeria* spp., and oocysts may be shed by kids as young as two weeks of age when kids are exposed to sporocysts at birth. This means that abdominal pain or diarrhea caused by coccidiosis may occur as early as one week of age, although this is not common.

Management and Environmental Factors. Clinical coccidiosis occurs more often in intensive management situations than in extensive ones because of the concentrating effects of confinement on both host and parasite. Dairy goat kids are commonly at risk when removed from their does at an early age and confined to group pens indoors. Most outbreaks of clinical coccidiosis occur around the time of weaning, particularly if kids are weaned abruptly and not offered solid feed *ad libitum* before termination of milk feeding.

Several factors may increase exposure to infective sporocysts at this time. Feeding young goats on the ground promotes ingestion of sporocysts. Poorly designed feeders in which goats can stand, climb, or defecate lead to contamination of feed and water sources. Watering systems that leak or overflow readily contribute to environmental moisture, which promotes sporulation. Overcrowding of pens or failure to segregate kids by age augments exposure to sporocysts and increases disease risk. When goats are kept on solid floors, the failure to maintain clean, dry bedding is a major factor in outbreaks of clinical disease. Even when floors are scraped clean, well-intentioned spraying or hosing of the pens may actually aggravate the problem because of the amount of moisture added to the atmosphere. If troughs and waterers are situated or hung so that they impede floor scraping, foci of heavy oocyst/sporocyst concentration may persist under or around them between cleanings.

Buildings that do not admit adequate sunlight also contribute to the persistence of oocysts, particularly in the winter months in temperate regions when days are short. Hot, humid weather is particularly conducive to sporocyst development and outbreaks of clinical coccidiosis are common in temperate regions during summer, especially because spring-born kids are being weaned during the hot, humid months.

Even when goats are managed extensively and the risk of coccidiosis is ostensibly less, it is important to scrutinize management practices for evidence of temporary mobbing that can predispose to outbreaks of coccidiosis. For example, Angora goats in Texas are managed extensively on range but coccidiosis can be a major problem in weaned kids. Kids are removed from dams, placed on solid feed for the first time, and housed in large pens. Despite the spaciousness of the pens, the stressed kids flock together in one area, leading to excessive buildup of oocysts and outbreaks of coccidiosis with mortality rates as high as 15% (Craig 1986). Outbreaks in adult Angoras are also seen when inclement weather occurs after shearing, and shorn goats are confined for two weeks to prevent losses due to hypothermia. In South Africa, the incidence of clinical coccidiosis is aggravated by drought when great numbers of grazing animals are transferred to small irrigated pastures or congregate to consume supplemental feed and water provided for them (van Tonder 1975).

In general, most exposures to coccidia cause subclinical infection and the acquisition of a protective though relative immunity. Most clinically affected individuals recover from clinical disease after a period of diarrhea as long as two weeks, and mortality rates do not usually exceed 10% when exposure to sporocysts has been gradual and continual before disease. When exposure to coccidial sporocysts is abrupt and intense, however, mortality rates in young goats can reach 50%. While the costs of treatment and death loss can be high, the major economic impact of coccidiosis in production animals may be reduced growth rates and weight gains after clinical or subclinical infection. In dairy goats, coccidiosis in weanlings can inhibit growth sufficiently so that spring-born kids will not reach breeding size by the fall of the same year and must be held over an additional year. It has been reported that the oral administration of the coccidiostat decoquinate (1 mg/kg bw) to young dairy goats from eight days prior to weaning through seventy-five days after weaning produced higher body weights at seven months of age and higher first lactation milk production at 100 and 200 days than controls (Morand-Fehr et al, 2002). In Angora goats, coccidiosis in weanlings may manifest as poor growth, poor hair coat, and increased susceptibility to pneumonia and other potentially fatal conditions.

Pathogenesis

The adverse effects of *Eimeria* infection in goats result from destruction of the gastrointestinal epithelium as these intracellular parasites progress through their complex life cycle in the digestive tract of the host. Multiple cycles of asexual and then sexual reproduction in the digestive epithelium result in successive waves of host cell disruption.

There are species-specific differences in the location of host cells invaded by various *Eimeria* spp. during their development cycles. For example, sporozooites of *E. ninakohlyakimovae*, considered the most pathogenic of the goat species, enter basal epithelial cells in the crypts of Lieberkuhn in villi of the small intestine. Many thousands of merozoites are produced in each schizont. These merozooites then invade epithelial cells in the large intestine. The subsequent gametogonous stages invade the ileum, cecum, and large intestine, where oocysts are produced. Because multiple infections are common in goats, disruption of gastrointestinal epithelium can be very widespread.

Diarrhea results from disruption and inflammation of the intestinal mucosa. In massive infections, severe hemorrhage into the intestinal lumen can result in death caused by blood loss. In the more typical acute form of the disease, fluid and electrolyte loss result from a compromise of the normal resorptive potential of the intestinal epithelium as well as leakage of plasma and lacteal constituents from the inflamed and disrupted mucosa. When extensive, these losses can lead to fatal systemic sequelae of dehydration, acidosis, and serum electrolyte derangement. Disruption of the mucosal integrity may also lead to increased susceptibility to secondary bacterial infection and resultant septicemia, thus increasing mortality rates. The ill thrift and poor growth commonly seen in the aftermath of clinical coccidiosis are manifestations of prolonged malabsorption and maldigestion associated with permanent damage to the intestinal mucosa. In many cases, regeneration of a normal epithelial lining is not complete and evidence of mucosal scarring or villous atrophy may be observed at necropsy in poorly doing animals.

Clinical Findings

Most goats with clinical coccidiosis are between three weeks and five months of age. However, cases have been confirmed in adults as old as seven years of age. Coccidiosis often occurs in conjunction with nematode infections, so attribution of clinical signs specifically to coccidiosis may be problematic because signs of gastrointestinal parasitism due to nematodes can be similar (Valentine et al. 2007).

Subclinical coccidiosis should be suspected when complaints of poor growth, weight loss, or loss of fecal pellet formation are reported for young, susceptible animals in management situations conducive to the persistence and multiplication of coccidia.

Clinical coccidiosis may develop within one to two weeks of ingestion of a large dose of infective sporocysts. Peracute cases, caused by severe blood loss in the intestinal lumen, may present as sudden death before signs of diarrhea or abdominal discomfort are seen. The intestinal lumen may be filled with blood due to massive destruction of the intestinal mucosa.

In acute cases, early signs include decreased appetite, listlessness, weakness, and abdominal pain that may be manifested by crying and frequent rising up and lying down. The feces may first be unpelleted, then pasty, and then, a watery yellowish-green to brown diarrhea develops. Fresh blood or melena may be seen. Tenesmus is less common than reported in cattle or sheep. The hindquarters and tail become stained and feces-coated as diarrhea persists. If dehydration becomes severe, animals become recumbent with cold extremities and subnormal temperature. They eventually become moribund and die. In Australia, polioencephalomalacia is reported to be a common sequela to coccidiosis in goats (Howe 1980). That disease, producing signs of neurological dysfunction, is discussed in Chapter 5.

Very young, highly susceptible animals may die of acute coccidiosis within one or two days of onset. Older or more resistant animals may exhibit diarrhea and weakness with resultant weight loss for as long as two weeks before spontaneously recovering. Animals that have recovered from clinical coccidiosis may develop ill thrift. They may be stunted, show a poor hair coat, and develop a pot-bellied appearance.

Clinical Pathology and Necropsy

The hemogram in coccidiosis may be normal, but a marked leukocytosis is possible when intestinal mucosal damage is extensive. Anemia is variable, depending on severity of disease, and may be masked by an increased packed cell volume caused by hemoconcentration associated with dehydration. Varying degrees of hyponatremia, hypocalcemia, hypophosphatemia, and metabolic acidosis can occur. Hyperkalemia has been reported in goats with coccidiosis and this may be caused by compensatory efforts to counter acidosis.

The use of fecal flotation methods to detect oocysts, though often useful, is not a wholly satisfactory approach to diagnosis of clinical coccidiosis. When oocysts are not found in the presence of active diarrhea, it may be because the affected individuals are in an early stage of infection. Intestinal disruption with resulting diarrhea can occur during the schizogony that precedes oocyst formation. In these cases, direct fecal smear instead of fecal flotation is employed to identify merozooites. Conversely, oocysts may be found routinely in the feces of all normal goats older than two to three weeks of age. Therefore, finding oocysts in the feces of diarrheic goats does not confirm coccidiosis as the cause of illness. Performing oocyst counts is of limited value, unless the oocysts of pathogenic species are morphologically identified and quantified, because some of the less pathogenic *Eimeria* spp. are prolific egg producers (Aumont et al. 1984; Yvore et al. 1985). If oocyst counts are undertaken, a modified McMaster technique should be used, with a flotation solution made of magnesium sulfate at a density of 1.18 (Yvore and Esnault 1987).

Necropsy examination offers more reliable indications of clinical coccidiosis (Figure 10.8). Gross lesions of enteritis seen in the gut mucosa may range from a mild catarrh to overt hemorrhage or necrosis. In peracute cases, the intestinal lumen may contain fresh blood. Thickening of the intestinal wall caused by edema is not uncommon. The most consistent and characteristic lesion is the occurrence of multiple raised, white nodules measuring between 1 and 6 mm in diameter on the intestinal mucosa, which may be apparent even when the intestine is viewed from the serosal side. These nodules represent sites of active gametogony and on smears or histologic examination

Figure 10.8. Intestinal lesions of coccidiosis in a goat. (Courtesy of Dr. Scott Schelling.)

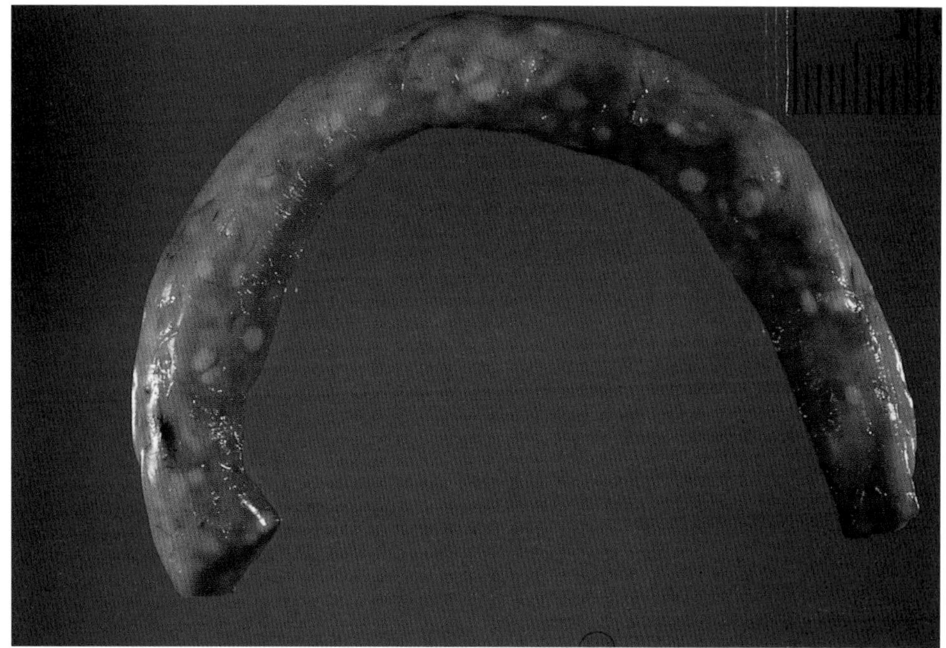

a

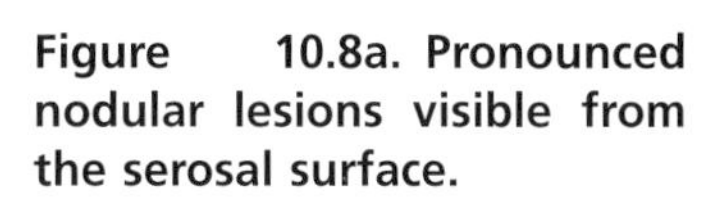

Figure 10.8a. Pronounced nodular lesions visible from the serosal surface.

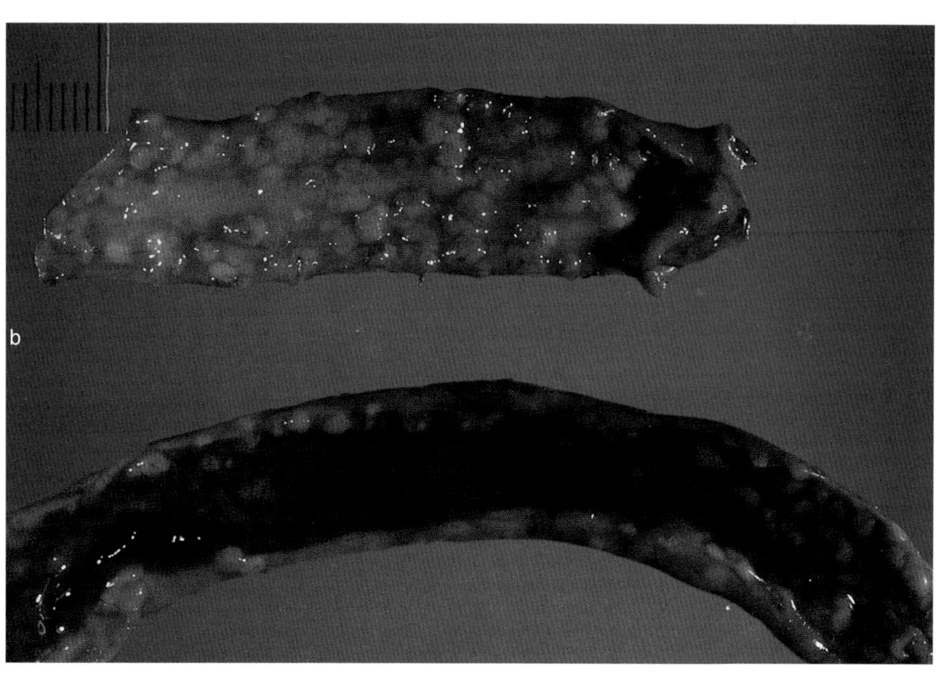

b

c

Figure 10.8b. Nodular lesions viewed from the mucosal surface.

Figure 10.8c. Intestinal lumen filled with blood. This is from a weanling goat that died acutely of anemia from severe coccidiosis before the clinical onset of diarrhea.

contain numerous macrogametes and oocysts. Lesions of enteritis and nodules may be seen in subclinical, peracute clinical, and acute clinical cases. The extent and severity of the lesions in conjunction with the history must be considered in establishing coccidiosis as the cause of death.

Lesions associated with coccidial infection have sporadically been reported in the abomasum of goats. Cysts, which appear on the mucosal surface as small whitish dots up to 1.5 mm in diameter, have been described and the condition has been referred to as globidiosis (Soliman 1960; Mehlhorn et al. 1984). Originally, *Globidia* was thought to be a distinct protozoal genus. It is now recognized that the protozoal structures seen histologically in the abomasa of goats and sheep are in fact large schizonts of an *Eimeria* species, most likely *E. gilruthi*. Some early reports attributed diarrhea, dehydration, and death in goats to abomasal globidiosis (Mugera and Bitakaramire 1968), but the infection is also recognized to occur in normal, healthy goats (Abdurahman et al. 1987). A recent report of clinical disease in a sheep with coccidial abomasitis due to *Eimeria* (*Globidium*) *gilruthi* suggests that the organism may indeed have pathogenic potential for goats as well (Maratea and Miller 2007).

Sporadic cases of hepato-biliary coccidiosis have also been reported in goats (Dai et al. 1991; Mahmoud et al. 1994; Schafer et al. 1995; Oruc 2007). Two types of lesions may be seen. In the biliary type, coccidial oocysts, schizonts, gametes, and gametocytes can be seen in the epithelium of the bile duct and the bile duct wall shows fibrosis. In the hepatic type, granulomata composed of oocysts and macrophages encapsulated in a fibrous capsule are present in the liver (Mahmoud et al. 1994).

Liver lesions may be severe, with large focal areas of necrosis reported (Schafer et al. 1995). Several species of *Eimeria* have been associated with these lesions. Clinical signs of diarrhea were reported in some of these cases, but since coccidial lesions were also present in the intestines, it was difficult to attribute the clinical disease to the liver involvement. A non-pathogenic coccidium has been identified in the gall bladder of a goat (Dubey 1986).

Diagnosis

The diagnosis of coccidiosis is presumptive, based on an appropriate signalment, history, clinical signs, and necropsy findings. In very young kids between one week and one month of age, other causes of abdominal pain and acute diarrhea must be differentiated. These include cryptosporidiosis, colibacillosis, enterotoxemia, salmonellosis, yersiniosis, viral enteritis, and dietary diarrhea. Abdominal pain alone would suggest abomasal bloat, mesenteric torsion, or other intestinal accidents if diarrhea does not develop. In cases of peracute death due to coccidiosis, the differential diagnosis includes enterotoxemia, bacterial septicemias, and plant and chemical toxins.

In weanlings two to five months of age, particularly those with access to pasture, kid yards, or poorly drained dry lots, helminthiasis is the major differential diagnosis for diarrhea. Gastrointestinal nematodiasis and paramphistomiasis should be considered. In fact, multiple parasitic infestations are common and it may be difficult to attribute diarrhea or ill thrift to coccidiosis alone. Other causes of diarrhea in this age group include simple indigestion and acute carbohydrate engorgement due to sudden feed changes or excessive grain feeding, as well as salmonellosis and enterotoxemia.

In subclinical coccidiosis, or after severe clinical coccidiosis, ill thrift or poor growth may be the primary clinical complaint in growing kids. Selenium deficiency or cobalt deficiency must be considered in these cases, particularly where soil deficiencies of these minerals are known to exist. Chronic helminthiasis must also be ruled out.

Treatment

Supportive care is the principal therapeutic intervention in active cases of coccidiosis. Diarrheic goats should be removed from the group and given oral or parenteral balanced electrolyte solutions depending on the degree of dehydration. In preweaned kids, milk should be fed only in small amounts, because disruption of the intestinal mucosa produces maldigestion and may promote osmotic diarrhea from undigested lactose. Weaned kids should be offered good quality grass hay and brought back on full feed gradually. Severely anemic kids with acute intestinal blood loss may require blood transfusions. Broad-spectrum antibiotics are indicated in severe cases to prevent bacterial septicemia secondary to disruption of the intestinal mucosal barrier. Probiotics have been recommended to help re-establish the normal gut flora (Bath et al. 2005).

The use of anti-coccidial drugs in active clinical cases may have limited value. Most anti-coccidial drugs are coccidiostats that inhibit but do not eliminate coccidial reproduction. These drugs usually act on early stages of the reproductive cycle. Animals already showing diarrhea have often progressed beyond the stages of infection where coccidiostats may prove beneficial. Nevertheless, goats are commonly infected with multiple species of *Eimeria* and some of these may still be in the early stages of development. In these cases, the duration of clinical disease may be shortened by treatment.

The main goal in administering coccidiostats is to reduce the number of additional cases developing in a group of animals at risk, rather than curing existing cases. Drugs reported for use in the treatment of caprine coccidiosis include sulfonamides, nitrofurazone, ionophores, amprolium, toltrazuril and diclazuril. Dosages and treatment regimens reported specifically for goats are summarized in Table 10.7

The sulfonamides and nitrofurazone may offer the added benefit of control of secondary bacterial infections. Because goats with clinical coccidiosis are often dehydrated, the sulfonamides must be used with care because nephrotoxicity can result from poor renal perfusion and decreased urine output. Sulfonamides are the oldest class of drugs used as coccidiostats and it is generally considered that resistance to sulfonamides is widespread among *Eimeria* spp. However, efficacy continues to be reported in some goats treated with sulfonamides. Sulfa drugs are available for oral and parenteral use. A variety of oral preparations can be given as boluses or added to feed or water. Nitrofurazones can produce neurotoxicity when overdosed, as

Table 10.7. Coccidiostats used in the treatment or prevention of caprine coccidiosis.

Drug used	*Treatment regimen*	*Prophylaxis regimen*	*Comments*	*References*
Sulfonamides				
Sulfadimethoxine	75 mg/kg bw orally for 4–5 days			Yvore 1984
	250 mg/kg bw orally once using a sustained-release bolus		Releases 50 mg/kg bw per day for 5 days	Yvore et al. 1986
Sulfadimidine	135 mg/kg bw orally for 4–5 days	55 g/ton of feed for at least 15 days		Yvore 1984, Radostits et al. 2007
Sulfaguanidine	280 mg/kg bw orally for 4 days			Vujic and Ilic 1985
Sulfaguanidine (or Sulfaquinoxaline) followed by Sulfathiazole (or Sulfadimethoxine)	1.3 g/kg bw orally for 4 days 1.1–2.2 g/kg bw orally for 4 days		Poor absorption from digestive tract	Guss 1977
Sulfamethazine		50 g/ton of feed		Shelton et al. 1982
Antibiotics				
Nitrofurazone	10–20 mg/kg bw orally for 5–7 days		No longer permitted for use in food producing animals in the US	Tarlatzis et al. 1955, 1957
Amprolium	10–20 mg/kg bw orally for 3–5 days			Yvore 1984
	50 mg/kg bw orally for 5 days			Swarup et al. 1982
		25–50 mg kg bw orally in feed or water continuously from 2 weeks to several months of age		Smith 1980
Ionophores				
Monensin		15–20 g/ton of feed		Shelton et al. 1982, Foreyt 1990
Lasalocid		20–30 g/ton of feed (1.1–2.2 mg/kg bw/day) continuously		Williams 1982
Salinomycin		100 ppm in concentrate fed for 3 weeks after weaning		Yvore 1984
Quinolones				
Decoquinate		0.5–1 mg/kg bw orally in feed; may be fed continuously		Foreyt et al. 1986
Triazinons				
Toltrazuril	20 mg/kg bw orally once	20 mg/kg bw orally once every 3–4 weeks		McKenna 1988
Diclazuril	1 mg/kg bw orally once	1 mg/kg bw orally once every 3–4 weeks	Recommended for use in goats but no dose given. Lamb dose provided here.	Harwood 2004
Clopidol and methylbenzoquate		12 mg/kg bw clopidol and 1 mg/kg bw methylbenzoquate/day for 5 weeks		Polack et al. 1987
Dapsone	80 mg/kg bw orally for 4 days			Devillard 1981
3,5, Dinitro-*O*-toluamide	100 mg/kg orally for 5 days			Dash and Misra 1988

ppm = parts per million.

may occur if the medicine is not properly mixed into milk or solid feeds. This drug is rarely used anymore in coccidiosis control. Note that in 2002, as a public health measure, all nitrofurans, including nitrofurazone, were banned in the United States for use in food-producing animals, because the nitrofurans have been identified as potential carcinogens.

Amprolium is a thiamine antagonist and works as a coccidiostat by blocking utilization of thiamine by coccidia. If amprolium is used for too long or at excessive doses, there is the potential for producing polioencephalomalacia in goats, though this should not discourage its proper usage. Polioencephalomalacia of ruminants may result from thiamine deficiency, as discussed further in Chapter 5. Amprolium is for oral use and is available as a liquid for addition to milk, milk replacer, or water, and in solid forms for addition to feeds.

The ionophores include monensin, lasalocid, and salinomycin; all have been used in goats. They are used mainly in solid feed in weaned animals. While monensin is used widely in poultry, cattle, and sheep, it is known to be toxic in horses and is potentially toxic in ruminants if overdosed. The lethal dosage LD_{50} in sheep is reported to be 12 mg/kg; in cattle, 22 to 80 mg/kg; and in goats 26.4 mg/kg. Muscle weakness and myoglobinuria are the clinical signs of toxicity in sheep (Langston et al. 1985). The cardiotoxicity of ionophores is discussed further in Chapter 8.

A new class of coccidiocidal drugs known as the symmetric triazinons emerged in the 1980s. They can disrupt all intracellular developmental stages of *Eimeria* and therefore can be more effective in the treatment of clinical coccidiosis than the coccidiostats, while also being useful for prophylaxis. Two drugs in this class are used in ruminants, toltrazuril and diclazuril, though neither is specifically approved for use in goats at this time. There are several reports on the use of toltrazuril in goats. In the earliest report, a single oral dose of 20 mg/kg produced a rapid, significant reduction in oocyst shedding that remained low for two to three weeks, suggesting that all developmental stages of the coccidia present were killed (Anonymous 1988a). In a later study, toltrazuril was administered orally at a dose of 25 mg/kg for two consecutive days to seven-week-old kids with clinical coccidiosis. Oocyst shedding was virtually eliminated and all treated kids became clinically normal (Ocal et al. 2007). In another study, the drug was given to four- to five-week-old kids at a lower dose of 10 mg/kg bw for two consecutive days (Slosarkova et al. 1998). Though oocyst counts in feces were reduced, considerable numbers of oocysts continued to be shed over the following three weeks and by five weeks were at higher levels than the pretreatment counts. Therefore, the higher doses of 20 to 25 mg/kg appear to be more effective in kids.

It is not clear that a second consecutive daily dose is required. In calves, a single dose of 20 mg/kg bw is considered to provide a full therapeutic effect. Diclazuril has been recommended for prophylactic use in goats. It is available as an oral suspension and is given as two doses two weeks apart (Harwood 2004). In lambs, the therapeutic and prophylactic doses of diclazuril are the same, 1 mg/kg bw, given at four to six weeks of age, with a second dose administered three weeks later for prophylactic use where there is high infection pressure.

In addition to the use of coccidiostats, implementing management changes is important in controlling outbreaks of coccidiosis. Attempts should be made to reduce exposure to infective sporocysts by removing contaminated bedding and feed, reducing the stocking rate, and moving animals to a new, uncontaminated environment.

Control

Under management conditions where outbreaks of coccidiosis can be reliably anticipated, measures should be taken to control coccidiosis before the observation of clinical disease. Proper control is a balancing act. The goals are to reduce oocyst numbers in the environment sufficiently to avoid massive challenge to susceptible animals while allowing sufficient exposure so that immunity and resistance can properly develop. This is accomplished by combining sound management and hygiene practices with the use of coccidiostats. In production systems where group housing of weanlings is unavoidable, control of coccidiosis without the use of coccidiostats is rarely achieved, even when management is excellent.

In attempting to maximize the immunologic resistance of the host, it is important to consider the mode of action of the various coccidiostats. The host immune response appears to be most stimulated by active schizogony, while most coccidiostats inhibit reproduction earlier in the infective cycle.

Sulfonamides, amprolium, and ionophores have been used as prophylactics and as therapeutics in goat-rearing programs with mixed success. The sulfonamides are folic acid antagonists, and are most inhibitory during the second schizogony. This late action allows for development of host immunity. However, as already mentioned, resistance to sulfas may be widespread. The ionophores primarily inhibit the early, asexual stages of coccidial development. However, they offer an added benefit of improved weight gains above and beyond their action as coccidiostats (Shelton et al. 1982). Unfortunately, outbreaks of clinical coccidiosis have been observed in young goats being fed lasalocid in their ration. This has been attributed to uneven consumption by individual goats, possible resistance to the drug, and failure to maintain good hygiene, in addition to feeding coccidiostats. Monensin was approved for use in nonlactating goats in the United States in 1989 as a feed additive at 20 grams/ton.

Decoquinate, a quinolone not used for treatment, has been found to be effective in preventing caprine coccidiosis. It works early in the *Eimeria* life cycle by inhibiting sporozoite development. Dose ranges from 0.3 to 4 mg/kg bw have been evaluated. All doses prevented clinical coccidiosis and allowed equal rates of weight gain. Doses at the higher end, however, resulted in a more rapid and pronounced decrease in the number of oocysts shed (Foreyt et al. 1986). In 2002, decoquinate was approved for use in non-lactating goats in the United States as an additive to milk replacers or feeds to be administered at a dose of 0.5 mg/kg bw (22.7 mg/100 lbs bw) for a minimum of twenty-eight days to control coccidiosis due to *E. ninakohlyakimovae* and *E. christenseni* (Vaughn 2002).

Coccidiostats are most often used between the ages of one and four months, usually in conjunction with grain feeding. However, in some intensive management situations, it may be necessary to begin use in the milk or milk replacer of pre-weaned kids. As discussed above in the treatment section, oral toltrazuril or diclazuril can also be highly effective for prevention of clinical coccidiosis in young kids if given at three- to four-week intervals through weaning.

Good hygiene and thoughtful management are essential to effective coccidiosis control. Weaning should be as unstressful as possible. To minimize weaning shock, kids should have access to grain well in advance of weaning. Whenever possible, dairy kids should be raised away from adults and housed individually or in small groups, segregated by age, and provided feed and water in devices that minimize contamination with feces. They should never be fed on the ground, and waterers must not leak or be liable to spillage.

Housing that allows shelter with ready access to sunlight is preferred. A successful system of weaned kid management using movable hutches is shown in Figure 10.9. No matter what type of housing is used, ground, floors, and bedding should not be allowed to become excessively wet. Adequate ground drainage, frequent floor scraping, and regular provision of clean bedding are necessary. Scraping floors and allowing them to dry is probably more effective in coccidia control than scraping followed by scrubbing or hosing because disinfectants are generally not effective, and excess moisture promotes sporulation. If disinfectants are used, products containing ammonia, particularly quarternary ammonium compounds, are the most effective.

In general, when proper control methods are implemented and goats are not exposed to new species of

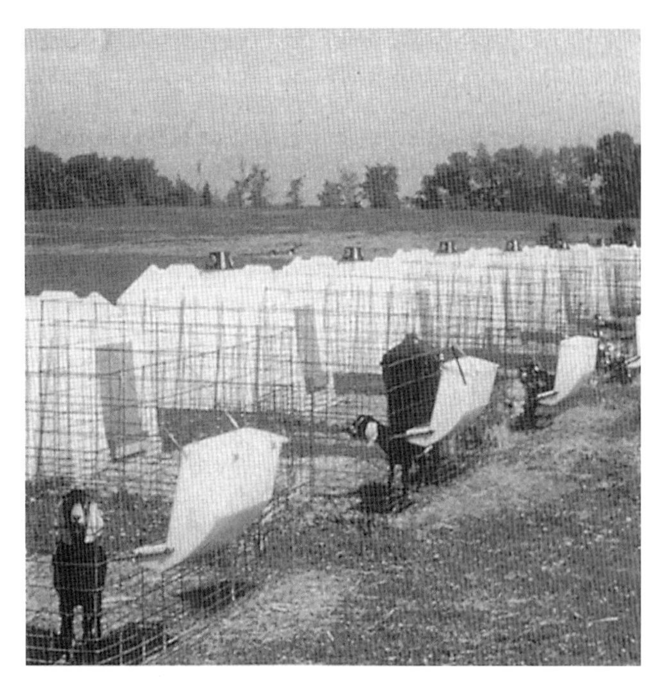

Figure 10.9. Movable hutches used in coccidiosis control. Fencing and hutches are moved every several weeks to minimize weanling exposure to oocyst buildup on the ground. (Courtesy of Vincent and Christine Maefsky, Poplar Hill Dairy Goat Farm, Scandia, Minnesota.)

Eimeria not previously experienced, immunity to reinfection is usually achieved by five months of age. Coccidiostat feeding may be terminated and, if possible, kids should be moved to uncontaminated housing at this time.

No vaccines are currently available for control of coccidiosis in ruminant animals, though live, multivalent, attenuated, coccidial oocyst vaccines are commercially available for poultry. There has been active research into the development of subunit vaccines for protozoa of veterinary importance, including the *Eimeria*, and these efforts have been reviewed (Jenkins 2001).

Cryptosporidiosis

First reported as a cause of fatal enteritis in goats in 1981, cryptosporidiosis has emerged as a major cause of diarrhea in kids younger than one month of age, particularly under intensive management conditions. Cryptosporidiosis is a zoonotic disease and has become an important and serious infection of patients with acquired immunodeficiency syndrome (AIDS) or other conditions involving immunosuppression.

Etiology

Cryptosporidiosis is caused by *Cryptosporidium* spp. which are small, protozoal parasites in the family Cryptosporidiidae in the phylum Apicomplexa. Though long considered to be members of the class

Coccidea, they are no longer considered to be coccidian parasites (Xiao and Cama 2007). The taxonomy of the *Cryptosporidium* genus is in flux as new molecular criteria become available to augment or replace the more traditional morphologic criteria of classification. Currently, fifteen *Cryptosporidium* species have been identified which infect a wide range of vertebrate hosts, including all the mammalian domestic livestock species; birds, including domestic poultry; reptiles, and fish. These fifteen species tend to be, but are not exclusively, host-specific. *C. parvum* infects domestic ruminants, including goats, sheep, and cattle as well as humans, and is the major focus of this discussion. Overviews of the taxonomy of the *Cryptosporidium* genus are available elsewhere (Fayer 2004; Xiao et al. 2004; Xiao and Cama 2007).

It is known that cryptosporidial oocysts are very resistant to environmental degradation, and many common disinfectants are reported to be ineffective in destroying them. Oocysts remained infective after eighteen hours of contact with iodophores, cresylic acid, sodium hypochlorite, benzalkonium chloride, and sodium hydroxide. Only 5% ammonia and 10% formol saline destroyed infectivity of oocysts (Campbell et al. 1982). Ammonium hydroxide, hydrogen peroxide, and chlorine dioxide are now also recognized to be effective disinfectants.

Epidemiology

Cryptosporidiosis occurs worldwide. In goats, kids from two days to three weeks old are mainly affected but older animals may also be affected. In outbreaks, especially in intensively managed herds, kid morbidity can approach 100% and mortality up to 40% has been reported.

The first reported field case of diarrhea attributed to cryptosporidiosis in a goat involved a four-week-old kid in Australia in 1978 (Mason et al. 1981). This was followed by a second Australian report in 1982 in which twenty-one of twenty-nine grazing goat kids developed diarrhea and three died. All kids examined were shedding cryptosporidial oocysts and tests for enteric viruses and K99+ *E. coli* were negative (Tzipori et al. 1982).

In Hungarian studies on the causes of diarrhea in kids younger than one month of age in large commercial dairy goat herds, cryptosporidia were isolated more frequently than rotavirus, coronavirus, adenovirus, or enterotoxigenic *E. coli*. In these studies, cryptosporidia were not identified in the feces of any normal goats, while all of the other agents mentioned were identifiable one or more times in non-diarrheic kids (Nagy et al. 1983, 1984). In a French survey, twenty-eight of forty-eight diarrheic kids (58%) on nine different premises had cryptosporidia detectable in feces or intestinal scrapings (Polack et al. 1983). A more extensive kid survey on twenty-four intensively managed dairy goat farms in France demonstrated an overall mortality rate from diarrhea of 10.3%, mostly during the first two weeks of life. Cryptosporidia were identified in feces of virtually all fatal diarrhea cases, but not in any non-diarrheic animals, save those recovering from diarrhea or those that subsequently developed diarrhea (Yvore et al. 1984). In contrast, cryptosporidia have been reported from feces of healthy kids in Tanzania (Matovelo et al. 1984) and Nigeria (Ayeni et al. 1985).

In diagnostic laboratory accessions seen from 1981 to 1985 in New Zealand, cryptosporidia were identified more frequently than any other single infectious agent, save *Eimeria* spp., in diarrheic kids younger than one month of age (Vickers 1986). Cryptosporidia also have been reported in association with diarrhea in a six-month-old goat in the Netherlands, four- to twenty-five-day-old kids in Italy, and a seven-day-old kid in conjunction with *Clostridium perfringens* in the United States (Ducatelle et al. 1983; Gialletti et al. 1986; Card et al. 1987). The author has confirmed cryptosporidiosis as a significant cause of diarrhea in young, intensively managed kids in a large goat herd in New York. More recently, major outbreaks of cryptosporidiosis affecting kids by the hundreds have been reported in herds from Oman (Johnson et al. 1999) and Turkey (Sevinc et al. 2005). In the Turkish incident, subclinically infected adult goats, insufficient colostrum intake in kids, and contamination of the kidding area were considered to contribute to the dramatic evolution of the outbreak.

Transmission is by the fecal-oral route from oocysts shed in the feces, and infections can spread quickly through group-housed kids once introduced into the group. It has been shown that goats may be infected with cryptosporidia isolated from calves and humans (Contrepois et al. 1984; Nagy et al. 1984). Colostrum-deprived kids develop more severe disease and a higher rate of mortality than colostrum-fed kids (Naciri et al. 1984). It is not yet clear if this is directly associated with *Cryptosporidium*-specific immunoglobulins or with other nonspecific nutritional or immune factors available from colostrum. The severity of disease does not appear to be affected by the state of the intestinal flora (Contrepois et al. 1984). While cryptosporidia are found infrequently in non-diarrheic kids during field investigations, experimental challenge can result in oocyst shedding in diarrhea-free kids, indicating that subclinical infections may occur (Nagy et al. 1984).

Pathogenesis

Cryptosporidium spp. are obligate, intracellular parasites. The only stage that occurs outside the host is the oocyst stage. The life cycle is similar in outline to the Eimeriidae, with some notable differences. Transmission is by the fecal oral route. Susceptible hosts ingest infective, sporulated oocysts which excyst and release sporozoites that invade intestinal enterocytes and undergo rapid asexual multiplication or schizogony. Meronts produced by schizogony release merozoites which invade new enterocytes. Sexual multiplication or gametogony also occurs in enterocytes, producing zygotes. Zygotes may form either thin-walled sporulated oocysts which rupture within the small intestine to release sporozoites that can further invade new host enterocytes (autoinfection) or a thick-walled sporulated oocyst that is passed in the feces as a source of infection to other animals.

Initially, these parasites of the gastrointestinal tract were considered to be extracellular, observed in close association with the brush border of the intestinal epithelial cells. Electron microscopic studies have confirmed that they are in fact intracellular, but extracytoplasmic, residing underneath the brush border of intestinal epithelial cells in a parasitophorous vacuole created from the host cell microvillous and plasma membranes.

The pathogenic effects of cryptosporidial infection are most likely due to the impairment of enterocyte function and integrity resulting from the rapid, cyclic reproduction of cryptosporidia that occurs within the brush border of enterocytes. In goats, infection leads to increased senescence of epithelial cells and villous atrophy in the ileum. The severity of these effects is related to the degree of infection (Matovelo et al. 1984). This can lead to both malabsorption and maldigestion, resulting in the clinical diarrhea observed. Prolonged weight loss may be associated with malabsorption. Steatorrhea caused by maldigestion has been documented in experimentally infected lambs (Contrepois et al. 1984). That diarrhea has been observed in kids as young as three to four days of age reflects the short life cycle of cryptosporidia. The prepatent period has been reported to be two to seven days in calves and two to five days in lambs (Radostits et al. 2007). Age-related immunity probably occurs, as clinical disease is far less common in older animals, but this immunity is not complete as oocysts are found in the feces of healthy adult goats (Castro-Hermida et al. 2007). Such goats can serve as a source of infection for kids. In ewes, it has been reported that there is a periparturient increase in the excretion of oocysts.

Clinical Findings

The most common presentation of cryptosporidiosis is an acute, white to yellow, watery diarrhea in kids younger than two weeks of age. The diarrhea may last from several days to two weeks, and may be mild to severe, presumably depending on the magnitude of the initial exposure to oocysts. Diarrhea may be persistent or recurrent. In addition to diarrhea, kids may show depression, inappetence, and a rough hair coat. Sequelae of dehydration, electrolyte imbalance, acidosis, and death may occur, depending on the severity of diarrhea and the time of intervention. Spontaneous recovery can also occur.

Explosive outbreaks of diarrhea with mortality rates of 10% to 20% have been observed in intensively managed dairy goat kids housed in groups indoors. Some of these outbreaks have begun toward the end of the kidding season, suggesting that environmental buildup of oocysts is contributory (Delafosse et al. 2006).

Two other syndromes of cryptosporidiosis have been reported from France (Polack and Perrin 1987). Progressive emaciation without diarrhea has been observed starting in one-week-old kids, and diarrhea has been noted beginning in six-week-old goats.

An atypical presentation of caprine cryptosporidiosis was reported from Oman (Johnson et al. 1999). Distinguishing features included clinical disease in adult goats as well as kids, and the limitation of cryptosporidiosis to goats, even though sheep, cows, and buffalo were in close proximity on the farm. No other enteric pathogens were identified during the outbreak. Morbidity approached 100% in goats under six months of age and mortality was high, with 37.8% of goats up to four weeks of age and 34.4% of goats between five and eight weeks of age dying.

Clinical Pathology and Necropsy

Current evidence suggests that cryptosporidial oocysts are not commonly shed in large numbers in the feces of healthy goats. Detection of oocysts in feces of diarrheic goats therefore is useful in supporting a diagnosis of cryptosporidiosis.

Direct fecal smears have been routinely used for examination because they are quick and easy to prepare. Oocysts, however, may be sparse, difficult to discover in fecal debris, or hard to distinguish from yeasts. Fecal flotation and sedimentation methods are preferable. Centrifugal flotation techniques including the use of potassium dichromate/saturated sucrose (sp. gr. $\geq$ 1.10), sucrose/phenol (sp. gr. = 1.27), and potassium iodomercurate (sp. gr. = 1.44) solutions have been reported. Yeasts do not float in the potassium dichromate/saturated sucrose solution (Willson and Acres 1982).

Concentrated oocysts can be viewed stained or unstained using direct light- or phase-contrast microscopy. The sample for examination should be taken from the meniscal surface using a wire loop, put on a slide, and covered with a coverslip. It is advisable to use high-power magnification, search the edges of the coverslip, and focus just below the coverslip because oocysts float up to its underside. A semi-quantitative flotation technique for counting oocysts in feces has been reported for use in calves (Anderson 1981) and applied to goats (Contrepois et al. 1984). Sedimentation using formalin-ethyl acetate solution with centrifugation at 1,700 × g or more also effectively concentrates oocysts (Kirkpatrick and Farrell 1984).

Numerous staining techniques have been used to assist in identifying cryptosporidia oocysts in feces. Currently, acid fast staining with modified Ziehl-Neelsen stains is generally favored. Oocysts stain pink to red with interior blue granules against a blue-green counterstained background. Auramine fluorescent stains or fluorescein isothiocyanate-labelled monoclonal antibodies are also being used. With these stains, oocysts display a yellow green fluorescence against a black background. Antigen based ELISA tests and PCR techniques are also available for detection of *C. parvum* oocysts in feces (Wright and Coop, 2007). Immunoassays are also available, but are more appropriate for surveillance studies than for case diagnosis because clinical disease generally precedes the immune response.

Gross lesions are nonspecific and unremarkable and may be limited to a mild to moderate enteritis most commonly located in the ileum. Smears should be made of the ileal mucosa for microscopic examination to detect oocysts. Histologically, sections of intestine reveal numerous small, round basophilic bodies of various sizes along the mucosal surface. These are the different endogenous stages of developing cryptosporidia in the brush border of the enterocytes. Free oocysts may also be seen in the intestinal lumen. Infection is accompanied by marked villous atrophy and villous fusion in the ileum and possibly the jejunum and large intestine. For accurate diagnosis, it is essential to fix fresh tissues in formalin immediately after death because autolysis of developing cryptosporidia and associated enterocytes is rapid. Oocysts in feces are more hardy, although freezing destroys them. If necessary, they may be preserved as long as 120 days by mixing one part feces with two parts of 2.5% potassium dichromate solution.

Diagnosis

A presumptive diagnosis of cryptosporidiosis is based on identifying oocysts in feces or various endogenous stages of the organism in intestinal smears or histologic sections. Since cryptosporidia may be present in association with other etiologic agents capable of producing diarrhea, laboratory evaluation for the various other bacterial, viral, and protozoal causes of kid diarrhea is indicated before a definitive diagnosis can be made. These are discussed later in the chapter in the section on the neonatal diarrhea complex, and a list of likely etiologic agents is provided in Table 10.3. Careful history taking is necessary to rule out dietary causes of diarrhea.

Treatment

Currently, treatment of cryptosporidiosis is limited to supportive care, particularly oral or parenteral fluid therapy, based on the severity of fluid and electrolyte loss. Nutritional management is an important consideration because maldigestion may be present. Diarrhea in cryptosporidiosis can last as long as two weeks. It is not possible to withhold milk for that period but regular milk feeding may result in aggravation of the diarrhea due to the osmotic influence of undigested lactose. Therefore, it is recommended to reduce the volume of milk fed per feeding while increasing the frequency of feeding. Lactose intolerance has been documented in a young goat in association with clinical cryptosporidiosis and feeding of lactase treated goat milk was reported to aid in recovery of the affected kid (Weese et al. 2000). Parenteral nutrition, though costly, could be considered in pet goats or other valuable individuals.

Reportedly, more than fifty anticoccidial, antibacterial, and antiparasitic drugs have been tested for therapeutic efficacy against cryptosporidiosis in numerous species and *in vitro*, and none were found effective (Tzipori 1983). More recently, some possible treatment options have emerged for use in goats and other ruminants, notably halofuginone lactate and paromomycin sulfate. Neither drug is approved for use in goats in the United States.

Preliminary results from a French field trial indicated that the anticoccidial drug halofuginone lactate was effective in arresting diarrhea and eliminating shedding of oocysts in goat kids with cryptosporidiosis (Naciri et al. 1989). The drug was given orally at a dose of 0.5 mg/kg daily for three to five days and the therapeutic response was marked compared with affected kids in the same flock treated with sulfonamides. Since that time, the therapeutic efficacy of halofuginone in cryptosporidiosis has been more widely recognized and the drug is now commercially available and approved for use in newborn calves in Europe for control of cryptosporidiosis. Available as an oral solution, it is given at a dose of 0.1 mg/kg bw for seven days beginning on the first or second day of life.

A cautionary note on the use of halofuginone is warranted. This drug has a very narrow margin of safety. It can be fatal when administered at three times the dose used. Animals should be weighed when possible to calculate an accurate dose and animals should be adequately hydrated before administration.

Paromomycin sulfate is an aminoglycoside antibiotic similar in structure to neomycin. It has been shown to have efficacy against *C. parvum* and is being used in human AIDS patients with cryptosporidiosis.

Several efficacy trials have been specifically carried out in experimentally infected (Mancassola et al. 1995) and naturally infected goats (Chartier et al. 1996; Johnson et al. 2000). In all studies, the drug was administered orally to kids at a dose of 100 mg/kg bw but for varying durations of ten, eleven, or twenty-one days. In all cases, there were marked reductions in oocyst shedding and clinical manifestations as compared to controls. When used for twenty-one days, in the face of a severe natural outbreak, treated animals showed no diarrhea and were negative for fecal oocysts on the day following cessation of treatment, while untreated controls in the same environment all developed diarrhea and had oocyst positive fecal samples (Johnson et al. 2000). Because the drug is given orally and is poorly absorbed from the alimentary tract, concerns about nephrotoxicity and ototoxicity associated with aminoglycoside administration, especially in diarrheic or dehydrated animals, are minimized.

There are also reports that decoquinate can reduce the severity of *C. parvum* infection and the number of oocysts shed in feces, though it does not prevent the development of clinical disease (Mancassola et al. 1997; Naciri et al. 1998; Ferre et al. 2005). In all these studies, the drug was administered orally to young kids for a period of twenty-one days at a dose of 2.5 mg/kg bw. In one study, however, the drug was also given to a group of pregnant does during their last three weeks of pregnancy, rather than to their kids. The positive effect on cryptosporidiosis in their kids was equivalent. The explanation was that treatment of the does suppressed the periparturient rise in oocyst shedding and therefore reduced environmental contamination and exposure of the newborn kids. Decoquinate is approved for use in the United States as an additive to feed or milk replacer for controlling coccidiosis in non-lactating goats as discussed in the preceding section of this chapter on coccidiosis.

The non-reducing oligosaccharide alpha-cyclodextrin has also been evaluated as a treatment for cryptosporidiosis in goats. In an experimental model, kids given 500 mg/kg bw orally for six days beginning on the day of experimental infection had a longer prepatent period, a reduction in the patent period, a decrease in the intensity of infection, and far fewer cases of diarrhea as compared with untreated neonatal kids (Castro-Hermida et al. 2004).

Control

The thrust of cryptosporidiosis control is in improved management and hygiene. Kids should be separated from does at birth and fed colostrum in clean nipple bottles. Goats that do not receive colostrum are more likely to develop cryptosporidiosis. Kids should be housed away from the adult herd and housed individually or in small groups. When kids are housed in groups, affected kids should be isolated at the first sign of diarrhea to reduce oocyst contamination of the environment. The author has had excellent results in checking the spread of cryptosporidiosis in groups of young kids at risk by practicing early removal and strict isolation of affected kids at the first sign of diarrhea. Outbreaks can be stopped without the use of drugs.

Excellent sanitation in housing, bedding, and feeding utensils is probably most critical in controlling the spread of cryptosporidiosis among susceptible kids (Thamsborg et al. 1990). Rodent control may also be indicated because there is evidence that oocysts derived from goats can infect mice, which in turn shed oocysts as well (Noordeen et al. 2002). In problem herds, water supplies should also be checked for contamination with *C. parvum* oocysts, because the risk of water-borne infection is recognized (Watanabe et al. 2005). Personnel handling diarrheic kids should not handle healthy kids. Hands should be washed thoroughly after handling sick kids because of the zoonotic potential of cryptosporidiosis. Because common disinfectants do not destroy cryptosporidia, steam cleaning or high pressure cold water spraying of pens or hutches between uses is recommended. No vaccine is currently available, though this is an area of active research (Sagodira et al. 1999; He et al. 2002). While no drugs are specifically approved for prophylactic use in goats, published reports indicate that halofuginone, paromomycin, or decoquinate can help control the disease in young kids, as discussed above in the treatment section.

HELMINTH DISEASES

Nematode Gastroenteritis

Nematode infection of the gastrointestinal tract is one of the most significant causes of wastage and decreased productivity in goats worldwide, especially under grazing conditions. The natural history of caprine nematodiasis is in many ways similar to that seen in cattle and sheep. Studies in the goat, however, suggest some important species differences in terms of parasite susceptibility, age-related immunity, and the pharmacokinetics of anthelmintic therapy. These differences must be understood and taken into account for effective control of nematode parasites in goats.

Etiology

A multitude of nematode parasites are at home in the gastrointestinal tract of goats. The major genera are first presented here in taxonomic family groups to facilitate discussion of common and distinct aspects of their life cycles. Subsequently, the individual species are discussed according to their locations in the caprine alimentary tract so that their pathophysiologic effects can be better understood. More detailed information about the biology of the various nematodes is available in standard veterinary parasitology texts (Soulsby 1982).

TRICHOSTRONGYLIDAE. The trichostrongyles are responsible for most of the disease and economic loss associated with nematode parasites in goats. Genera in this family include *Haemonchus*, *Trichostrongylus*, *Cooperia*, *Nematodirus*, *Marshallagia*, *Mecistocirrus*, *Ostertagia*, *Teladorsagia*, and *Camelostrongylus*. All have a direct life cycle. Adult nematodes in the alimentary tract of the host produce ova that are passed in the feces. First-stage larvae develop in ova within one day of passage to the external environment. For most species, first-stage larvae then break out of ova and molt to second-stage larvae. These molt one more time and become infective third-stage larvae. Development to the infective stage usually takes seven to ten days under favorable conditions but can vary according to environmental factors, mainly temperature and moisture.

Nematodirus spp. are distinguished from the other genera in that development to infective third-stage larvae occurs within the ova during the three-week period after passage in the feces. This adaptation enhances survivability over periods of adverse weather. In *Marshallagia* spp., larvae develop to the second stage before hatching from the ova.

Infective larvae of all genera are ingested by the host during consumption of contaminated feed. When goats are at pasture, infective larvae migrate to the tops of grasses during mornings and evenings, enhancing ingestion by grazing hosts. After ingestion, the larva travels to its predilection site in the alimentary tract. The larva then burrows into mucosal folds or digestive glands and molts within one to two days to a fourth-stage larva. This larva may remain in place for as long as ten days, and then returns to the mucosal surface to finally molt into an adult capable of producing ova to complete the life cycle. The average prepatent period is between three and four weeks.

Recently, two cases of human trichstrongylosis were reported in two suburban goat keepers in Australia who presented with abdominal pain and diarrhea. Eggs of *Trichostrongylus* spp. were identified from the patients and larvae of *T. colubriformis* from the goats. One patient had used goat manure as fertilizer on his vegetable garden (Ralph et al. 2006).

TRICHURIDAE. These parasites also have a direct life cycle. In *Trichuris* spp. of this family, known as whipworms, development to the third larval stage occurs within the egg and release of the larva does not occur until after ingestion by the host. Embryonation within the egg occurs after passage in the feces, taking three weeks or longer, depending on temperature and moisture conditions. Ingested eggs release larvae that penetrate the small intestine. Larvae develop for two to ten days before moving to the cecum for maturity to the adult stage. The prepatent period is seven to nine weeks.

OXYURIDAE. The members of this family that affect goats are *Skrjabinema* spp., referred to as pinworms. The life cycle is direct. Eggs ingested by the host hatch in the small intestine and larvae migrate to the large intestine to become adults within twenty-five days of infection. Eggs are fully embryonated and are deposited by the adult female pinworm on the perianal skin of the host.

STRONGYLIDAE. *Oesophagostomum* spp. in the family Strongylidae are referred to as nodular worms. They have a direct life cycle similar to the Trichostrongylidae except that infective larvae penetrate deep to the submucosa of the alimentary tract, reaching the lamina propria for development to fourth-stage larvae. This can occur anywhere from the pylorus to the rectum. After the molt, fourth-stage larvae return to the mucosal surface and migrate to the colon to develop into adults. The prepatent period is approximately six weeks. The characteristic nodules that occur in the intestine of affected animals due to *O. columbianum* are associated with a host reaction to the deeply burrowed infective larvae, not the surface feeding adults. The third-stage larvae of *Chabertia* spp. develop deep in the intestinal wall, but nodule formation is not a characteristic of chabertiosis. The prepatent period is approximately seven weeks.

ANCYCLOSTOMIDAE. This family includes the hookworms of goats, in the genera *Bunostomum* and *Gaigeria*. These nematodes have a direct life cycle, but a different route of transmission than the Trichostrongylidae. Infective larvae penetrate the skin or oral mucosa of the host. Such larvae enter the bloodstream via capillaries and end up in the lungs. They disrupt pulmonary capillaries and enter the alveoli, where they molt to fourth-stage larvae. These larvae are coughed up and swallowed. Migration to the small intestine and development of adults then occurs. The prepatent period is approximately nine to ten weeks, but adult worms may be present and feeding in the goat colon by four weeks after infection (Arantes et al. 1983).

STRONGYLOIDIDAE. *Strongyloides papillosus* is the sole caprine pathogen in this family. The life cycle is unique among the gastrointestinal nematodes. *S. papillosus* is parthenogenic—either free-living or parasitic development can occur. Under adverse environmental conditions, ova produced by parthenogenic females are passed in the host feces and develop only to infective third-stage larvae. Under more favorable environmental conditions, the free-living cycle is more common.

Ova are passed in the host feces again, but develop rapidly into sexually mature free-living males and females. After copulation, the females produce a single generation of infective larvae. In both cases, the resulting infective larvae must enter a suitable host to complete a subsequent life cycle. Infection of the host may occur by penetration of the skin, or the oral or esophageal mucosa. Penetrating larvae enter the bloodstream and localize in the lungs, where they enter the alveoli, migrate up the airways, and are swallowed. They mature to adults in the intestine. The prepatent period is six to seven days. In addition, transmission of infective larvae to neonates via the milk of infected dams has been documented to occur in goats, though transplacental transmission was not demonstrated (Moncol and Grice 1974; Yvore and Esnault 1986). Very young kids infected via milk or colostrum can pass ova in the feces, and *S. papillosus* may be the only gastrointestinal nematode found in preweaned kids.

GONGYLONEMATIDAE. *Gongylonema* spp. of the family Gongylonematidae (superfamily Spiruroidea) have an indirect life cycle. Eggs passed in feces of primary hosts such as the goat hatch after ingestion by coprophagous beetles. Infective larvae develop within the beetles for about thirty days. Goats are infected by eating beetles containing infective larvae.

Location of Nematodes in the Host

NEMATODES OF THE ESOPHAGUS AND RUMEN. Nematodes of the genus *Gongylonema*, *G. pulchrum*, *G. verrucosum*, and *G. monnigi* exist in the esophagus and forestomachs of the goat. Adult worms may be visible embedded in the mucosa and submucosa of the esophagus and rumen, but these parasites are essentially nonpathogenic and are of little clinical significance. Trematode parasites of the rumen, mainly *Paramphistomum* spp. and *Cotylophoron* spp., are more pathogenic, and are discussed later in this chapter.

NEMATODES OF THE ABOMASUM. The abomasal worms of goats regularly associated with morbidity, mortality, and production losses on a worldwide basis are *Haemonchus contortus*, *Teladorsagia circumcincta*, and *Trichostrongylus axei*. *H. contortus* is generally considered the most seriously pathogenic in goats. It is distinguished from the others in that the fourth-stage larvae and adults are voracious blood suckers. *Mecistocirrus digitatus*, like *H. contortus*, is an aggressive blood feeder and is a serious pathogen of goats in Central America and Southeast Asia.

Certain other abomasal worms affecting goats are less pathogenic or have a more limited geographic distribution. *Haemonchus longistipes* is a stomach worm of camelids in North Africa and India that occurs naturally in goats commingled with camels (Hussein et al. 1985). Pathogenicity for goats has been demonstrated experimentally (Arzoun et al. 1983). *H. placei*, usually associated with cattle and sheep, is found in the abomasum of goats in the Philippines (Tongson et al.1981).

Teladorsagia (Ostertagia) trifurcata often occurs in conjunction with *T. circumcincta*. Several species of *Ostertagia*, which are mainly associated with cattle, show variable infectivity for goats (Bisset 1980). *O. lyrata* has been found to occur naturally in New Zealand feral goats (Andrews 1973). Angora goats in Australia are readily infected with *O. ostertagi* when grazing contaminated paddocks (Le Jambre 1978). This parasite is also known to occur in goats in Chile, Cyprus, and the Ukraine.

Teladorsagia davtiani occurs primarily in goats in temperate regions. *Marshallagia marshalli* occurs in tropical and subtropical regions. *Marshallagia mongolica* infects goats, sheep, and camels in central Asia. *Camelostrongylus mentulatus* is a common, non-pathogenic abomasal worm primarily of camels in the Middle East and Australia that also can infect goats. All four species are morphologically similar to the *Ostertagia* and are considered to be minor pathogens.

Trichostrongylus axei is one of several important *Trichostrongylus* spp. to infect goats, but it is the only one found principally in the abomasum. It may also be found infrequently in the small intestine of the goat as well (Tongson et al. 1981; Akkaya 1998).

NEMATODES OF THE SMALL INTESTINE. The major pathogens of the small intestine of goats recognized worldwide are the black scour worms *Trichostrongylus colubriformis* and *T. vitrinus*, the small intestinal worm *Cooperia curticei*, the thin-necked worms *Nematodirus filicollis* and *N. spathiger*, and the hookworm *Bunostomum trigoncephalum*. This hookworm is an active blood sucker and may contribute significantly to the development of anemia. This is also true of the hookworm *Gaigeria pachyscelis*, which occurs in Indonesia, India, and Africa. As few as two dozen *G. pachyscelis* feeding in the proximal small intestine can lead to acute death from blood loss. *Strongyloides papillosus*, the threadworm of the small intestine, is moderately to markedly pathogenic in goats. In South Africa, field observations followed by experimental studies indicated that *S. papillosus* may be associated with severe clinical disease in young goats up to twelve months of age. Some of the signs observed were typical of gastrointestinal parasite infection such as abnormal feces or diarrhea, anorexia, cachexia, and dehydration, but other more dramatic and unexpected signs were also present including ataxia, stupor, nystagmus, and head pressing, as well as rupture of the liver (Pienaar et al. 1999).

Other nematodes of the caprine small intestine are geographically restricted or of limited pathogenicity. *Nematodirus oiratianus* and *N. abnormalis* are common caprine pathogens in cold regions of central Asia (Neiman 1977). *N. battus* has emerged as an important pathogen of lambs in the United Kingdom and North America, but there are no reports yet of disease in goats. *N. battus* was found in 5.8% of goat alimentary tracts examined at an abattoir in Nigeria (Nwosu et al. 1996). *Trichostrongylus falculatus* and *T. rugatus* infect goats in South Africa and Australia. *T. longispicularis* is primarily a parasite of cattle, but has been reported from a goat in Brazil (Lima and Guimaraes 1985).

Nematodes of the Cecum. The whipworm *Trichuris ovis* occurs worldwide in goats, but is not considered a primary cause of disease or production loss. It occurs commonly in mixed infections and may contribute to poor condition. Infections of goats with *T. ovis* and/or other *Trichuris* spp. have been reported to be more common during dry seasons in Brazil and Nigeria (Travassos et al. 1974; Okon 1974). *Trichuris* spp. burrow into the cecal mucosa and pierce vessels with their styletted mouth parts, subsequently feeding on the pools of blood created. The cecal worm *Skrjabinema ovis* occurs worldwide in goats but is generally considered nonpathogenic. A separate species, *S. caprae*, occurs in the United States. Adult forms of these small, nonpathogenic pinworms are sometimes present around the anus of goats, where they deposit their eggs. If observed, they may cause concern to owners.

Nematodes of the Colon. Adult *Oesophagostomum columbianum* reside in the colon, but the nodular lesions produced by infective larvae occur throughout the intestines. The parasite occurs worldwide. The remaining *Oesophagostomum* spp. that infect goats are not known to produce the characteristic intestinal nodule and are considered non-pathogenic. Experimental infection of goats with *O. venulosum* was reported to produce small nodular lesions in goats but this is generally not observed in natural infections (Goldberg 1952; Chhabra 1965). *Chabertia ovina* can contribute to clinical parasitism in goats worldwide. Morbidity caused by *Chabertia* infection alone is uncommon. However, in experimental challenge studies, *C. ovina* worm burdens of more than 800 were fatal to four- to six-month-old kids (Kostov 1982).

Epidemiology

The successful infection of goats by gastrointestinal nematodes and the completion of the parasitic life cycle depend on a variety of environmental, parasitic, and host-related factors and interactions.

Environmental-host Interactions. The feeding behavior of ruminant species is a major factor in the development of parasitism. Animals such as sheep and cattle that graze close to the ground are exposed to massive numbers of infective larvae. Free-ranging goats are less exposed to infective larvae because their feeding behavior includes a large component of browsing at levels well above the ground. In surveys of infection intensity in sheep and goats, where the animals are allowed to follow their natural feeding behaviors, sheep have been shown to carry heavier worm burdens than goats (Le Riche et al. 1973). Domesticated goats, however, are often managed in situations where access to browse is restricted and pasture grazing is obligatory. Under these conditions, goats may have equal or greater risk of nematode parasitism; this has been demonstrated experimentally in Australia (Le Jambre and Royal 1976).

Elimination characteristics also play a role. Splattering of naturally fluid cow feces when it hits the ground facilitates the dissemination of nematode ova on pasture. The fecal pellets of goats and sheep are not as accommodating, but natural disintegration of the feces with spreading of ova or larvae by heavy rain, melting snow, trampling by hooves, and the action of coprophagous beetles can achieve the same result, albeit more slowly. In addition, goats on lush pasture in spring, a time of increased ova production, often develop a more fluid manure that loses its pelleted character. Overt diarrhea caused by clinical parasitism also facilitates the dissemination of ova on herbage.

Lush, dense pasture in turn provides a protective umbrella for developing larvae, screening out direct sun to reduce desiccation. Direct sunlight has been shown to reduce the survival time of nematode larvae contained in goat fecal pellets (Tongson and Dimaculangan 1983). Survival time of infective larvae may also decrease in very hot weather due to the increased metabolic rate experienced by the larvae.

Overstocking and/or overgrazing of pastures generally promote increased parasitism. While intensive, rapid consumption of herbage may reduce survivability of ova and larvae by eliminating the protective plant growth, the total number of ova produced and deposited on the pasture each day increases directly with the number of animals present. Wild ruminants using pastures may also transmit nematodes to the goat, as demonstrated with *Camelostrongylus mentulatus* and *Trichostrongylus probolurus* transmitted to goats from blackbuck antelope (Thornton et al. 1973).

Management systems also play a role in the type and intensity of caprine nematodiasis, and a well-recognized advantage of confined housing systems is the marked reduction in nematode parasite loads. In a survey of forty-nine dairy goat farms in France, indoor housing was associated with a low incidence of clinical parasitism, attributable mainly to *Chabertia* and *Oesophagostomum*. In goats with access to yards, ostertagiasis was more common, and in pastured goats, haemonchosis was the predominant problem (Cabaret et al. 1986).

Environmental-parasite Interactions. Nematodes have evolved a number of adaptive strategies for surviving severe environmental stresses such as freezing, overheating, and desiccation. These include deep burrowing of larvae into soil during adverse seasons, delay of ova hatching until optimal conditions of temperature, moisture, and season are met, development of the infective larvae within the protective shell of the ova as is seen in *Nematodirus* spp., and the production of huge numbers of ova by a single female as is seen in *H. contortus*, which produces up to 10,000 eggs per day.

The most dramatic adaptation to hostile environments is hypobiosis, or arrested development. In hypobiosis, infective larvae consumed by the host during periods of environmental adversity remain voluntarily dormant and progress to adulthood only when environmental conditions favor development and survival of larvae outside the host. Host factors may also trigger renewed development as discussed below. In temperate regions, decreasing temperatures may signal the larva's commitment to hypobiosis, while in tropical regions with distinct seasons, hypobiosis is triggered by the onset of hot, arid conditions (Chiejina et al. 1988). Hypobiosis of *Haemonchus contortus* in goats in association with the hot, dry season has been reported from Kenya (Gatongi et al. 1998) and Togo (Bonfoh et al. 1995). Even in tropical regions where temperature and humidity conditions can support free-living larvae year-round, some degree of hypobiosis may occur in response to increasing moisture content of the soil (Ikeme et al. 1987).

Synchronous resumption of larval development in the host can lead to clinical disease, referred to as type II disease. Type II ostertagiasis has been reported in goats in Israel, with a significant increase in fecal egg counts occurring at the end of the hot dry summer and continuing through the subsequent cooler rainy season (Shimshony 1974). Type II infection also has been reported in goats in Spain with clinical signs occurring in January and February (Tarazona et al. 1982).

Environmental temperature is an important factor in the survival of nematode ova and free-living larvae. Various nematode ova in the feces of goats all died within six days at a temperature of 104°F (40°C). Ova survived and hatched optimally within eight to nine days at temperatures between 86°F and 95°F (30°C and 35°C). Hatching was delayed for fourteen days at temperatures between 68°F and 77°F (20°C and 25°C). At 32°F (0°C), ova remained alive but still did not hatch after thirty days (Tripathi 1980).

Some nematodes are best suited to tropical and subtropical conditions, notably *Haemonchus* spp., *Mecistocirrus digitatus*, and *Oesophagostomum columbianum*. *H. contortus* is representative of this group. No hatching of ova or larval development occurs when temperatures are 50°F (10°C) or below. The optimal conditions for development of *H. contortus* from ova to infective third-stage larvae are reported to be 28°C (82.4°F) with humidity greater than 70% (Rossanigo and Gruner 1995).

The ova are highly susceptible to desiccation and do not survive in regions where hot, dry summer follows winter rainfall, or where winters are intensely cold. Infective larvae, when developed, are more resistant to weather and can survive repeated periods of desiccation. Warm, humid regions of the world with summer rainfall and temperate regions with mild winters are conducive to development of infective larvae on pasture.

In *H. contortus*, hypobiosis largely replaces overwintering of free larvae as a means of survival for the species. This is true not only for tropical countries but also for cold, temperate regions. A recent report from Sweden indicated that *H. contortus* in sheep showed almost 100% arrested development in the early fourth larval stage as early as mid-summer, thus evolving a strategy to survive the long, cold winters entirely within the host as the arrested larval stage, and relying on the ewe to complete its life cycle with the periparturient resumption of egg-laying in the spring (Waller et al. 2004). The pattern of development of *Oesophagostomum columbianum* is similar to that of *H. contortus*.

Bunostomum trigonocephalum and *Gaigeria pachyscelis* are best suited to humid subtropical and warm temperate regions. They thrive under management conditions where housing and bedding are allowed to remain continuously damp because early larval stages are particularly susceptible to desiccation. Percutaneous penetration of larvae on the feet and legs of livestock is facilitated by grazing in wet herbage or housing in damp conditions.

Nematodes better adapted to cooler, temperate climates include *Teladorsagia* (*Ostertagia*) spp., *Trichostrongylus* spp., and *Chabertia ovina*. *Teladorsagia circumcincta* is the prototype of this group. *Trichostrongylus* spp. are more resistant to cold and desiccation than *H. contortus*, and are capable of overwintering. Ova accumulate on pasture until suitable conditions of moisture and temperature occur, at which time large numbers of infective larvae develop. Development occurs within four to six days at 80.6°F (27°C) but can take as long as one month when temperature and humidity are unfavorable. *Trichostrongylus* fare poorly in very hot, dry summer conditions. They are capable of hypobiosis as a survival mechanism.

Teladorsagia (*Ostertagia*) spp. are broadly adaptable, tolerating both colder winters and hotter, drier summers than *Trichostrongylus* spp. Overwintering of *Teladorsagia* (*Ostertagia*) larvae is successful as long as winters are not excessively dry. Survival is enhanced by slow release of infective larvae from disintegrating fecal pellets. This permits some larvae to persist on pasture as long as one year. Nevertheless, the *Teladorsagia* (*Ostertagia*) readily undergo hypobiosis when necessary. In regions of cold winter, larvae are conditioned to arrested development in the late autumn. In regions of hot, dry summer, larvae are conditioned in the spring.

Nematodirus spp. are well adapted to cold climates. They produce low numbers of ova, but survival rate is enhanced by the adaptation of larval development within the protective shell of the egg. They are extremely resistant to cold and dryness, and survive drought conditions. Hatching of ova of *N. filicollis* can begin in late autumn and continue through spring (Boag and Thomas 1975). *N. spathiger* does not show delayed hatching and behaves on pasture more like *Trichostrongylus* spp.

HOST-PARASITE INTERACTIONS. Two phenomena in the host-parasite relationship favor success for the parasite. These are hypobiosis and the periparturient egg rise phenomenon. The goat is not totally defenseless, however, and some host mechanisms are known to limit parasite infection. These are immunity, the phenomenon of self cure, and genetic resistance.

With regard to hypobiosis, environmental cues can trigger arrested development, as discussed in the preceding section. However, host factors may also trigger arrested development of ingested larvae. Host factors include immunity acquired from previous nematode infections, ingestion of large numbers of infective larvae, or a sizable pre-existing adult worm burden. Resumption of larval development also may be triggered by host factors, including depression of host immunity, removal of adult worm burdens by anthelmintic therapy, pregnancy-induced changes in hormone levels, and increased prolactin levels related to lactation. The latter two signals also are related to the phenomenon of periparturient egg rise.

The periparturient egg rise commonly observed in sheep results from maturation and ova production by previously arrested larvae, particularly of *H. contortus* and *T. circumcincta*. In temperate regions, when lambing occurs in the spring, ova deposited during the periparturient egg rise are largely responsible for the infections of grazing lambs that occur in summer. Overwintered larvae are usually killed off by the time lambs or kids are actively grazing. Lambs and kids in turn are more susceptible to infection than their older, possibly resistant dams. Lactation after pregnancy is a strong stimulus for renewed development of arrested larvae. Periparturient egg rise in goats has been documented. Fecal ova counts were highest in does one week after parturition and remained elevated for four weeks. This was independent of the season when they kidded, and no changes in fecal ova counts were observed in infected male goats sampled concurrently (Okon 1980). Increasing prolactin levels in goats have been reported to be associated with the periparturient egg rise (Chartier et al. 1998). It has also been postulated that a reduction in parasite-specific IgA antibodies in the dam associated with the transfer of maternal antibody to the colostrum around parturition may also facilitate the periparturient egg rise (Jeffcoate et al. 1992).

Immunity is an important host defense. While the neonate is immunologically naïve to parasites and colostral antibody does not appear to be protective, immunologic resistance to nematode parasites can develop over time and is enhanced by the continuous exposure to parasites. The development of resistance to infection with *Trichostrongylus colubriformis* in goats exposed to decreased weekly doses of infective larvae has been demonstrated experimentally (Pomroy and Charleston 1989).

The intensity of immunity with advancing age and parasite experience varies among domestic ruminant species. Goats show the weakest degree of immunity, sheep somewhat more, and cattle the most resistance to infection as adults. It is postulated that selection pressure on goats to develop parasite resistance is not as intense as in cattle and sheep because their browsing behavior in natural settings or under extensive range management systems does not demand strong resistance to parasite infection.

The greater susceptibility of goats is manifest in numerous studies. Significant worm burdens have been observed much earlier in kids than lambs, with worm burdens of more than 17,000 noted in kids between three and four weeks of age (McKenna 1984). When Merino sheep and Angora goats grazed the same contaminated pasture for four months, the goats had higher worm burdens of all species of gastrointestinal nematodes present except *Nematodirus* spp. (Le Jambre and Royal 1976). Adult goats carried mixed worm burdens similar in intensity to kids and yearlings in a survey of forty-seven dairy goat farms in New Zealand (Kettle et al. 1983). No difference in intensity of worm burdens or fecal egg counts was apparent between years one and two of pasturing when feral goats in New Zealand were pastured. In addition, when compared with sheep infections, worms infecting goats were more fecund, producing increased numbers of eggs per worm, and the return of high fecal egg counts was much quicker after anthelmintic therapy in goats than sheep (Brunsdon 1986). These findings suggest that direct extrapolation of sheep parasite control measures to goats may often be ineffective because of species differences in response to parasite infection. One practical consideration of these differences between goats and sheep is that adult goats represent a significant risk for the contamination of pastures and that goat parasite control programs, to be effective, must account for this risk (Hoste and Chartier 1998).

Any immunity to parasites that does develop in goats likely involves a complex interaction of mucosal and humoral antibody responses and cell mediated responses. For example, it was demonstrated that $CD4^+$ T lymphocytes in goats contribute to immunity against *H. contortus* gut antigens, but that antibody works synergistically with the CD4+ T lymphocytes to confer this immunity (Karanu et al. 1997). Nonspecific inflammatory mediators can also play a role (Smith 1988).

Immunity to parasites is not absolute. It predictably declines in the periparturient period, and may also be impaired by concurrent illness or malnutrition. It has been demonstrated by experimental challenge with *H. contortus* that goats on a low plane of nutrition subsequently pass more ova in the feces than better-fed goats (Preston and Allonby 1978). Goats with paratuberculosis are predisposed in increased worm burdens, and in Africa, goats with *Trypanosoma congolense* show increased susceptibility to *H. contortus* infection (Griffin et al. 1981).

The phenomenon of "self-cure" is known in sheep that ingest large numbers of infective larvae of *H. contortus* and subsequently expel their existing adult worm populations. Because these animals usually become immediately re-infected, the adaptive significance in terms of parasite control is unclear. Nevertheless, it does serve as an indicator of the potency of the immune response of the host to infection. There are two reports suggesting that self-cure is observed in goats (Fabiyi 1973; Preston and Allonby 1978). However, more recent and extensive field observations, as well as experimental studies, suggest that if self-cure does occur naturally in goats, the response is weaker and less reliable than that seen in sheep (Kettle et al. 1983; Brunsdon 1986; Watson and Hosking 1989). The failure of self-cure in pastured goats may lead to increased levels of sustained fecal egg counts and a resulting increased intensity of pasture contamination compared with sheep.

A final host defense against parasites is genetic resistance, the existence of which has been studied extensively in sheep (Courtney 1986; Gruner and Cabaret 1988). Evidence for genetic resistance in goats to helminths has been reported as well. In East Africa, imported Saanen goats showed more resistance to challenge with *H. contortus* than either of two indigenous breeds, the Galla and East African (Preston and Allonby 1978). It was postulated that the European dairy breed has been selected for resistance to *H. contortus* through generations of grazing behavior, while the indigenous breeds, as innate browsers, have not. In a later study, the Small East African goat breed was shown to be more resistant than the Galla breed based on significantly lower fecal egg counts in the post weaning period (Baker et al. 2001). In India, during a natural outbreak of haemonchosis after unexpected heavy rains, small grazing or pen-fed breeds such as the Black Bengal goat were far less affected than large, browsing goats such as the Beetal and Jamunapari (Yadav and Sengar 1982). Thai native goats demonstrated greater resistance to *H. contortus* infection based on fecal egg counts and worm counts on necropsy than Thai native (50%)-Anglo Nubian (50%) crosses (Pralomkarn et al. 1997).

In addition to breed differences, selection within breeds can also lead to greater resistance as indicated by long term studies involving large numbers of Creole goats in Guadeloupe (Mandonnet et al. 2001, 2006). Another extended study with cashmere goats in Scotland naturally exposed to mainly *Teladorsagia circumcincta* concluded that selection for reduced fecal egg counts was possible in breeding programs (Vagenas et al. 2002). Breeding for helminth resistance in small ruminants has been reviewed (Gruner, 1991; Baker 1998).

Hemoglobin type in sheep has been associated with resistance to helminth infection and this has also been studied in goats. Five hemoglobin phenotypes were identified in Red Sokoto goats in Nigeria and helminth egg counts on feces during the rainy season were correlated with these types. Significant differences in infection rates were observed, and hemoglobin types associated with high infection rates were less frequent in the older goat population than in the kid population, suggesting increased mortality among the more parasite-susceptible phenotypes (Buvanendran et al. 1981).

In summary, the development of gastrointestinal parasitism in goats depends on a complex interrelationship of parasite, host, and environmental factors, many known and some unknown. In general, the types and degree of parasitism that develop in goat populations may be predicted on the basis of geographic and climatic location, management system, and prevailing weather conditions. Nematodes, by evolving diverse strategies and rates of development, different mechanisms for feeding, and different predilection sites in the host alimentary tract, appear to have maximized their exploitation of the host, while minimizing competition among each other. This diversity encourages development of multiple nematode infections, which are the rule in goats.

The outcome of infection depends on host resistance, level of infection, variety and types of parasites involved, the development of parasite resistance to anthelmintics, and the extent of appropriate therapeutic intervention. Acute death, clinical disease, or subclinical infection with adverse effects on growth and lowered productivity are all possible outcomes. Worldwide, numerous studies on the causes of wastage in goats, particularly young goats, have confirmed that clinical gastrointestinal nematodiasis is a major cause of morbidity and mortality. However, specific studies concerning the impact of subclinical gastrointestinal nematodiasis on production parameters in dairy, fiber, and meat goats are comparatively scarce.

The impact of nematode parasites on dairy goat production is beginning to become clearer. One French study indicates that elimination of gastrointestinal nematodes in lactating does by treatment with thiabendazole resulted in a 17.6% increase in milk production compared with untreated control goats (Farizy and Taranchon 1970). More recent studies have revealed a number of interesting findings. Subclinical parasitism with *H. contortus* and *T. colubriformis* in lactating does resulted in a decrease in body condition score as well as a persistent decrease in milk yield ranging from 2.5% to 10% as compared to uninfected controls. However, when the highest producers were assessed separately from other infected does, reductions in milk output ranged between 13% to 25.1% and had lower fat content. It was concluded that high producing goats had less resistance and/or resilience to parasite infection than lower producing goats, leading to more severe depression of milk output (Hoste and Chartier 1993). Further studies reinforced these observations that resistance to parasite infection differed according to level of milk yield in lactating does (Chartier and Hoste 1997; Hoste and Chartier 1998a).

Pathogenesis

Various pathogenic mechanisms are involved in gastrointestinal nematodiasis depending on the genera involved. The principal effect of hematophagous worms on the host is a progressive debilitating anemia. Blood feeders include *Haemonchus contortus* and *Mecistocirrus digitatus* in the abomasum, *Bunostomum trigonocephalum* and *Gaigeria pachyscelis* in the intestine, and *Trichuris* spp. in the cecum. Each *H. contortus* adult in the abomasum may be responsible for the loss of 0.05 ml of blood per day, either by active feeding or by moving to new feeding sites and leaving old sites to continue hemorrhaging. Death caused by acute blood loss is possible when infection rates are high (more than 10,000 adults per host) and development of large adult populations is synchronous, as can happen after arrested development.

In less severe infections, three stages of anemia may be recognized in infected hosts (Dargie and Allonby 1975). In the initial stage of blood loss, packed cell volume (PCV) may decrease markedly because intraluminal blood loss in the alimentary tract is not a strong trigger for hematopoiesis. In experimental haemonchosis of goats the PCV decreased from a mean of 29% to 16% within nineteen days of infection with 9,000 to 12,000 larvae (Al-Quaisy et al. 1987). In the second stage, regenerative erythropoiesis begins and the PCV stabilizes, albeit at less than the normal level, for as long as six to fourteen weeks. During this time, however, iron stores in the host are reduced by loss in the feces. In the final stage, the PCV begins to decrease again as erythropoiesis is impaired by the progressive iron deficiency. Concurrently, a steady loss of serum proteins occurs as a result of parasite feeding. Serum albumin levels may be maintained initially due to replacement by tissue catabolism, but hypoalbuminemia eventually develops, accompanied by cachexia and clinical evidence of hypoproteinemia such as intermandibular edema.

The remainder of the nematode parasites of the caprine alimentary tract are not primarily blood feeders, though blood constituents are gradually lost in the process of feeding during chronic or large-scale infection. In these cases, anemia does not occur acutely or reach the severity seen with the blood feeders. In the field, however, this distinction may not be evident because mixed infections of hematophagous and nonhematophagous parasites often occur.

Infective larvae of *Trichostrongylus axei* develop to adults within the abomasal mucosa and the adults feed there and lead to erosion of the mucosal epithelium, catarrhal inflammation, hyperemia, edema, and diarrhea. Plasma loss from the mucosal damage contributes to the hypoproteinemia seen with this infection.

Infective larvae of *Teladorsagia (Ostertagia) circumcincta* enter the gastric glands of the abomasum to undergo the third and fourth molts to adulthood. When synchronous maturation of large numbers of arrested larvae occurs (type II ostertagiasis), a severe gastritis results. Gastric glands become hyperplastic, intercellular tight junctions are weakened, hydrochloric acid secretion diminishes, and the pH of stomach content increases. One result of the pH change is that pepsinogen is not converted to pepsin and pepsinogen may leak across the abomasal mucosa to the circulating blood. Increases in blood pepsinogen support a diagnosis of Type II ostertagiasis. Other plasma proteins also are leaked from the abomasum. Hypoproteinemia and diarrhea are cardinal signs of ostertagiasis.

The *Trichostrongylus* spp. that infect the intestine tunnel under the mucosal epithelium to feed. This results in a protein-losing enteropathy accompanied by diarrhea. Larval stages can be as destructive as adult worms. Over time, marked villous atrophy occurs. The pathogenesis of *Nematodirus* spp. is similar.

Oesophagostomum columbianum presents a unique situation in small ruminants. Infective larvae burrow into the submucosa of the small intestine, encyst for the third molt, and then return to the intestinal lumen to migrate to the colon for the final molt. In first-time infections, this process occurs unremarkably. In previously exposed, sensitized hosts, however, encysted third-stage larvae produce a dramatic local inflammatory response around the cyst, leading to the formation of caseating nodules. The larvae inside may die or resume migration at a much later time. Nodules may occasionally rupture serosally, causing peritonitis, adhesions, and partial or complete obstructions of the intestine. Even without rupture, widespread nodular formation may impair digestion, absorption, and passage of excreta. In addition, adult nodular worms can produce a severe catarrhal colitis with much mucus production. Diarrhea with mucus, weight loss, and hypoproteinemia occur in severe infections.

Anorexia with reduced feed intake is the most consistent finding in all forms of intestinal nematodiasis, and is accompanied by poor growth, decreased productivity, and weight loss. The causes of these host responses are complex and not fully understood. Failure of muscle growth in young animals results from a decrease in skeletal muscle synthesis, with a shift to increased albumin production by the liver to counteract ongoing protein loss. Muscle wasting in severely affected animals may be associated with muscle catabolism. In fiber-producing animals, fiber growth is also impaired by the shift in protein synthesis. In growing goats, bone growth is also compromised, possibly as a result of decreased intake of calcium and phosphorus and depletion from bones (Fitzsimmons 1966). The pathophysiological adaptations of the host to gastrointestinal parasitism have been reviewed (Hoste 2001).

Clinical Findings

Mixed parasitic infections are common and often it is not possible to attribute clinical signs to a single parasite. In general, infections with *Trichostrongylus*, *Teladorsagia (Ostertagia)*, *Cooperia*, and *Nematodirus* spp. produce a similar clinical picture. Young, grazing animals are most likely to be affected, particularly after weaning. A gradual, progressive loss of condition, poor growth, a dull attitude, and a decrease in feed intake are the most consistent findings. In more severe infections, a dark green to black diarrhea is evident, with staining of the hair and skin of the tail and perineal region. When the course is prolonged, intermandibular edema may develop secondary to hypoproteinemia. Chronically infected animals also develop a pot-bellied appearance, a rough, dry hair coat and flaky skin. Evidence of anemia is usually not pronounced. Deaths may be reported, and are usually spread out over a period of days or weeks. A more acute presentation may also be seen with type II disease when maturation of parasites resumes after arrested development.

Nodular worm (*O. columbianum*) infection may result in signs of abdominal pain such as hunched back and reluctance to move when nodule formation occurs and localized peritonitis results. Affected animals may be febrile. Occasionally, nodules may abscess and rupture. Pus may be passed per rectum if the rupture is intraluminal. Diffuse peritonitis may result if the rupture is intra-abdominal. In sheep, intussusceptions are reported sometimes in association with intestinal nodules, but this has not been reported in goats. When nodule formation is minimal, as in first time exposures, signs of *O. columbianum* infection may be limited to diarrhea in young kids, or in older animals, intermittent passage of soft, mucus-laden feces flecked with blood and progressive loss of condition. Excessively mucoid feces with occasional blood is also associated with *Chabertia ovina* infection. Anemia is uncommon.

When hematophagous parasites such as *H. contortus* infect goats, clinical evidence of anemia predominates. When infections are massive, peracute haemonchosis can occur, with animals dying of gastric hemorrhage. Acute and chronic forms are more common. Affected animals exhibit marked pallor of mucous membranes and conjunctivae, and respiratory and heart rates may be increased. Hemic murmurs may occasionally be heard. Intermandibular edema, or "bottle jaw," is common. Weakness, reluctance to move, and exercise intolerance are observed. Constipation is more common than diarrhea in uncomplicated haemonchosis. In prolonged disease, weight loss is also a common finding.

Diarrhea may be seen after constipation in hookworm infections. Restlessness and pruritus, particularly on the legs, may accompany skin penetration and migration of hookworm larvae in the host.

Clinical Pathology and Necropsy

In goats with clinical gastrointestinal nematodiasis, serum albumin is consistently below 2.5 g/dl and often less than 1.5 g/dl. Total serum or plasma protein is also usually low, but in chronic cases, may be normal due to concurrent hypergammaglobulinemia. Anemia is a variable but important finding. Packed cell volumes below 9% can occur in severe haemonchosis. In less severe or chronic infections, PCVs in the range of 15% to 25% are likely and red cells may by hypochromic due to iron deficiency. A mild to moderate anemia may occur during severe or prolonged infections with non–blood-feeding nematodes.

When larvae of abomasal nematodes develop in the gastric glands and cause gastric inflammation, serum pepsinogen levels may be increased. Serum pepsinogen levels between 400 and 3,500 mU tyrosine were measured in naturally infected goats with mixed trichostrongylid burdens, including some with type II ostertagiasis (Tarazona Vilas 1984). In experimental ostertagiasis, serum pepsinogen in non-infected goats remained below 800 mU while levels between 1,000 and 1,500 mU were seen beginning fifteen days after infection. In experimental haemonchosis, serum pepsinogen in non-infected control goats also remained less than 800 mU while infection produced levels between 1,000 and 3,500 mU three days after larval challenge (Kerboeuf and Godu, 1981). Because clinical disease may occur in type II infections before adult nematodes pass eggs in the feces, the estimation of pepsinogen may be a helpful diagnostic tool. These elevations can be highly variable in affected individuals, so several suspected animals should be tested to establish the presence of type II disease in the affected population. A slaughter house study in Sri Lanka demonstrated a strong correlation between increasing *H. contortus* abomasal worm burdens and increasing serum pepsinogen concentration in goats (Paranagama et al. 1999).

Baseline values for serum pepsinogen from normal, strongyle-free French Alpine and Saanen dairy goats have been reported (Chartier et al. 1993). Mean baseline serum pepsinogen for French Alpine goats under six months of age was 490 ± 175 mU tyr and for adults (more than twelve months of age) 825 ± 414 mU tyr. For Saanen goats it was 397 ± 135 mU tyr in young goats and 709 ± 274 mU tyr in adults. In addition to age and breed, farm and duration of lactation were identified as sources of variation. In general terms, serum pepsinogen levels above 1,000 mU tyr are indicative of significant abomasal strongylosis in goats.

Microscopic examination of feces for parasite ova by direct smear, flotation techniques, or quantitative methods can aid in diagnosis. Fecal specimens should be fresh or refrigerated. Most of the gastrointestinal nematodes have ova of approximately equal size (60 to 90 um long) and morphology, making specific etiologic diagnosis difficult. This requires *in vitro* cultivation of larvae and morphologic identification. Some infections, however, can be distinguished by ova structure. *Nematodirus* and *Marshallagia* spp. ova are distinctly larger than the rest, with average length of 160 to 180 um. *Trichuris* ova are barrel shaped, with obvious bipolar caps or plugs. *Skrjabinema ovis* and *S. papillosus* ova are smaller than average and contain fully developed embryos.

Ova may be counted by methods such as the McMaster technique, but direct correlations between egg counts and severity of infection do not always exist. The obvious example is type II disease in which serious damage to the abomasum may occur before adults even develop to produce ova. In severe *T. colubriformis* infection, marked clinical illness can result from larval feeding before patency of infection occurs (Fitzsimmons 1966). There also may be wide variation in the number of eggs produced by different species, and some prolific egg producers are not always the most serious pathogens. Precise parameters for ascribing significance to ova counts from goats, or using them as a basis for triggering therapeutic intervention, are not established, but a generally accepted guideline is that 0 to 500 eggs per gram (epg) represents a low parasite burden, 500 to 2,000 epg a moderate burden, and more than 2,000 epg a heavy burden. In a study from New Zealand, there was reasonable correlation between fecal egg counts and worm burdens in individual lambs within these three categories (McKenna 1981). In a Venezuelan study, a 10% to 30% mortality rate in goats was associated with *H. contortus* infection when fecal egg counts were in the range of 650 to 4,100 eggs per gram (Contreras 1976).

At necropsy, nematodiasis in general is suggested by emaciation with reduced fat reserves or serous atrophy of fat around the heart and kidneys. Subcutaneous edema may also be observed, especially in the intermandibular space, when hypoproteinemia is marked. In haemonchosis, the characteristic red- and white-striped females can be seen on the abomasal mucosa with careful inspection, although they may be absent in the extremely anemic goat at the time of death. Multiple sites of hemorrhage, ulceration, or both may be present. In *Teladorsagia* (*Ostertagia*) infection, the wall of the abomasum is edematous, and the mucosal surface has a grainy, "Moroccan leather" appearance caused by distension of gastric glands with developing larvae. An increase above the normal pH range of the abomasal content supports a diagnosis of severe type II disease.

For most of the intestinal worms, gross findings at necropsy are nonspecific, consisting only of catarrhal inflammation. The worms themselves are very difficult to see, especially in the small intestine, but may be larger in the large intestine. Preparation of mucosal impression smears and staining with aqueous iodine solution helps to establish the presence and intensity of the worm burden. A catarrhal enteritis and soft, unformed dark feces in the colon are consistent with most forms of nematodiasis. Transmural nodular lesions anywhere along the intestinal tract support the diagnosis of *O. columbianum* infection. Blood staining of intestinal content, particularly in the proximal small intestine, is suggestive of hookworm infection. Petechiation in the colon with edema and thickening of the colon wall are suggestive of *Chabertia ovina* infection. Extensive mucus covering the colonic mucosa is associated with adult *Oesophagostomum* spp. infection.

Diagnosis

Any combination of clinical signs of anemia, edema, poor body condition, and diarrhea should suggest gastrointestinal nematodiasis in goats. Evidence of increased fecal egg counts, heavy worm burdens in necropsied herd mates, or in the case of type II disease, characteristic Moroccan leather-type lesions of the abomasal mucosa, a preponderance of arrested fourth stage larvae, and/or increased serum pepsinogen levels, supports the diagnosis. When anemia is a predominant sign, various hemoparasites, hepatic fascioliasis, and cobalt or copper deficiency must also be considered in the differential diagnosis. Causes of anemia in goats are discussed in Chapter 7. In young goats, coccidiosis is the most important cause of diarrhea that must be differentiated from nematodiasis, but giardiasis and cryptosporidiosis should also be ruled out.

In certain regions, particularly Africa and southeast Asia, concurrent hemoparasite, gastrointestinal nematode, and liver trematode infections commonly occur in goats, so the clinician must look beyond gastrointestinal nematodiasis as the sole explanation for the clinical signs.

Subclinical parasitism often presents as poor growth in young animals or prolonged weight loss in adults with few additional clinical findings except in lactating goats, where a drop in milk production may be apparent. The differential diagnosis of progressive weight loss in goats is complex and is discussed separately in Chapter 15.

Treatment

Clinically affected individuals require supportive care to reverse the process of parasitic debilitation as well as anthelmintic therapy to eliminate existing infections. In severely debilitated goats, anthelmintics of low toxicity such as thiabendazole, fenbendazole, or ivermectin should be used because animals may be more susceptible to the adverse effects of drugs with a narrower margin of safety such as levamisole or organophosphate compounds.

Even when packed cell volumes are less than 10%, blood transfusions may not be a necessary aspect of therapy as long as animals are kept in quiet conditions of confinement with food and water provided. Perhaps more significant than anemia is the hypoalbuminemia. If serum albumin is below 1.5 g/dl, development of edema and anasarca will progress unchecked unless plasma or whole blood transfusions are administered to increase total serum protein. A good-quality, digestible hay or forage of high protein content should be fed during convalescence with a gradual supplementation of concentrate when available to restore body condition. Parenteral administration of iron as iron dextran may promote erythropoiesis because iron deficiency often results from prolonged parasitism.

A wide variety of anthelmintics have been used for treatment and prevention of gastrointestinal nematodiasis in goats. Some of the older drugs, notably the chlorinated hydrocarbons and organophasphates, are now rarely used because of toxicity and environmental safety issues. Other drugs are no longer available because markets for the products were limited and their distribution discontinued. Table 10.8 presents the anthelmintics that are currently in general use for goats, grouped according to anthelmintic class. Dosages appropriate for oral treatment of goats are given, because this is the preferred route of administration to delay development of resistance. Many of these anthelmintics, notably the benzimidazoles, also are useful in the treatment of cestode and trematode infections, nematode lungworm infections, and, in the case of the

Table 10.8. Dosages for various anthelmintics used orally in goats to treat gastrointestinal nematodiasis. (Dosing information for goats provided by Dr. Ray M. Kaplan, University of Georgia.)

Anthelmintic	*Goat oral dose (mg/kg)*	*Comments*
Benzimidazoles		
Thiabendazole	44	No longer marketed in US, but approved for use in goats.
Fenbendazole	10	
Oxfendazole	10	Basically the same drug as fenbendazole.
Albendazole	20	The recommended dose for nematodes is 20 mg/kg split into two equal doses (10 mg/kg each) given 12 hours apart. This is more effective than a single dose.
Macrocyclic lactones		
Ivermectin	0.4	
Doramectin	0.4	Doramectin has little efficacy advantage over ivermectin but has much longer persistence and can therefore promote resistance so its use in goats is discouraged.
Eprinomectin	0.4	Eprinomectin is available in the US only for topical administration.
Moxidectin	0.4	
Imidazothiazoles		
Levamisole	12	
Tetrahydropyrimidines		
Morantel tartrate	10	
Pyrantel tartrate	25	

macrocyclic lactones, arthropod parasites of the skin. The dosages and indications for these other infections are discussed in more detail in the pertinent sections of this book.

In most countries, the approved use of various anthelmintics in food producing animals is regulated by relevant government agencies. The list of drugs approved for use in goats varies considerably between countries as do the restrictions regarding slaughter withholding times and milk discard times after use.

In the United States, for example, only three anthelmintics, thiabendazole, fenbendazole, and morantel tartrate are approved for use in goats. Only thiabendazole is approved for use in lactating goats, with a milk discard time of ninety-six hours, but it is no longer marketed. In France, fenbendazole, oxfendazole, and febantel are approved for use in lactating goats with no milk discard required when prescribed doses are used. When resistance to these drugs has been documented by a veterinarian, then it is permitted for the veterinarian to use anthelmintics that are approved for use in lactating cattle with no withdrawal time, such as eprinomectin. However when used in goats, it is necessary to observe a seven-day milk withholding time in accordance with European Union "prescribing cascade" regulations. These regulations are akin to off-label, minor species drug use rules in the United States aimed at limiting the occurrence of drug residues in foods of animal origin.

Benzimidazoles and Pro-benzimidazoles. The benzimidazoles are a useful group of broad-spectrum anthelmintics, with the parent compound being thiabendazole. The pro-benzimidazoles, febantel, and thiophanate are broken down metabolically to benzimidazoles by the host. Both fenbendazole and the pro-benzimidazole febantel are metabolized in the goat to oxfendazole. In general, where resistance has not developed, these drugs are highly effective against adult and active immature stages of *Haemonchus*, *Teladorsagia* (*Ostertagia*), *Trichostrongylus*, *Cooperia*, and *Chabertia* spp., moderately effective against *Oesophagostomum*, *Nematodirus*, *Bunostomum*, *Gaigeria*, and *Strongyloides* spp., and poorly effective against *Trichuris* spp. (Bali and Singh 1977; Kirsch 1979; Sathianesan and Sundaram 1983).

Importantly, the newer compounds oxfendazole, febantel, fenbendazole, and albendazole are highly effective against arrested larvae of *Teladorsagia* (*Ostertagia*) and are useful in the control of type II disease. The benzimidazoles are ovicidal as well. This means that transfer to clean pastures after treatment can be made with minimal risk of contamination and subsequent re-infection.

The benzimidazoles, often referred to as "white drenches" due to their color, are only available for oral use, but a number of oral formulations are available including boluses, pastes, drenches, and feed or salt supplements. The spectrum of activity of these drugs can be a function of dose. Fenbendazole is effective against tapeworms in goats at 15 mg/kg but not at the usual sheep and cattle nematode dose of 5 mg/kg. Parbendazole is effective against *Oesophagostomum* and *Trichostrongylus* spp. at 10 mg/kg, *Teladorsagia* (*Ostertagia*) and *Strongyloides* spp. at 20 mg/kg, and *Nematodirus* spp. at 30 mg/kg (Theodorides et al. 1969). Whipworms that are not commonly killed at recommended doses of benzimidazoles often may be removed by doubling the recommended doses. Albendazole administered either in a single dose of 7.6 mg/kg or two daily doses of 3.8 mg/kg was highly effective against *Teladorsagia* (*Ostertagia*) and *Trichostrongylus* spp., but the latter dose regimen was less effective against *Oesophagostomum venulosum* and neither regimen was effective against *Nematodirus* spp. (Pomroy et al. 1988). A slow-release capsule formulation of albendazole has been evaluated in dairy goats (Chartier et al. 1996a). The capsule contains 3.85 g of the drug and is designed to release 36.7 mg/day for 105 days. This would provide at least 0.5 m/kg of albendazole for goats under 70 kg, which is sufficient to control *Teladorsagia circumcincta*, the dose-limiting species. For non-resistant parasite strains, the treatment eliminated 92% to 99% of existing infections and prevented new infections for eighty-five to ninety-one days post treatment.

As a group, these drugs are quite safe. Thiabendazole has been used safely in goats at doses up to 100 mg/kg (Bell et al. 1962). In toxicity studies of Angora goats, a death loss of 20% was observed at doses of 815 mg/kg (Snijders 1962). It has been suggested that the benzimidazoles can enhance the activity of thiaminase in the gut, thereby increasing the risk of polioencephalomalacia, but field confirmation is limited (Roberts and Boyd 1974). There is concern that overdosing with oxfendazole and its precursors, albendazole, fenbendazole, or febantel, can produce teratogenic effects, particularly if given in the first forty-five days of gestation; fetal defects have been observed in rats. Goats given either febantel or fenbendazole at 50 mg/kg during early pregnancy, however, had no embryotoxic or teratogenic effects (Savitskii 1984). Cambendazole and parbendazole have produced teratogenic effects in sheep in early gestation. This has not been substantiated in goats. However, cambendazole may be toxic when administered to goats on a high grain ration. Grain should be withheld for twenty-four hours before treatment (Howe 1984). Thiabendazole has antimycotic properties and is partially cleared in the milk. It can inhibit inoculation molds used in cheese making.

The pharmacokinetics of at least some benzimidazoles and thus the dose rates are different in goats than in sheep. At an oral dose of 5 mg/kg fenbendazole is absorbed relatively poorly from the gut of goats, with 43% of the dose excreted unchanged in the feces.

Peak mean plasma concentration was 0.13 µg/ml compared with 0.40 µg/ml in sheep (Short 1987). At a dose of 5 mg/kg, fenbendazole was undetectable in the milk of lactating does by forty-eight hours, and by seventy-two hours at a dose of 25 mg/kg (Waldhalm et al. 1989).

MACROCYCLIC LACTONES. The macrocyclic lactone anthelmintic class is comprised of avermectins and milbemycins, all of which are derived from soil microorganisms of the genus *Streptomyces*. They are often referred to as the "clear drenches." The commercially available products with use reported in goats include the avermectins ivermectin, doramectin, and eprinomectin, and the milbemycin moxidectin. Despite a comparatively high cost, avermectins are very popular with livestock owners because they have a very broad-spectrum of action against gastrointestinal and pulmonary nematodes including adult worms, infective larvae, and arrested or hypobiotic larvae, as well as activity against some ectoparasites, including mange mites and sucking lice. They also have a persistent effect, continuing to control new infections of gastrointestinal nematodes for up to several weeks following administration.

Ivermectin is the oldest compound in this class, the most studied and most widely used. The drug is available for oral, subcutaneous, or topical use. Pharmacokinetic studies indicate that the bioavailability of ivermectin in goats is less than that of sheep and cattle (Alvinerie et al. 1993; Lanusse et al. 1997; González et al. 2006). Accordingly, the current recommended dose for goats is 300 to 400 µg/kg bw, which is one and a half to two times the cattle and sheep dose (200 µg/kg). A double sheep dose requires an extension of the meat withdrawal time to fourteen days and a milk withdrawal of nine days (Baynes et al. 2000). The drug has a wide margin of safety. There are anecdotal reports of goat owners giving an entire tube of ivermectin paste formulated for an adult horse to a goat with no ill effect. Ivermectin, however, may be highly irritating to some individual goats when given subcutaneously. These goats may run around frantically after injection and attempt to rub the injection site vigorously against available objects. If the injection is given in the neck, they may throw their heads back, giving the suggestion of opisthotonos. However, the reaction invariably subsides within several minutes and no lasting local or systemic effects have been reported. The drug is highly lipophilic and as such, it concentrates in milk. Therefore it cannot be used in lactating animals, and if given subcutaneously in error, a meat withdrawal time of 35 days and milk withdrawal of 40 days are recommended (Baynes et al. 2000).

Eprinomectin is the least lipophilic of the macrocyclic lactones. Because of its partitioning profile between serum and milk, only 0.1% of the total topical dose is eliminated in the milk of cows and it is approved for use lactating dairy cattle with no milk withholding time worldwide. By contrast, 2.9% of the total subcutaneous dose of doramectin was recovered from milk, while 5.7% and 22.5% of an oral or subcutaneous dose of moxidectin were recovered from milk in goats (Carceles et al. 2001). Pharmacokinetic studies indicate that the systemic availability of eprinomectin is significantly lower in goats than in cattle (Alvinerie et al. 1999). Also, it has been noted that the mean residence time for the presence of eprinomectin in the lactating goat is markedly less (2.67 days) than in non-lactating goats (9.42 days) and that 0.3% to 0.5% of the total drug dose given is recovered in the milk with residues never exceeding the maximum acceptable limit set for cattle (Dupuy et al. 2001).

There is good evidence that the effective dose of eprinomectin in goats is 1 mg/kg, which is twice the established cattle dose of 0.5 mg/kg. In one study, at the dose of 0.5 mg/kg, applied topically, the drug had limited effectiveness against *T. colubriformis* in experimentally infected goats (Chartier et al. 1999), while in another study of naturally infected goats, fecal egg counts were reduced only 59.5% in adults and 89.9% in yearlings after topical treatment with the cattle dose (Gawor et al. 2000). In contrast, eprinomectin was 100% effective in eliminating existing worm burdens of *T. circumcincta* and *T. colubriformis* when given at a topical dose of 1 mg/kg (Chartier and Pors 2004). In an Italian study, reduction in fecal egg counts for naturally infected goats at seven days post treatment was 90% for goats receiving 0.5 mg/kg topically and 99.5% for goats receiving 1 mg/kg (Cringoli et al. 2004). Though eprinomectin is available only as a topical formulation, studies indicate that subcutaneous administration is two and a half times more efficient than topical administration in terms of the amount of drug present in the goat (Lespine et al. 2003). Moxidectin, though not approved in goats, has been reported to be effective at a dose of 0.2 mg/kg bw (Pomroy et al. 1992; Praslicka et al. 1994). At that dose, the subcutaneous route is preferred to the oral route in goats due to a superior pharmacokinetic profile of the parenteral route. If given orally to goats, the dose should be doubled to 0.4 mg/kg (Kaplan 2006).

A notable aspect of the macrocyclic lactones for use in grazing animals is their persistence of efficacy. Some studies have been done specifically on the persistence of eprinomectin in goats. In naturally infected goats in Italy with mixed infections of *H. contortus*, *T. circumcincta*, *T. colubriformis*, and *O. venulosum*, topical treatment with eprinomectin at 1 mg/kg resulted in fecal egg count reductions of 99.5% at seven days post treatment, 99.6% at fourteen days, 99.7% at twenty-one days, and 96.7% at twenty-eight days (Cringoli et al. 2004). In a Polish study, fecal egg count reductions of 97.6% in adult goats and 88.5% in yearling goats were recorded at fifty-six days after topical dosing at 1 mg/kg (Gawor et al. 2000).

Persistence of anthelmintic effect has also been assessed for doramectin and moxidectin in goats. Moxidectin given orally at 0.2 mg/kg bw was 99.7% effective against *H. contortus* at twenty-nine days post treatment and 100% at twenty-two days. There was also a high degree of protection at twenty-nine days (94.9%) against *Teladorsagia circumcincta* but no protective effect at all was seen against *Trichostrongylus colubriformis* (Torres-Acosta and Jacobs 1999). A failure to protect completely against *T. colubriformis* was also noted in goats with eprinomectin (Chartier et al. 1999). Doramectin at a dose of 0.2 mg/kg SQ protected goats against *H. contortus* for fourteen to twenty-five days post treatment. This was about half the time of protection recorded in cattle, suggesting that the proper doramectin dose for goats requires further calibration (Molina et al. 2005). While persistence of efficacy may be deemed desirable by producers because it potentially reduces the frequency of treatments, the downside of persistence is that it may contribute to the selection of resistant parasites.

Nematode resistance to the macrocyclic lactones in goats is now widely reported. Ivermectin- and moxidectin-resistant *Trichostrongylus* spp. and *Teladorsagia (Ostertagia)* spp. were identified by fecal egg count reduction tests and larval cultures in goats in Australia (Veale 2002). In another report from New Zealand, *Teladorsagia (Ostertagia)* spp. in goats were resistant to ivermectin and moxidectin each given orally at 0.2 mg/kg bw (Leathwick 1995). Resistance to eprinomectin has been recorded in *H. contortus* in dairy goats in Brazil. While eprinomectin had never previously been used in the herd, ivermectin and moxidectin had been used, indicating the development of cross resistance to this relatively new drug within its class (Chagas et al. 2007).

Cholinergic Agonists. There are two separate classes of anthelmintics that function as cholinergic agonists by interruption of nicotinic acetylcholine receptor functions in the nematode. These are the imidazothiazoles and the tetrahydropyrimidines. Levamisole, an imidazothiazole, is the most widely used drug in this group and may be commonly referred to as the "yellow drench." The spectrum of activity of these drugs against gastrointestinal nematodes is similar to that of the benzimidazoles and may be better than some of the benzimidazoles against *Nematodirus* and *Bunostomum* spp. However, there is minimal effect against arrested larvae and they are not ovicidal. They also have no activity against trematodes or cestodes. Levamisole is the L-isomer of tetramisole, which contains equal amounts of the D and L forms. Only the L form has anthelmintic properties. The racemic mixture was originally marketed as tetramisole at a recommended dose of 15 mg/kg. Currently, levamisole is marketed in the pure levo (L) form at a recommended dose of 8 mg/kg. The drug is available for either oral or subcutaneous use. An oral dose of 12 mg/kg has been established as the effective dose in goats (Coles et al. 1989).

The margin of safety is narrow for levamisole so it must be administered carefully. Even at recommended doses, some goats may demonstrate transient symptoms of depression, muscle fasciculation, salivation, or frothing at the mouth. Clinical signs of intoxication were consistently produced in Angora goats at a dose of 32 mg/kg and deaths occurred at 64 mg/kg (Smith and Bell 1971). Signs of overt toxicity include head shaking, lip smacking, increased salivation, muscle tremors, incoordination, hyperesthesia, clonic convulsions, increased respiratory rate, dyspnea, increased urination and defecation, collapse, and death. Many of these signs may be reversed by administration of atropine sulfate at intravenous doses up to 3 mg/kg, but death may still occur despite this intervention (Hsu 1980). Abortion has been ascribed to levamisole usage in goats at therapeutic levels but no direct link has been substantiated. Administration of levamisole orally at the recommended dose rate of 12 mg/kg bw is highly effective and not associated with any signs of toxicity (Chartier et al. 2000).

The pharmacokinetics of levamisole in goats are notably different than in sheep. Peak plasma concentrations are roughly equivalent in both species after subcutaneous or intramuscular administration but are only 59% of the ovine level in goats after oral administration. Subsequent plasma clearance is two to four times faster in the goat, depending on route of administration (Galtier et al. 1981). These differences have been cited as the cause of so-called treatment failures in the field (Gillham and Obendorf 1985). The elimination half-life of levamisole in goats is 222 minutes. The majority (55%) is excreted in urine, and 30% in feces. Less than 1% of the total dose is excreted in the milk (Nielsen and Rasmussen 1983). Goats exhibit a genetic polymorphism regarding the clearance rate of levamisole that may affect efficacy in field use (Babish et al. 1990).

The tetrahydropyrimidines include salts of pyrantel and morantel. Pyrantel tartrate at a dose of 25 mg/kg in goats was reported to be 98% to 100% effective against *Trichostrongylus, Ostertagia, Nematodirus, Bunostomum,* and *Strongyloides* spp., 97% effective against *Cooperia*, 91% against *Haemonchus*, and 70% against *Oesophagostomum* (Martinez Gomez 1968). However, in another experimental study in goats, the drug was highly effective against the abomasal worms *H. contortus* and *T. circumcincta*, but only 55% effective in goats against the intestinal worm, *T. colubriformis*, even at a dose of 40 mg/kg. This was due to host factors and not resistance in the parasite (Chartier et al. 1995). Morantel is a methyl analog of pyrantel and has become more commonly used. It can be used at a lesser dose than pyrantel (12.5 mg/kg) with equivalent efficacy against gastrointestinal nematodes (Anderson and Marais 1972). In experimental infections of goats and sheep, morantel citrate at an oral dose of 10 mg/kg was less effective against *Teladorsagia* (*Ostertagia*) spp. and *Trichostrongylus* spp. in goats than in sheep, suggesting that dosages specific for goats need to be established by pharmacokinetic studies (McKenna and Watson 1987; Elliot 1987). Morantel tartrate given orally at 10 mg/kg to goats was highly effective against *Haemonchus*, *Bunostomum*, and *Oesophagostomum* spp. but showed little effect against *Strongyloides papillosus* and *Trichuris* spp. (Chandrasekharan et al. 1973). Morantel is available as a sustained release bolus for continuous parasite control in cattle on pasture, but this formulation should not be used in goats or sheep.

When resistance is encountered to levamisole, it is presumed that such nematodes are also resistant to morantel; however, the converse may not be true. In an Australian study, trichostrongyles resistant to morantel remained susceptible to levamisole. It was recommended that morantel should be used in deworming programs until resistance is detected, at which time levamisole may be substituted for improved efficacy (Waller et al. 1986).

Organophosphates. Haloxon, coumaphos, and naphthalophos are the organophosphate anthelmintics that have received the most attention in goats. These drugs are most effective against *Haemonchus*, *Teladorsagia* (*Ostertagia*), and *Trichostrongylus* spp., moderately effective against *Nematodirus* spp., and have little or no efficacy against other gastrointestinal nematodes (Andersen and Christofferson 1973; McDougald et al. 1968). They have been available in drench, paste, bolus, and feed-additive formulations for oral use only. Coumaphos is also available as a topical pour-on, which should not be used in lactating does.

When used at prescribed doses, the acute toxicity potential of these compounds is low. However, haloxon has been demonstrated as a cause of delayed neurotoxicity in sheep, particularly Suffolk sheep and other breeds that may lack an esterase necessary to degrade haloxon. The condition manifests as progressive ataxia and paresis several weeks after administration of the drug. Since this discovery, haloxon has fallen into disfavor and has been removed from the market in many countries. There is no definitive evidence that the same syndrome occurs in goats, although there is the suggestion that it has been observed in Angora goats in Texas (Wilson et al. 1982).

Salicylanilides. These compounds, which include closantel, oxyclosanide, and rafoxanide, have efficacy primarily against trematodes and not nematodes and are discussed in more detail in the section on trematode infections of the liver. They are mentioned here because many show some efficacy against *H. contortus*. Because *H. contortus* resistance to other classes of broad-spectrum anthelmintics is increasing, salicylanilides may be useful in control of haemonchosis. In the humid tropics, haemonchosis and fascioliasis may be the primary parasite problems, making salicylanilides an appropriate therapeutic choice where resistance has not developed. Regarding toxicity, blindness caused by degeneration of the optic tracts has been reported in kids overdosed with closantel at four to thirteen times the recommended dose rate of 7.5 mg/kg (Button et al. 1986).

Miscellaneous Anthelmintics. Phenothiazine is one of the oldest drugs used in control of caprine nematode infection and it has been largely replaced by newer drugs. The drug is administered orally in a micronized form because small particle size increases efficacy. Bolus, drench, and powdered forms have been available and the powder has been incorporated into salt blocks for extended administration to inhibit nematode ova production. However, anthelmintic resistance is promoted by the practice and resistance of *H. contortus* in goats to phenothiazine was reported as early as 1967 (Colgazier et al. 1967).

Phenothiazine can produce photosensitization and abortion in goats. Phenothiazine sulfoxide produced in the alimentary tract is the photosensitizing agent. It is normally detoxified by the liver. However, in liver damage or with overdosing, the sulfoxide may concentrate in the skin and aqueous humor. Even at therapeutic doses, healthy Saanens and other light-skinned goats may show erythema and edema of the cornea and eyelids if exposed to direct sunlight after treatment. The same may occur to people handling the drug for administration to goats. The metabolites of phenothiazine excreted in urine and milk impart a pinkish color to these fluids and may stain the hair when animals lie in urine-soaked bedding. Abortion has been reported in goats given phenothiazine during the last three weeks of pregnancy (Osweiler et al. 1988).

Anthelmintic Resistance

Unfortunately, at present, there are no assurances that use of the anthelmintics just discussed will provide effective therapy for goats with clinical gastrointestinal nematodiasis. Parasite resistance to anthelmintics is widely recognized as a growing problem in the treatment and control of gastrointestinal nematodiasis in small ruminants (Coles 1986; Waller 1987; Wolstenholme et al. 2004; Kaplan 2006; Fleming et al. 2006). It has received more attention in sheep but is increasingly identified in goats. Early reports of the problem in goats were from Australia (Barton et al. 1985), New Zealand (Kettle et al. 1983), the United States (Uhlinger et al. 1988), France (Kerboeuf and Hubert 1985), and the United Kingdom (Scott et al. 1989).

In New Zealand surveys, the prevalence of nematode resistance was much higher on dairy goat farms than on sheep farms, as was the number of resistant species found. Based on post drenching larval cultures, resistant parasites included *Haemonchus*, *Teladorsagia* (*Ostertagia*), and *Trichostrongylus* spp. On some premises, the nematodes were resistant to anthelmintics in both the benzimidazole and cholinergic agonist classes. The degree of resistance on farms was positively correlated with the frequency of drenching, which was, on average, 12.5 times a year for kids and 13.4 times a year for adults (Kettle et al. 1983).

The anthelmintic resistance problem in goats has grown even more serious since the 1990s, with additional reports of benzimidazole resistant *Teladorsagia (Ostertagia)* spp. and *H. contortus* in goats in Scotland (Jackson et al. 1992) England and Wales (Hong et al. 1996), benzimidazole resistance for multiple trichostrongyles in goats in France (Beugnet 1992; Chartier et al. 1998a, 2001), avermectin resistance in *Teladorsagia* (*Ostertagia*) spp. of Angora goats in New Zealand (Badger and McKenna 1990) and trichostrongyles of dairy goats in Argentina (Aguirre et al. 2002).

Of greatest concern is the increased documentation of multiple anthelmintic resistance on goat farms involving two or more of the three major classes of broad spectrum anthelmintic drugs: the benzimidazoles; the cholinergic agonists such as levamisole (an imidazothiazole) and morantel (a tetrahydropyrimidine); and/or, the macrocyclic lactones, such as ivermectin (an avermectin) and moxidectin (a milbemycin).

Multiple resistance of one or more trichostrongyles to all three classes of broad-spectrum drugs has been reported in Saanen dairy goats (Watson and Hosking 1990) and purebred goats of unspecified breed in New Zealand (West et al. 2004), Angora goats in the United Kingdom (Coles et al. 1996), mixed breed meat goats in Virginia (Zajac and Gipson 2000), Spanish meat goats and Nubian cross dairy goats in Georgia (Terrill et al. 2001), and meat and dairy goats in Georgia and South Carolina (Mortensen et al. 2003).

In Kenya, resistance of *H. contortus* in goats was documented against benzimidazoles, levamisole, and a different third class of anthelmintic, the salicylanilides, represented by rafoxanide, while ivermectin remained effective (Waruiru et al. 1998). Notable with regard to the implications for international trade in livestock is a report of resistance to the three major classes of anthelmintic for *Trichostrongylus* spp. and *Teladorsagia (Ostertagia)* spp. in cashmere and Angora goats imported into the former Czechoslovakia from New Zealand (Varady et al. 1993). There is also a report from Switzerland on resistance of *H. contortus* to benzimidazoles and ivermectin in Boer goats imported from South Africa (Schnyder et al. 2005).

Some presumed cases of anthelmintic resistance may be in fact treatment failures that occur when anthelmintics are under dosed, or when doses prescribed for sheep are assumed to be effective in the goat. In an Australian study, *Haemonchus*, *Trichostrongylus*, and *Teladorsagia* (*Ostertagia*) nematodes in naturally infected dairy goats demonstrated marked apparent resistance to albendazole, fenbendazole, levamisole, morantel, naphthalophos, and phenothiazine used at prescribed sheep doses. However, when the surviving larvae were cultured and introduced into worm-free sheep, infections were effectively cleared by these same anthelmintics at the same doses (Hall et al. 1981). Similarly, in France, grazing goats treated with benzimidazoles continued to pass ova of *Haemonchus*, *Trichostrongylus*, and *Ostertagia*, while identically treated, commingled sheep had a total suppression of egg output (Kerboeuf and Hubert 1985). In the United States, thiabendazole administered at the same dose to commingled sheep and goats was moderately effective against *Haemonchus* in sheep but totally ineffective in goats (Andersen and Christofferson 1973). Similarly, the bioavailability of oxfendazole is reported to be less in goats than in sheep after a single equivalent oral dose (Bogan et al. 1987). Differences in pharmacokinetics and bioavailability between sheep and goats for other anthelmintics have been documented as well, such as for levamisole (Galtier et al. 1981), fenbendazole (Short 1987), albendazole (Hennessy et al. 1993), closantel (Hennessy et al. 1993a), and the macrocyclic lactones (Chartier et al. 2001a).

These results indicate that many anthelmintics do not achieve therapeutic levels in goats at commonly used sheep dosages. In fact, one study has definitively demonstrated that *Trichostrongylus* presumed to be resistant to levamisole in goats were indeed sensitive to levamisole *in vitro*. The presumed resistance was in essence a treatment failure because levamisole given to goats at the sheep dose of 7.5 mg/kg did not maintain adequate plasma levels for sufficient duration to be effective against this particular parasite (Gillham and Obendorf 1985).

The pharmacokinetic differences between sheep and goats for common anthelmintics have become widely acknowledged. Many authorities now routinely suggest that when goat doses for an anthelmintic are not specifically given, the sheep dose should be increased by one and a half to two times for use in goats, with the caveat that potentially toxic drugs such as levamisole should be given to goats only at a maximum of one and a half times the sheep dose per oral route (Smith 2005).

Over time, treatment failures contribute to the development of anthelmintic resistance, as suboptimal dosing favors the selection and survival of subpopulations of resistant parasites. Nematode parasites are also capable of developing an intrinsic resistance to anthelmintics that is genetically based. The mechanisms by which parasite resistance develops against different classes of anthelmintics in different species of nematodes are not fully understood, but some are known. Resistance to avermectins by *H. contortus* for example, is reported to be controlled by an autosomal, completely dominant gene in larvae, but in adult worms, its expression is sex-influenced, with males having lower resistance than females (Le Jambre et al. 2000). Benzimidazole resistance in trichostrongyles of small ruminants involves a mutation of phenylalanine to tyrosine at residue 200 of the isotype 1 β-tubulin gene and is a recessive trait (Elard and Humbert 1999).

It is clear that the use of any anthelmintic selects for populations of nematodes that can resist its lethal effects and that repeated use of that anthelmintic over time in a herd or flock results in the emergence of parasite populations that are widely resistant to that anthelmintic. The severity of the problem is exacerbated by the fact that when a population of parasites has evolved that shows resistance to a given anthelmintic, that population generally manifests resistance to all drugs in that anthelmintic class because they share a similar or identical mechanism of action. It is therefore necessary to switch to drugs from a different class to overcome a resistance problem, although there is no guarantee that populations resistant to other classes of drugs have not also evolved. In fact, as discussed above, there are already numerous reports of parasite populations in goats that have developed resistance to all three major classes of anthelmintic drugs.

Regrettably, anthelmintics have become a victim of their own success. When modern anthelmintics emerged in the 1960s and 1970s, they were so effective and relatively inexpensive that many producers came to depend on anthelmintics as the sole or predominant tool for parasite control, often applying frequent, repeated dosing on a calendar basis without regard to strategic or tactical justification. Such indiscriminate use was an engine driving the development of anthelmintic resistance, because repeated use of an anthelmintic selects for the survival of parasite populations that are resistant to it. There are now serious concerns that if anthelmintic resistance continues to spread, effective products will no longer be available in the near future. This concern is exacerbated by the fact that development of new classes or types of anthelmintics for use in ruminant livestock no longer appears to be a priority of the veterinary pharmaceutical companies (Geary et al. 1999). Therefore, many authorities are emphasizing techniques and practices that can be employed to slow the development of anthelmintic resistance and promote wise use of the anthelmintics that are still effective (Kaplan 2006; Van Wyk et al. 2006). A summary of these suggestions follows.

Manage the Introduction of New Stock. Resistant parasites are most often introduced into a herd or flock via the purchase of new stock. All new animals should be dewormed with double doses of broad-spectrum, nontoxic anthelmintics from at least two different classes before adding them to the existing herd or flock. They should be held in a dry lot for at least three days after treatment so that infective eggs not killed by non-ovicidal drugs are passed before turnout to pasture. Ideally, they should be held out for ten days until a follow-up fecal examination confirms that egg counts approach zero. These animals should be turned out to a dirty pasture so that any eggs from resistant worms that they may still be carrying will be diluted by eggs/larvae already on pasture.

Determine the Resistance Profile of the Herd. Given the current extent of anthelmintic resistance, particularly with regard to benzimidazoles, rational and effective use of anthelmintics requires knowledge of existing resistance patterns in a herd or flock. Several tools are available to accomplish this and the subject has been reviewed (Taylor et al. 2002; Coles et al. 2006). The most commonly used tests in small ruminants are the fecal egg count reduction test (FECRT) and the larval development assay (LDA) (Kaplan 2006).

As the name implies, the FECRT involves counting of parasite ova in feces before treatment with a specific class of anthelmintic, and then again at a prescribed time following treatment to determine response to therapy based on significant reduction of egg counts. The test is conducted as follows (Coles et al. 2006).

- Distribute goats into groups either randomly or balanced based on preliminary egg counts.
- Use animals three to six months of age or, if older, with egg counts greater than 150 eggs per gram (epg). Identify animals individually.
- Use at least ten animals per group if possible. The number of groups depends on the number of classes of anthelmintic to be tested. An untreated control group should be included to account for natural changes in egg counts possible during the period of the test.
- Collect 3 to 5 g of feces from each animal into separate containers, identifying samples to correlate with specific animals.
- Count eggs using the McMaster technique as soon as possible after collection.
- Only store at 4°C (39.2°F) for no more than twenty-four hours if samples will also be used for larval culture.
- Individually weigh animals and give the established or presumed caprine dose orally over the base of the tongue.

- Collect post treatment fecal samples at the following intervals: Levamisole group, three to seven days; benzimidazole group, eight to ten days; macrocyclic lactones group, fourteen to seventeen days, as discussed further below.
- Count eggs using the McMaster technique as soon as possible after collection.
- Greater than 95% reduction in fecal egg counts for a group indicates susceptibility of the parasites present and that the anthelmintic tested should still be useful for parasite control in the herd.
- When resistance is encountered, a composite fecal sample of 50 g from group members should be collected for larval culture and identification to determine the resistant species of parasites.

With regard to the timing of the post treatment collection of fecal samples, the intervals indicated above were proposed to make allowances for the temporary suppression of egg production which sometimes occurs after treatment even if adults are not killed. However, these proposed intervals are acknowledged to be best guesses (Coles et al. 2006). Where more than one anthelmintic type is being evaluated in a herd, the longer interval of fourteen days should be used with the understanding that levamisole does not have a high efficacy against intestinal L4 stages of nematode parasites. A post treatment interval of ten to eleven days may be best for assessment of levamisole by FECRT if multiple drugs are being evaluated simultaneously.

An alternative to FECRT is the microagar larval development assay (LDA), which is akin to antibiotic sensitivity testing. Eggs are harvested from the fecal sample and larvae are cultured from the eggs in microtiter plates with different anthelmintics added to the wells. Inhibition of larval growth indicates effectiveness of the anthelmintic, while development of the larvae indicates resistance. Surviving larvae are then identified by species. The LDA is more convenient for owners and practitioners because a single composite fecal sample from ten to twenty goats in the herd can be submitted one time for evaluation. The mean fecal egg count in the sample should be greater than 350 epg, but samples with a mean greater than 500 epg are preferred.

The one time cost for the LDA is fairly high, but when weighed against the time and expense of multiple sampling and egg counting needed to test for all three major anthelmintic classes using the FECRT, the cost is reasonable. In the United States, the LDA is offered by the University of Georgia under the original Australian marketed name, Drenchrite®, and information about the test and sample submissions is available at the website of the Southern Consortium for Small Ruminant Parasite Control (SCSRPC), www.scsrpc.org.

Administer and Dose Anthelmintics Appropriately. The persistence of infection after anthelmintic therapy is not always caused by the development of anthelmintic resistance. Inadequate or improper dosing is a major cause of treatment failure and may be due to several causes. Ideally, anthelmintics should be administered on a per weight basis to each animal. Practically, this is not commonly done, because weights are guessed or average doses administered when large numbers of animals require treatment. To minimize this problem, animals should be grouped according to size for drenching and the weight of the largest animal in the group accurately determined. All animals in the group should be given the dose calculated for the largest individual in the group. Doses specific for goats should be used when known based on scientific reports or proven, goat-specific manufacturers recommendations. However, if goat specific dosages are not available, then it is suggested that sheep dewormers be used at one and a half to two times the recommended sheep dose to account for pharmacokinetic differences in the two species (Smith 2005). For anthelmintics with potential toxicity, such as levamisole or moxidectin, only a one and a half time increase should be used.

Automatic dosing or drenching equipment should be checked before use to ensure the accuracy of doses dispensed. The tip of the drenching instrument should be carefully placed so that the anthelmintic is deposited over the base of the tongue. This facilitates passage of the drug directly into the rumen. If dispensed more anteriorly in the mouth, closure of the esophageal groove may be triggered and the drug will bypass the rumen, thus reducing its efficacy, especially in the case of benzimidazoles and macrocyclic lactones.

Holding animals off feed for twenty-four hours before drenching with benzimidazoles also helps to ensure that the drug is distributed properly and with the desired contact time. However, withholding feed is not advised for pregnant does due to the risk of inciting pregnancy toxemia. There is no added benefit to withholding feed with oral administration of levamisole or moxidectin (Kaplan 2006). Fasting for thirty-six hours before treatment was reported to not have any affect on the kinetic disposition, bioavailability, or retention time of ivermectin in goats (Escudero et al. 1997).

Another technique for extending contact time may be to repeat dosages of the anthelmintic at twelve-hour intervals, particularly when using benzimidazoles. In one study, two 10 mg/kg oral doses of fenbendazole given twelve hours apart produced a 92% reduction in fecal egg counts, whereas a single dose given to the same herd seven months earlier produced only a 50% reduction (Zajac and Gipson 2000).

These practices are important because the site of deposition of the drug can affect anthelmintic efficacy, particularly with the benzimidazoles. The effect of benzimidazoles is correlated with the contact time of parasite with drug. When these drugs are administered in the rumen and slowly absorbed into the bloodstream, the distribution and excretion phases are of appropriate length to ensure anthelmintic activity at prescribed doses. If the esophageal groove closes during administration of these drugs and they are deposited into the abomasum, then the periods of distribution and excretion, and hence, contact time with the parasites, are shortened and efficacy suffers.

Minimize Number of Treatments. The number of treatments administered during the course of a year should be kept to a minimum level because it has been demonstrated that the development of resistance correlates directly with the frequency of dosing. This underscores the importance of identifying and using strategic and tactical treatments based on the ecology of parasites and actual assessments of parasite burdens by techniques such as fecal egg counts rather than deworming simply on a calendar basis.

Consider Giving Two Anthelmintics at the Same Time. While drugs are still effective, treating simultaneously with two drugs from different classes of anthelmintics may delay the development of resistance (Kaplan 2006). Even when some resistance is present, there are reports that drugs may act synergistically to provide some protection even when alone, they are ineffective. In a report from Texas, Angora goats infected with *H. contortus* having known resistance to all three major classes of anthelmintics were treated with fenbendazole alone, levamisole alone, and the two in combination. Based on FECRT, the drugs together produced a 62% reduction in epg while fenbendazole alone produced a 1% reduction and levamisole alone a 23% reduction (Miller and Craig 1996). In another study of fiber goats in the former Czechoslovakia, resistance to all three classes of anthelmintic was well documented, but combination treatment of albendazole and levamisole completely cleared infections in Cashmere goats while a combination of albendazole, levamisole, and ivermectin completely cleared infection in Angora goats. The resistant nematodes were *Trichostrongylus* spp. and *Ostertagia* spp. (Varady et al. 1993).

Treat Selectively. A new emerging strategy for reducing the rate of development of anthelmintic resistance in a herd is to target specific animals within the herd for anthelmintic treatment rather than treating the whole herd. There are two key principles underlying this approach. The first is that only a comparatively small percentage of animals in any given herd is responsible for the bulk of the parasite load, with an estimated 20% to 30% of the animals harboring 80% of the worms (Kaplan 2006). The second is that by not treating the remainder of the herd, the untreated animals will deposit significant numbers of eggs from parasites not selected for resistance by treatment onto pastures and thereby dilute the population of eggs and infective larvae from resistant worms. These populations of non-resistant eggs and infective larvae are referred to as refugia and are considered by some to be the most potent factor in mitigating the development of anthelmintic resistance (Van Wyk 2001).

Because the animals harboring the largest number of worms are the most likely to develop signs of parasitism, various techniques may be employed to identify those animals in the herd and treat them selectively. In the case of *Haemonchus contortus*, which produces anemia in affected animals, a screening system based on assessment of the color of the conjunctiva was developed in South Africa, known as the FAMACHA© system. The development, application, and impact of the FAMACHA© system have been reviewed (Van Wyk and Bath 2002). The system was specifically designed for use with sheep. A laminated card depicts the color of sheep ocular mucous membranes representing five different categories of anemia from none to severe associated with membrane colors from red (1) to white (5). The card is brought to the field and animals' membranes are matched to the card. Only sheep having scores consistent with anemia—scores of 4 and 5 or 3, 4, and 5, as reported in different studies—are treated. The assessment may be repeated during the grazing season with treatments repeated on anemic animals. This selective deworming based on clinical signs leaves the clinically unaffected and less infected animals to continue to shed eggs of mainly non-resistant parasites onto pastures, and contribute to the pasture load of eggs and larvae in refugia. In South African reports, relatively few individual animals require repeated treatments within a flock over one season and those that do are candidates for culling if efforts to select for parasite resistance are undertaken.

The FAMACHA© scoring card has been evaluated for use in goats by comparison of scores with packed cell volumes and/or fecal egg counts and its reliability in goats has been validated in South Africa (Vatta et al. 2001; Jeyakumar 2007), the United States (Kaplan et al. 2004; Burke et al. 2007), Germany (Koopmann et al. 2006), Kenya (Ejlertsen et al. 2006), Brazil (Molento et al. 2004), and Guadeloupe (Mahieu et al. 2007). The FAMACHA© system has been recognized as particularly useful for the southern United States where *Haemonchus contortus* is the predominant pathogenic nematode confronting the growing meat goat industry. Use of FAMACHA© in the southern United States is being strongly promoted by the Southern Consortium for Small Ruminant Parasite Control (SCSRPC) and the group provides access to abundant information about FAMACHA© and other aspects of parasite control to minimize anthelmintic resistance at their Website www.scsrpc.org.

Veterinarians must work closely with producers, who should be specifically trained on the use of FAMACHA©. Faulty interpretation of charts and improper selection of animals for treatments could lead to unexpected deaths if severe anemia is overlooked. In addition, in some areas, hemoparasites may also contribute to anemia, thereby confounding the interpretation of anemia scores and diminishing the expected response to anthelmintic therapy. Producers also must understand that the system applies only to gastrointestinal parasitism caused by *H. contortus*. The other clinically important trichostrongyles are not hematophagous and therefore do not produce anemia as a criterion for selection. In those cases, if the principle of selective treatment is going to be applied, then other parameters for selection must be used, such as individual fecal egg counts, total protein measurements, body condition scores, or the presence of diarrhea in animals unlikely to have other gastrointestinal diseases.

For dairy goats, it may be possible to apply selective treatment on the basis of age and production level. Epidemiologic studies in France indicate that in dairy herds, goats in first lactation and multiparous does with the highest level of milk production before the beginning of the grazing season have the highest burdens of and impact from parasitism compared to herd mates (Hoste and Chartier 1993, 1998a). In a controlled trial, a dairy herd was divided into two balanced groups with all goats in one group treated once with oxfendazole during the grazing season but only first lactation does and heavy producers treated similarly in the second group, with the groups grazed on separate pastures after treatment and monitored monthly. The results indicated a similar level of egg excretion in the two groups as well as similar milk production for both years of the experiment, indicating that similar benefits were achieved by selective treatment with the added benefits of lower treatment costs and some mitigation of the development of parasite resistance in the herd (Hoste et al. 2002).

Rotate Dewormers Rationally. Finally, despite a widespread conviction that rotation of anthelmintics reduces the development of resistance, experimental data suggest that resistance occurs as rapidly with use of multiple anthelmintics as with a single anthelmintic (Le Jambre et al. 1978). Therefore, it is suggested that only a single anthelmintic be used during the entire course of a seasonal exposure to infective larvae. Where larvae are present throughout the year, the anthelmintic may be used until evidence of resistance appears. When subsequent changes are made, the change should be to an anthelmintic of a different chemical class.

Prevention and Control

Over the years, much emphasis has been placed on the strategy of modifying livestock management practices to minimize the animals' exposure to parasites, based on knowledge of life cycles and ecological behavior of those parasites (Baker 1975; Schillhorn van Veen 1982). A seminal notion of parasite control is that gastrointestinal nematodes are primarily a disease of pastures that also involve livestock. With this concept in mind, grazing management control strategies are often developed with the goal of reducing the build up of infective larvae on pasture or when possible, eliminating animal contact with pasture. The role of epidemiological knowledge and grazing management for helminth control in small ruminants has been reviewed (Barger 1999; Waller 2006).

Total confinement or zero-grazing systems are the most aggressive strategy for eliminating the use of pasture. They are most suitable to intensive management systems, such as goat dairying, under conditions in which adequate volumes of stored feed can be grown, processed, and brought to confined goats under economically favorable conditions. When zero grazing is carried out, goats should be housed in a roomy, comfortable, well lit barn or have access to dry lots for general welfare, exercise, and exposure to sunlight. In tropical and subtropical regions, where infective larvae may be continuously present on herbage, goats are often housed in pens with slatted floors, raised off the ground (Figure 10.10). This system reduces parasite exposure, predation, and theft. Many of these animals, however, are fed with fresh herbage cut and carried

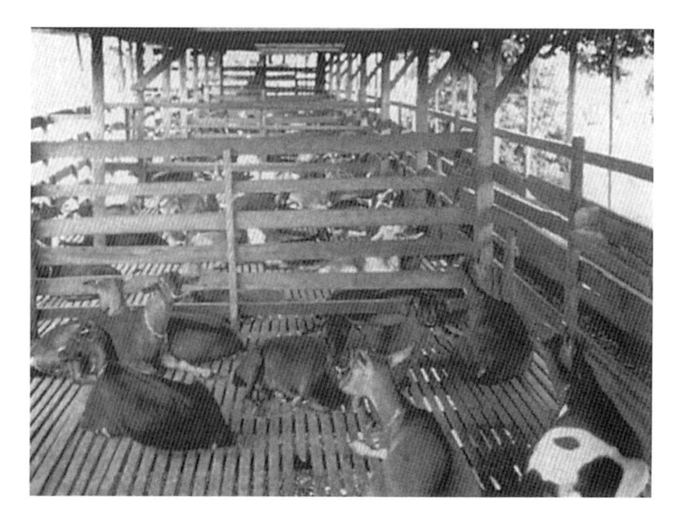

Figure 10.10. In the tropics, goats are often housed in raised pens on slatted floors as a means of controlling gastrointestinal parasitism. If the goats are fed fresh-cut herbage, however, they may still be exposed to infective larvae. (Courtesy of Dr. David M. Sherman.)

daily by caretakers. These feedstuffs may be contaminated with infective larvae from free-ranging goats, sheep, or cattle, and it cannot be safely assumed that penned goats are in fact parasite-free. A Brazilian study has indicated that maintaining goats on raised, slatted floors did not reduce worm burdens compared with goats maintained in corrals with beaten earth floors (Alberto Fagonde Costa and Da Silva Vieira 1987). To be effective, forages must be stored or processed to eliminate the presence of viable larvae. At the least, sun drying of fresh cut grasses before feeding may reduce viable larvae on herbage and improve its dry matter content (Siamba 1990).

In intensive management systems in temperate regions, goats are often continuously housed in barns on solid floors, fed stored feeds such as hay and silage, and allowed exercise in well-drained dry lots. Under these conditions, goats, in most cases, can be maintained relatively free of gastrointestinal nematode parasites, although certain species, e.g., *Skrjabinema*, *Trichuris*, and *Capillaria*, are adapted to successful transmission away from moist herbage. To be totally effective, confinement should be absolute for all age groups in the herd. However, a drawback of total confinement systems is that, if not carefully managed, the advantages gained by controlling nematodiasis may be lost to an increase in coccidiosis and respiratory problems.

Many small dairy herd owners practice only semiconfinement rearing, turning goats out on pasture after winter confinement. These pastures may contain some level of overwintering parasite larvae if stocked with goats the year before. Harsh winters with extended periods of cold or freezing weather sharply reduce larvae on pasture, but even under such conditions, a small proportion of larvae may still survive. After mild winters, the population of overwintering larvae is greater and goats turned out in spring can become infected. By late summer, when weaned kids begin grazing in earnest, pastures can be heavily infected.

Under conditions of seasonal pasturing, two strategic worming interventions may be justified and beneficial, based on the prevailing herd situation. Pregnant does should be dewormed within one month of kidding to minimize the exposure of kids to infective larvae associated with the periparturient egg rise, and all goats, including kids, should be treated with anthelmintics before turn out in the spring. Drugs employed should be effective against both adult and arrested larval stages. When possible, in temperate climates, spring turnout should be onto pastures not grazed by goats or sheep for a full year. In tropical climates, a few months may suffice. Monitoring of infection levels by fecal egg counts from composite fecal samples should be done periodically during the grazing period to determine the need for tactical anthelmintic therapy.

Some strategies for pasture management can reduce parasite burdens and risk to goats in spring. Pasture rotation is important and should be practiced when there is sufficient pasture area available. Avoid using the same pastures for goats two years in a row. Grazing cattle or horses the preceding year, growing and harvesting a hay or grain crop or leaving the land fallow are some options to reduce the risk of dangerous overwintering larvae on a given pasture. Other tools include: maintaining forage height greater than two inches, providing areas of browse within pastures or along fence lines for goats, maintaining a low stocking rate, grazing goats along with cattle, avoiding creation of wet patches associated with leaky waterers, and fencing off of naturally occurring wet patches in pasture (Hale et al. 2007)

In some situations, goats are grazed year-round, but confined at night in corrals for protection. In such a system in Tanzania, with a single rainy season, significant, superior weight gains were achieved in grazing goats when a strategic anthelmintic treatment was administered at the end of the rainy season (Connor et al. 1990).

In extensive grazing systems, continuous or prolonged grazing is the fundamental management scheme, as is often the case in fiber or meat goat production. The extent and severity of parasite infection depends on multiple factors including stocking rates, herbage quantity and quality, season, and weather conditions. For example, Angora goats on the Edwards Plateau in west Texas exhibit a low prevalence of *H. contortus* infection, probably because range is extensive, browse is abundant, and rainfall is limited. When these goats are moved to east Texas and forced to graze intensively on improved pasture with little browse, and much more rainfall, clinical haemonchosis is widespread (Craig 1982).

Careful observation and monitoring of body condition, fecal consistency, and fecal ova counts are advisable in grazing animals to identify the effects of management and weather changes on the incidence of parasitic infection. In the case of haemonchosis, if 5% to 10% of the herd have fecal egg counts of 500 eggs per gram of feces or more, then tactical treatment is justified before the onset of clinical signs. Where *H. contortus* is the principal concern, FAMACHA© scores can be used for monitoring and/or planning intervention.

When the predominant parasites and their behavior are well known, problems may be anticipated without monitoring. In Texas, tactical anthelmintic therapy has been automatically given to grazing Angora goats after heavy rains on the reasonable presumption that acute haemonchosis is likely to ensue because of rapid, synchronous larval development. The use of tactical treatments must be weighed against concerns of promoting anthelmintic resistance. For best effect, tactical treatments should be accompanied by movement of stock to clean pastures to avoid immediate re-infection on contaminated herbage. If strip grazing is practiced, care must be taken that restricted grazing areas are of sufficient size for the animal population. Otherwise, the rate and intensity of larval buildup may be severe enough that the presumed beneficial effect of strip grazing is negated. The smaller the strip, the more frequently animals should be moved.

Drought affects the use of pastures. Management changes made in response to drought, such as congregation of animals for supplemental feeding and watering, may precipitate an increased incidence of parasitism. Supplemental feed should be fed in feeders, not from the ground, and should be provided at multiple sites, spread out to avoid the intensification of parasite ova in places of high animal density. This is even more important with point source water supplies. If runoff or seepage from tanks or troughs is not properly avoided or drained away, heavy contamination of the soil with infective larvae can occur at points where goats congregate to drink.

In tropical regions, extensive grazing is often practiced and the lack of seasonal changes in temperature and humidity allows infective larvae to be continuously present in the environment. In this situation, the frequent, regular use of anthelmintics is often practiced to limit resident worm populations and minimize the effects of parasitism in goats. This approach is labor-intensive and costly, and can accelerate the development of drug resistance. If such suppressive treatment regimens are necessary, it may be helpful to use limited-spectrum anthelmintics when the local parasite population permits it. For example, salicylanilides could be useful where the primary nematode problem is *H. contortus* and broad-spectrum therapy is not required. Three week treatment intervals are suggested so that larvae ingested since the preceding treatment will not have yet matured to adulthood and begun producing ova. Rotation of anthelmintics among the different classes of available drugs should be kept to a minimum, because too frequent rotation of drugs within an active season or cycle of parasite development can itself promote resistance. Also, when haemonchosis is the main concern, as it often is in tropical environments, selective deworming based on FAMACHA© scores can help keep parasites under control while reducing the use of anthelmintics and increasing the proportion of larvae from non-resistant larvae on pasture (in refugia). Whenever local conditions allow, producers should be encouraged to raise goats in confinement in raised pens on slotted floors, and not feed them fresh cut herbage. Effective grazing systems have been developed for the tropics wherein small ruminants are moved to a new area of pasture after three to four days of grazing and not returned to the previous area for about one month (Barger 1999; Waller 2006). A longer rest period is required in cooler climates, because the larvae survive longer on pasture.

Where grazing of goats is practiced, mixed grazing of different livestock species is being recommended as a means of parasite control on the presumption that even though cross-species transmission can occur, the parasites infecting one species are less suited to an alternative host and will therefore result in a less severe infection. The net effect is one of dilution of the parasites most infective for each host species. Another effect is less competition for available herbage and browse among grazing animals with different feeding preferences, leading to a better plane of nutrition for all. In Texas, goats make up 20% to 40% of the grazing population and may be mixed with sheep, cattle, deer, or any combination of the three. Mixed grazing, however, does open the door to potential cross transmission of other diseases such as paratuberculosis.

In the face of growing anthelmintic resistance, other approaches to parasite control are also being adopted or explored. Selective deworming is one such approach, aimed at increasing the number of non-resistant parasites in refugia, as discussed above. Other approaches include breeding and selecting stock for parasite resistance, using forages with anthelmintic properties, administering copper oxide wires, and using anti-nematodal fungi. They are discussed briefly as follows.

Resistance can be defined as the ability of an animal to suppress establishment and/or subsequent development of worm infection. As discussed earlier, there is good evidence of a genetic basis for helminth resistance in small ruminants and some heritability estimates have been reported for different breeds of goats relative to different parasites under a variety of environmental conditions. At present, there is little documentation in the literature that farmers are applying selective breeding to their herds and flocks for improved parasite control, but the experimental evidence indicates that it has potential as a useful parasite management tool and no doubt some are practicing it. Owners can select a breed with known resistance characteristics, or they can attempt selective breeding for resistance within their own herds. Veterinarians can work with farmers on the development of these breeding programs. In the published studies, various criteria or markers were used as a basis for selection, including fecal egg counts; packed cell volume; total protein; serum pepsinogen; body condition scoring; or FAMACHA© score based on the type of goat, production system, predominant parasites, and other factors. One important caveat in such an undertaking is that correlations of parasite resistance to other desirable production traits have not been well studied in goats and the risk exists that selection for parasite resistance might also select for loss of desirable production traits. Breeding schemes for small ruminants relative to the development of resistance or resilience to endoparasites in the tropics have been reviewed (Baker and Gray 2004).

Host nutrition can play a significant role in mitigating the effects of parasites. Adequate and proper nutrition, particularly the provision of supplemental protein, can boost host resilience in the face of parasite infestation, and help minimize the adverse affects of the parasite burden (Coop and Kyriazakis 2001). Furthermore, some feeds may have a direct anthelmintic effect, for example, forages high in condensed tannins such as sulla (*Hedysarum coronarium*), birdsfoot trefoil (*Lotus corniculatus*), big trefoil (*Lotus pedunculatus*), sainfoin (*Onobrychis viciafolia*), and sericea lespedeza (*Lespedeza cuneata*). Several controlled studies have demonstrated the capacity of condensed tannin forages to produce an anthelmintic effect on trichostrongyles in goats compared to other forages. These studies include the grazing of sericea lespedeza at pasture in Oklahoma (Min et al. 2004) as well as the feeding of sericea lespedeza as pellets or hay in Georgia (Shaik et al. 2006; Terrill et al. 2007). The latter work indicated that the anthelmintic effect is retained through drying, pelleting, and storage of the forage. The mitigating effects produced included a direct anthelmintic effect on the adult worms in the gastrointestinal tract as well as a reduction in parasite egg viability and/or larval development in feces (Shaik et al. 2006). Sericea lespedeza is well suited to the growing conditions of the southern United States and offers a possible adjunct to anthelmintic therapy for parasite control in that region, where the number of goats raised for meat has increased dramatically in recent years, along with a growing problem of gastrointestinal nematodiasis.

Other studies demonstrating anthelmintic effects against trichostrongyles in goats involved the feeding of sainfoin as hay in France (Paolini et al. 2003, 2005) and the feeding of dried leaves of *Acacia karoo* in Zimbabwe (Kahiya et al. 2003).

Another aspect of nutrition with the potential to be exploited for parasite control relates to observations that macrominerals and trace elements may modify the host-parasite relationship. In particular, copper, in the form of copper oxide wire particles (COWP), was demonstrated to have anthelmintic activity against some nematodes in experimentally infected sheep, notably *H. contortus* (Bang et al., 1990). Subsequently a number of studies with COWP have been carried out in goats (Chartier et al. 2000a; Martínez Ortiz de Montellano et al. 2007; Burke et al. 2007a). A recent summary of the outcome of COWP trials in the United States is available on the Internet (Hale et al. 2007).

The source of COWP in these studies is generally a commercially available 2 g gelatin capsule containing COWP with a 1.7 g copper metal content that is marketed for control of copper deficiency and congenital swayback in lambs. Others have used 12.5 or 25 g COWP boluses marketed for cows, but the boluses are repackaged into small gelatin capsules to produce a dosage suitable for small ruminants (Hale et al. 2007). The results of these studies have been varied. The main anthelmintic effect is directed against *H. contortus* as measured by reductions in fecal egg counts or parasite counts at necropsy. Little or no effect has been reported against other abomasal or intestinal trichostrongyles such as *Teladorsagia circumcincta* or *Trichostrongylus colubriformis* in goats. Duration of effect in pastured goats appears to be about three to four weeks, possibly up to six weeks, and the effects are more evident in young goats than adults.

Potential toxicity is a concern, though goats are less susceptible to copper toxicity than sheep. Copper oxide is preferred over other copper salts because of its limited absorption from intestine, thus reducing the risk of toxicity. Dosage is empirical but is generally reported as 0.5 grams for kids and 2 grams for adults. Dosing can be repeated during the grazing season in kids up to a maximum of 2 g total dose. It has been suggested that COWP be administered selectively to heavily parasitized goats based on FAMACHA© scores or other parameters rather than dosing the whole flock because of concerns for development of resistance to COWP. However, the mechanisms of action for COWP are unknown, so risk of resistance is unclear. What is clear is that COWP can be a useful adjunct to parasite control where *H. contortus* is the main concern, but it must be coupled with other interventions in an integrated parasite management program to be most beneficial.

Biological control of parasitic nematodes using nematophagous fungi is another tool currently under evaluation. A number of such fungi, which naturally occur in soil and feces, are known to kill infective third-stage and second-stage larvae, thus reducing the larval burdens in pastures. Some of these fungi, most notably *Duddingtonia flagrans*, are also capable of surviving passage through the alimentary tract of livestock. Therefore, research has been conducted in a variety of livestock species to determine if feeding spores of *D. flagrans* can reduce the number of free living stages of gastrointestinal nematodes in feces and therefore pastures.

Results in species other than goats have been variable but promising. Several experimental studies have now been carried out in goats in the laboratory or in pilot trials (Paraud and Chartier 2003; Waghorn et al. 2003; Terrill et al. 2004; Paraud et al. 2005) which indicate, in general, that the fungus is capable of reducing the number of developing larvae of important parasitic nematodes in the goat. In a field trial (Paraud et al. 2007), young grazing goats in France were given a daily oral dose rate of 10^6 spores/kg body weight for just over three months via inclusion in a mineral mix. Compared to controls, kids receiving the spores showed lower fecal egg counts and serum pepsinogen levels at the end of the grazing season as well as a higher growth rate. Technical challenges regarding the growth of fungal spores in sufficient quantities for commercial markets and challenges in how to reliably and conveniently administer the fungus have slowed the development of marketable, commercial products.

As the prospects for reliable anthelmintic efficacy continue to decline in the face of growing anthelmintic resistance, producers and their veterinarians will have to develop integrated parasite management plans that use a variety of strategies, tools, and practices which are appropriate to the management system, environment, climate, and production goals of the farm under consideration.

Currently, no vaccines are available for controlling gastrointestinal nematodiasis in goats, although the area is one of intense research investigation. One promising focus is the use of parasite gut membrane proteins as antigens for control of *Haemonchus contortus* and other trichostrongyles (Knox, 2000; Knox et al. 2003). There are also preliminary reports on new classes of anthelmintically active compounds. The cyclooctadepsipeptides have a distinctly different mechanism of action than the existing anthelmintic classes (Harder and Samson-Himmelstjerna 2002). Two compounds from this new class have been shown experimentally to possess resistance-breaking properties against benzimidazole-, levamisole- and ivermectin-resistant *H. contortus* from sheep (Samson-Himmelstjerna et al. 2005). Another new class of anthelmintic with a novel mechanism of action, the amino-acetonitrile derivatives, has recently been described and shows efficacy against a broad range of nematodes, including those resistant to existing classes of anthelmintics (Kaminsky et al. 2008). It is not clear if or when commercial products based on these newly reported classes might be available or if resistance will develop against them.

Paramphistomiasis

Paramphistomes are trematode parasites commonly referred to as rumen flukes, stomach flukes, or conical flukes. Adult flukes may be present in the rumen of goats in large numbers, but are essentially nonpathogenic. Clinical paramphistomiasis is associated primarily with the immature forms that feed voraciously in the small intestine before moving to the rumen to mature.

Etiology

Numerous genera in the family Paramphistomatidae infect domestic ruminants. In goats, *Paramphistomum cervi*, *P. explanatum*, *Fischoederius elongatus*, *Gastrothylax crumenifer*, and *Cotylophoron cotylophorum* are found. More recently, *C. travassosi*, *C. bareilliensis*, and *C. fullerborni* also have been reported from goats in Brazil (Cavalcante et al. 2000) and *Paramphistomum daubneyi* from goats in France (Silvestre et al. 2000). These trematodes all have a similar, indirect life cycle involving water snails as intermediate hosts (Soulsby 1982). The size of mature flukes ranges from 5 to 20 mm, making them visible to the unaided eye. They are pink to red. One paramphistome of Asia, *Gigantocotyle explanatum*, migrates to and matures in the bile ducts. It is essentially non-pathogenic, and should not be confused with the pathogenic liver fluke *Dicrocoelium dendriticum*.

Adult paramphistomes inhabit the rumen and lay clear, operculated eggs that are passed in the feces. When feces are passed into water, miracidia develop from these eggs over a period of twelve to twenty-one days, depending on temperature. Swimming miracidia enter water snails of various genera, including *Planorbis*, *Bulinus*, *Lymnaea*, and others. Mature sporocysts containing rediae develop in snails over a period of eleven days. Rediae are released within the snail and after an additional maturation of ten days, contain multiple cercariae. In turn, cercariae are released from rediae and mature within the snail for approximately thirteen more days. Mature cercariae are released from snails into water under stimulation of strong sunlight. Liberated cercariae attach to herbage and encyst as metacercariae, remaining viable for as long as three months.

When ruminants ingest contaminated herbage, metacercariae excyst in the small intestine where they feed aggressively and mature for a period of six to eight weeks. Young flukes then migrate anteriorly to the rumen where they undergo additional maturation after attachment to the rumen mucosa, begin laying eggs, and complete the life cycle. Migration to the rumen and subsequent development in that organ can be delayed or prolonged up to several additional months when fluke infestations are heavy.

Development of flukes varies in goats, cattle, and sheep. After experimental infection of the three ruminants with metacercariae of *P. microbothrium*, migration of maturing flukes from the intestine to the rumen was virtually complete in sheep and cattle by thirty-four days after challenge, but was just beginning in goats at that point, and subsequent egg laying began two weeks later in goats than cattle or sheep (Horak 1967). This prolonged residence of maturing paramphistomes in the small intestine may contribute to increased pathogenicity of the fluke in the goat.

Epidemiology

Though paramphistome infection of domestic ruminants occurs throughout the world, reports of clinical disease have been limited to Africa, Asia, Australasia, eastern Europe, Russia, and the Mediterranean countries (Horak 1971). While most reports involve cattle and sheep, reports of caprine paramphistomiasis from India (Katiyar and Varshney 1963; Chhabra et al. 1978; Rao and Sikdar 1981), Sardinia (Deiana et al. 1962), Bulgaria (Denev et al. 1985), and Pakistan (Mohiuddin et al. 1982) suggest that goats are at risk wherever sheep and cattle are affected. However, one abattoir survey from Iran (Moghaddar and Khanitapeh 2003) identified paramphistome infection in sheep up to 4% but no infection in goats, while a survey in the former Zaire (Chartier et al. 1990) showed an infection rate of 54% in sheep but only 14.8% in goats, so species differences in exposure or response to exposure may occur.

In general, outbreaks of paramphistomiasis are increased during dry seasons when snail and livestock populations become concentrated around shrinking natural water sources with restricted grazing and browsing (Horak 1971). Animals grazing in low-lying, poorly drained, swampy areas or with access to irrigation ditches and other standing water supplies are at high risk of infection caused by increased contact with metacercariae produced by water snails.

In north central India, most outbreaks are seen in small ruminants between late September and January after the rains that promote increases in snail populations. During subsequent dry periods of decreased forage availability, goats may be fed rice paddy straw and other grasses grown underwater that contain large numbers of metacercariae. The disease can be costly. Morbidity rates in goats in India during such outbreaks have been reported in the range of 35% to 79% and fatality rates in the range of 45% to 88% (Katiyar and Varshney 1963). Slaughterhouse surveys in the region show that mature rumen fluke burdens are highest from March to October and lowest from November to February, while immature fluke burdens are highest from September to April, the time period correlating to clinical outbreaks (Gupta et al. 1985).

Pathogenesis

The immature fluke developing in the upper small intestine is most responsible for the pathologic effects of paramphistome infection. These immature flukes embed deeply in the intestinal mucosa via suckers and feed by drawing a plug of mucosa into the sucker. This mucosal plug becomes necrotic and sloughs, leaving an erosion and petechiation. The pathogenicity of the paramphistomes is correlated directly with the immature fluke burden. It is estimated that attachment of 50,000 immature flukes would completely denude the upper 3 m of small intestine, where most paramphistome infections are confined during the developmental stage. Worm burdens of this intensity occur under natural conditions. Large numbers of simultaneously feeding, immature flukes cause marked intestinal irritation and mucosal disruption, leading to hypoproteinemia, diarrhea, and general debilitation.

Clinical Signs

The clinical signs of paramphistomiasis are similar to those of nematode gastroenteritis and the two diseases commonly occur together. Young goats are more frequently and seriously affected than older goats. Affected goats are listless and have diminished appetite. They may be polydipsic, and stand for long periods with their muzzles in the water. They will show a fluid diarrhea that may be projectile at first but later may just drip from the rectum, staining the hindquarters. The diarrhea may contain mucus, epithelial shreds, and immature flukes. It has a characteristic and pronounced fetid odor. Intermandibular edema is pronounced and may extend over the face and brisket. Anemia, if present, is usually mild or moderate. The course of the disease is approximately five to ten days in goats. During that time the animals lose weight, get progressively weaker, and eventually die. They may pass nothing but copious mucus from the rectum in the terminal stages. A prolonged form may occur where animals survive but persist in the cachexic state.

Clinical Pathology and Necropsy

Marked hypoproteinemia and hypoalbuminemia occur. Anemia may also be present. Because clinical disease is caused by immature non-egg laying flukes, fecal sedimentation techniques for egg identification have little value because false-negative results would be common. As an alternative to checking for ova, diarrheic feces can be passed through a sieve with 53 μ apertures and the residue examined either microscopically or macroscopically against a black background for immature flukes that are commonly passed in the feces. The immature flukes are pinkish-white with a large prominent sucker (Horak 1971).

At necropsy, the carcass is thin and the hindquarters are soiled with diarrheic feces. Subcutaneous edema, ascites, hydrothorax, hydropericardium, and lung edema may be present. Significant gross lesions of the alimentary tract are limited to the pyloric portion of the abomasum and the first 2 to 3 m of the small intestine. The abomasal folds are enlarged and edematous and immature flukes may be seen attached to the mucosa, which also contains numerous erosions and petechia. The affected intestine is thickened and edematous. The pitted mucosal surface is covered with catarrhal exudate. Careful inspection may reveal flukes deeply embedded in the mucosa, with only the external ends present in the lumen. The mucosa in this affected region appears corrugated with many elevated ridges and multiple foci of hemorrhage. Immature flukes may also be found free in the gut lumen. Mature flukes may be present in the rumen and omasum. Multiple intestinal diverticula measuring 2 cm in diameter have been reported as an unusual finding associated with paramphistomiasis (Prajapati et al. 1982).

Histologically, affected areas of intestine show hypertrophy, edema, inflammatory cellular infiltrates, and fibrosis in the mucosa and submucosa (Sharma Deorani and Katiyar 1967). Histopathologic effects of adult flukes in the rumen are limited to epithelial desquamation of the papillae (Singh et al. 1984).

Diagnosis

Presumptive diagnosis is difficult because of the clinical similarity of paramphistomiasis to nematode gastroenteritis. Haemonchosis is more likely to produce anemia and less likely to produce diarrhea. However, other trichostrongyle infections may mimic paramphistomiasis exactly. Definitive diagnosis depends on ruling out nematode gastroenteritis by fecal flotation or necropsy and ruling in paramphistomiasis by identification of immature flukes in feces or at necropsy. Chronic fascioliasis must also be considered in the differential diagnosis. It occurs under similar environmental circumstances and may appear similar to the chronic form of paramphistomiasis.

Treatment

Elimination of the immature flukes with appropriate anthelmintic therapy is the major therapeutic objective and is life saving if treatment is started early in the course of disease. Animals must be removed from the source of infection before treatment or they will be immediately reinfected. Morantel citrate at a dose of 6 mg of morantel base/kg bw has recently been shown to be 99.5% effective against immature paramphistomes (Srivastava et al. 1989). Other drugs with a reported efficacy of more than 95% against immature flukes in sheep and goats include bithionol (25 to 100 mg/kg), niclofolan (6 mg/kg), niclosamide (50 to 100 mg/kg), and resorantel (65 mg/kg) (Rolfe and Boray 1988). Resorantel is also 100% effective against adult paramphistomes in goats (Sahai and Prasad 1975). Oxyclozanide (15 mg/kg) has a slightly less consistent efficacy range of 85% to 100% against immature flukes, but is also 100% effective against adult flukes. A new tertiary butylbenzathiole has been shown to be 99.7% effective against immature flukes and 100% effective against mature ones (Rolfe and Boray 1988). In general, the benzimidazoles are minimally effective against paramphistomes despite their relative effectiveness against liver flukes. Bithional may be toxic to goats at the higher end of the effective dose range (Boray 1985).

Directing treatment toward adult flukes is controversial. It has no direct benefit in the face of clinical outbreaks. Elimination of adult flukes reduces fecal egg counts and subsequent infection of snails, thereby reducing the general environmental burden of paramphistomes. Elimination of adult flukes, however, may also reduce the level of immunity that they induce in infected hosts, thereby increasing the risk of clinical disease in subsequent exposures (Horak 1971).

Control

The major thrust in the prevention of paramphistomiasis is to keep grazing animals away from areas with heavy concentrations of infected snails and from herbage contaminated with metacercariae. This means avoiding low-lying, poorly drained, or swampy areas, ponds, ditches, and paddy fields. Small ruminants should not be grazed with cattle under such circumstances, because the latter are known to shed large numbers of eggs and promote increased infection of snails.

Forages from contaminated areas can be used safely if ensiled or made into hay before feeding. When local conditions do not permit restricted grazing or harvesting, molluscicides may be used to reduce snail populations, but the relative cost-effectiveness of this remains to be proven. Water for drinking can be pumped from contaminated areas, treated with molluscicides, and provided in raised troughs, but this too is capital-intensive.

Strategic use of anthelmintics can be helpful in controlling paramphistomiasis. In India it is recommended that livestock be treated in June and August to reduce mature fluke burdens and thereby reduce egg laying, and in November, January, and March to control immature flukes (Gupta et al. 1985).

Though not yet available for widespread practical application, immunization may be a major future tool in paramphistomiasis control. Oral vaccination with irradiated metacercariae significantly reduced paramphistome burdens in goats on subsequent challenge compared with unvaccinated control goats (Horak 1967; Hafeez and Rao 1981).

Intestinal Cestodiasis or Tapeworms

Intestinal tapeworms occur in goats throughout the world. Relative to gastrointestinal nematodiasis, cestodiasis in goats usually has little clinical or economic significance. However, goat owners are often keenly aware of tapeworms because the proglottids, or egg packets, shed by the adult worm in the goat's feces are visible to the naked eye.

Etiology and pathogenesis

The major intestinal tapeworm of goats worldwide is *Moniezia expansa*, though other *Moniezia* spp. may also infect goats. *Avitellina* spp. occur in goats in Europe, Africa, and Asia, often in conjunction with *Moniezia* spp., and are sometimes the predominant cestode (Raina 1973). *Thysaniezia giardi* infects goats in Europe, the former USSR, Africa, India, and North America. *Stilesia globipuncta* occurs in goats and other ruminants mainly in tropical regions of Africa and Asia. It is potentially the most pathogenic of the ruminant tapeworms, producing inflammatory nodules at the sites of attachment in the duodenal and jejunal mucosa that can lead to enteritis and diarrhea. Nevertheless, clinical illness in goats attributable to *Stilesia* infection is poorly documented.

Another *Stilesia* tapeworm, *S. hepatica*, occurs in the bile ducts of ruminants in Africa and Asia and several new or additional *Stilesia* spp. have been identified from goats in India in recent years. *Thysanosoma actinioides*, the fringed tapeworm, can be found in the small intestine, though it is more commonly located in the bile and pancreatic ducts. It occurs only in western North America and South America. Principally a tapeworm of sheep and deer, its prevalence in goats is poorly documented. There is one slaughter survey from Mexico in which the fringed tapeworm was found on average in about 1.5% of the livers of goats examined as compared to about 15% for sheep livers (Cuéllar Ordaz 1980). It has been cited as a caprine parasite in the United States as well (Guss 1977). The liver tapeworms are discussed in detail in Chapter 11.

These anoplocephalid tapeworms all use ruminants as definitive hosts and various species of oribatid or psocid mites as intermediate hosts. Adult tapeworms developing in the goat intestine can be up to several meters long (Figure 10.11). They consist of a head or scolex and short neck followed by a long, segmented body composed of proglottids. The most posterior proglottids are packed with eggs. These gravid segments separate from the worm and are passed in the feces. These egg packets are white and 1 to 1.5 cm in length. They are visible in the fecal pellets and have the appearance of rice (Figure 10.12). The proglottid casing gradually disintegrates and oribatid or psocid mites, common in soils and on herbages, ingest the eggs. Infective cysticercoids develop within these arthropod intermediate hosts over a period of four months. Infective mites are consumed by ruminants while they feed. Cysticercoids are released from the ingested mites in the intestine and mature tapeworms begin to develop. The prepatent period in the goat is around forty days for *Moniezia* spp.

The goat also serves as an intermediate host for a number of cestode parasites that use canids as definitive hosts. In many cases, these infections are more economically and clinically significant than the adult tapeworm infections just listed above. All of these intermediate metacestode infections are addressed elsewhere in this text, in conjunction with the organ system most often affected. A summary overview of the various cestode infections is given in Table 10.9.

Light infestations of goats by the common tapeworms are generally nonpathogenic (Soulsby 1982; Williams and Schillhorn van Veen 1985). This is largely because tapeworms do not feed destructively with active mouthparts, but rather absorb nutrients from the intestinal lumen through their integument. In goats, at least fifty worms are required to produce deleterious effects. Several hundred may be present in an individual goat (Guss 1977). They may compete significantly for nutrients with the host, leading to ill thrift. They may produce luminal distension in the intestine resulting in a distended, pot-bellied appearance. Their presence may prolong transit time of

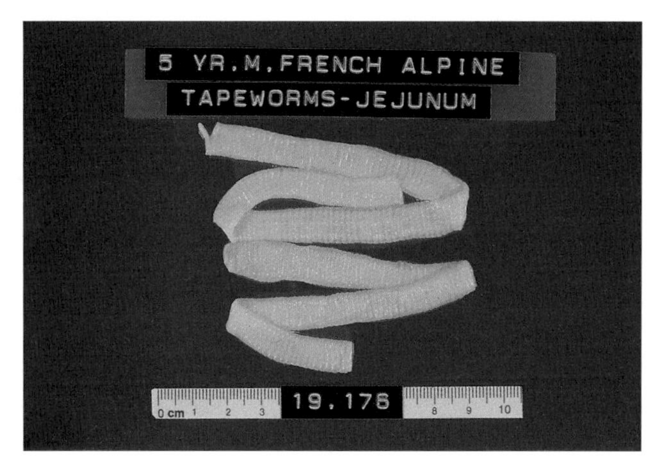

Figure 10.11. Adult Moniezia tapeworm from the intestine of a goat. (Courtesy of Dr. T.P. O'Leary.)

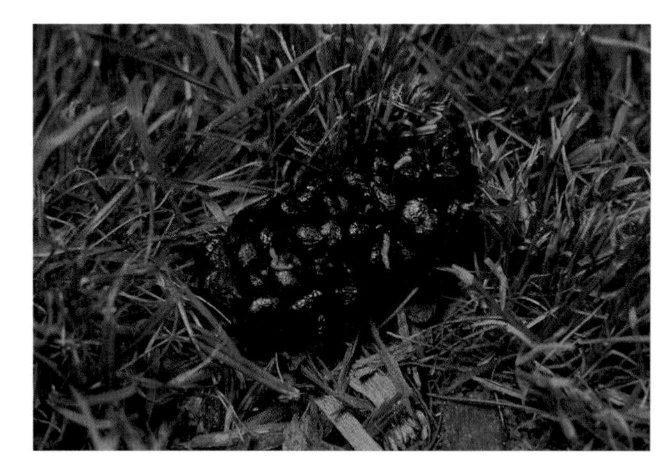

Figure 10.12. Tapeworm proglottids in goat feces. (Reproduced by permission of Dr. C.S.F. Williams.)

Table 10.9. Overview of cestode infections of goats.

Cestode	*Definitive host*	*Intermediate hosts*	*Form in goat*	*Locations in goat*	*Impact*
Moniezia expansa, other *Moniezia* spp.	Goats, other ruminants	Mites	Adult tapeworm	Intestine	Usually nonpathogenic
Avitellina spp.	Goats, other ruminants	Mites	Adult tapeworm	Intestine	Usually nonpathogenic
Thysaniezia spp.	Goats, other ruminants	Mites	Adult tapeworm	Intestine	Usually nonpathogenic
Stilesia globipunctata	Goats, other ruminants	Mites	Adult tapeworm	Intestine	Occasionally diarrhea
Stilesia hepatica	Goats, other ruminants	Mites	Adult tapeworm	Bile ducts	Liver condemnations
Thysanosoma actinoides	Goats, other ruminants	Mites	Adult tapeworm	Bile ducts	Liver condemnations
Taenia multiceps	Canids	Goats, other ungulates, humans	Metacestode cysts	Brain, spinal cord, muscle	Coenurosis, lameness, trim at slaughter, zoonosis*
Taenia hydatigena	Canids	Goats, other ruminants, pigs	Metacestode cysts	Liver, mesentery, omentum	Liver condemnation, trim at slaughter
Taenia ovis	Canids	Goats and more commonly sheep	Metacestode cysts	Heart, diaphragm, other muscle	Trim or condemnation at slaughter
Echinococcus granulosus	Canids	Goats, other ungulates, man	Metacestode (hydatid) cysts	Liver, lungs, CNS, bone, muscle	Liver disease, slaughter condemnation, zoonosis*

*Zoonotic potential of these cestodes does not derive from contact with goats or other intermediate host ruminants but from contact with feces of definitive host canids.
CNS = central nervous system.

ingesta in the gut. In feedlot lambs on grain rations, this is believed to promote the development of clostridial enterotoxemia. A similar interaction has not been described in goats. Massive tapeworm infections may sometimes even occlude the intestinal lumen. This results in signs of colic and may lead to spontaneous rupture of the intestine in young lambs and kids with dire consequences.

Epidemiology

Infections are most often observed in young kids at pasture during their first summer grazing season. Pasturing is not a prerequisite for infection, however, because the infective mites may be present in the barnyard or on carried forage. The pattern of infection may vary with climate and geography. In Nigeria, no seasonal variation was seen in the incidence of sheep and goat tapeworms in the dry savannah and desert regions, while the incidence was increased during the rainy season in the rain forest zone (Enyenihi et al. 1975). A natural resistance to cestode infection develops with age, and in populations of goats with constant exposure to tapeworms, worm burdens are always less severe in older goats.

Because tapeworms are often derived at pasture, heavy tapeworm burdens may also be a sentinel for heavy nematode infections. Therefore, when owners notice tapeworm proglottids in goat feces, deworming for tapeworms may be used as an opportunity to treat more serious nematode infections when broad-spectrum anthelmintics are used. Multiple parasitic infections are the rule, not the exception, in goats.

Clinical Signs

When clinical disease is associated with tapeworms, it usually involves young goats under six months of age. Affected animals may show poor growth rates and a pot-bellied appearance. Proglottids are present in voided feces that are usually normal in appearance, but may be soft or unpelleted. Constipation may also occur. In complete luminal obstruction caused by tapeworms, kids have symptoms of colic and decreased fecal output. Animals that have ruptured the intestine may be profoundly depressed, or found moribund or dead.

Clinical Pathology and Necropsy

In addition to proglottids in the feces, characteristic tapeworm eggs may be detected by fecal flotation methods because proglottids sometimes degenerate before being shed. *Moniezia expansa* ova are distinctly triangular. There are no other specific clinical chemistry or hematologic abnormalities associated with tapeworms.

At necropsy, the long, white-segmented tapeworms are strikingly obvious in the lumen of the small intestine. In obstructions, they pack the lumen, and may be free in the abdominal cavity when rupture of the intestine has occurred.

Diagnosis

Tapeworm infections are definitively diagnosed by the presence of proglottids in the feces or worms in the intestine. Attributing disease to tapeworm infection is more problematic. It is essential that nematode parasitism, paramphistomiasis, and liver fluke disease all be thoroughly ruled out before clinical disease is ascribed to tapeworms.

Treatment

A wide range of anthelmintics are currently available for eliminating adult tapeworms in goats. Oral niclosamide (50 mg/kg bw) is highly effective and has a wide margin of safety; it is nontoxic at five times the recommended dose. Praziquantel (5 mg/kg bw) is also effective, but the injectable form can be highly irritating to goats at the injection site. Oral febantel (5 mg/kg) is effective against *Moniezia expansa* and a range of nematodes. The newer benzimidazoles are also effective against tapeworms and nematodes. These include mebendazole (15 mg/kg), fenbendazole (15 mg/kg), cambendazole (20 mg/kg), and oxfendazole (10 mg/kg). Albendazole (10 mg/kg) is effective against tapeworms, nematodes, and the adult liver fluke *Fasciola hepatica*. Cautions associated with the use of benzimidazoles are discussed in the section on treatment of nematode gastroenteritis.

Older treatments for tapeworms in goats include copper sulfate, nicotine sulfate, and phenothiazine with lead arsenate. Though reasonably effective, these compounds all are potentially toxic if misused or improperly dosed, and their use is discouraged.

Control

It is difficult to justify a preventive program aimed at adult tapeworm control on economic grounds because the clinical impact on goats is usually minimal. When the appropriate broad-spectrum anthelmintics are used for nematode parasite control, however, tapeworm control can be included in the program as a bonus. The group of major concern in both cases is the young goat on pasture for the first time. Given current concerns about the development of anthelmintic resistance in nematode parasites, it would not be prudent to administer benzimidazoles expressly for the control of tapeworms unless there was also some strategic or tactical justification for their use against gastrointestinal nematodes at the same time.

Controlling the intermediate host mites is difficult because these arthropods are ubiquitous and often present in enormous concentrations. Plowing and reseeding are considered to reduce mite populations at pasture, but the overall effect on tapeworm populations in goats is questionable. Pasture rotation with at least a one-year layoff may be helpful because mite populations decrease over winter.

METABOLIC DISEASES

Bloat

Ruminal tympany, or bloat, is less common in goats than cattle and sheep. When it occurs, however, it must be considered a medical emergency as in other ruminant species. Frothy (primary, or nutritional) bloat is more likely to be encountered than free gas (secondary) bloat.

Etiology and Pathogenesis

Gas production is a normal outcome of rumen fermentive activity. Ordinarily, gas rises to the dorsal sac of the rumen and is discharged by the orderly process of rumination and eructation. Frothy bloat derives from nutritional causes. Under certain dietary conditions, such as the feeding of legumes or finely ground grains, gas bubbling through the rumen content can no longer freely coalesce in the dorsal sac but rather is trapped in a stable foam in the liquid phase of the rumen content. Certain species of bacteria that proliferate in the rumen when carbohydrate-rich diets are fed can produce an insoluble slime that increases rumen fluid viscosity and helps trap rumen gas in the stable foam (Radostits et al. 2007). Stable foam cannot be freely eructated and a progressive distension of the rumen ensues as additional gas becomes trapped. This progressive ruminal distension can be fatal as a result of subsequent respiratory and cardiovascular compromise. Experimentally in goats it has been documented that ruminal insufflation leads to decreased cardiac output, increased blood pressure, and increased total peripheral resistance due to obstruction of venous return by the distended rumen (Reschly and Dale 1970).

Free gas or secondary bloat occurs when gas accumulating normally in the dorsal sac of the rumen cannot be expelled because of extraruminal obstructions to outflow. When free gas cannot be eructated, progressive ruminal distension ensues with consequences similar to those just described.

Epidemiology

Bloat occurs in goats throughout the world. All goats with a mature functional rumen are at risk. Factors that have been identified as predisposing goats to frothy bloat include unaccustomed ingestion of lush legumes such as clover or alfalfa, either as green feeds or as new hay, recent turnout to legume pastures, and even turnout to grass pastures if they are wet. As such, bloat may have a seasonal occurrence in the spring. Feeding of garden greens as treats to goats on a dry hay diet is a frequent cause of bloat in Australia (King 1980b). Sudden access to grain either as concentrate feed or from gleaning of grain fields can also lead to frothy bloat. Turnout to grain fields results in a seasonal increase of bloat in the fall.

Free gas bloat occurs only sporadically in goats, usually secondary to esophageal choke. Pieces of apple or carrot are common foreign bodies. A cud can lodge in the esophagus, particularly in debilitated or sick animals and in animals with inadequate water supply. Internal abscesses in the anterior abdomen or mediastinum associated with caseous lymphadenitis or other causes can also produce secondary or free gas bloat by compression of the cardia or esophagus.

Clinical Signs

Frothy bloat can occur within hours of exposure to the offending feed or feeding situation. Many cases of bloat are first recognized by finding animals dead at pasture. In the initial stages of the disease, affected animals become anxious and uncomfortable and stop eating. The most characteristic sign is a progressive distension of the abdomen, particularly apparent on the left side and high in the left paralumbar fossa. Percussion of this area reveals the tight, tympanic feel of the distended rumen and a drum-like sound. As the distension progresses, animals become more uncomfortable, stamping their feet, vocalizing, salivating, urinating frequently, and moving with a stilted gait. Without intervention, these animals become recumbent, exhibit marked, labored respiration, and die within one hour.

In free gas bloat, signs are similar. Salivation is more pronounced if the esophageal obstruction is high and complete and saliva cannot be passed to the rumen. If intraluminal obstruction is not complete, or if the pressure of accumulating gas in the rumen can override an extraluminal obstruction, gas is intermittently expelled and the abdominal distension caused by the rumen may be less pronounced with less severe tympany. Such cases often result in a prolonged bloating that is not immediately life-threatening.

Clinical Pathology and Necropsy

Because of the acute nature of bloat, laboratory investigations are not performed. Necropsy is commonly employed in the diagnosis of bloat because the condition often proceeds to the fatal stage without detection. In a fresh necropsy of a case of frothy bloat, the ruminal distension is obvious and large amounts of froth are present within the rumen. In free gas bloat, rumen distension is present but the rumen does not contain froth. Careful inspection of the alimentary tract and surrounding structures from the mouth through the forestomachs should identify the source of secondary obstruction leading to free gas bloat. When animals are found several hours after death, diagnosis becomes more problematic, particularly in warm weather. Rumen distension with gas caused by the continued fermentive action of rumen flora after death eventually produces bloat in all carcasses. Froth also breaks down after death, causing frothy bloat to appear as free gas bloat. Examination of the carcass may help to establish the presence of antemortem bloat. In bloat cases, there is congestion of tissues in the anterior portions of the carcass and blanching or paleness of tissues in the caudal portions, reflecting peripheral vascular changes induced by the distended rumen. A line of demarcation "bloat line") between red congested esophageal mucosa in the cervical region and pale mucosa in the thoracic esophagus may be noted.

Diagnosis

Bloat is easily confirmed by physical examination. It is important to determine whether the condition is primary or secondary because this affects treatment and subsequent management decisions. The difficulty in the diagnosis of bloat comes when animals are found dead. Because bloat may be a normal post mortem change, it is necessary to rule out all possible causes of sudden death under the circumstances that the animal is found.

Treatment

Timely intervention is essential. Simple passage of a stomach tube, though often effective in relieving free gas bloat, does not correct frothy bloat unless the foam is first broken down. Cooking oils or mineral oil given orally in a dose range of 100 to 200 cc can be effective but may not work as rapidly as some of the commercial anti-frothing agents available. If given as a drench, care must be taken to avoid aspiration pneumonia. Linseed oil should not be used because it is associated with indigestion in goats. Oil of turpentine is a common home remedy. Though effective, it can taint meat and milk for five days after use.

There are a number of commercial, surface-acting (surfactant) agents that are also effective in degrading foam and results may be seen within minutes. Poloxalene is available as a concentrate to be diluted for use as a drench. It is dosed at a rate of 100 mg of poloxalene per kg bw. Dioctyl sodium sulfosuccinate (DSS) (15 to 30 ml dose), polymerized methyl silicone (10 to 15 ml dose), and docusate sodium (1.4 g dose) are other effective compounds. When large numbers of animals are affected and treatment time becomes a critical factor, anti-frothing agents can be injected directly into the rumen through the distended left paralumbar fossa using an 18-gauge needle rather than administering them orally by stomach tube. Polymerized methyl silicone works more effectively than poloxalene when given by this route. The newer, alcohol ethoxylate detergent products are more effective in controlling frothy bloat associated with grain ingestion than poloxalene and the other products, which perform best with legume-induced bloat.

Forced exercise after administering oils or surfactants helps break down foam and promotes expulsion of gas. If animals are recumbent, rolling the goat or massaging the rumen may help distribute the oil and break down the foam. A stomach tube should be passed to facilitate gas removal as the foam breaks down.

Trocharization of the rumen through the left paralumbar fossa can be life saving in goats in the terminal stages of bloat. However, this invasive treatment should be reserved for the most advanced cases due to the potential sequelae of peritonitis and prolonged rumen dysfunction. Goats trocharized for relief of bloat should be placed on a three- to five-day course of broad-spectrum antibiotic therapy after the procedure.

Control

Because goats are generally not managed in feedlots, control of feedlot bloat is not a major concern. When goats are fed grain, concentrate feeds should not be too finely ground and should not be abruptly introduced into the ration. For goats that show a tendency to bloat when fed grain, top dressing of the grain with vegetable oils can be helpful, as can the addition of poloxalene to mineral supplements or mineral blocks.

If grazing of legume pastures is an integral part of the goat management system, the risk of bloat can be high. A number of interventions have been described for cattle and/or sheep to reduce that risk. They include daily drenching of individual animals with oils before turn out, including anti-frothing agents such as poloxalene in feed or mineral supplements, feeding the ionophores monensin or lasalocid or administering a sustained release monensin capsule, and spraying oils or fats directly onto pasture. Managing the pasture itself can also be of value; interventions include sowing grasses with legumes, using forage types high in condensed tannins, strip grazing, and swathing and wilting alfalfa for twenty-four hours before turning animals out onto pasture. All these techniques and interventions are discussed in more detail elsewhere (Radostits et al. 2007).

The most fundamental intervention for controlling pasture bloat in goats is to adapt them gradually to pastures in spring, turning them out initially for short periods on a full stomach of hay to limit pasture consumption. A similar recommendation applies to animals turned out to glean grain fields in the fall. Whenever green feeds are fed, dry hay should be available simultaneously to avoid overconsumption of green feeds. To help control pasture bloat, poloxalene can be added to feed or mineral supplements to achieve a dose of 10 to 20 mg/kg bw. The supplementation should begin one to two weeks before turnout on pasture. If goats are being fed monensin or lasalocid for control of coccidiosis at recommended doses, they may appreciate some additional benefit in bloat control, as the ionophore antibiotics can reduce the incidence of bloat. The ionophores inhibit rumen bacteria, which produce large amounts of gas-trapping mucus and increase the rumen production of propionic acid, resulting in a decrease in the acetate:propionate ratio and a reduction in the amount of carbon dioxide and methane produced.

Rumen Impaction

Rumen distension secondary to impaction has been caused in the goat by sand ingestion and by prolonged feeding of low-energy, high-fiber diets, such as horse feed containing more than 25% oats in conjunction with poor quality grass hay (Guss 1977). It has also been associated with the feeding of bread, pollard, pellets, wheat, corn, or barley in excessive proportions of the total ration (King 1980). In northern India, rumen impaction in goats and other ruminants is more common in the hot, dry summer season when green fodders are unavailable, water is scarce, and the diet is composed mainly of low-grade, dry roughages (Prasad and Rekib 1979). The distension is primarily on the left, in the ventral abdomen, and ballotment reveals a firm, doughy consistency to the rumen content.

In recent years, the global proliferation of plastic bags in commerce and their careless disposal in the environment have become an important cause of ruminal impaction in goats. This is particularly the case in developing countries where flocks of goats may be brought to trash bins or garbage dumps to forage or when drought drives goats to eat items in the environment not normally consumed. Reports of rumen impaction due to plastic bags in goats have come from Nigeria (Otesile and Akpokodje 1991; Remi-Adewunmi et al. 2004), Jordan (Hailat et al. 1998), the Sudan (Abdel-Mageed et al. 1991), and South Africa (Donkin and Boyazoglu 2004). There is some indication that goats develop pica for plastic bags and consume them preferentially (Abdel-Mageed et al. 1991). Other foreign materials reported in association with rumen impaction in goats include cloth, leather, twine, and rope.

In addition to developing a firm, distended rumen, animals with rumen impaction become dull and listless, appetite is reduced, and milk production falls off. Cud chewing ceases, there may be mild bloating, and the feces may become scant, dry and mucus-covered. Progressive weight loss and debilitation ensue if the condition is not recognized and treated.

For sand impaction, one week of daily drenching with 60 g of magnesium sulfate is recommended. Each drench should be followed by manual kneading of the lower left abdomen to break up impaction. If impaction persists, rumenotomy may be required. Up to 20 pounds (9.1 kg) of sand have been removed from a goat rumen (King 1980b). Animals should be fed in racks or troughs off of the ground when possible. For fibrous impactions, daily oral dosing with mineral oil and dioctyl sodium sulfosuccinate (DSS) may soften impactions, but rumenotomy may be necessary. When fibrous impactions are diagnosed, the ration needs to be evaluated and corrected to provide more digestible energy and less fiber. Rumenotomy is required for the treatment of goats with rumen impaction due to plastic bags.

DISEASES OF MIXED ETIOLOGY

Neonatal Diarrhea Complex

Etiology and Epidemiology

Diarrheal disease is documented as a very frequent cause of kid loss throughout the world (Sherman 1987). A high incidence of diarrheal disease is associated with intensive rearing of kids under conditions of overcrowding and poor sanitation. Though less common under extensive management conditions, the incidence can increase when kidding seasons coincide with periods of extreme weather conditions, especially excessive heat, excessive cold, or heavy rains.

Much has been and continues to be presumed about the causes of neonatal kid diarrhea, based on the widespread information available from calf and lamb studies. As a result, colibacillosis, caused by *E. coli*, is often considered to be the most common cause of diarrhea in young kids. The few epidemiologic studies actually carried out in kids, however, suggest that the nature and frequency of the various etiologic agents of diarrhea may differ considerably in the goat compared with calves and lambs, or remain unknown. In a New Zealand study, up to 72% of the diarrhea cases in kids younger than one month of age remained undiagnosed regarding specific etiology (Vickers 1986).

The generally held presumption that *E. coli* is a major cause of diarrhea in kids is challenged by several studies (Nagy et al. 1983; Yvore et al. 1984; Polack et al. 1989; Muñoz et al. 1996). In these field surveys and diagnostic laboratory investigations, cryptosporidiosis is the most commonly diagnosed cause of diarrhea in kids younger than one month of age, and particularly in kids younger than fifteen days of age. The organism is rarely isolated from nondiarrheic kids. Cryptosporidiosis can occur alone or in conjunction with other presumed pathogenic bacteria, viruses, and protozoa.

The virulence attributes of gastrointestinal *Escherichia coli* isolates of veterinary significance have been reviewed (DebRoy and Maddox 2001). There are four main types of *E. coli* that can potentially be associated with diarrhea in kids: enterotoxigenic *E. coli* (ETEC); enteropathogenic *E. coli* (EPEC); enterohemorrhagic *E. coli* (EHEC); and necrotoxigenic *E. coli* (NTEC). Their characteristics and role in neonatal diarrhea complex of goat kids are as follows.

The enterotoxigenic *E. coli* (ETEC) are characterized by the production of heat stable and heat labile enterotoxins and the possession of adherence structures, known as pili or fimbriae, which allow the bacteria to colonize the intestinal lining where the enterotoxin can exert its effect on villous and crypt epithelial cells, producing a hypersecretory diarrhea. The ETEC are noninvasive and produce minimal lesions in the gut.

Though a major cause of diarrhea in neonatal calves, ETEC have been infrequently identified as a cause of neonatal kid diarrhea. In a Hungarian study, the adherence pilus K99 (now also referred to as F5), that is most frequently associated with ETEC in calves, was rarely identified in kids, though it was actively screened for. In fact, it was found in non-diarrheic kids more often than in diarrheic kids (Nagy et al. 1987).

More recently, a number of studies from Spain have provided additional information on the relationship of various *E. coli* types and diarrhea in kids. In one study, 210 strains of *E. coli* were cultured from diarrheic kids up to three weeks of age on fourteen farms. None of the strains produced the F5 or F41 fimbrial antigens associated with ETEC in calves. Eighteen of the isolates produced F17 fimbrial antigen, but none of these F17 isolates produced enterotoxin (Cid et al. 1993). A subsequent report indicated that F17-positive *E. coli* isolated from diarrheic kids and lambs in Spain had the phenotypic characteristic of septicemic strains and not enterotoxigenic strains (Cid 1999). In another study, no *E. coli* possessing either the F5 or the F41 fimbriae typical of ruminant ETEC were identified from fecal samples of seventeen diarrheic kids up to four weeks of age on seven farms (Orden et al. 2002). In a different investigation, only three of fifty-five *E. coli* isolates from fifty-five diarrheic kids produced toxins of any kind. One was a verotoxin and two were cytotoxic necrotizing factor 2 (CNF2), generally associated with septicemic strains. None of the isolates produced enterotoxin and it was concluded that most *E. coli* associated with diarrhea in kids were non-toxigenic (Cid et al. 1996).

There is one Spanish study in which fimbriated *E. coli* were found frequently in diarrheic kids and lambs but their significance was unclear because the same organisms were recovered with similar frequency from non-diarrheic kids and lambs and none of the fimbriated isolates produced enterotoxins (Muñoz et al. 1996). Furthermore, the fimbriated *E. coli* were present in kids and lambs at approximately equal frequencies among the age groups—one to five days, six to ten days, eleven to fifteen days, and sixteen to forty-five days—whereas in calves, ETEC are most often found in the first few days of life. Notably, the predominant pathogen isolated from diarrheic kids in this survey was *Cryptosporidium parvum*. It occurred mainly in kids one to ten days of age and was not isolated from any non-diarrheic kids.

In contrast to the Spanish studies, there are reports from Greece which suggest that ETEC are a common cause of diarrhea in newborn kids (Kritas 2002; Kritas et al. 2003). Isolates from kids on dairy goat farms with diarrhea in the first few days of life were confirmed as having F5 (K99) and F4 (K88) fimbriae. However, the isolates were not tested for enterotoxin and the presence of other possible pathogens, e.g., rotaviruses, was not investigated, so the etiologic role of ETEC in these outbreaks was not definitively established. The most convincing evidence offered for ETEC as the etiologic agent was that vaccination of does with a subunit vaccine containing K88 and K99 pilus antigens substantially reduced the occurrence and severity of diarrhea in newborn kids receiving colostrum as compared to kids of unvaccinated does in a controlled study (Kritas et al. 2003). More goat-specific epidemiologic investigations and laboratory confirmations are required to better clarify the role of ETEC in neonatal diarrhea of kids.

The enteropathogenic *E. coli* (EPEC) are also known as adhering and effacing *E. coli* (AEEC). They are characterized by the possession of the *eae* gene which encodes intimin, an outer membrane protein that mediates intimate bacterial adhesion to host enterocytes. A second *espB* gene may also be involved in adhesion but is not present in all isolates containing the *eae* gene. The adhering and effacing *E. coli* produce characteristic attachment and effacing lesions of the gut mucosa, involving destruction of the brush border of enterocytes, but are usually non-invasive.

Spanish studies on the prevalence and characteristics of AEEC in goats indicate that healthy kids and adults have a higher prevalence of AEEC than diarrheic kids, but there are differences in the characteristics of the AEEC organisms. AEEC from healthy kids and adults possess both the *eae* and *espB* genes and produced verotoxin, while the isolates from diarrheic kids possessed only the *eae* gene and did not produce verotoxin. All kids sampled were ≤ four weeks old and the prevalence of AEEC was highest in diarrheic kids eight to fourteen days of age (Cid et al. 1996; Fuente et al. 2002). Six types of the *eae* gene are known, and the AEEC associated with diarrhea in kids most often possessed the *eaeβ* type (Orden et al. 2003). In Canada, an AEEC was identified in a ten-day-old diarrheic kid from a herd of French Alpine dairy goats in which twenty-one of thirty-four kids died over a period of three weeks with profuse diarrhea and dehydration beginning at one week of age. The organism did not possess fimbrial antigens nor did it produce either enterotoxins or verotoxin, but it was *eae* gene positive (Drolet et al. 1994).

The enterohemorrhagic *E. coli* (EHEC) are characterized by production of verotoxin, a toxin similar to the shiga toxin of *Shigella dysenteriae*. Some but not all EHEC are also attaching and effacing and possess the *eae* gene. Those possessing the gene are considered more likely to be pathogenic to humans. Virulence factors and the epidemiology of EHEC have been reviewed (Caprioli et al. 2005).

Though sometimes associated with diarrhea in ruminant hosts, the greater significance of the EHEC is in their zoonotic potential. *E. coli* O157:H7 is the most well known EHEC, although there are numerous other enterohemorrhagic serotypes as well. *E. coli* O157:H7 is associated with diarrhea, hemorrhagic colitis, thrombocytopenic purpura, and hemolytic uremic syndrome in humans. Cattle are considered the main reservoir of the organism and there is widespread public health concern about the transmission of *E. coli* O157:H7 to humans through foods of bovine origin. However, other livestock, including goats, can harbor verotoxigenic *E. coli*.

E. coli O157:H7 has been isolated from goats on commercial farms (Dontorou et al. 2004) and tourist farms (Pritchard et al. 2000), at agricultural fairs (Keen et al. 2006), and in petting zoos (DebRoy and Roberts 2006). It has been associated with hemorrhagic colitis and hemolytic uremic syndrome in humans through foods of caprine origin, including unpasteurized milk (Bielaszewska et al. 1997; McIntyre et al. 2002) and fresh unpasteurized goat cheese (Espié et al. 2006) and possibly by direct contact with goats or goat feces (Pritchard et al. 2000; Heuvelink et al. 2002).

EHEC serovars other than O157 are found more commonly in goats. For instance, a fatal case of diarrhea in a two-month old goat was confirmed as being due to a verotoxic *E. coli* serotype O103:H2 (Duhamel et al. 1992). In a German study, seventy verotoxin-producing strains were isolated from ninety-three healthy goats from six farms. None was O157 and only one possessed the *eae* gene (Zschöck et al. 2000). In another German study, thirty-seven of sixty-six healthy goats yielded verotoxin-producing strains and none was 0157. The predominant serotype (70%) was O5:H⁻ with single isolates of O82:H8, O87:H21, O5:H10, and O74:H⁻, as well as nine untypeable strains also recorded (Beutin et al. 1993). In a Spanish study of healthy and diarrheic goats, verotoxin-producing *E. coli* were isolated more frequently from the feces of healthy goats than diarrheic goats. No O157 serotypes were identified but 12% of the isolates from goats represented serotypes known to be pathogenic for humans: O5:H⁻, O26:H11, O91:H⁻, O128:H2, and O128:H⁻. It was concluded that verotoxigenic *E. coli* are not strongly associated with diarrhea in kids, but that goats can serve as an important source of EHEC infection for humans (Orden et al. 2003a). In a survey of twelve dairy goat farms in Spain, verotoxigenic *E. coli* were more prevalent in adult goats than kids, no strains were *eae* positive, and 16% of the strains isolated from healthy goats belonged to serotypes associated with disease in humans, again indicating that goats can be an important reservoir of EHEC (Cortés et al. 2005).

Other pathogenic *E. coli* that can infect ruminant neonates are primarily associated with septicemia rather than enteritis. Some of these may be necrotoxigenic strains of *E. coli* (NTEC) that produce cytotoxic necrotizing factor. Others may belong to known invasive serotypes. In colisepticemia, invasive strains of *E. coli* gain entrance to the bloodstream and produce clinical disease through the effects of bacteremia and endotoxemia. Diarrhea may be part of the clinical syndrome, but is not the primary problem. Colisepticemia occurs most commonly in neonates that have not received adequate passive immunity through consumption of the dam's colostrum. The condition is discussed further in Chapter 7 in the section on failure of passive transfer of maternal antibody.

A poorly understood disease known locally as "chevreau mou" in France or "floppy kid syndrome" in North America was first recognized as a cause of diarrhea in kids in intensive management systems in winter in France. Affected kids were usually three to four days of age and showed severe generalized weakness, distension of the forestomachs with undigested milk, and sometimes diarrhea (Garcin 1982). The condition was originally thought to be a form of colisepticemia because of its similar clinical presentation to the condition known in lambs in the UK as "watery mouth" (Savey 1985; Eales 1986). However, a similar condition was later observed in Canada in kids nine to ten days old and reported to be associated with metabolic acidosis without dehydration (Tremblay et al. 1991). Currently, floppy kid syndrome is recognized as a form of metabolic acidosis associated with high concentrations of D-lactate in the plasma (Bleul et al. 2006) and diarrhea is no longer considered to be part of the case definition (Rowe 2006). The underlying cause of the syndrome remains unknown but there is currently no evidence that it has an infectious etiology. The condition is discussed further in Chapter 19 as a metabolic disease.

In a New Zealand study, *Clostridium perfringens* types C and D were rarely identified as causes of diarrhea in kids. Enterotoxemia is considered to more commonly assume the neurologic or sudden death forms than the enteric form in New Zealand (Vickers 1986).

Rotaviruses have been identified from diarrheic kids for thirty years, and serologic surveys indicate a high prevalence of infection in goats in some countries—for example 60% in Japan (Takahashi et al. 1979), 41% in Turkey (Gumusova et al. 2007), and 25.7% in Italy (Iovane et al. 1988). It is reported to be the most common enteric virus of goats in New Zealand, and it is believed to cause profuse diarrhea either alone or in combination with *E. coli* and/or cryptosporidia (Thompson 2001).

However, the epidemiology of rotavirus as a cause of neonatal diarrhea in kids still requires further clarification. In an early report from the UK rotavirus particles were identified from the diarrheic feces of several four-month-old goatlings (Scott et al. 1978). If the virus was indeed responsible for the diarrhea, this would be in marked contrast to rotavirus infection in calves and lambs, where clinical diarrhea is unusual in individuals older than three weeks of age. In France, rotaviruses were identified readily from non-diarrheic kids with almost equal frequency as diarrheic kids, raising questions about their pathogenicity in goats (Yvore et al. 1984).

Rotaviruses are now known to belong to seven different serogroups, A through G, based on the cross reactivity of antibodies to the major inner capsid protein, VP6. Group A rotaviruses are most commonly associated with diarrhea in farm animals. Rotavirus A was identified as the cause of diarrhea in twelve- to sixteen-week-old Saanen kids in South Africa (Costa Mendes et al. 1994). The presence of rotavirus A was also confirmed in Canada in one- to two-week-old goat kids with diarrhea in conjunction with cryptosporidial infection. Rotavirus A was considered to be contributory to the diarrhea because villous atrophy was more pronounced histologically in kids with dual infection than in kids with cryptosporidiosis alone (Sanford et al. 1991). In contrast, no association between group A rotavirus and diarrhea in kids could be made in a Spanish goat herd where rotavirus was identified in the feces of five times as many normal kids as diarrheic kids (Muñoz et al. 1994).

Group B rotavirus was identified in Spain as the sole cause of severe diarrhea, dehydration, and prostration in kids two to three days of age and affecting 22.6% of kids on the farm (Muñoz et al. 1995). In a broader survey of diarrheic and healthy kids on sixteen goat farms in Spain, group A, B, and C rotaviruses were identified. Group A rotaviruses were identified in healthy kids more often than diarrheic kids, while group C rotavirus was identified in healthy kids only. An association between infection and diarrhea was established only for the group B rotaviruses (Muñoz et al. 1996).

Coronavirus is a major cause of diarrhea in calves, but information on coronavirus infection in goats is limited. A seroprevalence study in five provinces in Turkey found 41% of goats sampled positive for bovine coronavirus (Gumusova et al. 2007). There are no published reports of diarrhea outbreaks in kids confirmed as due solely to coronavirus. Some disease investigations in diarrheic kids have actively screened for the presence of coronavirus as an etiologic agent. Either coronavirus was not found at all (Muñoz et al. 1996) or it was present at a low prevalence, almost always in mixed infections with other likely causative agents, notably cryptosporidia or enterotoxigenic *E. coli* (Nagy et al. 1983; Ozmen et al. 2006). These findings suggest that coronavirus is a possible but unlikely contributor to the neonatal disease complex in kids.

Adenoviruses are not commonly associated with diarrhea in kids. Adenoviruses were identified in diarrheic goats in Hungary (Nagy et al. 1983). They also have been isolated from the intestine of two goats in Nigeria that died of peste des petits ruminants (PPR) (Gibbs et al. 1977) as well as from goats in Senegal during PPR outbreaks (Nguyen et al. 1988). Because PPR is a major, known cause of diarrhea, it is difficult to ascribe significance to the adenovirus. Also, a new serotype of adenovirus was isolated from a three-week-old kid with diarrhea and respiratory disease in California (Lehmkuhl et al. 2001). It was one of about fifty kids from a 900-doe herd showing similar signs.

Yersinia spp., *Giardia*, and *Campylobacter jejuni* were confirmed as causes of diarrhea in New Zealand (Vickers 1986). *Campylobacter jejuni* has also been isolated from diarrheic feces of kids in Nigeria (Adetosoye and Adeniran 1987) and Canada (Prescott and Bruin-Mosch 1981). Again, the role of this organism remains equivocal because, in the Canadian study, *C. jejuni* was also isolated from the feces of normal goats.

Infection with the flagellated protozoa *Giardia duodenalis* (syn. *G. intestinalis*, *G. lamblia*) has been reported from most continents and has been identified in all the common agricultural animals, but its role in disease remains controversial (Radostits et al. 2007). Cysts of *G. duodenalis* are frequently found in the feces of healthy animals, and when present in diarrheic animals, they are often present with other potential etiologic agents, so attribution of pathogenicity remains equivocal. This reflects the situation in goats as well. Several prevalence studies have been reported. In Spain, 19.8% of adult goats were infected in one survey and 33% in another (Castro-Hermida et al. 2007a, 2007b). In pregnant does, shedding of cysts in feces increased seven to ten times in the three weeks around kidding time (Castro-Hermida et al. 2005). In France, goats on 100% of twenty farms shed *G. duodenalis* cysts and on-farm prevalence ranged from 10% to 80%, with an overall rate of 38%. Prevalence was highest in kids six to eight months of age (Castro-Hermida et al. 2005a). In Romania, 16% to 18% of adult goats were infected in both pasture and housed environments, while 10% to 50% of kids were infected, with pastured kids having higher prevalence than intensively reared kids (Suteu et al. 1987).

Experimental infection of goats has been reported, indicating that *G. duodenalis* is capable of producing enteric disease by itself, though only three of eight challenged kids developed loose stool, depression, and decreased appetite (Koudela and Vítovec 1998). In reports of naturally occurring infection associated with diarrheal disease, *G. duodenalis* is usually identified in association with other potential etiologic agents such as *Cryptosporidium parvum* (Sutherland 1982; Sutherland and Clarkson 1984; Ozmen et al. 2006) or coccidia and trichostrongyles (Suteu et al. 1987). It is reasonable to consider *G. duodenalis* as a pathogen when found in kids with diarrhea, but additional potential causes should be investigated and the presence of the organism in adults does not necessarily mean that the organism will cause problems in kids. When *Giardia* is present in herds, however, managers and veterinarians must be cognizant of the fact that the organism has zoonotic potential as a cause of diarrhea in humans.

Caprine herpesvirus infection has been associated with diarrhea in kids. Herpesvirus infection was first recognized in California in 1972 in association with a severe generalized infection of one- to two-week-old French Alpine kids, causing increased morbidity and mortality rates (Saito 1974). A similar outbreak of disease characterized by fever and ulcerative enteritis with high mortality in kids was recorded in dairy goats in Switzerland in 1978 (Mettler et al. 1979). Affected kids show signs of weakness, dyspnea, cyanosis, abdominal pain, diarrhea, nasal discharge, and oral erosions. Not all signs are present in all individual kids. The disease has a fatal course of one to four days. Necrosis and ulceration of the digestive tract, especially the cecum and colon, are prominent necropsy findings. More detailed information on other manifestations of herpesvirus infection in goats is found in Chapter 12 and elsewhere in this text.

These limited studies suggest that the conventional wisdom about the etiologic basis of infectious diarrhea in young goat kids, largely extrapolated from experience with calves and lambs, bears additional examination. Enterotoxigenic *E. coli* may be involved less often than is generally assumed. Veterinarians working up diarrhea outbreaks in kids should specifically seek to establish the presence and characteristics of ETEC but should also be looking to identify other likely bacterial, viral, protozoal, and/or non-infectious causes of diarrhea in young goats. *Cryptosporidium parvum* appears to be a more significant cause of diarrhea in the first week of age, with rotaviruses also playing a potentially important role. Multiple agents may be present and their contributory importance and possible interactions need to be further clarified. More local diagnostic surveys should be undertaken wherever goats are raised because appropriate recommendations for treatment and control may depend on more accurate knowledge of causative agents.

Infectious agents may not always be involved in diarrhea of young kids. Many cases may be nutritionally based and difficult to diagnose at post mortem without adequate feeding and management history which may be difficult to obtain after the fact.

Nutritional causes of diarrhea in young kids are often associated with husbandry and feeding practices. Problems identified include overfeeding of milk, using poor quality milk replacers, suddenly changing the feeding routine, and switching to cow milk replacers. Incorrect mixing and dispensing of milk replacer by a malfunctioning automatic feeder has been reported as a cause of kid diarrhea (Lane 1987). These situations may produce noninfectious diarrhea, or predispose to the proliferation of pathogenic bacteria in the abomasum, rumen, or intestine.

When kids reach one month of age, the common causes of diarrhea are better established. Coccidiosis is likely the most common and helminthiasis the second most common prevailing identifiable cause of diarrhea in weaned, growing kids worldwide. Other well-known causes of diarrhea in older kids also include enterotoxemia caused by *Clostridium perfringens* type D, salmonellosis, yersiniosis, peste des petits ruminants, and indigestion associated with the transition to solid feeds. These are either more sporadic or more geographically restricted than coccidiosis and helminthiasis.

Pathogenesis

Diarrhea, as a pathophysiologic process, results in dehydration, acidosis, and electrolyte depletion, and in neonates, is also associated with hypoglycemia. These physiologic derangements, when unchecked, are often fatal. Certain agents such as *Salmonella* spp. and *Clostridium perfringens*, though primarily enteric pathogens, can cause marked, concurrent systemic effects in addition to diarrhea as a result of bacteremia and toxemia respectively. Certain agents may produce clinical effects in multiple organ systems as exemplified by the pneumoenteritis syndrome seen in peste des petits ruminants.

Clinical Findings

In the case of diseases limited to the gastrointestinal tract such as cryptosporidiosis, enteropathogenic colibacillosis, and the enteric viruses, diarrhea is the predominant clinical sign. The character of diarrheic feces in kids can vary considerably from pasty white to loose, yellowish green, to watery brown and it is inadvisable to ascribe too much diagnostic significance to the color or consistency of feces in a given case, especially because mixed etiologies are possible. Streaking of feces with blood may also be seen with a variety of causative agents. Regardless of cause, there may be some degree of abdominal discomfort, possible abdominal distension, and probable loss of appetite in association with diarrhea. Giardiasis has been reported to assume a chronic form in kids and lambs lasting several weeks with gassy, watery brown feces (Ozmen et al. 2006).

If diarrhea is prolonged or severe, then dehydration ensues. Dehydrated animals become depressed, the mouth is dry, and they gradually lose the sucking reflex. They grow progressively weaker until they are unable to stand. Loss of body fluid produces hypovolemia and poor peripheral circulation. Extremities feel cold, the eyeballs become sunken, and the body temperature may become subnormal. Electrolyte and acid-base imbalances resulting from diarrhea may lead to neurologic disturbances including hyperesthesia and opisthotonus or terminal convulsions. Loss of bicarbonate in the diarrheic feces and a build up of L-lactate due to the poor peripheral perfusion associated with dehydration combine to produce a severe metabolic acidosis in diarrheic, dehydrated kids, which is life threatening.

Clinical Pathology and Necropsy

Measurement of packed cell volume, total plasma protein, serum sodium, potassium, bicarbonate, blood glucose, and blood gases are useful in determining the severity of electrolyte deficits, acidosis, and hypoglycemia in neonatal diarrhea cases. In the field, however, useful estimates of these deficits can also be gauged based on the severity of clinical dehydration. In general, diarrheic kids have a hyperkalemic, metabolic acidosis with a high serum anion gap.

Submission of diarrheic feces to a diagnostic laboratory for etiologic evaluation is encouraged. At the very minimum, samples from kids younger than three weeks of age should be evaluated for cryptosporidia, enterotoxigenic and enteropathogenic *E. coli*, *Salmonella*, rotavirus, and coronavirus. In kids older than three weeks of age, additional evaluations should include coccidiosis, giardiasis, enterotoxemia, and yersiniosis. Samples should be collected within twelve to twenty-four hours of the onset of diarrhea, because the viruses may be rapidly cleared from the gut. A volume of 5 to 10 cc of fresh, diarrheic feces should be submitted under refrigeration. If such volumes are unavailable and rectal swabs are used, they should be shipped to the lab in a suitable bacterial transport medium. Also, fresh fecal smears prepared on glass slides can be valuable in the diagnosis of cryptosporidiosis and enteric viruses by acid-fast staining and fluorescent antibody testing, respectively. Survival of cryptosporidial oocysts in fresh feces is poor. While viruses can be identified in fresh feces by electron microscopy, such equipment is not always available. Many virulence factors associated with the various types of *E. coli* can be identified using molecular techniques such as gene probes and multiplex PCR to help characterize isolates from neonatal diarrhea cases. These techniques have been reviewed (DebRoy and Maddox 2001).

At necropsy, a loop of bowel can be ligated and removed and submitted to the lab unopened under refrigeration. Formalinized tissues from major organs and various portions of the gastrointestinal tract should also be submitted for histopathologic evaluation. Gross lesions may be found at necropsy in the case of coccidiosis, salmonellosis, yersiniosis, enterotoxemia, and some forms of gastrointestinal nematodiasis, and these lesions are discussed under each of these disease headings elsewhere in the chapter. The remainder of the causes of diarrhea in young kids may produce little or no gross abnormalities beyond some gaseous distension of the bowel and slight hyperemia. Histological evaluation can be helpful in some of these cases and immunohistochemistry is now also available for identification of some enteric pathogens, for example *Cryptosporidium* and *Giardia*.

Diagnosis

Definitive diagnosis of the causes of diarrhea in young kids may require exhaustive and costly bacteriologic, virologic, and parasitologic testing in the diagnostic laboratory. A list of likely causes of diarrhea in young kids based on age is given in Table 10.3 to serve as a general diagnostic guideline.

Treatment

Many of the common causes of diarrhea are self-limiting, and the major goals of therapy are to keep the kid physiologically intact while the diarrhea runs its course. Implementation of this strategy includes moving the kid to a warm, dry place to maintain proper body temperature and providing appropriate fluid therapy to counter dehydration, electrolyte depletion, hypoglycemia, and acidosis. Oral or parenteral therapy can be used depending on the severity of disease. Oral fluids can be used in kids up to 7% dehydration, but they should receive intravenous fluids with bicarbonate supplementation if dehydration level exceeds 8%. Many commercial preparations are manufactured for oral rehydration therapy in diarrheic animals and are increasingly available worldwide. Effective oral rehydration preparations should contain sodium chloride, potassium chloride, sodium bicarbonate, glucose, and glycine. The basic intravenous fluids should contain equal volumes of isotonic saline, isotonic sodium bicarbonate, and isotonic dextrose, but additional amounts of isotonic bicarbonate (1.3%) likely need to be given to correct the bicarbonate deficit associated with severe diarrhea. Additional details on the management of parenteral therapy in diarrheic neonates is available elsewhere (Radostits et al. 2007).

The feeding of milk or milk replacer products should be approached cautiously during the acute phase of diarrhea. Because there likely will be some derangement of digestive function, lactose in milk-based feeds may remain undigested in the gut and promote a hyperosmotic diarrhea on top of the existing enteritis. Alternating oral electrolyte solutions with small feedings of milk is a reasonable approach. The use of commercial, lactose-free milk products or the addition of lactase to goat milk before feeding to kids may also be useful. Kids should be brought back on milk gradually as diarrhea improves. In diarrhea that lasts for more than several days, it is necessary to feed milk products to avoid starvation. The strategy then becomes to decrease the volume fed per feeding and to increase the number of feedings. In this manner, the residual digestive capacity of the gut may not be overwhelmed.

A variety of oral antidiarrheal medications and intestinal protectants such as bismuth subsalicylate or kaolin/pectin have been used in kids. They may be helpful, but no efficacy trials have ever been reported in goats. Similarly, oral yogurt or lyophilized *lactobacillus* cultures are given empirically to restore a more normal gut flora.

Whenever possible, antibiotic therapy for diarrhea should be based on culture and sensitivity tests. When bacterial causes of diarrhea are strongly suspected and sensitivity testing is not possible, then broad-spectrum oral or parenteral antibiotic therapy such as trimethoprim/sulfa may be indicated. More details on specific antibiotic choices are given in the separate discussions of each bacterial disease elsewhere in this chapter. Antibiotics are also indicated prophylactically in scouring kids to protect against secondary bacterial pneumonias that are common in debilitated kids. Antibiotics are sometimes used indiscriminately by goat owners in lieu of diagnostic veterinary services, and client education is an important part of managing diarrhea outbreaks.

Control

Regardless of the etiologic cause, one of the most effective means of controlling the spread of diarrhea in kid populations in the face of an outbreak is to immediately and strictly isolate affected kids at the first sign of diarrhea. When possible, other exposed kids should be moved to a clean pen or at least temporarily removed from diarrhea-contaminated pens to permit disinfection. In the case of viral enteritides and cryptosporidiosis, where effective therapeutic agents may not be available, the use of isolation and sanitation as control measures becomes critical.

As with other species, diarrhea in kids is likely to be more common in intensive rearing operations. In these situations, kids should be born in clean, draft-free quarters and not allowed to become chilled. They should receive adequate colostrum as early in life as possible, at least before six hours of age. Colostrum banks may be helpful in ensuring an adequate supply of colostrum. Outbreaks of diarrhea often occur at the end of the kidding season, indicating that there is a progressive build up of pathogens over time and that better sanitation is needed in kidding areas, kid housing areas, and feeding equipment.

Vaccination of the doe in the four to six weeks before kidding may improve the concentration and specificity of protective antibodies available in the colostrum. Vaccination of the dam with *Clostridium perfringens* types C and D is already justified. Bovine K99+ *E. coli* vaccines have been demonstrated to produce increased K99 specific antibody in doe serum and colostrum (Contrepois and Guillimin 1984). More recently, a subunit vaccine for pigs containing K88 and K99 pilus antigens reduced diarrhea in a herd when does were vaccinated and kids consumed their colostrum (Kritas et al. 2003). The economic justification for using such vaccines depends on confirmation that enterotoxigenic E. coli are involved in diarrheal outbreaks on the farm or in the veterinarian's practice area. It is also unknown if bovine rotavirus and coronavirus vaccines are effective in the control of diarrhea in young goats. In endemic areas, vaccination of goats for peste des petits ruminants is justified.

Kids should be housed separately or in small groups of approximately equal age. Bedding should be clean and dry. Regardless of feeding system, all utensils and equipment should be cleaned and disinfected between feedings. In *ad libitum* feeding systems, a small amount of formalin has been added to milk to inhibit bacterial overgrowth in the milk and the kids' gastrointestinal tract. Kids should be offered access to hay soon after birth and a grain ration offered by week two to initiate good rumen development and a normal flora, and to avoid subsequent weaning shock. When possible, kid pens should be organized so feed can be fed in trays or buckets outside the pen to avoid fecal contamination of feedstuffs.

REFERENCES

Abdel-Ghani, M., Mohomed, A.H. and Yassein, S.: Occurrence of salmonellae in sheep and goats in Egypt. J. Egypt Vet. Med. Assoc., 47:161–170, 1987.

Abdel-Mageed, A.B., Abbas, B. and Oehme, F.W.: The pathogenesis of foreign body-pica syndrome in goats. Agri-Practice, 12(2):31–35, 1991.

Abdin-Bey, M.R. and Ramadan, R.O.: Retrospective study of hernias in goats. Sci. J. King Faisal Univ., 2(1):77–88, 2001.

Abdurahman, O.S., Hilali, M. and Jarplid, B.: A light and electron microscopic study on abomasal globidiosis in Somali goats. Acta Vet. Scand., 28:181–187, 1987.

Abu Elzein, E.M.E., et al.: Severe PPR infection in gazelles kept under semi-free range conditions. J. Vet. Med. B, 51:68–71, 2004.

Adesiyun, A.A. and Lombin, L.H.: Multiplication of *Yersinia enterocolitica*, *Staphylococcus aureus*, and *Escherichia coli* in caprine colostrum and experimental mastitis in does. Isr. J. Vet. Med., 45:1–11, 1989.

Adetosoye, A.I. and Adeniran, M.O.A.: *Campylobacter* enteritis in animals in Ile-Ife, Oyo State, Nigeria. Rev. Élev. Méd. Vét. Pays. Trop., 40:39–40, 1987.

Afshar, A. and Myers, D.J.: Simple and rapid dot-enzyme immunoassay for visual detection of rinderpest antibodies in bovine and caprine sera. Trop. Anim. Health Prod., 18:209–216, 1986.

Aguirre, D.H., Cafrune, M.M., Vinabal, A.E. and Salatin, A. O.: Epidemiological and therapeutics aspects of goat gastrointestinal nematodiasis in a subtropical area of Argentina. Rev. Invest. Agropecuarias, 31(1):25–39, 2002.

Akkaya, H.: Investigations on the trichostrongylid nematodes of hair goats slaughtered in Istanbul. Acta Parasitol. Turcica., 22(1):77–87, 1998.

Al-Ani, F.K., Khamas, W.A., Al-Qudah, K.M. and Al-Rawashdeh, O.: Occurrence of congenital anomalies in Shami breed goats: 211 cases investigated in 19 herds. Small Rumin. Res., 28(3):225–232, 1998.

Albert, K.: Abortion and mortality due to *Yersinia pseudotuberculosis* in a herd of goats. Tierarzt. Umschau, 43:718–720, 1988.

Alberto Fagonde Costa, C. and Da Silva Vieira, L.: Influencia do aprisco de piso ripado suspenso sobre a incidencia de nematodeos intestinais em caprinos. Rev. Cabra Bodes, 3:10, 1987.

Alhendi, A.B., Ramadan, R.O. and Moudawi, M.M.: Treating a goat tongue strangulation. Large Anim. Pract., 20(2);40, 1999.

Ali, B. El H.: A natural outbreak of rinderpest involving sheep, goats and cattle in Sudan. Bull. Epizoot. Dis. Afr., 21:421–428, 1973.

Ali, M.A., Ahmed, J.U. and Rahman, M.H.: Congenital atresia ani in kids, Bang. Vet. J., 10:67–68, 1976.

Alibasoglu, M., Erturk, E. and Yucel, N.: Turkiyede rastlanan ilk keci paratuberkuloz olaylari uzerinde patolojik incelemeler. Veteriner. Fakult. Dergisi, 20:43–63, 1973.

Allison, M.J., Hammond, A.C. and Jones, R.J.: Detection of ruminal bacteria that degrade toxic dihydroxypyridine compounds produced from mimosine. Appl. Environ. Microbiol., 56(3):590–594, 1990.

Al-Quaisy, H.H.K., Al-Zubaidy, A.J., Altaif, K.I. and Makkawi, T.A.: The pathogenicity of haemonchosis in sheep and goats in Iraq: 1. Clinical, parasitological and haematological findings. Vet. Parasitol., 24:221–228, 1987.

Alvinerie, M., Sutra, J.F. and Galtier, P.: Ivermectin in goat plasma and milk after subcutaneous injection. Vet. Res., 24:417–421, 1993.

Alvinerie, M., Lacoste, E., Sutra, J.F. and Chartier, C.: Some pharmacokinetic parameters of eprinomectin in goats following pour-on administration. Vet. Res. Commun., 23(7):449–455, 1999.

Andersen, F.L. and Christofferson, P.V.: Efficacy of haloxon and thiabendazole against gastrointestinal nematodes in sheep and goats in the Edwards plateau area of Texas. Am. J. Vet. Res., 34:1395–1398, 1973.

Anderson, B.: Patterns of shedding of cryptosporidial oocysts in Idaho calves. J. Am. Vet. Med. Assoc., 178:982–984, 1981.

Anderson, P.J.S. and Marais, F.S.: The anthelmintic efficacy of morantel tartrate in sheep and goats. J. S. Afr. Vet. Med. Assoc., 43:271–285, 1972.

Andrews, A.H., Giles, C.J. and Thomsett, L.R.: Suspected poisoning of a goat by giant hogweed. Vet. Rec., 116:205–207, 1985.

Andrews, J.R.H.: A host-parasite checklist of helminths of wild ruminants in New Zealand. N. Z. Vet. J., 21:43–47, 1973.

Anonymous: Gladiolus poisoning a painful death. Goat Health Prod., 2(4):7–8, 1988.

Anonymous: New drug for coccidiosis. N. Z. Goat Health Prod., 2(3):7, 1988a.

Arantes, I.G., Do Nascimento, A.A. and Pereira, O. da C.: *Gaigeria pachyscelis*. A morphological study of larval and young adult parasites in goats. Arq. Inst. Biol. São Paulo, Braz., 50:21–37, 1983.

Arnold, T. et al.: Prevalence of *Yersinia enterocolitica* in goat herds from northern Germany. J. Vet. Med. B, 53:382–386, 2006.

Arora, A.K.: Recovery of *Salmonella* serotypes from various sources in slaughtered goats. Indian J. Public Health, 22:305–306, 1978.

Arora, A.K.: The effect of stress on the carrier state of *Salmonella typhimurium* in goats. Vet. Arhiv., 53:181–187, 1983.

Arzoun, I.H., Hussein, H.S. and Hussein, M.F.: The pathogenesis of experimental *Haemonchus longistipes* infection in goats. J. Comp. Pathol., 93:619–628, 1983.

Aumont, G., Yvore, P. and Esnault, A.: Experimental coccidiosis in goats. 1. Experimental model. Effects of parasitism on the feeding behaviour and the growth of animals; intestinal lesions. Ann. Res. Vét., 15:467–473, 1984.

Australian Veterinary Emergency Plan: Disease Strategy Bluetongue. Ausvetplan, Agriculture and Resource Management Council of Australia and New Zealand, 1996. pp. 49. http://www.animalhealthaustralia.com.au/fms/Animal%20Health%20Australia/AUSVETPLAN/btvfinal.pdf.

Ayeni, A.O., Olubunmi, P.A. and Abe, J.O.: The occurrence and effect of *Cryptosporidium* species on livestock in Ile-Ife, Nigeria. Trop. Vet., 3:96–100, 1985.

Babish, J.G., et al.: Toxicity and tissue residue depletion of levamisole hydrochloride in young goats. Am. J. Vet. Res., 51:1126–1130, 1990.

Backx, A. Heutink, C.G., Van Rooij, E.M.A. and Van Rijn, P.A.: Clinical signs of bluetongue virus serotype 8 infection in sheep and goats. Vet. Rec., 161(17):591–593, 2007.

Badger, S.B. and McKenna, P.B.: Resistance to ivermectin in a field strain of *Ostertagia* spp. in goats. N. Z. Vet. J., 38:72–74, 1990.

Baker, J.C. and Sherman, D.M.: Lymphosarcoma in a Nubian goat. Vet. Med. Small Anim. Clin., 77:557–559, 1982.

Baker, N.F.: Control of parasitic gastroenteritis in goats. J. Am. Vet. Med. Assoc., 167:1069–1075, 1975.

Baker, R.L.: Genetic resistance to endoparasites in sheep and goats. A review of genetic resistance to gastrointestinal nematode parasites in sheep and goats in the tropics and evidence for resistance in some sheep and goat breeds in sub-humid coastal Kenya. Anim. Genet. Resour. Inf., 24:13–30, 1998.

Baker, R.L., Audho, J.O., Aduda, E.O. and Thorpe, W.: Genetic resistance to gastro-intestinal nematode parasites in Galla and Small East African goats in the sub-humid tropics. Anim. Sci., 73(1):61–70, 2001.

Baker, R.L. and Gray, G.D.: Appropriate breeds and breeding schemes for sheep and goats in the tropics. ACIAR Monograph Series: Worm control for small ruminants in tropical Asia. Australian Centre for International Agricultural Research (ACIAR), Canberra, Australia:, pp. 63–95, 2004.

Bali, M.K. and Singh, R.P.: Efficacy of fenbendazole suspension (Hoechst) in goat nematodiasis. Haryana Agric. Univ. J. Res., 7:155–157, 1977.

Bandyopadhyay, P.K.: A new coccidium *Eimeria sundarbanensis* n. sp. (Protozoa: Apicomplexa: Sporozoea) from *Capra hircus* (Mammalia: Artiodactyla). Protistology, 3(4):223–225, 2004.

Banerjee, K., Gupta N.P. and Goverdhan M.K.: Viral infections in laboratory personnel. Indian J. Med. Res., 69:363–373, 1979.

Bang, K.S., Familton, A.S. and Sykes, A.R.: Effect of copper oxide wire particle treatment on establishment of major gastrointestinal nematodes in lambs. Res. Vet. Sci., 39(2):132–137, 1990.

Barger, I.A.: The role of epidemiological knowledge and grazing management for helminth control in small ruminants. Internat. J. Parasitol., 29:41–47, 1999.

Barri, M.E.S., El Dirdiri, N.I., Abu Damir, H. and Idris, O.F.: Toxicity of *Abrus precatorius* in Nubian goats. Vet. Hum. Toxicol., 32:541–545, 1990.

Barron, N.S.: Entero-toxaemia in goats. Vet. Rec., 54:82, 1942.

Barton, N.J., et al.: Anthelmintic resistance in nematode parasites of goats. Aust. Vet. J., 62:224–227, 1985.

Barzilai, E. and Tadmor, A.: Multiplication of bluetongue virus in goats following experimental infection. Refuah Vet., 28:11–19, 1971.

Bassissi, M.F., Alvinerie, M. and Lespine, A.: Macrocyclic lactones: distribution in plasma lipoproteins of several animal species including humans. Comp. Biochem. Physiol. C, 138(4):437–444, 2004.

Bastianello, S.S.: A survey of neoplasia in domestic species over a 40-year period from 1935 to 1974 in the Republic of South Africa. III. Tumours occurring in pigs and goats. Onderstepoort J. Vet. Res., 50(1):25–28, 1983.

Bath, G.F.: Abomasal phytobezoariasis of goats and sheep. J. S. Afr. Vet. Med. Assoc., 49:133, 1978.

Bath, G.F. and Bergh, T.: A specific form of abomasal phytobezoar in goats and sheep. J. S. Afr. Vet. Assoc., 50:69–72, 1979.

Bath, G.F., van Wyk, J.A. and Pettey, K.P.: Control measures for some important and unusual goat diseases in southern Africa. Small Rumin. Res., 60:127–140, 2005.

Baynes, R.E., et al.: Extralabel use of ivermectin and moxidectin in food animals. J. Am. Vet. Med. Assoc., 217(5):668–671, 2000.

Bell, F.R. and Lawn, A.M.: The pattern of rumination behaviour in housed goats. Br. J. Anim. Behav., 5:85–89, 1957.

Bell, R.R., Galvin, T.J. and Turk, R.D.: Anthelmintics for ruminants VI. Thiabendazole. Am. J. Vet. Res., 23:195–200, 1962.

Benzie, D. and Phillipson, A.T.: The Alimentary Tract of the Ruminant. Edinburgh, Oliver and Boyd. 1957.

Beugnet, F.: Presence of benzimidazole-resistant strains of gastro-intestinal strongyles in sheep and goats, west of Lyon. Rev. Med. Vét., 143(6):529–533, 1992.

Beutin, L., et al.: Prevalence and some properties of verotoxin (Shiga-like toxin) producing *Escherichia coli* in seven different species of healthy domestic animals. J. Clin. Microbiol., 31(9):2483–2488, 1993.

Bhattacharya, A.N.: Research on goat nutrition and management in Mediterranean, Middle East and adjacent Arab countries. J. Dairy Sci., 63:1681–1700, 1980.

Bidjeh, K. Ouagal, M., Diallo, A. and Bornarel, P.: Transmission of rinderpest virus strains of different virulence to goats in Chad. Annal. Méd. Vét., 141:1, 65–69. 1997.

Bielaszewska M., et al.: Human *Escherichia coli* O157:H7 infection associated with the consumption of unpasteurized goat's milk, Epidemiol. Infect., 119:299–305, 1997.

Billington, S.J., et al.: *Clostridium perfringens* type E animal enteritis isolates with highly conserved, silent enterotoxin gene sequences. Infect. Immun. 66(9):4531–4536, 1998.

Bisset, S.A.: Goats and sheep as hosts for some common cattle trichostrongylids. Vet. Parasitol. 7:363–368, 1980.

Blackwell, T.E.: Enteritis and diarrhea. Vet. Clin. N. Am., Large Anim. Pract., 5:557–570, 1983.

Blackwell, T.E. and Butler, D.G.: Clinical signs, treatment, and postmortem lesions in dairy goats, with enterotoxemia: 13 cases (1979–1982), J. Am. Vet. Med. Assoc., 200:214–217, 1992.

Blackwell, T.E., Butler, D.G. and Bell, J.A.: Enterotoxemia in the goat: the humoral response and local tissue reaction following vaccination with two different bacterin-toxoids. Can. J. Comp. Med., 47:127–132, 1983.

Blackwell, T.E., Butler, D.G., Prescott, J.F. and Wilcock, B.P.: Differences in signs and lesions in sheep and goats with enterotoxemia induced by intraduodenal infusion of *Clostridium perfringens* type D. Am. J. Vet. Res., 52:1147–1152, 1991.

Bleul, U., et al.: Floppy kid syndrome caused by D-lactic acidosis in goat kids. J. Vet. Intern. Med., 20(4):1003–1008, 2006.

Boag, B. and Thomas, R.J.: Epidemiological studies on *Nematodirus* species in sheep. Res. Vet. Sci., 19(3):263–268, 1975.

Bogan, J., Benoit, E. and Delatour, P.: Pharmacokinetics of oxfendazole in goats: a comparison with sheep. J. Vet. Pharmacol. Ther., 10:305–309, 1987.

Bonfoh, B., et al.: Epidemiology of gastrointestinal nematodes in small ruminants in the plateaux region of Togo. Rev. Élev. Méd. Vét. Pays. Trop., 48(4):321–326, 1995.

Bonneau, K.R., DeMaula, C.D., Mullens, B.A. and MacLachlan, N.J.: Duration of viraemia infectious to *Culicoides sonorensis* in bluetongue virus-infected cattle and sheep. Vet. Microbiol., 88(2):115–125, 2002.

Boray, J.C.: Flukes of domestic animals. In: Parasites, Pests and Predators. S.M. Gafaar, W.E. Howard and R.E. Marsh, eds. Amsterdam, Elsevier, 1985.

Boughton, I.B. and Hardy, W.T.: Infectious entero-toxemia (milk colic) of lambs and kids. Tex. Agric. Exp. Sta. Bull., 598:5–20, 1941.

Brooker, J.D., et al.: *Streptococcus caprinus* sp. nov., a tannin-resistant ruminal bacterium from feral goats. Lett. Appl. Microbiol., 18(6):313–318, 1994.

Brooks, M.E. and Entessar, F.: Anomalous *Clostridium welchii* type B strains isolated in Iran. Br. Vet. J., 113:506–508, 1957.

Brosh, A., Sneh, B. and Shkolnik, A.: Effect of severe dehydration and rapid rehydration on the activity of the rumen microbial population of black Bedouin goats. J. Agric. Sci., Camb., 100:413–421, 1983.

Brown, C.C., Mariner, J.C. and Olander, H.J.: An immunohistochemical study of the pneumonia caused by peste des petits ruminants virus. Vet. Pathol., 28(2): 166–170, 1991.

Brown, L.E. and Johnson, W.L.: Comparative intake and digestibility of forages and byproducts by goats and sheep. A review. Int. Goat Sheep Res., 2:212–226, 1984.

Brumbaugh, G.W., Edwards, J.F., Roussel, A.J. and Thomson, T.D.: Effect of monensin sodium on histological lesions of naturally occurring bovine paratuberculosis. J. Comp. Pathol., 123(1):22–28, 2000.

Brunsdon, R.V.: Comparative epidemiology of nematode infections in sheep and goats grazed together. In: Proc. 16th Seminar, Sheep and Beef Cattle Soc., Palmerston North, N. Z. Vet. Assoc., pp. 25–33, 1986.

Buddle, B.M., et al.: A goat mortality study in the southern North Island. N. Z. Vet. J., 36:167–170, 1988.

Bulgin, M.A. and Anderson, B.C.: Salmonellosis in goats. J. Am. Vet. Med. Assoc., 178:720–723, 1981.

Burke, J.M., et al.: Accuracy of the FAMACHA system for on-farm use by sheep and goat producers in the southeastern United States. Vet. Parasitol., 147:89–95, 2007.

Burke, J.M., et al.: Use of copper oxide wire particles to control gastrointestinal nematodes in goats. J. Anim. Sci., 85(10):2753–2761, 2007a.

Burnside, D.M. and Rowley, B.O.: Evaluation of an enzyme-linked immunosorbent assay for diagnosis of paratuberculosis in goats. Am. J. Vet. Res., 55(4):465–466, 1994.

Button, C., Jerrett, I., Alexander, P. and Mizon, W.: Blindness in kids associated with overdosage of closantel. Aust. Vet. J., 64:226, 1986.

Buvanendran, V., Sooriyamoorthy, T., Ogunsusi, R.A. and Adu, I.F.: Haemoglobin polymorphism and resistance to helminths in Red Sokoto goats. Trop. Anim. Health Prod., 13:217–221, 1981.

Cabaret, J., Anjorand, N. and Leclerc, C.: Dairy goat farms in Touraine. I. Management, parasitism and estimation of disease in adult goats. Rech. Méd. Vét., 162:575–585, 1986.

Campbell, I., et al.: Effect of disinfectants on survival of *Cryptosporidium* oocysts. Vet. Rec., 111:414–415, 1982.

Cao, G.R., English, P.B., Filippich, L.J. and Inglis, S.: Experimentally induced lactic acidosis in the goat. Aust. Vet. J., 64:367–370, 1987.

Cappucci, D.T., et al.: Caprine mastitis associated with *Yersinia pseudotuberculosis.* J. Am. Vet. Med. Assoc., 173:1589–1590, 1978.

Caprioli, A., Morabito, S., Brugere, H. and Oswald, E.: Enterohaemorrhagic *Escherichia coli*: emerging issues on virulence and modes of transmission. Vet. Res., 36:3, 289–311, 2005.

Carceles, C.M., et al.: Milk kinetics of moxidectin and doramectin in goats. Res. Vet. Sci., 70(3):227–231, 2001.

Card, C.E., Perdrizet, J.A., Georgi, M.E. and Shin, S.J.: Cryptosporidiosis associated with bacterial enteritis in a goat kid. J. Am. Vet. Med. Assoc., 191:69–70, 1987.

Casteel, S. and Wagstaff, J.: *Rhododendron macrophyllum* poisoning in a group of goats and sheep. Vet. Hum. Toxicol., 31:176–177, 1989.

Castle, E.J.: The rate of passage of foodstuffs through the alimentary tract of the goat. 1. Studies on adult animals fed on hay and concentrates. Br. J. Nutr., 10:15–23, 1956.

Castle, E.J.: The rate of passage of foodstuffs through the alimentary tract of the goat. 2. Studies on growing kids. Br. J. Nutr., 10:115–125, 1956a.

Castle, E.J.: The rate of passage of foodstuffs through the alimentary tract of the goat. 3. The intestines. Br. J. Nutr., 10:338–346, 1956b.

Castro, A., et al.: Serum biochemistry values in normal pygmy goats. Am. J. Vet. Res., 38:2085–2087, 1977.

Castro, A., et al.: Serum electrolytes in normal pygmy goats. Am. J. Vet. Res., 38:663–664, 1977a.

Castro-Hermida, J.A., et al.: Efficacy of alpha-cyclodextrin against experimental cryptosporidiosis in neonatal goats. Vet. Parasitol., 120(1/2):35–41, 2004.

Castro-Hermida, J.A., et al.: *Giardia duodenalis* and *Cryptosporidium parvum* infections in adult goats and their implications for neonatal kids. Vet. Rec., 157(20):623–627, 2005.

Castro-Hermida, J.A., et al.: Prevalence of *Giardia duodenalis* and *Cryptosporidium parvum* in goat kids in western France. Small Rumin. Res., 56(1/3):259–264, 2005a.

Castro-Hermida, J.A., et al.: Occurrence of *Cryptosporidium parvum* and *Giardia duodenalis* in healthy adult domestic ruminants. Parasitol. Res., 101(5):1443–1448, 2007.

Castro-Hermida, J.A., et al.: Occurrence of *Cryptosporidium parvum* and *Giardia duodenalis* in healthy adult domestic ruminants. Parasitol. Res. 101(5):1443–1448, 2007a.

Castro-Hermida, J.A., Gonzalez-Warleta, M. and Mezo, M.: Natural infection by *Cryptosporidium parvum* and *Giardia duodenalis* in sheep and goats in Galicia (NW Spain). Small Rumin. Res., 72(2/3):96–100, 2007b.

Cavalcante, A.C.R., Rosa, J.S., Vieira, L. da S. and Pinheiro, R.R.: Infection by Paramphistomidae in goats from Sobral, Ceara, Brazil. Rev. Bra. Med. Vet., 22(6):255–257, 2000.

Cegarra, I.J. and Lewis, R.E.: Contrast study of the gastrointestinal tract in the goat *(Capra hircus).* Am. J. Vet. Res., 38:1121–1128, 1977.

Chagas, A.C., et al.: Anthelmintic action of eprinomectin in lactating Anglo-Nubian goats in Brazil. Parasitol. Res., 100(2):391–394, 2007.

Chandra, M., et al.: Study on prevalence of *Salmonella* infection in goats. Small Rumin. Res., 65(1/2):24–30, 2006.

Chandrasekharan, K., Sundaram, R.K. and Peter, C.T.: A clinical study on the anthelmintic activity of morantel tartrate (Banminth II) in calves and kids. Kerala J. Vet. Sci., 4:59–62, 1973.

Chartier, C. and Hoste, H.: Response to challenge infection with *Haemonchus contortus* and *Trichostrongylus colubriformis* in dairy goats. Differences between high and low-producers. Vet. Parasitol., 73(3/4):267–276, 1997.

Chartier, C. and Pors, I.: Duration of activity of topical eprinomectin against experimental infections with *Teladorsagia circumcincta* and *Trichostrongylus colubriformis* in goats. Vet. Parasitol., 125(3/4):415–419, 2004.

Chartier, C., Benoit, C. and Pellet, M.-P.: Serum pepsinogen concentrations in strongyle-free French dairy goats. Prev. Vet. Med., 16:255–261, 1993.

Chartier, C., Bushu, M. and Lubingo, M.: Principal helminths of small ruminants in Ituri (High Zaire). Ann. Soc. Belg. Med. Trop., 70(1):65–75, 1990.

Chartier, C., et al.: Periparturient rise in fecal egg counts associated with prolactin concentration increase in French Alpine dairy goats. Parasitol. Res., 84(10):806–810, 1998.

Chartier, C., et al.: Prevalence of anthelmintic resistant nematodes in sheep and goats in western France. Small Rumin. Res., 29(1):33–41, 1998a.

Chartier, C., Etter, E., Pors, I. and Alvinerie, M.: Activity of eprinomectin in goats against experimental infections with *Haemonchus contortus*, *Teladorsagia circumcincta* and *Trichostrongylus colubriformis*. Vet. Rec., 144(4):99–100, 1999.

Chartier, C., et al.: Efficacy of copper oxide needles for the control of nematode parasites in dairy goats. Vet. Res. Commun., 24(6):389–399, 2000a.

Chartier, C., et al.: Prevalence of anthelmintic resistance in gastrointestinal nematodes of dairy goats under extensive management conditions in southwestern France. J. Helminthol., 75(4):325–330, 2001.

Chartier, C., Lespine, A., Hoste, H. and Alvinerie, M.: Endectocides in goats: pharmacology, efficacy and conditions of use in the context of anthelmintic resistance. 8emes Rencontres autour des Recherches sur les Ruminants, Paris, France, 5–6 decembre 2001. Institut National de la Recherche Agronomique, Paris, France: pp. 181–186, 2001a.

Chartier, C., Mallereau, M. and Naciri, M.: Prophylaxis using paromomycin of natural cryptosporidial infection in neonatal kids. Prev. Vet. Med., 25(3/4):357–361, 1996.

Chartier, C., Pors, I. and Benoit, C.: Efficacy of pyrantel tartrate against experimental infections with *Haemonchus contortus*, *Teladorsagia circumcincta* and *Trichostrongylus colubriformis* in goats. Vet. Parasitol., 59(1):69–73, 1995.

Chartier, C., Pors, I., Bernard, N. and Hubert, J.: Efficacy of an albendazole slow-release capsule for the control of susceptible or resistant nematode parasites of dairy goats. Vet. Parasitol. 67(3/4):197–206, 1996a.

Chartier, C., Pors, I., Sutra, J.F. and Alvinerie, M.: Efficacy and pharmacokinetics of levamisole hydrochloride in goats with nematode infections. Vet. Rec., 146:12, 350–351, 2000.

Chatelain, E.: Atlas d'Anatomie de la Chèvre. Paris, Institut National Recherche Agronomique, 1987.

Chaudhari, A.Q., Fawi, M.T. and Obeid, H.J.: First report of Johne's disease in the Sudan. Vet. Rec., 76:246–247, 1964.

Chennells, D.: Bloat in kids. Goat Vet. Soc. J., 2:16–17, 1981.

Chhabra, R.C.: Studies on some aspects of *Oesophagostomum venulosum* (Nematoda). Indian Vet. J., 42:577–580, 1965.

Chhabra, R.C., Gill, B.S. and Dutt, S.C.: Paramphistomiasis of sheep and goats in the Punjab state and its treatment. Indian J. Parasitol., 2:43–45, 1978.

Chhabra, R.C. and Pandey, V.S.: Coccidia of goats in Zimbabwe. Vet. Parasitol., 39:199–205, 1991.

Chhadha, B.P. and Gahlot, T.K.: Positive contrast radiography of gastrointestinal tract in goats. Indian J. Vet. Surg., 27(1):37–38, 2006.

Chiejina, S.N., Fakae, B.B. and Eze, B.O.: Arrested development of gastrointestinal trichostrongylids in goats in Nigeria. Vet. Parasitol., 28:103–113, 1988.

Chiodini R.J., et al.: Possible role of mycobacteria in inflammatory bowel disease. I. An unclassified *Mycobacterium* species isolated from patients with Crohn's disease. Dig. Dis. Sci., 29(12):1073–1079, 1984.

Christie, A.B., Chen, T.H. and Elberg, S.S.: Plague in camels and goats: their role in human epidemics. J. Infect. Dis., 141:724–726, 1980.

Chungath, J.J., Radhakrishnan, K., Ommer, P.A. and Paily, L.: Histological studies on caprine forestomach. Kerala J. Vet. Sci., 16:41–46, 1985.

Church, D.C.: The Ruminant Animal: Digestive Physiology and Nutrition. Prospect Heights IL., Waveland Press Inc., p. 564, 1993.

Cid, D., Ruiz Santa Quiteria, J.A., Fuente, R. de la: F17 fimbriae in *Escherichia coli* from lambs and kids. Vet. Rec., 132(10):251, 1993.

Cid, D., et al.: Serogroups, toxins and antibiotic resistance of *Escherichia coli* strains isolated from diarrhoeic goat kids in Spain. Vet. Microbiol., 53(3/4):349–354, 1996.

Cid, D., et al.: Characterization of nonenterotoxigenic *Escherichia coli* strains producing F17 fimbriae isolated from diarrheic lambs and goat kids. J. Clin. Microbiol., 37(5):1370–1375, 1999.

Coles, G.C.: Anthelmintic resistance in sheep. Vet. Clin. North Am. Food Anim. Pract., 2:423–432, 1986.

Coles, G.C., Giordano, D.J. and Tritschler, J.P.: Efficacy of levamisole against immature and mature nematodes in goats with induced infections. Am. J. Vet. Res., 50(7):1074–1075, 1989.

Coles, G.C., Warren, A.K. and Best, J.R.: Triple resistant *Ostertagia* from Angora goats. Vet. Rec., 139(12):299–300, 1996.

Coles, G.C., et al.: The detection of anthelmintic resistance in nematodes of veterinary importance. Vet. Parasitol., 136(3/4):167–185, 2006.

Collins, D.M., Gabric, D.M. and Lisle, G.E.: Identification of two groups of *Mycobacterium paratuberculosis* strains by restriction endonuclease analysis and DNA hybridization. J. Clin. Microbiol., 28(7):1591–1596, 1990.

Collins, M.T., et al.: Enhanced radiometric detection of *Mycobacterium paratuberculosis* by using filter-concentrated bovine fecal specimens. J. Clin. Microbiol., 28(11):2514–2519, 1990a.

Colgazier, M.L., Enzie, F.D. and Lehmann, R.P.: Strain variation in the response of *Haemonchus contortus* in sheep and goats given phenothiazine: efficacy of N.F. and purified products on pure parasitic infections. Am. J. Vet. Res., 28:1711–1722, 1967.

Colmeiro, A.: Personal communication, Manager of Business Development, CZ Veterinaria, S.A., Pontevedra, Spain. February, 2008.

Connor, R.J., Munyuku, A.P., Mackyao, E. and Halliwell, R.W.: Helminthosis in goats in southern Tanzania: investigations on epidemiology and control. Trop. Anim. Health Prod., 22:1–6, 1990.

Constantinescu, G.M.: Guide to Regional Ruminant Anatomy Based on the Dissection of the Goat. Iowa State University Press, Ames, p. 243, 2001.

Contrepois, M. and Guillimin, P.: Vaccination anti-*Escherichia coli* K99 chez la chèvre. In: Les Maladies de la Chèvre, Les Colloques de l'INRA, No. 28. P. Yvore and G. Perrin, eds. Paris. Institut National de la Recherche Agronomique, pp. 473–476, 1984.

Contrepois, M., et al.: Cryptosporidiose expérimentale chez des chevreaux et des agneaux axéniques. In: Les Maladies de la Chèvre, Les Colloques de l'INRA, No. 28. P. Yvore and G. Perrin, eds. Paris. Institut National de la Recherche Agronomique, pp. 453–463, 1984.

Contreras, J.A., Lopez, W. and Sanchez, J.: *Haemonchus* infection in goats. Rev. Vet. Venez., 40:91–97, 1976.

Coop, R.L. and Kyriazakis, I.: Influence of host nutrition on the development and consequences of nematode parasitism in ruminants. Trends Parasitol., 17(7):325–330, 2001.

Corbera, J.A., Arencibia, A., Morales, I. and Gutierrez, C.: Congenital duplication of the caudal region (monocephalus dipygus) in a kid goat. Anat. Histol. Embryol., 34(1):61–63, 2005.

Corpa, J.M., Pérez, V., Sánchez M.A. and García Marín, J.F.: Control of paratuberculosis (Johne's disease) in goats by vaccination of adult animals. Vet. Rec., 146:195–196, 2000.

Cortés, C., et al.: Serotypes, virulence genes and intimin types of verotoxin-producing *Escherichia coli* and enteropathogenic *E. coli* isolated from healthy dairy goats in Spain. Vet. Microbiol., 110(1/2), 67–76, 2005.

Costa Mendes, V.M., et al.: Rotavirus in Saanen goats. J. So. Afr. Vet. Assoc., 65(3):132–133, 1994.

Courtney, C.H.: Host genetic factors in helminth control of sheep. Vet. Clin. North Am., Food Anim. Pract., 2:433–438, 1986.

Craig, D.R., Roth, L. and Smith, M.C.: Lymphosarcoma in goats. Comp. Contin. Educ. Pract. Vet., 8:S190–S197, 1986.

Craig, T.M.: Parasitism of Texas Angora goats. Proc. III International Conf. Goat Prod. Dis., Tucson, Arizona, pp. 72–76, 1982.

Craig, T.M.: Epidemiology and control of coccidia in goats. Vet. Clin. North Am., Food Anim. Pract., 2:389–395, 1986.

Cringoli, G., et al.: Effectiveness of eprinomectin pour-on against gastrointestinal nematodes of naturally infected goats. Small Rumin. Res., 55(1/3):209–213, 2004.

Cronje, P.B.: Ruminant Physiology: Digestion, Metabolism, Growth and Reproduction, New York, CABI Publishing, p. 496, 2000.

Cuéllar Ordaz, J.A.: Pathological effect of *Thysanosoma actinioides* and its incidence during winter (1978–1979) and spring (1979) in sheep and goats slaughtered at the municipal abattoir in Tlalnepantla, Mexico State. Vet. Mex., 11(2):47–48, 1980.

Dai, Y.B., Lin, M.C., Zhang, S.X. and Fu, A.Q.: Hepatic coccidiosis in the goat. Int. J. Parasitol. 21(3): 381–382, 1991.

DaMassa, A.J., Brooks, D.L. and Adler, H.E.: Caprine mycoplasmosis: widespread infection in goats with *Mycoplasma mycoides* subsp *mycoides* (large colony type). Am. J. Vet. Res., 44:322–325, 1983.

Dargie, J.M. and Allonby, E.W.: Pathophysiology of single and challenge infection of *Haemonchus contortus* in Merino sheep: Studies on red cell kinetics and the "self cure" phenomenon. Int. J. Parasitol., 5:147–157, 1975.

Dash, B. and Misra, S.C.: Efficacy of zonamix against experimental coccidiosis in kids. Indian Vet. J., 65:981–984, 1988.

Daube, G., et al.: Typing of *Clostridium perfringens* by *in vitro* amplification of toxin genes. J. Appl. Bacteriol., 77:650–655, 1994.

Davies, F.G.: Nairobi sheep disease. Parassitologia, 39(2):95–98, 1997.

DeBey, B.M., Blanchard, P.C. and Durfee, P.T.: Abomasal bloat associated with *Sarcina*-like bacteria in goat kids. J. Am. Vet. Med. Assoc., 209(8):1468–1469, 1996.

DebRoy, C. and Maddox, C.W.: Identification of virulence attributes of gastrointestinal *Escherichia coli* isolates of veterinary significance. Anim. Health Res. Rev., 2(2):129–140, 2001.

DebRoy, C. and Roberts, E.: Screening petting zoo animals for the presence of potentially pathogenic *Escherichia coli*. J. Vet. Diagn. Invest., 18(6):597–600, 2006.

Deiana, S., Lei, G.M. and Arru, E.: Catarrhal enteritis due to *Paramphistomum cervi* in goats in Sardinia. Vet. Ital., 13:1029–1039, 1962.

Delafosse, A., et al.: Herd-level risk factors for *Cryptosporidium* infection in dairy-goat kids in western France. Prev. Vet. Med., 77(1/2):109–121, 2006.

Delahaye, J.: Maladies, Prévention, Traitements. In: La Chèvre. E. Quittet, ed. Paris, La Maison Rustique, 1975.

Deligaris, N.M.: Contribution à l'etude de l'entérotoxémie des petits ruminants. Types du *Clostridium perfringens* qui sont responsables de la maladie en Grèce. Hellenike Kteniatrike, 21:74–76, 1978.

DeMaula, C.D., Leutenegger, C.M., Bonneau, K.R. and MacLachlan, N.J.: The role of endothelial cell-derived inflammatory and vasoactive mediators in the pathogenesis of bluetongue. Virology, 296(2):330–337, 2002.

Demment, M.W. and Longhurst, W.M.: Browsers and grazers: Constraints on feeding ecology imposed by gut morphology and body size. Proc. IV International Conf. Goats, Brasilia, EMBRAPA-DDT, pp. 989–1004, 1987.

Denev, I., Kostrov, R. and Tonchev, T.: Attempted eradication of *Fasciola hepatica* and *Paramphistomum microbothrium* in small domestic ruminants and in the environment. Vet. Sbirka, 83:37–39, 1985.

Dercksen, D., et al.: First outbreak of bluetongue in goats in the Netherlands. Tijdschr. Diergeneeskd., 132(20):786–790, 2007.

Desenclos, J.C., et al.: Large outbreak of *Salmonella enterica* serotype *paratyphi B* infection caused by a goats' milk cheese, France, 1993: a case finding and epidemiological study. Brit. Med. J. (Clin. Res. Ed.), 312(7023):91–94, 1996.

Devendra, C. and Burns, M.: Goat Production in the Tropics. 2nd edition. Slough. Commonwealth Agricultural Bureaux. 1983.

Devendra, C.: Feed resources and their relevance in feeding systems for goats in developing countries. Proc. IV International Conf. Goats, Brasilia, EMBRAPA-DDT, pp. 1037–1062, 1987.

Devillard, J.P.: Coccidiose de la chèvre. Bull. Group. Tech. Vét., No. 3:94–98, 1981.

Dhar, P., et al.: Recent epidemiology of peste des petits ruminants virus (PPRV). Vet. Microbiol., 88:153–159, 2002.

Diallo, A., et al.: The threat of peste des petits ruminants: progress in vaccine development for disease control. Vaccine., 25(30):5591–5597, 2007.

Diaz-Aparicio, E., Jaramillo-Meza, L., Aguilar-Romero, F. and Sergio-Cardenas, L.: Isolation and identification of *Salmonella* in goats from Mexico. Tec. Pec. Mex., 25:49–52, 1987.

Dimareli-Malli, Z., et al.: Statistical evaluation of ELISA methods for testing caprine paratuberculosis. Internat. J. Appl. Res. Vet. Med., 2(1):10–16, 2004.

Dobereiner, J., Stolf, L. and Tokarnia, C.H.: Poisonous plants affecting goats. Proc. IV International Conf. Goats, Brasilia, EMBRAPA-DDT, pp. 473–487, 1987.

Donkin, E.F. and Boyazoglu, P.A.: Diseases and mortality of adult goats in a South African milk goat herd. S. Afr. J. Anim. Sci., 34(Suppl. 1):254–257, 2004.

Dontorou, A., et al.: Isolation of a rare *Escherichia coli* O157: H7 strain from farm animals in Greece. Comp. Immunol. Microbiol. Infect. Dis., 27(3):201–207, 2004.

Drahn, F.: Futtervergiftungen bei Ziegen. Mh. Vet. Med., 6:29–30, 1951.

Dray, T.: *Clostridium perfringens* type A and β2 toxin associated with enterotoxemia in a 5-week-old goat. Can. Vet. J., 45:251–253, 2004.

Drolet, R., Fairbrother, J.M. and Vaillancourt, D.: Attaching and effacing *Escherichia coli* in a goat with diarrhea. Can. Vet. J., 35(2):122–123, 1994.

Dubey, J.P.: Coccidiosis in the gall bladder of a goat. Proc. Helminthol. Soc. Wash., 53:277–281, 1986.

Ducatelle, R., et al.: Cryptosporidiosis in goats and in mouflon sheep. Vlaams Diergeneesk. Tijdschr., 52:7–17, 1983.

Duhamel, G.E., Moxley, R.A., Maddox, C.W. and Erickson, E.D.: Enteric infection of a goat with enterohemorrhagic *Escherichia coli* (O103:H2). J. Vet. Diagn. Investig., 4(2):197–200, 1992.

Dunbar, R.: Scapegoat for a thousand deserts. New Scientist, 104:30–33, 1984.

Dupuy, J., Chartier, C., Sutra, J.F. and Alvinerie, M.: Eprinomectin in dairy goats: dose influence on plasma levels and excretion in milk. Parasitol. Res., 87(4):294–298, 2001.

Dziuk, H.E. and McCauley, E.H.: Comparison of ruminoreticular motility patterns in cattle, sheep, and goats. Am. J. Physiol., 209:324–328, 1965.

Eales, F.A., et al.: A field study of watery mouth: clinical, epidemiological, biochemical, haematological and bacteriological observations. Vet. Rec., 119:543–547, 1986.

Eamens, G.J., et al.: Comparative sensitivity of various faecal culture methods and ELISA in dairy cattle herds with endemic Johne's disease. Vet. Microbiol., 77(3/4):357–367, 2000.

Eamens, G.J., Walker, D.M., Porter, N.S. and Fell, S.A.: Pooled faecal culture for the detection of *Mycobacterium avium* subsp. *paratuberculosis* in goats. Aust. Vet. J., 85(6):243–251, 2007.

East, N.E.: Pregnancy toxemia, abortions and periparturient diseases. Vet. Clin. N. Am. Large Anim. Pract., 5:601–618, 1983.

Eckburg, P.B. and Relman, D.A.: The role of microbes in Crohn's disease. Clin. Inf. Dis., 44:254–262, 2007.

Ejlertsen, M., Githigia, S.M., Otieno, R.O. and Thamsborg, S.M.: Accuracy of an anaemia scoring chart applied on goats in sub-humid Kenya and its potential for control of *Haemonchus contortus* infections. Vet. Parasitol., 141(3/4):291–301, 2006.

El Aich, A. and Waterhouse, A.: Small ruminants in environmental conservation. Sm. Rum. Res., 34(3):271–287, 1999.

Elard, L. and Humbert, J.F.: Importance of the mutation of amino acid 200 of the isotype 1 beta-tubulin gene in the benzimidazole resistance of the small-ruminant parasite *Teladorsagia circumcincta*. Parasitol. Res., 85(6):452–456, 1999.

El Dirdiri, N.I., Barakat, S.E.M. and Adam, S.E.I.: The combined toxicity of *Aristolochia bracteata* and *Cadaba rotundifolia* to goats. Vet. Hum. Toxicol., 29:133–137, 1987.

El Sayed, N.Y., Abdelbari, E.M., Mahmoud, O.M. and Adam, S.E.I.: The toxicity of *Cassia senna* to Nubian goats. Vet. Q., 5:80–85, 1983.

Elliot, D.C.: Removal of *Haemonchus contortus*, *Ostertagia circumcincta*, and *Trichostrongylus* spp. from goats by morantel citrate, levamisole hydrochloride, fenbendazole, and oxfendazole. N. Z. Vet. J., 35:208–210, 1987.

Elliott, H.: Bluetongue disease: background to the outbreak in NW Europe. Goat Vet. Soc. J., 23:31–39, 2007.

Emele-Nwaubani, J.C. and Ihemelandu, E.C.: Anodontia of the incisor and canine teeth in a cryptorchid West African dwarf goat. Trop. Vet., 2:172–174, 1984.

Enyenihi, U.K., Okon, E.D. and Fabiyi, J.P.: Tapeworm infections of small ruminants in Nigeria. Bull. Anim. Health Prod. Afr., 23:289–295, 1975.

Erdenebaatar, J., et al.: Enzyme-linked immunosorbent assay to differentiate the antibody responses of animals infected with *Brucella* species from those of animals infected with *Yersinia enterocolitica* O9. Clin. Diag. Lab. Immunol. 10(4):710–714, 2003.

Escudero, E., Carceles, C.M., Galtier, P. and Alvinerie, M.: Influence of fasting on the pharmacokinetics of ivermectin in goats. J. Vet. Pharmacol. Ther., 20(Supplement 1):71–72, 1997.

Espié, E., et al.: *Escherichia coli* O157 outbreak associated with fresh unpasteurized goats' cheese. Epidemiol. Infect., 134(1):143–146, 2006.

Espié, E. and Vaillant, V.: International outbreak of *Salmonella* Stourbridge infection, April- July 2005: results of epidemiological, food and veterinary investigations in France. Eurosurveillance, 10(8): E050811.3., August 11, 2005. http://www.eurosurveillance.org/ew/2005/050811.asp#3.

Estevez-Denaives, I., Hernandez-Castro, R., Trujillo-Garcia, A.M. and Chavez-Gris, G.: Detection of *Mycobacterium avium* subsp. *paratuberculosis* in goat and sheep flocks in Mexico. Small Rumin. Res., 72(2/3):209–213, 2007.

Ezeifeka, G.O., Umoh, J.U., Belino, E.D. and Ezeokoli, C.D.: Complement fixing antibodies to Orungo virus in food animals of northern Nigeria. Int. J. Zoon., 11:149–154, 1984.

Ezeokoli, C.D., et al.: Clinical and epidemiological features of peste des petits ruminants in Sokoto Red goats. Rev. Élev. Méd. Vét. Pays. Trop., 39:269–273, 1986.

Fabiyi, J.P.: Seasonal fluctuations of nematode infestations in goats in the savannah belt of Nigeria. Bull. Epizoot. Dis. Afr., 21:277–286, 1973.

Falade, S.: Isolation of *Salmonella poona* from diarrhoeic Nigerian goats. Vet. Rec., 99:419, 1976.

Faraj, M.K., Abd. A.A. and Abdal-Karim, A.K.: *Salmonella* serotypes from animals slaughtered in Baghdad (Iraq). Haryana Vet., 22:122–123, 1983.

Farizy, P. and Taranchon, P.: Intérêt d'un traitement anthelminthique au thiabendazole chez la chèvre en lactation. Rec. Méd. Vét., 146:251–260, 1970.

Fayer, R.: *Cryptosporidium*: a water-borne zoonotic parasite. Vet. Parasitol., 126: 37–56, 2004.

Fernandez Miyakawa, M.E. and Uzal, F.A.: The early effects of *Clostridium perfringens* type D epsilon toxin in ligated intestinal loops of goats and sheep. Vet. Res. Commun., 27:231–241, 2003.

Ferre, I., et al.: Effect of different decoquinate treatments on cryptosporidiosis in naturally infected cashmere goat kids. Vet. Rec., 157(9):261–262, 2005.

Fitzsimmons, W.M.: Experimental *Trichostrongylus colubriformis* infection in the goat. Res. Vet. Sci., 7:101–111, 1966.

Fleming, S.A., et al.: Anthelmintic resistance of gastrointestinal parasites in small ruminants. J. Vet. Intern. Med., 20:435–444, 2006.

Fleming, S.A., Dallman, M.J. and Sedlacek, D.L.: Esophageal obstruction as a sequela to ruptured esophagus in a goat. J. Am. Vet. Med. Assoc., 195:1598–1600, 1989.

Fodstad, F.H. and Gunnarsson, E.: Post-mortem examination in the diagnosis of Johne's disease in goats. Acta Vet. Scand., 20:157–167, 1979.

Food and Agriculture Organization: The Pan-African Rinderpest campaign. Report, Conf. FAO, 23rd Sess., Nov 9–28, 1985, Rome, Italy, pp. 46–47, 1985.

Foreyt, W.J., Hancock, D. and Wescott, R.B.: Prevention and control of coccidiosis in goats with decoquinate. Am. J. Vet. Res., 47:333–335, 1986.

Foreyt, W.J.: Coccidiosis and cryptosporidiosis in sheep and goats. Vet. Clin. N. Am. Food Anim. Pract., 6:655–670, 1990.

Fuente, R. de la, et al.: Prevalence and characteristics of attaching and effacing strains of *Escherichia coli* isolated from diarrhoeic and healthy sheep and goats. Am. J. Vet. Res., 63:2, 262–266, 2002.

Furley, C.W., Taylor, W.P. and Obi, T.U.: An outbreak of peste des petits ruminants in a zoological collection. Vet. Rec., 121:443–447, 1987.

Galal, M., Adam, S.E.I., Maglad, M.A. and Wasfi, I.A.: The effects of *Cassia italica* on goats and sheep. Acta Vet. Beograd, 35:163–174, 1985.

Galtier, P., Escoula, L., Camguilhem, R. and Alvinerie, M.: Comparative bioavailability of levamisole in non lactating ewes and goats. Ann. Rech. Vét., 12:109–115, 1981.

Garcin, D.V.: Réflexion sur la maladie du chevreau "mou." La Chèvre, No. 129:11, 1982.

Garg, D.N. and Sharma, V.K.: The detection of nasal carriers of *Salmonella* and other enterobacteria amongst young farm animals. Zentrlbl. Bakt. Parasit. Infekt. Hyg., 243A:542–546, 1979.

Gargadennec, L. and Lalanne, A.: La peste des petits ruminants. Bull. Serv. Zootech. Epizoot. Afr. Occ. Fr., 5:16–21, 1942.

Gatongi, P.M., et al.: Hypobiosis of *Haemonchus contortus* in natural infections of sheep and goats in a semi-arid area of Kenya. Vet. Parasitol., 77(1):49–61. 1998.

Gawor, J., Borecka, A. and Malczewski, A.: Use of eprinomectin (Eprinex Pour-On) to control natural infection by gastro-intestinal nematodes in goats. Medycyna Weterynaryjna, 56(6):398–400, 2000.

Geary, T.G., Sangster, N.C. and Thompson, D.P.: Frontiers in anthelmintic pharmacology. Vet. Parasitol. 84(3/4):275–295, 1999.

Geoffroy, F.: Étude comparée du comportement alimentaire et merycique de deux petits ruminants: la chèvre et le mouton. Ann. Zootech., 23:63–73, 1974.

Gezon, H.M., et al.: Identification and control of paratuberculosis in a large goat herd. Am. J. Vet. Res., 49:1817–1823, 1988.

Gialletti, L., Grelloni, V., Rossanigo, E.C. and Fioroni, A.: Diagnosi di criptosporidiosi in alcuni allevamenti dell'Italia centrale. Atti Soc. Ital. Sci. Vet., 39:751–753, 1986.

Gibb, M.C.: Lily of the valley poisoning in an Angora goat. N. Z. Vet. J., 35:59, 1987.

Gibbs, E.P.J. and Greiner, E.C.: The epidemiology of bluetongue. Comp. Immun. Microbiol. Infect. Dis., 17(3/4):207–220, 1994.

Gibbs, E.P.J. and Lawman, M.J.P.: Infection of British deer and farm animals with epizootic haemorrhagic disease of deer virus. J. Comp. Pathol., 87:335–343, 1977.

Gibbs, E.P.J., Taylor, W.P. and Lawman, M.J.P.: The isolation of adenoviruses from goats affected with peste des petits ruminants in Nigeria. Res. Vet. Sci., 23:331–335, 1977.

Gibbs, E.P.J., Taylor, W.P., Lawman, M.J.P. and Bryant, J.: Classification of peste des petits ruminants virus as the fourth member of the genus *Morbillivirus*. Intervirology, 11:268–274, 1979.

Gibson, D.A.: An outbreak of *Salmonella dublin* infection in goats. Vet. Rec., 69:1026–1028, 1957.

Gilbert, M., Jolivet-Renaud, C. and Popoff, M.R.: Beta2 toxin, a novel toxin produced by *Clostridium perfringens*. Gene, 203:65–73, 1997.

Gillham, R.J. and Obendorf, D.L.: Therapeutic failure of levamisole in dairy goats. Aust. Vet. J., 62:426–427, 1985.

Goldberg, A.: Effects of the nematode *Oesophagostomum venulosum* on sheep and goats. J. Parasitol., 38(1):35–47, 1952.

Gomez-Tejedor, C.: Brief overview of the bluetongue situation in Mediterranean Europe, 1998–2004. Vet. Ital., 40(3):57–60, 2004.

González, A., et al.: Pharmacokinetics of a novel formulation of ivermectin after administration to goats. Am. J. Vet. Res. 67(2):323–328, 2006.

Goudswaard, J.: Studies on the incidence of *Mycobacterium johnei* in the organs of experimentally infected goats. Neth. J. Vet. Sci., 4:65–75, 1971.

Government of Norway: Central Bureau of Statistics. Sjukdommer hos sau og geit. In: Veterinaerstatistikk 1983. Oslo, Norway; Statistisk Sentrabyra, 1985.

Grant, I.R., Ball, H.J. and Rowe, M.T.: Effect of higher pasteurization temperatures, and longer holding times at 72 degrees C, on the inactivation of *Mycobacterium paratuberculosis* in milk. Lett. Appl. Microbiol., 28(6):461–465, 1999.

Grant, I.R., Rowe, M.T., Dundee, L. and Hitchings, E.: *Mycobacterium avium* ssp. *paratuberculosis*: its incidence, heat resistance and detection in milk and dairy products. Internat. J. Dairy Technol. 54(1):2–13, 2001.

Grant, I.R.: *Mycobacterium avium* ssp. *paratuberculosis* in foods: current evidence and potential consequences. Int. J. Dairy Technol. 59(2):112–117, 2006.

Green, D.S., Green, M.J., Hillyer, M.H. and Morgan, K.L.: Injection site reactions and antibody responses in sheep and goats after the use of multivalent clostridial vaccines. Vet. Rec., 120:435–439, 1987.

Greig, A., et al.: Epidemiological study of paratuberculosis in wild rabbits in Scotland. J. Clin. Microbiol., 37:1746–1751, 1999.

Griffin, L., Allonby, E.W. and Preston, J.M.: The interaction of *Trypanosoma congolense* and *Haemonchus contortus* infections in 2 breeds of goat. 1. Parasitology. J. Comp. Pathol., 91:85–95, 1981.

Groocock, C.M.: Nairobi sheep disease. In: Foreign Animal Diseases. Richmond, VA, United States Animal Health Association, 1998.

Gruner, L.: Breeding for helminth resistance in sheep and goats. In, Breeding for disease resistance in farm animals. CAB International, Wallingford, UK, pp. 187–200, 1991.

Gruner, L. and Cabaret, J.: Resistance of sheep and goats to helminth infections: A genetic basis. In: Increasing Small Ruminant Productivity in Semi-arid Areas. E.F. and F.S. Thomson, Dordrecht, Kluwer Academic Publishers, 1988.

Gueltekin, M.: Observations on anatomic differences in gut compartments between Angora goats and sheep and comparative studies on the structure of abomasal glands in different animals. Vet. Publ. No. 68, Ankara Univ., Yeni Desen Press, Ankara, Turkey, 1953.

Gumber, S., Eamens, G. and Whittington, R.J.: Evaluation of a Pourquier ELISA kit in relation to agar gel immunodiffusion (AGID) test for assessment of the humoral immune response in sheep and goats with and without *Mycobacterium paratuberculosis* infection. Vet. Microbiol., 115(1/3):91–101, 2006.

Gumusova, O.S., Yazici, Z., Albayrak, H. and Cakiroglu, D.: First report of bovine rotavirus and bovine coronavirus seroprevalence in goats in Turkey. Vet. Glasnik, 61(1/2):75–79, 2007.

Gunning, O.V.: Poisoning in goats by black nightshade *(Solanum nigrum)*. Br. Vet. J., 105:473–474, 1949.

Gupta, P.D.: Incidence of salmonella in beef and goat meat in West Bengal and its public health importance. Indian J. Anim. Health, 13:161–163, 1974.

Gupta, R.P., Chaudhri, S.S., Ruprah, N.S. and Yadav, C.L.: Epizootiology of paramphistomiasis in Haryana state. Indian J. Anim. Sci., 55:14–19, 1985.

Guss, S.B.: Management and Diseases of Dairy Goats. Scottsdale, Dairy Goat Journal Publishing Co., 1977.

Habel, R.E.: Ruminant digestive system. In: Sisson and Grossman's Anatomy of Domestic Animals, 5th edition, volume I. R. Getty, ed. Philadelphia, W.B. Saunders Co. 1975.

Haddow, J.R. and Idnani, J.A.: Goat dermatitis: A new virus disease of goats in India. Indian Vet. J., 24:332–337, 1948.

Hafeez, M. and Rao, B.V.: Studies on amphistomiasis in Andhra Pradesh (India). VI. Immunization of lambs and kids with gamma irradiated metacercariae of *Cercaria indicae* XXVI. J. Helminthol., 55:29–32, 1981.

Haibel, G.K.: Intestinal adenocarcinoma in a goat. J. Am. Vet. Med. Assoc., 196:326–328, 1990.

Hailat, N., et al.: Pathology of the rumen in goats caused by plastic foreign bodies with reference to its prevalence in Jordan. Small Rumin. Res., 30(2):77–83, 1998.

Hale, M., Burke, J., Miller, J. and Terrill, T.: Tools for managing internal parasites in small ruminants: copper wire particles. ATTRA—National Sustainable Agriculture Information Service, Fayetteville, AR, 8 pp, 2007. http://www.attra.ncat.org/attra-pub/PDF/copper_wire.pdf.

Hall, A.: Digestive disorders—part 1. Diagnosing bloat, compaction and peritonitis. Dairy Goat Guide, 6:17–18, 1983.

Hall, C.A., Ritchie, L. and McDonell, P.A.: Investigations for anthelmintic resistance in gastrointestinal nematodes from goats. Res. Vet. Sci., 31:116–119, 1981.

Hamdy, F.M. and Dardiri, A.H.: Response of white-tailed deer to infection with peste des petits ruminants virus. J. Wildlife Dis., 12:516–522, 1976.

Hamdy, F.M., et al.: Etiology of the stomatitis pneumoenteritis complex in Nigerian dwarf goats. Can. J. Comp. Med., 40:276–284, 1976.

Harder, A., Samson-Himmelstjerna, G. von: Cyclooctadepsipeptides—a new class of anthelmintically active compounds. Parasitol. Res., 88(6):481–488, 2002.

Harding, H.P.: Experimental infection with *Mycobacterium johnei:* the histopathology of infection in experimental goats. J. Comp. Pathol., 67:37–52, 1957.

Hardy, W.T. and Price, D.A.: Soremuzzle of sheep. J. Am. Vet. Med. Assoc., 120:23–25, 1952.

Harris, N.B. and Barletta, R.G.: *Mycobacterium avium* subsp. *paratuberculosis* in veterinary medicine. Clin. Microbiol. Rev., 14(3):489–512, 2001.

Harwood, D.: Diseases of dairy goats. In Practice, 26(5):248–259, 2004.

He, H.X., et al.: Studies on nucleic acid vaccine of *Cryptosporidium parvum*. J. Jilin Agric. Univ., 24(3):75–79, 2002.

Hennessy, D.R., Sangster, N.C., Steel, J.W. and Collins, G.H.: Comparative pharmacokinetic behaviour of albendazole in sheep and goats. Internat. J. Parasitol., 23(3):321–325, 1993.

Hennessy, D.R., Sangster, N.C., Steel, J.W. and Collins, G.H.: Comparative pharmacokinetic disposition of closantel in sheep and goats. J. Vet. Pharmacol. Ther., 16(3):254–260, 1993a.

Herholz, C., et al.: Prevalence of β2-toxigenic *Clostridium perfringens* in horses with intestinal disorders. J. Clin. Microbiol., 37(2):358–361, 1999.

Hermon-Taylor, J. and Bull, T.: Crohn's disease caused by *Mycobacterium avium* subspecies *paratuberculosis*: a public health tragedy whose resolution is long overdue. J. Med. Microbiol., 51(1):3–6, 2002.

Hermon-Taylor, J., et al.: Causation of Crohn's disease by *Mycobacterium avium* subsp. *paratuberculosis*. Can J. Gastroenterol., 14(6):521–539, 2000.

Heuvelink, A.E. et al.: *Escherichia coli* O157 infection associated with a petting zoo. Epidemiol. Infect., 129(2):295–302, 2002.

Hines, M.E., II, et al.: Experimental challenge models for Johne's disease: a review and proposed international guidelines. Vet. Microbiol., 122(3/4):197–222, 2007.

Hodges, R.T., Carman, M.G. and Mortimer, W.J.: Serotypes of *Yersinia pseudotuberculosis* recovered from domestic livestock. N. Z. Vet. J., 32:11–13, 1984.

Hofmann, R.R.: Morphophysiological evolutionary adaptations of the ruminant digestive system. In: Aspects of Digestive Physiology in Ruminants. A. Dobson and M.J. Dobson, eds. Ithaca, Comstock Publishing Associates, pp. 1–20, 1988.

Hollands, R.D. and Hughes, M.-C.: *Pieris formosanum* poisoning in the goat. Vet. Rec., 118:407–408, 1986.

Holstad, G., et al.: *Mycobacterium avium* subspecies *paratuberculosis*—a review of present research in Norway. Acta Vet. Scand., 44(3/4):269–272, 2003.

Hong, C., Hunt, K.R. and Coles, G.C.: Occurrence of anthelmintic resistant nematodes on sheep farms in England and goat farms in England and Wales. Vet. Rec., 139(4):83–86, 1996.

Horak, I.G.: Host parasite relationships of *Paramphistomum microbothrium* Fischoeder, 1901, in experimentally infected ruminants with particular reference to sheep. Onderstepoort J. Vet. Res., 34:451–540, 1967.

Horak, I.G.: Paramphistomiasis of domestic ruminants. Adv. Parasitol., 9:33–72, 1971.

Horenstein, L. and Elias, E.: Ventral uterina (histerocoele) in the goat: a case report. Isr. J. Vet. Med., 43:86, 1987.

Hornitzky, M.A.Z., Romalis, L.F., Ross, A.D. and Sheldrake, R.F.: Comparison of counter immunoelectrophoresis with mouse protection assay in the detection of epsilon toxin in the intestinal contents of goats. Aust. Vet. J., 66:121–122, 1989.

Horowitz, A. and Venzke, W.G.: Distribution of blood vessels to the postdiaphragmatic digestive tract of the goat: celiac trunk-gastroduodenal and splenic tributaries of the portal vein. Am. J. Vet. Res., 27:1293–1315, 1966.

Hoste, H.: Adaptive physiological processes in the host during gastrointestinal parasitism. Int. J. Parasitol., 31: 231–244, 2001.

Hoste, H. and Chartier, C.: Comparison of the effects on milk production of concurrent infection with *Haemonchus contortus* and *Trichostrongylus colubriformis* in high- and low-producing dairy goats. Am. J. Vet. Res., 54(11):1886–1893, 1993.

Hoste, H. and Chartier, C.: Goat resistance to trichostrongyle infections of the gastro-intestinal tract. Point Vét., 29(189):161–166, 1998.

Hoste, H. and Chartier, C.: Response to challenge infection with *Haemonchus contortus* and *Trichostrongylus colubriformis* in dairy goats. Consequences on milk production. Vet. Parasitol., 74(1):43–54, 1998a.

Hoste, H., Le Frileux, Y. and Pommaret, A.: Comparison of selective and systematic treatments to control nematode infection of the digestive tract in dairy goats. Vet. Parasitol., 106:345–355, 2002.

Howe, P.A.: Coccidiosis in goats. In: Proceedings, Refresher Course for Veterinarians, Post-Graduate Committee in Veterinary Science, University of Sydney, 52:285–290, 1980.

Howe, P.A.: Diseases of Goats. Number 5 in The T. G. Hungerford Vade Mecum Series for Domestic Animals. The University of Sydney Post-Graduate Foundation in Veterinary Science. 1984.

Hsu, W.H.: Toxicity and drug interactions of levamisole. J. Am. Vet. Med. Assoc., 176:1166–1169, 1980.

Hubbert, W.T.: Yersiniosis in mammals and birds in the United States. Am. J. Trop. Med. Hyg., 21:458–463, 1972.

Hughes, D. and Jensen, N.: *Yersinia enterocolitica* in raw goat's milk. Appl. Environ. Microbiol., 41:309–310, 1981.

Hussein, H.S., Arzoun, I.H. and Hussein, M.F.: *Haemonchus longistipes* (Railliet and Henry, 1909) in goats in the Sudan. J. Helminthol., 59:79–81, 1985.

Hutchinson, L.J., Weinstock, D. and Byler, L.I.: Case report—management of paratuberculosis in a dairy goat herd. Bov. Pract., 38(2):142–146, 2004.

Iggo, A.: Central nervous control of gastric movements in sheep and goats. J. Physiol., 131:248–256, 1956.

Ikeme, M.M., Iskander, F. and Chong, L.C.: Seasonal changes in the prevalence of *Haemonchus* and *Trichostrongylus* hypobiotic larvae in tracer goats in Malaysia. Trop. Anim. Health Prod., 19:184–190, 1987.

Inverso, M., Lukas, G.N. and Weidenbach, S.J.: Caprine bluetongue virus isolations. Am. J. Vet. Res., 41:277–278, 1980.

Iovane, G., Pagnini, P., Martone, F. and Bonaduce, A.: Presence and distribution of serum antibodies against rotavirus in sheep and goats in southern Italy. Acta Med. Vet., 34(1):3–9, 1988.

Isawa, K., Tajimi, A. and Nishihara, N.: The excessive salivation of goats caused by some Japanese isolates of blackpatch disease fungus *(Rhizoctonia leguminicola)* of leguminous forage. Bull. Natl. Inst. Anim. Husb. Summaries, 24:10, 1971.

Jackson, F., et al.: Prevalence of anthelmintic-resistant nematodes in fibre-producing goats in Scotland. Vet. Rec., 131(13):282–285, 1992.

Janakiraman, D. and Rajendran, M.P.: The significance of isolation of *Salmonella* from goats used for the production of freeze-dried rinderpest goat-tissue vaccine. Indian J. Anim. Sci., 43:220–223, 1973.

Jeffcoate, J.A., et al.: Pathophysiology of the periparturient egg rise in sheep: a possible role for IgA. Res. Vet. Sci., 53(2):212–218, 1992.

Jenkins, M.C.: Advances and prospects for subunit vaccines against protozoa of veterinary importance. Vet. Parasitol., 101:291–310, 2001.

Jeyakumar, C.S.: A preliminary report on the use of FAMACHA© for haemonchosis in goats in the Eastern Cape Province of South Africa during the late autumn/early winter period. J. S. Afr. Vet. Assoc., 78(2):90–91, 2007.

Johne, H.A. and Frothingham, L.: Ein eigenthümlicher Fall von Tuberculose beim Rind. Deut. Z. Tier. Verg. Pathol., 21:438–454, 1895.

Johnson, E.H., et al.: Atypical outbreak of caprine cryptosporidiosis in the Sultanate of Oman. Vet. Rec., 145(18):521–524, 1999.

Johnson, E.H., et al.: Confirmation of the prophylactic value of paromomycin in a natural outbreak of caprine cryptosporidiosis. Vet. Res. Commun., 24(1):63–67, 2000.

Johnson, E.H., Nyack, B. and Marsh, A.: Surgical repair of atresia ani and rectovaginal fistula in a goat. Vet. Med. Sm. Anim. Clin., 75:1833–1834, 1980.

Jones, R.J.: The value of *Leucaena leucocephala* as a feed for ruminants in the tropics. World Anim. Rev., 31:13–23, 1979.

Jones, R.J. and Megarrity, R.G.: Comparative toxicity responses of goats fed on *Leucaena leucocephala* in Australia and Hawaii. Aust. J. Agric. Res., 34:781–790, 1983.

Jones, R.J. and Megarrity, R.G.: Successful transfer of DHP-degrading bacteria from Hawaiian goats to Australian ruminants to overcome the toxicity of *Leucaena.* Aust. Vet. J., 63:259–262, 1986.

Jones, T.O.: Caprine mastitis associated with *Yersinia pseudotuberculosis* infection. Vet. Rec., 110:231, 1982.

Jorgensen, P.H., Halliwell, R.W. and Honhold, N.: Prevalence of serum antibodies to bluetongue virus in indigenous goats in Zimbabwe revealed by a blocking enzyme-linked immunosorbent assay. Trop. Anim. Health Prod., 21:58, 1989.

Jung, S.H. Kim, C.S and Huh, C.K.: Development of the esophagus of fetuses and neonates in Korean native goats. Korean J. Vet. Res., 34(4):679–686, 1994.

Kahiya, C., Mukaratirwa, S. and Thamsborg, S.M.: Effects of *Acacia nilotica* and *Acacia karoo* diets on *Haemonchus contortus* infection in goats. Vet. Parasitol., 115(3):265–274, 2003.

Kaminsky, R., et al.: A new class of anthelmintics effective against drug-resistant nematodes. Nature, 452(7184):176–180, March 13, 2008.

Kaneko, J.J.: Appendixes. In: Clinical Biochemistry of Domestic Animals. 3rd Ed. J.J. Kaneko, ed. New York, Academic Press, 1980.

Kanyari, P.W.N.: Coccidiosis in goats and aspects of epidemiology. Aust. Vet. J., 65:257–258, 1988.

Kaplan, R.M.: Update on parasite control in small ruminants 2006—Addressing the challenges posed by multiple-drug resistant worms. Proceedings, 39th Annual Convention, American Association of Bovine Practitioners, AABP, Auburn, AL, pp. 196–206, 2006.

Kaplan, R.M., et al.: Validation of the FAMACHA© eye color chart for detecting clinical anemia in sheep and goats on farms in the southern United States. Vet. Parasitol., 123:105–120, 2004.

Kapur, M.P., Kalra, D.S. and Randhawa, A.S.: Occurrence of *Salmonella* serotypes in goats. Indian Vet. J., 50:859–862, 1973.

Karanu, F.N., et al.: CD4+ T lymphocytes contribute to protective immunity induced in sheep and goats by *Haemonchus contortus* gut antigens. Parasite Immunol., 19(10):435–445 1997.

Karstad, L., Nestel, B. and Graham, M. (eds.): Wildlife Disease Research and Economic Development. Ottawa, International Development Research Centre, 1981.

Katiyar, R.D.: A report on plant poisoning in sheep and goats. Livestock Adviser, 6:57–62, 1981.

Katiyar, R.D. and Varshney, T.R.: Amphistomiasis in sheep and goats in Uttar Pradesh. Indian J. Vet. Sci. Anim. Husb., 33:94–98, 1963.

Keen, J.E., et al.: Shiga-toxigenic *Escherichia coli* O157 in agricultural fair livestock, United States. Emer. Infect. Dis., 12(5):780–786, 2006.

Kerboeuf, D. and Godu, J.: Les strongyloses gastrointestinales, données épidémiologiques et diagnostic chez les caprins. Bull. Group. Tech. Vét., 3:67–84, 1981.

Kerboeuf, D. and Hubert, J.: Benzimidazole resistance in field strains of nematodes from goats in France. Vet. Rec., 116:133, 1985.

Kettle, P.R., Vlassof, A., Reid, T.C. and Horton, C.T.: A survey of nematode control measures used by milking goat farmers and of anthelmintic resistance on their farms. N. Z. Vet. J., 31:139–143, 1983.

Kimberling, C.V.: Jensen and Swift's Diseases of Sheep. 3rd Edition. Philadelphia, Lea and Febiger, 1988.

King, N.B.: Goat practice—summer management problems. In: Proceedings, Refresher Course for Veterinarians, Post-Graduate Committee in Veterinary Science, University of Sydney, 52:39–46, 1980.

King, N.B.: Pregnancy toxemia and enterotoxemia. In: Proceedings, Refresher Course for Veterinarians, Post-Graduate Committee in Veterinary Science, University of Sydney, 52:209–212, 1980a.

King, N.B.: Metabolic diseases. In: Proceedings, Refresher Course for Veterinarians, Post-Graduate Committee in Veterinary Science, University of Sydney, 52:203–207, 1980b.

Kirkland, P.D.: Bluetongue viruses, vectors and surveillance in Australia—the current situation and unique features. Vet. Ital., 40(3):47–50, 2004.

Kirkpatrick, C.E. and Farrell, J.P.: Cryptosporidiosis. Comp. Cont. Educ. Pract. Vet., 6:S154–S164, 1984.

Kirsch, R.: The activity of Panacur in goats naturally or experimentally infected with gastro-intestinal nematodes. Blauen Hefte Tierarzt, 59:453–458, 1979.

Knight, A.P.: Rhododendron and laurel poisoning. Comp. Cont. Educ. Pract. Vet., 9:F26–F27, 1987.

Knox, D.P.: Development of vaccines against gastrointestinal nematodes. Parasitol., 120:43–61, 2000.

Knox, D.P., et al.: The nature and prospects for gut membrane proteins as vaccine candidates for *Haemonchus contortus* and other ruminant trichostrongyloids. Int. J. Parasitol., 33(11):1129–1137, 2003.

Kock, R.A., et al.: Re-infection of wildlife populations with rinderpest virus on the periphery of the Somali ecosystem in East Africa. Prev. Vet. Med., 75(1/2):63–80, 2006.

Kohler, B.: Bluetongue. In: Applied Veterinary Epidemiology. T. Blaha, ed. Amsterdam, Elsevier, 1989.

Kojouri, G.A.: A new treatment of abomasal tympany in goat kids. Animal health: a breakpoint in economic development? The 11th International Conference of the Association of Institutions for Tropical Veterinary Medicine and 16th Veterinary Association Malaysia Congress, 23–27 August 2004, Petaling Jaya, Malaysia. pp. 281–282, 2004.

Komarov, A. and Goldsmit, L.: A disease similar to blue tongue in cattle and sheep in Israel. Refuah Vet., 8:96–100, 1951.

Komolafe, O.O., Ugwu, H.O. and Ebirim, R.A.: An investigation into the possible role of peridomestic rats in the epizootiology of peste des petits ruminants in goats. Bull. Anim. Health Prod. Afr., 35:207–210, 1987.

Koopmann, R., Holst, C. and Epe, C.: Experiences with the FAMACHA© Eye Colour Chart for identifying sheep and goats targeted for anthelmintic treatment. Berliner und Münchener Tierärztliche Wochenschrift. 119(9/10):436–442, 2006.

Kostov, R.: Experimental infection of lambs and kids with *Chabertia ovina*. Nauchni Trudove Raionen Nachnoizsl. Veterinarnomed. Inst., Veliko Turnovo, 2:99–108, 1982.

Koudela, B. and Vitovec, J.: Experimental giardiasis in goat kids. Vet. Parasitol., 74(1):9–18, 1998.

Krametter, R., Bagó, Z., Floeck, M. and Baumgartner, W.: Abdominal mesothelioma in a goat. N. Z. Vet. J., 52(5):293–296, 2004.

Kritas, S.K.: Prevention of scours in neonatal kids after oral administration of an organic acid solution. J. Vet. Med. Series A, 49(1):23–26, 2002.

Kritas, S.K., et al.: Prevention of scours in neonatal kids after modification of management and experimental vaccination against *Escherichia coli*. Small Rumin. Res., 50(1/2):51–56, 2003.

Krogstad, O., Tiege, J. and Lassen, J.: *Yersinia enterocolitica* type 2 associated with disease in goat. Acta Vet. Scand., 13:594–596, 1972.

Krogstad, O.: *Yersinia enterocolitica* infection in goat. Acta Vet. Scand., 15:597–608, 1974.

Kruze, J., Salgado, M. and Collins, M.T.: Paratuberculosis in Chilean dairy goat herds. Arch. Med. Vet., 39(2):147–152, 2007.

Kumar, A. and Misra, D.S.: Drug-resistant and R-factor-bearing *Escherichia coli* and *Salmonella* in goats and pigs. Indian J. Anim. Sci., 53:683–686, 1983.

Kumar, R., Prasad, M.C. and Paliwal, O.P.: Paratuberculosis in goats—a retrospective study. Indian Vet. J., 65:582–584, 1988.

Kumar, S., Saxena, S.P. and Gupta, B.K.: Carrier rate of salmonellas in sheep and goats and its public health significance. J. Hyg. Camb., 71:43–47, 1973.

Kwon, O.D. et al.: Electrolyte changes of blood and rumen juice in experimental abomasal diseases in goats. Korean J. Vet. Clin. Med., 14(2):258–262, 1997.

Lager, I.A.: Bluetongue virus in South America: overview of viruses, vectors, surveillance and unique features. Vet. Ital., 40(3):89–93, 2004.

Lãnada, E.B., Morris, R.S., Jackson, R. and Fenwick, S.G.: A cohort study of *Yersinia* infection in goats. Aust. Vet. J. 83(9):567–571, 2005.

Lane, R.H.: A case of scours in goat kids. N. Z. Vet. J., 35:58–59, 1987.

Lane, V.M. and Anderson, B.C.: Adenocarcinoma of the mouth of a goat. J. Am. Vet. Med. Assoc., 183:1099–1100, 1983.

Langston, V.C., Galey, F., Lovell, R. and Buck, W.B.: Toxicity and therapeutics of monensin: a review. Vet. Med., 80:75–84, 1985.

Lanusse, C., et al.: Comparative plasma disposition kinetics of ivermectin, moxidectin and doramectin in cattle. J. Vet. Pharmacol. Ther., 20:91–99, 1997.

Leathwick, D.M.: A case of moxidectin failing to control ivermectin resistant *Ostertagia* species in goats. Vet. Rec., 136(17):443–444, 1995.

Lee K.W., et al.: Seroprevalence of *Mycobacterium avium* subspecies *paratuberculosis* in Korean black goats (*Capra hircus aegagrus*). J. Vet. Med. Sci., 68(12):1379–1381, 2006.

Lehmkuhl, H.D., DeBey, B.M. and Cutlip, R.C.: A new serotype adenovirus isolated from a goat in the United States. J. Vet. Diagn. Investig., 13(3):195–200, 2001.

Le Jambre, L.F.: *Ostertagia ostertagi* infections in Angora goats. Vet. Parasitol, 4:299–303, 1978.

Le Jambre, L.F. and Royal, W.M.: A comparison of worm burdens in grazing Merino sheep and Angora goats. Australian Vet. J., 52:181–183, 1976.

Le Jambre, L.F., Gill, J.H., Lenane, I.J. and Baker, P.: Inheritance of avermectin resistance in *Haemonchus contortus*. Internat. J. Parasitol., 30(1):105–111, 2000.

Le Jambre, L.F., Southcott, W.H. and Dash, K.M.: Development of simultaneous resistance in *Ostertagia circumcincta* to thiabendazole, morantel tartrate, and levamisole. Int. J. Parasitol., 8:443–447, 1978.

Le Riche, P.D., Efstathiou, G.C., Altan, Y. and Campbell, J.B.: A helminth survey of sheep and goats in Cyprus. Part II. Age distribution and the severity of infection with gastro-intestinal parasites. J. Helminth., 47:251–262, 1973.

Lefèvre, P.C.: Peste des Petits Ruminants et Infection Bovipestique des Ovins et Caprins. Maisons-Alfort, Institut d'Élevage et de Médecine Vétérinaire des Pays Tropicaux. 1982.

Lefèvre, P.C. and Calvez, D.: La fièvre catarrhale du mouton (bluetongue) en Afrique intertropicale: influence des facteurs écologiques sur la prévalence de l'infection. Rev. Élev. Méd. Vét. Pays. Trop., 39:263–268, 1986.

Lenghaus, C., Badman, R.T. and Gillick, J.C.: Johne's disease in goats. Aust. Vet. J., 53:460, 1977.

Leon Vizcaino L., et al.: Observaciones sobre la paratuberculosis caprina en España meridional. Arch. Zootecnia, 33:205–217, 1984.

Leondidis, S., et al.: Abortion and losses of newborn lambs and kids due to *Salmonella* spp. In: Priority Aspects of Salmonellosis Research. H.E. Larsen, ed. Luxembourg, Commission of the European Communities, 1984.

Lespine, A., Sutra, J.F., Dupuy, J. and Alvinerie, M.: Eprinomectin in goat: assessment of subcutaneous administration. Parasitol. Res., 89(2):120–122, 2003.

Levi, M.L.: Experimental study of Johne's disease in goats. J. Comp. Pathol., 58:38–63, 1948.

Levi, M.L.: *Salmonella dublin* infection in young goats. Vet. Rec., 61:555–557, 1949.

Libeau, J. and Scott, G.R.: Rinderpest in eastern Africa today. Bull. Epizoot. Dis. Afr., 8:7–12, 1960.

Liebermann, H.: Nairobi sheep disease. In: Applied Veterinary Epidemiology. T. Blaha, ed. Amsterdam, Elsevier, 1989.

Lima, J.D.: Prevalence of coccidia in domestic goats from Illinois, Indiana, Missouri, and Wisconsin. Int. Sheep Goat Res., 1:234–241, 1980.

Lima, W.D.S. and Guimaraes, M.P.: First description of *Trichostrongylus longispicularis* parasitizing a goat *(Capra hircus)* in the State of Minas Gerais, Brazil. Arq. Bras. Med. Vet. Zootec., 37:515–516, 1985.

Lopez, A.C. and Botija, C.S.: L'épizootie de fièvre catarrhale ovine en Espagne (blue tongue). Bull. Off. Int. Epizoot., 50:65–93, 1958.

Luedke, A.J. and Anakwenze, E.I.: Bluetongue virus in goats. Am. J. Vet. Res., 33:1739–1745, 1972.

Luedke, A.J., Jochim, M.M. and Jones, R.H.: Bluetongue in cattle: effects of *Culicoides variipennis*-transmitted bluetongue virus on pregnant heifers and their calves. Am. J. Vet. Res., 38(11):1687–1695, 1977.

Luedke, A.J., Jochim, M.M. and Jones, R.H.: Bluetongue in cattle: effects of vector-transmitted bluetongue virus on calves previously infected in utero. Am. J. Vet. Res., 38(11): 1697–1700, 1977a.

Macadam, I.: Transmission of rinderpest from goats to cattle in Tanzania. Bull. Epizoot. Dis. Afr., 16:53–60, 1968.

MacLachlan, N.J. and Osburn, B.I.: Impact of bluetongue virus infection on the international movement and trade of ruminants, J. Am. Vet. Med. Assoc., 228(9):1346–1349, 2006.

MacLachlan, N.J., et al.: Detection of bluetongue virus in the blood of inoculated calves: comparison of virus isolation, PCR assay, and *in vitro* feeding of *Culicoides variipennis*. Arch. Virol., 136(1/2):1–8, 1994.

Maddy, K.T.: Traumatic gastritis in sheep and goats. J. Am. Vet. Med. Assoc., 124:124–125, 1954.

Mago, M.L., Ahuja, S., Singh, H. and Saxena, S.N.: Prevalence of multiple drug resistance against *Salmonella* strains isolated from animals in India during 1973–77: a five year study. Indian Vet. J., 59:754–759, 1982.

Mahieu, M., et al.: Evaluation of targeted drenching using Famacha© method in Creole goat: reduction of anthelmintic use, and effects on kid production and pasture contamination. Vet. Parasitol., 146(1/2):135–147, 2007.

Mahmoud, O.M., Haroun, E.M. and Sulman, A.: Hepatobiliary coccidiosis in a dairy goat. Vet. Parasitol., 53(1/2): 15–21, 1994.

Mancassola, R., Reperant, J.M., Naciri, M. and Chartier, C.: Chemoprophylaxis of *Cryptosporidium parvum* infection with paromomycin in kids and immunological study. Antimicrob. Agents Chemother., 39(1):75–78, 1995.

Mancassola, R., Richard, A. and Naciri, M.: Evaluation of decoquinate to treat experimental cryptosporidiosis in kids. Vet. Parasitol., 69(1/2):31–37, 1997.

Mandonnet, N., et al.: Assessment of genetic variability of resistance to gastrointestinal nematode parasites in Creole goats in the humid tropics. J. Anim. Sci., 79: 7, 1706–1712, 2001.

Mandonnet, N., et al.: Genetic variability in resistance to gastro-intestinal strongyles during early lactation in Creole goats. Anim. Sci., 82(3):283–287, 2006.

Manning, E.J.B., Cushing, H.F., Hietala, S. and Wolf, C.B.: Impact of *Corynebacterium pseudotuberculosis* infection on serologic surveillance for Johne's disease in goats. J. Vet. Diagn. Invest., 19(2):187–190, 2007.

Manning, E.J.B., Steinberg, H., Krebs, V. and Collins, M.T.: Diagnostic testing patterns of natural *Mycobacterium paratuberculosis* infection in pygmy goats. Can. J. Vet. Res., 67:213–218, 2003.

Maratea, K.A. and Miller, M.A.: Abomasal coccidiosis associated with proliferative abomasitis in a sheep. J. Vet. Diagn. Investig., 19(1):118–121, 2007.

Marczinke, B.I. and Nichol, S.T.: Nairobi sheep disease virus, an important tick-borne pathogen of sheep and goats in Africa is also present in Asia. Virol., 303:146–151, 2002.

Mariner, J.C., et al.: Comparison of the effect of various chemical stabilizers and lyophilization cycles on the thermostability of a Vero cell-adapted rinderpest vaccine. Vet. Microbiol., 21:195–209, 1990.

Mariner, J.C., et al.: The serological response to a thermostable Vero cell-adapted rinderpest vaccine under field conditions in Niger. Vet. Microbiol., 22:119–127, 1990a.

Martinez Gomez, F.: Experiencias con el tartrato de pirantel en el tratamiento de las parasitosis gastrointestinales de la cabra. Rev. Iber. Parasitol., 28:67–76, 1968.

Martínez Ortiz de Montellano, C., et al.: Combining the effects of supplementary feeding and copper oxide needles for the control of gastrointestinal nematodes in browsing goats. Vet. Parasitol., 146:66–76, 2007.

Mason, R.W., Hartley, W.J. and Tilt, L.: Intestinal cryptosporidiosis in a kid goat. Australian Vet. J., 57:386–388, 1981.

Matovelo, J.A., Landsverk, T. and Amaya Posada, G.: Cryptosporidiosis in Tanzanian goat kids: Scanning and transmission electron microscopic observations. Acta Vet. Scand., 25:322–326, 1984.

McDougald, L.R.: Attempted cross-transmission of coccidia between sheep and goats and description of *E. ovinoidalis* sp. J. Protozool. 26:109–113, 1979.

McDougald, L.R., White, R.G. and Hansen, M.F.: Efficacy of naphthalophos and coumaphos against nematodes of goats. Am. J. Vet. Res., 29:1077–1079, 1968.

McFadyean, J. and Sheather, A.L.: Johne's disease: the experimental transmission of the disease to cattle, sheep and goats with notes regarding the occurrence of natural cases in sheep and goats. J. Comp. Pathol. Ther., 29:62–94, 1916.

McIntyre, L., et al.: *Escherichia coli* O157 outbreak associated with the ingestion of unpasteurized goat's milk in British Columbia, 2001. Canada Communicable Disease Report, 28(1):6–8, 2002. http://dsp-psd.pwgsc.gc.ca/Collection/H12-21-28-1.pdf

McKenna, P.B.: The diagnostic value and interpretation of faecal egg counts in sheep. N.Z. Vet. J., 29:129–132, 1981.

McKenna, P.B.: Gastro-intestinal parasitism and "anthelmintic resistance" in goats. Surveillance N.Z., 11:2–4, 1984.

McKenna, P.B.: The efficacy of toltrazuril against naturally-acquired coccidial infections in goats. Vet. Med. Rev., 59(2):157–161, 1988.

McKenna, P.B. and Watson, T.G.: The comparative efficacy of four broad spectrum anthelmintics against some experimentally induced trichostrongylid infections in sheep and goats. N. Z. Vet. J., 35:192–195, 1987.

McOrist, S. and Miller, G.T.: Salmonellosis in transported feral goats. Aust. Vet. J., 57:389–390, 1981.

McQueen, D.S. and Russell, E.G.: Culture of *Mycobacterium paratuberculosis* from bovine foetuses. Aust. Vet. J., 55:203–204, 1979.

McSweeney, C.S.: A comparative study of the anatomy of the omasum in domesticated ruminants. Aust. Vet. J., 65:205–207, 1988.

Meer, R.R. and Songer, J.G.: Multiplex polymerase chain reaction assay for genotyping *Clostridium perfringens*. Am. J. Vet. Res., 58(7):702–705, 1997.

Mehlhorn, H., Senaud, J. and Heydorn, A.O.: Two types of globidium-cysts of goats. Zeitschrift fur Parasitenkunde. 70(6):731–737, 1984.

Memon, M.A., Schelling, S.H. and Sherman, D.M.: Mucinous adenocarcinoma of the ovary as a cause of ascites in a goat. J. Am. Vet. Med. Assoc., 206(3):362–364, 1995.

Merrill, L.B. and Taylor, C.A.: Diet selection, grazing habits, and the place of goats in range management. In: Goat Production. C. Gall, ed. London, Academic Press. 1981.

Mettler, F., Engels, M., Wild, P. and Bivetti, A.: Herpesvirus-Infektion bei Zicklein in der Schweiz. Schweiz Arch. Tierheilk., 121:655–662, 1979.

Mikhail, M., Brugere, H., Le Bars, H. and Colvin, H.W.: Stimulated esophageal groove closure in adult goats. Am. J. Vet. Res., 49:1713–1715, 1988.

Milhaud, G., Zundel, E. and Crombet, M.: Étude expérimentale de la fluorose caprine. I-Protocole expérimental, comportement des animaux, lésions dentaires. Rec. Méd. Vét., 156:37–46, 1980.

Miller, D.K. and Craig, T.M.: Use of anthelmintic combinations against multiple resistant *Haemonchus contortus* in Angora goats. Small Rumin. Res., 19(3):281–283, 1996.

Milner, A.R., Mack, W.N. and Coates, K.J.: A modified ELISA for the detection of goats infected with *Mycobacterium paratuberculosis*. Aust. Vet. J. 66(9):305–306, 1989.

Min, B.R., Pomroy, W.E., Hart, S.P. and Sahlu, T.: The effect of short-term consumption of a forage containing condensed tannins on gastro-intestinal nematode parasite infections in grazing wether goats. Small Rumin. Res. 51:279–283, 2004.

Misk, N.A., Youssef, H.A. and Ali, M.A.: Ventral abdominal herniation at the level of the udder in a goat. Vet. Med. Rev., No. 2, pp. 200–202, 1986.

Misri, J., Vihan, V.S. and Kumar, A.: Toxicity studies on *Prosopis juliflora* in goats—haematobiochemical and pathological profile. Indian J. Anim. Sci., 73(4):349–352, 2003.

Mitchell, W.C.: Intussusception in goats. Vet. Med. Sm. Anim. Clin., 78:1918, 1983.

Mittal, K.R. and Tizzard, I.R.: Studies on the relationship between *Yersinia enterocolitica* IX and *Brucella abortus* agglutinins in naturally infected animals. Res. Vet. Sci., 28:311–314, 1980.

Moghaddar, N. and Khanitapeh, N.: Prevalence of paramphistomes in sheep and goat in the Fars province of Iran. Iran. J. Vet. Res., 4(2)(Ser.8):166–170, 2003.

Mohan Kumar, O.R. and Christopher, K.J.: An outbreak of rinderpest in goats. Indian Vet. J., 62:909–910, 1985.

Mohiuddin, A., Khan, M.M., Mughal, F.A. and Sheikh, M.A.: Incidence of amphistomiasis in sheep and goats of different ages in Sind. Pak. Vet. J., 2:17–18, 1982.

Molento, M.B., et al.: Famacha guide as an individual clinic parameter for *Haemonchus contortus* infection in small ruminants. Ciencia Rural., 34(4):1139–1145, 2004.

Molina, A., Morera, L. and Llanes, D.: Enzyme-linked immunosorbent assay for detection of antibodies against *Mycobacterium paratuberculosis* in goats. Am. J. Vet. Res. 52(6):863–868, 1991.

Molina, J.M., et al.: Persistent efficacy of doramectin against *Haemonchus contortus* in goats. Vet. Rec., 156(14):448–450, 2005.

Molina Caballero, J.M., et al.: Use of an enzyme-linked immunosorbent assay for serodiagnosis of clinical paratuberculosis in goats. Study by Western blotting of false-positive reactions. Rev. Sci. Tech. Off. Int. Epiz. 12(2):629–638, 1993.

Moncol, D.J. and Grice, M.J.: Transmammary passage of *Strongyloides papillosis* in the goat and sheep. In: Proceedings, Helminth. Soc. Wash., 41:1–4, 1974.

Montgomery, E.: On a tick-borne gastro-enteritis of sheep and goats occurring in British East Africa. J. Comp. Pathol. Therap., 30:28–57, 1917.

Morand-Fehr, P.: Nutrition and feeding of goats: Application to temperate climatic conditions. In: Goat Production. C. Gall, ed. London. Academic Press. 1981.

Morand-Fehr, P., Hervieu, J., Bas, P. and Sauvant, D.: Feeding of young goats. Proc. III International Conf. Goat Prod. Dis., Tucson, Arizona, pp. 90–104, 1982.

Morand-Fehr, P., Richard, A., Tessier, J. and Hervieu, J.: Effects of decoquinate on the growth and milk performance of young female goats. Small Rumin. Res., 45(2):109–114, 2002.

Morin, M.: Johne's disease (paratuberculosis) in goats: a report of eight cases in Quebec. Can. Vet. J., 23:55–58, 1982.

Morita, M., Nakamatsu, M. and Goto, M.: Pathological studies on pseudotuberculosis caused by *Yersinia (Pasteurella) pseudotuberculosis*. IV. A spontaneous case in the goat. Jpn. J. Vet. Sci., 35:193–198, 1973.

Mortensen, L.L., et al.: Evaluation of prevalence and clinical implications of anthelmintic resistance in gastrointestinal nematodes in goats. J. Am. Vet. Med. Assoc., 223(4):495–500, 2003.

Moser C.L.: Johne's disease (paratuberculosis) in a goat. Can. Vet. J., 23:63–66, 1982.

Mugera, G.M. and Bitakaramire, P.: Gastroenteritis in Kenya goats caused by *Globidium gilruthi.* Vet. Rec., 82:595–597, 1968.

Mugera, G.M. and Nderito, P.: *Cestrum* poisoning in Kenya livestock. Bull. Epizoot. Dis. Afr., 16:501–506, 1968.

Mukaratirwa, S. and Sayi, S.T.: Partial facial duplication (diprosopus) in a goat kid. J. S. Afr. Vet. Assoc., 77(1):42–44, 2006.

Mukherjee, G.S. and Sinha, P.K.: Incidence of rumen protozoa in Black Bengal goats. Indian J. Anim. Health, 29(1):73–75, 1990.

Munjal, S.K. Tripathi, B.N. and Paliwal, O.P.: Progressive immunopathological changes during early stages of experimental infection of goats with *Mycobacterium avium* subspecies *paratuberculosis*. Vet. Pathol., 42(4):427–436, 2005.

Munjal, S.K., et al.: Evaluation of a LAM ELISA for diagnosis of paratuberculosis in sheep and goats. Vet. Microbiol., 103(1/2):107–114, 2004.

Muñoz, M., Lanza, I., Alvarez, M. and Carmenes, P.: Rotavirus excretion by kids in a naturally infected goat herd. Small Rumin. Res., 14(1):83–89, 1994.

Muñoz, M., Álvarez, M., Lanza, I. and Cármenes, P.: An outbreak of diarrhoea associated with atypical rotaviruses in goat kids. Res. Vet. Sci., 59(2):180–182, 1995.

Muñoz, M., Álvarez, M., Lanza, I. and Cármenes, P.: Role of enteric pathogens in the aetiology of neonatal diarrhoea in lambs and goat kids in Spain. Epidemiol. Infect., 117(1):203–211, 1996.

Mwangi, E. and Swallow, B.: Invasion of *Prosopis juliflora* and local livelihoods: Case study from the lake Baringo area of Kenya. ICRAF Working Paper—no. 3. Nairobi: World Agroforestry Centre, p. 42, June 2005.

Nabbut, N.H. and Al-Nakhli, H.M: Incidence of *Salmonellae* in lymph nodes, spleens and feces of sheep and goats slaughtered in the Riyadh public abattoir. J. Food Protect., 45:1314–1317, 1982.

Nabbut, N.H., Barbour, E.K. and Al-Nakhli, H.M.: *In vitro* susceptibility of salmonellae to eight antimicrobial agents. Zentrlbl. Bakt. Parasit. Infekt. Hyg., 251A:190–195, 1981.

Naciri, M., Mancassola, R. and Richard, A.: Study of the efficacy of decoquinate (Deccox 6Reg.) in the prevention of experimental cryptosporidiosis in goats. Bulletin des G.T.V., 3:47–52, 1998.

Naciri, M., Yvore, P. and Levieux, D.: Cryptosporidiose expérimentale du chevreau. Influence de la prise du colostrum. Essais de traitements. In: Les Maladies de la Chèvre, Les Colloques de l'INRA, No. 28. P. Yvore and G. Perrin, eds. Paris. Institut National de la Recherche Agronomique, pp. 465–471, 1984.

Naciri, M., Yvore, P., Polack, B. and Martin, F.X.: Essai du lactate d'halofuginone dans le traitement de la cryptosporidiose chez le chevreau. Abstracts, 2e Colloque International de Niort, Pathologie Caprine et Productions. Station Régionale de Pathologie Caprine, Niort, France, p. 25, June 1989.

Nagaratnam, W. and Ratnatunga, P.C.C.: Incidence of *Salmonella* amongst cattle and goats brought for slaughter. Ceylon Vet. J., 19:69–71, 1971.

Nagy, B., Nagy, G., Palfi, V. and Bozso, M.: Occurrence of cryptosporidia, rotaviruses, coronavirus-like particles, and K99+ *Escherichia coli* in goat kids and lambs. Proc. 3rd Internat. Symp. Vet. Lab. Diag., Ames, Iowa, pp. 525–531, 1983.

Nagy, B., et al.: Studies on cryptosporidial infection of goat kids. In: Les Maladies de la Chèvre, Les Colloques de l'INRA, No. 28. P. Yvore and G. Perrin, eds. Paris. Institut National de la Récherche Agronomique, pp. 443–451, 1984.

Nagy, B., et al.: Infectious gastrointestinal diseases of young goats. Proc. IV International Conf. Goats, Brasilia, EMBRAPA-DDT, pp. 373–388, 1987.

Nakamatsu, M., Fujimoto, V. and Satoh, H.: The pathological study of paratuberculosis in goats centered around the formation of remote lesions. Jpn. J. Vet. Res., 16:103–119, 1968.

National Research Council of the National Academies. Diagnosis and Control of Johne's Disease. Committee on Diagnosis and Control of Johne's Disease. Board of Agriculture and Natural Resources. Washington DC,

National Academies Press. 244 pp, 2003. http://www.nap.edu/catalog.php?record_id=10625#toc.
Nawar, S.M.A.: Micromorphological studies on the salivary glands of the goat. Vet. Med. J., 28:329–339, 1980.
Nayak, N.C. and Bhowmik, M.K.: Naturally occurring necrobacillosis in goats. Indian J. Anim. Sci., 58:783–786, 1988.
Naylor, R.D., Martin, P.K. and Sharpe, R.T.: Detection of *Clostridium perfringens* epsilon toxin by ELISA. Res. Vet. Sci., 42:255–256, 1987.
Neiman, P.K.: The biology of *Nematodirus* parasites of goats in southern Kirgiziya. Byull. Vsesoyuznogo Inst. Gelminologii, 21:50–53, 1977.
Nesbakken, T. *Yersinia enterocolitica*. Chapter 14, In: Emerging foodborne pathogens. Cambridge, UK, Woodhead Publishing Ltd., pp. 373–405, 2006.
Nguyen B.V., Leforban Y., Gillet J.P. and Thery P: Identification of ovine adenovirus type 5 in goats in Senegal. Rev. Élev. Méd. Vét. Pays Trop., 41:35–39, 1988.
Nielsen, P. and Rasmussen, F.: Pharmacokinetics of levamisole in goats and pigs. In: Veterinary Pharmacology and Toxicology. Y. Ruckebusch, P.L. Toutain and G.D. Koritz, eds. Westport, Connecticut, AVI Publishing Co., 1983.
Nikolaou, K., et al.: Prevalence of anti-*Yersinia* outer protein antibodies in goats in Lower Saxony. J. Vet. Med. B, 52:17–24, 2005.
Noordeen, F., et al.: Infectivity of *Cryptosporidium parvum* isolated from asymptomatic adult goats to mice and goat kids. Vet. Parasitol. 103(3):217–225, 2002.
Norton, C.C.: Coccidia of the domestic goat *Capra hircus*, with notes on *Eimeria ovinoidalis* and *E. bakuensis* (syn. *E. ovina*) from the sheep *Ovis aries*. Parasitology, 92:279–289, 1986.
Nwosu, C.O., Ogunrinade, A.F. and Fagbemi, B.O.: Prevalence and seasonal changes in the gastro-intestinal helminths of Nigerian goats. J. Helminthol., 70(4):329–333, 1996.
Obi, T.U., Ojo, M.O., Taylor, W.P. and Rowe, L..: Studies on the epidemiology of peste des petits ruminants in southern Nigeria. Trop. Vet., 1:209–217, 1983.
Obi, T.U., Taylor, W.P. and Ojo, M.O.: Prevalence of bluetongue virus precipitating antibodies in sheep and goats in southern Nigeria. Trop. Vet., 1:205–208, 1983a.
Obi, T.U., Rowe, L.W. and Taylor, W.P.: Serological studies with peste des petits ruminants and rinderpest viruses in Nigeria. Trop. Anim. Health Prod., 16:115–118, 1984.
Obwolo, M.J.: A review of yersiniosis (*Yersinia pseudotuberculosis* infection). Vet. Bull., 46:167–171, 1976.
Ocal, N., Yagc, B.B., Duru, S.Y. and Kul, O.: Toltrazuril treatment for acute clinical coccidiosis in hair goat kids: clinical, pathological, haematologic and biochemical findings. Medycyna Weterynaryjna. 63(7):805–809, 2007.
OIE: Manual of Diagnostic Techniques and Vaccine for Terrestrial Animals. 5th Ed. Chapter 2.1.5. Peste des petits ruminants. Paris, Office Internationale des Epizooties, 2004. http://www.oie.int/eng/normes/mmanual/A_00028.htm.
OIE: Manual of Diagnostic Techniques and Vaccine for Terrestrial Animals. 5th Ed. Chapter 2.1.9. Bluetongue. Paris, Office Internationale des Epizooties, 2004a. http://www.oie.int/eng/normes/mmanual/A_00032.htm.
OIE: Manual of Diagnostic Techniques and Vaccine for Terrestrial Animals. 5th Ed. Chapter 2.10.2. Bunyaviral diseases of animals. Paris, Office Internationale des Epizooties, 2004b. http://www.oie.int/eng/normes/mmanual/A_00128.htm.
OIE: Terrestrial Animal Health Code. Chapter 2.2.13. Bluetongue. Paris, Office Internationale des Epizooties, 2007. http://www.oie.int/eng/normes/mcode/en_chapitre_2.2.13.htm.
Okon, E.D.: *Trichuris* infection in Nigerian goats. J. Nigerian Vet. Med. Assoc., 3:17–20, 1974.
Okon, E.D.: Effects of parturition on faecal strongyle egg output in Nigerian goats. Bull. Anim. Health Prod. Afr., 28:155–158, 1980.
Omar, A.R. and Fatimah, I.: Primary salivary gland tumour in a goat. Kajian Vet., Malaysia, 13:37–39, 1981.
Orden, J.A., Ruiz-Santa-Quiteria, J.A., Cid, D. and Fuente, R. de la: Presence and enterotoxigenicity of F5 and F41 *Escherichia coli* strains isolated from diarrhoeic small ruminants in Spain. Small Rumin. Res., 44(2):159–161, 2002.
Orden, J.A., et al.: Typing of the *eae* and *espB* genes of attaching and effacing *Escherichia coli* isolates from ruminants. Vet. Microbiol., 96(2):203–215, 2003.
Orden, J.A., et al.: Prevalence and characterization of Vero cytotoxin-producing *Escherichia coli* isolated from diarrhoeic and healthy sheep and goats. Epidemiol. Infect., 130(2):313–321, 2003a.
O'Reilly, C.E., et al.: Surveillance of bulk raw and commercially pasteurized cows' milk from approved Irish liquid-milk pasteurization plants to determine the incidence of *Mycobacterium paratuberculosis*. Appl. Environ. Microbiol. 70(9):5138–5144, 2004.
Orr, M., Craighead, L. and Cameron, S.: Yersiniosis outbreak in goat weanlings. Surveillance N.Z., 14:10–11, 1987.
Orr, M., Craighead, L., Kyle, B. and Mackintosh, C.: The isolation of *Yersinia* species from the faeces of farmed goats. Surveillance, 17(2):27–28, 1990.
Oruc, E.: Histopathological findings in naturally occurring biliary coccidiosis in a goat kid. Vet. Rec. 160(3):93, 2007.
Osburn, B.I., et al.: Epizootiologic study of bluetongue: virologic and serologic results. Am. J. Vet. Res., 42:884–887, 1981.
Osweiler, G.D., Carson, T.L., Buck, W.B. and Van Gelder, G.A.: Clinical and Diagnostic Veterinary Toxicology, 3rd Ed. Dubuque, Kendall/Hunt Publishing Co. 1988.
Otesile, E.B., Ahmed, G. and Adetosoye, A.I.: Experimental infection of Red Sokoto goats with *Salmonella typhimurium*. Revue Élev. Méd. vét Pays trop., 43(1):49–53, 1990.
Otesile, E.B. and Akpokodje, J.U.: Fatal ruminal impaction in West African dwarf goat and sheep. Trop. Vet., 9:9–11, 1991.
Owen-Smith, N. and Cooper, S.M.: Foraging strategies of browsing ungulates: Comparisons between goats and African wild ruminants. Proc. IV International Conf. Goats, Brasilia, EMBRAPA-DDT, pp. 957–969, 1987.
Oxer, D.T.: Enterotoxaemia in goats. Aust. Vet. J., 32:62–66, 1956.
Ozmen, O., Yukari, B.A., Haligur, M. and Sahinduran, S.: Observations and immunohistochemical detection of Coronavirus, *Cryptosporidium parvum* and *Giardia intestina-*

lis in neonatal diarrhoea in lambs and kids. SAT, Schweizer Arch. Tierheilk., 148(7):357–364, 2006.

Panter, K.E., Keeler, R.F., Bunch, T.D. and Callan, R.J.: Congenital skeletal malformations and cleft palate induced in goats by ingestion of *Lupinus*, *Conium* and *Nicotiana* species. Toxicon (Oxford), 28(12):1377–1385, 1990.

Panter, K.E., Gardner, D.R. and Molyneux, R.J.: Comparison of toxic and teratogenic effects of *Lupinus formosus*, *L. arbustus* and *L. caudatus* in goats. J. Nat. Toxins. 3(2):83–93, 1994.

Paolini, V., Dorchies, P., Hoste, H.: Effects of sainfoin hay on gastrointestinal infection with nematodes in goats. Vet. Rec., 152(19):600–601, 2003.

Paolini, V., et al.: Effects of the repeated distribution of sainfoin hay on the resistance and the resilience of goats naturally infected with gastrointestinal nematodes. Vet. Parasitol., 127:277–283, 2005.

Paranagama, W.D., et al.: Evaluation of serum pepsinogen concentration as a diagnostic aid in haemonchosis of goats. Trop. Agric. Res., 11:372–379, 1999.

Paraud, C. and Chartier, C.: Biological control of infective larvae of a gastro-intestinal nematode (*Teladorsagia circumcincta*) and a small lungworm (*Muellerius capillaris*) by *Duddingtonia flagrans* in goat faeces. Parasitol. Res., 89:102–106, 2003.

Paraud, C., et al.: Administration of *Duddingtonia flagrans* chlamydospores to goats to control gastro-intestinal nematodes: dose trials. Vet. Res., 36:157–166, 2005.

Paraud, C., Pors, I. and Chartier, C.: Efficiency of feeding *Duddingtonia flagrans* chlamydospores to control nematode parasites of first-season grazing goats in France. Vet. Res. Commun., 31(3):305–315, 2007.

Pathak, D.C. and Datta, B.M.: The effects of oral administration of sodium selenite on clinical signs and mortality. Indian Vet. J., 61:845–846, 1984.

Patnaik, R.K.: Epidemic of goat dermatitis in India. Trop. Anim. Health Prod., 18:137–138, 1986.

Patterson, D.S.P. and Allen, W.M.: Chronic mycobacterial enteritis in ruminants as a model of Crohn's disease. Proc. R. Soc. Med., 65(11):998–1001, 1972.

Perera, L.P., Peiris, J.S.M. and Weilgama, D.J.: Nairobi sheep disease virus isolated from *Haemaphysalis intermedia* ticks collected in Sri Lanka. Ann. Trop. Med. Parasitol., 90:91–93, 1996.

Pfister, J.A., Hansen, D. and Malechek, J.C.: Surgical establishment and maintenance of esophageal fistulae in small ruminants. Small Rumin. Res., 3(1):47–56, 1990.

Philip, P.J.: Surgical treatment for anal and anorectal agenesis in animals. Kerala J. Vet. Sci., 4:1–6, 1973.

Phukan, A., Dutta, G.N., Devriese, L.A. and Das, B.C.: Experimental production of *Clostridium perfringens* type A and type D infections in goats. Indian Vet. J., 74(10):821–823, 1997.

Pienaar, J.G., et al.: Experimental studies with *Strongyloides papillosus* in goats. Onderstepoort J. Vet. Res., 66:191–235, 1999.

Pinsent, J. and Cottom, D.S.: Metabolic diseases of goats. Goat Vet. Soc. J., 8:40–42, 1987.

Plowright, W. and Ferris, R.D.: Studies with rinderpest virus in tissue culture: the use of attenuated culture virus as a vaccine for cattle. Res. Vet. Sci., 3:172–182, 1962.

Plowright, W.: The duration of immunity in cattle following inoculation of rinderpest cell culture vaccine. J. Hyg., 92:285–296, 1984.

Polack, B. and Perrin, G.: La cryptosporidiose du chevreau. Bull. Group. Tech. Vét., 3:45–46, 1987.

Polack, B., Chermette, R., Savey, M. and Bussieras, J.: Les cryptosporidies en France: techniques usuelles d'identification et résultats préliminaires d'enquêtes épidémiologiques. Point Vét., 15:41–46, 1983.

Polack, B., Guerrault, P., Perrin, G. and Gaillard-Perrin, G.: Pathologie néonatale du chevreau en Poitou-Charentes. Abstracts, 2e Colloque International de Niort, Pathologie Caprine et Productions. Station Régionale de Pathologie Caprine, Niort, France, p. 20, June 1989.

Polack, B., Perrin, G. and Yvore, P.: Utilisation d'aliments médicamenteux dans la prévention de la coccidiose de la chevrette. Bull. Group. Tech. Vét., No. 3:59–62, 1987.

Polydorou, K.: Annual Report of the Department of Veterinary Services for the Year 1983. Nicosia, Cyprus, Ministry of Agriculture and Natural Resources, 1984.

Pomroy, W.E. and Charleston, W.A.G.: Development of resistance to *Trichostrongylus colubriformis* in goats. Vet. Parasitol., 33:283–288, 1989.

Pomroy, W.E., Gething, M.A. and Charleston, W.A.G.: The efficacy of albendazole against some gastrointestinal nematodes in goats. N. Z. Vet. J., 36:105–107, 1988.

Pomroy, W.E., et al.: Multiple resistance in goat-derived *Ostertagia* and the efficacy of moxidectin and combinations of other anthelmintics. N. Z. Vet. J. 40(2):76–78, 1992.

Popesko P.: Atlas of Topographical Anatomy of Domestic Animals, new revised English edition, Bratislava, Vydavatelstvo Priroda, 2008.

Pralomkarn, W., et al.: Genetic resistance of three genotypes of goats to experimental infection with *Haemonchus contortus*. Vet. Parasitol., 68(1/2):79–90, 1997.

Prajapati, K.S., Avsatthi, B.L. and Patel, A.I.: Multiple intestinal diverticuli in goat associated with immature amphistomiaisis. Indian J. Parasitol., 6:291–292, 1982.

Prasad, J. and Rekib, A.: Studies on dietetic abnormalities in ruminants. I-Seasonal dynamics and etio-diagnosis of primary anorexia. Indian Vet. Med. J., 3:171–175, 1979.

Prasad, J., Gupta, S.C., Karnani, L.K. and Rekib, A.: Note on the utilization of Para grass *(Brachiaria mutica)* in goats. Indian J. Anim. Sci., 51:673–674, 1981.

Praslicka, J., Varady, M. and Corba, J.: Persistent infection with multiple anthelmintic-resistant gastrointestinal nematodes in Cashmere goats. Vet. Res. Commun., 18(6):443–446, 1994.

Prescott, J.F. and Bruin-Mosch, C.W.: Carriage of *Campylobacter jejuni* in healthy and diarrheic animals. Am. J. Vet. Res., 42:164–165, 1981.

Preston, J.M. and Allonby, E.W.: The influence of breed on the susceptibility of sheep and goats to a single experimental infection with *Haemonchus contortus*. Vet. Rec., 103:509–512, 1978.

Pritchard, G.C., et al.: Verocytotoxin-producing *Escherichia coli* O157 on a farm open to the public: outbreak investigation and longitudinal bacteriological study, Vet. Rec., 147:259–264, 2000.

Purohit, R.K., Chouhan, D.S., Purohit, N.R. and Sharma, S. S.: Abomasal impaction in goat with metallic particles. Indian J. Vet. Surg., 7:63–64, 1986.

Purse, B.V., et al.: Climate change and the recent emergence of bluetongue in Europe. Nat. Rev. Microbiol. 3(2):171–181, 2005.

Quarmby, W.B.: An investigation into enterotoxaemia in goats. Vet. Rec., 58:541–582, 1946.

Quarmby, W.B.: Enterotoxaemia in goats. Vet. Rec., 59:196, 1947.

Raats, J.G. and Clarke, B.K.: Remote control collection of oesophageal fistula samples in goats. Small Rumin. Res., 7(3):245–251, 1992.

Raats, J.G., Webber, L. Tainton, N.M. and Pepe, D.: An evaluation of the equipment for the oesophageal fistula valve technique. Small Rumin. Res., 21(3):213–216, 1996.

Radostits, O.M., Gay, C.C., Hinchcliff, K.W. and Constable, P.D.: Veterinary Medicine. A textbook of the diseases of cattle, horse, sheep, pigs and goats. 10th Ed, Edinburgh, Saunders Elsevier, 2007.

Rai, G.S. and Pandey, M.D.: Development and capacities of different segments of gastrointestinal tract of goat. Indian Vet. J., 55:195–198, 1978.

Raina, M.K.: Incidence of infection of sheep and goat with *Avitellina* Gough, 1911, *Stilesia* Railliet, 1893, and *Moniezia* Blanchard, 1891, in Kashmir. J. Sci., Univ. Kashmir, 1:59–62, 1973.

Rajan, A., Maryamma, K.I. and Nair, M.K.: Mortality in goats. A study based on post mortem observations. Kerala J. Vet. Sci., 7:79–83, 1976.

Rajukumar, K. Tripathi, B.N., Kurade, N.P. and Parihar, N.S.: An enzyme-linked immunosorbent assay using immuno-affinity-purified antigen in the diagnosis of caprine para-tuberculosis and its comparison with conventional ELISAs. Vet. Res. Commun., 25(7):539–553, 2001.

Ralph, A., O'Sullivan, M.V.N., Sangster, N.C. and Walker, J.C.: Abdominal pain and eosinophilia in suburban goat keepers—trichostrongylosis. Med. J. Austral., 184(9): 467–469, 2006.

Ramadan, R.O.: Megaesophagus in a goat. Agri-Practice, 14(1):26–28, 1993.

Ramesh Babu, N.G. and Rajesekhar, M.: Prevalence of rinderpest antibodies in sheep and goats in southern India. Vet. Rec., 123:595–597, 1988.

Ramirez Casillas, C., Gonzalez Sanchez, R. and de Lucas Tron, J.: Evaluacion de tres metodos de diagnostico para la deteccion de paratuberculosis en cabras. Tec. Pec. Mex., 47:128–132, 1984.

Ramirez, P.C., et al.: Encuesta serologica en ovinos y caprinos para determinar la presencia de la enfermedd de Johne en Mexico. Rev. Latinoam. Microbiol., 25:56, 1983.

Rao, J.R. and Sikdar, A.: Immature amphistomiasis in sheep and goat. Pathogenicity, treatment and control. Livestock Adviser, 6:39–42, 1981.

Razavi, S.M. and Hassanvand, A.: A survey on prevalence of different *Eimeria* species in goats in Shiraz suburbs. J. Fac. Vet. Med. Univ. Tehran, 61(4):373–376, 2007.

Reece, W.O.: Dukes' Physiology of Domestic Animals, 12th Ed., Ithaca, NY, Cornell University Press, 1024 pp., 2004.

Remi-Adewunmi, B.D., Gyang, E.O. and Osinowo, A.O.: Abattoir survey of foreign body rumen impaction small ruminants. Nigerian Vet. J., 25(2):32–38, 2004.

Reschly, L.J. and Dale, H.E.: Effects of ruminal insufflation on the circulatory system of the anesthetized goat. Am. J. Vet. Res., 31:279–283, 1970.

Ribelin, W.E., Fukushima, K. and Still, P.E.: The toxicity of ochratoxin to ruminants. Can. J. Comp. Med., 42:172–176, 1978.

Ridell, M.: Studies on corynebacterial precipitinogens common to mycobacteria, nocardiae and rhodochrous. Int. Arch. Allergy Appl. Immunol., 55:468–475, 1977.

Ridges, A.P. and Singleton, A.G.: Some quantitative aspects of digestion in goats. J. Physiol., 161:1–9, 1962.

Ris, D.R., Hamel, K.L. and Weaver, A.M.: Natural transmission of Johne's disease to feral goats. N. Z. Vet. J., 36:98–99, 1988.

Roberts, G.W. and Boyd, J.W.: Cerebrocortical necrosis in ruminants. Occurrence of thiaminase in the gut of normal and affected animals and its effect on thiamine status. J. Comp. Pathol., 84:365–374, 1974.

Roeder, P.L.: Personal communication, Taurus Animal Health, Hampshire, U.K., 2007.

Roeder, P.L.: Eradicating pathogens: the animal story. Br. Med. J. 331(7527):1262–1264, 2005.

Roeder, P.L. and Obi, T.U.: Recognizing *peste des petits ruminants*: a field manual. FAO Animal Health Manual 5, Rome, Italy, Food and Agricultural Organization of the United Nations, pp. 28, 1999.

Roeder, P.L., Abraham, G., Kenfe, G. and Barrett, T.: Peste des petits ruminants in Ethiopian goats. Trop. Anim. Health Prod., 26:69–73, 1994.

Roeder, P.L., Taylor, W.P. and Rweyemamu, M.M.: Rinderpest in the twentieth and twenty-first centuries. In: Rinderpest and peste des petits ruminants: virus plagues of large and small ruminants. T. Barrett, P.-P. Pastoret and W.P. Taylor, eds. Elsevier, Netherlands, pp. 105–142, 2005.

Roeder, P.L., et al.: Failure to establish congenital bluetongue virus infection by infecting cows in early pregnancy. Vet. Rec., 128(13):301–304, 1991.

Rolfe, P.F. and Boray, J.C.: Chemotherapy of paramphistomosis in sheep. Aust. Vet. J., 65:148–150, 1988.

Ross, J.D.: Herd health program for Angora goats. In: Current Veterinary Therapy, Food Animal Practice. 1st Ed. Edited by J.L. Howard. Philadelphia, W.B. Saunders Co., 1981.

Rossanigo, C.E. and Gruner, L.: Moisture and temperature requirements in faeces for the development of free-living stages of gastrointestinal nematodes of sheep, cattle and deer. J. Helminthol., 69:357–362, 1995.

Rossiter, P.B., et al.: Re-emergence of rinderpest as a threat in East Africa since 1979. Vet. Rec., 113:459–461, 1983.

Rossiter, P.B., et al.: Neutralising antibodies to rinderpest virus in wild animal sera collected in Kenya between 1970 and 1981. Prev. Vet. Med., 1:257–264, 1983a.

Rossiter, P.B., Jessett, D.M. and Taylor, W.P.: Neutralising antibodies to rinderpest virus in sheep and goats in western Kenya. Vet. Rec., 111:504–505, 1982.

Rossiter, P.B., et al.: Cattle plague in Shangri-La: observations on a severe outbreak of rinderpest in northern Pakistan 1994–1995. Vet. Rec., 143(2):39–42, 1998.

Rothel, J.S., et al.: A sandwich enzyme immunoassay for bovine interferon-gamma and its use for the detection of tuberculosis in cattle. Aust. Vet J., 67(4):134–137, 1990.

Rowe, J.D.: Floppy kid syndrome. Proceedings of the North American Veterinary Conference, Large Animal Edition, Volume 20, Orlando, Florida, USA, 7–11 January, 2006. The North American Veterinary Conference, Gainesville, USA: p. 284, 2006.

Rowland, A.C., Scott, G.R., Ramachandran, S. and Hill, D.H.: A comparative study of peste des petits ruminants and kata in West African dwarf goats. Trop. Anim. Health Prod., 3:241–245, 1971.

Roztocil, V., Chaudhari, A.Q. and El Mouty, I.A.: Induced traumatic reticulo-peritonitis in goats. Vet. Rec., 83:667–673, 1968.

Rudge, M.R.: Dental and periodontal abnormalities in two populations of feral goats (*Capra hircus* L.) in New Zealand. N.Z. J. Sci., 13:260–267, 1970.

Russell, W.C.: Type A enterotoxemia in captive wild goats. J. Am. Vet. Med. Assoc., 157:643–646, 1970.

Saegerman, C., Berkvens, D. and Mellor, P.S.: Bluetongue epidemiology in the European Union. Emer. Inf. Dis., 14(4):539–544, 2008.

Sagodira S., et al.: Protection of kids against *Cryptosporidium parvum* infection after immunization of dams with CP15-DNA. Vaccine, 17(19):2346–55, 1999.

Sahai, B.N. and Prasad, K.D.: Anthelmintic efficacy of terenol against immature and mature *Cotylophoron cotylophorum* in goats. Riv. Parasitol., 36:171–176, 1975.

Saito, J.K., et al.: A new herpesvirus isolate from goats: preliminary report. Am. J. Vet. Res., 35:847–848, 1974.

Salgado, M., Kruze, J., and Collins, M.T.: Diagnosis of paratuberculosis by fecal culture and ELISA on milk and serum samples in two types of Chilean dairy goat herds. J. Vet. Diagn. Invest., 19:1, 99–102, 2007.

Salgado, M., Manning, E.J.B. and Collins, M.T.: Performance of a Johne's disease enzyme linked immunosorbent assay adapted for milk samples from goats. J. Vet. Diagn. Invest., 17(4):350–354, 2005.

Samson-Himmelstjerna, G. von, Harder, A., Sangster, N.C. and Coles, G.C.: Efficacy of two cyclooctadepsipeptides, PF1022A and emodepside, against anthelmintic-resistant nematodes in sheep and cattle. Parasitology, 130(3):343–347, 2005.

Sanchis, R. and Cornille, Y.: *Salmonella abortusovis* infection of a male goat. Rec. Med. Vet., 131:473–475, 1980.

Sanford, S.E., Josephson, G.K.A., Rehmtulla, A.J. and Baker, K.C.: Cryptosporidiosis, rotaviral, and combined cryptosporidial and rotaviral infections in goat kids. Can. Vet. J., 32(10):626, 1991.

Sapre, S.N.: An outbreak of blue tongue in goats and sheep in Maharashtra state, India. Vet. Rev., 15:69–71, 1964.

Sathianesan, V. and Sundaram, R.K.: Comparative efficacy of four newer anthelmintics against *Trichuris globulosa* in experimentally infected goats. Kerala J. Vet. Sci., 14:1–8, 1983.

Savey, M.: La maladie ovine du "watery mouth," un modèle pour comprendre le "chevreau mou"?, Point Vét., 17:738–740, 1985.

Savitskii, S.V.: Embryonic and teratogenic action of rintal, morantel tartrate, pyrantel tartrate and panacur in goats and sheep. In: Diagnostika bolznei zhivotnikh i profilaktika ikh na fermakh i kompleksakh. Sbornik Nauchykh Trudov, USSR, pp. 113–115, 1984.

Saxegaard, F.: Experimental infection of calves with an apparently specific goat-pathogenic strain of *Mycobacterium paratuberculosis.* J. Comp. Pathol., 102:149–156, 1990.

Saxegaard, F. and Fodstad, F.H.: Control of paratuberculosis (Johne's disease) in goats by vaccination. Vet. Rec., 116:439–441, 1985.

Schafer, K.A., Stevenson, G.W. and Kazacos, K.R.: Hepatic coccidiosis associated with hepatic necrosis in a goat. Vet. Pathol. 32(6):723–727 1995.

Scharfe, S. and Elze, K.: Enzootic occurrence of lamb dysentery in two herds of goats. Praktische Tierarzt., 76(9):769–774, 1995.

Schillhorn van Veen, T.W.: Role of parasitism in goat management. Proc. III International Conf. Goat Prod. Dis., Tucson, Arizona, pp. 85–89, 1982.

Schnyder, M., et al.: Multiple anthelmintic resistance in *Haemonchus contortus* isolated from South African Boer goats in Switzerland. Vet. Parasitol., 128(3/4):285–290, 2005.

Schroeder, C., et al.: Diagnosis, epidemiology, signs and pathology of paratuberculosis in a goat herd in Germany. Tierärztliche Praxis., 29:1, 19–26, 2001.

Scott, A.C., Luddington, J., Lucas, M. and Gilbert, F.R.: Rotavirus in goats. Vet. Rec., 103:145, 1978.

Scott, E.W., Bairden, K., Holmes, P.H. and McKellar, Q.A.: Benzimidazole resistance in nematodes of goats. Vet. Rec., 124:492, 1989.

Scott, G.R.: Rinderpest and peste des petits ruminants. In: Virus Diseases of Food Animals. A World Geography of Epidemiology and Control. Vol. II, Disease Monographs. E.P.J. Gibbs, ed. London, Academic Press, pp. 401–432, 1981.

Scott, G.R.: Rinderpest in the 1980's. Prog. Vet. Microbiol. Immunol., 1:145–174, 1985.

Scott, G.R.: The incidence of rinderpest in sheep and goats. Bull. Epizoot. Dis. Afr., 3:117–118, 1955.

Scott, G.R.: The risk associated with the importation of meat from countries where rinderpest control measures are still required. Bull. Epizoot. Dis. Afr., 5:11–13, 1957.

Seimiya, Y.M., et al.: Caprine enteritis associated with *Yersinia pseudotuberculosis* infection. J. Vet. Med. Sci., 67(9):887–890, 2005.

Seth, D.N., et al: A note on the rate of secretion of parotid saliva in sheep and goat. Indian J. Anim. Sci., 46:660–663, 1976.

Sevinc, F., Simsek, A. and Uslu, U.: Massive *Cryptosporidium parvum* infection associated with an outbreak of diarrhoea in neonatal goat kids. Turk. J. Vet. Anim. Sci., 29(6):1317–1320, 2005.

Shaik, S.A., et al.: Sericea lespedeza hay as a natural deworming agent against gastrointestinal nematode infection in goats. Elsevier, Amsterdam, Netherlands: 139(1/3):150–157, 2006.

Shaila, M.S., et al.: Geographic distribution and epidemiology of peste des petits ruminants viruses. Virus Res., 43:149–153, 1996.

Shanks, P.I.: Enterotoxaemia in goats. Vet. Rec., 61:262–263, 1949.

Sharma, A.K., Tripathi, B.N., Verma, J.C., and Parihar, N.S.: Experimental *Salmonella enterica* subspecies *enterica* serovar Typhimurium infection in Indian goats: clinical, serological, bacteriological and pathological studies. Small Rumin. Res., 42(2):125–134, 2001.

Sharma, K.B. and Ranka, A.K.: Foreign body syndrome in goats—a report of five cases. Indian Vet. J., 55:413–414, 1978.

Sharma Deorani, V.P. and Katiyar, R.D.: Studies on the pathogenicity due to immature amphistomes among sheep and goats. Indian Vet. J., 44:199–205, 1967.

Shaw, J.M.: Suspected cyanide poisoning in two goats caused by ingestion of crab apple leaves and fruits. Vet. Rec., 119:242–243, 1986.

Shelton, M., Thompson, P. and Snowder, G.: Effect of monensin and sulfamethiazine on performance and naturally occurring coccidiosis in kid goats. Southwest. Vet., 35:27–32, 1982.

Sherman, D.M.: Duodenal obstruction by a phytobezoar in a goat. J. Am. Vet. Med. Assoc., 178:139–140, 1981.

Sherman, D.M. and Gezon, H.M.: Comparison of agar gel immunodiffusion and fecal culture for identification of goats with paratuberculosis. J. Am. Vet. Med. Assoc., 177:1208–1211, 1980.

Sherman, D.M. and Robinson, R.A.: Clinical examination of sheep and goats. Vet. Clin. N. Am. Large Anim. Pract., 5:409–426, 1983.

Sherman, D.M.: Causes of kid morbidity and mortality: An overview. Proc. IV International Conf. Goats, Brasilia, EMBRAPA-DDT, 1987, pp. 335–354.

Shihabudheen, P.K., Pillai, U.N. and Kumar, S.A.: Serum biochemical, physico-chemical and microbial changes in rumen liquor of experimental acidosis in goats. Indian Vet. J., 83(3):267–270, 2006.

Shimshony, A.: Bluetongue in Israel—a brief historical review. Vet. Ital. 40(3):116–118, 2004.

Shimshony, A.: Observations on parasitic gastroenteritis in goats in northern Israel. I. Clinical and helminthological findings. Refuah Vet., 31:63–75, 1974.

Shimshony, A. and Bar Moshe, B.: A case of Johne's disease in an Israeli Saanen goat. Refuah Vet., *29*:35–37, 1972.

Shlosberg, A.: Acute copper poisoning in a herd of goats. Refuah Vet., 35:15, 1978.

Short, C.R., et al.: Disposition of fenbendazole in the goat. Am. J. Vet. Res., 48:811–815, 1987.

Siamba, D.M.: Personal communication, Maseno, Kenya, June, 1990.

Sigurðardóttir, Ó.G., Bakke-McKellep, A.M., Djønne, B. and Evensen Ø.: *Mycobacterium avium* subsp. *paratuberculosis* enters the small intestinal mucosa of goat kids in areas with and without Peyer's patches as demonstrated with the everted sleeve method. Comp. Immunol. Microbiol. Inf. Dis., 28(3):223–230, 2005.

Silva, A.C. and Lima, J.D.: *Eimeria minasensis* n. sp. (Apicomplexa: Eimeriidae) in the domestic goat *Capra hircus*, from Brazil. Memorias do Instituto Oswaldo Cruz. 93(6):741–744, 1998.

Silvestre, A., Sauve, C. and Cabaret, J.: Caprine *Paramphistomum daubneyi* (Trematoda) infection in Europe. Vet. Rec., 146(23):674–675, 2000.

Singh, R.P., Sahai, B.N. and Jha, G.J.: Histopathology of the duodenum and rumen of goats during experimental infections with *Paramphistomum cervi.* Vet. Parasitol., 15:39–46, 1984.

Singh, U.M., Tripathi, B.N. and Paliwal, O.P.: Status of caprine paratuberculosis at organised and unorganised farms of Nepal. Indian J. Anim. Sci., 77(9):852–854, 2007.

Sinha, M.N.: The incidence of clostridial species in the alimentary tract of apparently healthy goats. Kajian Vet. Malaysia-Singapore, 2:171–175, 1970.

Slee, K.J. and Button, C.: Enteritis in sheep, goats, and pigs due to *Yersinia pseudotuberculosis* infection. Aust. Vet. J., 67:320–322, 1990.

Slee, K.J. and Button, C.: Enteritis in sheep and goats due to *Yersinia enterocolitica* infection. Aust. Vet. J., 67:396–398, 1990a.

Slocombe, R.F.: Combined streptomycin-isoniazid-rifampin therapy in the treatment of Johne's disease in a goat. Can. Vet. J., 23:160–163, 1982.

Slosarkova, S., Chroust, K. and Skrivanek, M.: Effects of toltrazuril and monensin in kids naturally infected with coccidia. Vet. Med., 43(8):239–244, 1998.

Sly, L.I., Cahill, M.M., Osawa, R. and Fujisawa, T.: The tannin-degrading species *Streptococcus gallolyticus* and *Streptococcus caprinus* are subjective synonyms. Int. J. Syst. Bacteriol., 47(3):893–894, 1997.

Smith, G.W., Rotstein, D.S. and Brownie, C.F.: Abdominal fat necrosis in a pygmy goat associated with fescue toxicosis. J. Vet. Diagn. Invest., 16(4):356–359, 2004.

Smith, H.V. and Klose, J.B.: Responses of goats to clostridial vaccines. Victorian Vet. Proc., p. 86, 1980.

Smith, J.P. and Bell, R.R.: Toxicity of the levo form of tetramisole in Angora goats. Am. J. Vet. Res., 32:871–873, 1971.

Smith, M.C.: Japanese pieris poisoning in the goat. J. Am. Vet. Med. Assoc., 173:78–79, 1978.

Smith, M.C.: Fetal mummification in a goat due to Japanese pieris *(Pieris japonica)* poisoning. Cornell Vet., 69:85–87, 1979.

Smith, M.C.: Coccidiosis in goats. Dairy Goat J., 58(4):80–82, 1980.

Smith, M.C.: Diagnosis, treatment, and prevention of common small ruminant parasites. In: Proceedings, 38th Annual Convention, American Association of Bovine Practitioners, pp. 123–127, 2005.

Smith, W.D.: Mechanisms of immunity to gastrointestinal nematodes of sheep. In: Increasing Small Ruminant Productivity in Semi-arid Areas. E.F. and F.S. Thomson, eds. Dordrecht, Kluwer Academic Publishers, pp. 275–286, 1988.

Snijders, A.J.: Thiabendazole trials on Angora goats. IV Pan-Am. Cong. Vet. Med. Zootech., Mexico City, Nov, pp. 51–56, 1962.

Sockett, D.C., Carr, D.J. and Collins, M.T.: Evaluation of conventional and radiometric fecal culture and a commercial DNA probe for diagnosis of *Mycobacterium paratuberculosis* infection in cattle. Can. J. Vet. Res., 56(2):148–153, 1992.

Soe, A.K. and Pomroy, W.E.: New species of *Eimeria* (Apicomplexa: Eimeriidae) from the domesticated goat *Capra hircus* in New Zealand. Systemic Parasitol., 23:195–202, 1992.

Soliman, K.N.: Globidium infections in the Sudan with special reference to *Globidium gilruthi* (Chatton, 1910) in sheep and goats. J. Parasitol., 46:29–32, 1960.

Songer, J.G.: Clostridial enteric diseases of domestic animals. Clin. Microbiol. Rev., 9(2):216–234, 1996.

Soulsby, E.J.L.: Helminths, Arthropods and Protozoa of Domesticated Animals. 7th Ed. Philadelphia, Lea and Febiger, 1982.

Spruell, J.: Malarial catarrhal fever (bluetongue) of sheep in South Africa. J. Comp. Pathol., 18:321–337, 1905.

Sreenivasulu, D., Subba Rao, M.V., Reddy, Y.N. and Gard, G.P.: Overview of bluetongue disease, viruses, vectors, surveillance and unique features: the Indian sub-continent and adjacent regions. Vet. Ital., 40(3):73–77, 2004.

Srivastava, P.S., Sinha, S.R.P. and Rama, S.P.: Efficacy of morantel citrate (banminth) against spontaneous immature amphistomiasis in indigenous goats. Indian Vet. J., 66:400–404, 1989.

Stehman, S.M.: Paratuberculosis in small ruminants, deer and South American camelids, Vet. Clin. N. Am., Food Anim. Pract., 12(2):441–455, 1996.

Stehman, S.M.: Advances in identifying and controlling paratuberculosis. Proceedings, 7th International Conference on Goats. International Goat Association, Tours, France, 15–21, pp. 273–277, May 2000. http://www.iga-goatworld.org/Conferences/7th_Tours/Advan_paratuberculosis_%5BStehman,%20S%5D.pdf.

Stevens, E.T. and Thomson, D.U.: Siderophore receptor and porin protein technology for control of *Salmonella* and *Escherichia coli* 0157:H7 in cattle. In: Proceedings, 38th Annual Convention, American Association of Bovine Practitioners, pp. 25–29, 2005.

Stewart, D.J., et al.: A long-term study in Angora goats experimentally infected with *Mycobacterium avium* subsp. *paratuberculosis*: clinical disease, faecal culture and immunological studies. Vet. Microbiol., 113(1/2):13–24, 2006.

Storset, A.K., et al.: Subclinical paratuberculosis in goats following experimental infection: an immunological and microbiological study. Vet. Immunol. Immunopathol., 80(3/4):271–287, 2001.

Stott, J.L., et al.: Epizootiological study of bluetongue virus infection in California livestock: an overview. In: Bluetongue and Related Orbiviruses. T.L. Barber and M.M. Jochim, eds. New York, Alan R. Liss Inc., 1985.

Straube, E.F. and McGregor, B.A.: Johne's disease in a goat. Australian Vet. J., 59:62, 1982.

Subasinghe, D.H.A. and Ramakrishnaswamy, A.: Salmonellosis in Sri Lanka: Isolation of *Salmonellae* from goats slaughtered at an abattoir. Sri Lanka Vet. J., 31:40–42, 1983.

Subramanian, G. and Srivastava, V.K.: A note on the species of *Setaria* Viborg 1795 reported from sheep and goats with a description of the parasite found in the peritoneum of goat. Riv. Parassitol., 34:59–62, 1973.

Sulochana, S. and Sudharma, D.: Isolation of *Yersinia pseudotuberculosis* from cases of abortion in goats. Kerala J. Vet. Sci., 16:139–142, 1985.

Sumberg, J.E. and Mack, S.D.: Village production of West African dwarf goats and sheep in Nigeria. Trop. Anim. Health Prod., 17:135–140, 1985.

Suteu, E., Rotaru, O. and Cozma, V.: Report of *Giardia* infection of goats in Romania. Seminarul. Actualitati in patologia animalelor domestice. Cluj-Napoca, 18–19 iunie 1987. Institutul Agronomic, Cluj-Napoca, Romania:, pp. 217–222, 1987.

Sutherland, R.J.: Giardiasis in Saanen goats. Surveillance. 9(4):25, 1982.

Sutherland, R.J. and Clarkson, A.R.: Giardiasis in intensively reared Saanen kids. N. Z. Vet. J., 32(3):34–35, 1984.

Swarup, D., Parai, T.P. and Lal, M.: Therapeutic efficacy of amprolium hydrochloride (Amprolsol 20% MSD) against coccidiosis in Pashmina kids. Indian Vet. J., 59:69–70, 1982.

Tabachnick, W.J.: *Culicoides* and the global epidemiology of bluetongue virus infection. Vet. Ital., 40(3):145–150, 2004.

Takahashi, E., et al.: Antibody to rotavirus in various animal species. Natl. Inst. Anim. Health Q., 19(1/2):72–73, 1979.

Tamarin, R. and Landau, M.: Congenital and uterine infection with *Mycobacterium johnei* in sheep. Refuah Vet., 18:43–44, 1961.

Tamate, H.: The anatomical studies of the stomach of the goat. I. The post natal development of the stomach with special reference to the weaning and prolonged suckling. Tohoku J. Agric. Res., 7:209–229, 1956.

Tamate, H.: The anatomical studies of the stomach of the goat. II. The post-natal changes in the capacities and the relative sizes of the four divisions of the stomach. Tohoku J. Agric. Res., 8:65–77, 1957.

Tanwar, R.K. and Mathur, P.D.: Biochemical and microbial changes in experimentally induced rumen acidosis in goats. Indian J. Anim. Sci., 53:271–274, 1983.

Tanwar, R.K. and Saxena, A.K.: Radiographic detection of foreign bodies. Vet. Med., 79:1195–1197, 1984.

Tarazona Vilas, J.M.: Parasitic gastroenteritis in goats in Spain. In: Les Maladies de la Chèvre, Les Colloques de l'INRA, No. 28. P. Yvore and G. Perrin, eds. Paris. Institut National de la Récherche Agronomique. pp. 507–512, 1984.

Tarazona, J.M., Sanz Pastor, A., Babin, M.M. and Dominguez, T.: Caprine trichostrongylidosis. III. Provisional epidemiological model. Anales INIA, Serie Ganadera, Spain, 14:125–132, 1982.

Tarlatzis, C., Panetsos, A. and Dragonas, P.: Furacin in the treatment of ovine and caprine coccidiosis. J. Am. Vet. Med. Assoc., 126:391–392, 1955.

Tarlatzis, C., Panetsos, A. and Dragonas, P.: Further experiences with furacin in treatment of ovine and caprine coccidiosis. J. Am. Vet. Med. Assoc., 131:474, 1957.

Tarlatzis, C.B., Frangopoulos, A. and Stoforos, E.: Gangrenous mastitis of ewes and goats and the identification of the causal agent *Clostridium perfringens* type C. Delt. hellen. kten. Hetair., 50:88–95, 1963.

Taylor, M.A., Hunt, K.R. and Goodyear, K.L.: Anthelmintic resistance detection methods. Vet. Parasitol., 103(3):183–194, 2002.

Taylor, W.P.: Serological studies with the virus of peste des petits ruminants in Nigeria. Res. Vet. Sci., 26:236–242, 1979.

Taylor, W.P. and Barrett, T.: Rinderpest and peste des petits ruminants, In: Diseases of Sheep, 4th Ed, I.D. Aitken, ed. Blackwell Publishing, Oxford, UK, 2007.

Taylor, W.P., et al.: Peste des petits ruminants has been widely present in southern India since, if not before, the late 1980s. Prev. Vet. Med., 52(3/4):305–312, 2001.

Tenter, A.M., et al.: The conceptual basis for a new classification of the coccidia. Int. J. Parasitol., 32:595–616, 2002.

Terrill, T.H., et al.: Anthelmintic resistance on goat farms in Georgia: efficacy of anthelmintics against gastrointestinal nematodes in two selected goat herds. Vet. Parasitol., 97(4):261–268, 2001.

Terrill, T.H., et al.: Capability of the nematode-trapping fungus *Duddingtonia flagrans* to reduce infective larvae of gastrointestinal nematodes in goat faeces in the southeastern United States: dose titration and dose time interval studies. Vet. Parasitol., 120(4):285–296, 2004.

Terrill, T.H., et al.: Effect of pelleting on efficacy of sericea lespedeza hay as a natural dewormer in goats. Vet Parasitol., 146(1/2): 117–122, 2007.

Thamsborg, S.M., Jorgensen, R.J. and Henriksen, S.A.: Cryptosporidiosis in kids of dairy goats. Vet. Rec., 127(25/26): 627–628, 1990.

Theodorides, V.J., Scott, G.C. and Laderman, M.: Efficacy of parbendazole against gastrointestinal nematodes in goats. Am. J. Vet. Res., 30:1887–1890, 1969.

Thomas, G.W.: Paratuberculosis in a large goat herd. Vet. Rec., 113:464–466, 1983.

Thompson, J.: Artificial kid rearing. Proc. 17th Seminar, Sheep and Beef Cattle Soc., N.Z. Vet. Assoc., Wellington, pp. 6–10, 1987.

Thompson, K.G., Enteric diseases of goats. Proc. Course Goat Husbandry Medicine, Publ. No. 106, Vet. Cont. Ed., Massey Univ., Palmerston North, NZ, pp. 78–85, 1985.

Thompson, K.G.: Some diseases of importance in goats as seen by animal health laboratories. Proc. 16th Seminar, Sheep and Beef Cattle Soc. N.Z. Vet. Assoc., Palmerston North, N.Z., 1986.

Thompson, K.G.: Infectious diseases of goats in New Zealand. Surveillance., 28(2):3–7, 2001.

Thoresen, O.F. and Olsaker, I.: Distribution and hybridization patterns of the insertion element IS900 in clinical isolates of *Mycobacterium paratuberculosis*. Vet. Microbiol., 40:293–303, 1994.

Thornton, J.E., Galvin, T.J., Bell, R.R. and Ramsey, C.W.: Transmissibility of gastrointestinal nematodes from blackbuck antelope to cattle, sheep, and goats. J. Am. Vet. Med. Assoc., 163:554–555, 1973.

Tongson, M.S. and Dimaculangan, A.M.: Comparative viability of strongyle ova in goat feces exposed and unexposed to sunlight. Philip. J. Vet. Med., 22:38–47, 1983.

Tongson, M.S., Manuel, M.F. and Eduardo, S.L.: Parasitic fauna of goats in the Philippines. Philip. J. Vet. Med., 20:1–37, 1981.

Tontis, A. and König, H.: Zur Paratuberkulose der Ziege. Schweizer Archiv Tierheilk., 120:527–531, 1978.

Torres-Acosta, J.F.J. and Jacobs, D.E.: Duration of activity of oral moxidectin against *Haemonchus contortus*, *Teladorsagia circumcincta* and *Trichostrongylus colubriformis* in goats. Vet. Rec., 144(23):648–649, 1999.

Travassos, T.E., Pereira, I.H.O., Leite, A.C.R. and Tavares, H.P.: The epizootiology of the helminthiases of goats in the bush of Pernambuco. Cong. Brasil. Med. Vet., 14:153, São Paulo, 1974.

Tremblay, R.R.M., Butler, D.G., Allen, J.W. and Hoffman, A.M.: Metabolic acidosis without dehydration in seven goat kids. Can. Vet. J., 32(5):308–310, 1991.

Tripathi, J.C.: Effect of different temperatures on the eggs of gastrointestinal nematodes of goats under controlled conditions. Indian Vet. J., 57:719–722, 1980.

Tustin, R.C., Thornton, D.J. and Kleu, C.B.: An outbreak of *Cotyledon orbiculata* L. poisoning in a flock of Angora goat rams. J. S. Afr. Vet. Med. Assoc., 55:181–184, 1984.

Twort, F.W. and Ingram, G.L.: A monograph on Johne's disease. Baillière, Tindall and Cox, London, 1913.

Tzipori, S., Larsen, J., Smith, M. and Luefl, R.: Diarrhoea in goat kids attributed to cryprosporidium infection. Vet. Rec., 111:35–36, 1982.

Tzipori, S.: Cryptosporidiosis in animals and humans. Microbiol. Rev., 47:84–96, 1983.

Uhlinger, C., Fetrow, J. and Johnstone, C.: A field evaluation of benzimidazole and nonbenzimidazole drugs in a herd of dairy goats. J. Vet. Intern. Med., 2:113–116, 1988.

Ullrich, N.A., Grumbein, S. and Coles, B.: Paratuberculosis (Johne's disease) in goats. Vet. Med. Sm. Anim. Clin., *77*:1101–1104, 1982.

Uzal, F.A. and Kelly, W.R.: Protection of goats against experimental enterotoxaemia by vaccination with *Clostridium perfringens* type D epsilon toxoid. Vet. Rec., 142(26):722–725, 1998.

Uzal, F.A., et al.: Detection by polymerase chain reaction of *Clostridium perfringens* producing epsilon toxin in faeces and in gastrointestinal contents of goats. Lett. Appl. Microbiol., 23(1):13–17, 1996.

Uzal, F.A., Glastonbury, J.R.W., Kelly, W.R. and Thomas, R.: Caprine enterotoxaemia associated with cerebral microangiopathy. Vet. Rec., 141(9):224–226, 1997.

Uzal, F.A., Bodero, D.A.V., Kelly, W.R. and Nielsen, K.: Variability of serum antibody responses of goat kids to a commercial *Clostridium perfringens* epsilon toxoid vacine. Vet. Rec., 143:472–474, 1998.

Uzal, F.A., et al.: Comparison of four techniques for the detection of *Clostridium perfringens* type D epsilon toxin in intestinal contents and other body fluids of sheep and goats. J. Vet. Diagn. Invest., 15:94–99, 2003.

Vagenas, D., et al.: Genetic control of resistance to gastrointestinal parasites in crossbred cashmere-producing goats: responses to selection, genetic parameters and relationships with production traits. Anim. Sci., 74(2):199–208, 2002.

Valentine, B.A., Cebra, C.K. and Taylor, G.H.: Fatal gastrointestinal parasitism in goats: 31 cases (2001–2006). J. Am. Vet. Med. Assoc., 231(7):1098–1103, 2007.

Valheim, M., et al.: Lesions in subclinical paratuberculosis of goats are associated with persistent gut-associated lymphoid tissue. J. Comp. Pathol., 127(2/3):194–202, 2002.

Valheim, M., et al.: Characterization of macrophages and occurrence of T cells in intestinal lesions of subclinical paratuberculosis in goats. J. Comp. Pathol., 131(2/3):221–232, 2004.

Van Metre, D.C., Tyler, J.W. and Stehman, S.M.: Diagnosis of enteric disease in small ruminants. Vet. Clin. N. Am. Food Anim. Pract., 16(1):87–115, 2000.

Van Soest, P.J.: Interactions of feeding behavior and forage composition. Proc. IV International Conf. Goats, Brasilia, EMBRAPA-DDT, pp. 971–987, 1987.

Van Soest, P.J.: Nutritional ecology of the ruminant, 2nd Ed. Cornell University Press, Ithaca, NY, pg. 203, 1994.

van Tonder, E.M.: Notes on some disease problems in Angora goats in South Africa. Vet. Med. Rev., 1/2:109–138, 1975.

van Tonder, E.M., Kellerman, G.E. and Bolton, T.F.W.: An outbreak of diphtheria in Boergoat kids. J. S. Afr. Vet. Assoc., 47:123–124, 1976.

Van Wyk, J.A.: Refugia—overlooked as perhaps the most potent factor concerning the development of anthelmintic resistance. Onderstepoort J. Vet. Res., 68(1):55–67, 2001.

Van Wyk, J.A. and Bath, G.F.: The FAMACHA© system for managing haemonchosis in sheep and goats by clinically identifying individual animals for treatment. Vet. Res., 33(5):509–529, 2002.

Van Wyk, J.A., Hoste, H., Kaplan, R.M. and Besier, R.B.: Targeted selective treatment for worm management—how do we sell rational programs to farmers? Vet. Parasitol., 139(4):336–346, 2006.

Varady, M., Praslicka, J., Corba, J. and Vesely, L.: Multiple anthelmintic resistance of nematodes in imported goats. Vet. Rec. 132(15):387–388, 1993.

Vatta, A.F., et al.: Testing for clinical anaemia caused by *Haemonchus* spp. in goats farmed under resource-poor conditions in South Africa using an eye colour chart developed for sheep. Vet. Parasitol. 99(1):1–14, 2001.

Vaughn, S.D.: New Animal Drugs For Use in Animal Feeds; Decoquinate. Federal Register, 67(234):72370–72373, 2002. http://www.fda.gov/OHRMS/DOCKETS/98fr/02–30863.htm.

Veale, P.I.: Resistance to macrocyclic lactones in nematodes of goats. Australian Vet. J., 80(5):303–304, 2002.

Verma, D.N., Pant, H.C., Rai, G.S. and Rawat, J.S.: Concentration of VFA and lactic acid in the rumen of goat. Indian Vet. J., 52:442–444, 1975.

Vickers, M.C.: Enteric infections in young goats and their control. Proc. 16th Seminar, Sheep and Beef Cattle Soc., N.Z. Vet. Assoc., Palmerston North, pp. 46–55, 1986.

Visser, I.J.R., van den Hoven, R. Vos, J.H. and van den Ingh, T.S.G.A.M.: *Pieris japonica* (pieris)-intoxicatie bij tweegeiten. Tijdschr. Diergeneeskd., 113:185–189, 1988.

Von Rotz, A., Corboz, L., and Waldvogel, A.: *Clostridium perfringens* typ D-enterotoxämie der Ziege in der Schweiz. Pathologisch-anatomische und bakteriologische Untersuchungen. Schweiz. Arch. Tierheilk., 126:359–364, 1984.

Vujic, B. and Ilic, G.: Study of the most important diseases of goats: coccidiosis. Veterinarski Glasnik, 39:799–810, 1985.

Wafula, J.S. and Wamwayi, H.M.: Development and distribution of rinderpest virus antigen in experimentally infected goats. Vet. Rec., 123:199–200, 1988.

Waghorn, T.S., Leathwick, D.M., Chen, L.Y. and Skipp, R.A.: Efficacy of the nematode-trapping fungus *Duddingtonia flagrans* against three species of gastro-intestinal nematodes in laboratory faecal cultures from sheep and goats. Vet. Parasitol., 118:227–234, 2003.

Waldhalm, S.J., Criss, E.A., Neff-Davis, C.A. and Huber, W.G.: Fenbendazole clearance from goat milk. Small Rumin. Res., 2:79–84, 1989.

Walker, S.J. and Gilmour, A.: The incidence of *Yersinia enterocolitica* and *Yersinia enterocolitica*-like bacteria in goats milk in Northern Ireland. Let. Appl. Microbiol., 3:49–52, 1986.

Waller, P.J.: Anthelmintic resistance and the future for roundworm control. Vet. Parasitol., 25:177–191, 1987.

Waller, P.J.: Sustainable nematode parasite control strategies for ruminant livestock by grazing management and biological control. Anim. Feed Sci. Technol., 126(3/4):277–289, 2006.

Waller, P.J., Dobson, R.J., Obendorf, D.L. and Gillham, R.J.: Resistance of *Trichostrongylus colubriformis* to levamisole and morantel: differences in relation to selection history. Vet. Parasitol., 21:255–263, 1986.

Waller, P.J., Rudby-Martin, L., Ljungstrom, B.L. and Rydzyk, A.: The epidemiology of abomasal nematodes of sheep in Sweden, with particular reference to overwinter survival strategies. Vet. Parasitol., 122:207–220, 2004.

Walton, T.E.: The history of bluetongue and a current global overview. Vet. Ital., 40(3):31–38, 2004.

Wanasinghe, D.D.: An outbreak of enterotoxaemia due to *Clostridium welchii* type D in goats. Ceylon Vet. J., 21:62–65, 1973.

Warren, A.L., Uzal, F.A., Blackall, L.L. and Kelly, W.R.: PCR detection of *Clostridium perfringens* type D in formalin-fixed, paraffin-embedded tissues of goats and sheep. Lett. Appl. Microbiol. 29(1):15–19, 1999.

Waruiru, R.M., Kogi, J.K., Weda, E.H. and Ngotho, J.W.: Multiple anthelmintic resistance on a goat farm in Kenya. Vet. Parasitol., 75(2/3):191–197, 1998.

Washburn, K.E., et al.: Honey mesquite toxicosis in a goat. J. Am. Vet. Med. Assoc., 220(12):1837–1839, 2002.

Watanabe, Y.; Kimura, K.; Yang C.H. and Ooi H.K.: Detection of *Cryptosporidium* sp. oocyst and *Giardia* sp. cyst in faucet water samples from cattle and goat farms in Taiwan. J. Vet. Med. Sci. 67(12):1285–1287, 2005.

Waters, M., et al.: Genotyping and phenotyping of beta2-toxigenic *Clostridium perfringens* fecal isolates associated with gastrointestinal diseases in piglets. J. Clin. Microbiol., 41(8):3584–3591, 2003.

Watson, T.G. and Hosking, B.C.: Observations on resistance and "self-cure" to nematode parasites exhibited by grazing lambs and Saanen kids. Proceedings, N. Z. Soc. Anim. Prod., 49:179–182, 1989.

Watson, T.G. and Hosking, B.C.: Evidence for multiple anthelmintic resistance in two nematode parasite genera on a Saanen goat dairy. N. Z. Vet. J., 38:50–53, 1990.

Weese, J., Kenney, D.G. and O'Connor, A.: Secondary lactose intolerance in a neonatal goat. J. Am. Vet. Med. Assoc., 217(3):372–375, 2000.

West, D.M., Pomroy, W.E. and Leathwick, D.M.: Multiple resistance in *Trichostrongylus* and *Teladorsagia* (*Ostertagia*) in goats to oxfendazole, levamisole and moxidectin, and inefficacy of trichlorphon. N. Z. Vet. J., 52(5), 298–299, 2004.

West, G., et al.: Paratuberculosis in California dairy goats. Calif. Vet., 33:28–31, 1979.

West, G.A., Dale, T. and Mayhew, R.F.: Left displacement of the abomasum in a goat. Vet. Med. Small Anim. Clin., 78:1919–1921, 1983.

Whitlock, R.H., et al.: Johne's disease: the effect of feeding monensin to reduce the bioburden of *Mycobacterium avium* subspecies *paratuberculosis* in neonatal calves. Proceedings, 38th Annual Convention, American Association of Bovine Practitioners, 24–26 September, 2005. American Association of Bovine Practitioners, Stillwater, USA: pp. 191–192, 2005.

Whittington, R.J., Eamens, G.J. and Cousins, D.V.: Specificity of absorbed ELISA and agar gel immuno-diffusion tests for paratuberculosis in goats with observations about use of these tests in infected goats. Aust. Vet. J., 81(1/2):71–75, 2003.

Whittington, R.J., et al.: Evaluation of modified BACTEC 12B radiometric medium and solid media for culture of *Mycobacterium avium* subsp. *paratuberculosis* from sheep. J. Clin. Microbiol. 37:1077–1083, 1999.

Whittington, R.J., et al.: Survival and dormancy of *Mycobacterium avium* subsp. *paratuberculosis* in the environment. Appl. Environ. Microbiol., 70(5):2989–3004, 2004.

Williams, C.S.F.: Dairy goat herd health management. In: Current Veterinary Therapy, Food Animal Practice, 2nd edition. J.L. Howard, ed. Philadelphia, W.B. Saunders Co., pp. 181–184, 1982.

Williams, J.F. and Schillhorn van Veen, T.W.: Tapeworms. In: Parasites, Pests and Predators. S.M. Gafaar, W.E. Howard and R.E. Marsh, eds. Amsterdam, Elsevier, 1985.

Willson, P.J. and Acres, S.D.: A comparison of dichromate solution floatation and fecal smears for diagnosis of cryptosporidiosis in calves. Can. Vet. J., 23:240–246, 1982.

Wilson, R.D., Witzel, D.A. and Verlander, J.M.: Somatosensory-evoked response of ataxic Angora goats in suspected haloxon-delayed neurotoxicity. Am. J. Vet. Res., 43:2224–2226, 1982.

Wirth, H.J.: Diseases of goats commonly seen in Victoria. In: Proceedings, Refresher Course for Veterinarians, Post-Graduate Committee in Veterinary Science, University of Sydney, 52:377–395, 1980.

Witte, S.T., Sponenberg, D.P. and Collins, T.C.: Abortion and early neonatal death of kids attributed to intrauterine *Yersinia pseudotuberculosis* infection. J. Am. Vet. Med. Assoc., 187:834, 1985.

Woldemariam, E., Molla, B., Alemayehu, D. and Muckle, A.: Prevalence and distribution of *Salmonella* in apparently healthy slaughtered sheep and goats in Debre Zeit, Ethiopia. Small Rumin. Res., 58(1):19–24, 2005.

Wolstenholme, A.J., et al.: Drug resistance in veterinary helminths. Trends Parasitol., 20(10):469–476, 2004.

Worrall, E.E., Litamoi, J.K., Seck, B.M. and Ayelet, G.: *Xerovac*: an ultra rapid method for the dehydration and preservation of live attenuated Rinderpest and Peste des Petits ruminants vaccines. Vaccine. 19(7/8):834–839, 2000.

Wright, S.E. and Coop, R.L.: Cryptosporidiosis and coccidiosis. In: Diseases of Sheep, 4th Ed., I.D. Aitken, ed. Blackwell Publishing, Oxford, pp. 179–185, 2007.

Xenos, G., et al.: Paratuberculosis in sheep and goats in certain regions of northern and central Greece. In: Paratuberculosis, Diagnostic Methods, Their Practical Application and Experience with Vaccination. J. Berg Jorgensen and O. Aalund, eds. Luxembourg, Commission of the European Communities, 1984.

Xiao, L.H. and Cama, V.: Cryptosporidium. Chapter 142. In. Manual of Clinical Microbiology, 9th Edition. Vol. 2, Murray, P.R., Ed., Washington DC, ASM Press, pp. 2122–2132, 2007.

Xiao, L.H., Fayer, R., Ryan, U. and Upton, S.J.: *Cryptosporidium* taxonomy: recent advances and implications for public health. Clin. Microbiol. Rev., 17(1):72–97, 2004.

Yadav, S.C. and Sengar, O.P.S.: Breed variations in the gastrointestinal parasitism of Indian goats. Proc. III International Conf. Goat Prod. Dis., Tucson, Arizona, pp. 342, 1982.

Yalcin, N. and Des Francs, E.: L'entérite paratuberculeuse caprine. Rec. Méd. Vét., 146:807–811, 1970.

Yvore, P.: Les coccidioses caprines. In: Les Maladies de la Chèvre, Les Colloques de l'INRA, No. 28. P. Yvore and G. Perrin, eds. Paris. Institut National de la Recherche Agronomique. pp. 479–485, 1984.

Yvore, P. and Esnault, A.: Transmission of *Strongyloides papillosus* to kids through the milk of their dams. Bull. Mensuel Soc. Vét. Prat. Fr., 70(8):479–483, 1986.

Yvore, P. and Esnault, A.: Interpreting fecal examinations for ovine and caprine coccidial infection. Vet. Med., 82:740–743, 1987.

Yvore, P., et al.: Enquête épidémiologique sur les diarrhées neonatales des chevreaux dans les élevages de Touraine. In: Les Maladies de la Chèvre, Les Colloques de l'INRA, No. 28. P. Yvore and G. Perrin, eds. Paris. Institut National de la Recherche Agronomique, pp. 437–442, 1984.

Yvore, P., et al.: La coccidiose caprine effet de contaminations mono ou multispécifiques. Rec. Méd. Vét., 161:347–351, 1985.

Yvore, P., Esnault, A., Naciri, M. and Guillimin, P.: Essais de traitement de la coccidiose du chevreau par administration unique d'oblets à la sulfademethoxine. Bull. Mensuel Soc. Vét. Prat. Fr., *70*:233–240, 1986.

Zahinuddin, M. and Sinha, R.P.: Effects of antituberculosis agents on *Mycobacterium johnei* in infected goats. Indian Vet. J., 61:574–577, 1984.

Zajac, A.M. and Gipson, T.A.: Multiple anthelmintic resistance in a goat herd. Vet. Parasitol., 87(2/3):163–172, 2000.

Zdragas, A., Petsaga-Tsimperi, V. and Tsakos, P: Investigation of the incidence of *Salmonella* spp. in the diarrhoeic syndrome of young ruminants. Deltion tes Ellenikes Kteniatrikes Etaireias, 51(4):288–292, 2000.

Zschöck, M., Hamann, H.P., Kloppert, B. and Wolter, W.: Shiga-toxin-producing *Escherichia coli* in faeces of healthy dairy cows, sheep and goats: prevalence and virulence properties. Lett. Appl. Microbiol. 31(3):203–208, 2000.

Zwart, D. and Macadam, I.: Transmission of rinderpest by contact from cattle to sheep and goats. Res. Vet. Sci., 8:37–47, 1967.

Zwart, D. and Macadam, I.: Observations on rinderpest in sheep and goats and transmission to cattle. Res. Vet. Sci., 8:53–57, 1967a.

11

Liver and Pancreas

Several common goat diseases principally involve the liver and may produce a considerable amount of economic loss (Sriraman et al. 1982). The most important hepatic diseases are fluke infestations and pregnancy toxemia. Pregnancy toxemia is discussed in Chapter 19. Copper toxicity, which produces hemolytic anemia and toxic hepatitis, is discussed in Chapter 7. All other liver diseases are discussed in this chapter. Pancreatic disease in goats is limited to pancreatic fluke infestations that are most often subclinical in nature.

BACKGROUND INFORMATION OF CLINICAL IMPORTANCE

Anatomy and Physiology

Liver

The caprine liver comprises four distinct lobes: the right, left, quadrate, and caudate. It is located in the dorsal two-thirds of the right anterior abdomen, in contact with the diaphragm and the abdominal wall from the seventh to last rib (Figure 11.1). Dorsally, the liver is covered by the lung as far caudally as the ninth rib space, but the liver is percussible or accessible for biopsy between the ventral lung border and the costochondral junctions in the seventh through ninth rib spaces. The gallbladder extends below the ventral border of the liver.

Structural variation has been reported in the biliary apparatus of the goat. The cystic duct from the gallbladder enters the right hepatic duct in about half of goats examined, while in the other half, it enters at the junction of the left and right hepatic ducts so that the common bile duct is not preceded by a common hepatic duct (Robinson and Dunphy 1962). The distribution of the various branches of the hepatic veins of the goat has also been identified as distinct from the arrangement traditionally described for all ruminants (Brikas and Tsiamitas 1980).

Pancreas

The pancreas is located in close association with the portal vein in the craniodorsal abdomen to the right of the midline. It is composed of a larger right lobe, extending along the descending duodenum, and a smaller left lobe (Lukens 1938; Naranjo et al. 1986). The pancreatic duct enters the common bile duct

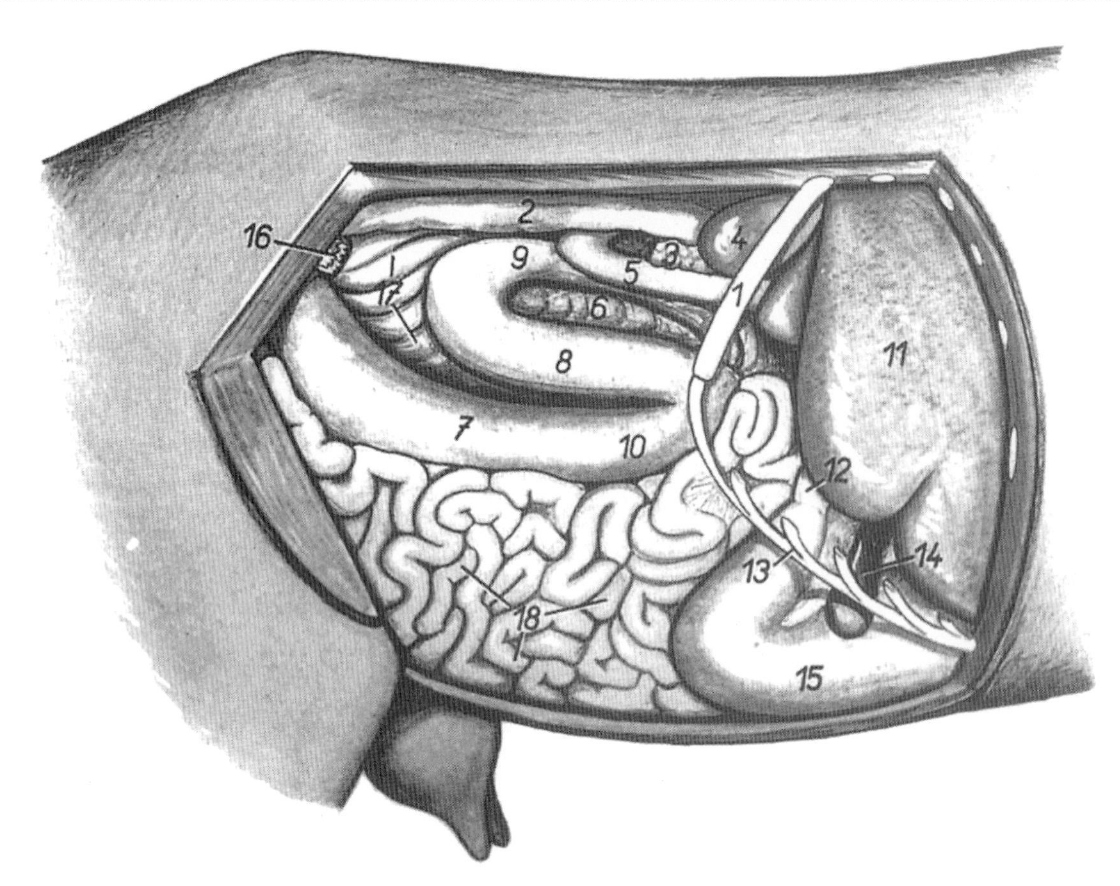

Figure 11.1. Location of the liver in the abdomen of the goat and relationship to other visceral structures. 1, thirteenth rib; 2, descending colon; 3, pancreas, right lobe; 4, right kidney; 5, descending part of duodenum; 6, distal loop of ascending colon; 7, cecum; 8 to 10, proximal loop of ascending colon (8, middle gyrus; 9, dorsal gyrus; 10, ventral gyrus); 11, liver; 12, cranial part of duodenum; 13, costal arch; 14, gallbladder; 15, abomasum; 16, ovary and uterine tube; 17, spiral loop of colon; 18, jejunum. (Reproduced with permission from Popesko P.: Atlas of Topographical Anatomy of Domestic Animals, new revised English edition, Vydavatelstvo Priroda, Bratislava, 2008, www.priroda.sk.)

(Robinson and Dunphy 1961). Histologically, the structure of the goat pancreas is similar to that of other domestic ruminants (Reddy and Eliot 1985; Lone et al. 1989).

Clinical Pathology

Enzymology

Hepatic parenchymal disease that causes a disruption of hepatocytes can lead to measurably increased serum levels of a number of intracellular hepatic enzymes in goats. Information about normal serum levels of these enzymes and their variation in goats due to age, breed, and sex is given in Table 11.1.

Increases in aspartate aminotransferase (AST) and lactate dehydrogenase (LDH) are not liver-specific, and also result from muscle cell damage as discussed in Chapter 4. Basal levels of sorbitol dehydrogenase (SDH) in goat liver and serum are much higher than those reported for cattle and sheep.

It is advised that alanine aminotransferase (ALT), formerly serum glutamic pyruvic transaminase (SGPT), commonly used as an indicator of hepatic disease in dogs and cats, not be used in the evaluation of liver disease in ruminants because the livers of cattle and sheep contain low levels of ALT (Cornelius 1980). This is also true in goats. Changes in serum ALT concentrations are highly variable and unpredictable in response to hepatic injury (Hanifa Moursi et al. 1979; Abu Damir et al. 1982; Jones and Shah 1982; Clark et al. 1984; Shimizu et al. 1986; El Dirdiri et al. 1987).

Concentrations of liver-specific enzymes are generally higher in acute liver disease than chronic liver disease and may be within normal limits in the later stages of prolonged hepatic disease, so careful interpretation of laboratory values in conjunction with clinical findings is essential.

Biliary stasis or obstruction can occur concurrently or independently of parenchymal damage, and different enzymes are used to evaluate cholestasis, namely,

Table 11.1. Some normal values reported for liver-associated enzymes and other blood parameters associated with liver disease.

Enzyme	*Unit*	*Goat description (number of animals)*	*Mean ± S.D.*	*Range*	*Reference*
Alanine aminotransferase (ALT, SGPT)	IU/l	General values		24.0–83.0	Kaneko 1980
	IU/l	Adult, lactating F, Saanen and Alpine (79)	18.7 ± 3.1	12.5–24.9	Ridoux et al. 1981
	IU/l	Adult, lactating F, Saanen only (25)	20 ± 3.6		Ridoux et al. 1981
	IU/l	Adult, lactating F, Alpine only (54)	18.1 ± 2.7		Ridoux et al. 1981
Albumin	g/dl	General values		2.7–3.9	Kaneko 1980
	g/dl	General values		2.3–3.6	Kahn 2005
Alkaline phosphatase (AP)	IU/l	General values	219 ± 76	93–387	Kaneko 1980
	IU/l	Adult, lactating F, Saanen and Alpine (63)	184 ± 120	0.0–424	Ridoux et al. 1981
Ammonia	mmol/l	Adult Nubian goats (11)		40.2–43.7	Ali and Abu Samra 1987
Arginase	IU/l	0.5 to 2.5 yr, F, breed not stated (<28)	13.21	0.0–23	Adam et al. 1974
	IU/l	0.5 to 2.5 yr, M, breed not stated (<28)	14.87	0.0–20	Adam et al. 1974
Aspartate aminotransferase (AST, SGOT)	IU/l	General values		167.0–513.0	Kaneko 1980
	IU/l	4-month-old adult MC, F, Saanen—feral (5)	70 ± 13		Kramer and Carthew 1985
	IU/l	All ages, M, MC, F, pygmy (53)	32.3 ± 10.1		Castro et al. 1977
	IU/l	Adult, lactating F, Saanen and Alpine (80)	43.6 ± 9.9	23.8–63.4	Ridoux et al. 1981
	IU/l	Adult, lactating F, Saanen only (25)	51.7 ± 8.7		Ridoux et al. 1981
	IU/l	Adult, lactating F, Alpine only (55)	39.8 ± 8		Ridoux et al. 1981
Bilirubin, Total	mg/dl	General values		0.0–0.1	Kaneko 1980
	mg/dl	4–6 yr, F, pygmy (7)	0.2 ± 0.05		Castro et al. 1977
	mg/dl	2–3 yr, F, pygmy (17)	0.4 ± 0.1		Castro et al. 1977
	mg/dl	1–2 yr, F, pygmy (7)	0.8 ± 0.3		Castro et al. 1977
	mg/dl	<1 yr, F, pygmy (10)	0.5 ± 0.1		Castro et al. 1977
	mg/dl	All ages, F, pygmy (41)	0.4 ± 0.2		Castro et al. 1977
	mg/dl	All ages, M, pygmy (7)	0.5 ± 0.2		Castro et al. 1977
	mg/dl	All ages, MC, pygmy (5)	0.7 ± 0.1		Castro et al. 1977
	mg/dl	Adult, lactating F, Saanen and Alpine (89)	0.24 ± 0.08		Ridoux et al. 1981
	mg/dl	<1 yr, lactating F, Saanen and Alpine (30)	0.26 ± 0.06		Ridoux et al. 1981
	mg/dl	>1 yr, lactating F, Saanen and Alpine (59)	0.23 ± 0.09		Ridoux et al. 1981
	mg/dl	Adult, lactating F, Saanen only (25)	0.21 ± 0.07		Ridoux et al. 1981
	mg/dl	Adult, lactating F, Alpine only (64)	0.25 ± 0.08		Ridoux et al. 1981
Cholesterol	mg/dl	General values		65–136	Kahn 2005
Glucose	mg/dl	General values		48–76	Kahn 2005
	mg/dl	General values		50–75	Kaneko 1980

Table 11.1. *Continued*

Enzyme	*Unit*	*Goat description (number of animals)*	*Mean ± S.D.*	*Range*	*Reference*
Glutamate dehydrogenase	IU/l	4-month-old adult MC and F, Saanen—feral (5)	3.4 ± 0.6		Kramer and Carthew 1985
Gamma glutamyl transferase	IU/l	4-month-old adult MC and F, Saanen—feral (5)	32 ± 4.4		Kramer and Carthew 1985
Isocitrate dehydrogenase	IU/l	Adult, lactating and nonlactating F, Alpine (104)		2.3–14.8	Garnier et al. 1984
Lactate dehydrogenase	IU/l	Not specified	281 ± 71	123–392	Kaneko 1980
	IU/l	All ages, M, MC, F, pygmy (53)	289.9 ± 80.9		Castro et al. 1977
	IU/l	All ages, F, pygmy (41)	302.4 ± 83.6		Castro et al. 1977
	IU/l	All ages, M, pygmy (7)	225.7 ± 20		Castro et al. 1977
	IU/l	All ages, MC, pygmy (5)	239.8 ± 35.9		Castro et al. 1977
	IU/l	Adult, nonlactating F, Alpine (35)		217–417	Garnier et al. 1984
	IU/l	Adult, lactating F, Alpine (70)		300–586	Garnier et al. 1984
Ornithine carbamyl transferase	IU/l	Adult, lactating F, Saanen and Alpine (69)	13.4 ± 5.5	2.4–23.4	Ridoux et al. 1981
	IU/l	<1 yr, lactating F, Saanen and Alpine (27)	14.8 ± 4.7		Ridoux et al. 1981
	IU/l	>1 yr, lactating F, Saanen and Alpine (42)	12.2 ± 5.3		Ridoux et al. 1981
	IU/l	Adult, lactating F, Saanen only (23)	15.8 ± 4.3		Ridoux et al. 1981
	IU/l	Adult, lactating F, Alpine only (46)	11.9 ± 5.1		Ridoux et al. 1981
Sorbitol dehydrogenase	IU/l	Not specified	19.4 ± 3.6	14.0–23.6	Kaneko 1980
	IU/l	4-month-old adult, MC and F, Saanen—feral (5)	37 ± 7.2		Kramer and Carthew 1985
	IU/l	Adult, lactating and nonlactating F, Alpine (105)		2.6–11.6	Garnier et al. 1984

F = female, M = male, MC = castrated male, IU = international units.

alkaline phosphatase (AP) and gamma glutamyl transferase (GGT). Increases in serum AP or GGT are associated with irritation or destruction of biliary epithelium and can occur in obstructive conditions of the biliary system, such as fascioliasis. While serum elevations of GGT are essentially liver-specific, AP occurs in other tissues, especially bone, and serum concentrations may be elevated in young, growing animals because of normal osteoblastic activity or secondary to pathologic conditions of bone unrelated to biliary disease, as discussed in Chapter 4. Thus, serum GGT is the preferred test for assessment of biliary integrity in goats. While the goat kidney contains high levels of GGT, the enzyme is passed in the urine in association with renal damage and does not enter the blood.

Total bilirubin concentration in the serum of normal goats is generally reported to be in the range of 0.0 to 0.1 mg/dl (Kaneko 1980). Higher bilirubin concentrations in the range of 0.2 to 0.8, however, have been reported in normal pygmy goats, with values varying with both age and sex (Castro et al. 1977). As in cattle and sheep, circulating bilirubin levels increase only modestly in the face of severe, generalized hepatic disease (Sen et al. 1976). The most dramatic increases in serum or plasma bilirubin in the goat are due to hemolytic crises rather than liver dysfunction (Wasfi and Adam 1976).

Serum bile acids can be a useful indicator of liver dysfunction and may be a more reliable indicator of liver disease than either circulating bilirubin levels or transaminase activities (Kaneko 1980). Because the liver is responsible for the uptake, conjugation, and secretion of bile acids, there is a decreased secretion of bile acids into bile with liver dysfunction and an associated increase in blood concentrations. However, to date there has been little reported use of bile acids for diagnostic purposes in goats. Serum bile acid concentrations have been reported for normal goats before, during, and after fasting, with no fasting effect on serum bile acid concentrations noted (Rudolph et al. 2000).

Serum cholesterol levels have been used as an indicator of liver dysfunction in various species, but there are few reports in goats on variation of serum cholesterol levels in disease. Serum cholesterol levels in goats have been reported in relation to various physiological and nutritional states including pregnancy, lactation, fasting, and diet, but the results of similar studies are sometimes contradictory, so it appears that more assessment is needed before serum cholesterol levels will be a useful diagnostic tool in goat medicine.

Liver Function Tests

Galactose elimination, a liver function test used in humans, is not appropriate in goats due to a high percentage of galactose loss in the urine (Treacher 1972). Sulfobromophthalein (Bromsulphalein, BSP) clearance is used to evaluate liver function in ruminants and other species. A delay in the clearance of this dye from the blood by the liver suggests functional impairment or decreased flow of bile. Focal liver diseases, such as abscesses, do not interfere with BSP clearance. Prolongation of clearance time in the goat is most often seen with generalized hepatic lipidosis (fatty liver) secondary to pregnancy toxemia, with chronic, toxic hepatitis, or with biliary obstruction. The T1/2 for BSP clearance in normal goats was reported as 2.13 ± 0.19 minutes (Sen et al. 1976). It increased to 4.04 ± 0.24 minutes subsequent to a single dose of carbon tetrachloride, to 16.5 minutes after repeated doses of carbon tetrachloride, and to more than 34 minutes after bile duct ligation.

In another study, Lal et al. (1991) used percent retention of BSP rather than BSP clearance to assess liver function. Normal goats had a mean % retention time of 4.2 ± 0.34 at ten minutes after intravenous injection of BSP dye at a dose of 5 mg/kg bw. Twelve hours after the induction of ruminal acidosis by feeding of wheat, % retention of BSP in those goats increased to 15 ± 1.08.

Other Laboratory Tests

The liver is the primary site of albumin production, and hepatic insufficiency leads to hypoalbuminemia. Normal serum albumin levels in the goat are reported in the range of 2.7 to 3.9 g/dl (Kaneko 1980). Hepatic dysfunction can also cause hypoglycemia. Normal blood glucose levels in the goat are reported in the range of 50 to 75 mg/dl (Kaneko 1980). When goats are in negative energy balance, such as occurs in pregnancy toxemia or lactational ketosis, the liver produces increased ketone bodies that are detectable in serum, milk, or urine. Blood ammonia levels may be elevated in goats with generalized liver disease, particularly when neurologic signs are present, but it is not a consistently reported finding. In a case of hepatic encephalopathy associated with paratuberculosis in a goat, blood ammonia concentration was reported at 230 µmol/l compared to a value of 27 µmol/l in a healthy control goat (Rubin et al. 1999), while in a case of hepatoencephalopathy associated with portocaval shunt in a goat, plasma ammonia concentration reached 599 µg/dl (352 µmol/l) with a normal reference value range given as 25.5 to 109 µg/dl (15 to 64 µmol/l) (Humann-Ziehank et al. 2001).

Beyond the identification of ketone bodies in urine, interpretation of urinalysis in goats for diagnosing liver disease has received little attention. Normal goat urine does not contain bilirubin, so presumably, evidence of conjugated bilirubin in the urine may indicate obstructive liver disease or severe hemolytic disease. The absence of urobilinogen would suggest complete biliary obstruction, while increases in urobilinogen could represent active hepatocellular disease.

Diagnostic Procedures

Biopsy

Liver biopsy can be an aid in the diagnosis of suspected hepatic disease, particularly in cases of chronic liver disease when clinical findings suggest hepatic involvement but clinical chemistry results are equivocal. A prolonged BSP clearance time may also be justification for liver biopsy to determine the basis of impaired function. In focal hepatic disease, the liver biopsy may be misleading because a circumscribed lesion may be missed altogether.

Access to the liver for obtaining a biopsy sample is limited in the goat, and when possible, ultrasound needle guidance is desirable. Unguided liver biopsies should be performed cautiously, using a transthoracic approach. Tranquilization of excitable individuals may be helpful. With the animal standing, the preferred site for introduction of the biopsy instrument is the right ninth intercostal space (Fetcher 1983). Entry should be dorsal to a line drawn from the point of the elbow to the craniodorsal angle of the paralumbar fossa. Entering at the eighth intercostal space can cause a puncture of the caudal lung lobe, while use of the tenth space may put the biopsy instrument behind the caudal edge of the liver. The correct site should be surgically prepared and a local anesthetic applied. The biopsy instrument must traverse the caudal thorax and penetrate the diaphragm before entering the liver. The instrument should be directed anteriorly after passing through the intercostal muscle to avoid puncture of the gallbladder, especially if the animal has been anorexic and the gallbladder is distended. It should not be necessary to introduce the biopsy instrument to a depth more than 3 to 4 cm because the transthoracic space in this area is less than 2 cm and the liver thickness is approximately 4 to 5 cm.

Ultrasound

Ultrasonography can be helpful in identifying uncommon mass lesions in the liver such as abscesses, hydatid cysts, and rarely neoplasms. It has also been reported to be useful in the diagnosis of fatty liver in goats, with affected livers showing multiple hyperechoic foci of fatty infiltration distributed throughout an isoechoic liver parenchyma (Gonenci et al. 2003). When available, ultrasonography can be particularly helpful in performing accurate liver biopsies.

Cholecystography

Intravenous cholecystography has been performed successfully in goats using 20 ml of intravenous contrast material (biligrafin). In normal goats, the gallbladder can be visualized thirty to sixty minutes after injecting contrast media. It is located between the caudal border of the eighth rib and the cranial border of the twelfth rib, 6 to 8 cm below the vertebral column. In goats with liver disease, visualization may be delayed and the position of the gallbladder may shift subject to hepatomegaly (Singh et al. 1990).

DIAGNOSIS OF HEPATIC DISEASE BY PRESENTING SIGN

Abdominal Pain

Pressure on the liver capsule from parenchymal swelling such as occurs in acute diffuse hepatitis or trauma to the capsule itself can cause liver-associated pain. If severe, the animal may adopt a guarded, tucked-up stance with an arched back and be reluctant to move. This, of course, can also occur as a result of nonhepatic causes of abdominal pain, so pain must be localized to the liver by palpation over the right anterior ventrolateral aspect of the abdomen and the last few ribs. The most commonly reported causes of hepatic pain in goats are the acute forms of liver fluke disease and acute toxic hepatitis.

Anemia

Liver-associated causes of anemia are limited to the parasitic diseases, chronic copper toxicity, and some experimentally induced plant poisonings. In acute liver fluke disease, the cause of anemia is severe hemorrhage into the peritoneal cavity associated with large numbers of larvae penetrating the liver capsule. In chronic fascioliasis, the anemia is caused by mechanical trauma and feeding activity of adult *Fasciola* spp. within the biliary tree resulting in continuous blood loss. Anemia is accompanied by hypoproteinemia in these chronic cases.

Anorexia

Loss of appetite is a consistent finding in diffuse liver disease but is nonspecific.

Ascites and/or Edema

Hypoproteinemia is a common outcome of chronic liver disease and the most common clinical manifestation of liver-related hypoproteinemia is intermandibular edema, often seen in chronic liver fluke disease. However, nonhepatic causes of hypoproteinemia, most notably gastrointestinal helminthiasis, also produce the same sign.

Generalized ascites as a result of caprine liver disease is uncommon. One exception is a disease known as "waterpens" or "water belly" seen in goats and sheep in South Africa grazing the plant *Galenia africana* (kraalbos). At necropsy, there is severe ascites and evidence of liver and cardiac disease. It is unclear if ascites is caused by a primary cardiac or primary hepatic abnormality (van der Lugt et al. 1988). Experimental challenge studies with toxic plant extracts indicate that the hepatic lesions precede the cardiac lesions in the development of the condition (van der Lugt et al. 1992).

In Texas, consumption of the range plant *Sartwellia flaveriae* by Angora goats leads to marked ascites, abdominal distension, and weight loss associated with hepatic cirrhosis (Mathews 1940). Although a rare occurrence, bile duct carcinoma has also been reported as a cause of ascites in a goat in India (Chauhan and Singh 1969).

Bleeding Tendency

Coagulopathies are uncommon in goats and are rarely associated with liver problems. Only three reported instances of prolonged clotting time in goats have been associated with hepatic disease (Bassir and Bababunmi 1972; Saad et al. 1972; Jones and Shah 1982).

Diarrhea and Constipation

Diarrhea can occur in chronic fascioliasis. Diarrhea occurs in hepatotoxic plant poisonings, but concurrent enteritis also may be responsible for the diarrhea. Constipation is characteristic of *Lantana* poisoning in goats and other ruminants.

Alternating diarrhea and constipation have been associated with liver disease in large animals due to decreases in bile salt excretion and reflex intestinal activity associated with liver distension. This pattern is not well documented in goats with hepatitis.

Jaundice

Hyperbilirubinemia caused by obstructive biliary conditions is rare in goats. Jaundice is most likely to result from hemolytic anemia and primarily involves increases in indirect unconjugated bilirubin. Table 7.6 in Chapter 7 lists the hemolytic causes of jaundice. Chronic copper poisoning produces both liver damage and hemolytic anemia with resultant jaundice, but the condition is rare in goats, which are much more tolerant of copper than sheep. The plant *Acanthospermum hispidum*, common in the Sudan, also produces both hepatic necrosis and hemolytic anemia in goats (Ali and Adam 1978).

No cases have been reported of complete, extrahepatic biliary obstruction in goats. Nonhemolytic jaundice may occur in Rift Valley fever and Wesselsbron disease in Africa, and has been reported sporadically in goats in association with other diverse causes including aflatoxicosis (Wanasinghe 1974), suspect halothane toxicity (O'Brien et al. 1986), sawfly larvae poisoning (Thamsborg et al. 1987), hepatic fibrosarcoma (Higgins et al. 1985), and consumption of the plants sacahuiste *(Nolina texana)* in Texas (Mathews 1940a) and signal grass *(Brachiaria decumbens)* in Malaysia and Nigeria (Mazni et al. 1985; Opasina 1985). In general, the occurrence of jaundice in caprine liver disease carries an unfavorable prognosis.

Neurologic Signs

Altered states of mentation and other neurologic signs are often seen in goats with diffuse liver disease and are associated with disruptions in normal liver metabolism. The pathogenesis of this hepatoencephalopathy is not completely understood, but is presumed to be multi-factorial. Prevailing theories include: ammonia acting as a neurotoxin possibly in synergy with other toxins, alteration in monoamine neurotransmitters as a result of altered aromatic amino acid metabolism, imbalances in the amino acid neurotransmitters glutamate and γ-aminobutyric acid, and/or increased cerebral concentrations of an endogenous benzodiazepine-like substance (Maddison 1992). There is general consensus that ammonia plays a key role, especially since therapeutic interventions that decrease blood and CSF ammonia levels usually mitigate the neurologic signs associated with hepatic encephalopathy (Katayama 2004).

Clinical presentations associated with hepatoencephalopathy range from signs of hypoexcitablity including depression, head pressing, generalized weakness, ataxia, and coma, to signs of hyperexcitability such as hyperesthesia, muscle tremors, and convulsions.

While all the causes of diffuse liver disease in goats have the potential to produce neurologic signs, the most common causes are pregnancy toxemia and toxic hepatitis. The known causes of toxic hepatitis in goats are discussed later in this chapter.

Nonhepatic causes of neurologic signs are numerous in goats and must be differentiated from hepatoencephalopathy. Primary neurologic diseases are discussed in Chapter 5.

Photodermatitis

Hepatic or secondary photosensitization occurs in goats. Signs of photosensitization are varied and include uneasiness and pruritus with much scratching and rubbing activity, severe dermatitis with erythema, extensive subcutaneous edema, and eventual ulceration and sloughing of skin. Ophthalmia with excessive lacrimation, photophobia, and corneal cloudiness may also occur. The dermatitis and edema are particularly evident on the head and ears. In some outbreaks, jaundice is seen in conjunction with signs of photodermatitis. Secondary blindness, pyoderma, loss of body condition, and occasional deaths are possible sequelae. Light-colored animals are more severely affected.

Photosensitization associated with hepatotoxicity has been reported in goats consuming a variety of plants around the world, including sacahuiste weed *(Nolina texana)* (Mathews 1940a), green oats *(Avena sativa)* and wheat (Schmidt 1931), lechuguilla *(Agave lecheguilla)* (Mathews 1937), and kleingrass *(Panicum coloratum)* (Bailey 1986) in the United States; signal grass *(Brachiaria decumbens)* in Malaysia and Nigeria (Mazni et al. 1985; Opasina 1985); caltrop *(Tribulus terrestris)* in South Africa (Kellerman et al. 1980); and caltrop, boobiala tree *(Myoporum tetrandrum)*, and Ellangowan poison bush *(M. deserti)* in Australia (Allen et al. 1978; Glastonbury and Boal 1985; Jacob and Peet 1987). Additional details are given in the discussion of toxic hepatitis at the end of this chapter. Primary, nonhepatic photodermatitis also occurs in goats and must be differentiated from the hepatic form. It is discussed in Chapter 2.

Weight Loss

Chronic liver fluke disease is important in the differential diagnosis for wasting in goats. Weight loss may be the only sign associated with liver abscesses. It is one of many signs associated with a wide range of hepatotoxic plants that cause prolonged hepatic insufficiency.

Yawning

Occasional yawning in goats is normal. Repeated yawning may suggest liver disease in goats as in other species, although the causal relationship is not clear.

Goats with pregnancy toxemia or other causes of hepatic lipidosis are most likely to exhibit repeated yawning.

SPECIFIC DISEASES OF THE LIVER

VIRAL DISEASES

Rift Valley Fever

This arthropod-borne virus disease of ruminants, camels, and humans is thus far limited to Africa and the Arabian peninsula. The disease is characterized by acute, severe hepatic necrosis with abortion in pregnant dams and high mortality in neonatal animals. Goats are generally considered to be less susceptible than cattle or sheep, but there is a high variability between breeds.

Etiology

The causative agent is an enveloped, single-stranded RNA phlebovirus in the *Bunyaviridae* family. The virus is very stable near neutral pH in blood or serum and also in aerosol. It is killed by 2% sodium orthophenylphenate and 4% sodium carbonate disinfectants. There is only a single serotype of the infective agent, though differences in pathogenicity have been noted between isolates (Swanepoel et al. 1986). Phylogenetic analysis of the virus indicates two distinct lineages for the RVF virus—one Egyptian and the other sub-Saharan (Sall et al. 1997). However, there are two distinct groupings within the sub-Saharan viruses, one West African and the other central and southern African, now including the viruses from the Arabian peninsula.

Epidemiology

Rift Valley fever (RVF) was first identified in Kenya's Rift Valley in 1930, although there are earlier descriptions of what could well have been RVF. The disease was historically limited to East and Central sub-Saharan Africa and was first recognized in southern Africa in the 1950s. However, later outbreaks in Egypt, Senegal, and Mauritania indicated its potential for further spread (Ksiazek et al. 1989; Lancelot et al. 1989). It is now known to occur throughout Africa, including the island of Madagascar. In 2000, the disease was confirmed for the first time outside of Africa, on the Arabian peninsula in Yemen and Saudi Arabia, and it affected large numbers of livestock and humans, with more than 120 human deaths (Al-Afaleq et al. 2003; Anyamba et al. 2006).

The RVF virus is transmitted to susceptible hosts during feeding by infected mosquitoes in the genera *Aedes, Culex, Mansonia, Eretmapodites, Coquillettidia,* and *Anopheles,* and possibly by other insects. The *Aedes* mosquitoes are capable of transovarial transmission of the virus, and their eggs can survive desiccation well, thus sustaining infection even for decades. Viremic ruminants and humans can also contribute to the spread and amplification of infection. Direct transmission from infected animals to people can occur by aerosols of blood at the time of slaughter as well as by ingestion of blood and milk.

Epizootics often follow periods of heavy rainfall; the rain facilitates the hatching of previously laid, dormant, infected mosquito eggs resulting in sudden increases in infected *Aedes* mosquito populations. These initiate infection which is then amplified markedly by *Culex* and other species of mosquitoes whose population increases lag somewhat behind those of the *Aedes* mosquitoes.

Two additional factors that contribute to epizootics are heavy winds that blow infected insects into previously uninfected areas and transport of infected livestock into such areas. Places with extensive irrigation networks or standing water, warm climate, suitable arthropod populations, and susceptible ruminant and human populations are most prone to epizootic occurrences (Wittmann 1989). An RVF epizootic which affected the contiguous areas of the Northeastern province of Kenya, the south of Somalia, and southern Ethiopia in 1997–1998 is estimated to have affected more than a half million small ruminants and sickened 89,000 people, leading to possibly 450 human deaths in Kenya alone. A similar, severe RVF outbreak occurred in Kenya and Tanzania in late 2006 through early 2007 and spread later in the year into Sudan.

It is now well documented that RVF epizootics in the Horn of Africa are associated with the El Nino-Southern Oscillation (ENSO) phenomenon. These warm ENSO events are known to increase precipitation in portions of East Africa. Retrospective studies on data from 1950 through 1998 demonstrated that an analytical model which included measurements of southern oscillation indices, equatorial sea surface temperatures in the Pacific and Indian Oceans, and satellite derived vegetation indices in East Africa would have accurately predicted 100% of the RVF epizootics that occurred during that forty-eight-year period (Linthicum et al. 1999). Such predictive epidemiological tools can be extremely useful for instituting timely and effective disease control programs.

Pathogenesis

After infection, there is a viremia with fever and leukopenia. Despite the destruction of liver cells by rapidly multiplying virus, localization of virus in tissues does not occur to any great extent, and blood always contains the highest levels of virus. A carrier state does not develop in ruminants. Lesions are limited to the liver and are characterized by focal hepatic necrosis. Experimental infections in goats have been described (Easterday et al. 1962).

Clinical Findings

The incubation period is as short as twelve hours in kids and as long as forty-eight hours in adult goats. Adult animals are always less severely affected than young stock. In epizootics involving goats, the predominant effects are abortion in pregnant does and death in kids younger than one week of age. Many infections in non-gravid individuals are subclinical.

While peracute death with no prodromal signs is most likely in neonatal kids, some young kids may show fever up to 108.0°F (42.2°C), accompanied by listlessness and inappetence. Death may occur within the next several days.

The acute form of the disease is more likely in older kids and some adults, though it is seen less frequently than in sheep. In addition to fever and depression, variable signs may include icterus, vomiting, hemorrhagic diarrhea, unsteady gait, catarrhal stomatitis, and skin necrosis on the udder or scrotum, with death in one to four days.

Except for abortion in pregnant does, most affected adult goats are likely to show only subacute disease, with fever in the range of 104°F to 106.2°F (40°C to 41.2°C), dullness, and inappetence for one to three days. Mortality rates are low in adult goats. Breeds of imported goats are more likely to show overt signs of disease than indigenous breeds.

Clinical Pathology and Necropsy

Leukopenia is common in the early stages of disease. Virus isolation in cell culture is possible from blood of live, febrile goats; or liver, spleen, and brain of fatal cases; and organs of aborted fetuses. When immediate submission to the laboratory is not possible, samples should be frozen at –94°F (–70°C). Alternatively, immunofluorescence can be used to identify RVF virus antigen on impression smears of liver, spleen, and brain. Other techniques available for detection of viral antigen include agar gel immunodiffusion (AGID), complement fixation, and reverse transcriptase polymerase chain reaction (RT-PCR)(OIE 2004).

After outbreaks, seroconversion can be documented using indirect enzyme-linked immunoabsorbent assay or other serologic methods in serum samples taken three weeks apart. An IgM capture ELISA can diagnose RVF on a single blood sample taken early in infection. Other tests that can be used to assess seroconversion in paired samples are virus neutralization, hemagglutination inhibition, and complement fixation (OIE 2004).

At necropsy, the liver may be friable and appear moderately enlarged, soft, and pale with focal areas of subcapsular hemorrhage. On cut section, 1 to 2 mm gray-yellow necrotic foci are distributed throughout the parenchyma. Other possible findings include visceral and serosal hemorrhage, icterus, hemorrhagic gastritis, and enteritis. Similar lesions may be seen in aborted fetuses.

Histologically, the liver lesion is one of focal centrilobular or midzonal necrosis of small groups of hepatocytes. As lesions progress, they may become confluent and involve a large portion of the lobule. Eosinophilic, intranuclear inclusion bodies surrounded by marginated chromatin are common in degenerating hepatocytes in advanced lesions.

Diagnosis

Definitive diagnosis is by virus isolation or the demonstration of virus genome and by confirmation of seroconversion in affected goats. In those parts of Africa where both diseases occur, RVF must be differentiated from Wesselsbron disease, a liver disease that is also described in this chapter. In sheep, bluetongue is considered in the differential diagnosis but bluetongue is almost always asymptomatic in indigenous goats. When people handling livestock complain of influenza-like illness during epizootics of animal disease, the diagnoses of Rift Valley fever or Wesselsbron disease should be pursued vigorously.

Treatment

The antiviral drug ribivarin is the drug of choice for bunyavirus infections in humans, but no recommendations for use in animals are made. The intravenous or intraperitoneal administration of 10 to 30 ml of serum from convalescent sheep to one- to three-day-old lambs reduced mortality, even when lambs were already showing signs of illness (Bennett et al. 1965).

Control

In endemic areas, an attenuated live vaccine, prepared from the mouse-brain-adapted Smithburn strain, is available. The vaccine is recommended for use in cattle, sheep, and goats, but should not be used in pregnant animals, because viremia, abortion, fetal death, and fetal anomalies occur, especially in sheep. Immunity lasts at least two years and is generally considered to be lifelong.

Vaccination should not be undertaken during an epizootic of RVF. If deemed necessary, then needles must be used on a single animal only, and then replaced, because needle passage of the disease during periods of active transmission is quite likely and can further spread the disease and extend the duration of the outbreak.

Formalin-inactivated vaccines are available for use in nonendemic areas but they are less effective, especially in cattle. Work is ongoing in the development of newer live vaccines with less objectionable side effects.

Mosquito control is problematic but there are some indications that insecticidal fogging and the use of *Bacillus thuringensis* might have potential for control in the face of an epidemic. Movement of animals out of known mosquito breeding areas after heavy rainfall, for example into cooler highland areas, might reduce the incidence of disease. During epizootic outbreaks, movement of nonvaccinated animals should be restricted.

In recent years, the use of historic and real-time climate data and vegetation indices obtained by satellite imaging have allowed for the reliable prediction of RVF epizootics two to five months in advance of the first clinical cases (Linthicum et al. 1999; Anyamba et al. 2002). In 2006, the Food and Agriculture Organization of the United Nations (FAO), through its Emergency Prevention System (EMPRES), was able to accurately predict the RVF epidemic in Kenya and Tanzania about two months before it occurred (FAO 2006). It has now been demonstrated during the 2006–2007 Kenyan epidemic that participatory disease surveillance techniques are capable of providing strong support to systems based on satellite imaging for predicting the emergence of epidemic RVF in Kenya (Jost 2007). These are very useful tools for allowing the implementation of disease response plans, including vaccination, before the onset of disease.

Most human cases can be related to direct contact with blood or tissues of infected animals, or inhalation of aerosols associated with such tissues. While the disease in humans is usually inapparent or produces transient flu-like symptoms, in a subset of patients, the disease can be fatal following signs of hemorrhage, encephalitis, and/or severe hepatic disease. Retinal damage and visual impairment is a common sequel to acute human infection. Veterinarians should take suitable precautions against infection when performing examinations or necropsies and advise against slaughter and consumption of meat from suspected cases (Davies 2006). Consumption of raw milk in areas undergoing an active outbreak is unwise. Vaccination with a killed vaccine should also be considered by people such as veterinarians and laboratory workers with a high risk of exposure.

Wesselsbron Disease

This mosquito-borne virus disease of domestic livestock is enzootic in south, central, and west Africa. Largely asymptomatic in adults, it primarily causes abortion and neonatal mortality. It is important in the differential diagnosis of Rift Valley fever. It occasionally infects humans.

Etiology and Epidemiology

The causative agent is an enveloped, single-stranded RNA, group B flavivirus in the *Togaviridae* family. The disease was first identified in the Wesselsbron district of the Orange Free State in South Africa in 1955. *Aedes caballus* and *A. circumluteolus* mosquitoes are the primary disease transmitters, but contact and aerosol transmission have also been reported (Barnard 1986).

Cattle, sheep, and goats are principally affected, but the mammalian host range is wide and includes humans. There is serological evidence of infection throughout southern, central, and western Africa but disease incidence is low. Epizootic outbreaks occur in South Africa in association with heavy rainfall, which favor increased vector mosquito activity. Cattle may be a natural reservoir of the disease. The virus is isolated from some wild rodents and birds, including ostriches, but their role as reservoirs is debatable.

Pathogenesis

Infection is followed after a short incubation period by viremia with fever. The virus shows a predilection for the liver, and even when clinical disease is not observed, focal necrosis of the liver occurs, as demonstrated in experimental infection of adult goats (Coetzer and Theodoridis 1982). Kids are more severely affected than adults (Theodoridis and Coetzer 1980). Increased levels of antibody are detectable within three weeks of infection.

Clinical Findings

In epizootics of Wesselsbron disease, clinical signs in adults are usually limited to abortion in pregnant does and ewes, with nonpregnant females and males showing no clinical effects. Kids and lambs, especially if less than four weeks of age, can die suddenly or soon after showing some weakness, loss of appetite, increased respiratory rate, icterus, and fever up to 105.8°F (41°C). Lamb mortality as high as 30% has been documented.

Clinical Pathology and Necropsy.

When laboratory support is available, intracerebral inoculation of infant mice with liver or brain of affected kids and subsequent identification of the virus by serum neutralization should be attempted. Alternately, immunohistochemical staining of formalin-fixed liver specimens using polyclonal antibody against Wesselsbron virus also has been reported in diagnosis of field cases and experimental infections (van der Lugt et al. 1995). In lieu of virus or antigen identification, seroconversion can be documented using the hemagglutination inhibition (HI) assay in acute and convalescent serum samples taken three weeks apart. An antibody detection ELISA has also been developed. It is reported to be more sensitive than hemagglutination inhibition and less cross reactive to other flaviviruses (Williams et al. 1997), but to date, the HI test is still routinely used.

At necropsy, the liver may be slightly swollen and yellow to orange brown in color. In some animals, slight hydropericardium and ascites, lymphadenopathy, splenomegaly, serosal hemorrhage, and jaundice may be seen. Histologically, the liver lesions are characterized by small, focal areas of necrosis and a pronounced, nodular Kupffer cell reaction (Coetzer and Theodoridis 1982). Eosinophilic intranuclear inclusions are sometimes seen. Lymphoid tissues may show pyknotic lymphocytes and lymphoid hyperplasia. Neutrophilic infiltration of the red pulp of the spleen may occur. Myocardial necrosis has been noted in some goats.

Diagnosis

Wesselsbron disease and Rift Valley fever present a similar clinical picture in goats. It is important to make a specific etiologic diagnosis because the zoonotic implications of Rift Valley fever are much more profound. Virus isolation is the ideal method. Intraperitoneal inoculation of suckling or weaned mice or hamsters leads to death of the lab animals in three to four days when RVF virus is present in the inoculum, but not in the case of Wesselsbron disease virus. Serology and histopathology can also be helpful in differentiating the two diseases.

Treatment and Control

There is no treatment for this virus disease. An attenuated live virus vaccine produced in South Africa is in use in enzootic areas. Pregnant animals and those younger than six months of age should not be vaccinated because the vaccine itself can cause abortion or illness in young stock. It is recommended that flocks be vaccinated in the spring three to six weeks before mating because disease usually occurs in late summer and autumn. Vaccine should not be used in the face of an outbreak. Immunity, which develops three weeks after vaccination, is considered to be lifelong. Removing animals to high ground after heavy rains in anticipation of increased mosquito activity in low, wet areas may reduce the risk of disease.

BACTERIAL DISEASES

Bacteria are an uncommon cause of clinical liver disease in goats. Infectious necrotic hepatitis, or black disease caused by *Clostridium novyi*, is uncommon in goats as compared to sheep. The disease is discussed later in the chapter in the section on fascioliasis, which predisposes to its occurrence. In this section, liver abscesses, which tend to be subclinical but can cause economic wastage due to liver condemnations, are discussed.

Liver Abscesses

The syndrome of liver abscesses secondary to rumenitis that is well documented in feedlot cattle on high energy rations has not been reported in goats thus far, even though there is increased interest in raising goats for meat under intensive or semi-intensive conditions. Sporadic cases of subclinical liver abscesses, however, do occur in goats and cause economic loss through liver condemnation at slaughter.

Etiology

A variety of organisms have been reported from caprine liver abscesses. *Corynebacterium pseudotuberculosis* is most common. *Arcanobacterium pyogenes* and *Escherichia coli* are also common. Other sporadic isolates include *Proteus* spp., *Mannheimia haemolytica, Staphylococcus epidermidis, S. aureus, Rhodococcus equi, Erysipelothrix rhusiopathiae,* and the yeast *Candida krusei* (Whitford and Jones 1974; Eamens et al. 1988; Panebianco and Santagada 1989; Santa Rosa et al. 1989). The common isolate from bovine liver abscesses, *Fusobacterium necrophorum,* is not reported from the goat.

Epidemiology and Pathogenesis

No particular management, feed, or breed factors have been identified in the development of caprine liver abscesses. Reports of caprine liver abscess have come from Brazil (Santa Rosa et al. 1989), Botswana (Diteko et al. 1988), and Australia (Carrigan et al. 1988). In the Brazilian study, 2.5% of a necropsy study population showed liver abscesses. A greater proportion of adult goats was affected than young. Concurrent disease problems were always found, including caseous lymphadenitis, bronchopneumonia, rumen abscesses, peritonitis, and omphalophlebitis, among others. The association with concurrent infections suggests that liver abscesses probably occur from lymphatic or hematogenous spread from other loci of infection, but spread by parasite migrations through the liver is another possible cause.

Das and Misra (1992) induced ruminal acidosis in goats by feeding high levels of rice and demonstrated that serum concentrations of the liver enzymes AST, ALT, and GDH increased twenty-four hours following induction of rumen acidosis. They concluded that as in other species, ruminal acidosis can disrupt ruminal epithelial integrity and lead to entry of bacteria and fungi into the portal circulation, predisposing to the development of liver abscesses. This suggests that efforts to feed concentrates to meat goats under intensive conditions could lead to increased occurrence of liver abscesses.

Clinical Findings

There is one case reported from Trinidad in which an approximately two-year-old Anglo Nubian doe with chronic weight loss was found to have a liver abscess caused by *Rhodococcus equi* as the principal necropsy finding (Ojo et al. 1993). In all other reports

Table 11.2. Helminth parasites of the liver, pancreas, and related blood vessels.*

Scientific name	*Common names*	*Location in goat*	*Geographic distribution*	*Clinical effects*
Fasciola hepatica	Common liver fluke	Liver parenchyma, bile ducts	Worldwide	Acute death; marked anemia, edema, emaciation
Fasciola gigantica	Giant liver fluke	Liver parenchyma bile ducts	Africa, Asia	Acute death; marked anemia, edema, emaciation
Fascioloides magna	Giant liver fluke; large American liver fluke	Liver parenchyma	North America	Acute death
Dicrocoelium dendriticum	Lesser liver fluke; lancet fluke	Bile ducts	Europe, Asia, North America	Marked anemia, edema, emaciation
Eurytrema pancreaticum	Pancreatic fluke	Pancreatic ducts, bile ducts, duodenum	Eastern Asia, Brazil	Ill thrift
Stilesia hepatica	Liver tapeworm	Biliary ducts	Africa	Nonpathogenic; liver condemnation
Thysanosoma actinoides	Fringed tapeworm	Bile ducts, also small intestine	Western United States, South America	Nonpathogenic; liver condemnation

*For schistosomes of the liver and related vessels see Chapter 8, Table 8.3.

to date, liver abscess in goats is either a subclinical finding or only one of several disease findings that could account for weight loss.

Clinical Pathology and Necropsy

Though not specifically reported in goats, elevation of liver-specific enzyme concentrations in the serum resulting from destruction of hepatocytes by expanding abscesses might occur. Abscesses may be detectable by ultrasonographic study of the liver but would need to be differentiated from metacestode cysts. At necropsy, abscesses may be single or multiple, measure up to 5 cm in diameter, and contain purulent or caseous material.

Treatment and Control

There are no specific treatment or control recommendations. Appropriate therapy of concurrent disease problems may lead to some improvement in affected individuals. Efforts to control caseous lymphadenitis and omphalophlebitis in goats may be instrumental in reducing the frequency of liver abscesses. If concentrates are fed to meat goats, they should be introduced gradually into the forage-based diet and not provided in excessive amounts. The inclusion of antacids or buffers such as sodium bicarbonate in the ration is also indicated to reduce the risk of ruminal acidosis which could lead to liver abscesses.

PARASITIC DISEASES

In addition to the parasitic diseases of the liver discussed below, the liver may be the site of various *Schistosoma* spp. infections which can produce disease as discussed in Chapter 8. (See Table 8.3.) A summary of parasites affecting the liver, pancreas, and related blood vessels of goats is given in Table 11.2.

Stilesia and *Thysanosoma* Tapeworm Infections

The goat is a definitive host for the tapeworm, *Stilesia hepatica*, which occurs extensively throughout Africa and Asia. The adult tapeworm may be found in the bile duct in large numbers. Adult *Stilesia hepatica* measure 20 to 50 cm long and 3 mm wide. The life cycle probably involves oribatid mites as an intermediate host. Eggs are passed in the feces of the goat.

This tapeworm is considered nonpathogenic in the living animal. However, large numbers of adult tapeworms may induce sufficient bile duct thickening that affected livers are condemned during meat inspection. In one study in Zimbabwe, 18.75% of communal goats had their livers condemned at slaughter and 72.9% of these condemnations were due to *Stilesia hepatica* (Chambers 1990). Praziquantel orally at 15 mg/kg is effective in eliminating *S. hepatica* in sheep but there are no reports on its use in goats for *Stilesia* infections.

The goat is infrequently infected with *Thysanosoma actinoides*, the fringed tapeworm of North and South America that is commonly found in the bile ducts, pancreatic ducts, and small intestine of sheep, cattle, and deer. Clinical disease in goats caused by this tapeworm infection is poorly documented.

Echinococcosis or Hydatid Disease

Clinical hydatid disease is uncommon in goats, but hydatid cysts in liver and other tissues at slaughter are widespread and cause condemnations and economic loss.

The adult tapeworm, *Echinococcus granulosus*, is found in the intestine of carnivores, particularly dogs. Eggs are passed in the feces and are ingested by goats, other ungulates, or humans. In these intermediate hosts, the ingested eggs release oncospheres that enter intestinal venules or lacteals and migrate via the circulation to liver or lung. The metacestode stage, known as the hydatid cyst, develops in these organs over a period of several months. Brood capsules containing protoscolices develop within some cysts. Occasionally cysts rupture and the released protoscolices produce additional daughter cysts within the intermediate host. When dogs eat viscera containing protoscolices, these evaginate and mature to adults in the intestine in about seven weeks, completing the life cycle.

Echinococcus granulosus occurs essentially worldwide. However, there are noted areas of so-called hyperendemicity where the disease occurs frequently and represents a public health concern. These areas include much of northern and eastern Africa, the Mediterranean region, Eastern Europe, Central Asia, parts of China, and the cone of South America (Lightowlers 2002). The disease also occurs in eastern Australia and the western United States, where sheep are common. Infections are likely to occur in those places where ruminant livestock and domestic and wild canids commingle.

Newer studies of genome patterns indicate that there are numerous distinct strains of *E. granulosis*. The so-called sheep strain (G1) and the so-called camel strain (G6) affect goats (Schantz 2006). The prevalence of disease is increased when carnivore populations are high and no efforts are made to segregate domestic and wild carnivores from livestock or their grazing areas. The feeding of ruminant offal to dogs also enhances completion of the life cycle. Increases in prevalence of hydatid disease in livestock occur after rainy periods, presumably because the rain widely disseminates eggs in feces on grazing land or in water supplies.

Prevalence data of hydatid disease in goats is available from abattoir and post mortem surveys around the world. The prevalence range in endemic regions is 0.26% to 6.5% (Pandey 1971; Rahman et al. 1975; Naus 1982; Al-Yaman et al. 1985; Lorenzini and Ruggieri 1987). Hydatid cysts are most common in the liver, lung, and spleen, but may be found in other organs at slaughter or necropsy. In some places, lung cysts are more common than liver cysts in goats. More information on hydatid cysts in goat lung is given in Chapter 9.

Hydatid cysts may average 5 to 10 cm in diameter and contain a yellowish, serum-like fluid and may have a granular inner wall containing multiple brood capsules. Hydatid "sand," which is an accumulation of detached brood capsules, may be seen in the cyst fluid. Hydatid cysts should be differentiated from *Cysticercus tenuicollis* cysts as discussed below. Cysts containing nymphs of the canid nasal parasite, *Linguatula serrata*, also have been found in the liver, lungs, and mesenteric lymph nodes of goats in Bangladesh (Rahman et al. 1980).

In the last twenty years ELISA and immunoblot assays have been developed to diagnose Echinococcosis in livestock, but due to a high number of false-negative and false-positive results, these assays remain unsuitable for surveillance of echinococcal infections (Moro and Schantz 2006). Various imaging techniques can be used to identify hydatid cysts, including ultrasound, computed tomography (CT), and magnetic resonance imaging (MRI).

There is no practical or economical treatment for hydatid cysts in ruminants. Control efforts involve disruption of the carnivore/ruminant life cycle. The principal efforts should be directed at eliminating the feeding of livestock offal to dogs, encouraging burial of livestock carcasses or viscera, and using routine anthelmintic therapy in dogs to reduce adult tapeworm populations. There has been notable progress in the development of effective vaccines for controlling hydatid cysts. Though not yet commercially available, a recombinant DNA vaccine based on the oncospheric protein EG95 has been shown to be effective in protecting cattle, sheep, and goats against hydatid disease with immunity lasting for at least one year (Dalton and Mulcahy 2001; Lightowlers 2002).

Echinococcosis is a serious zoonotic disease. Humans are infected by ingestion of tapeworm eggs shed by canids. International efforts to reduce hydatidosis, especially with regard to its zoonotic potential, have been reviewed (Moro and Schantz 2006).

Cysticercosis

Etiology

Adult *Taenia hydatigena* tapeworms are found in the intestine of dogs, coyotes, wolves, and other carnivores. The eggs are passed in the feces and ingested by goats, sheep, and other domestic and wild ruminants. Eggs hatch in the small intestine of the intermediate hosts and enter the blood. Upon reaching the liver, the embryos leave the portal vasculature and migrate through the hepatic parenchyma to the peritoneal cavity, causing distinct hemorrhagic tracts in the liver. The metacestode, which is the developmental phase

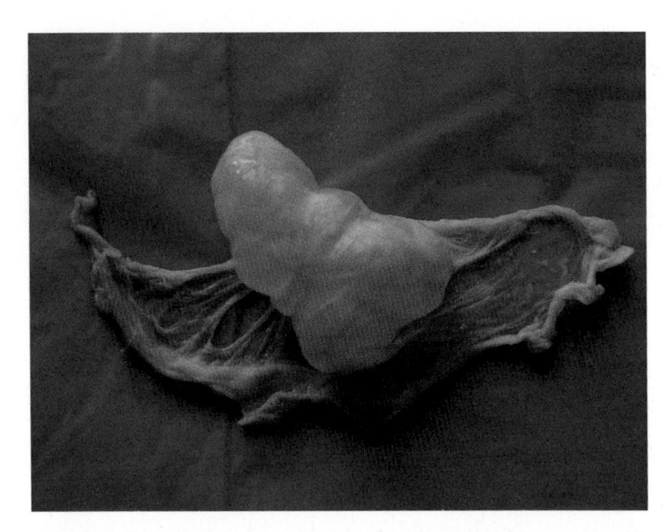

Figure 11.2. Cysticercus metacestode (*Cysticercus tenuicollis*) of the canid tapeworm, *Taenia hydatigena*, attached to the mesentery of a goat. (Courtesy of Dr. Jaroslaw Kaba, Faculty of Veterinary Medicine, Warsaw University of Life Sciences, Warsaw, Poland.)

that occurs in ruminants, is a bladderworm called *Cysticercus tenuicollis*. It matures over a period of five to eight weeks, and is found attached to the mesentery, omentum, and serosal surface of abdominal organs (Figure 11.2). Occasionally, migration out of the liver is not achieved and the cysticercus is found in the liver itself. Aberrant migrations sometimes occur with cysticercus found in the lungs or other organs.

Epidemiology

Factors that promote the infection of goats with *Cysticercus tenuicollis* from contact with canids are similar to those described above for echinoccocosis. Cysticercosis occurs worldwide. Reported prevalence in slaughtered goats around the world ranges from 0.2% in Australia to 23.3% in Nigeria (Rahman et al. 1975; McKenzie et al. 1979; Akinboade and Ajiboye 1983; Sanyal and Sinha 1983).

Pathogenesis

The migration of embryos of *T. hydatigena* in the liver produces parenchymal damage and the creation of blood-filled tracts. When many embryos are migrating, acute, fatal hepatic insufficiency may occur in goats (Everett and de Gruchy 1982). Less severe migrations of embryos may still lead to liver condemnations in otherwise healthy animals, as the blood-filled tracts become fibrotic over time. Occasionally, peritonitis is associated with migration out of the liver and into the peritoneal cavity. The mature cysts in the mesentery, omentum, or liver usually do not produce any clinical disease.

Clinical Findings

Acute cysticercosis may produce signs of depression, weakness, anorexia, and possibly collapse and death caused by hepatic insufficiency. Signs consistent with pneumonia, peritonitis, and/or anemia can occur as a result of aberrant migration in the lungs and abdominal viscera with resulting hemorrhage. Fever may be recorded if peritonitis occurs. Signs usually occur between seven and twenty days after exposure (Pathak and Guar 1981). Chronic cysticercosis is usually asymptomatic.

Clinical Pathology and Necropsy

Experimentally, goats infected with eggs of *T. hydatigena* showed marked elevations of ornithine carbamyltransferase (OCT) and AST ten days after infection, but this is not specific for cysticercosis (Pathak and Gaur 1981a). Indirect hemagglutination and complement absorption tests have been used in the diagnosis of caprine cysticercosis (Varma et al. 1973, 1974). Radiography or ultrasonography can be useful in identifying hepatic or peritoneal cysts. In human medicine, CT and MRI are also used to identify cysts, and these techniques could be applicable to veterinary medicine as well.

At necropsy, *C. tenuicollis* cysts may be present in the liver, but are common in the mesentery, omentum, and serosal surface of peritoneal viscera. Increased volumes of serofibrinous fluid may be present in the peritoneal cavity. Mature cysticerci have a smooth inner surface and contain only a single invaginated scolex, in contrast to hydatid cysts.

Acute cysticercosis is recognized by the presence of tubular, red, blood-filled tracts 2 to 4 mm in diameter in the liver, as shown in Figure 11.3. More chronic lesions may appear white as leukocytes fill the tracts and fibrosis occurs.

Treatment

Praziquantel, at a single, oral dose of 60 mg/kg, was reported as 93% to 100% effective in removing *C. tenuicollis* from sheep and goats in China (Li and Li 1986).

Control

Control measures involve disruption of the carnivore/ruminant life cycle as described above for echinococcosis. As with echinococcosis, there has been a considerable effort to develop effective recombinant protein vaccines to control cysticercosis, with good progress reported for vaccines against *T. ovis* but not yet specifically *T. hydatigenea* (Lightowlers et al. 2000)

Fascioliasis

Fascioliasis is the most common liver fluke disease of goats worldwide. In certain regions, chronic fascio-

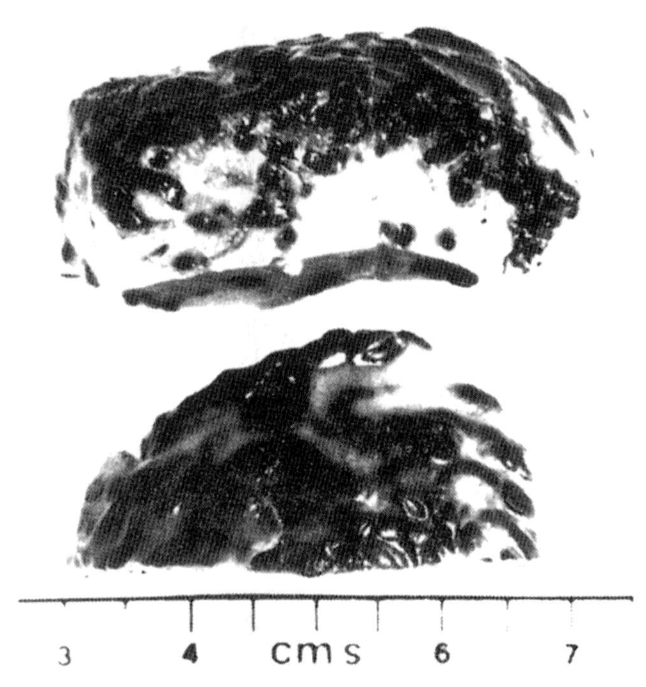

Figure 11.3. Blood-filled tracts in the liver due to migration of embryos of *Taenia hydatigena.* (From Everett and de Gruchy 1982).

liasis represents a major constraint on goat production.

Etiology

There are two *Fasciola* species that infect goats. *F. hepatica* is smaller, with an adult length of 18 to 32 mm and a width of 7 to 14 mm. *F. gigantica* is longer, with an adult length of 24 to 76 mm and a width of 5 to 13 mm.

Fasciola spp. have an indirect life cycle, with water snails of the superfamily *Lymnaeidae* acting as the intermediate host. More than fifteen species of these snails serve as hosts for *F. hepatica* worldwide, and at least thirteen for *F. gigantica*, with some overlap. When *Fasciola* are introduced into new areas by importation of livestock, local species of *Lymnaeidae* may serve as suitable, adaptive, intermediate hosts. Infected snails introduced into a new area may also act as the source of new infections.

Adult flukes reside within the biliary tract of definitive hosts such as goats and lay eggs that are passed via the bile duct to the feces. Egg production is substantial, with a mean of 303,000 eggs found in the gallbladders of infected, slaughtered goats (Jimenez-Albarran and Guevara-Pozo 1977). Eggs passed in feces hatch within ten to twelve days, releasing miracidia that invade intermediate host snails. Eggs hatch optimally at a temperature of 79°F (26°C), while temperatures must be at least 50°F (10°C) for miracidia to survive, invade snails, and develop further. Within the snail, the miracidium undergoes subsequent multiplications through sporocyst, rediae, daughter rediae, and cercariae stages. The average time from infection of snails to shedding of cercariae is five to eight weeks but can be as short as twenty-one days or prolonged as much as ten months under adverse conditions.

When cercariae are shed by snails, they swim to a nearby plant, attach to herbage, encyst, and become infective metacercariae that are then ingested by grazing vertebrate hosts. The ingested metacercariae excyst, penetrate the intestinal wall, and migrate through the abdominal cavity to the liver. They then penetrate the liver capsule and migrate through the liver parenchyma to the bile ducts, where they mature. They reach the bile ducts about six to seven weeks after infection. Maturation within the bile ducts to egg-laying adults requires an additional two to four weeks. Adult flukes may remain in situ for months to years.

Occasionally, flukes are found in aberrant organ locations such as kidney and lungs, caused by inaccurate migration out of the intestine (Charan and Iyer 1972; Haroun et al. 1989).

Epidemiology

Fascioliasis occurs principally in domestic ruminants, but other nonruminant livestock, numerous wild mammals, and marsupials also can be infected and may serve as reservoir hosts. Humans can contract fascioliasis from ingesting fresh plants contaminated with metacercariae.

The distribution of *F. hepatica* is cosmopolitan, and reports of fascioliasis in goats come from around the world (Rafyi and Eslami 1971; Jimenez-Albarran and Guevara-Pozo 1977; Chevis 1980; Quittet 1980; Vasquez-Vasquez 1980; El Moukdad 1981; Leathers et al. 1982; Bendezu et al. 1983; Anwar and Chaudhri 1984; Fernandes and Hamann 1985; Liakos 1985; Thompson 1986; Campano 1987; Wang et al. 1987; Molan and Saeed 1988). Prevalence varies considerably. No liver flukes were identified in an abattoir study in Queensland, Australia (McKenzie et al. 1979). Approximately 4% of sheep and goat livers were infected in a Mexican study (Vasquez-Vasquez 1980), while as many as 79% of sheep and goat livers inspected in Pakistan had *F. hepatica* (Anwar and Chaudhri 1984).

The distribution of *F. gigantica* is more limited, primarily to the tropical regions of Asia and Africa, and the Middle East. Caprine infection with *F. gigantica* has been reported from all these regions (Fabiyi 1970; Rafyi and Eslami 1971; Charan and Iyer 1972; Tager-Kagan, 1978; Assoku 1981; El Moukdad 1981; Nooruddin et al. 1987). In a year-long Indian abattoir survey, 14.7% of goat livers were infected with *F. gigantica* and 22.3% of potentially marketable liver was condemned (Pachauri et al. 1988).

Besides a suitable snail host, the key element that regulates the occurrence of fascioliasis is a suitable combination of moisture and temperature that allows persistent surface wetness on pasture for the snail and the free-living stages of the parasite to thrive. The relationship of infection rate to weather conditions is sufficiently well known that meteorological calculation of increased fascioliasis risk is done to determine the need for timing of prophylaxis (Soulsby 1982). These forecasting techniques were first applied in Europe but are now being applied elsewhere, including North America (Malone and Zukowski 1992), South America (Fuentes et al. 1999), and Africa (Yilma and Malone 1998).

Low-lying, poorly drained, persistently marshy, or swampy areas in warm climates grazed by ruminants are ideal for completion of the life cycle of *Fasciola* spp. Water sources, however, do not need to be permanent. Intermittent flooding of fields by overflow of streams or frequent irrigation can facilitate infection because snails can burrow into mud and survive temporary dry periods. Irrigation canals and ditches can be an important point of infection for goats and sheep in dry regions where fresh herbage and water may only be available at certain periods of the year along the snail-infested irrigation channels.

In temperate regions, infection of snails typically peaks in late spring and early summer, leading to peak pasture contamination with infective metacercariae in late summer and early fall. Peak incidence of clinical disease in ruminants is then seen in late fall and winter. Where winters are not extremely cold or excessively dry, some snails and eggs survive winter and recommence development in early spring so that a less significant cycle of infection with metacercariae occurs on pastures in late spring and early summer as well. In tropical regions, metacercariae can be present all year long, and there is no well-defined season for clinical outbreaks in ruminants. Grazing is not a prerequisite for infection if stabled animals are fed fresh green herbage contaminated with metacercariae. Feeding fresh cut grass to penned goats is a typical husbandry practice in much of Asia.

Goats, like sheep, do not develop as strong an immunity to *Fasciola* infection as cattle, and remain largely susceptible to re-infection. However, some immunity does develop as evidenced by reduced size and numbers of flukes recovered from repeated challenge infections (Reddington et al. 1986; El Sanhouri et al. 1987; Haroun et al. 1989).

Pathogenesis

There is little or no damage produced during migration of metacercariae through the intestinal wall or the peritoneal cavity. The potential for damage begins when metacercariae penetrate the liver capsule and begin migration through the parenchyma. When large numbers invade simultaneously, as may happen in the early fall, a traumatic hepatitis ensues and is recognized clinically as acute fascioliasis. When moderate numbers invade over an extended period of time, then subacute fascioliasis can occur. One thousand infective metacercariae can produce fatal acute fascioliasis in goats and 200 can produce severe subacute fascioliasis. *Fasciola gigantica* is more pathogenic to goats than *F. hepatica*, and goats may be more susceptible to *F. gigantica* than sheep (Ogunrinade 1984).

In acute fascioliasis, there is marked disruption of liver parenchyma with extensive hemorrhage. The liver capsule may rupture, leading to severe intra-abdominal bleeding and death. Even without fatal hemorrhage, animals may die within a few days as a result of hepatic insufficiency from parenchymal damage. In the subacute form, invading metacercariae still produce migratory tracts, hemorrhage, and necrosis within the liver and lead to a more prolonged clinical picture of hepatic insufficiency. Extensive fibrosis occurs in the liver during subsequent attempts at healing.

Acute fascioliasis is not commonly seen in goats and the reason is not clear. It may be related to feeding behavior because goats are not intensive grazers, and may not ingest sufficient numbers of metacercariae in short periods to produce severe acute reactions.

Chronic fascioliasis occurs after arrival and maturation of flukes in the bile ducts. Persistence of adult flukes in the biliary tree results in hyperplastic cholangitis with ongoing loss of plasma proteins caused by increased permeability of the biliary mucosa. Feeding activity and movement of flukes within the biliary tree produces chronic blood loss. Under natural circumstances of exposure, individual animals may simultaneously experience acute, subacute, and chronic fascioliasis.

In sheep, infectious necrotic hepatitis, or black disease, is a common complication of fascioliasis. In these cases, *Clostridium novyi* organisms already present in the liver suddenly proliferate in the anaerobic environment of necrotic tissue created by migrating fluke larvae. The release of toxins by proliferating bacteria produces an acute, fatal toxemia. The prevalence of this disease in goats is poorly documented, but it is considered to be a serious potential risk in areas of Australia and New Zealand where goat populations are expanding into traditional sheep-raising areas (Pauling 1986). In Australia, black disease has been documented in Angora goats. It occurs seasonally between February and June in well-conditioned goats between nine months and four years of age. It is presumed that goats are less frequently affected than sheep because of their browsing habits. The prevalence in goats increases when they are forced to graze in wet areas during drought because *C. novyi* is a soil-borne organism (King 1980). Black disease was also confirmed in goats in the Sudan, where eighteen normal appearing animals in a herd of 435 were found dead overnight. At necrospy, all the goats were heavily infested with *F. gigantica* and the presence of *C. novyi* Type B was established (Hamid et al. 1991). Where there is concern of the risk of black disease, goats can be vaccinated against *C. novyi*, which is included in many of the commercially available, multivalent, clostridial vaccines.

Clinical Findings

Acute fascioliasis, though uncommon, may present as sudden death or as progressive weakness, depression, anorexia, and pallor lasting as long as three days and resulting in death. Before death, pain may be elicited by deep palpation over the liver. Subacute fascioliasis may show similar signs for as long as several weeks. Black disease usually presents as sudden death with no other signs except some possible frothing at the mouth and nostrils.

Chronic fascioliasis is the most common presentation. The history may include a period of depression, poor appetite, lethargy, and weight loss for one month or longer. In prolonged cases, some animals have diarrhea. There may also be a complaint of decreased milk production in milking does. Physical findings include poor body condition, rough hair coat, pale mucous membranes, and tachycardia. Intermandibular edema, or bottle jaw, frequently occurs in long-standing cases and is highly suggestive of chronic fascioliasis.

Clinical Pathology and Necropsy

Acute fascioliasis is most often diagnosed at necropsy. In subacute disease, the hemogram may document normochromic anemia, eosinophilia, and possibly neutrophilia. Hypoalbuminemia and increases in serum concentration of liver-related enzymes may be noted in the chemistry profile.

Normocytic or macrocytic anemia, hemoglobinemia, hypoalbuminemia, and eosinophilia can be expected in chronic fascioliasis. Total protein may be in the normal range as a result of accompanying hypergammaglobulinemia. Increases in liver-specific enzymes in the blood occur less reliably in chronic fascioliasis, although increases in GDH and OCT have been reported to occur even when flukes are present only in the biliary tree (Treacher et al. 1974).

In chronic fascioliasis, fluke eggs can be found in the feces of goats. Sedimentation methods for fecal examination are preferred to flotation methods. Eggs are yellow colored, ovoid, and operculated at one end. Eggs of *F. gigantica* are slightly larger than eggs of *F. hepatica*. Where rumen flukes occur, their eggs must be differentiated from those of liver flukes.

Because acute fascioliasis occurs during the prepatent period of infection, detection of ova in feces is not a useful aid for identification of early infections with *F. hepatica* or *F. gigantica*. This inability to detect prepatent infections has spurred a good deal of research in the area of serodiagnosis over the last two decades. The main focus has been to isolate and characterize parasite antigens suitable for use in serodiagnostic tests such as ELISA to detect anti-fasciola antibodies in infected animals. One category has been the so-called excretory-secretory antigens of *Fasciola* spp., including cathepsins. These antigens have been derived directly from flukes and purified, or more recently, obtained through use of recombinant DNA technology. ELISA assays using such antigens have been able to detect circulating IgG against *F. hepatica* and F. *gigantica* as early as one week post infection (Paz-Silva et al. 2005), but more commonly three to seven weeks post infection (Cornelissen et al. 2001, Mezo et al. 2003, Yadav et al. 2005).

However, there are still some constraints with serodiagnostic tests. Though it is becoming less common as antigen purification techniques improve, cross reactivity still may occur with other helminths sharing similar antigens, notably paramphistomes. Also, detectable antibodies persist even after effective treatment of fascioliasis, making interpretation of test results difficult. A commercial ELISA test kit for identifying prepatent fascioliasis in cattle and sheep is currently available in Europe and Australia.

Necropsy in acute fascioliasis demonstrates a swollen, traumatized, friable liver with multiple perforations of the capsule and subcapsular hemorrhage. Fibrin tags may be present on the liver surface and blood accumulated in the peritoneal cavity. Migrating flukes are not easily seen on cut surface of the liver parenchyma, but may be visualized by shaking a piece of liver in a pan of water and looking for the larvae to settle out at the bottom.

When black disease complicates acute fascioliasis, signs of clostridial toxemia may be evident. These include blackening of the subcutaneous blood vessels observed as the skin is reflected, serosanguinous pericardial and peritoneal effusions, and patchy areas of liver necrosis with reddish borders. These reddened edges are likely sites for isolation of *Clostridium novyi*.

In chronic fascioliasis the carcass is emaciated, subcutaneous edema may be present, and organs are pale. The liver may be cirrhotic and irregularly nodular and the capsule opaque in areas. On cut surfaces, there is extensive fibrosis of the parenchyma. Bile ducts are thickened and fibrosed, but mineralization is uncommon. Upwards of one hundred adult flukes may be found in the cystic biliary ducts and gallbladder. They may be expressed by squeezing on cut sections of liver.

Flukes have also been found in the pancreatic duct of goats at necropsy (Leathers et al. 1982).

Diagnosis

Acute fascioliasis is one of many potential causes of sudden death in goats, as discussed in Chapter 16. Definitive diagnosis is by necropsy. Chronic fascioliasis is most easily confused with gastrointestinal nematodiasis, and, in practice, concurrent nematode and trematode infections are common in goats. Schistosomosis, as discussed in Chapter 8, can also present similarly to chronic fascioliasis. When chronic weight loss is the major complaint or presenting sign, a wide variety of other diseases needs to be considered, as discussed in Chapter 15.

Treatment

The choice of therapy largely depends on the stage of infection requiring treatment (Boray 1985). Carbon tetrachloride, hexachloroethane, bromsalans, oxyclozanide, niclofolan, and albendazole are only effective on mature flukes, ten weeks of age or older. Nitroxynil and clioxanide are moderately effective in flukes from eight to nine weeks of age and highly effective against mature flukes. Brotianide and rafoxanide are most effective against flukes eight weeks and older but only have 50% to 90% effectiveness against flukes six to seven weeks of age. Clorsulon is effective against all flukes two weeks of age and older. Triclabendazole and diamphenethide are effective against flukes from one day of age through maturity. This information is summarized in Table 11.3.

Other considerations in drug selection include safety, cost, regulatory concerns, and lactation and pregnancy status. The earliest available treatments, namely, carbon tetrachloride and hexachloroethane, are themselves hepatotoxic and can cause mortality in goats. These products may still be available in some developing countries where liver flukes exist. Though inexpensive, the use of these products should be discouraged. Brom-

Table 11.3. Summary of information on flukicides used in goats.

Flukicide	*Class of drug*	*Reported doses (mg/kg bw)*	*Effective against*			*Withholding times (days)*	
			Immature flukes 1–6 weeks old	*Immature flukes 6–10 weeks old*	*Adult flukes >10 weeks*	*Meat*	*Milk*
Triclabendazole	Bezimidizole	***5–15 PO***	+	+	+	28	X
Diamphenethide	Aromatic amine	***150 PO***	+	+	±	7	X
Clorsulon	Sulfonamide	***7 PO***	±	+	+	8	4
Closantel	Salicylanilide	***10–20 PO***	–	±	+	28–42	X
Rafoxanide	Salicylanilide	***7.5 PO***	–	±	+	28	X
Brotianide	Salicylanilide	7.5 PO	–	±	+	21	X
Clioxanide	Salicylanilide	20	–	±	+	?	?
Nitroxynil	Substituted phenol	***15 SQ***	–	±	+	30–60	X
Albendazole	Benzimidazole	***7.5–15 PO***	–	–	+	14	3
Niclofolan	Substituted phenol	***0.8 SQ, 2–4 PO***	–	–	+	?	?
Oxyclozanide	Salicylanilide	***15 PO***	–	–	+	28	X
Bromsalans	Salicylanilide	20	–	–	+	?	?
Bromophenophos	Organophosphate	***16.5 PO***	–	–	+	21	7
Hexachloroethane	Chlorinated Hydrocarbon	200–300	–	–	+	?	?
Carbon tetrachloride	Chlorinated Hydrocarbon	80 PO	–	–	+	?	?

Doses in bold italic are reported in the literature specifically for goats. Other doses are those reported for sheep because goat-specific information was not found in the literature. Similarly, very little goat-specific information is available for meat and milk withholding times following use of these flukicides. Times given are for cattle and/or sheep and come from European and Australian reports. They are to be used as general guidelines. Regulatory authorities should be contacted in individual countries to determine if there is goat-specific information available on the use and withholding times for these products. X = not suitable for use in lactating animals; – = not effective; ± = variably effective, tending to be more effective at the older range of the category; + = effective; PO = orally, SQ = subcutaneously; ? = no information found.

salans, which are substituted salicylanilides, can be toxic when combined with benzimidazoles, and should be used cautiously in goats. Diamphenethide is expensive and may be cost prohibitive for widespread use in commercial flocks. Only albendazole and clorsulon are available for treatment of fascioliasis in the United States and neither one is specifically approved for use in goats. The use of flukicides in lactating goats is problematic. Few products are specifically approved for use in lactating animals of any species, and withholding times for the same products may vary between countries. As a rule of thumb, if flukicides are used which are approved for other lactating species but not goats, then milk should be discarded for at least the time recommended for the other species, or for seven days, whichever is longer.

Specific doses for goats are established for a number of flukicides for use against *F. hepatica*. Albendazole orally at 15 mg/kg was 95.9% effective against adult flukes and produced no signs of toxicity, even when given at 75 mg/kg (Foreyt 1988). In France, it is marketed for goats at a dose of 7.5 mg/kg orally. Diamphenethide given orally at 150 mg/kg removed 87.5% of juvenile and adult flukes. Treated animals included pregnant does and no adverse reactions were observed (Wang et al. 1987). In another goat study, the drug was 84% effective against one-week-old larvae and 97% effective against three-week-old larvae (Hughes et al. 1974).

Oral triclabendazole completely eliminated ova shedding in chronically infected goats at a dose of 5 mg/kg (Wolff et al. 1983). It is commercially marketed in drench or bolus form in some countries for oral use in goats at a dose of 10 mg/kg. In sheep, it has been shown that the lower dose kills flukes only as young as two weeks of age, whereas the higher dose is effective on flukes as young as one day of age.

Niclofolan was 90% effective against *F. hepatica* when given subcutaneously at a dose of 0.8 mg/kg in goats, with no adverse effects (Girardi et al. 1979). In China, it is used in goats at 2 to 4 mg/kg given orally (Weng 1983). Closantel effectively eliminated *F. hepatica* in goats at an orally administered dose of 10 mg/kg (Lee et al. 1996) but a dose of 20 mg/kg was required for 100% elimination of *F. gigantica* (Yadav et al. 1995).

Rafoxanide was reported to be 100% effective against *F. hepatica* in goats at a dose of 7.5 mg/kg orally (Campos Ruelas et al. 1976). Nitroxynil was 89% effective against six-week-old larvae at a subcutaneous dose of 15 mg/kg (Hughes et al. 1973). Closantel, rafoxanide, and nitroxynil are also effective against *Haemonchus contortus* in goats.

Clorsulon given to goats orally at a dose of 7 mg/kg reduced fluke numbers and fecal egg counts by 98% (Sundlof et al. 1991). Oral bromophenophos at 16.5 mg/kg eliminated all adult *F. gigantica* in goats but was only 50% effective against immature forms. Doubling the dose had little additional effect (Qadir 1979, 1981).

In many regions of the world where goats are kept, access to veterinary products may be limited and local treatments are employed. In a controlled study in Sudan, oral administration of extracts from either the local shrub *Albizia anthelmintica* or the local tree *Balanites aegyptiaca* showed reduction in liver fluke counts relative to untreated controls of 95.5% and 93.2%, respectively (Koko et al. 2000).

In most cases, drugs and dosages effective against *F. hepatica* are effective against *F. gigantica*. Acute and subacute fascioliasis are best treated with either diamphenethide or triclabendazole. All animals at risk should be treated whether they are showing signs at the time of first diagnosis or not. The prognoses in acute and subacute fascioliasis are poor.

The prospects are much better in treating chronic fascioliasis. Any of the drugs effective against mature flukes can be used in these cases. However, if drugs not effective against immature forms are used, then animals should be retreated at an interval appropriate for that drug to eliminate subsequently maturing larvae. Early response to treatment can be demonstrated by eliminating ova shedding. It may take one month or longer for erythrocyte and protein parameters to return to normal in treated goats.

In the last twenty years, parasite resistance to anthelmintics has emerged as a major challenge to treatment and control of parasitic diseases. The problem of resistance has been most pronounced in relation to treatment of gastrointestinal nematode parasites and is discussed further in Chapter 10. However, there have also been reports of anthelmintic resistance in liver flukes. The main problem, reported from a number of countries, is with triclabendazole, but failures of treatment with closantel have also been reported from Australia.

Because triclabendazole is effective against flukes at all stages of development, it has become the most widely used drug for fascioliasis and this has contributed to the development of resistance. Resistance may first be recognized as a failure for the drug to kill the youngest stages of the fluke. This may be manifested as the reappearance of fluke eggs in the feces sooner after treatment than normally expected. Gradually, as resistance grows stronger, more mature flukes survive treatment as well (Abbot et al. 2004).

There are no *in vitro* tests for evaluating resistance to flukicides (Coles et al. 2006). When resistance is suspected, other flukicides should be used. Because most other flukicides are not effective against young flukes, the treatment may need to be at a more frequent interval than when using triclabendazole.

Abbot et al. (2004) discourage the use of combination fluke and worm products because they can lead to off target selection for resistance to broad-spectrum anthelmintics in nematodes, or fasciolicide resistance in *F. hepatica*. However, in the case of closantel-benzimidazole combinations, there may actually be synergistic activity that can enhance their activity against resistant *F. hepatica* (and *H. contortus*) and slow the emergence of resistance to either class of compound.

Control

The objective of control is to limit fluke burdens in grazing animals. This is accomplished mainly by strategic use of flukicides and by keeping grazing animals out of environments likely to contain infective metacercariae from associated snail populations. Snail control is another tool, but may be difficult to achieve.

Pasture contamination by metacercariae is a dynamic process largely dependent on weather conditions. When calculated, the meteorological index can be helpful in determining the amount of tactical control necessary to avoid clinical disease and production loss on a seasonal basis (Urquhart et al. 1988). At the minimum, in temperate regions or arid zones, flukicide treatments should be administered strategically once in the early spring before turnout to pasture using an adult flukicide. Goats should be retreated in the autumn to kill developing and adult flukes picked up over the grazing season. An anthelmintic that kills immature and mature flukes should be used.

In tropical settings, particularly when year-round grazing occurs, treatment every eight to ten weeks with triclabendazole or diamphenethide may be indicated. This facilitates destruction of all ages of immature flukes within the prepatent period to eliminate egg production while controlling both acute and chronic fascioliasis in the goat. Egg production can also be controlled by using rafoxanide or closantel at five- or six-week intervals, but the risk of acute fascioliasis is still high because immature larvae are not killed. Such intensive control measures are effective in reducing pasture burdens and may not have to be repeated in subsequent years. When goats are part of mixed grazing systems, all potential hosts need to be treated simultaneously. When flukicides are used frequently, the potential for anthelmintic resistance should be monitored by fecal examinations for fluke eggs.

Limiting access of goats to snail populations is an adjunct to the use of flukicides. High-risk areas such as low-lying, marshy portions of grazing land, drainage ditches, irrigation channels, or stagnant ponds should be identified and drained or fenced off when possible. Cutting back vegetation at the edges of standing water makes the environment less amenable to snails. High-risk situations should also be identified such as intensified grazing by animals near water after drought or at the end of the grazing season when forage is in short supply. Housed goats should not be offered freshly cut herbage likely to be contaminated with metacercariae.

When mild winters and warm, moist summers promote high snail populations, the application of molluscicides to snail habitat could be considered. Copper sulfate in solutions of 1:100,000 to 1:5,000,000 or as a powder at 10 to 35 kg/hectare is effective in destruction of snails and their eggs (Soulsby 1982). Applications in spring kill overwintered snails and applications in summer and fall kill newly developed snails. Goats are less susceptible to copper toxicity than sheep, but caution should still be taken in turning goats out on copper-treated pastures before a dilution by rain has occurred. There are environmental concerns related to the use of molluscicides which may be toxic to fish and other species. Check local regulations before use. Biological control strategies using ducks and competitive non-host snail populations have also been applied for snail control with some success.

Fascioloidosis

Fascioloides magna, also known as the large American liver fluke, is a more important cause of morbidity in goats than fascioliasis in certain parts of North America and Europe.

Etiology and Pathogenesis

Adult *Fascioloides magna* are larger than *F. hepatica* and *F. gigantica*. The length is 23 to 100 mm and the width 11 to 26 mm. They are ovoid and pink-colored. Eggs are not found in goat feces for reasons described below.

This fluke has an indirect life cycle. The intermediate hosts are snails of various genera including *Fossaria, Galba (Lymnaea), Pseudosuccinia*, and *Stagnicola*. These snails tolerate a wider range of habitat, temperature, and moisture conditions than the snail hosts of *Fasciola* spp. The normal definitive hosts are members of the family Cervidae, including various deer, elk, and moose. Abnormal hosts include the large Bovidae such as bison, yak and cattle, as well as goats and sheep.

The adult fluke resides in the bile ducts of definitive hosts and lays eggs that are passed to the outside in the feces. Eggs hatch after four weeks and miracidia invade the intermediate host snails. Development to cercariae takes an additional seven to eight weeks. Voided cercariae encyst on vegetation. These encysted metacercariae are quite resistant to desiccation. When consumed by definitive hosts such as deer, the metacercariae penetrate the intestine, migrate through the peritoneal cavity, invade the liver, migrate through the parenchyma, and finally form encapsulated cysts.

These cysts communicate with the biliary tree so that mature flukes can pass eggs out through the bile. The prepatent period is thirty to thirty-two weeks.

In cattle, a similar pattern is followed except that cysts rarely communicate with the biliary tree. Eggs, then, are not passed and the life cycle is not completed. Adult flukes reach maturity in thirty-two to forty-four weeks and the cysts become thick-walled and fibrotic.

In goats and sheep, migrating larvae rarely form cysts. Instead, they continue to wander aimlessly through the liver parenchyma, causing considerable damage and hepatic dysfunction. Peritonitis and hemorrhage into the abdominal cavity can also contribute to disease severity. Even a single wandering fluke can be potentially fatal to goats. Clinical disease usually occurs three to six months after exposure (Foreyt and Leathers 1980). Ova are rarely if ever passed in the feces of infected goats so microscopic examination of feces does not aid in the diagnosis.

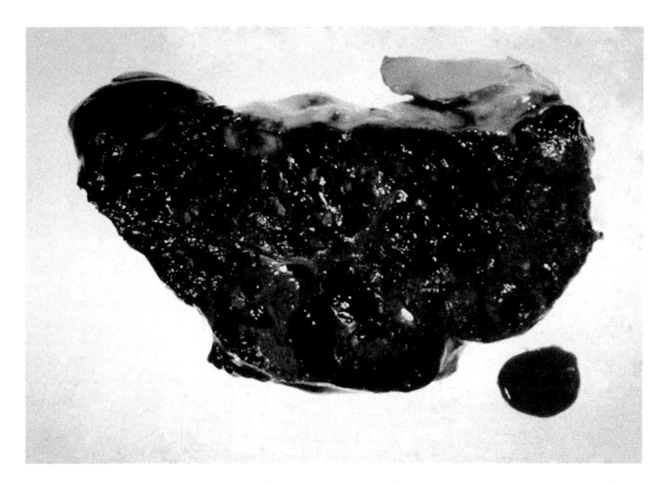

Figure 11.4. *Fascioloides magna* fluke and cross section of a necrotic goat liver through which it migrated. (Courtesy Dr. M.C. Smith.)

Epidemiology

Fascioloides magna is native to North America and is concentrated particularly in the Great Lakes region, the Gulf coast, and the Rocky Mountains and Pacific Northwest, including western Canada. The parasite was introduced into Europe with game deer and has become well established, particularly in Eastern Europe, including Italy, Germany, Austria, Slovenia, the Czech Republic, Slovakia, and Hungary.

Goats become infected with *F. magna* when they feed in areas also inhabited by deer or elk (wapiti) and intermediate host snails. Though the risk is increased when these areas are marshy, the requirement for standing water is not as strict as for fascioliasis. In the Great Lakes region, small ruminants become infected in late August or September and clinical disease is usually seen in January and February.

Clinical Findings

The most frequent presentation is sudden death. There are no descriptions of subacute disease in goats. In sheep, animals so affected show depression, pallor, weakness, anorexia, and abdominal pain that is accentuated by palpation over the liver.

Clinical Pathology and Necropsy

Animals seen before death may have increases in serum concentrations of liver-related enzymes. Necropsy reveals extensive liver damage characterized by necrosis and numerous hemorrhagic tracts throughout the liver parenchyma (Figure 11.4). These tracts are characteristically black in color due to accumulation of black iron porphyrin pigment. The pigment may also be seen in mesenteric nodes. Though rare, cysts containing live or dead flukes may be found in the livers of goats (Olsen 1949).

Diagnosis

Diagnosis is based on a history of sudden death and characteristic lesions in the liver at necropsy. Differential diagnosis must include acute fascioliasis, cysticercosis, toxic hepatitis, and in younger animals, haemonchosis and coccidiosis. Other causes of sudden death are reviewed in Chapter 16.

Treatment

Treatment is difficult because clinical disease is caused by immature flukes that can induce serious or fatal illness when present even in small numbers. This means that useful drugs must approach 100% efficacy against immature flukes. Albendazole administered orally to goats at 15 mg/kg was reported to be 99% effective against flukes eight weeks of age or older (Foreyt and Foreyt 1980). The use of albendazole during the first months of pregnancy may carry some risk to the fetus.

Other flukicides have not been evaluated specifically for *F. magna* infection in goats. Closantel was 95% to 98% effective in sheep at a dose of 15 mg/kg orally or 7.5 mg/kg intramuscularly (Stromberg et al. 1985). Clorsulon was not effective against immature *F. magna* in sheep at a single oral dose of 15 mg/kg (Conboy et al. 1988), but was 92% effective against eight-week-old larvae in sheep at a dose of 21 mg/kg (Foreyt 1988a). Oral rafoxanide at 15 mg/kg has been reported to be effective in red deer (Rajsky et al. 2002). No products are approved for use against *F. magna* in the United States.

Control

Control of fascioloidiasis is complicated by the need to control wild animal definitive hosts and an ecologically diverse, intermediate host snail population. In endemic areas where cases have occurred, intensive management without pasturing should be considered for dairy goats. This is obviously difficult for extensively managed fiber-producing goats. Avoidance of marshy pastures and attempts to fence off deer may be helpful. When exposure cannot be controlled, reduction of fluke loads in goats can be undertaken. In northern climes, prophylactic treatment with albendazole is administered after the first killing frost and repeated one month later to help reduce clinical losses.

Lancet Fluke Infection

Dicrocoelium dendriticum, the lancet fluke, generally produces a chronic form of liver fluke disease in goats that is less severe than that produced by *Fasciola* spp. It has a cosmopolitan distribution.

Etiology

Dicrocoelium dendriticum is a small liver fluke measuring 6 to 10 mm in length and 1.5 to 2.5 mm in width. It has an indirect life cycle involving two intermediate hosts: terrestrial snails and ants. Forty species of snails from nine families may serve as primary intermediate hosts but all secondary host ant species are of the subfamily Formicinae (Boray 1985). Goats, sheep, and cattle are the common definitive hosts, but other livestock species and wild mammals and humans can be infected.

Adult flukes reside in the bile ducts and excrete eggs to the outside in feces. Eggs are ingested by snails where they develop into cercariae. Cercariae are expelled by snails in slime balls and are ingested by ants. Infectious metacercariae develop in the ants and are neuropathogenic, causing ants to remain paralyzed on herbage during peak times of livestock grazing. Infected ants are ingested by grazing livestock and the young flukes excyst from metacercariae in the small intestine of the definitive host. In contrast with the *Fasciolidae*, these immature flukes do not migrate through the peritoneal cavity and liver parenchyma. Instead, they enter the hepatic biliary system directly through the common bile duct via the small intestinal lumen. The prepatent period for *D. dendriticum* is eight to twelve weeks.

Epidemiology

Dicrocoelium dendriticum infection is common in North America, Europe, Asia, North Africa, and the Middle East. Prevalence in goat populations is reported as high as 45% in endemic areas (Manas-Almendros et al. 1978). It is less common in South America and is not found in Australia, New Zealand, and much of Africa. *Dicrocoelium hospes*, a cattle fluke of West and East Africa, has been reported in goats in Niger and Nigeria (Tager-Kagan 1979; Schillhorn van Veen et al. 1980).

Numerous habitats are potentially contaminated with *D. dendriticum* because snail hosts are numerous, terrestrial ant populations are widespread, and many wild mammals serve as reservoir hosts. Grazing areas near forests are particularly high-risk sites. The fluke eggs are also resistant to desiccation and freezing. Hibernating ants can maintain metacercarial infections so that grazing stock are at risk from the beginning of spring grazing.

Pathogenesis

These flukes are less pathogenic than the *Fascioloidae* because they do not migrate through liver parenchyma. *Dicrocoelium dendriticum* infection, which may involve thousands of flukes per goat, can cause progressive inflammation of the entire biliary tree and potentially lead to fibrosis, biliary cirrhosis, and hepatic insufficiency.

Clinical Findings

Dicrocoelium dendriticum may be a subclinical infection or produce a disease syndrome similar to chronic fascioliasis. Affected goats have a history of weight loss. They appear thin and depressed and may show signs of anemia and hypoproteinemia, including pallor and intermandibular edema.

Clinical Pathology and Necropsy

Identification of lancet fluke eggs in the feces of goats is the most reliable means of diagnosis. The dark brown, operculated eggs are much smaller than those of *F. hepatica* or *F. gigantica* and can be found by both fecal flotation and sedimentation methods. *Dicrocoelium dendriticum* infection may produce elevated serum levels of GGT and AP caused by biliary inflammation. Anemia and hypoproteinemia are evidenced in the hemogram.

At necropsy, adult lancet flukes are found in the bile ducts. In early cases there is thickening of the biliary ducts. In severe, chronic infections, biliary fibrosis, cirrhosis, and scarring of the liver surface may be noted. The comparative liver pathology of *D. dendriticum* and *F. hepatica* in goats has been described (Rahko 1972).

A paramphistome parasite of the bile duct of buffalo and cattle in Asia, *Gigantocotyle explanatum*, sometimes is found in the bile duct of goats (Upadhyay et al. 1986). It should be differentiated from *D. dendriticum*, which has a similar appearance.

Diagnosis

Lancet fluke disease must be differentiated from chronic fascioliasis, gastrointestinal helminthiasis, paratuberculosis, and other causes of chronic wasting, as discussed in Chapter 15.

Treatment

In France, albendazole is marketed for use against the lancet fluke at 15 mg/kg orally with a precaution against use during the first three months of pregnancy. Thiophanate is marketed at 50 mg/kg orally with a milk withdrawal time of three days. Diamphenethide at 220 to 330 mg/kg orally is highly effective, with no toxic side effects noted (Devillard and Villemin 1976). Drugs reported to have an efficacy of 90% or greater in sheep include thiabendazole at 200 mg/kg, fenbendazole at 100 mg/kg, praziquantel at 50 mg/kg, and netobimin at 20 mg/kg (Boray 1985; Sanz et al. 1987). Note that some of these doses exceed the routine doses used in helminthiasis. Brotianide was found to be ineffective in goats at oral doses as high as 22.5 mg/kg (Shahlapour et al. 1986).

Control

Control measures are complicated by the existence of two intermediate hosts, and strategic anthelmintic therapy may be the only practical control method. In endemic areas in temperate regions, goats should be treated in the autumn to reduce adult fluke burdens before the winter feeding season begins. In tropical and subtropical areas, year-round, repetitive treatments timed within the prepatent period of the flukes reduce fluke burdens and pasture contamination.

Pancreatic Flukes

Eurytrema spp., or pancreatic flukes, produce mostly subclinical infections in goats. The presence of *Eurytrema* eggs in feces may confuse the diagnosis of the more clinically important lancet fluke, *D. dendriticum*.

Eurytrema pancreaticum is widely distributed throughout Asia and also in Brazil. The fluke has a similar life cycle to *D. dendriticum* with different snails serving as primary intermediate hosts, and grasshoppers instead of ants serving as secondary intermediate hosts. The definitive hosts are goats, sheep, cattle, buffalo, and humans. The young flukes ascend the pancreatic duct, but occasionally mature in the bile duct or duodenum. This fluke is wider and spinier than *D. dendriticum*. The prepatent period is eleven to fifteen weeks. Other species of *Eurytrema* reported from goats include *E. cladorchis* in China and Nepal (Chongti and Tongmin 1980; Mahato 1987) and *E. coelomaticum* from Taiwan and Brazil (Shien et al. 1978; Fernandes and Hamann 1985).

Pancreatic fluke infestations are usually subclinical but heavy infections may contribute to emaciation. A case of sudden death in a cachexic adult goat in Nepal was caused by rupture of the gastroepiploic vein that contained *E. cladorchis* (Mahato 1987).

At necropsy, pancreatic flukes may be found in the duodenum and bile ducts, but most commonly in the pancreatic ducts. These ducts may show catarrhal inflammation and thickening and the pancreas itself may show focal areas of atrophy and fibrosis. The severity of lesions increases with the number of flukes present (Shien et al. 1979).

Praziquantel given two consecutive days at 20 mg/kg orally is effective against *Eurytrema* spp. in goats (Kono et al. 1986). Triclabendazole (Kono et al. 1986), niclofolan (Weng 1983), and nitroxynil (Suh 1983) are not effective.

NUTRITIONAL AND METABOLIC DISEASES

White Liver Disease

White liver disease, a manifestation of cobalt deficiency known for some time in sheep, has been reported in goats only in New Zealand and Oman, though it may be under-diagnosed in other regions where cobalt deficient soils occur. It is characterized by progressive emaciation and hepatic lipodystrophy that gives the liver a grayish appearance at necropsy.

Etiology and Pathogenesis

Cobalt deficiency in ruminants is a well-known condition associated with grazing of cobalt deficient soils. It results in chronic wasting with anemia and hypoproteinemia. However, the specific manifestation of white liver disease apparently occurs only in sheep and goats.

Cobalt is used in the rumen by microflora to produce cyanocobalamin, or vitamin B_{12}, which serves as a coenzyme to methylmalonyl-CoA mutase in the citric acid cycle facilitating the conversion of propionic acid to glucose via succinate in the liver. When small ruminants are cobalt deficient or are fed high carbohydrate diets that exceed the capacity of the liver to convert propionate to succinate, these animals may accumulate methylmalonyl-CoA or methylmalonic acid in the tissues and convert it to branched chain fatty acids that accumulate in hepatocytes. This conversion to branched chain fatty acids does not occur in cattle or deer and white liver disease as a manifestation of cobalt deficiency is not observed in these species (Black et al. 1988).

Epidemiology

Cobalt deficiency in livestock associated with cobalt deficient soils has been reported from New Zealand, Australia, Europe, and northeastern North America. Ovine white liver disease has been specifically reported from New Zealand, Australia, Brazil, the UK, Holland, Switzerland, and Norway. For a long time, caprine white liver disease had been reported only from New Zealand (Pearson, 1987; Black et al. 1988) but more recently the disease also was confirmed in goats in Oman (Johnson et al. 1999). It is reasonable to assume that the disease occurs in goats where it is found in sheep but may be overlooked because clinically, the disease can mimic gastrointestinal helminthiasis.

Reported cases of white liver disease from New Zealand involve young Angora or Angora-cross goats between four and eighteen months of age, but mostly between four and six months of age. Grass pastures appear to be more conducive to deficiency in goats than legume pastures, and lush pasture may also predispose to the condition. The diagnosis in Oman derived from slaughterhouse samples of goat livers that showed hepatic lipidosis and low cobalt concentrations. The management of these goats while alive was unreported.

Clinical Findings

The principal complaint in cobalt deficiency is chronic ill thrift. Affected goats are thin, weak, and listless, with decreased appetite, pale mucous membranes, and submandibular edema. Diarrhea may be seen. White liver disease in sheep is associated with photosensitization, but this has not yet been reported in goats.

Clinical Pathology and Necropsy

A macrocytic, normochromic anemia and hypoalbuminemia are common findings. The cases of caprine white liver disease reported from New Zealand were confirmed on the basis of serum vitamin B_{12} levels antemortem or liver levels at necropsy using normal values established for sheep. Adequate serum levels are reported as more than 400 pmol/l and adequate liver levels as more than 200 nmol/kg. In Oman, confirmation was based on analysis of liver cobalt concentrations, which in affected goats were 0.08 ± 0.02 ppm dry matter as compared to 0.53 ± 0.11 ppm dry matter in livers of normal control goats. Standard reference values for liver cobalt in normal goats are not reported. In cattle and sheep the normal range is 0.15 to 0.20 ppm dry matter and 0.02 to 0.06 ppm dry matter in cobalt deficient animals (Johnson et al. 1999).

Necropsy findings include an emaciated carcass and a pale-colored liver. Histologically, there is widespread fatty change in the liver with many hepatocytes containing single, large fat globules in the cytoplasm, mild to moderate bile duct proliferation, portal fibroplasia, and sinusoidal accumulations of macrophages containing periodic acid-Schiff (PAS)-positive ceroid material.

Diagnosis

All causes of prolonged weight loss must be considered in the diagnosis, as discussed in Chapter 15. Because young goats often have gastrointestinal helminthiasis that appears clinically similar, cobalt deficiency as a concurrent or underlying condition should not be neglected, even when evidence of helminthiasis is found on fecal flotation or necropsy.

Treatment

For young stock, intramuscular injection of vitamin B_{12} at a weekly dose of 100 µg, or for adults, 300 µg has been used to ameliorate signs of white liver disease in affected herds. Also, sheep respond to daily oral supplementation of cobalt at 1 mg/head/day (or 7 mg/head/week) given until there is noticeable improvement.

Control

Deficient pastures may be top-dressed with cobalt as cobalt sulfate at a rate of 350 g/ha annually, but animals should be supplemented nutritionally in the short term, because pasture uptake is not immediate. When pasture treatment is not possible, cobalt should be supplemented in the diet. For sheep the recommendation is 0.1 mg/head/day. Commercially available cobalt pellets given orally to sheep provide continuous release of cobalt for as long as three years, as long as they remain in the rumen (Kimberling 1988). They are of particular value in extensive grazing systems where pasture top-dressing of cobalt or regular feed supplementation is impractical.

TOXICOLOGIC DISEASES

Numerous drugs, chemicals, plants, and fungal mycotoxins have been reported to cause toxic hepatitis specifically in goats. Recognition of toxic hepatitis and identification of the specific cause can be a difficult challenge to the practitioner, requiring careful history taking, thorough environmental examination, complete physical examination, and often, laboratory support. The following discussion is divided into two parts. The first is a general discussion of the salient features of toxic hepatitis in goats. This is followed by brief descriptions of the specific known causes of the condition.

General Features of Toxic Hepatitis

Diffuse destruction of liver parenchyma from various chemicals and drugs occurs sporadically in goats. Predisposing factors include overdosage of drugs, inappropriate uses of drugs, idiosyncratic reactions, unsuspected exposures, and predispositions to toxicity.

Patterns of poisoning by plants are variable. In some cases, goats are offered poisonous plants unknowingly in the form of garden cuttings. Occasionally, poisonous plants are incorporated into hay, but not usually at concentrations capable of producing widespread toxicity. In grazing situations, the potential toxicity of plants may be altered by weather conditions or the occurrence of fungal parasites on plants that enhance toxicity. Many poisonous plants are unpalatable to goats under normal circumstances and will not be eaten readily. However, when drought or overgrazing occurs, goats may be compelled to eat toxic plants, and in fact, may be more likely to eat them than sheep and cattle due to their inherently diverse feeding behavior.

The development of hepatotoxicity is related to the dose of toxin, the action of the toxin, the duration of exposure, and the ability of the goat to detoxify the toxic agent. Drugs and chemicals tend to produce acute toxicity after a single exposure, while most plant poisonings involve long-term feeding or grazing of the offending plant. With some plants, chronic disease develops gradually, while with others, the plant toxicity is cumulative, and there is an extended period of normality before acute disease occurs.

Biotransformation of toxic compounds to inactive metabolites occurs primarily in the liver and involves microsomal enzyme systems, particularly mixed function oxidases, and the hemoprotein cytochrome P-450. Marked differences in various detoxifying activities occur among the ruminant livestock species (Patterson and Roberts 1970; Dalvi et al. 1987). Hepatic microsomal protein content of goats is equivalent to that of cattle but significantly less than in sheep. The content of cytochrome P-450 is equivalent to cattle but significantly more than in sheep, and goats have a significantly higher level of activity for the drug-metabolizing enzyme benzphetamine *N*-demethylase than either cattle or sheep. These findings suggest a basis for understanding the known variation in susceptibility to some toxic agents in goats, sheep, and cattle, and serve as a caution against presuming equivalent toxicities in goats for various xenobiotics based on their effects in sheep or cattle (Al-Qarawi and Ali 2003; Szotáková et al. 2004; Dacasto et al. 2005). Age can be a factor in biotransformation capacity as well. Livers of newborn goats exhibited very low activities of drug-metabolizing enzymes relative to six-week-old and adult goats (Eltom et al. 1993).

In general terms, hepatotoxins manifest their toxicity by one or more of the following mechanisms: centrilobular necrosis, midzonal necrosis, periportal necrosis, cholestasis, biliary hyperplasia, or venous occlusion. Acute, often fatal hepatic insufficiency can result when the initial toxic effects are severe. In less severe or in chronic poisonings, lesions of ongoing hepatic necrosis are mixed with evidence of attempts to heal, mainly characterized by fibrosis, leading over the long term to cirrhosis. Many of the hepatotoxic agents, particularly plants, exert toxic effects in other organs as well, particularly the kidney, lung, and the alimentary tract when toxins are ingested.

The clinical findings in toxic hepatitis of goats vary with the cause. In general, depression and anorexia are the most consistent findings. Signs of hepatoencephalopathy, including weakness, ataxia, head pressing, torticollis, coma, and convulsions are common. Evidence of liver pain, characterized by an arched back and resistance to liver palpation, are common in acute toxicities. Jaundice is a less common finding than might be expected. Signs of photodermatitis may be observed in some plant poisonings. Because many hepatotoxic agents affect other organs as well, many clinical signs may be noted that are not hepatic in origin. Common findings in this category include dyspnea, diarrhea, and signs of renal failure.

In acute toxicity, serum levels of liver-associated enzymes are elevated. Liver specific enzymes should be measured, because some toxic agents also damage muscle, causing increases in AST. Elevations of total bilirubin are not consistent in acute caprine hepatotoxicity. When elevations are observed, assessment of erythrocyte parameters is indicated to determine if concurrent hemolysis is occurring.

Evaluation of liver function by BSP clearance and characterization of lesions by biopsy are helpful in confirming the presence of toxic hepatitis in poisonings over the long term because levels of liver-specific enzymes in the serum may not be pronounced in chronic disease. Anemia, hypoproteinemia, and hypoalbuminemia are common in chronic liver disease, but are by no means specific for hepatic dysfunction. When neurologic signs are observed, elevated blood ammonia levels are helpful in distinguishing hepatoencephalopathy from primary neurologic disease.

At necropsy, in acute toxic hepatitis, the liver is swollen with rounded edges. On cut surface the lobular pattern of the parenchyma is accentuated by the presence of centrilobular necrosis and vascular congestion. When jaundice is present, organs and body fat appear yellow. Edema, and less often, ascites may be seen when hypoproteinemia has had an opportunity to develop or when there is concurrent congestive heart failure. In many instances, the toxicity of hepatotoxic agents is not limited to the liver and multiple organ involvement is common. Gastroenteritis is common with ingested toxins and kidney lesions are frequent, presumably resulting from the toxin-filtering and concentrating action of the kidney. The rumen content should be examined for evidence of hepatotoxic plants.

Definitive diagnosis of toxicity can be difficult. Success depends on careful history taking to identify all possible exposures to toxins and environmental examination to determine the presence of chemicals or plants unrecognized by the animal caretaker. Although toxic principles of many poisonous plants are identifiable by laboratory methods, these methods are often expensive and not widely available for diagnostic use. Identifying the plant itself in the rumen content or feed or on grazing lands may be sufficient to make a presumptive diagnosis. The ability to identify fragments of toxic plants in rumen content is a valuable skill.

Specific treatments for toxic hepatitis are limited. Animals should be removed from risk of additional exposure when possible. In known, acute, oral toxicities, administering activated charcoal at a dose of 500 g for an adult goat may inhibit additional uptake of toxin from the gut. In individual, valuable animals, rumenotomy might be attempted early in the course of disease to remove ingesta that may contain toxins. Supportive care includes fluids supplemented with glucose to counter dehydration and likely hypoglycemia, feeding low protein diets to suppress additional hyperammonemia, and controlling seizures. When photosensitization is present, animals should be kept out of direct sun, given corticosteroids to ameliorate the photodermatitis, and placed on antibiotics to prevent secondary pyodermas. In many cases of toxic hepatitis, animals that recover from acute disease may never return to full health or production potential due to permanent liver damage. The prognosis, therefore, should always be guarded.

Controlling toxic hepatitis depends on identifying the toxic agent and preventing additional exposure. This includes accurate dosing of medications such as ivermectin, substituting newer drugs for carbon tetrachloride in the treatment of liver flukes, restricting grazing of goats to avoid toxic plants, avoiding overgrazing, providing supplemental feed during periods of drought, and recognizing periods of enhanced toxicity in certain plants. Obviously, accomplishing many of these goals is problematic. Additional recognition of environmental agents toxic to goats, particularly plants, and increased understanding of the patterns of occurrence of poisonings will lead to more specific recommendations for control.

Chemical and Drug-related Causes of Toxic Hepatitis

Carbon Tetrachloride

Carbon tetrachloride administered as a flukicide can be hepatotoxic, even at the recommended dose of 1 ml/10 kg bw (Jones and Shah 1982). Overdosing can lead to acute death from respiratory arrest or a more prolonged three- to seven-day course involving hepatic and renal insufficiency. The sensitivity of goats to carbon tetrachloride toxicity was increased when animals were first treated with the chlorinated hydrocarbon insecticide dieldrin (Abdelsalam et al. 1982).

Hexachloroethane

Idiosyncratic reactions to routinely used drugs may occur as reported in the case of Jamunapari goats in India given standard doses of hexachloroethane for treatment of liver flukes (Vihan 1987). Early signs of toxicity included rumen atony, bloat, diarrhea, and dyspnea, followed by depression, staggering gait, muscle spasms, and convulsions. Necropsy lesions included hepatic necrosis, renal tubular degeneration, pulmonary edema, desquamation of forestomach mucosa, and generalized hemorrhage. Such reactions have also been reported in cattle and sheep.

Halothane

Though no longer in common use in the United States, halothane gas anesthesia was used commonly in goats without incident. Nevertheless, there are two separate reports of presumed halothane toxicity producing massive hepatic necrosis with clinical signs of hepatoencephalopathy in the days immediately after anesthesia (Fetcher 1985; O'Brien et al. 1986). Although the exact mechanism remains unclear, it was postulated that a combination of prolonged anesthesia, hypoxia, and hypotension led to reductive rather than oxidative metabolism of halothane in the liver, resulting in production of hepatotoxic rather than inert metabolites. In a subsequent study, careful monitoring of clinical enzymology in goats under halothane anesthesia for no more than two hours and histologic examination of liver samples one and two months later did not indicate any evidence of liver damage or dysfunction (McEwen et al. 2000).

Iron

Iron toxicity, caused by extralabel administration of an equine hematinic product to cattle, was reproduced experimentally in goats given the same product (Ruhr et al. 1983). The product was formulated for intravenous use, but given intramuscularly at approximately five times the recommended horse dosage. Signs included respiratory distress, weakness, jaundice, recumbency, and convulsions. There was severe hepatic necrosis at necropsy.

Ivermectin

Ivermectin, given subcutaneously at twenty-five times the recommended dose (5 mg/kg versus 0.2 mg/kg), produced acute collapse, hyperexcitability, and death, or a three- to four-day course of anorexia, weakness, recumbency, apparent blindness, coma, and death in Nubian goats. The principal post mortem lesion was a multifocal, nonsuppurative, necrotizing hepatitis (Ali and Abu Samra 1987). In another study, East African goats were given eight times the recommended dose and showed no adverse effects except for some immediate, transient irritation at the subcutaneous injection site (Njanja et al. 1985).

Copper

Chronic copper toxicity has been documented in young goats fed calf milk replacers containing copper

(Belford and Raven 1986; Humphries et al. 1987). Chronic copper toxicity can cause hemolytic anemia as well as liver damage, though recently there has been a documented occurrence of chronic copper toxicosis in a dairy goat herd that showed no icterus or other signs of anemia (Cornish et al. 2007). Copper toxicity is discussed in more detail in Chapter 7.

Plants Causing Toxic Hepatitis

Caltrop

Geeldikkop, a hepatogenous photosensitization disease associated with grazing of *Tribulus terrestris*, or caltrop, a nutritious annual herb, causes severe economic loss in goat and sheep operations in South Africa (Kellerman et al. 1980). The condition has also been reported from Australia (Glastonbury and Boal 1985; Jacob and Peet 1987), Iran (Amjadi 1977), Argentina (Tapia et al. 1994), and California (McDonough et al. 1994). The plant, also known as puncture vine, yellow vine, and goathead, is found in warm, temperate, and tropical regions throughout the world. The disease is seasonal; the plant becomes toxic when wilted in hot, dry weather after summer rains. The hepatotoxicity and photosensitization are believed to be caused by steroidal saponins contained in the plant (Kellerman et al. 1991). Their toxic effect is enhanced when the plant is wilted. It has also been proposed that the presence of sporidesmin, a mycotoxin of *Pithomyces chartarum*, a fungus that grows on caltrops under the weather conditions described, may enhance the toxic effects of the steroidal saponins of *T. terrestris*. The clinical and pathological effects of experimental poisoning of goats with *T. terrestris* have been described (Aslani et al. 2004).

Sacahuiste

Sacahuiste *(Nolina texana)* poisoning occurs in Texas and other portions of the southwestern United States only during a brief, three-week period in spring when this common range plant is bearing buds, blooms, or ripe fruit, because the leaves are not toxic. The period of blooming often coincides with a period of feed scarcity on rangeland, so consumption by goats, sheep, and cattle is likely. Clinical signs include anorexia, depression, jaundice, dark yellow urine, purplish discoloration of the hoof, and photosensitization. The latter is more likely when green feed is available because sacahuiste blooms contain little chlorophyll (Mathews 1940a).

Lechuguilla

Agave lecheguilla, or lechuguilla, is another important cause of caprine hepatogenous photosensitization in Texas, New Mexico, and northern Mexico during drought conditions, especially in the spring. The disease is known locally as "goat fever" or "swellhead." The plant is believed to contain two photosensitizing toxins, one of which is a saponin. Signs include depression, loss of appetite, jaundice, yellow ocular and nasal discharge, photosensitization with swelling of the face and ears, and coma. Morbidity and mortality rates of 5% to 30% can occur (Mathews 1937).

Spurge

Poisoning by the spurge, *Phyllanthus abnormis*, occurs only in Texas in areas of sandy soil during drought periods when livestock eat young green plants. The toxin is degraded by drying. Goats are less susceptible than cattle, but can develop signs of listlessness, anorexia, unthriftiness, and diarrhea. There is severe fatty degeneration of the liver at necropsy (Mathews 1945).

Lantana

Lantana camara, which contains hepatotoxic lantadenes, is an important cause of poisoning in cattle and sheep in Australia, India, Mexico, and the United States. The shrub occurs commonly in many tropical and subtropical regions of the world and it may be consumed in large amounts during periods of drought. The toxic syndrome is characterized by photosensitization, jaundice, rumen atony, and constipation. At necropsy, the carcass is icteric, the liver swollen and dark brown to black in color, and the gall bladder is distended. Enlarged kidneys and congested lungs may also be noted. Lantana poisoning with characteristic photosensitization has been reported to occur in goats in coastal eastern Australia (Seawright 1984). A naturally occurring case in a Boer kid was reported from South Africa in which there was icterus, dehydration, and constipation but no photosensitization (Ide and Tutt 1998). Attempts to reproduce the disease experimentally in goats caused hepatotoxicity with jaundice and some deaths, but no photosensitization in one study (Lin et al. 1985) and no clinical signs at all except loss of appetite in another (Lal and Kalra 1960). More recently an experimental challenge in India produced both jaundice and photosensitization (Ali et al. 1995). Additional documentation and description of field outbreaks in goats would be useful.

Pyrrolizidine alkaloid toxicity

In contrast with cattle and horses, but similarly to sheep, goats are relatively resistant to pyrrolizidine alkaloid toxicosis commonly associated with ingestion of *Senecio* spp., *Crotalaria* spp., and *Heliotropium* spp. of plants. This resistance is not absolute, but dose-dependent. Experimentally, signs and lesions typical of pyrrolizidine alkaloid toxicity were produced in goats by prolonged feeding of tansy ragwort *(S. jacobaea)* at total doses of 125% to 400% of bw, compared with lethal doses in horses and cattle of 5% to 20% of bw (Goeger et al. 1982). Experimental challenge of goats with *Crotalaria saltiana* (Barri et al. 1984) and *Heliotropium ovalifolium* (Abu Damir et al. 1982) have also been reported. While toxicity was produced in both cases, hepatic lesions consistent with pyrrolizidine alkaloid toxicity, namely megalocytosis, biliary hyperplasia, portal fibrosis, and veno-occlusive disease, were absent or scarce. The toxic effects in goats challenged with these plants were presumed to be caused by toxic constituents other than pyrrolizidine alkaloids.

It is unlikely that under normal grazing conditions, goats would eat sufficient amounts of *Senecio* during the period of availability of the plant to produce severe, fatal, clinical disease. However, some hepatotoxicity can occur with chronic consumption and may impair growth and production. The use of goats and sheep to clear *Senecio longilobus* and *S. spartoides* from Texas rangeland to make it safe for cattle has been recommended (Dollahite 1972).

Even though goats may not become ill from long-term consumption of plants containing pyrrolizidine alkaloids, these hepatotoxins can be passed into the milk. Rats fed milk from goats receiving a ration containing 25% tansy ragwort developed liver lesions characteristic of pyrrolizidine alkaloid toxicosis, though calves did not (Goeger et al. 1982a). Human poisoning by such a mechanism of relay toxicity from goat milk has not been reported.

Miscellaneous Plant Poisonings

A large body of research on plant poisonings in goats comes from the Sudan. The plants have been evaluated because they are commonly suspected to be involved in natural outbreaks of livestock poisoning, often under drought conditions. Plants found in the Sudan that were demonstrated experimentally to be hepatotoxic to goats include *Heliotropium ovalifolium* (Abu Damir et al. 1982), *Crotalaria saltiana* (Barri et al. 1984), *Acanthospermum hispidum* (Ali and Adam 1978), *Jatropha aceroides, J. glauca, Solanum dubium, Lagenaria siceraria, Citrullus colocynthis* (Barri et al. 1983), *Aristolochia bracteata, Cadaba rotundifolia* (El Dirdiri et al. 1987), *Ipomoea carnea* (Abu Damir et al. 1987), *Indigofera hochstetteri* (Suliman et al. 1983), *Capparis tomentosa* (Ahmed and Adam 1980), and *Tephrosia apollinea* (Suliman et al. 1982).

In Brazil, extracts of the fruit of *Sessea brasiliensis* caused anorexia, incoordination, hyperexcitability, opisthotonos and death in goats within twenty-eight to ninety-two hours. Centrilobular necrosis and fatty degeneration of the liver were observed at necropsy. *Vernonia mollissima*, another Brazilian plant toxic to sheep and cattle, produced depression, staggering gait, recumbency with paddling, and death within fifty-five hours when fed to goats. Hepatic necrosis and renal damage were the predominant necropsy findings (Dobereiner et al. 1987).

In New Zealand, *Vestia foetida* (Solanaceae) was reported to have caused severe periacinar necrosis and fatty change in the liver. Two young goats were observed consuming the plant. Following consumption the goats had clinical signs of mydriasis, loss of menace response, ataxia, muscle fasciculations, recumbency, and malodorous breath indicative of the crushed leaves of the plant. One responded to treatment with diazepam and vitamins and the other died. Necropsy revealed the liver lesions as well as fatty nephrosis (McKeough et al. 2005).

Hepatotoxicity has been observed in goats and cattle in Western Australia eating the leaves of *Myoporum* spp., including the Boobialla tree and Ellangowan poison bush. The toxic principle is a furanoid sesquiterpene essential oil that produces midzonal and centrilobular necrosis of the liver (Allen et al. 1978). Clinical signs include photosensitization, hemorrhage, dyspnea, and death.

Other sporadic causes of hepatogenous photosensitization reported in goats include kleingrass (*Panicum* spp.) in the United States (Smith 1981) and signal grass *(Brachiaria decumbens)* in Nigeria (Opasina 1985) and Malaysia (Mazni et al. 1985).

The indolizidine alkaloids present in *Oxytropis* species can cause liver damage with vacuolation of liver observed histologically (Li et al. 2005). The clinical effects of *Oxytropis* spp. consumption are discussed in more detail in Chapter 5 relative to locoism.

Fungal and Mycotoxic Causes of Toxic Hepatitis

In South Africa, hepatotoxicity with photosensitization has been caused by a mycotoxin of the fungus *Drechslera campanulata* found growing on green oats (*Avena sativa*) grazed by Boer goats. Clinical signs developed within eight days of the onset of grazing and included photodermatitis with edema of the head, diarrhea, and a 3.5% mortality rate (Schneider et al. 1985).

Aflatoxicosis has been reported in Sri Lanka in young goats receiving a concentrate supplement containing coconut meal contaminated with *Aspergillus flavus*. Clinical cases were observed over a seven-month period and mortality rate was high. Jaundice was the most prominent sign, accompanied by lethargy, anorexia, a serous nasal discharge, and hypothermia terminally after a course of five to seven days. The livers were firm, congested, and fibrosed, and the gallbladder distended with tarry bile. There was biliary hyperplasia and periportal fibrosis microscopically. Similar findings have been reproduced experimentally in goats (Samarajeewa et al. 1975; Miller et al. 1984). Decreased milk production has been demonstrated in aflatoxicosis and is correlated with the dosage of aflatoxin fed to goats (Hassan et al. 1985).

"Hard yellow liver" or hepatic fatty cirrhosis is a sporadic disease of grazing goats, sheep, cattle, and deer in west and south Texas causing chronic weight loss, neurologic signs, and terminal hepatic coma. At necropsy there is hepatic lipidosis and cirrhosis (Bailey 1985). The definitive cause is unknown. It was hypothesized that a mycotoxin, roridin A, extracted from *Phomopsis* fungus growing on grasses in endemic regions was responsible for the disease (Samples et al. 1984). However, administration of purified roridin A to sheep for sixty days failed to produce liver lesions typical of the disease (Thormahlen et al. 1994), and the etiology remains unclear. The epizootiologic and clinical features of the condition have been reviewed (Helman et al. 1993).

The hepatic form of lupinosis, a mycotoxicosis associated with *Diaporthe toxica* (formerly *Phomopsis leptostromiformis)* fungus on lupine plants, is an important disease of cattle and sheep in Europe, South Africa, and Australia. It has been produced experimentally in goats, but natural occurrence is poorly documented (Marasas 1974).

NEOPLASTIC DISEASES

Hepatic neoplasms are rare in goats. Two cases of hepatocellular carcinoma have been reported. One was an incidental finding from a four-year-old Angora goat detected during meat inspection (Rousseaux 1984). The other was in a ten-year-old Nubian male presenting in a thin and moribund state. This goat had a pheochromocytoma and a leiomyoma in addition to the hepatocellular carcinoma, and attribution of clinical signs to the liver tumor would be difficult (Lairmore et al. 1987). A case of primary hepatic fibrosarcoma has been reported in a Toggenburg goat (Higgins et al. 1985). Two cases of bile duct carcinoma have also been reported in goats, with metastases to the lungs (Chauhan and Singh 1969; Paikne 1970). One case presented with weight loss and ascites, the other was an incidental finding at slaughter. Two additional cases of malignant cholangiocarcinoma in goats without metastases have been reported (Rodriguez et al. 1996; Domínguez et al. 2001) as well as one benign cholangioma identified in a healthy-appearing goat during slaughter inspection (Puette and Hafner 1995). Lymphosarcoma has been identified in both diffuse and nodular forms in the livers of affected goats at necropsy (Craig et al. 1986).

DIABETES MELLITUS

There is one report of diabetes mellitus in a pygmy goat secondary to a hyperplastic pars distalis of the pituitary gland. It was hypothesized that the abnormal pituitary was excreting excessive amounts of growth hormone which led to permanent stimulation of the insulin-producing islet cells of the pancreas, resulting in their exhaustion and degeneration and the associated clinical manifestation of diabetes mellitus. The affected goat showed chronic, pronounced weight loss, polydipsia, polyuria, hyperglycemia, glucosuria, and ketonuria. Fasting insulin concentration was 5.5 μIU/ml as compared to a normal level of 45 ± 9 μIU/ml in healthy goats (Lutz et al. 1994).

There is one other report of diabetes mellitus in a goat of unknown cause (Akdoğan Kaymaz et al. 2001). Otherwise, the disease is considered rare in this species, though diabetes mellitus has been induced in goats experimentally using alloxan (Schwalm 1975; Prasad et al. 1985; Kaul and Prasad 1990) or streptozotocin (Cheema et al. 2000; Rubina Mushtaq and Cheema 2001).

REFERENCES

Abbot, K.A., Taylor, M.A. and Stubbings, L.A.: Sustainable Worm Control Strategies for Sheep. A Technical Manual for Veterinary Surgeons and Advisors. National Sheep Association, Worcestershire, UK, pp. 34–36, 2004.

Abdelsalam, E.B., Adam, S.E.I. and Tartour, G.: Modification of the hepatotoxicity of carbon tetrachloride and chloroform in goats by pre-treatment with dieldrin and phenobarbitone. Zbl. Vet. Med. A., 29:142–148, 1982.

Abu Damir, H., Adam, S.E.I. and Tartour, G.: The effects of *Heliotropium ovalifolium* on goats and sheep. Br. Vet. J., 138:463–472, 1982.

Abu Damir, H., Adam, S.E.I. and Tartour, G.: The effects of *Ipomoea carnea* on goats and sheep. Vet. Hum. Toxicol., 29:316–319, 1987.

Adam, S.E.I., Obeid, H.M., Ashour, N. and Tartour, G.: Serum enzyme activities and haematology of normal and diseased ruminants in the Sudan. Acta Vet. Brno., 43:225–231, 1974.

Ahmed, O.M.M. and Adam, S.E.I.: The toxicity of *Capparis tomentosa* in goats. J. Comp. Pathol., 90:187–195, 1980.

Akdoğan Kaymaz, A., Bakirel, U., Gürel, A. and Tan, H.: Idiopathic diabetes mellitus in a goat. Istanbul Univ. Vet. Fac. Derg., 27(1):7–12, 2001.

Akinboade, O.A. and Ajiboye, A.: Studies on cysticercosis of small ruminants in Nigeria. Int. J. Zoon., 10:164–166, 1983.

Al-Afaleq, A.I., Abu Elzein, E.M.E., Mousa, S.M. and Abbas, A. M.: A retrospective study of Rift Valley fever in Saudi Arabia. Rev. Sci. Tech. Off. Int. Epiz., 22(3): 867–871, 2003.

Ali, B. and Adam, S.E.I.: Effects of *Acanthospermum hispidum* on goats. J. Comp. Pathol., 88:533–544, 1978.

Ali, B.H. and Abu Samra, M.T.: Some clinico-pathological observations in Nubian goats treated with ivermectin. Rev. Élev. Méd. Vét. Pays. Trop., 40:141–145, 1987.

Ali, M.K., Pramanik, A.K., Guha, C. and Mitra, M.: Clinical and haematological studies in *Lantana camara* poisoning in goats. Indian Vet. J. 72(12):1262–1264, 1995.

Allen, J.G., Seawright, A.A. and Hrdlicka, J.: The toxicity of *Myoporum tetrandrum* (Boobialla) and myoporaceous furanoid essential oils for ruminants. Aust. Vet. J., 54:287–292, 1978.

Al-Qarawi, A.A. and Ali, B.H.: Variations in the normal activity of esterases in plasma and liver of camels (*Camelus dromedarius*), cattle (*Bos indicus*), sheep (*Ovis aries*) and goats (*Capra hircus*). J. Vet. Med. A 50:201–203, 2003.

Al-Yaman, F.M., Assaf, L., Hailat, N. and Abdel-Hafez, S.K.: Prevalence of hydatidosis in slaughtered animals from North Jordan. Ann. Trop. Med. Parasitol., 79:501–506, 1985.

Amjadi, A.R., Ahourai, P. and Baharsefat, M.: First report of geeldikkop in sheep in Iran. Acrh. Inst. Razi., 29:71–78, 1977.

Anwar, M. and Chaudhri, A.Q.: Incidence of fascioliasis in sheep and goats of Faisalabad. Pak. Vet. J., 4:35–36, 1984.

Anyamba, A., et al.: Mapping potential risk of Rift Valley fever outbreaks in African savannas using vegetation index time series data. Photogrammetric Eng. Remote Sens., 68(2):137–145, 2002.

Anyamba, A., et al.: Rift Valley fever potential, Arabian peninsula. Emerg. Inf. Dis., 12(3):518–520, 2006.

Aslani, M.R., et al.: Experimental *Tribulus terrestris* poisoning in goats. Small Rumin. Res., 51:261–267, 2004.

Assoku, R.K.G.: Studies of parasitic helminths of sheep and goats in Ghana. Bull. Anim. Health Prod. Afr., 29:1–10, 1981.

Bailey, E.M.: Hepatic fatty cirrhosis (hard yellow liver) of domestic and wild ruminants. Proc. Australia-USA poisonous plant symposium. Brisbane, May 14–18. Yeerongpilly, Queensland, Australia, Animal Research Institute. 1985. pp. 541–549, 1984.

Bailey, E.M.: Principal poisonous plants in the southwestern United States. In: Current Veterinary Therapy, Food Animal Practice, 2nd Ed. J.L. Howard, ed. Philadelphia, W.B. Saunders Co., pp. 412–420, 1986.

Barnard, B.J.H.: Wesselsbron disease. In: Current Veterinary Therapy, Food Animal Practice, 2nd Ed. J.L. Howard, ed. Philadelphia, W.B. Saunders Co., pp. 520–521, 1986.

Barri, M.E.S., Adam, S.E.I. and Omer, O.H.: Effects of *Crotalaria saltiana* on Nubian goats. Vet. Hum. Toxicol., 26:476–480, 1984.

Barri, M.E.S., et al.: Toxicity of five Sudanese plants to young ruminants. J. Comp. Pathol., 93:559–575, 1983.

Bassir, O. and Bababunmi, E.A.: Liver function and histology in various species of animal treated with non-lethal doses of aflatoxin B_1. J. Pathol., 108:85–90, 1972.

Belford, C.J. and Raven, C.R.: Chronic copper poisoning in Angora kids. Surveillance, N.Z., 13:4–5, 1986.

Bendezu, P., et al.: *Fasciola hepatica* and other helminths in goats in Puerto Rico. J. Agri. Univ. Puerto Rico, 67:501–506, 1983.

Bennett, D.G., Block, R.D. and Gerone, P.J.: Protection of mice and lambs against pantropic Rift Valley fever virus using immune serum. Am. J. Vet. Res., 26:57–61, 1965.

Black, H., Hutton, J.B., Sutherland, R.J. and James, M.P.: White liver disease in goats. N. Z. Vet. J., 36:15–17, 1988.

Boray, J.C.: Flukes of domestic animals. In: Parasites, Pests and Predators. S.M. Gaafar, W.E. Howard, and R.E. Marsh, eds. Amsterdam, Elsevier, 1985.

Brikas, P. and Tsiamitas, C.: Anatomic arrangement of the hepatic veins in the goat. Am. J. Vet. Res., 41:796–797, 1980.

Campano, S.: The presence of parasites in goats in Chile, 1977–1985. Proc. IV International Conf. Goats, Brasilia, EMBRAPA-DDT, p. 1355, 1987.

Campos Ruelas, R., et al.: Valoracion de la efectividad del MK-990 (Rafoxanide) en la fasciolasis y hemoncosis caprina. Tec. Pec. Mex., 30:76–79, 1976.

Carrigan, J.J., Links, I.J. and Morton, A.G.: *Rhodococcus equi* infection in goats. Australian Vet. J., 65:331–332, 1988.

Castro, A., et al.: Serum biochemistry values in normal pygmy goats. Am. J. Vet. Res., 38:2085–2087, 1977.

Chambers, P.G.: Carcass condemnations of communal goats at meat inspection in Zimbabwe. Zimb. Vet. J., 21(1):44–45.1990.

Charan, K. and Iyer, P.K.R.: The occurrence of *Fasciola gigantica* in the kidney of a goat *(Capra hircus).* Indian Vet. J., 49:1062–1063, 1972.

Chauhan, H.V. and Singh, C.M.: Bile duct carcinoma in a goat with metastasis in the lungs. Indian Vet. J., 46:945–947, 1969.

Cheema, A.M., Sadya Javaid and Rubina Mushtaq: Streptozotocin induced hypoinsulinaemia on structural aspects of thyroid gland in dwarf goat. Punjab Univ. J. Zool., 15:161–170, 2000.

Chevis, R.A.F.: Internal parasites of goats and their control. In: Proceedings, Refresher Course for Veterinarians, Post-Graduate Committee in Veterinary Science, University of Sydney, 52:179–186, 1980.

Chongti, T. and Tongmin, L.: Investigations on eurytremosis of cattle and goats in mountainous regions of North Fujian. Acta Zool. Sin., 26:42–51, 1980.

Clark, J.D., Hatch, R.C., Miller, D.M. and Jain, A.V.: Caprine aflatoxicosis: experimental disease and clinical pathologic changes. Am. J. Vet. Res., 45:1132–1135, 1984.

Coetzer, J.A.W. and Theodoridis, A.: Clinical and pathological studies in adult sheep and goats experimentally infected with Wesselsbron disease virus. Onderstepoort J. Vet. Res., 49:19–22, 1982.

Coles, G.C., et al.: The detection of anthelmintic resistance in nematodes of veterinary importance. Vet. Parasitol., 136:167–185, 2006.

Conboy, G.A., Stromberg, B.E. and Schlotthauer, J.C.: Efficacy of clorsulon against *Fascioloides magna* infection in sheep. J. Am. Vet. Med. Assoc., 192:910–912, 1988.

Cornelissen, J.B.W.J., et al: Early immunodiagnosis of fasciolosis in ruminants using recombinant *Fasciola hepatica* cathepsin L-like protease. Int. J. Parasitol., 31(7):728–737, 2001.

Cornelius, C.F.: Liver function. In: Clinical Biochemistry of Domestic Animals, 3rd Ed. J.J. Kaneko, ed. New York, Academic Press, 1980.

Cornish, J., et al.: Copper toxicosis in a dairy goat herd. J. Am. Vet. Med. Assoc., 231(4):586–589, 2007.

Craig, D.R., Roth, L. and Smith, M.C.: Lymphosarcoma in goats. Comp. Cont. Educ. Pract. Vet., 8:S190–S197, 1986.

Dacasto, M., et al.: Effect of breed and gender on bovine liver cytochrome P450 3A (CYP3A) expression and inter-species comparison with other domestic ruminants. Vet. Res., 36:179–190, 2005.

Dalton, J.P. and Mulcahy, G.: Parasite vaccines—a reality? Vet. Parasitol., 98:149–167, 2001.

Dalvi, R.R., Nunn, V.A. and Juskevich, J.: Hepatic cytochrome P-450 dependent drug metabolizing activity in rats, rabbits and several food-producing species. J. Vet. Pharmacol. Ther., 10:164–168, 1987.

Das S.K. and Misra, S.K.: Liver function in experimental rumen acidosis in goats. Indian J. Anim. Sci., 62(3):243–244, 1992.

Davies, F.G.: Risk of a Rift Valley fever epidemic at the haj in Mecca, Saudi Arabia Rev. Sci. Tech. Off. Int. Epiz., 25(1):137–147, 2006.

Devillard, J.P. and Villemin, P.: Treatment of dicrocoeliasis in the goat with diamphenethide. Bull. Mensual Soc. Vet. Prat. Fr., 60:563–577, 1976.

Diteko, T., Winnen, G.M. and Manth, L.M.: Isolations of *Rhodococcus (Corynebacterium) equi* from goats in Botswana. Zimbabwe Vet. J., 19:11–15, 1988.

Dobereiner, J., Stolf, L. and Tokarnia, C.H.: Poisonous plants affecting goats. Proc. IV International Conf. Goats, Brasilia, EMBRAPA-DDT, pp. 473–487, 1987.

Dollahite, J.W.: The use of sheep and goats to control *Senecio* poisoning in cattle. Southwest Vet., 25:223–226, 1972.

Domínguez, M.C., Chávez, G., Trigo, F.J. and Rosales, M.L.: Concurrent cholangiocarcinoma, peritonitis, paratuberculosis, and aspergillosis in a goat. Can. Vet. J., 42:884–885, 2001.

Eamens, G.J., Turner, M.J. and Catt, R.E.: Serotypes of *Erysipelothrix rhusiopathiae* in Australian pigs, small ruminants, poultry, and captive wild birds and animals. Aust. Vet. J., 65:249–252, 1988.

Easterday, B.C., Murphy, L.C. and Bennett, D.G.: Experimental Rift Valley fever in calves, goats and pigs. Am. J. Vet. Res., 23:1224–1230, 1962.

El Dirdiri, N.I., Barakat, S.E.M. and Adam, S.E.I.: The combined toxicity of *Aristolochia bracteata* and *Cadaba rotundifolia* to goats. Vet. Hum. Toxicol., 29:133–137, 1987.

El Moukdad, A.R.: Occurrence of helminths among goats in Syria. Berl. Munch. Tierärzttiche Wschr., 94:85–87, 1981.

El Sanhouri, A.A., Haroun E.M., Gameel, A.A. and Bushara, H.O.: Protective effect of irradiated metacercariae of *Fasciola gigantica* and irradiated cercariae of *Schistosoma bovis* against fascioliasis in goats. Trop. Anim. Health Prod., 19:245–249, 1987.

Eltom, S.E., Babish, J.G. and Schwark, W.S.: The postnatal development of drug-metabolizing enzymes in hepatic, pulmonary and renal tissues of the goat. J. Vet. Pharm. Ther., 16(2):152–163, 1993.

Everett, G. and de Gruchy, P.H.: Hepatic cysticercosis. Vet. Rec., 111:565, 1982.

Fabiyi, J.P.: An investigation into the incidence of goat helminth parasites in the Zaria area of Nigeria. Bull. Epiz. Dis. Afr., 18:29–34, 1970.

FAO: Possible RVF activity in the Horn of Africa. EMPRES Watch, November, 2006, pp. 1–7. http://www.fao.org/docs/eims/upload/217874/EW_hornafrica_nov06_rvf.pdf.

Fernandes, B.F. and Hamann, W.: Parasites of goats in Parana state. Arquiv. Biol. Technol., 28:597–599, 1985.

Fetcher, A.: Liver diseases of sheep and goats. Vet. Clin. North Am., Large Anim. Pract., 5:525–538, 1983.

Fetcher, A.: Halothane-associated hepatotoxicity in a young goat. Agri-Practice, 6(5):30–32, 1985.

Foreyt, W.J.: Efficacy and safety of albendazole against experimentally induced *Fasciola hepatica* infection in goats. Vet. Parasitol., 26:261–264, 1988.

Foreyt, W.J.: Evaluation of clorsulon against immature *Fascioloides magna* in cattle and sheep. Am. J. Vet. Res., 49:1004–1006, 1988a.

Foreyt, W.J. and Foreyt, K.M.: Albendazole treatment of experimental induced *Fascioloides magna* infection in goats. Vet. Med. Small Anim. Clin., 75:1441–1444, 1980.

Foreyt, W.J. and Leathers, C.W.: Experimental infection of domestic goats with *Fascioloides magna.* Am. J. Vet. Res., 41:883–884, 1980.

Fuentes M.V., et al.: Analysis of climatic data and forecast indices for human fascioliasis at very high altitude. Ann. Trop. Med. Parasitol., 93(8):835–850, 1999.

Garnier, F., Benoit, E., Jacquet, J.P. and Delatour, P.: Blood enzymology in the goat: Usual values of CPK, LDH, ICDH, and SDH. Ann. Rech. Vét., 15:55–58, 1984.

Girardi, C., Lanfranchi, P., Abate, O. and Pau, S.: Severe outbreak of fascioliasis in a herd of goats. Ann. Fac. Med. Vet. Torino, 26:428–442, 1979.

Glastonbury, J.R.W. and Boal, G.K.: Geeldikkop in goats. Aust. Vet. J., 62:62–63, 1985.

Goeger, D.E., Cheeke, P.R., Schmitz, J.A. and Buhler, D.R.: Toxicity of tansy ragwort *(Senecio jacobaea)* to goats. Am. J. Vet. Res., 43:252–254, 1982.

Goeger, D.E., Cheeke, P.R., Schmitz, J.A. and Buhler, D.R.: Effect of feeding milk from goats fed tansy ragwort *(Senecio jacobaea)* to rats and calves. Am. J. Vet. Res., 43:1631–1633, 1982a.

Gonenci, R., et al.: Subclinical fatty liver syndrome in Damascus goats. Indian Vet. J., 80(8):739–742, 2003.

Hamid M.E., Mohamed, G.E., Abu Samra, M.T. and Hamad. A.A.: First report of infectious necrotic hepatitis (black disease) among Nubian goats in Sudan. Rev. Élev. Méd. Vét. Pays. Trop., 44(3):273–275, 1991.

Hanifa Moursi, S.A., Atef, M. and Al-Khayyat, A.A.: Hepatoxicity of chloramphenicol in normal goats by the assay of serum enzyme activity. Zbl. Vet. Med. A., 26:715–720, 1979.

Haroun, E.M., El Sanhouri, A.A. and Gameel, A.A.: Response of goats to repeated infections with *Fasciola gigantica.* Vet. Parasitol., 30:287–296, 1989.

Hassan, G.A., et al.: Effect of aflatoxins on milk yield, plasma cortisol and blood haematological characteristics in lactating goats. Indian J. Anim. Sci., 55:5–10, 1985.

Helman, R.G., Adams, L.G. and Bridges, C.H.: Hepatic fatty cirrhosis in ruminants from western Texas. J. Am. Vet. Med. Assoc., 202(1):129–132, 1993.

Higgins, R.J., Rae, A. and Abraham, A.: Primary hepatic fibrosarcoma in a Toggenburg goat. Vet. Rec., 116:444, 1985.

Hughes, D.L., Treacher, R.J. and Harness, E.: Plasma enzyme changes in goats infected with *Fasciola hepatica* and the effect of nitroxynil. Res. Vet. Sci., 15:249–255, 1973.

Hughes, D.L., Treacher, R.J. and Harness, E.: The anthelmintic activity of diamphenethide against immature *Fasciola hepatica* in goats and the course of experimental infections as demonstrated by plasma enzyme changes. Res. Vet. Sci., 17:302–311, 1974.

Humann-Ziehank, E., Bruegmann, M. and Ganter, M.: Hepatoencephalopathy in a goat: clinical manifestation of an intrahepatic porto-systemic shunt. Small Rumin. Res., 42(2):157–162, 2001.

Humphries, W.R., Morrice, P.C. and Mitchell, A.N.: Copper poisoning in Angora goats. Vet. Rec., *121*:231, 1987.

Ide, A. and Tutt, C.L.C.: Acute *Lantana camara* poisoning in a Boer goat kid. J. S. Afr. Vet. Assoc. 69(1):30–32, 1998.

Jacob, R.H. and Peet, R.L.: Poisoning of sheep and goats by *Tribulis terrestris* (caltrop). Aust. Vet. J., 64:288–289, 1987.

Jimenez-Albarran, M. and Guevara-Pozo, D.: Experimental studies on the biology of *Fasciola hepatica:* I. Number and viability of *Fasciola hepatica* recovered from the bile ducts of cattle, sheep and goats. Rev. Iber. Parasitol., 37:291–300, 1977.

Johnson, E.H., Muirhead, D.E., Annamalai, K., King, G.J., Al-Busaidy, R. and Hameed, M.S.: Hepatic lipidosis associated with cobalt deficiency in Omani goats. Vet. Res. Commun. 23(4): 215–221, 1999.

Jones, B.-E.V. and Shah, M.: Clinico-chemical changes in goats given carbon tetrachloride. Nord. Vet. Med., 34:25–32, 1982.

Jost, C.: Personal communication, Dr. Christine Jost, Research Scientist, International Livestock Research Institute, Nairobi, Kenya, 2007.

Kaneko, J.J.: Appendixes. In: Clinical Biochemistry of Domestic Animals. 3rd Ed. J.J. Kaneko, ed. New York, Academic Press, 1980.

Katayama, K.: Ammonia metabolism and hepatic encephalopathy. Hepatol. Res., 30 (Suppl.):S71-S78, 2004.

Kaul, P.L. and Prasad, M.C.: Effect of alloxan diabetes on experimental atherosclerosis in goats. Indian J. Anim. Sci., 60(8): 933–938, 1990.

Kellerman, T.S., et al.: Photosensitivity in South Africa. II. The experimental production of the ovine hepatogenous photosensitivity disease geeldikkop (tribulosis ovis) by the simultaneous ingestion of *Tribulus terrestris* plants and cultures of *Pithomyces chartarum* containing the mycotoxin sporidesmin. Onderstepoort J. Vet. Res., 47:231–261, 1980.

Kellerman, T.S., et al.: Photosensitivity in South Africa. VI. The experimental induction of geeldikkop (photosensitive dermatitis) in sheep with crude steroidal saponins from *Tribulus terrestris*. Onderstepoort J. Vet. Res., 58(1):47–53, 1991.

Kimberling, C.V.: Jensen and Swift's Diseases of Sheep, 3rd Ed. Philadelphia, Lea and Febiger, 1988.

King, N.B.: Clostridial diseases. In: Proceedings, Refresher Course for Veterinarians, Post-Graduate Committee in Veterinary Science, University of Sydney, 52:217–219, 1980.

Koko, W.S., Galal, M. and Khalid, H.S.: Fasciolicidal efficacy of *Albizia anthelmintica* and *Balanites aegyptiaca* compared with albendazole. J. Ethnopharmacol. 71(1–2):247–52, 2000.

Kono, I., et al.: The pathological studies on anthelmintic effects of praziquantel and triclabendazole against *Eurytrema coelomaticum* in experimentally infected goats. Bull. Fac. Agric. Iwate Univ., 36:183–190, 1986.

Kramer, J.W. and Carthew, G.C.: Serum and tissue enzyme profiles of goats. N. Z. Vet. J., 33:91–93, 1985.

Ksiazek, T.G., et al.: Rift Valley fever among domestic animals in the recent West African outbreak. Res. Virol., 140:67–77, 1989.

Lairmore, M.D., Knight, A.P., and DeMartini, J.C.: Three primary neoplasms in a goat: Hepatocellular carcinoma, phaeochromocytoma and leiomyoma. J. Comp. Pathol., 97:267–271, 1987.

Lal, M. and Kalra, D.B.: Lantana poisoning in domesticated animals. Indian Vet. J., 37:265–269, 1960.

Lal, S.B., Sharma, M.C. and Pandey, N.N.: Utility of bromosulphophthalein per cent retention test in acidotic goats for diagnosing liver disorder. Indian J. Anim. Sci., 61(1):69–70, 1991.

Lancelot, R., et al.: Épidémiologie descriptive de la fièvre de la vallée du Rift chez les petits ruminants dans le Sud de la Mauritanie après l'hivernage. Rev. Élev. Méd. Vét. Pays. Trop., 42:485–491, 1989.

Leathers, C.W., Foreyt, W.J., Fetcher, A. and Foreyt, K.M.: Clinical fascioliasis in domestic goats in Montana. J. Am. Vet. Med. Assoc., 180:1451–1454, 1982.

Lee, C.G., Cho, S.H., Kim, J.T. and Lee, C.Y.: Efficacy of closantel against *Fasciola hepatica* in Korean native goats. Vet. Parasitol., 65(3/4):307–311, 1996.

Li, Q.F. et al.: The test of *Oxytropis glacialis* poisoning in goats. Chinese J. Vet. Sci., 25(5):511–513, 2005.

Li, W.X. and Li, Z.S.: The treatment of distomiasis and *Cysticercus tenuicollis* in sheep and goats with praziquantel. Chin. J. Vet. Med., 12:6–8, 1986.

Liakos, D.V.: Epidemiological survey of parasitoses of sheep and goats. Ellenike Kteniatrike, 28:271–278, 1985.

Lightowlers, M.W., et al.: Vaccination against cysticercosis and hydatid disease. Parasitol. Today, 16(5):191–196, 2000.

Lightowlers, M.W.: Vaccination against hydatid disease. Dev. Biol., 110:81–87, 2002.

Lin, S.C., et al.: Studies on the hepatogenous photosensitization of cattle in Taiwan. IV. Experimental *Lantana camara* poisoning in white Taiwan native hybrid goats. Taiwan J. Vet. Med. Anim. Husb., 45:81–91, 1985.

Linthicum, K.J., et al.: Climate and satellite indicators to forecast Rift Valley fever epidemics in Kenya. Science, 285(5426):397–400, 1999.

Lone, T.K., Prasad, G. and Sinha, R.D.: Histological studies on the exocrine pancreas of goat *(Capra hircus)*. Indian Vet. J., 66:333–335, 1989.

Lorenzini, R. and Ruggieri, A.: Distribution of echinococcosis/hydatidosis in Italy. J. Helminthol., 61:261–267, 1987.

Lukens, F.D.W.: Pancreatectomy in the goat. Am. J. Physiol., 122:729–733, 1938.

Lutz, T.A., Rossi, R., Caplazi, P. and Ossent, P.: Secondary diabetes mellitus in a pygmy goat. Vet. Rec., 135:93, 1994.

Maddison, J.E.: Hepatic encephalopathy: Current concepts of the pathogenesis. J. Vet. Internal Med., 6:341–353, 1992.

Mahato, S.N.: A fatal case of *Eurytrema cladorchis* infection in a goat in Nepal. Indian J. Anim. Sci., 57:1103–1104, 1987.

Malone, J B. and Zukowski, S.H.: Geographic models and control of cattle liver flukes in the southern USA. Parasitology Today, 8:266–270, 1992.

Manas-Almendros, I., et al.: Frequency in dicrocoeliasis among cattle, sheep and goats in Granada province, Spain. Rev. Iberica Parasitol., 38:751–773, 1978.

Marasas, W.F.O.: *Phomopsis leptostromiformis.* In: Mycotoxins. I.F.H. Purchase, ed. Amsterdam, Elsevier Sci. Publ. Co., pp. 111–127, 1974.

Mathews, F.P.: Lechuguilla *(Agave lecheguilla)* poisoning in sheep, goats and laboratory animals. Texas Agric. Exp. Sta. Bull., 554, 1937.

Mathews, F.P.: The toxicity of *Sartwellia flaveriae* to goats. J. Agric. Res., 61:287–292, 1940.

Mathews, F.P.: Poisoning in sheep and goats by sacahuiste *(Nolina texana)* buds and blooms. Bull. Tex. Agric. Exp. Sta., 585:5–19, 1940a.

Mathews, F.P.: The toxicity of a spurge *(Phyllanthus abnormis)* for cattle, sheep, and goats. Cornell Vet., 35:336–346, 1945.

Mazni, O.A., Sharif, H., Khusahry, M.Y.M. and Vance, H.N.: Photosensitization in goats grazed on *Brachiaria decumbens.* MARDI Res. Bull. (Malaysia), 13:203–206, 1985.

McDonough, S.P., et al.: Hepatogenous photosensitization of sheep in California associated with ingestion of *Tribulus terrestris* (puncture vine). J. Vet. Diagn. Invest., 6(3):392–395, 1994.

McEwen, M.M., et al.: Hepatic effects of halothane and isoflurane anesthesia in goats. J. Am. Vet. Med. Assoc., 217(11):1697–1700, 2000.

McKenzie, R.A., Green, P.E., Thornton, A.M. and Blackall, P.J.: Feral goats and infectious disease: An abattoir survey. Aust. Vet. J., 55:441–442, 1979.

McKeough, V.L., Collett, M.G. and Parton, K.H.: Suspected *Vestia foetida* poisoning in young goats. N.Z. Vet. J., 53: 5, 352–355, 2005.

Mezo, J., González-Warleta, M. and Ubeira, F.M.: Optimized serodiagnosis of sheep fascioliasis by fast-d protein liquid chromatography fractionation of *Fasciola hepatica* excretory-secretory antigens. J. Parasitol., 89(4):843–849, 2003.

Miller, D.M., Clark, J.D., Hatch, R.C. and Jain, A.V.: Caprine aflatoxicosis: serum electrophoresis and pathologic changes. Am. J. Vet. Res., 45:1136–1141, 1984.

Molan, A.L. and Saeed, I.S.: A survey of hepatic and pulmonary helminths and cestode larval stages in goats and cows of Arbil Province. J. Agric. Water Resources Res. Anim. Prod., 7:105–114, 1988.

Moro, P.L. and Schantz, P.M. Echinococcosis: historical landmarks and progress in research and control. Ann. Trop. Med. Parasitol. 100(8): 703–714, 2006.

Naranjo, J.A., et al.: Surgical preparation for the study of pancreatic exocrine secretion in the conscious preruminant goat. Lab. Anim., 20:231–233, 1986.

Naus, A.H.: Diseases present in Chilean goats. Proc., 3rd Internat. Conf. Goat Prod. Disease. Scottsdale, AZ, Dairy Goat Journal Publishing Co., p. 343, 1982.

Njanja, J.C., Bell, J.F. and Wescott, R.B.: Apparent lack of toxicity in adult East African goats on parenterally administered ivermectin. Bull. Anim. Health Prod. Afr., 33:123–127, 1985.

Nooruddin, M., Baki, M.A. and Mondal, M.M.H.: Pathology of *Fasciola gigantica* infection in the livers of goats. Livestock Advisor, 12:43–45, 1987.

O'Brien, T.D., et al.: Hepatic necrosis following halothane anesthesia in goats. J. Am. Vet. Med. Assoc., 189:1591–1595, 1986.

Ogunrinade, A.F.: Infectivity and pathogenicity of *Fasciola gigantica* in West African Dwarf sheep and goats. Trop. Anim. Health Prod., 16:161–166, 1984.

OIE: Chapter 2.1.8., Rift Valley Fever. In: Manual of Diagnostic Tests and Vaccines for Terrestrial Animals, 5th Ed. Paris, Office International des Epizooties, 2004. http://www.oie.int/eng/normes/mmanual/A_00031.htm.

Ojo, M.O. et al.: Isolation of *Rhodococcus equi* from the liver abscess of a goat in Trinidad. Can. Vet. J. 34:504, 1993.

Olsen, O.W.: White-tailed deer as a reservoir host of the large American liver fluke. Vet. Med., 44:26–30, 1949.

Opasina, B.A.: Photosensitization jaundice syndrome in West African dwarf sheep and goats grazed on *Brachiaria decumbens.* Trop. Grasslands, 19:120–123, 1985.

Pachauri, S.P., Yadav, T.S. and Swarup, D.: Studies on the epidemiology and economic impact of fascioliasis in goat. Internat. J. Anim. Sci., 3:171–176, 1988.

Paikne, D.L.: Cholangiocellular carcinoma with pulmonary metastasis in goat. Indian Vet. J., 47:1043–1045, 1970.

Pandey, V.S.: Pathologic observations on echinococcosis due to *Echinococcus granulosus* in the goat and the dog. An. Med. Vet., 115:519–527, 1971.

Panebianco, A. and Santagada, G.: Plurivisceral candidiasis due to *Candida krusei* in a goat. Obiet. Document. Vet., 10:49–52, 1989.

Pathak, K.M.L. and Gaur, S.N.S.: Clinical signs associated with experimental *Cysticercus tenuicollis* infection in kids. Haryana Vet., 20:22–23, 1981.

Pathak, K.M.L. and Gaur, S.N.S.: Serum levels of GOT, GPT, and OCT enzymes in goats infected with *Cysticercus tenuicollis.* Vet. Parasitol., *8*:95–97, 1981a.

Patterson, D.S.P. and Roberts, B.A.: The comparison of liver microsomes and levels of detoxicating enzymes in 9 animal species. Res. Vet. Sci., 11:399–401, 1970.

Pauling, B.A.: Clostridial diseases and vaccination of goats. Proc. 16th Seminar, Sheep and Beef Cattle Soc., N.Z. Vet. Assoc., Palmerston North, N.Z., pp. 56–72, 1986.

Paz-Silva, A., et al.: Isolation, identification and expression of a *Fasciola hepatica* cDNA encoding a 2.9-kDa recombinant protein for the diagnosis of ovine fasciolosis. Parasitol. Res., 95:129–135, 2005.

Pearson, A.B.: White liver disease and pestivirus in goat kids. Surveillance, N.Z., 14:21, 1987.

Prasad, M.C., Kaul, P.L. and Iyer, P.K.R.: Alloxan diabetes in goats: clinical and pathomorphological studies. Indian Vet. J., 62(10):832–836, 1985.

Puette, M. and Hafner, S.: Cholangioma in a goat. J. Vet. Diagn. Invest., 7:574–575, 1995.

Qadir, A.N.M.A.: Comparative anthelmintic efficiency of Acedist, a new compound and Bilevon against *Fasciola gigantica* infection in goats. Indian Vet. J., 56:429–431, 1979.

Qadir, A.N.M.A.: Anthelmintic efficiency of Acedist (bromophenophos), a new fasciolicide against immature *Fasciola gigantica* in goats. Indian Vet. J., 58:197–198, 1981.

Quittet, E. (ed.): La Chèvre. Guide de l'Éleveur. Paris, La Maison Rustique, 1980.

Rafyi, A. and Eslami, H.: *Fasciola* infections in Iran. Cahiers Med. Vet., 40:277–282, 1971.

Rahko, T.: Studies on the pathology of dicrocoeliaisis and fascioliasis in the goat. II. The histopathology of the liver and bile ducts. Acta Vet. Scand., 13:554–562, 1972.

Rahman, A., Ahmed, M.U. and Mia, A.S.: Diseases of goats diagnosed in slaughterhouses in Bangladesh. Trop. Anim. Health Prod., 7:164, 1975.

Rahman, M.H., Mondal, M.M.H. and Haq, S.: On the occurrence of *Linguatula serrata* in goats and cattle of Mymensingh District Bangladesh. Bangladesh Vet. J., 14:41–44, 1980.

Rajsky, D., et al.: Control of fascioloidosis (*Fascioloides magna* Bassi, 1875) in red deer and roe deer. Helminthologia, 39(2):67–70, 2002.

Reddington, J.J., Leid, R.W. and Westcott, R.B.: The susceptibility of the goat to *Fasciola hepatica* infections. Vet. Parasitol., 19:145–150, 1986.

Reddy, S. and Elliott, R.B.: Insulin, glucagon, pancreatic polypeptide hormone and somatostatin in the goat pancreas: Demonstration by immunocytochemistry. Aust. J. Biol. Sci., 38:59–66, 1985.

Ridoux, R., Siliart, B. and Andre, F.: Biochemical parameters of the milking goat. I. Determination of some reference values. Rec. Méd. Vét., 157:357–361, 1981.

Robinson, T.M. and Dunphy, J.E.: Effects of incomplete obstruction of the common bile duct. Arch. Surg., 83:18–26, 1961.

Robinson, T.M. and Dunphy, J.E.: An experimental study of the effect of pancreatic juice on the gall bladder. Gastroenterology, 42:36–47, 1962.

Rodríguez, F., et al.: Cholangiocarcinoma in a goat. Vet. Rec., 139:143–144, 1996.

Rousseaux, C.G.: Hepatocellular carcinoma in a goat. Aust. Vet. J., 61:193, 1984.

Rubin, J.L., et al.: Hepatic encephalopathy associated with paratuberculosis in a goat. J. Am. Vet. Med. Assoc., 215(2):236–238, 1999.

Rubina Mushtaq and Cheema, A.M.: Metabolite alterations in principal insulin target tissues following induced hypoinsulinaemia in male dwarf goats. Punjab Univ. J. Zool., 16:137–146, 2001.

Rudolph, W.G., Gonzalez V.A.M. and Contreras T.M.A.: Blood bile acid and cholesterol concentration before, during and after fasting in the goat. Avances en Ciencias Vet., 15(1/2):3–8, 2000.

Ruhr, L.P., Nicholson, S.S., Confer, A.W. and Blakewood, B. W.: Acute intoxication from a hematinic in calves. J. Am. Vet. Med. Assoc., 182:616–618, 1983.

Saad, A.D., Alencar-Filho, R.A. de., Andrada, S.O. and Aguiar, A.A.: Experimental *Sessea brasiliensis* poisoning of goats, sheep and pigeons. Rev. Med. Vet. São Paulo, 8:27–51, 1972.

Sall, A.A., et al.: Variability of the NS(S) protein among Rift Valley fever virus isolates. J. Gen. Virol., 78:2853–2858, 1997.

Samarajeewa, U., Arseculeratne, S.N. and Tennekoon, G.E.: Spontaneous and experimental aflatoxicosis in goats. Res. Vet. Sci., 19:269–277, 1975.

Samples, D., Hill, D.W., Bridges, C.H. and Camp, B.J.: Isolation of a mycotoxin (roridin A) from *Phomopsis* spp. Vet. Hum. Toxicol., 26:21–23, 1984.

Santa Rosa, J., Johnson, E.H., Alves, F.S.F. and Santos, L.F.L.: A retrospective study of hepatic abscesses in goats: Pathological and microbiological findings. Br. Vet. J., 145:73–76, 1989.

Sanyal, P.K. and Sinha, P.K.: Caprine metacestodiasis: Incidence in West Bengal. Haryana Vet., 22:38–40, 1983.

Sanz, F., et al.: An evaluation of the efficacy of netobimin against *Dicrocoelium dendriticum* in sheep. Vet. Rec., 120:57–58, 1987.

Schantz, P.M.: Progress in diagnosis, treatment and elimination of echinococcosis and cysticercosis. Parasitol. Int., 55:S7–S13, 2006.

Schillhorn van Veen, T.W., Folaranmi, D.O.B., Usman, S. and Ishaya, T.: Incidence of liver fluke infections (*Fasciola gigantica* and *Dicrocoelium hospes*) in ruminants in northern Nigeria. Trop. Anim. Health Prod., 12:97–104, 1980.

Schmidt, H.: Swellhead in sheep and goats. Texas Agric. Exp. Sta. Ann. Rept., 44:11, 1931.

Schneider, D.J., Marasas, W.F.O., Collett, M.G. and Van der Westhuizen, G.C.A.: An experimental mycotoxicosis in sheep and goats caused by *Drechslera campanulata,* a fungal pathogen of green oats. Onderstepoort J. Vet. Res., 52:93–100, 1985.

Schwalm, J.W. Insulin studies in ruminants with emphasis on ketosis in dairy cows and experimental diabetes in fed and fasted goats. Dissertation Abstracts International. 36B(3):992, 1975.

Seawright, A.A.: Goats and poisonous plants. In: Proceedings, Refresher Course for Veterinarians, Post-Graduate Committee in Veterinary Science, University of Sydney, 73:544–547, 1984.

Sen, M.M., Rahman, A. and Mia, A.S.: Liver function tests in goat. Indian Vet. J., 53:504–507, 1976.

Shahlapour, A.A., Rahnou, M.N. and Nazary, J.H.: Observations on the efficiency of thiabendazole, albendazole and brotianide against natural dicrocoeliasis in sheep and goats in Iran. Arch. Inst. Razi., 36, 37:63–68, 1986.

Shien, Y.S., Liu, J.J. and Huang, S.W.: Studies on eurytremiasis. I. Investigation on the infection status of eurytremes in cattle and goats as well as identification of flukes isolated in Taiwan. J. Chin. Soc. Vet. Sci., 4:35–39, 1978.

Shien, Y.S., Yang, P.C., Liu, J.J. and Huang, S.W.: Studies on eurytremiasis. II. Pathological study of the pancreas of cattle and goats naturally infected with *Eurytrema pancreaticum.* J. Chin. Soc. Vet. Sci., 5:133–138, 1979.

Shimizu, T., et al.: Hepatic and spinal lesions in goats chronically intoxicated with cycasin. Jpn. J. Vet. Sci., 48:1291–1295, 1986.

Singh, G.R., Setia, H.C., Pandey, N.N. and Mogha, I.V.: Cholecystography in goats. Indian J. Anim. Sci., 60:766–768, 1990.

Smith, M.C.: Caprine dermatologic problems: a review. J. Am. Vet. Med. Assoc., 178:724–729, 1981.

Soulsby, E.J.L.: Helminths, Arthropods, and Protozoa of Domesticated Animals, 7th Ed. Philadelphia, Lea and Febiger, 1982.

Sriraman, P. K., Rama Rao, P. and Gopal Naidu, N.R.: Goat mortality in Andhra Pradesh. Indian Vet. J., 59:96–99, 1982.

Stromberg, B.E., et al.: Activity of closantel against experimentally induced *Fascioloides magna* infection in sheep. Am. J. Vet. Res., 46:2527–2529, 1985.

Suh, M.D.: Anthelmintic efficacy of nitroxynil against *Fasciola hepatica, Eurytrema pancreaticum,* and *Paramphistomum* in Korean native goats. Korean J. Vet. Res., 23:199–203, 1983.

Suliman, H.B., Wasfi, I.A. and Adam, S.E.I.: The toxic effects of *Tephrosia apollinea* on goats. J. Comp. Pathol., 92:309–315, 1982.

Suliman, H.B., Wasfi, I.A., Tartour, G. and Adam, S.E.I.: The effects of *Indigofera hochstetteri* on goats. Rev. Élev. Méd. vét. Pays. Trop., 36:393–402, 1983.

Sundlof, S.F., et al.: Efficacy of clorsulon for the treatment of experimentally induced infections of *Fasciola hepatica* in goats. Am. J. Vet. Res., 52(1):111–114, 1991.

Swanepoel R., et al.: Comparative pathogenicity and antigenic cross-reactivity of Rift Valley fever and other African phleboviruses in sheep. J. Hyg. (Camb.), 97:331–346, 1986.

Szotáková, B., et al.: Comparison of *in vitro* activities of biotransformation enzymes in pig, cattle, goat and sheep. Res. Vet. Sci., 76(1):43–51, 2004.

Tager-Kagan, P.: Contribution à l'étude de la fasciolose au Niger. Rev. Élev. Méd. vét. Pays. trop., 31:437–442, 1978.

Tager-Kagan, P.: Dicrocoeliasis due to *Dicrocoelium hospes* in Niger. Rev. Élev. Méd. Vét. Pays. Trop., 32:53–55, 1979.

Tapia, M.O., Giordano, M.A. and Gueper, H.G.: An outbreak of hepatogenous photosensitization in sheep grazing *Tribulus terrestris* in Argentina. Vet. Hum. Toxicol. 36(4): 311–313, 1994.

Thamsborg, S.M., Jorgensen, R.J. and Brummerstedt, E.: Sawfly poisoning in sheep and goats. Vet. Rec., 121:253–255, 1987.

Theodoridis, A. and Coetzer, J.A.W.: Wesselsbron disease: Virological and serological studies in experimentally infected sheep and goats. Onderstepoort J. Vet. Res., 47:221–229, 1980.

Thompson, K.G.: Some diseases of importance in goats as seen by animal health laboratories. Proc. 16th Seminar, Sheep and Beef Cattle Soc., N.Z. Vet. Assoc., Palmerston North, N.Z., pp. 39–45, 1986.

Thormahlen, K.A., Garland, T. and Bailey, E.M.: The subchronic toxicity of Roridin A in sheep. In: Plant Associated Toxins: Agricultural, Phytochemical and Ecological Aspects. Colegate, S.M., and Dorling P.R., eds. Wallingford, UK, CAB International, pp. 561–566, 1994.

Treacher, R.J.: Galactose elimination as a liver function test in goats. Res. Vet. Sci., 13:427–430, 1972.

Treacher, R.J., Hughes, D.L. and Harness, E.: The detection of liver cell damage by plasma enzyme changes in goats given immature *Fasciola hepatica* directly into the biliary system. Br. Vet. J., 130:xii–xv. 1974.

Upadhyay, D.S., Swarup, D. and Bhatia, B.B.: A note on biliary amphistomiasis in goats. Indian J. Vet. Med., 6:134–135, 1986.

Urquhart, G.M., et al.: Veterinary Parasitology. Essex, England, Longman Scientific and Technical, 1988.

van der Lugt J.J., Coetzer, J.A.W., Smit, M.M.E. and Cilliers, C.: The diagnosis of Wesselsbron disease in a new-born lamb by immunohistochemical staining of viral antigen. Onderstepoort J. Vet. Res., 62(2):143–146, 1995.

van der Lugt J.J., et al.: *Galenia africana* L. Poisoning in sheep and goats: hepatic and cardiac changes. Onderstepoort J. Vet. Res., 59(4):323–333, 1992.

van der Lugt, J.J., Fourie, N. and Schultz, R.A.: *Galenia africana* L. (Aizoaceae) poisoning in sheep. J. S. Afr. Vet. Assoc., 59:99, 1988.

Varma, T.L., Kulshrespha, S.B. and Rao, B.V.: Indirect hemagglutination test in the diagnosis of cysticercosis caused by *Cysticercus tenuicollis* infection in sheep and goats. Riv. Parasitol., 35:103–111, 1974.

Varma, T.L., Kulshrespha, S.B., Rao, B.V. and Kumar, S.: The conglutinating complement absorption test for the serodiagnosis of *Cysticercus tenuicollis* infection in sheep and goats. J. Helminthol., 47:191–197, 1973.

Vasquez-Vasquez, M.T.: Economic losses through condemnation of *Fasciola hepatica*-infected livers in cattle and goats slaughtered in Milpa Alta abattoir, Mexico. Vet. Mex., 11:51–52, 1980.

Vihan, V.S.: Hexachloroethane toxicity in goats. Indian Vet. J., 64:180–181, 1987.

Wanasinghe, D.D.: A suspected outbreak of aflatoxicosis among goats in Sri Lanka. Ceylon Vet. J., 22:64–65, 1974.

Wang, P.Y., et al.: Regional trials of diamfenetide against *Fasciola hepatica* in naturally infected sheep and goats. Chinese J. Vet. Sci. Tech., 8:17–19, 1987.

Wasfi, I.A. and Adam, S.E.I.: The effects of intravenous injection of small amounts of copper sulphate in Nubian goats. J. Comp. Pathol., 86:387–391, 1976.

Weng, Y.L.: Experiment on the treatment of fascioliasis in milk goats with Chinese-made niclofolan. Chin. J. Vet. Med., 9:16–18, 1983.

Whitford, H.W. and Jones, L.P.: *Corynebacterium equi* infection in the goat. Southwest. Vet., 27:261–262, 1974.

Williams, R., et al.: Comparison of ELISA and HI for detection of antibodies against Wesselsbron disease virus. Onderstepoort J. Vet. Res. 64:4, 245–250, 1997.

Wittmann, W.: Rift Valley fever. In: Applied Veterinary Epidemiology. T. Blaha, ed. Amsterdam, Elsevier, pp. 44–46, 1989.

Wolff, K., Eckert, J., Schneiter, G. and Lutz, H.: Efficacy of triclabendazole against *Fasciola hepatica* in sheep and goats. Vet. Parasitol., 13:145–150, 1983.

Yadav, C.L., Uppal, R.P., and Gupta, S.C.: Efficacy of closantel against experimental infections of *Fasciola gigantica* and *Haemonchus contortus* in goats. Indian Vet. J., 72(12):1251–1254, 1995.

Yadav, S.C., et al.: *Fasciola gigantica* cathepsin-L cysteine proteinase in the detection of early experimental fasciolosis in ruminants. Parasitol. Res., 97:527–534, 2005.

Yilma, J.M. and Malone, J.B.: A geographic information system forecast model for strategic control of fascioliasis in Ethiopia. Vet. Parasitol., 78:103–127, 1998.

12

Urinary System

OVERVIEW OF CONDITIONS AFFECTING THE CAPRINE URINARY SYSTEM

Clinical disease of the urinary system is uncommon in goats, with the exception of obstructive urolithiasis. This condition occurs frequently in males, especially castrated males. Urolithiasis is discussed in detail later in the chapter.

Subclinical and Clinical Conditions of the Kidney

Despite the low prevalence of clinical renal disease, pathologic lesions of the kidneys are not unusual in normal goats at slaughter. In an Indian study, 71% of all kidneys examined showed histologic abnormality, even when the kidneys were grossly normal. Nephrosis was the most common descriptive finding (Sankarappa and Rao 1982). In contrast, gross morphologic changes have been found in only 1.5% to 3% of kidneys examined at slaughter (Khanna and Iyer 1971; Tomar 1984; Babu and Paliwal 1988). Interstitial nephritis of unknown etiology is the most common histologic lesion in these kidneys, followed by nephrocalcinosis. The most common gross abnormalities are congenital polycystic kidneys and white spots on the kidney surface. White spots are sometimes caused by leptospirosis infection (Kharole and Rao 1968; Khanna and Iyer 1971), and in one case, by *Encephalitozoon (Nosema) cuniculi*, a protozoal parasite uncommon in goats (Khanna and Iyer 1971a).

Spontaneous glomerulonephritis occurs in goats, but is rarely recognized clinically. The glomerular lesion contains heavy deposition of immunoglobulin G and complement but the antibody is not directed against basement membrane. The inciting cause of the immune mediated lesion is not known (Lerner et al. 1968). Glomerulonephritis has also been reported as an incidental necropsy finding in goats with a primary diagnosis of mycoplasma pneumonia.

A subclinical condition known first as symmetrical cortical siderosis and later as "cloisonné kidney" has been observed in goats in Iraq (Zahawi 1957) and India (Kharole 1967) and in castrated male Angora goats in Texas (Light 1960; Thompson et al. 1961; Grossman and Altman 1969). The kidney cortices are diffusely pigmented dark brown to black with the pigmentation stopping abruptly at the corticomedullary junction. The pigmentation is associated with thickening of the basement membranes of those portions of the proximal convoluted tubules present in the renal cortex. The lesion is frequently associated with renal hemosiderosis and the affected basement membranes stain variably for iron. While a number of explanations for the etiology of this subclinical condition have been offered, the actual cause remains unknown (Hatipoglu and Erer 2001).

Pyelonephritis is infrequently reported in goats and may be caused by organisms other than *Corynebacterium renale*, such as *Arcanobacterium pyogenes* (Gajendragad et al. 1983). The relatively low prevalence of post partum uterine infections in goats as compared with cattle may in part account for the lower prevalence of this ascending kidney infection in goats.

The kidneys have filtering and excretory functions. As a result, toxins may concentrate in the kidneys, causing toxic nephropathy. A diverse group of metals, chemicals, plants, fungi, and drugs have been reported to produce renal lesions in the goat, either experimentally or in spontaneous cases. Despite this extensive documentation there is scant information on the antemortem effects of various toxins on renal function, clinicopathologic abnormalities, and relevant clinical signs.

The metals reported to cause toxic nephropathy include arsenic (Biswas et al. 2000), cadmium (Bose et al. 2001), copper (Humphries et al. 1987; Belford et al. 1989), iron (Ruhr et al. 1983), lead (Gouda et al. 1985), mercury (Pathak and Bhowmik 1998), and selenium (Hosseinion et al. 1972; Qin et al. 1994). Chemicals include aldrin (Singh et al. 1985), chlorpyrifos compounds (Mohamed et al. 1990), diesel fuel (Toofanian et al. 1979), ethylene glycol (Boermans et al. 1988), fenvalerate (Mohamed and Adam 1990), hexachloroethane (Vihan 1987), kerosene (Aslani et al, 2000) sevin (Wahbi et al. 1987), and uranyl nitrate (Dash and Joshi 1989).

Plants causing toxic nephropathy in goats include *Acanthospermum hispidum* (Ali and Adam 1978), *Agave lechequilla* (Mathews 1937), *Amaranthus* spp. (Gonzalez 1983), *Aristolochia bracteata* (El Dirdiri et al. 1987), *Azadirachta indica* (Ali 1987), *Cadaba rotundifolia* (El Dirdiri et al. 1987), *Capparis tomentosa* (Ahmed and Adam 1980), *Cestrum taurantiacum* (Mugera and Nderito 1968), *Citrullus colocynthis* (Barri et al. 1983), *Crotalaria saltiana* (Barri et al. 1984), *Gutierrezia microcephala* (Mathews 1936), *Heliotropium ovalifolium* (Abu Damir et al. 1982), *Indigofera hochstetteri* (Suliman et al. 1983), *Ipomoea carnea* (Abu Damir et al. 1987), *Jatrophia* spp. (Barri et al. 1983), *Lagenaria siceraria* (Barri et al. 1983), *Lantana camara* (Ide and Tutt 1998), *Narthecium ossifragum* (Flåøyen et al. 1997), *Nolina texana* (Mathews 1940), *Palicourea aenofusca* (Dobereiner et al. 1987), *Pennisetum clandestinum* (Peet et al. 1990), *Pieris japonica* (Visser et al. 1988), *Senecio jacobaea* (Goeger et al. 1982), *Solanum dubium* (Barri et al. 1983), *Tephrosia apollinea* (Suliman et al. 1982), *Tribulus terrestris* (Jacob and Peet 1987), and *Vestia foetida* (McKeough et al. 2005).

Fungi causing nephropathy include *Drechslera campanulata* (Schneider et al. 1985) and *Aspergillus flavus* (Samarajeewa et al. 1975). *Aspergillus* and *Penicillium* fungi are frequent feed contaminants. Experimentally it was shown that ochratoxin, a metabolite of some species of these fungi, produced marked nephrotoxicity, especially in the proximal convoluted tubules when administered intravenously (Maryamma and Krishnan Nair 1990). Ingestion of sawfly larvae also produced renal lesions in goats (Thamsborg et al. 1987).

Halothane (O'Brien et al. 1987), imidocarb dipropri-onate (Corrier and Adams 1976), and furazolidone (Ali et al. 1984) are drugs documented to have caused lesions in the caprine kidney. The aminoglycosides are known to be nephrotoxic in various animals when used at high doses for prolonged periods of time, or if there are underlying conditions predisposing to renal damage such as dehydration. Gentamicin was shown to produce subclinical nephrotoxicity in goats, as evidenced by decreased urine specific gravity, proteinuria, presence of granular epithelial casts in urine, and increased urine alkaline phosphatase when the drug was given intramuscularly at a dose of 35 mg/kg bw divided in two daily doses for ten days (Kumar and Pandey 1994).

Several infectious diseases that affect primarily other organ systems also may produce renal lesions and severe kidney dysfunction. They are discussed in detail elsewhere in this book. Cowdriosis, or heartwater, discussed further in Chapter 8, produces renal ischemia that leads to tubular nephrosis (Prozesky and Du Plessis 1985). Chronic trypanosomosis, discussed further in Chapter 7, can produce mononuclear infiltrates and amyloid deposits in goat kidneys (Bungener and Mehlitz 1976). Leptospirosis, discussed in Chapters 7 and 13, may cause interstitial nephritis.

Renal failure can occur as a result of massive hemolysis or muscle necrosis because hemoglobin or myoglobin accumulates in the renal tubules. Therefore, parenteral fluid administration to promote diuresis is an important aspect of therapy for the hemolytic anemias and for nutritional muscular dystrophy. Pregnancy toxemia, a nutritional/metabolic disease, can produce fatty infiltration of the kidney proximal tubular epithelium (Tontis and Zwahlen 1987).

Conditions of the Urinary System Distal to the Kidney

Pathologic conditions of the ureters and bladder are infrequent in goats, including cystitis, a comparatively common disease in cows. There are two reports of multiple leiomyomas in the bladder wall seen at necropsy. No clinical signs attributable to the tumors were reported (Jackson 1936; Lairmore et al. 1987). There are two additional reports of leiomyoma of the urinary bladder in goats as well as a transitional cell papilloma of the urinary bladder identified during abattoir inspections (Timurkaan et al. 2001; Raoofi et al. 2007).

The principal condition affecting the urethra is obstructive urolithiasis in male goats. Ulcerative posthitis affecting the preputial opening and causing dysuria is more common in sheep but also occurs in bucks and especially wethers. It is discussed in detail in this chapter.

Malformations of the urethra also occur and are most commonly reported in newborn and young kids that present with dysuria. Abnormalities may include atresia, hypospadias, diverticulum, and/or dilatation of the urethra, usually at or near the prepuce (Karras et al. 1992, Klc et al. 2005). These abnormalities are often associated with the intersex condition in goats. Vaginitis in does and balanoposthitis in bucks are caused by herpesvirus infection and are spread venereally as discussed in this chapter. *Mycoplasma* infections are also associated with vaginitis.

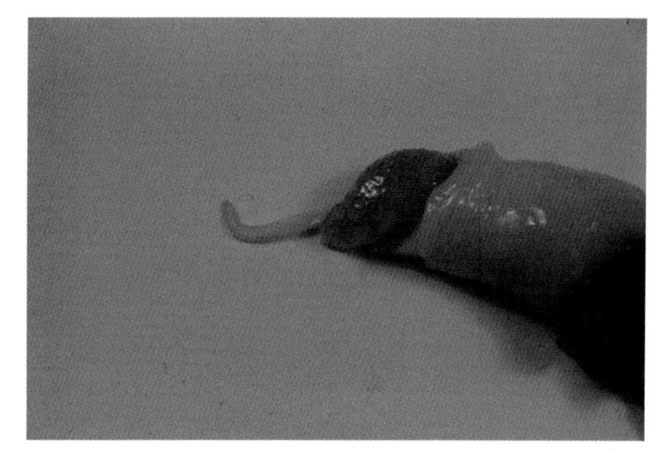

Figure 12.1. Urethral process of the buck extending beyond the glans penis. (Reproduced by permission of Dr. C.S.F. Williams.)

BACKGROUND INFORMATION OF CLINICAL IMPORTANCE

Anatomy

The comparative anatomy of the ruminant urinary tracts has been reported (Nickel et al. 1973; Sisson 1975; Barone 1978). The paired kidneys of the goat are smooth, elliptically bean-shaped, and located retroperitoneally in the abdomen. They are normally surrounded by perirenal fat, more abundantly so on the left. In the adult, they each weigh 100 to 160 g and are 6 to 7 cm in length. The location of the right kidney is fixed in the dorsal abdomen, occurring at the level of vertebrae T_{13} to L_3. The left kidney is located more caudally at L_4 to L_5 with its lateral aspect in contact with the dorsal sac of the rumen. It is frequently pushed to the right of the abdominal midline by a full rumen.

The right ureter follows the vena cava dorsal to the left kidney. The left ureter begins to the right of the median plane, courses ventral to the right ureter, and then crosses back to the left to enter the bladder. The ureters pass obliquely through the bladder wall and enter the dorsum of the bladder in the trigone region. The ureteral openings are 1 to 1.5 cm apart. The urinary bladder is ovoid and extends into the abdominal cavity when full. It lies ventral to the uterus in the doe. Cystocentesis is difficult, even when the bladder is full, because of the depth of the caudal abdomen.

The penis is fibroelastic in character as in other ruminants and similarly possesses a sigmoid flexure. Paired retractor penis muscles run laterally to the penis and attach proximal to the sigmoid flexure. The action of these muscles makes exteriorization of the penis from the prepuce for clinical examination difficult.

As is the case in sheep, the pars spongiosa of the penile urethra extends well beyond the glans penis for a length of approximately 2.5 cm, forming a vermiform appendage with erectile capacity known as the urethral process (Ghoshal and Bal 1976) (Figure 12.1). While the urethral process in sheep is attached to the left side of the glans, it is median in position in the goat. The process is folded back inside the prepuce when the penis is flaccid but becomes rigid and extended when the penis is erect. During ejaculation, the process rotates spirally and is believed to spray semen on the external uterine orifice or possibly even enter the external os of the cervix. At birth, the urethral process is adhered to the preputial mucosa and gradually separates under the influence of testosterone.

Urinary calculi are commonly trapped in the urethral process, causing obstruction of urine flow. This is particularly true in castrated males, where the urethral diameter may be reduced and the urethral process remains adhered to the preputial mucosa because of loss of the developmental effects of testosterone. The urethral process is commonly removed as part of the medicosurgical management of obstructive urolithiasis to restore urine flow. There is no evidence that removal of the urethral process impairs fertility in goats.

Male goats possess a urethral recess projecting caudodorsally from the spongy portion of the urethra in the region of the ischial arch (Figure 12.2). The paired bulbourethral glands empty their secretions into this recess, which is 0.5 cm deep. In earlier descriptions, the urethral recess was referred to as the urethral diverticulum (Hinkle et al. 1978; Garrett 1987). This structure assumes clinical importance in attempts to catheterize the urethra retrograde to the bladder during clinical management of obstructive urolithiasis. As the catheter moves dorsally up the urethra in the perineal region and begins to arch cranially over the pubis, the tip invariably becomes lodged in the urethral recess and will not pass to the bladder. Ignorance of the presence of the recess may lead to forceful manipulation of

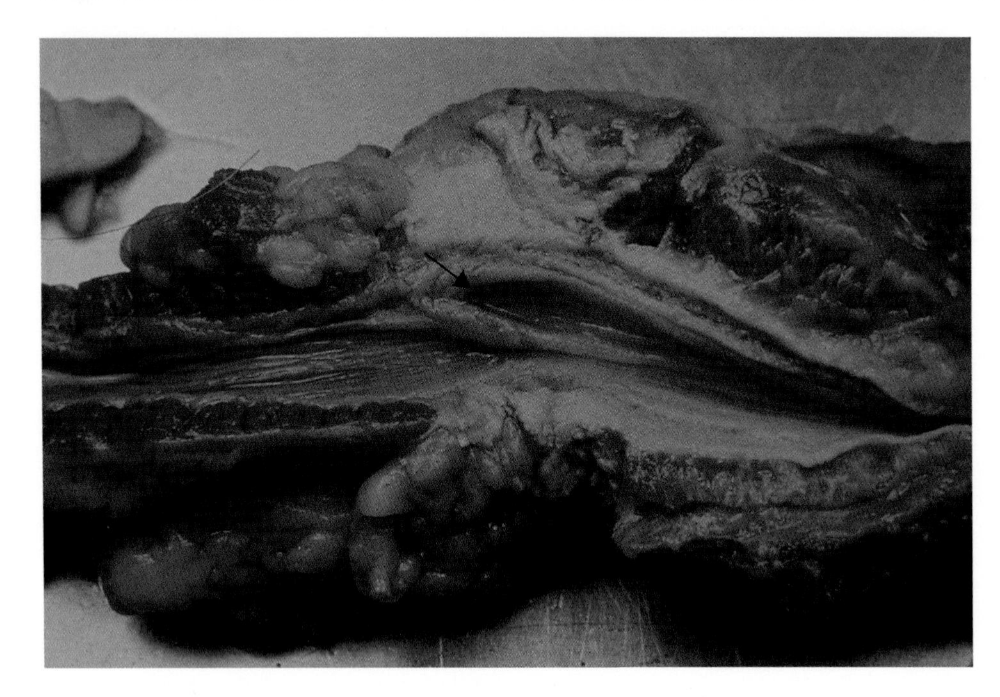

Figure 12.2. Urethral recess (arrow) of the buck at the ischial arch. (Reproduced by permission of Dr. C.S.F. Williams).

the catheter to reach the bladder. This can cause tearing of the urethral recess with subsequent accumulation of urine in perineal tissues or trauma, scarring, and contracture of the urethra.

In contrast to the male urethra, the female urethra is short and straight, with an average adult length of 5 to 6 cm. The external urethral opening is on the floor of the vestibule approximately 2 to 3 cm inside the vulva. There is a suburethral diverticulum approximately 0.5 cm deep just inside the external urethral orifice, ventral to the urethra, which must be avoided for successful catheterization of the bladder. The doe has no vestibular glands.

Physiology

As in other species, the kidney serves multiple functions, including water and electrolyte balance, nutrient conservation, maintenance of normal blood pH levels, and regulation of nitrogenous wastes. The kidney also has endocrine functions. It responds to antidiuretic hormone (ADH) for control of water balance, aldosterone for sodium and potassium regulation, and parathyroid hormone to increase excretion of phosphorus. It also produces erythropoietin for stimulation of erythropoiesis, participates in the activation of vitamin D, and produces renin in response to decreased renal perfusion to activate angiotensin. Limited physiologic data reported for the goat is provided in Table 12.1.

The excretion of inulin, creatinine, sodium sulfanilate (SS), and phenolsulfonphthalein (PSP) have been evaluated to assess caprine renal function (Brown et al. 1990). Creatinine clearance was determined not to be a reliable measure of glomerular filtration rate (GFR) in goats, primarily because of the existence of a tubular secretory mechanism for creatinine excretion in this species. Clearance of SS exceeds inulin clearance because of the existence of a secretory mechanism for SS in the proximal portion of the nephron. In addition, SS may be eliminated by routes other than the kidney in the goat. The clearance of PSP also exceeds inulin clearance, presumably because of excretion of PSP both by glomerular filtration and tubular secretion.

Even though SS and PSP clearance from plasma are not exact measurements of GFR, the use of these tests to assess renal function is attractive in that urine samples are not required to interpret results. This is important in goats because collecting urine by catheterization can be problematic, especially in males.

Maturation of the caprine kidney may affect functional studies. The efficiency of renal function is relatively low in the newborn kid but reaches adult capacity by two weeks of age, as indicated by increases in GFR and clearance of *p*-aminohippurate (Friis 1983). Tubular function increases more than glomerular function postnatally.

Goats show marked adaptation to conditions of poor nutrient availability and lack of water. Desert breeds such as the black Bedouin goat have a superior ability to conserve urea under adverse dietary conditions. In comparative studies with Swiss Saanen goats, both breeds could significantly increase the tubular reabsorption of urea when fed low-protein diets, but the Bedouin goat possessed a superior capacity to reduce GFR, thus lowering the amount of urea filtered by the kidney (Silanikove 1984). Urea thus conserved is available to the rumen microflora for protein anabolism.

Table 12.1. Physiologic parameters of caprine renal function.

Parameter	*Type of goat*	*Special conditions*	*Unit of measurement*	*Reported value*	*Reference*
Aldosterone in plasma	Adult Bedouin	Normal hydration	ng%	5.5 ± 4.3	Wittenberg et al. 1986
	Adult Bedouin	Water deprived	ng%	13.9 ± 2.3	Wittenberg et al. 1986
Clearance of creatinine	Young adult, mixed breed	Normal, conscious	ml/mn/kg bw	1.97 ± 0.09	Brown et al. 1990
Clearance of inulin	Young adult, mixed breed	Normal, conscious	ml/mn/kg bw	2.26 ± 0.08	Brown et al. 1990
Clearance of phenolsulphonphthalein	Young adult, mixed breed	Normal, conscious	ml/mn/kg bw	6.88 ± 0.39	Brown et al. 1990
Clearance of sodium sulfanilate	Young adult, mixed breed	Normal, conscious	ml/mn/kg bw	3.71 ± 0.39	Brown et al. 1990
Effective renal plasma flow (ERPF)	General	—	ml/mn/M^2	493	Fletcher et al. 1964
	Adult Bedouin	Fully hydrated	ml/mn	344 ± 146	Wittenberg et al. 1986
Filtration fraction	General	—	—	0.18	Fletcher et al. 1964
Glomerular filtration rate (GFR)	General	—	ml/mn/m^2	86	Fletcher et al. 1964
	Not specified	1–3 days of age	ml/mn/kg bw	2.1 ± 0.6	Friis 1983
	Not specified	14–20 days of age	ml/mn/kg bw	3.3 ± 0.2	Friis 1983
	Not specified	69–78 days of age	ml/mn/kg bw	2.8 ± 0.5	Friis 1983
	Adult Bedouin	Normal diet	l/day/kg bw	4.85 ± 0.3	Silanikove 1984
	Adult Bedouin	low-protein diet	l/day/kg bw	2.26 ± 0.1	Silanikove 1984
	Adult Bedouin	Fully hydrated	ml/mn	76 ± 29	Wittenberg et al. 1986
	Adult Saanen	Normal diet	l/day/kg bw	6.61 ± 0.4	Silanikove 1984
	Adult Saanen	Low-protein diet	l/day/kg bw	4.14 ± 0.3	Silanikove 1984
Maximum tubular reabsorption rate (T_{max})	General	—	mg/mn/M^2	248	Fletcher et al. 1964
Urine chloride	Adult Saanen	Normal diet	mEq/l	209 ± 55	Silanikove 1984
	Adult Saanen	Low-protein diet	mEq/l	366 ± 37	Silanikove 1984
Urine creatinine	General	—	mg/kg/day	10	Brooks et al. 1984
Urine flow	General	—	ml/day/kg bw	10–40	Brooks et al. 1984
	Adult Bedouin	Normal diet	ml/day/kg bw	16.7 ± 3.7	Silanikove 1984
	Adult Bedouin	Low-protein diet	ml/day/kg bw	2.4 ± 0.07	Silanikove 1984
	Adult Bedouin	Fully hydrated	ml/mn	0.74 ± 0.4	Wittenberg et al. 1986
	Adult Saanen	Normal diet	ml/day/kg bw	26.3 ± 5.9	Silanikove 1984
	Adult Saanen	Low-protein diet	ml/day/kg bw	4.8 ± 0.26	Silanikove 1984
Urine osmolality	Adult Saanen	Normal diet	mOsm/kg	1745 ± 183	Silanikove 1984
	Adult Saanen	Low-protein diet	mOsm/kg	1523 ± 171	Silanikove 1984
	Adult East African	Water deprivation	mOsm/kg	2800–3000	Maloiy 1974
Urine potassium	Adult Saanen	Low-protein diet	mEq/l	342 ± 55	Silanikove 1984
	Adult Saanen	Normal diet	mEq/l	528 ± 47	Silanikove 1984
Urine sodium	Adult Saanen	Normal diet	mEq/l	135 ± 32	Silanikove 1984
	Adult Saanen	Low-protein diet	mEq/l	46 ±31	Silanikove 1984
Urine urea	General	—	mg/kg/day	230	Brooks et al. 1984
	Adult Saanen	Normal diet	mM/l	968 ± 84	Silanikove 1984
	Adult Saanen	Low-protein diet	mM/l	241 ± 39	Silanikove 1984

Typically, desert goats may go without water for two to four days. When offered water, they can consume as much as 40% of their dehydrated bw at one time. The rumen and kidneys work in concert to conserve water so consumed. Five hours after drinking, more than 80% of water taken in remains in the rumen. Effective renal blood flow, GFR, and urine output drop markedly, and urine flow remains below levels recorded in dehydrated goats, even four hours after drinking. At the same time, urine sodium concentration drops to half of that observed in dehydrated goats. There is a concomitant drop in urine potassium and chloride concentrations. Thus, the rumen acts as a water reservoir that is protected by renal conservation of sodium, chloride, and water (Choshniak et al. 1984; Wittenberg et al. 1986; Shaham et al. 1994).

Cold exposure causes goats to reduce their water intake. In lactating goats, there appears to be no compensatory reaction by the kidney, and circulating ADH levels remain similar to those of goats in a thermoneutral environment. The net result is a decrease in milk production as a method of water conservation (Thomson et al. 1980). When goats are exposed to heat stress and/or deprived of water, circulating ADH levels increase and the kidney actively participates in water conservation (Olsson and Dahlborn 1989; Mengistu et al. 2007). In one study, excretion of ADH in the urine increased eight-fold after forty-eight hours of dehydration (Lishajko and Andersson 1975).

Diagnostic Methods and Clinical Pathology

Examination of the Penis

Clinical management of obstructive urolithiasis requires examination of the penis. This can be difficult for several reasons. Cases often involve a young, castrated male with a small, poorly developed penis and residual adhesions between the penis and prepuce, making it difficult to manually extend the penis from the sheath. Obstructed goats are often in pain and resist manipulation. Sedation can assist in examination but must be used cautiously when animals are severely uremic.

A common approach to examination is to sit the animal on its rump, which pushes the penis forward in the sheath. The penis is then grasped just behind the sigmoid flexure and pushed forward until the glans and free portion of the penis breach the preputial orifice. The free portion of the penis is then wrapped securely, but carefully, with a length of gauze to pull the penis farther forward and immobilize it. Use of the gauze helps to resist the opposing action of the retractor penis muscles. Successful examination in this manner usually requires at least one assistant, especially if partial catheterization is to be attempted. This technique can also be applied with the goat in lateral recumbency. In this case, the goat may be easier to restrain, but it may be more difficult to achieve extension of the penis.

An alternative method for exteriorizing the penis is to position the goat on its back with an assistant pulling both the animal's hind limbs forward as close to its ears as possible. This straightens the penis and controls kicking. The technique works better with intact male goats than with wethers, where the penis may be adhered to the prepuce (Pieterse 1994).

In cattle and sheep, the internal pudendal nerve block, though sometimes considered difficult to perform, is used for anesthesia of the penis and relaxation of the retractor penis muscle to facilitate clinical manipulation (Hofmeyr 1987). While the internal pudendal nerve also controls the retractor penis muscle in goats, the nerve block may not produce the desired effect, because the preputial muscles are under separate neurologic control and their persistent contraction may still inhibit protrusion of the penis (Prakash and Kumar 1983). Alternatively, epidural anesthesia administered at the lumbosacral junction can be used to facilitate examination, but the concomitant loss of locomotor function may complicate patient management.

Chemical restraint and tranquilization are useful adjuncts to examination. Diazepam given intravenously at a total dose of 5 to 15 mg provides patient relaxation and lowers resistance to manipulation. Xylazine at a dose of 0.05 mg/kg bw intravenously provides similar effects. Xylazine should be used with caution in obstructed goats. The drug elevates blood glucose, thereby promoting diuresis. Increased urine production is undesirable if the obstruction is not successfully relieved. Acepromazine maleate at 0.1 mg/kg intravenously may promote relaxation of the retractor penis muscle but the results are variable and the potential for phimosis exists. Propryonylpromazine at a dose of 1 mg/kg intramuscularly facilitates protrusion of the penis of goats in lateral recumbency, but spontaneous protrusion from the sheath did not occur (Schöntag 1984).

Once the penis has been exteriorized, partial catheterization of the urethra may be attempted when indicated. This is made easier by amputation of the urethral process, but passage through the sigmoid flexure is still problematic. The urethral recess at the level of the ischial arch makes introduction of the catheter into the bladder practically impossible. These constraints should be recognized to avoid unnecessary effort and trauma. Retractor penis myotomy performed at the median raphe 5 cm ventral to the anus may allow maximal straightening of the penis to assist in getting the catheter past the sigmoid flexure. Normal penis function was reported after reapposition of the muscles and healing (Shokry and Al-Saadi 1980).

Urine Collection

In cattle and sheep, urination can be induced by manual stimulation of the prepuce (male cattle) or skin in the perineal region (cows) or by holding off the nostrils (sheep). None of these techniques is effective in goats. Male goats may urinate frequently during the breeding season as part of mating behavior but patience is a virtue when waiting for a urine sample from a doe. Goats often urinate immediately after rising from extended recumbency, so the sampler should be prepared with a urine cup at appropriate moments. Introducing the goat to a new pen or stall may promote urination but this is unreliable. If able, bucks often urinate after release from restraint for examination.

Catheterization of the female for urine collection is simpler than in the male so long as the suburethral diverticulum at the external urethral orifice is avoided. A 12 French catheter can be used in an adult doe. Experience in other species suggests that administration of bethanecol, a parasympathomimetic drug, at a dose of 75 mcg/kg subcutaneously may stimulate urination in goats and not alter the composition of the urine.

For continuous collection of urine, pediatric urine bags have been sutured to the perineal region of female goats and a harness constructed to hold the collected urine (Mount 1984).

Clinical Chemistry and Urinalysis

Normal blood urea nitrogen (BUN) levels are in the range of 10 to 28 mg/dl, normal creatinine levels from 0.9 to 1.8 mg/dl, and normal uric acid levels from 0.33 to 1 mg/dl. Breed, sex, and age variations in these normal parameters have not been identified in goats.

Measurement of gamma glutamyl transferase (GGT) in urine is being used in other species as an indicator of renal damage in the proximal tubular epithelium. There is one report of its application in goats. In a study on the nephrotoxic effects of the plant *Narthecium ossifragum* on goats in Norway, normal, control goats had a mean urine GGT concentration of 18.8 U/l with a range of 10 to 25 U/l and a urine alkaline phosphatase concentration of 11.8 U/l, with a range of 5 to 19 U/l (Wisløff et al. 2003).

General values for urinalysis in the goat are given in Table 12.2. Breed, sex, and age variations are not reported for urinalysis in normal goats. However, urine osmolarity has been demonstrated to progressively decrease in advancing pregnancy in goats and increase again with the onset of lactation (Olsson et al. 1982).

Table 12.2. Normal caprine urinalysis values.

Parameter	*Normal value*
Color	Pale yellow
Turbidity	Clear
Specific gravity	1–1.05
pH level	Alkaline (7.2–8)
Glucose	Negative
Ketones	Negative
Bilirubin	Negative
Occult blood	Negative
Protein	Negative to trace
Sediment (observed per high-powered field)	
Red blood cells	<5
White blood cells	<5
Epithelial cells	Occasional
Fat droplets	Rare
Crystals	Rare
Casts	Occasional hyaline
Sperm	Variable
Gamma glutamyl transferase (U/l)	18.8 (10–25)
Alkaline phosphatase (U/l)	11.8 (5–19)

Imaging Techniques

Plain survey radiographs are usually of little value as aids in diagnosing urinary tract conditions in goats, but may occasionally reveal cystic calculi (Figure 12.3). Contrast studies are often more helpful. Intravenous pyelography in the goat has been described (Cegarra and Lewis 1977). Sedation with xylazine facilitates the procedure. Ideally, goats should be fasted for forty-eight hours to reduce rumen size, but this can be detrimental to sick goats. Sodium iothalamate is given at a dose of 2 ml/kg intravenously in goats up to 28 kg, while in heavier goats the calculated dose is reduced to 75%. The kidneys are opacified within twenty seconds of injection and the entire urinary tract opacified within fifteen minutes. The technique is helpful in identifying congenital renal abnormalities and the presence and extent of uroliths, especially in the bladder.

Cystourethrography in the goat has also been described, requiring catheterization of the bladder under fluoroscopic guidance. The technique has proven useful for establishing the presence and character of cystic calculi (van Weeren et al 1987). A triple contrast cystography technique, with the addition of pneumoperitoneum, has also been described for use in the goat and is recommended for detailed evaluation of the mucosal surface of the bladder (Tayal et al. 1984).

In a review of twenty-six cases of obstructive urolithiasis, including twenty goats, positive normograde cystourethrography through a tube cystostomy catheter offered the best visualization of the lower urinary tract structures for assessing and subsequently

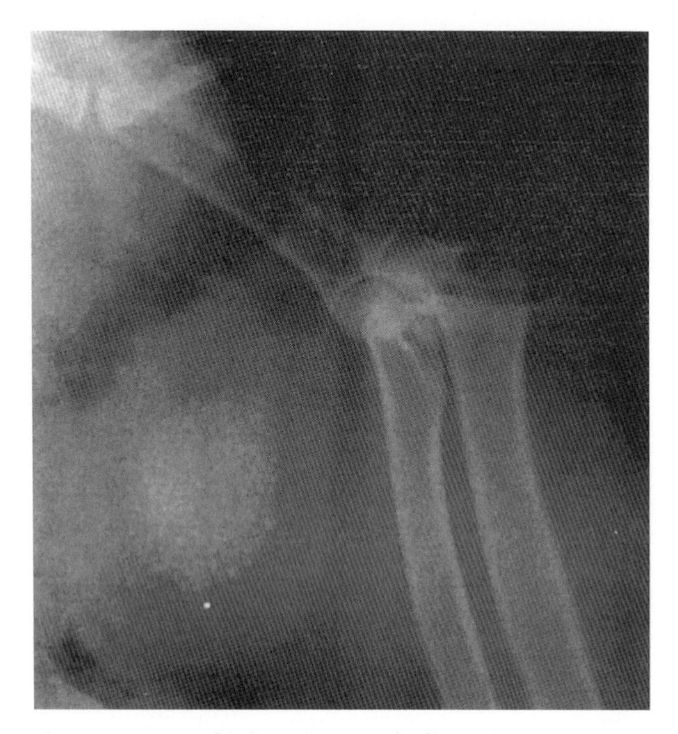

Figure 12.3. Multiple urinary calculi present in a goat urinary bladder as seen by plain radiography. This is an unusually diagnostic film. Contrast studies are often required to identify cystic calculi. (Courtesy of the Cummings School of Veterinary Medicine at Tufts University.)

managing the obstructive lesion (Palmer et al. 1998). In that same review, survey radiographs obtained in twenty-three patients with obstructive urolithiasis were diagnostic for urinary calculi in only one animal.

In recent years, ultrasonography has proven to be a rapid, useful technique in the diagnosis of urinary tract disease. Cystic calculi are readily identifiable by ultrasound and the technique is more reliable than survey radiography (Figure 12.4). A recent, illustrated discussion of ultrasound techniques used for examination of the urinary tract in small animals is very applicable to the goat (Widmer et al. 2004).

Kidney Biopsy

Percutaneous biopsy of the right kidney can be accomplished in some goats. The right kidney is readily palpable in the abdomen of thin goats in the anterior portion of the right paralumbar fossa just medial to the last rib. It can be captured manually, retracted caudally, and held in a fixed position in the right paralumbar fossa during the biopsy procedure. A Vim-Silverman needle is used for the procedure. A series of 300 right kidney biopsies was performed in this manner in thin Angora goats, with bleeding complications noted in fewer than 1% of the goats. This procedure would be more difficult in larger, well-fleshed goats. In dogs, it is reported that kidney biopsies obtained with lapar-

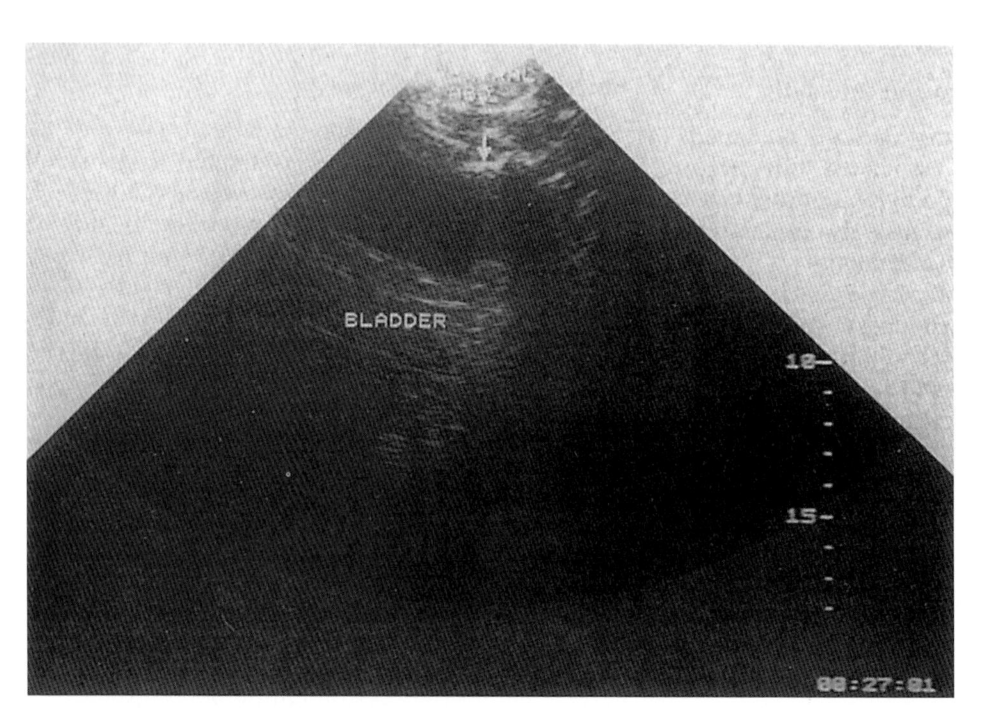

Figure 12.4. Urinary calculi (arrow at top of picture) in a goat urinary bladder as seen by ultrasound. (Courtesy of the Cummings School of Veterinary Medicine at Tufts University.)

ascopy are of higher quality than those obtained with ultrasound guidance in terms of the number of intact glomeruli in the biopsy specimen (Rawlings et al. 2003).

DIAGNOSIS OF URINARY TRACT DISEASE BY PRESENTING SIGN

Abdominal Distension

Rupture of the urinary bladder with passage of urine into the abdominal cavity secondary to obstructive urolithiasis is the most common cause of abdominal distension related to the urinary system. In rare cases, the ureter may rupture instead of or in addition to the bladder. Either condition is more likely observed in males than females. The contour of abdominal distension is bilateral and ventral. A similar "pot bellied" appearance may be seen in normal pygmy goats, obstructions of the forestomachs, gastrointestinal parasitism, infectious peritonitis, and reproductive conditions leading to distension of the uterus.

There is one case report of congenital polycystic disease affecting the kidneys and liver of a one-month-old pygmy goat. The animal presented with a history of progressive abdominal distension from birth and subsequently, hematuria (Newman et al. 2000). Congenital polycystic disease in goats is extremely rare; there is only one other case report in a Nubian kid (Krotec et al. 1996).

Subcutaneous Swelling

Rupture of the urethra secondary to obstructive urolithiasis leads to subcutaneous pooling of urine in either the perineal or preputial region. Leakage of urine into the perineal region can also result from trauma to the urethra at the urethral recess from careless or forceful attempts at bladder catheterization.

Focal swelling on the ventral aspect of the prepuce also is seen in cases of congenital urethral diverticulum in young males. This infrequent lesion consists of single or multiple outpocketings of the penile urethra, sometimes in association with a bipartite or split scrotum. Urine is not free in the subcutis, but does pool in the diverticulum. Contrast urethrography can be used to confirm the diagnosis and successful surgical correction of the defect has been reported (Gahlot et al. 1982; Fuller et al. 1992).

Hypospadias, a more extreme form of congenital urethral defect, is seen in young phenotypically male goats (Eaton 1943). These animals may be genetically female intersexes, as discussed in Chapter 13. In hypospadias, the urethra remains open on the ventral surface of the penis and is visible externally on the preputial midline. Urine may seep constantly from the opening. Phenotypically male goats showing this condition are probably infertile. In ulcerative posthitis, preputial swelling may result from accumulation of urine in the preputial space because inflammation and scabbing of the preputial orifice do not permit extension of the penis or passage of urine.

Balanoposthitis can occur in venereal caprine herpesvirus infection, causing edematous swelling of the prepuce in bucks.

Hypoproteinemia from any cause may cause subcutaneous ventral edema. The prepuce may be involved in this swelling.

Abnormal Appearing Vulva and Vagina

Hyperemia and swelling occur normally during estrus, and a clear to cloudy mucous discharge may be observed. The normal discharge of late estrus is white and tenacious and full of neutrophils. It is easily misinterpreted as pus by the inexperienced observer.

The intersex condition is common in goats and much variation in the structure of the external genitalia can be observed in affected female phenotypes. A bulbous or projecting vulva and an enlarged or protruding clitoris are indicative of the intersex condition. Additional internal abnormalities in the genitourinary organs may accompany these external signs.

Caprine herpes vulvovaginitis produces vulvar edema and erythema and a cloudy to gray or yellow vulvar discharge, in addition to vesicular lesions and erosions as discussed later in this chapter.

Granular vulvovaginitis can result from *Mycoplasma* spp. infections as discussed further in Chapter 13. Ulcerative vulvitis with purulent vulvar discharge caused by *Arcanobacterium pyogenes* and *Staphylococcus* spp. also occurs in goats.

Abnormal Appearance of Urine or Abnormal Urinalysis

Normal urine is clear and pale to dark yellow. Cloudy urine suggests inflammation associated with pyelonephritis, cystitis, or possibly vulvovaginitis. When inflammation is severe, the urine may also contain visible clumps of inflammatory cells and debris.

Pink to red urine usually indicates either hematuria or hemoglobinuria, though phenothiazine-based drugs can also turn the urine pink. Hematuria can occur in association with obstructive urolithiasis, pyelonephritis, cystitis, or, as in a case known to the author, by an infiltrative carcinoma at the neck of the urinary bladder. It has also been reported in goats with nephritis caused by consumption of broomweed *(Gutierrezia microcephala)* during drought in the southwestern United States (Mathews 1936). Bloody urine may also be found in the bladder in goats dead of anthrax. There is a case report of two kid goats with red urine from excessive water consumption leading to hypotonicity, hemolysis, and hemoglobinuria (Middleton et al. 1997).

Additional causes of hemoglobinuria secondary to hemolytic anemia are discussed in Chapter 7.

Brown urine results from myoglobinuria. In goats this may be seen in nutritional muscular dystrophy and in certain plant poisonings resulting in muscle necrosis. Brownish yellow urine can occur with bilirubinuria. Causes of bilirubinuria are poorly documented in goats.

Proteinuria caused by proteins other than myoglobin and hemoglobin does not alter the color of urine, but often accompanies inflammatory conditions of the urogenital tract. Post partum does may also have protein in the urine as a contaminant from normal discharge of lochia. Bacterial endotoxemia can result in proteinuria.

Persistent, elevated proteinuria, in conjunction with prolonged weight loss, is a hallmark of renal amyloidosis, which is the deposition of fibrillar amyloid protein in the kidney, mainly in the glomeruli. The condition is not common in small ruminants, but when it occurs, it is most likely associated with the AA form of amyloid which derives from serum amyloid A (SAA), an acute phase protein involved in cholesterol transport but also as a chemoattractant in the inflammatory process. Chronic inflammation leads to increased concentrations of SAA and the cleavage of certain isoforms of SAA, the fragments of which tend to form fibrillar aggregates (amyloid) that are deposited systemically, but mainly in the kidney, liver, and spleen (Ménusa et al. 2003). In goats, amyloidoisis has been most frequently seen in hyperimmunized animals that are used for commercial antibody production and thereby subjected to chronic stimulation of the immune system (Gezon et al. 1988). In addition, sporadic cases of amyloidosis involving the kidney and/or liver have been reported in relation to other chronic diseases of goats, including caseous lymphadenitis (Tham and Bunn 1992), caprine arthritis encephalitis (Crawford et al. 1980), contagious agalactia (Ménusa et al. 2003), and chronic arthritis presumably due to *Erysipelothrix rhusiopathiae* (Wessels 2003).

Marked ketonuria may be seen in pregnant does and is virtually diagnostic for pregnancy toxemia in the nonlactating, pregnant doe. It can also occur in lactational ketosis.

Glucosuria is recorded in enterotoxemia caused by *Clostridium perfringens* type D. Glucose may occur in the urine of goats stressed by other serious disease problems, including convulsions from any cause. Iatrogenic causes of glucosuria include xylazine and parenterally administered dextrose. Goats on aspirin therapy or those grazing *Salix* spp. may have false positive glucose tests caused by salicylates in urine (Wilkinson 1969).

Crystalluria can be observed in conjunction with or before clinical obstructive urolithiasis, or after consumption of ethylene glycol or plants high in oxalates.

Casts in the urine reflect tubular damage in the kidney, usually because of poor renal perfusion, toxins, or drugs. Increased white cells, red cells, and epithelial cells in the sediment indicate inflammation. Urine of sexually active bucks can normally contain sperm.

Anuria, Oliguria, or Polyuria

Male goats with obstructive urolithiasis may produce no urine, but dysuria is more common. Instances of anuric renal failure are poorly documented in goats. In most documented cases of toxic nephropathy, affected goats were oliguric initially and later polyuric. Oak toxicity is a common cause of nephrosis with polyuria in cattle and sheep. Goats are considered highly resistant to oak poisoning though there is one documented case in a goat herd (Katiyar 1981).

Dysuria, Pollakiuria, and Stranguria

Abnormal behavior related to urination in goats is most commonly associated with obstructive urolithiasis in males. The signs are described later in this chapter.

In ulcerative posthitis cases, scabbing over of the preputial orifice can also lead to dysuria in males. "Hair rings," or accumulations of loosely matted hairs encircling the penis behind the glans, have been recorded in feral goats in Australia (Figure 12.5) (Tarigan et al. 1990). These also could be associated with dysuria.

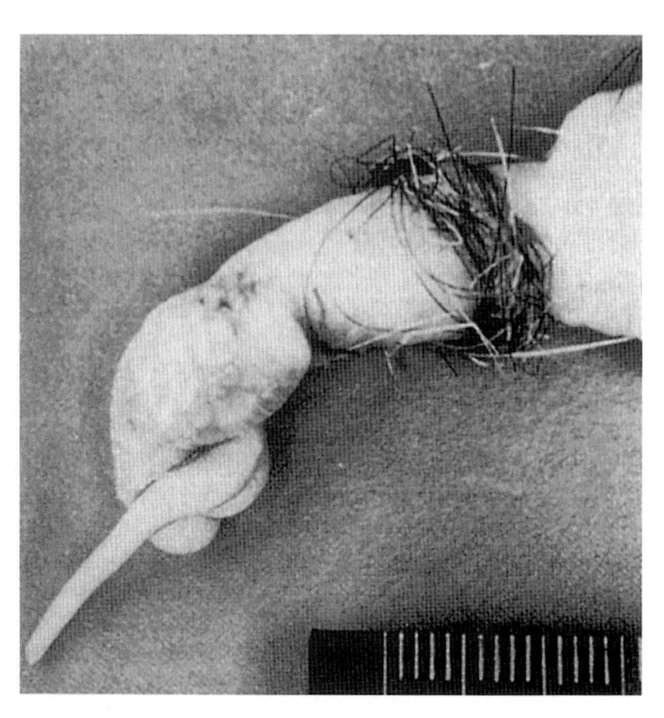

Figure 12.5. Hair ring encircling the penis of a goat. This can lead to dysuria. (From Tarigan et al. 1990.)

In females, abnormal urination occurs with cystitis and may also occur in cases of vulvovaginitis. Stranguria was observed in a doe with obstructive uropathy from trauma and adhesions of the urinary tract secondary to dystocia (Morin and Badertscher 1990). Pollakiuria, or frequent urination, can be associated with hydrometra in does and has also been reported in a case of uterine enlargement due to neoplasia (Pfister et al. 2007).

Malignant enzootic dysuria has been reported in grazing goats, sheep, and especially cattle in Morocco. The condition is considered to be most likely caused by consumption of leaves, buds, or acorns of *Quercus suber*, the cork tree, common in the Mediterranean countries. In addition to dysuria, affected animals show poor body condition, hypothermia, muzzle lesions, purulent nasal discharge, and recurring keratitis and conjunctivitis. Death can occur in two to four weeks, but more prolonged cases also occur (Mahin and Chadli 1982).

Uremia

Uremia is a systemic, toxic condition associated with the failure to remove the products of protein metabolism from the body via the urinary tract. The origins of uremia can be pre-renal, renal, or post renal. Elevated concentrations of urea nitrogen in the blood or plasma are the main laboratory indicator of uremia, also referred to as azotemia. Pre-renal uremia is associated mainly with dehydration or poor renal perfusion which may result from a variety of causes unrelated to the urinary system.

In cattle, very high levels of BUN can occur in the absence of primary renal disease (Divers et al 1982). Therefore, marked azotemia must be interpreted cautiously. Experimental evidence suggests that this is also true in goats. Induction of pyloric stenosis by ligation resulted in serum urea levels of 353 mg/dl with no evidence of impaired renal function. The increase correlated with a decrease in effective renal blood flow (Jorna 1978).

Uremia of renal origin is associated with decreased renal function or outright kidney failure. Naturally occurring, clinical cases in goats are not widely documented or reported, though they undoubtedly occur. Experiments involving partial or total nephrectomy in goats provide indications of the clinical manifestations of uremia of renal origin in the species.

Experimentally, five of nine goats subjected to subtotal nephrectomy survived for fifty-two weeks without clinical signs, while four died within eight days. All goats with total bilateral nephrectomy were terminally ill within eight days. Clinical signs included decreased appetite, rumen atony, depression, weakness, excess salivation, wiry pulse and jerky respiration, subnormal temperature, recumbency, convulsions, and coma. The degree of azotemia was not measured (Vyas et al. 1978).

Hypocalcemia, hyperphosphatemia, and hypermagnesemia have been recorded in toxic nephrosis in the goat. Hyperkalemia is not a consistent finding. In experimental lead poisoning, hypokalemia was observed along with hypocalcemia and hyperphosphatemia (Gouda et al. 1985). There is one reported case of renal (uremic) encephalopathy in a two-year-old male goat in which spongiform lesions of the brain were observed. The cause of the underlying nephrosis was not determined but the brain lesions were considered to be secondary to the uremia (Radi et al. 2005).

In goats, most reported clinical cases of uremia are post renal in origin and are associated with obstructive urolithiasis. The condition is discussed in more detail later in the chapter.

SPECIFIC DISEASES OF THE URINARY SYSTEM

INFECTIOUS DISEASES

Caprine Herpesvirus Vulvovaginitis and Balanoposthitis

In the goat, an alphaherpesvirus, caprine herpesvirus-1 (CpHV-1), has been identified as the cause of a venereally transmitted vulvovaginitis and balanoposthitis. The same agent has been implicated in epizootics of fatal viremia involving kids one-to two-weeks of age and abortion in does. It has also been isolated in conjunction with *Mannheimia (Pasteurella) haemolytica* from an outbreak of severe pneumonia of goats. CpHV-1 infection should be viewed as an emerging disease of growing importance in goats, especially in Mediterranean countries. The respiratory form, the viremic kid form, and the abortion form are discussed further in Chapters 9, 10, and 13, respectively.

Etiology

CpHV-1 is an icosahedral, double-stranded, linear DNA virus measuring 135 nm in diameter. It is sensitive to lipid solvents and trypsin and is inactivated at a pH value of 3 and at a temperature of 122°F (50°C). It can be cultivated on a variety of cell culture types and is cytopathic (Berrios and McKercher 1975). The biological and physicochemical properties of the virus have been described (Engels et al. 1983).

In early reports of disease, CpHV-1 was sometimes referred to as bovine herpesvirus type 6 but it is now recognized as a distinct entity, CpHV-1. Still, CpHV-1 belongs to an important group of alphaherpesviruses pathogenic to ruminants and closely related to each other. This group includes bovine herpesvirus-1 (BoHV-1), the cause of infectious bovine rhinotracheitis and infectious pustular vulvovaginitis in cattle, bovine herpesvirus-5 (BoHV-5), which causes bovine encephalitis, bubaline herpesvirus-1, associated with subclinical genital infections in water buffalo, cervid herpesvirus-1, which causes an ocular syndrome in red deer, cervid herpesvirus-2, associated with subclinical genital infections in reindeer, and elk herpesvirus-1, associated with subclinical genital infections in elk.

The relatedness of these viruses has practical significance relative to disease diagnosis and control. Cross-species infections occur, though rarely. This has been investigated under experimental conditions, as reviewed by Thiry et al. (2006). Because of the antigenic similarity of these alphaherpesviruses, most serologic tests of antibody detection cannot distinguish reliably among them, as discussed further below in the clinical pathology section. Also, if multiple infections occur, recombination between these related viruses is theoretically possible, though it has not yet been confirmed between CpHV-1 and BoHV-1 (Meurens et al. 2004). Of greatest concern is that goats and other ruminants may serve as reservoirs for BoHV-1, and thereby confound national and international efforts to eradicate infectious bovine rhinotracheitis in cattle. This underscores the need for diagnostic tests that can reliably discriminate among the alphaherpesviruses. The molecular and epidemiological relationships of the alphaherpesviruses have been recently reviewed (Thiry et al. 2006).

Goats have been experimentally infected with BoHV-1, resulting in mild clinical signs, high levels of BoHV-1 excretion for several days during primary infection, an antibody response, and establishment of latent infection in the trigeminal ganglia of the challenged goats (Six et al. 2001). These latent infections could be reactivated by treatment of the goats with high doses of dexamethasone.

Conversely, calves experimentally challenged with CpHV-1 also became infected. They did not manifest any clinical signs but they did excrete CpHV-1 virus and produce an antibody response. Latent infection in the trigeminal ganglia was established as demonstrated by PCR, but could not be reactivated (Six et al. 2001).

Naturally occurring infections of goats with BoHV-1 have also been reported. In 1972, it was reported that the virus was isolated from nasal and ocular swabs from two goats in Maryland with fever and signs of respiratory disease (Mohanty et al. 1972). The BoHV-1 virus was also isolated from four goats in Washington state, one with clinical signs of vulvovaginitis, two with pneumonia, and one with a wart-like lesion. All these goats had commingled with cattle. The isolates were found to be more closely related to bovine vaccine strains of BoHV-1 than to CpHV-1 on the basis of restriction endonuclease analysis (Whetstone and Evermann 1988).

Recently, a gammaherpesvirus, known as caprine herpesvirus-2, was isolated from goats and characterized (Li et al. 2001). It has been shown to cause malignant catarrhal fever in whitetail deer (*Odocoileus virginianus*)(Li et al. 2003). In a more recent report, a putative case of malignant catarrhal fever in a pygmy goat was described (Twomey et al. 2006). The goat, which was kept with sheep, had a multisystemic necrotizing vasculitis and the gammaherpesvirus, ovine herpesvirus-2 (OvHV-2), was identified in the goat's tissues by PCR. The gammaherpesviruses are biologically distinct from the alphaherpesviruses and are not considered further here.

Epidemiology

The isolation and identification of CpHV-1 in association with naturally occurring disease was first reported from California in 1974 in cases of severe systemic infection of goat kids (Saito et al. 1974). Vulvovaginitis caused by CpHV-1 was first observed in Saanen does in New Zealand in 1981 and then in Australia in 1986 (Horner et al. 1982; Grewal and Wells 1986). Posthitis in males was identified in New Zealand in 1982, in Australia in 1984 (Tarigan et al. 1987), and more recently in bucks in California from herds experiencing abortions due to CpHV-1 (Uzal et al. 2004). Typical of herpesviruses, CpHV-1 infection demonstrates latency and recrudescence. In one New Zealand goat herd, the genital form of the disease was reported to reoccur a year after the first outbreak (Horner 1982).

Transmission of the genital disease is presumed to be venereal, but bucks need not be infected or have active lesions to spread the disease from infected to noninfected does mechanically. Increases in clinical prevalence or seroconversion can occur after the onset of the breeding season, suggesting either venereal transmission of new infections or recrudescence of latent infections secondary to stress associated with estrus and/or breeding activity. Clinical signs of vulvovaginitis in does have been reported to appear within eleven days of introduction of teaser bucks (Horner et al. 1982).

There is growing evidence of widespread CpHV-1 infection in world goat populations. Serologic evidence of CpHV-1 infection has been reported from Norway, northern Ireland, Spain, Italy, Turkey, Greece, and Syria (Kao et al. 1985; Thiry et al. 2006). In Greece, neutralizing antibodies were identified in 52.6% of 795 goats from various locations in the country (Koptopoulos et al. 1988). The Mediterranean region in general has a high seroprevalence of CpHV-1 infection in goats. As of 2006, CpHV-1 infection had not yet been identified in Belgium or the UK (Thiry et al. 2006). The infection recently has been identified in France (Thiry et al. 2008)

Pathogenesis

Genital infections in goats have been established experimentally by intranasal and intravaginal inoculation, but the pathogenesis appears to vary with the route of introduction. With intranasal challenge, virus first replicates locally, producing epithelial lesions in the nasal cavity. This is followed by viremia, as evidenced by the presence of virus in the buffy coat, and then infection of the genital tract, where virus produces characteristic lesions in the external genitalia and is shed in high titer (Tempesta et al. 1999). The viremia associated with intranasal inoculation has also been demonstrated experimentally by recovery of virus or its detection by PCR assay from the dead fetuses of pregnant does (Tempesta et al. 2004). Case reports of natural infections indicate that abortion in does due to CpHV-1 as well as the fatal syndrome observed in one- to two-week old kids are also the result of viremia, as aborted fetuses (Williams et al. 1997; Chénier et al. 2004; Uzal et al. 2004) and dead kids (Roperto et al. 2000) demonstrate the presence of CpHV-1 virus or viral DNA in multiple organs.

When goats were experimentally infected intravaginally, successful infection was manifested by genital lesions and recovery of virus from vaginal swabs for five to seven days post infection. However, no virus was identified from ocular, nasal, or rectal swabs or buffy coat, suggesting that genital infections can be established without an associated viremia (Tempesta et al. 2000).

As is characteristic of herpesviruses in other species, CpHV-1 results in latent infections with the capacity for recrudescence. The presence of virus in the sacral ganglia of latently infected goats has been confirmed by PCR assay (Tempesta et al. 1999a). Experimentally, recrudescence with viral shedding has been induced by repeated administration of high doses of dexamethasone over several days (Buonavoglia et al. 1996). In natural infections, recrudescence occurs in infected does in association with estrus, but primarily in does with low neutralizing antibody titers (Tempesta et al. 1998, 2005). Because recrudescence is associated with viral shedding, this suggests that the condition could spread rapidly through goat herds during the breeding season.

CpHV-1 was isolated from the lungs of goats in a naturally occurring outbreak of severe, fatal pneumonia in New Zealand in 1986. However, *Mannheimia (Pasteurella) haemolytica* was isolated from affected lungs in addition to CpHV-1 (Buddle et al. 1990). Experimental follow-up challenge studies were undertaken to clarify the etiologic role of CpHV-1 in these cases. Challenge with CpHV-1 alone did not produce pneumonia, while challenge with *M. haemolytica* alone or *M. haemolytica* with CpHV-1 did (Buddle et al. 1990a). CpHV-1 readily proliferated in the upper respiratory tract and lungs of the challenged goats, but its role in the pathogenesis of pneumonia remains unclear.

Clinical Findings

All goats of breeding age are susceptible to the genital form of disease. Clinical cases occur most frequently in epidemic form shortly after the onset of the breeding season. This reflects the presumption that hormonal changes associated with the onset of estrus trigger recrudescence of virus shedding in latently infected does, which may then be spread to susceptible does by breeding bucks.

The initial signs of vulvovaginitis in does are vulvar edema and hyperemia with possibly a slight amount of blood-stained discharge. No systemic signs of disease are observed. Over the next several days, a more copious yellow to gray discharge may develop, and multiple, focal, shallow erosions appear on the vulvar and vaginal mucosa. These erosions may be covered with yellow to red-brown necrotic scabs. The vulva is painful to the touch and dysuria is possible though not often reported. Lesions usually heal spontaneously within two weeks. Reproductive performance and conception rates are not affected, though animals that experienced the disease may have subsequent recurrences of lesions due to recrudescence of latent infections, usually at the next breeding season. Males used in breeding may or may not show lesions. When present, lesions consist of penile hyperemia and focal, punctate, epithelial erosions on the penis, and more frequently, the prepuce (Figure 12.6). A preputial discharge may also be present.

Clinical Pathology and Necropsy

The virus can be isolated from vaginal or preputial swabs of acute lesions for confirmation of CpHV-1 infection. Rising titers to CpHV-1 can be detected in both clinical and subclinical infections immediately after an outbreak of vulvovaginitis and balanoposthitis. Acute and convalescent serum sampling should be initiated early in the course of disease, because titers may begin to decline again by three weeks after onset of disease. Serum neutralization titers in infected goats range from 1:4 to greater than 1:256.

While a rise in titer using serum neutralization or ELISA techniques is certainly indicative of CpHV-1 infection, definitive diagnosis of CpHV-1 infection cannot be made by serologic methods because of the common cross reactivity of the alphaherpesviruses and the fact that cross-species infection can also occur, particularly with regard to BoHV-1. A blocking ELISA based on the B glycoprotein of BoHV-1 has been reported to be a good screening test for tentative identification of CpHV-1 in goat herds (Keuser et al. 2004).

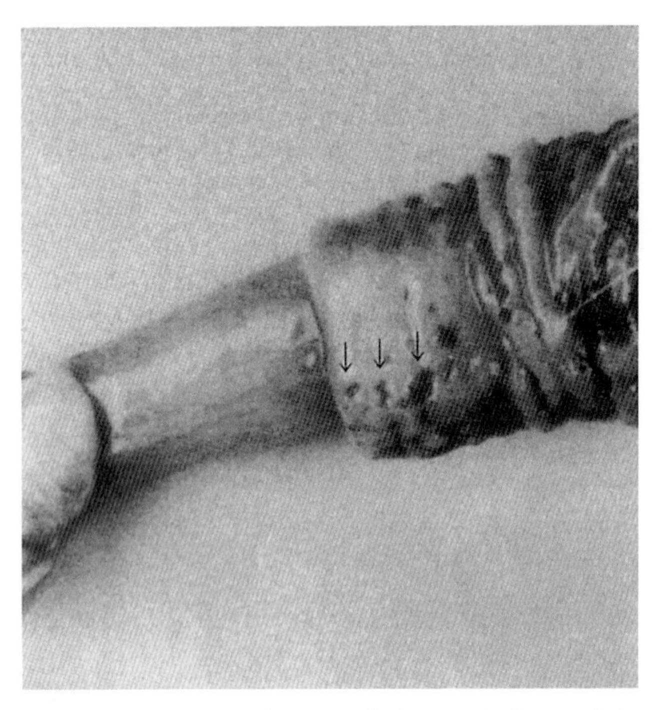

Figure 12.6. Erosive lesions of the penis (arrows) in balanoposthitis caused by caprine herpesvirus. (From Tarigan et al. 1987.)

Confirmation can be achieved by following up with double seroneutralization tests using BoHV-1 and CpHV-1 antigens and finding higher titers to the CpHV-1 antigen (Thiry et al. 2008).

Definitive diagnosis depends on virus isolation with precise characterization of the virus or detection of CpHV-1 viral DNA in tissues by appropriate means. Current techniques used for detection or characterization of the CpHV-1 virus include restriction endonuclease analysis (REA), real-time polymerase chain reaction (RT-PCR) (Elia et al. 2008), and an immunofluorescence assay able to differentiate five related alphaherpesviruses in infected cells (Thiry et al. 2006).

Necropsy diagnosis of the genital form of CpHV-1 infection is rarely required or undertaken. However, necropsy is most valuable in the diagnosis of other forms of the disease, notably abortion and death of kids one to two weeks of age. Virus isolation and viral DNA identification techniques should be conducted on tissues of aborted fetuses and dead kids.

Diagnosis

Normal estrus produces some degree of hyperemia and edema of the vulva and should not be confused with the early signs of CpHV-1 infection. Granular vulvovaginitis caused by various *Mycoplasma* spp. must be differentiated from CpHV-1 infection. Granular vulvovaginitis is reported most often from India and Nigeria (Singh et al. 1975; Singh and Rajya 1977; Tiwana et al. 1984; Chima et al. 1986). The condition is discussed more in Chapter 13. An ulcerative vulvitis with copious purulent vaginal discharge has been reported in Nigerian goats. *Arcanobacterium pyogenes* and *Staphylococcus* spp. were isolated (Ihemelandu 1972).

Treatment

There is no practical, specific treatment for CpHV-1 infection. However, there is a recent report of the use of the human antiviral drug cidofovir in goats. The drug, administered intravaginally, inhibited onset of local vaginal lesions in does and reduced viral shedding (Tempesta et al. 2007). Does and bucks with the genital form usually heal spontaneously within two weeks, though recurrent lesions are possible. Risk of secondary bacterial infections may be controlled by administration of prophylactic antibiotics.

Control

Efforts to eradicate genital CpHV-1 infection from infected flocks have been proposed based on the assumption that the disease is venereally transmitted. The evidence for this was that kids born to seropositive does and left to nurse on them did not acquire infection by passage through the birth canal, nursing, or close contact. Therefore, it was proposed that gradual elimination of infection from known infected flocks could be achieved according to the following recommendations (Horner 1988): Kids should be separated from older animals before they become sexually active and maintained as a separate group. Only seronegative bucks or teasers should be used for mating in this separate kid group. Buck kids tested before four months of age may have maternal antibody present and should be retested at a later age. At the same time, the mature, source herd should be serotested regularly and positive animals culled at detection. No new animals should be introduced into the herd that have not first been found seronegative.

Since those recommendations were made, it has been demonstrated, at least experimentally, that goats infected with CpHV-1 by the intranasal route can develop vulvovaginitis and shed virus from the genital tract (Tempesta et al. 1999). A better understanding of the transmission of CpHV-1 under field conditions is required to develop updated recommendations for management interventions to control CpHV-1 in infected herds.

Currently, there are no commercial vaccines available for controlling CpHV-1 infection. However, some experimental efforts have been reported that show promise. A β-propiolactone inactivated CpHV-1 vaccine given either subcutaneously or intravaginally protected does from clinical signs of vulvovaginitis when they were subsequently challenged intravaginally with CpHV-1 (Tempesta et al. 2001; Camero et al. 2007). A commercially available, live, attenuated, glycoprotein E-negative, BoHV-1 virus vaccine has been reported to be safe for use in goats and demonstrated partial efficacy against subsequent challenge with CpHV-1 (Thiry et al. 2006a). Additional evaluation of the vaccine against CpHV-1 is ongoing.

Ulcerative Posthitis

Though principally a disease of sheep, this infectious, inflammatory condition of the prepuce and penis is sometimes seen in castrated male goats as well. The condition is also known as enzootic posthitis, sheath rot, or pizzle rot.

Etiology and Pathogenesis

The disease is associated with the Gram-positive, diphtheroid bacterium *Corynebacterium renale*, which is capable of hydrolyzing urea. The organism is present in the prepuce of infected animals and is believed to be transmitted venereally or by insects. However, presence of the organism in the sheath alone is not sufficient to produce clinical disease. The feeding of a high protein diet increases urine urea content and thereby provides a substrate for the production of large quantities of ammonia by *C. renale.* The ammonia is believed to irritate the preputial mucosa and skin around the preputial orifice. The condition is more common in wethers than in intact males, probably because of the hypoplastic nature of the penis in castrated males. In wethers, the preputial and penile mucosa do not completely separate and urination frequently occurs without exteriorization of the penis from the prepuce. This promotes urine pooling in the preputial space and allows more complete degradation of urea by *C. renale.* Another contributing factor may be excessive hair or wool at the preputial orifice, causing the area to remain moist with urine and allowing prolonged bacterial activity on urea substrate.

Epizootiology

The disease in goats has been reported only from the United States, though the potential for it to occur elsewhere exists, because it is seen in sheep in Australia, the United Kingdom, and Spain (Loste et al. 2005). While the disease is known to be venereally transmitted by rams to ewes in some flocks, there are no reports of the condition affecting does.

The principal report of posthitis in goats comes from south central Texas where Angora wethers may be kept to advanced ages for mohair production (Shelton and Livingston 1975). The condition was observed in a large flock of wethers on rangeland containing guajillo *(Acacia angustissima).* Guajillo, a leguminous shrub, has a protein content in the range of 22% to 27% and is readily consumed by goats. Morbidity was estimated at 10% and no mortality was directly attributable to the problem.

The author has observed ulcerative posthitis in wethers in a different context. Affected goats were castrated males of dairy breeds kept to advanced age for the purpose of commercial antibody production. These animals were maintained on a commercial dairy ration containing 16% protein. Morbidity was low and the condition was not severe, but obvious swelling and inflammation were evident around the preputial orifice.

Clinical Findings

The condition may be mild to severe. In the mild form, signs are limited to a swelling of the prepuce readily noted in short-haired dairy wethers or detected in long-haired Angora wethers at shearing time. In severe cases, swelling and inflammation interfere with normal urination and signs of straining are present. These animals may kick at the abdomen, show a stiff gait or an arched back, and may lie down and rise repeatedly. Examination of the ventral abdomen reveals scabs or ulcers on the skin dorsal to and surrounding the prepuce and preputial orifice. The orifice itself may be distorted, reduced in diameter, or completely scabbed over. The sheath may be filled with urine, and exudate may be expressed by applying pressure to the prepuce. Fistulous tracts may be present. The preputial cavity and the penis may show severe ulceration and possibly maggot infestation. Animals with complete occlusion of the preputial orifice may die of uremia.

Clinical Pathology and Necropsy

Swabs of the preputial cavity should allow isolation of *C. renale.* Animals with extensive ulceration inside the prepuce and on the penis may die. Necropsy demonstrates extensive exudation within the preputial cavity and ulcers and scar tissue on the mucosa. The urethral process may be necrotic and ulcers present on the glans penis.

Diagnosis

On rare occasions, goats may show scabby lesions of contagious ecthyma on the prepuce, but similar lesions also likely would be found elsewhere on the face and body. Ulcerative dermatosis, a similar viral disease of sheep, is not reported in goats. Obstructive disease of the gastrointestinal tract and obstructive urolithiasis must be considered in the differential diagnosis of goats with signs of straining or abdominal discomfort.

Treatment

Affected animals should be separated from the herd or flock and the high protein component of their

. Clipping hair from around the pre- improve the rate of healing. Reestab- of the urethral orifice is the first in animals unable to urinate. Lesions be debrided and topical treatment begun. *C. renale* is usually sensitive to penicillins, ampicillins, and cephalosporins. As these antibiotics are excreted in urine, systemic treatment will also provide local therapy. Intramammary infusion tubes designed for mastitis treatment are convenient vehicles for administering these antibiotics into the preputial cavity, though care should be taken not to transmit infection to unaffected herd mates. Repeated daily treatment with ophthalmic ointment containing bacitracin, neomycin, and prednisolone applied topically to the prepuce has also been reported to be effective as an ancillary treatment in sheep (Loste et al. 2005). In severe exudative cases, opening the prepuce surgically with a scissors along the ventrum is indicated for salvage. Except in the most severe cases, the prognosis for recovery is good.

Control

Dietary protein should be limited to a level consistent with the nutritional requirement of the animals. This may be problematic under range conditions. Preputial hair should be kept clipped to reduce urine accumulation. Animals with external lesions identified at shearing time should be treated topically with antiseptics or antibiotics to control lesions and reduce spread in the flock. Implantation of wethers with 70 to 100 mg of testosterone at three-month intervals has been effective in controlling ulcerative posthitis, but this method has not been evaluated in goats (Kimberling 1988). Castration using the so-called short scrotum technique has also been suggested because it renders wethers infertile but allows the urethra and penis to mature under the influence of testosterone. In this technique, both testes are pushed up into the inguinal canal or inguinal region and a rubber ring is applied around the neck of the scrotum below the testes. There are animal welfare concerns associated with the use of this technique (Molony et al. 2002).

NUTRITIONAL AND METABOLIC DISEASES

Obstructive Urolithiasis

In goats, clinical obstructive urolithiasis is most frequently seen in young, castrated males and the calculi are usually comprised of phosphate salts, especially calcium phosphate (apatite) and magnesium ammonium phosphate (struvite). Goats kept as pets are at high risk for developing the condition due primarily to the feeding of excessive grain in the diet. The case management and treatment options of goats kept as pets may differ considerably from those for goats kept as livestock.

Etiology and Pathogenesis

Obstructive urolithiasis is the inability to normally void urine because of obstruction of the urinary outflow tract by calculi. The formation of urinary calculi results from the interaction of numerous physiological, nutritional, and management-related factors. The tendency for urinary calculi to become lodged in the urethra derives from anatomic factors and castration practices in male ruminants. Factors predisposing to urinary calculi formation in livestock have been well reviewed (Radostits et al. 2007).

The urine is a highly saturated solution of mineral solutes. Under normal circumstances, these solutes usually remain in solution. However, numerous factors can predispose to precipitation of minerals from urine leading to calculi formation. These include increased urine concentration from decreased water intake or increased insensible water loss, urine stasis, increases in urine pH that favor precipitation of phosphate calculi, increased mineral concentration in the urine related to diet composition, and decreases in the concentration of protective colloids in the urine that ordinarily inhibit precipitation by transforming the urine into a stable gel.

Calculus composition frequently reflects diet. Silicate calculi are common where grass and cereal hays are the main dietary constituents, particularly in arid regions. Forages high in oxalates promote oxalate calculi, with certain plants such as *Halogeton* contributing significantly to the problem. Subterranean clover is high in calcium and extensive grazing may lead to calcium carbonate stones. Grain rations, or concentrates, are commonly high in phosphorus and relatively low in calcium. This imbalance promotes the formation of phosphate calculi, as frequently seen in feedlot steers and wethers on fattening diets. The calculogenic potential of such diets is increased when the concentrate is also high in magnesium.

In goats, several relationships of diet to calculus formation have been observed in the field or confirmed experimentally. Obstructive urolithiasis caused by magnesium ammonium phosphate (struvite) calculi was observed in Brazilian goats fed a concentrate ration of three parts corn to one part cottonseed meal (Unanian et al. 1982) and in Australian Angora goats fed a pelleted feedlot fattening ration with a calcium-to-phosphorus ratio of 1:15 (Bellenger et al. 1981). Goats fed rations containing magnesium in excess of 0.6% developed struvite crystals or calculi even when the calcium-to-phosphorus ratio was properly balanced (James and Chandran 1975; James and Mukundan 1978). Experimentally, phosphate calculi were consistently produced in goats fed a ground corn and soybean meal ration supplemented with 3.5% K_2HPO_4 (Sato and Omori 1977).

There are additional factors in the actual formation of calculi. A nidus may be necessary for calculus formation to occur. Desquamated epithelial cells in the urinary bladder are commonly considered to function as a nidus. Factors which may contribute to increased desquamation of epithelial cells include vitamin A deficiency and infections of the urinary tract. A role for vitamin A deficiency in obstructive urolithiasis has been specifically confirmed in goats (Schmidt 1941). Desquamated epithelium in sufficient quantity may obstruct the urethra, even without the formation of mineral calculi. Infections can alter urine pH, which may promote precipitation of mineral salts.

Once calculus formation is initiated, growth occurs by the process of concretion. Increased mucoproteins in the urine serve as a matrix and favor concretion. The feeding of high concentrate rations, particularly in pelleted form, promotes an increase in urine mucoproteins.

Obstruction is not a necessary result of calculus formation, but is predisposed by anatomic factors. Obstructive urolithiasis is rarely seen in female ruminants despite the fact that calculi can and do form. The short, straight urethra allows calculi to pass easily with the urine. In contrast, the long, convoluted course of the urethra through the sigmoid flexure of the penis, ending in the small urethral process, provides ample opportunity for even small calculi to become lodged in the male urethra. This tendency is aggravated by early castration of male ruminants that results in penile hypoplasia with attendant reduction in urethral bore size, and failure of the maturing urethral process to separate completely from its distal attachment to the preputial mucosa. The effect of castration on reduced urethral diameter has been documented in goats (Kumar et al. 1982). Exogenous estrogens either in the diet or from growth-promoting implants can also lead to reduced urethral diameter by promoting swelling of the surrounding accessory sex glands in the pelvic region.

When complete obstruction of the urethra occurs, forceful attempts to urinate produce little or no voided urine. Animals so affected soon become azotemic because of decreased renal function, secondary hydroureter, and hydronephrosis.

Unless the obstruction is relieved spontaneously or by intervention, the urinary bladder or the urethra will eventually rupture. In the former case, abdominal distension may result as urine fills the peritoneal cavity. In the latter case, urine fills the subcutaneous space in the perineal or preputial region depending on the site of urethral rupture. At this point, the uremic process accelerates and, without veterinary intervention, the animal ultimately dies.

Epidemiology

Obstructive urolithiasis is a well recognized, highly prevalent, and costly disease of fattening steers and sheep wethers maintained in feedlot conditions and fed high concentrate rations. Goats are rarely managed in similar intensified fattening situations, and therefore the disease is far less prevalent in the caprine species, though growing interest in commercial goat meat production could alter this situation.

In the United States and Europe, most affected goats are young males, often castrated, and frequently maintained as pets (Craig et al. 1987; van Weeren et al. 1987a). A retrospective study of thirty-eight cases of caprine obstructive urolithiasis seen at Tufts University in Massachusetts showed twenty-four affected goats to be castrated males and fourteen to be intact males, with no female cases seen. The average age of affected goats was twenty-seven months, with a range of two months to twelve years. Many of these goats were obese, and virtually all were on high grain diets providing energy in excess of their metabolic needs as inactive pets. There was an increased prevalence in summer and winter, times when dehydration is more likely to occur. Phosphatic calculi (struvite and apatite) were most common and occurred in the form of either sand or sediment. Calcium carbonate calculi were less frequently identified, larger, and more likely to occur as stones. More recent case reviews from a number of veterinary teaching hospitals or referral centers report similar findings, with young, castrated male goats representing the most common signalment for obstructive urolithiasis, and virtually no cases involving females (Ewoldt et al. 2006; George et al. 2007). Pet goats are increasingly represented in these case populations, at least in the United States.

In Texas, obstructive urolithiasis is recognized as a potential problem in young Angora males being raised for sale as replacement breeding stock. To promote growth and condition in time for sale before the breeding season, these animals are fed a pelleted ration comprised of sorghum or corn, cottonseed hulls, and alfalfa. The diet is recognized as highly calculogenic and obstructive urolithiasis is avoided by appropriate adjustment of the calcium-to-phosphorus ratio and addition of salt and urinary acidifiers.

In Brazil, urolithiasis occurs sporadically in the Northeast region when goats are managed intensively and fed corn and cottonseed concentrates (Unanian and Silva 1987). In Queensland, Australia, Angora goats were most commonly reported to experience obstructive urolithiasis because of greater access to grain and formulated feedstuffs (Manning and Blaney 1986). Urolithiasis in goats occurs elsewhere in the world but contributing factors are not always evident or reported.

Clinical Findings

In the first phase of obstruction, male goats show restlessness and anxiety. Tail twitching is an early sign. There may be excessive vocalizing and animals strain frequently and forcefully to urinate, often stretching their bodies out to full length with a dip to the back, followed by arching. Marked abdominal press may produce some degree of rectal prolapse. Inexperienced owners may assume that the animals are constipated and medicate goats inappropriately rather than seeking veterinary attention. Palpation of the urethra on the median raphe in the perineal region reveals distension and pulsation during straining. Drops of bloody urine and/or crystals may be seen attached to preputial hairs. Animals with partial obstruction may be able to void small intermittent streams of urine, but show discomfort.

Careful examination of the urethra should be undertaken in an attempt to locate the site of obstruction. Visualization of the urethral process may reveal calculi at this common site of blockage (Figure 12.7). Deep palpation of the urethra along the prepuce and perineum may indicate pain or swelling at more proximal sites of obstruction such as the sigmoid flexure.

When the obstruction goes uncorrected, rupture of the bladder or urethra usually results within twenty-four to forty-eight hours. Rupture relieves pressure and may produce alleviation of discomfort and anxiety so that the animal resumes a more normal attitude, at least until the signs of uremia supervene. Inexperienced owners may interpret this as a resolution of the problem rather than a progression of the problem, and thereby delay seeking veterinary attention. If it is the urethra that ruptures, then subcutaneous filling of the preputial or perineal region becomes noticeable. In rupture of the urinary bladder, bilateral, ventral abdominal distension develops, but progresses more slowly and may be more difficult to detect, especially in obese goats or pygmy goats that already have distended appearing abdomens.

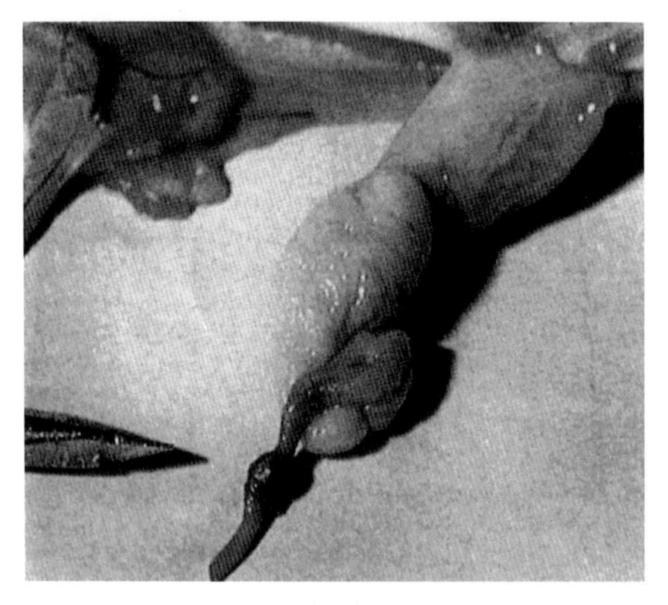

Figure 12.7. A common site of urethral obstruction with calculi is at the urethral process. The lesion pictured is highly unusual in that the obstruction at the urethral process is a lead shotgun pellet rather than mineral calculi as is usually the case. (From Blackwell and Dale 1983.)

Ensuing uremia causes affected goats to become anorexic, weak, and depressed. Advanced cases often present in a moribund state and the condition is fatal if left untreated. The entire clinical course is usually two to five days.

Clinical Pathology, Radiology, and Necropsy

The most consistently reported abnormality of clinical chemistry in goats with obstructive urolithiasis is azotemia. This is reflected in the chemistry profile as high levels of blood urea nitrogen and serum creatinine. These levels may climb even higher if rupture of the bladder or urethra occurs. Levels of BUN in affected goats have been reported in the range of 11.7 to 47.5 mmol/l (70 to 285 mg/dl) (van Weeren et al. 1987). Recently, a summary of biochemical abnormalities in 107 goats with uroliths was reported (George et al. 2007). Compared to control goats, goats with urolithiasis had higher mean BUN, creatinine, total CO_2, glucose, and potassium concentrations, and lower phosphorus concentrations. Hypochloremic metabolic alkalosis was the most common acid-base disorder. Rupture of the bladder or urethra was associated with an increased prevalence of hyperkalemia and hyponatremia. Hypophosphatemia was an unexpected finding in this series of cases, because among the domestic species, with the exception of horses, hyperphosphatemia is usually associated with postrenal obstruction or ruptured bladder.

Urine sediment should be examined whenever a urine sample can be obtained. Marked crystalluria supports the diagnosis of obstructive urolithiasis. Aspiration of subcutaneous or peritoneal fluid can be helpful, though confirming that the fluid is urine can be problematic. It has been reported that urine can accumulate in the abdomen, even in the absence of bladder rupture, presumably due to passage of urine through an intact but compromised bladder wall under intense pressure (Ewoldt et al. 2006). Some obstructed goats develop hydronephrosis or leak urine around the kidney. A urea nitrogen or creatinine level equal to or greater than that of blood suggests that the abdominal fluid is urine. An odor of urine may be helpful in field diagnosis.

Plain radiographs only rarely reveal cystic or urethral calculi and their use in cases of obstructive urolithiasis is not considered to be cost-effective, whereas contrast studies can be very effective both as diagnostic aids and in case management. In one retrospective study involving twenty-one goats with urolithiasis, the most useful imaging technique was normograde contrast cystourethrography performed through a tube cystostomy catheter placed as part of the surgical treatment for the cases involved (Palmer et al. 1998). Plain radiographs and excretory urethrography offered little diagnostic assistance in those cases. Ultrasonography also provides a rapid, noninvasive, and safe means of assessing the extent and location of calculi.

At necropsy, careful dissection of the urinary tract reveals the presence of calculi, urethral trauma (Figure 12.8), and bladder or urethral rupture. Calculi may be present in the bladder or renal pelvis as an incidental finding in goats dying of causes other than obstructive urolithiasis, and their presence suggests the need for reviewing nutritional management in the source herd. Calculi obtained during case management or at necropsy should be submitted for chemical analysis.

Diagnosis

Diagnosis is based on the characteristic signalment, history, and clinical signs of obstructive urolithiasis. During the early stages, when straining is present, gastrointestinal obstructions should be considered. When stranguria is recognized, cystitis and ulcerative posthitis must be ruled out. When the bladder or urethra has ruptured and signs of uremia predominate, other causes of profound depression and weakness must be considered, especially hepatoencephalopathy and enterotoxemia. Confirmation of the presence of urine in the abdomen or subcutaneously quickly narrows the diagnosis.

Treatment

The approach to treatment depends on the stage of the disease, the nature and extent of calculi present, the intended long-term use of the animal, and frequently, financial constraints. When conservative treatment does not alleviate the condition and surgical intervention becomes necessary, a guarded prognosis should be given for successful long-term outcome. This is particularly true for intact breeding bucks and goats maintained as pets.

Medical Management. If cases are seen before rupture of the bladder or urethra occurs, conservative management can be attempted. If calculi are lodged in the urethral process, the process can be amputated to reestablish patency. When sandy material or sludge is present in the urethral process, it sometimes can be successfully milked out without removing the process itself. Such efforts require exteriorization of the penis from the sheath. This can be facilitated by the cooperation of a capable assistant as described earlier in the chapter for examination of the penis and by tranquilization of the animal, using diazepam, at a dose range of 0.1 to 0.5 mg/kg intravenously or acepromazine (0.05 to 0.1 mg/kg intravenously). Alternatively, for better analgesia and relaxation of the retractor penis muscle, lumbosacral epidural anesthesia can be

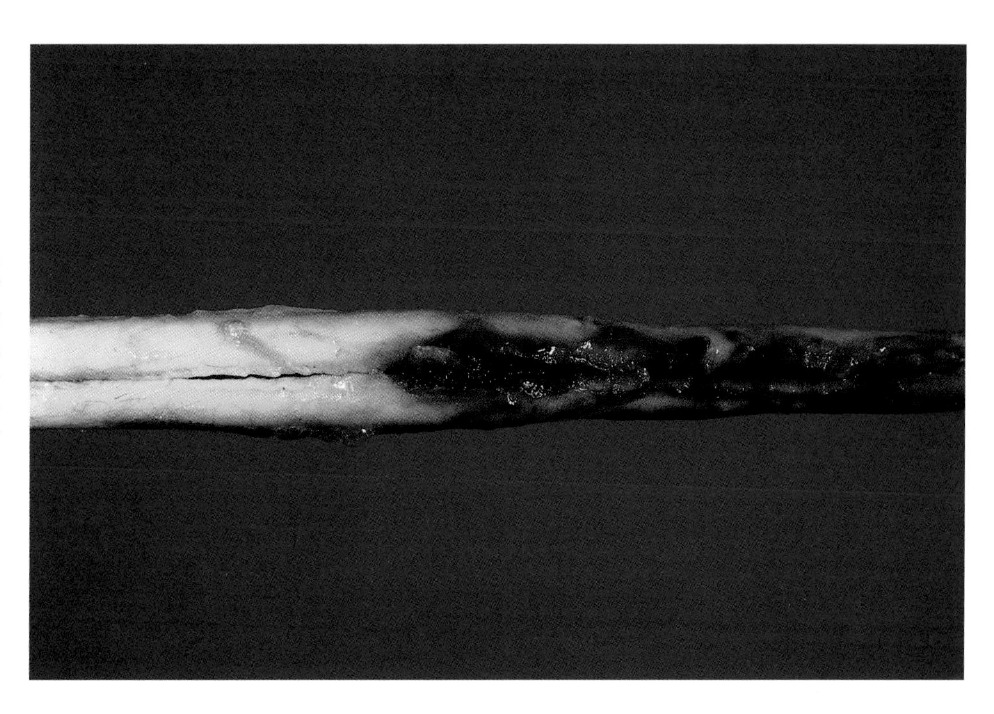

Figure 12.8. Necrosis, inflammation, and hemorrhage of the penile urethra at the site of an obstructive calculi in a young wether viewed at necropsy. (Courtesy of the Cummings School of Veterinary Medicine at Tufts University.)

employed, using 2% lidocaine at a dose of 0.1 to 0.2 ml/kg bw administered into the epidural space at the lumbosacral junction. The maximum dose of lidocaine should not exceed 15 ml (Van Metre et al. 1996).

Amputation of the urethral process should be viewed as a short-term, temporary solution or as a salvage operation, because the likelihood of recurrence of obstructive urolithiasis is high after removal of the urethral process. This is exemplified in one retrospective study from North Carolina, where, in fourteen of sixteen cases (87.5%), urethral process amputation with medical therapy either did not relieve the obstruction or provided relief of less than thirty-six hours (Haven et al. 1992).

If calculi are lodged proximal to the urethral process, attempts can be made to pass a catheter far enough into the urethra to permit infusions of sterile saline in attempts to distend the urethra and dislodge the offending calculi (urohydropulsion). This procedure is frequently unsuccessful and often traumatic, and may result in urethral rupture or stricture, especially if attempts to force the catheter past the urethral diverticulum are made. Recently the use of urethroscopy in association with laser lithotripsy has been reported to fracture and clear calculi from the distal urethra in three goats for which urohydropulsion was not successful (Halland et al. 2002).

When urohydropulsion fails, tranquilizers and antispasmodics may help to promote urethral relaxation and facilitate natural expulsion of the calculus by the pressure of attempted urination. Diazepam, at a dose range of 0.1 to 0.5 mg/kg intravenously, acepromazine (0.1 mg/kg intravenously), or aminopromazine (2 mg/kg intramuscularly) each have been used for this purpose, with variable results. Xylazine hydrochloride should not be used in these cases because its hyperglycemic effect promotes diuresis, and increases in urine production are problematic in a goat with urinary tract obstruction.

Surgical Management. When conservative treatment fails, then some sort of surgical intervention, or euthanasia, becomes necessary. Detailed descriptions of the surgical procedures discussed here are beyond the scope of this book and are available in current veterinary surgery texts (Tibary and Van Metre 2004) as well as on the Internet in the "hot topics" section of the Website of the American Association of Small Ruminant Practitioners (www.aasrp.org). The surgical procedures discussed here include perineal urethrostomy, penile amputation, ischial urethrostomy, ischial urethrotomy, surgical tube cystostomy, and marsupialization of the bladder. Prepubic urethrostomy, used in feline practice as a salvage technique for obstructive disease of the pelvic urethra, is also sometimes used in goats with favorable results, but is not discussed further here (Stone et al. 1997).

Before any surgery is attempted, particularly if general anesthesia will be involved, the patient should be evaluated for hydration status, uremia, and electrolyte imbalances, and these should be addressed through appropriate fluid therapy. Because goats with obstructive urolithiasis tend to be hyperkalemic, hypochloremic, and hyponatremic, sterile physiologic saline solution is a good empirical choice of intravenous fluid if laboratory assessment is not available (Van Metre et al. 1996). With regard to evaluating the suitability of cases for surgery and the associated prognosis, it has been reported that an intact urethral process, the absence of fluid in the abdomen, and serum potassium concentrations less than 5.2 mEq/L at admission were all associated with greater survival following surgical tube cystostomy (Ewoldt et al. 2006).

It should be noted that bladder rupture in and of itself does not necessarily require surgery. If urine outflow can be established by conservative means, the bladder defect, which often seals with fibrin or by adhesions, may heal spontaneously. This is more true of rents in the dorsal bladder wall than the ventral wall.

If the bladder has ruptured, urine should be drained from the abdomen via abdominocentesis to slow the uremic process if surgery is delayed. This should not be accomplished too abruptly, because it could predispose to hypovolemic shock when blood which was displaced by the fluid pressure of uroperitoneum returns to the visceral vasculature from the general circulation. If the urethra has ruptured, multiple, small stab incisions can be made in the skin over the areas of urine accumulation to allow drainage.

When the decision is made that surgery is required for satisfactory case management, then the surgical approach selected depends to a great extent on the intended use of the animal and the estimated overall cost of the surgery, hospitalization, and aftercare. Clear and careful client communication is critical in these cases, because uncomplicated, fully satisfactory recoveries cannot be guaranteed and misunderstandings or false expectations about the ultimate outcome can lead to poor veterinarian-client relations, especially when pet goats or breeding bucks are involved.

For commercial wethers or intact males destined for slaughter, two relatively simple and low cost salvage procedures are commonly in use—perineal urethrostomy and penile amputation. When performing perineal urethrostomy, a site as low on the perineum as possible should be selected for the incision for two reasons. First, it reduces the extent of subsequent urine scald. Second, the procedure is prone to failure due to stricture of the surgically created urethral opening. If that occurs, the surgery can be repeated at a site higher on the perineum to extend the salvage period for the animal. Additional salvage procedures which have been used in goats or sheep include ischial urethrostomy and ischial urethrotomy. Ischial urethrostomy offers an advantage over perineal urethrostomy in that the pelvic urethra is exteriorized instead of the penile urethra. The wider bore of the pelvic urethra reduces the likelihood of stricture at the stoma site.

For breeding bucks, surgical tube cystostomy has emerged as the preferred surgical approach for retaining breeding capacity (Van Metre and Fubini 2006). In this procedure, a paramedian abdominal approach is made and the bladder exteriorized so that a cystostomy can be performed to remove calculi from the bladder, and to place an indwelling balloon type (Foley) catheter which is exteriorized through a second stab incision and sutured in place (Figure 12.9). Ruptures of the bladder can also be repaired during this procedure if required. Antibiotic treatment should be initiated prior to surgery and continued for one week after the cystostomy catheter is finally removed, because cystitis is a potential complication of this procedure.

Recently, in a report on the outcomes of fifty goats and thirteen sheep treated for obstructive urolithiasis with surgical tube cystostomy, forty-eight of sixty-three cases (76%) were discharged from the hospital with normal urethral urination. At six-month follow up, thirty-four cases could be located and twenty-two (65%) of these had no recurrence of urethral obstruction. While some animals were lost to long-term follow up, at twelve months up to seventy-two months after discharge, eighteen of twenty animals (90%) identified as still alive had no recurrence of urethral obstruction (Ewoldt et al. 2006).

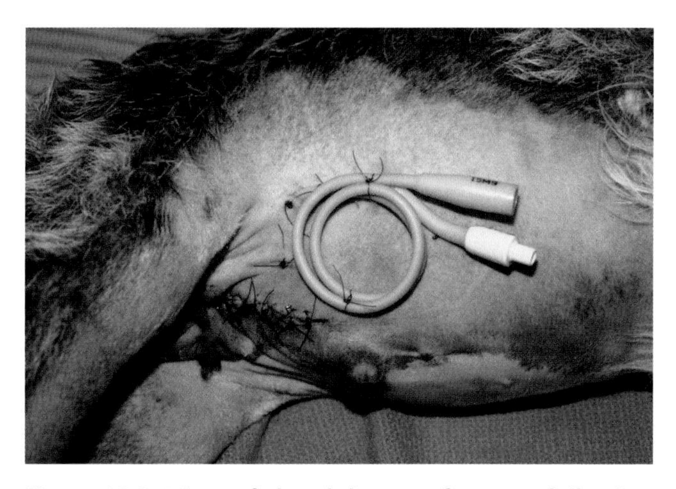

Figure 12.9. View of the abdomen of a goat following surgical tube cystostomy for treatment of obstructive urolithiasis. Note the Foley catheter secured to the skin distal to its emergence from the urinary bladder through a paramedian stab incision. The primary cystostomy incision is lateral to the prepuce. (Photo courtesy of Dr. Peter Rakestraw.)

Early reports of surgical tube cystostomy often included antegrade flushing of the urethra as part of the surgical procedure, but more recently, flushing has been seen as potentially traumatic, contributing to prolonged surgical time and unnecessary. In the report of Ewoldt et al. (2006), calculi present in the bladder were removed, but no urethral flushing was done. Reestablishment of urethral patency was allowed to occur spontaneously after surgery.

In such cases, the indwelling catheter is left open after surgery to allow urine outflow. Then, beginning on the fourth day after surgery, the catheter is periodically occluded to determine if the animal is able to pass urine through the urethra. If the animal continues to display stranguria or failure to urinate, then the catheter is reopened to allow urine outflow and occluded again periodically until the patient can urinate freely. Once that occurs, the catheter is left in place for an additional three days and then removed, allowing the cystostomy site to heal on its own. Rakestraw et al. (1995) reported that the mean time until animals could urinate freely following surgery was eleven and a half days, with a mean time of fourteen and a half days until the cystostomy tube was removed. The principle behind this approach is that diversion of urine outflow through the catheter avoids repeated trauma to the urethra caused by straining, and thereby allows the urethra to relax and heal, with a strong likelihood that calculi present in the distal urethra will ultimately dissolve or dislodge spontaneously.

Of course a successful outcome is not guaranteed in these cases. Obstruction of the catheter itself with clotted blood, calculi, or sludge can occur. Therefore, it is suggested that larger bore catheters, 18 to 24 or larger French, be used (Van Metre and Fubini 2006). In addition, catheters have been reported to malfunction, with the balloon not retaining its inflation. This has been associated with catheters that have been reused after autoclaving and it is therefore recommended that for tube cystostomy, only new catheters be used. Animals may also chew on catheters and dislodge or damage them, so application of Elizabethan restraint collars is indicated post surgically.

Even when the animal recovers successfully from the procedure, maintenance of reproduction in breeding bucks is not assured as evidenced by the reported case of erection failure associated with vascular occlusion of the corpus cavernosum penis in a goat three months after surgical tube cystostomy. The vascular lesion was believed to be associated with trauma from the inciting urethral obstruction and not the surgical procedure (Todhunter et al. 1996). Nevertheless the ultimate goal of retaining breeding function was not realized.

Anti-inflammatory drugs post surgically should be used to facilitate urethral healing. Flunixin meglumine at a dose of 1.1 mg/kg bw BID intravenously for three to five days and then 0.5 mg/kg SID IM for an additional three to five days has been reported. Acepromazine can be given to promote relaxation of the urethra post surgically. A low dose of 0.02 mg/kg bw given subcutaneously two or three times a day has been used (Ewoldt et al. 2006).

Efforts to dissolve existing calculi have also been employed to improve outcomes. In one case, irrigation of the bladder through the cystostomy catheter with the chemolytic solution hemiacidrin was reported for dissolution of calculi (Streeter et al. 2002). Hemiacidrin is an acidic solution of citric acid, magnesium carbonate, and glucono-delta-lactone used effectively for dissolution of calcium phosphate and magnesium ammonium phosphate uroliths in human medicine. In the case of the goat, 30 ml of hemiacidrin was infused into the bladder via the cystostomy catheter and then the catheter was occluded for thirty minutes, after which the infusion was allowed to drain out. This was repeated four times a day for three days and appeared to be effective in dissolving existing calculi based on ultrasound evaluation. Because the report only involved one case, additional assessment on the use of hemiacidrin as an adjunct to cystostomy for treatment of caprine urolithiasis is needed.

Acetic acid solution is also used for daily infusion into the bladder through the cystostomy tube post surgically (Tibary and Van Metre 2004). One drop of glacial acetic acid in 500 ml of nonbuffered sterile saline produces a solution in the desired pH range of 4.5 to 5.5, 60–150 ml of which can be infused and left for one to two hours before draining (Van Metre et al. 1996a). The pH should be checked before use.

Cystostomy combined with antegrade and retrograde flushing of the urethra but without tube placement was also reported to offer good results (Haven et al. 1993) but the procedure has some disadvantages, including the risk of urethral rupture during flushing, the need for an assistant to accomplish retrograde urethral flushing, and a potentially prolonged surgical time, since it can sometimes take two to three hours of repetitive flushing to fully clear the urethra of obstruction (Van Metre et al. 1996a). The technique has largely been displaced by surgical tube cystostomy.

Ultrasound-guided percutaneous tube cystostomy has been assessed as a surgical treatment option and found to be unsatisfactory. In a series of ten cases, all required a second surgery, five because of tube displacement from the bladder, four because of persistent or recurrent obstructive urolithiasis, and one because of subsequent urethral rupture (Fortier et al. 2004). While surgical tube cystostomy takes longer and is more costly than percutaneous tube cystostomy, the long-term outcome is much better.

Another alternative surgical procedure for breeding animals is urethrotomy in those cases in which a discrete single stone can be located by palpation or imaging studies and can be accessed and removed via an incision through the urethra. Success depends in large part on the accuracy of determining that only a single calculus is involved. Urethral stricture at the surgery site is a serious potential complication.

For pet goats, surgical tube cystostomy or marsupialization of the bladder are considered satisfactory surgical approaches. The former is likely to produce a more desirable outcome, but the latter is cheaper, a consideration for many owners. In one study of surgically managed obstructive urolithiasis cases, goats with bladder marsupialization had a median duration of hospitalization less than one-fourth the duration of goats with surgical tube cystostomy and at two-thirds the cost (Fortier et al. 2004) The main objection to marsupialization is that the permanent stoma on the ventral abdomen is associated with chronic urine scald which requires regular attention by the owner, including clipping the hair around the site, washing, and applying petroleum jelly or other salves. Surgical placement of the stoma as far forward on the ventral abdomen as is possible without causing undue tension or strain on the bladder itself helps to obviate this problem.

Other complications of marsupialization may include prolapse of the urinary bladder mucosa, stricture of the stoma, and possibly cystitis. In one report of nineteen cases of obstructive urolithiasis corrected by bladder marsupialization, eighteen of nineteen goats survived the procedure. At follow up between one and fifty-nine months after surgery, one animal had developed cystitis and one had a closure of the stoma due to fibrosis. While all the surviving goats had urine scald associated with the stoma site, fifteen of seventeen owners were satisfied with the procedure and its outcome. The two dissatisfied owners cited odor and urine scald as their objections (May et al. 1998). In that study, the median hospitalization time associated with the procedure was four days (range one to ten days) as compared to a mean hospitalization time of fourteen ± ten days in a report on a case series of sixty-three small ruminants treated by tube cystostomy (Ewoldt et al. 2006).

Before the techniques of surgical tube cystostomy and bladder marsupialization were refined and successfully applied in goats, perineal urethrostomy was often the intervention used for managing obstructive urolithiasis in pet goats. However, with the advent of these improved procedures, perineal urethrostomy should not be recommended for goats kept as pets due to the likelihood of recurrence, associated expense of additional corrective procedures, and owner dissatisfaction.

If owners insist on this salvage procedure for financial reasons, it should be made clear that long-term prospects for return to normalcy are poor because strictures of the urethra at the urethrostomy site are common. In a study from the Netherlands on perineal urethrostomy in twenty-eight goats and sheep, ten died or were euthanized in the immediate post surgical period. Of the eighteen that left the hospital, only eight had no additional problems on extended follow-up. Most of the others re-obstructed and were destroyed or required second or even third operations (van Weeren et al 1987a). Even when patency is maintained after urethrostomy, persistent problems with urine scalding on the perineum and hind limbs often make the outcome undesirable to owners.

Regardless of the type of surgical management selected, certain considerations of post surgical management apply. Animals need to be monitored for abnormalities associated with uremia and treated with appropriate fluid and electrolytes as needed. Antibiotic therapy is indicated to prevent cystitis or ascending infection. Procaine penicillin G at 22,000 IU/kg intramuscularly BID, or ampicillin at 15 mg/kg TID subcutaneously have been used effectively. In the case of surgical tube cystostomy, continuation of antibiotic therapy for one week after removal of the tube is recommended.

In bladder marsupialization, antibiotics should be given for one week post surgery. While there may be an inclination to keep the animals on antibiotics for prolonged periods because the bladder is open to contamination through the stoma, this is not recommended. One reason is that the occurrence of cystitis is facilitated by urine stasis and there is no stasis when the urine can passage continuously from the bladder stoma. Second, prolonged antibiotic use may promote selection of highly resistant bacteria so that if cystitis does occur, treatment options will be limited. As such, infections that occur in marsupialized animals should be treated as they occur, preferably with antibiotic selection guided by culture and sensitivity. Marsupialized animals should be housed in clean, dry quarters when returned home.

Whenever possible, calculi removed at time of surgery or by conservative treatment should be submitted to a suitable laboratory for structural analysis. This permits appropriate dietary and management recommendations to be made for preventing new calculi on the basis of their composition.

Control

Prevention of obstructive urolithiasis depends primarily on inhibiting the formation of calculi through ion aggregation in the urine. There are three main points of control to achieve this goal: increasing urine output, acidifying the urine, and reducing the presence of calculogenic solutes in the urine. Each will be discussed separately but in practice, they are combined to successfully control the disease.

Increasing Urine Output. The solutes in concentrated urine are more likely to precipitate and form uroliths than the solutes in dilute urine, so efforts to increase water intake and promote diuresis are critically important. Access to a clean, reliable, and adequate water supply must be assured. Goats can be particularly finicky about drinking water that is contaminated with feces, feed, or other foreign materials, so care in placement and cleanliness of waterers is important. Goats are also very hierarchical and some dominant animals may keep others away from waterers, so adequate space at the water source is also a consideration. Heating water supplies in the winter and shading then in the summer may also promote consumption. For pet goats, owners may try adding flavored, sugared drink powders to encourage water consumption.

A key intervention to stimulate water consumption and to dilute the urine is the feeding of increased salt in the ration. Sodium chloride should be fed at a rate of 3% to 5% of the total dry matter intake, which can be estimated at about 2% of bodyweight, so that a 40-kg wether would eat about 0.8 kg dry matter and require between 24 and 40 g of sodium chloride per day. Goats may be unwilling to consume this level of salt reliably if offered free choice or in a lick, so if necessary, it should be incorporated directly into the ration. One approach is to put the salt into solution and spray it onto the hay.

Acidify Urine. Ruminant urine is normally alkaline and the alkaline pH favors the formation of calculi. Acidification of urine can increase the solubility of uroliths composed of magnesium ammonium phosphate (struvite), calcium phosphate (apatite), and calcium carbonate, and thereby inhibit their precipitation from the urine. There is also evidence in sheep that silicate urolith formation can be suppressed by urinary acidification (Stewart et al. 1991). Addition of anionic salts such as ammonium chloride to the ration can be helpful in this regard (Stratton-Phelps and House 2004). The daily dose can be calculated as either 0.5% to 1% of the total dry matter intake, 2% of the concentrate ration, or 200 to 300 mg/kg/bw/day. Ammonium sulfate has been used in place of ammonium chloride at a rate of 0.6% to 0.7% of the total ration. However, feeding of ammonium sulfate has been associated with cases of polioencephalomalacia in lambs (Jeffrey et al. 1994). Ammonium chloride is not very palatable to goats, so free choice feeding is not likely to be successful. It may be necessary to add the ammonium chloride to some concentrate feed to encourage consumption, remembering that concentrate feed itself is calculogenic and should be limited in the diet. Alternately, for individual animals, it can be mixed with a sugar solution, honey, or syrup, and administered as a drench.

Urinary acidifiers are not a panacea. Under experimental conditions in Brazil, ammonium chloride given to goats on a calculogenic diet at a rate of 0.5% of the concentrate ration did not prevent the occurrence of calculi (Unanian et al. 1985). It is also possible that goats may become refractory to the urinary acidifying effects of anion supplementation and the urine pH may gradually revert to the alkaline range (Stratton-Phelps and House 2004). In addition, it has been suggested that long-term use of ammonium chloride can lead to bone resorption in goats (Vagg and Payne 1970).

Reduce Calculogenic Solutes in Urine. Dietary management is key to reducing the solutes in urine that lead to urolith formation. Dietary changes need to be linked to the particular type of urolith affecting the animal or herd.

The occurrence of phosphate calculi such as struvite is closely associated with the feeding of rations containing high levels of cereal grains which are high in phosphorous content. There is a tendency for pet goat owners to feed grain to their animals well beyond the goat's metabolic needs, which may require no more than a maintenance diet. Grain feeding to pet goats should be sharply curtailed and grass hay or oat hay should be promoted as the basis of the diet.

The feeding of pelleted rations reduces saliva production and with it, the excretion of phosphorus through the saliva and alimentary tract. As a result, phosphorus secretion via the kidney increases. Therefore, herds in which phosphate calculi are a problem should not be fed pelleted rations. Another concern relative to phosphatic calculi is the calcium-to-phosphorus ratio in the diet. Calcium inhibits phosphorus absorption from the gut, so if the ratio of calcium to phosphorus in the diet is too low, then more phosphorus is absorbed and ultimately excreted in the urine. Ideally, the calcium-to-phosphorus ratio in the diet should be in the range of 2:1 to 2.5:1.

Magnesium can also play a role in the development of phosphatic calculi. Even when the calcium-to-phosphorus ratio is in the desired range, excess magnesium in the diet can lead to the development of calcium phosphate, or apatite calculi. With the calcium-to-phosphorus ratio maintained at 2:1, magnesium content in the total ration should not exceed 0.3% on a dry matter basis.

When calculi occur in preweaned goats fed milk replacer, constituent analysis of the milk replacer is warranted. Some milk replacers have a Ca-to-P ratio of only 1:1 that may require supplementation of calcium to kids. In addition, increased magnesium content of 0.6% in milk replacer was identified as contributory to the formation of calcium apatite calculi in calves, while a magnesium content of 0.1% produced no abnormalities (Petersson et al. 1988). The calculogenic effect of high magnesium content in the ration is exacerbated by high phosphorus content, but countered by high calcium content (Kallfelz et al. 1987).

The occurrence of calcium carbonate uroliths is associated with the feeding of alfalfa or other legume hays, which are high in calcium content, or the grazing of clover pastures. Mature breeding bucks, wethers, and pet goats—the main candidates for urolithiasis—are unlikely to require calcium in their diets at the level provided by legume hays. Therefore, a high-quality grass hay should be substituted in herds with urolith problems.

Silica calculi are seen most often in extensively grazed ruminants where the range grasses contain high silicate content. Therefore, dietary management options are limited. Ensuring adequate access to water and supplemental feeding of salt may be helpful.

Some other control interventions merit consideration. Feeding animals frequently or on an *ad libitum* basis rather than only once or twice per day may be helpful. Large meals can draw extracellular fluid into the rumen, resulting in transient increases in urine concentration that can promote calculus formation. This effect is less pronounced with smaller, more frequent feedings. Ensuring adequate vitamin A in the diet is also advised.

Delaying castration may be another management tool for reducing the prevalence of obstructive urolithiasis. However, the early precocity of goats requires that castration be performed by three months of age to avoid unwanted sexual activity unless assured separation of males from females can be achieved past that age.

Oxalate Toxicity

Like other ruminants, goats are susceptible to oxalate toxicity from consumption of oxalate-containing plants or chemical compounds such as ethylene glycol that produce oxalates as metabolites. However, reports of naturally occurring disease in goats are uncommon as compared with sheep (Kimberling 1988).

Etiology and Epidemiology

Oxalate toxicity results from consuming large quantities of plants containing increased levels of sodium or potassium oxalate. Plants in the genus *Rumex*, such as sorrel and dock, and the family *Chenopodiaceae* are well known as oxalate accumulators. The most commonly involved species are *Halogeton glomeratus* (halogeton) and *Sarcobatus vermiculatus* (greasewood) found in the semiarid grazing areas of the western United

States and *Oxalis* spp. (soursob) in Australia. Numerous other plants are also recognized as containing soluble oxalates but are less frequently involved in poisoning of livestock (Osweiler et al. 1985).

In goats, clinical oxalate toxicity has been diagnosed after consumption of *Amaranthus* spp. (pigweed) in Mexico (Gonzalez 1983). In Australia, goats died after grazing almost exclusively *Pennisetum clandestinum*, or Kikuyu grass. Though it was not the primary lesion, the affected goats had nephrosis with tubular casts containing calcium oxalate crystals (Peet et al. 1990). Goats maintained as pets or on hobby farms may be at increased risk if they are fed certain garden cuttings. Rhubarb and spinach ingestion have been associated with oxalate toxicity of goats in Australia (Baxendell 1988).

In addition, oxalates may be found in some manmade chemical products or be derived from other products by metabolism in the body. Ethylene glycol poisoning, likely resulting from automotive antifreeze ingestion, has been reported in goats (Boermans et al. 1988). Excessive administration of ascorbic acid, a metabolic precursor of oxalate, was believed to be responsible for a case of oxalate nephrotoxicosis in a ten-year-old Toggenburg doe (Adair and Adams 1990). The goat received 108 g of ascorbic acid over a six-day period before the onset of azotemia.

Pathogenesis

When small quantities of oxalates are consumed by ruminants, most of the oxalates are either destroyed in the rumen or combined with free calcium and excreted in the feces. A small quantity may be directly absorbed into the blood. When large quantities are consumed, the amount of oxalate absorbed increases. When in the blood, oxalates combine with calcium ions to form calcium oxalate. This causes a decrease of serum calcium levels, sometimes as much as 50%, and leads to a clinical syndrome of neuromuscular dysfunction similar to that seen in milk fever in cattle. Because calcium oxalate is insoluble, crystal formation ensues, with crystals accumulating both in the systemic vasculature and in the renal tubules. Renal tubular damage can cause severe renal insufficiency.

Ethylene glycol, the active ingredient in engine antifreeze products, is less toxic to ruminants than monogastrics or preruminants because much of it is degraded by rumen microflora after ingestion. However, when sufficient quantities are consumed, absorption and subsequent metabolism to toxic intermediates such as oxalic acid can occur. Unmetabolized ethylene glycol can act directly on the central nervous system as a depressant. Pathophysiologic changes induced by ethylene glycol toxicity include hypocalcemia, increased serum osmolarity, acidosis, renal tubular dysfunction, and uremia, though death is not necessarily related to the degree of uremia.

Clinical Findings

Oxalate toxicity is an acute poisoning with clinical signs developing within several hours of ingestion of offending plants. Affected goats exhibit incoordination, muscular trembling, hyperexcitability, and restlessness, followed by weakness, recumbency, and torticollis. Coma ensues and death often occurs within hours of the onset of clinical signs.

In the one reported case of ethylene glycol toxicosis in a goat (Boermans et al. 1988), the affected goat initially showed polydipsia, constipation, corneal opacity, and a progressive incoordination, especially in the hind limbs. This was followed by depression and increasing salivation. On the fifth day, before death, clonic-tonic convulsions were observed accompanied by blindness, vertical nystagmus, decreased rumen motility, diarrhea, and a subnormal temperature.

Clinical Pathology and Necropsy

Hypocalcemia may be detectable in affected goats, but the degree and occurrence are variable. Hyperphosphatemia and hypermagnesemia also may occur. A moderate to severe azotemia is usually present. Urine samples may demonstrate proteinuria and crystalluria. A characteristic rectangular parallelepiped shape for calcium oxalate dihydrate crystals found in the urine of a goat have been reported (Clark et al. 1999). When oxalate toxicity is suspect, oxalate levels should be measured in suspected plants, if available.

Oxalate toxicity is most accurately diagnosed at necropsy. The rumen content should be carefully inspected for evidence of oxalate-containing plants, and oxalate concentration of the rumen content can be measured. In affected goats, the rumen oxalate content ranged from 0.5% to 1.8% (Gonzalez 1983). Inflammation and hemorrhage of the gastric and intestinal mucosa and serosa, hydrothorax, and ascites are common but nonspecific findings. The kidneys are edematous and swollen.

A characteristic but inconsistent finding is a clearly demarcated yellow to yellow-green, streaked appearance of the renal cortex on visual inspection, with the medulla remaining red-brown. Kidney oxalate content in affected goats ranged from 2.9% to 7.1%. Histologically, the renal tubules are dilated and filled with birefringent oxalate crystals. These crystals may also be found in vessel walls, especially in the rumen vasculature. Similar histologic renal lesions are observed in ethylene glycol toxicosis. Glycolic acid, a stable metabolite of ethylene glycol, can be measured in serum, urine, and ocular fluid post mortem to support the diagnosis of ethylene glycol toxicosis.

Diagnosis

Diagnosis is based on a history of exposure, clinical signs, and often oxalate crystals in the renal tubules at necropsy. In the live animal, other causes of hypocalcemia, both metabolic and nutritional, must be ruled out. When signs of excitation or convulsions occur, primary neurologic diseases must be considered. The differential diagnosis for convulsions is given in Chapter 5.

Treatment

The prognosis for recovery is guarded once clinical signs appear. Animals at risk should be removed from the offending source of oxalates and alternate food sources provided. Subcutaneous administration of 50 to 100 ml of calcium borogluconate helps to counter the potential hypocalcemia of animals at risk. Severely affected individuals may require intravenously administered calcium salts and intravenously administered fluid therapy to counter the accumulation of oxalate crystals in renal tubules and the development of severe nephrosis. Oral administration of large quantities of water may be beneficial when there are economic constraints to therapy.

In ethylene glycol toxicosis, the prognosis is poor once signs appear. If the ingestion is recognized before signs begin, oral administration of activated charcoal (0.75–2.0 g/kg bw in water) may be beneficial in detoxification. When signs are present, intravenous fluid therapy should include sodium bicarbonate to counter the severe acidosis. Calcium borogluconate is also indicated to counter hypocalcemia. Neurologic signs may be controlled with diazepam. The administration of ethanol intravenously to serve as a competitive inhibitor of ethylene glycol metabolism in the liver has been used as an effective therapy in dogs and cats but has not been reported in ruminants. The dose in dogs is 5.5 ml of 20% ethanol per kg given intravenously every four hours.

Control

Controlling oxalate toxicity involves avoiding grazing animals on range with heavy cover of oxalate-containing plants. When such grazing is necessary, supplementary feed should be provided for at least the first few days to allow time for the rumen flora to adapt to more efficient degradation of oxalates. A good calcium source such as dicalcium phosphate helps to form calcium oxalate in the alimentary tract, thereby limiting absorption of oxalate.

Oak Poisoning

Oak poisoning (*Quercus* spp.), which is caused by ingesting large quantities of young leaves, blossoms, buds, stems, or acorns, produces considerable morbidity and mortality in cattle and sheep. The toxic principle is believed to be a gallotannin and it produces a severe intestinal irritation and a characteristic nephrosis. Animals show depression, abdominal cramping, and constipation followed by bloody, mucoid feces, and they often succumb to uremia.

Goats appear highly resistant to oak toxicity, possibly because of comparatively increased levels of tannase enzymes in the rumen mucosa. It has been demonstrated *in vitro* that infusion of tannin into goat rumen fluid increases fermentation activity while it depresses activity in sheep rumen fluid (Narjisse and El Hansali 1985). Goats are routinely used to clear scrub oak from pastures to make them safe for sheep and cattle.

The only report of spontaneous oak poisoning in goats involved consumption of *Quercus floribunda* in Sikkim. Affected animals showed signs of abdominal pain and constipation followed by hemorrhagic diarrhea and death (Katiyar 1981). In experiments, clinical signs of oak poisoning typically seen in cattle were produced in goats when they were fed a diet consisting almost exclusively of fresh shin oak *(Quercus havardi)* for an extended period (Dollahite 1961). In an unrelated study, goats fed 1 kg of dry oak leaves daily for three days showed no ill effects and it was concluded that goats can browse oak with impunity. In this same study, however, oral administration of tannic acid (1 liter of a 7% solution) resulted in an acute hemolytic crisis with hemoglobinuria. A regenerative response developed seven to fourteen days later, with macrocytes and reticulocytes observed. A transient thrombocytopenia also occurred seventy-two hours after administering tannic acid (Begovic et al. 1978).

If oak poisoning is suspected in goats, the animals should be removed from the source of oak and treated with oral purgatives including mineral oil and/or magnesium sulfate. Intravenous fluid therapy may be required to correct dehydration and acidosis.

THE ADRENAL GLANDS

Anatomy

The paired adrenal glands, or suprarenal glands, are found in proximity to the kidneys. The left adrenal gland is found anterior to the cranial pole of the left kidney and the right adrenal gland is found medial to the right kidney. The glands average 2 to 3 cm in length and 1 cm in width, with the left larger than the right. The gland is composed of a capsule, a cortex, and a medulla. The zona fasciculata of the cortex is the thickest portion of the gland and is consistently thicker in females than in males (Prasad and Sinha 1981). Accessory adrenal cortical nodules occur in goats and may be located intracapsularly or extracapsularly. These represent cortical cells separated from the germinal cortex during embryonic development (Prasad and Sinha 1980). Extracapsular nodules are usually close to the main glands.

Physiology

The endocrine and physiologic functions of the adrenal gland in the goat are essentially similar to those in other domestic ruminants, and mammals in general. Seasonal variations of corticoid levels in Angora goats have been measured. The baseline plasma level is quite variable, with range of means between 2.2 and 10.6 ng/ml. A distinct increase is noted, however, in the autumn months associated with breeding season in females. Mean autumn corticoid levels in does reach 18 ng/ml with individual measurements as high as 26 ng/ml, while the mean in males remains less than 10 ng/ml (Wentzel et al. 1979).

Pathology

Neoplasia occurs in the caprine adrenal gland. Adrenal cortical adenomas have been identified at necropsy in a high percentage of castrated male goats older than four and a half years of age. The tumor is virtually nonexistent in females and intact males. Castration is thought to predispose the goat to the tumor (Richter 1958; Altman et al. 1969). The tumor has been recognized more frequently in Angora goats than in dairy breeds, but this probably reflects that Angora wethers are more likely to be maintained for production to advanced age than castrated dairy goats. No clinical syndromes have been associated with these tumors, except for one reported case in which a six-year-old castrated Toggenburg wether was presented for udder enlargement and lactation and subsequently diagnosed with adrenal cortical adenoma post mortem. Ante mortem, the goat had increased serum concentrations of estradiol 17β, incomplete suppression of cortisol secretion by dexamethasone, and an exaggerated response to ACTH administration (Löfstedt et al. 1997).

Less common are tumors of the medulla. There is one published report of a pheochromocytoma identified in the adrenal medulla of a ten-year-old Nubian buck at necropsy. Again, no clinical signs were associated with the tumor ante mortem (Lairmore et al. 1987). The author has seen similar gross and histologic lesions at necropsy in the adrenal medullae of aged goats, but the existence of functional pheochromocytomas that secrete excessive epinephrine and produce hypertension in living goats still remains to be documented.

There is a report of presumed hereditary caprine pheochromocytoma from Finland in which the tumor was identified in a doe, its dam, and its granddam at ages 10, 13, and 15, respectively. All three goats were said to have shown repeated, sudden attacks of nervousness and anxiety (De Gritz 1997). There is also a report of two does, aged twenty years and ten years, that were presented for lactation though neither had been bred. The abnormal lactation in both does was attributed to acidophilic pituitary adenomas, but both goats also coincidentally had pheochromocytomas (Miller et al. 1997)

Histologically, evidence of adrenal cortical hyperplasia associated with stress in chronic disease has been reported in goats with chronic paratuberculosis (Rajan et al. 1980) and prolonged trypanosomosis (Mutayoba et al. 1988).

Clinical Disease

Classic types of hyperadrenocorticism (Cushing's syndrome) or hypoadrenocorticism (Addison's disease) have not been recognized in goats. Hyperadrenocorticism, however, is believed to play a role in the complex pathophysiology of a distinct form of noninfectious abortion peculiar to the Angora goat in South Africa (Wentzel et al. 1975). Affected does that abort the characteristic edematous fetuses associated with this condition show adrenal cortical hyperplasia histologically and maintain high adrenal corticosteroid levels throughout gestation, whereas normal does show a drop in corticosteroid levels in the third trimester. This condition, inherited abortion of Angoras, is discussed further in Chapter 13.

It is well recognized that as a breed, Angora goats do not handle stress as well as other goat breeds or sheep. In South Africa, death of Angora goats stressed during periods of unexpected cold weather is a major constraint on production. These stress-related deaths are associated with hypoglycemia. Van Rensburg (1971) reported that selection of Angora goats for fine mohair production was linked to selection for reduced adrenal function. This has prompted a good deal of research to determine what role the adrenal gland might play in the hypoglycemia seen in stressed and dying Angora goats.

Experimentally, Angora goats given insulin to lower their blood glucose did not, when compared to Boer goats and Merino sheep, respond with the appropriately increased cortisol production necessary for gluconeogenesis and restoration of blood sugar under stress conditions (Englebrecht et al. 2000). Furthermore, it was demonstrated in that study using adrenal cell cultures that the adrenocorticotropic hormone receptor on the adrenocortical cell membrane of Angora goats cannot adequately stimulate the cAMP signaling mechanism required for enhanced glucocorticoid production under stress. In addition, it was reported that the activity of the cytochrome P450c17 enzyme in Angora goats differed from that in Boer goats and Merino sheep and that difference may contribute to the lowered production of glucocorticoids in Angora goats (Engelbrecht and Swart 2000).

REFERENCES

Abu Damir, H., Adam, S.E.I. and Tartour, G.: The effects of *Heliotropium ovalifolium* on goats and sheep. Br. Vet. J., 138:463–472, 1982.

Abu Damir, H., Adam, S.E.I. and Tartour, G.: The effects of *Ipomoea carnea* on goats and sheep. Vet. Hum. Toxicol., 29:316–319, 1987.

Adair, H.S. and Adams, W.H.: Ascorbic acid as suspected cause of oxalate nephrotoxicosis in a goat. J. Am. Vet. Med. Assoc., 197:1626–1628, 1990.

Ahmed, O.M.M. and Adam, S.E.I.: The toxicity of *Capparis tomentosa* in goats. J. Comp. Pathol., 90:187–195, 1980.

Ali, B. and Adam, S.E.I.: Effects of *Acanthospermum hispidum* on goats. J. Comp. Pathol., 88:533–544, 1978.

Ali, B.H., Hassan, T., Wasfi, I.A. and Mustafa, A.I.: Toxicity of furazolidine to Nubian goats. Vet. Hum. Toxicol., 26:197–200, 1984.

Ali, B.H.: The toxicity of *Azadirachta indica* leaves in goats and guinea pigs. Vet. Hum. Toxicol., 29:16–19, 1987.

Altman, N.H., Streett, C.S. and Terner, J.Y.: Castration and its relationship to tumors of the adrenal gland in the goat. Am. J. Vet. Res., 30:583–589, 1969.

Aslani, M.R., Movassaghi, A.R., Mohri, M. and Vojdani, M.: Experimental kerosene poisoning in goats. Vet. Hum. Toxicol., 42(6):354–355, 2000.

Babu, N.S. and Paliwal, O.P.: Spontaneously occurring renal lesions in sheep and goats. Indian Vet. J., 65:868–871, 1988.

Barone, R.: Anatomie Comparée des Mammifères Domestiques, Volume 3, Splanchnologie. Lyon, École Nationale Vétérinaire, 1978.

Barri, M.E.S., Adam, S.E.I. and Omer, O.H.: Effects of *Crotalaria saltiana* on Nubian goats. Vet. Hum. Toxicol., 26:476–480, 1984.

Barri, M.E.S., et al.: Toxicity of five Sudanese plants to young ruminants. J. Comp. Pathol., 93:559–575, 1983.

Baxendell, S.A.: The Diagnosis of the Diseases of Goats. Sydney South, Post-Graduate Committee in Veterinary Science, 1988.

Begovic, S., Duaic, E., Sacirbegovic, A. and Tafro, A.: Study of etiology and pathogenesis of function disturbances of haematopoietic system in alimentary intoxications with tannins. Veterinaria, Yugoslavia, 27(4):459–470, 1978.

Belford, C.J., Raven, C.R. and Black, H.: Chronic copper poisoning in Angora kids. N.Z. Vet. J., 37(4):152–154, 1989.

Bellenger, C.R., Rutar, A.J., Ilkiw, J.E. and Salamon, S.: Urolithiasis in goats. Aust. Vet. J., 57:56, 1981.

Berrios, P.E. and McKercher, D.G.: Characterization of a caprine herpesvirus. Am. J. Vet. Res., 36:1755–1762, 1975.

Biswas, U., et al.: Chronic toxicity of arsenic in goats: clinicobiochemical changes, pathomorphology and tissue residues. Small Rumin. Res. 38(3):229–235, 2000.

Blackwell, J.G. and Dale, A.W.: A lead pellet as the cause of urethral obstruction in a goat. Vet. Med. Small Anim. Clin., 78:597–598, 1983.

Boermans, H.J., Ruegg, P.L. and Leach, M.: Ethylene glycol toxicosis in a pygmy goat. J. Am. Vet. Med. Assoc., 193:694–695, 1988.

Bose, S.K. Bhowmik, M.K. and Roy, M.M. Pathomorphology and tissue residues of cadmium in goat exposed to chronic cadmium toxicity. Indian Vet. J., 78(10):886–889, 2001.

Brooks, D.L., Tilman, P.C. and Niemi, S.M.: Ungulates as laboratory animals. In: Laboratory Animal Medicine. J.G. Fox, B.J. Cohen, and F.M. Loew, eds. Orlando, Academic Press, 1984.

Brown, S.A., Groves, C., Barsanti, J.A. and Finco, D.R.: Determination of excretion of inulin, creatinine, sodium sulfanilate, and phenolsulphonphthalein to assess renal function in goats. Am. J. Vet. Res., 51:581–586, 1990.

Buddle, B.M., et al.: A caprine pneumonia outbreak associated with caprine herpesvirus and *Pasteurella haemolytica* respiratory infections. N.Z. Vet. J., 38:28–31, 1990.

Buddle, B.M., et al.: Experimental respiratory infection of goats with caprine herpesvirus and *Pasteurella haemolytica.* N.Z. Vet. J., 38:22–27, 1990a.

Bungener, W. and Mehlitz, D.: Experimentelle Trypanosomeninfektion bei kamerun-Zwergziegen: Histopathologische Befunde. Tropenmed. Parasitol., 27:405–410, 1976.

Buonavoglia, C., et al.: Reactivation of caprine herpesvirus 1 in latently infected goats. Comp. Immunol. Microbiol. Infect. Dis., 19(4):275–281, 1996.

Camero, M., et al.: Intravaginal administration of an inactivated vaccine prevents lesions induced by caprine herpesvirus-1 in goats. Vaccine. 25(9):1658–1661, 2007.

Cegarra, I.J. and Lewis, R.E.: Excretory urography in the goat *(Capra hircus).* Am. J. Vet. Res., 38:1129–1132, 1977.

Chénier, S., Montpetit, C. and Hélle, P.: Caprine herpesvirus-1 abortion storm in a goat herd in Quebec. Can. Vet. J. 45:241–243, 2004.

Chima, J.C., Erno, H. and Ojo, M.O.: Characterization and identification of caprine genital mycoplasmas. Acta Vet. Scand., 27:531–539, 1986.

Choshniak, I., Wittenberg, C., Rosenfeld, J. and Shkolnik, A.: Rapid rehydration and kidney function in the black Bedouin goat. Physiol. Zool., 57:573–579, 1984.

Clark, P., Swenson, C.L., Osborne, C.A. and Ulrich L.K.: Calcium oxalate crystalluria in a goat. J. Am. Vet. Med. Assoc., 215(1):77–78, 1999.

Corrier, D.E. and Adams, L.G.: Clinical, histologic, and histochemical study of imidocarb diproprionate toxicosis in goats. Am. J. Vet. Res., 37:811–816, 1976.

Craig, D.R., Stephan, M. and Pankowski, R.L.: Urolithiasis: A retrospective study in sheep and goats. J. Am. Vet. Med. Assoc., 190:1609, 1987.

Crawford, T.B., et al.: The connective tissue component of the caprine arthritis-encephalitis syndrome. Am. J. Pathol. 100(2):443–454, 1980.

Dash, P.K. and Joshi, H.C.: Clinico-biochemical studies on acute toxic nephropathy in goats due to uranyl nitrate. Vet. Hum. Toxicol., 31:5–9, 1989.

De Gritz, B.G.: Hereditary caprine phaeochromocytoma. J. Vet. Med. A, 44:313–316, 1997.

Divers, T.J., Crowell, W.A., Duncan, J.R., and Whitlock, R.H.: Acute renal disorders in cattle: a retrospective study of 22 cases. J. Am. Vet. Med. Assoc., 181:694–699, 1982.

Dobereiner, J., Stolf, L., Tokarnia, C.H.: Poisonous plants affecting goats. Proceedings, Fourth International Conf. Goats, Brasilia, EMBRAPA-DDT, pp. 473–487, 1987.

Dollahite, J.W.: Shin oak *(Quercus havardi)* poisoning in cattle. Southwest Vet., 14:198–201, 1961.

Eaton, O.N.: An anatomical study of hermaphrodism in goats. Am. J. Vet. Res., 4:333–343, 1943.

El Dirdiri, N.I., Barakat, S.E.M. and Adam, S.E.I.: The combined toxicity of *Aristolochia bracteata* and *Cadaba rotundifolia* to goats. Vet. Hum. Toxicol., 29:133–137, 1987.

Elia, G., et al.: Development of a real-time PCR for the detection and quantitation of caprine herpesvirus 1 in goats. J. Virol. Methods, 148(1/2):155–160, 2008.

Engelbrecht, Y. and Swart, P.: Adrenal function in Angora goats: a comparative study of adrenal steroidogenesis in Angora goats, Boer goats and Merino sheep. J. Anim. Sci., 78:1036–1046, 2000.

Engelbrecht, Y., Herselman, T., Louw, A. and Swart, P.: Investigation of the primary cause of hypoadrenocorticism in South African Angora goats (*Capra aegagrus*): A comparison with Boer goats (*Capra hircus*) and Merino sheep (*Ovis aries*). J. Anim. Sci., 78:371–379, 2000.

Engels, M., Gelderblom, H., Darai, G. and Ludwig, H.: Goat herpesviruses: biological and physicochemical properties. J. Gen. Virol., 64:2237–2247, 1983.

Ewoldt, J.M., Anderson, D.E., Miesner, M.D and Saville, W.J.: Short- and long-term outcome and factors predicting survival after surgical tube cystostomy for treatment of obstructive urolithiasis in small ruminants. Vet. Surg., 35:417–422, 2006.

Flåøyen, A., et al.: Nephrotoxicity in goats caused by dosing with a water extract from the stems of *Narthecium ossifragum* plants. Vet. Res. Commun. 21(7):499–506, 1997.

Fletcher, W.S., Rogers, A.L. and Donaldson, S.S.: The use of the goat as an experimental animal. Lab. Anim. Care, 14:65–90, 1964.

Fortier, L.A., Gregg, A.J., Erb, H.N. and Fubini, S.L.: Caprine obstructive urolithiasis: requirement for a second surgical intervention and mortality after percutaneous tube cystostomy, surgical tube cystostomy or urinary bladder marsupialization. Vet. Surg., 33:661–667, 2004.

Friis, C.: Postnatal development of renal function in goats. In: Veterinary Pharmacology and Toxicology. Y. Ruckenbusch, P.L. Toutain and G.D. Koritz, eds. Westport, Conn., AVI Publishing Co., 1983.

Fuller, D.T. Baird, A.N. Morris, E.L. and Kraemer, D.C. What is your diagnosis? [Hypospadias and urethral diverticulum in goat]. J. Am. Vet. Med. Assoc., 201(9):1431–1432, 1992.

Gahlot, T.K., Ranka, A.K., Chouhan, D.S., and Choudhary, R.J.: Congenital urethral diverticulum in male goat *(Capra hircus)*—Surgical management. Indian J. Vet. Surg., 3:95–97, 1982.

Gajendragad, M.R., Kumar, A.A. and Biswas, J.C.: Unilateral pyonephrosis in a Pashmina goat. Indian Vet. J., 60:494, 1983.

Garrett, P.D.: Urethral recess in male goats, sheep, cattle, and swine. J. Am. Vet. Med. Assoc., 191:689–691, 1987.

George, J.W., Hird, D.W. and George L.W.: Serum biochemical abnormalities in goats with uroliths: 107 cases (1992–2003). J. Am. Vet. Med. Assoc., 230(1):101–106, 2007.

Gezon, H.M., et al.: Identification and control of paratuberculosis in a large goat herd. Am. J. Vet. Res., 49:1817–1823, 1988.

Ghoshal, N.G. and Bal, H.S.: Histomorphology of the urethral process of the goat *(Capra hircus)*. Acta Anat., 94:567–573, 1976.

Goeger, D.E., Cheeke, P.R., Schmitz, J.A. and Buhler, D.R.: Toxicity of tansy ragwort *(Senecio jacobaea)* to goats. Am. J. Vet. Res., 43:252–254, 1982.

Gonzalez, S.C.: Nefrosis tubular toxica en ovinos y caprinos asociada a la ingestion de plantas del genero *Amaranthus* spp. Vet. Mex., 14:247–251, 1983.

Gouda, I.M., et al.: Changes in some liver functions in experimentally lead-poisoned goats. Arch. Exp. Veterinarmed., 39:257–267, 1985.

Grewal, A.S. and Wells, R.: Vulvovaginitis of goats due to a herpesvirus. Aust. Vet. J., 63:79–82, 1986.

Grossman, I.W. and Altman, N.H.: Caprine cloisonné renal lesion. Arch. Pathol., 88:609–612, 1969.

Halland S.K., House, J.K. and George L.W.: Urethroscopy and laser lithotripsy for the diagnosis and treatment of obstructive urolithiasis in goats and pot-bellied pigs. J. Am. Vet. Med. Assoc., 220(12):1831–1834, 2002.

Hatipoglu, F. and Erer, H.: Lesions of cloisonné kidney in sheep: report on four cases. Rev. Méd. Vét. 152(4):311–315, 2001.

Haven, M.L., Bowman, K.F., Engelbert, T.A. and Blikslager A.T.: Surgical management of urolithiasis in small ruminants. Cornell Vet., 83:47–55, 1993.

Hinkle, R.F., Howard, J.L. and Stowater, J.L.: An anatomic barrier to urethral catheterization in the male goat. J. Am. Vet. Med. Assoc., 173:1584–1585, 1978.

Hofmeyr, C.F.B.: Ruminant Urogenital Surgery. Ames, Iowa, Iowa State University Press, 1987.

Horner, G.W.: Caprine herpesvirus: eradication from infected flocks. Surveillance, N.Z., 15:18, 1988.

Horner, G.W., Hunter, R., and Day, A.M.: An outbreak of vulvovaginitis in goats caused by a caprine herpesvirus. N.Z. Vet. J., 30:150–152, 1982.

Horner, G.W.: Caprine herpesvirus reappears. Surveillance, N.Z., 9:24, 1982.

Hosseinion, M., et al.: Selenium poisoning in a mixed flock of sheep and goats in Iran. Trop. Anim. Health Prod., 4:173–174, 1972.

Humphries, W.R., Morrice, P.C., and Mitchell, A.N.: Copper poisoning in Angora goats. Vet. Rec., 121:231, 1987.

Ide, A. and Tutt, C.L.C.: Acute *Lantana camara* poisoning in a Boer goat kid. J. S. Afr. Vet. Assoc., 69(1):30–32, 1998.

Ihemelandu, E.C.: Ulcerative vulvitis in goats. Vet. Rec., 91:197, 1972.

Jackson, C.: The incidence and pathology of tumours of domesticated animals in South Africa. Onderstepoort J. Vet. Sci., 6:3–399, 1936.

Jacob, R.H. and Peet, R.L.: Poisoning of sheep and goats by *Tribulis terrestris* (caltrop). Aust. Vet. J., 64:288–289, 1987.

James, C.S. and Chandran, K.: Enquiry into the role of minerals in experimental urolithiasis in goats. Indian Vet. J., 52:251–258, 1975.

James, C.S. and Mukundan, G.: Suitability of jack tree leaves *(Artocarpous)* as a fodder for stall-fed goats. Indian Vet. J., 55:716–721, 1978.

Jeffrey, M., et al.: Polioencephalomalacia associated with the ingestion of ammonium sulphate by sheep and cattle. Vet. Rec., 134(14):343–348, 1994.

Jorna, T. The renal blood flow in ruminants with pyloric stenosis. Faculteit der Diergeneeskunde, Rijksuniversiteit de Utrecht, the Netherlands, 1978. (Thesis.)

Kallfelz, F.A., et al.: Dietary magnesium and urolithiasis in growing calves. Cornell Vet., 77:33–45, 1987.

Kao, M., et al.: Goat herpesvirus infection: a survey on specific antibodies in different countries. In: Immunity to Herpesvirus Infections of Domestic Animals. P.P. Pastoret, E. Thiry, and J. Saliki, eds. Luxembourg, CEC, 1985.

Karras, S., Modransky, P. and Welker, B.: Surgical correction of urethral dilatation in an intersex goat. J. Am. Vet. Med. Assoc., 201(10):1584–1586, 1992.

Katiyar, R.D.: A report on plant poisoning in sheep and goats. Livestock Adviser, 6:57–62, 1981.

Keuser, V., et al.: Isolation of caprine herpesvirus type 1 in Spain. Vet. Rec., 154:395–399, 2004.

Khanna, R.S. and Iyer, P.K.R.: Suspected leptospirosis in goats. Indian J. Med. Res., 59:1588–1592, 1971.

Khanna, R.S. and Iyer, P.K.R.: A case of *Nosema cuniculi* infection in a goat. Indian J. Med. Res., 59:993–995, 1971a.

Kharole, M.U. Symmetrical cortical siderosis. Indian Vet. J., 44: 1030–1032, 1967.

Kharole, M.U. and Rao, U.R.K.: Leptospirosis in goats in India. Indian Vet. J., 45:14–18, 1968.

Kimberling, C.V.: Jensen and Swift's Diseases of Sheep. 3rd Ed. Philadelphia, Lea and Febiger, 1988.

Klc, E., et al.: Preputial aplasia, urethral diverticulum, and distal urethral atresia in kids. Kafkas Universitesi Veteriner Fakultesi Dergisi, 11(1):73–76, 2005.

Koptopoulos, G., Papanastasopoulou, M., Papadopoulos, O. and Ludwig, H.: The epizootiology of caprine herpesvirus (BHV6) infections in goat populations in Greece. Comp. Immunol. Microbiol. Infect. Dis., 11:199–205, 1988.

Krotec, K., Smith Meyer, B., Freeman, W. and Hamir, A.N.: Congenital cystic disease of the liver, pancreas, and kidney in a Nubian goat (*Capra hircus*). Vet. Pathol. 33:6, 708–710, 1996.

Kumar, R. and Pandey, N.N.: Biomedical profile of gentamicin intoxication in goats. Indian J. Anim. Sci., 64(11):1147–1150, 1994.

Kumar, R.K., et al.: Effect of castration on urethra and accessory sex glands in goats. Indian Vet. J., 59:304–308, 1982.

Lairmore, M.D., Knight, A.P. and DeMartini, J.C.: Three primary neoplasms in a goat: hepatocellular carcinoma, phaeochromocytoma and leiomyoma. J. Comp. Pathol., 97:267–271, 1987.

Lerner, R.A., Dixon, F.J., and Lee, S.: Spontaneous glomerulonephritis in sheep. II. Studies on natural history, occurrence in other species, and pathogenesis. Am. J. Pathol., 53:501–512, 1968.

Li, H., et al.: Caprine herpesvirus-2-associated malignant catarrhal fever in white-tailed deer (*Odocoileus virginianus*). J. Vet. Diagn. Investig., 15(1):46–49, 2003.

Li, H., Keller, J., Knowles, D.P. and Crawford, T.B.: Recognition of another member of the malignant catarrhal fever virus group: an endemic gammaherpesvirus in domestic goats. J. Gen. Virol., 82:227–232, 2001.

Light, F.W.: Pigmented thickening of the basement membranes of the renal tubules of the goat (cloisonné kidney). Lab Invest., 9:228–238, 1960.

Lishajko, F. and Andersson, B.: Recovery of ADH activity in the urine of goats under normal and stimulated conditions. Acta Physiol. Scand., 95:102–109, 1975.

Löfstedt, R.M., Laarveld, B. And Ihle, S.L.: Adrenal neoplasia causing lactation in a castrated male goat. J. Vet. Intern. Med., 8(5):382–384, 1994.

Loste, A., et al.: High prevalence of ulcerative posthitis in rasa Aragonesa rams associated with a legume-rich diet. J. Vet. Med. A, 52:176–179, 2005.

Mahin, L. and Chadli, M.: Malignant enzootic dysuria, a disease of unknown aetiology in domestic ruminants in Morocco. Proceedings, Twelfth World Cong. Dis. Cattle, the Netherlands. Vol. II, pp. 1021–1024, 1982.

Maloiy, G.M.O.: Digestion and renal function in East African goats and haired sheep. East Afr. Agric. For. J., 40:177–188, 1974.

Manning, R.A. and Blaney, B.J.: Epidemiological aspects of urolithiasis in domestic animals in Queensland. Aust. Vet. J., 63:423–424, 1986.

Maryamma, K.I. and Krishnan Nair, M.: Ultrastructural pathology of the kidney in experimental ochratoxicosis in goats. Indian J. Anim. Sci., 60(6):623–627, 1990.

Mathews, F.P.: The toxicity of broomweed *(Gutierrezia microcephala)* for sheep, cattle and goats. J. Am. Vet. Med. Assoc., 88:55–61, 1936.

Mathews, F.P.: Lechuguilla *(Agave lecheguilla)* poisoning in sheep, goats and laboratory animals. Tex. Agric. Exp. Stn. Bull., 554, 1937.

Mathews, F.P.: Poisoning in sheep and goats by sacahuiste *(Nolina texana)* buds and blooms. Bull. Tex. Agric. Exp. Stn., 585:5–19, 1940.

May, K.A., et al.: Urinary bladder marsupialization for treatment of obstructive urolithiasis in male goats. Vet. Surg., 27:583–588, 1998.

McKeough, V.L., Collett, M.G. and Parton, K.H.: Suspected *Vestia foetida* poisoning in young goats. N.Z. Vet. J., 53(5):352–355, 2005.

Mengistu, U., Dahlborn, K. and Olsson, K.: Effects of intermittent watering on water balance and feed intake in male Ethiopian Somali goats. Small Rumin. Res., 67(1):45–54, 2007.

Ménusa, C., et al.: Pathology of AA amyloidosis in domestic sheep and goats. Vet. Pathol., 40:71–80, 2003.

Meurens, F., et al.: Interspecific recombination between two ruminant alphaherpesviruses, bovine herpesviruses 1 and 5. J. Virol., 78(18):9828–9836, 2004.

Middleton, J.R., Katz, L., Angelos, J.A. and Tyler, J.W.: Hemolysis associated with water administration using a nipple bottle for human infants in juvenile Pygmy goats. J. Vet. Intern. Med., 11(6):382–384, 1997.

Miller, C.C., Williamson, L.H., Miller-Liebl, D.M. and Thompson, F.N.: Lactation associated with acidophilic pituitary adenoma, pheochromocytoma and cystic endometrial hyperplasia in two goats. J. Am. Vet. Med. Assoc., 210(3):378–381, 1997.

Mohamed, O.S.A., Adam, S.E.I. and El Dirdiri, N.I.: The combined effect of dursban and reldan on Nubian goats. Vet. Hum. Toxicol. 32:47–48, 1990.

Mohamed, O.S.A. and Adam, S.E.I.: Toxicity of sumicidin (fenvalerate) to Nubian goats. J. Comp. Pathol., 102:1–6, 1990.

Mohanty, S.B., Lillie, M.G., Corselius, N.P. and Beck, J.D.: Natural infection with infectious bovine rhinotracheitis virus in goats. J. Am. Vet. Med. Assoc., 160:879–880, 1972.

Molony, V., Kent, J.E. and McKendrick, I.J.: Validation of a method for assessment of an acute pain in lambs. Appl. Anim. Behav. Sci. 76:215–238, 2002.

Morin, D.E. and Badertscher, R.R.: Ultrasonographic diagnosis of obstructive uropathy in a caprine doe. J. Am. Vet. Med. Assoc., 197:378–380, 1990.

Mount, M.E.: Diagnostic value of urinary dialkyl phosphate measurement in goats exposed to diazinon. Am. J. Vet. Res., 45:817–824, 1984.

Mugera, G.M. and Nderito, P.: *Cestrum* poisoning in Kenya livestock. Bull. Epizoot. Dis. Afr., 16:501–506, 1968.

Mutayoba, B.M., Gombe, S., Kaaya, G.P. and Waindi, E.N.: Effect of chronic experimental *Trypanosoma congolense* infection on the ovaries, pituitary, thyroid and adrenal glands in female goats. Res. Vet. Sci., 44:140–146, 1988.

Narjisse, H. and El Hansali, M.: Effect of tannins on nitrogen balance and microbial activity of rumen fluid in sheep and goats. Ann. Zootech., 34:482, 1985.

Newman, S.J., Leichner, T., Crisman, M. and Ramos, J.: Congenital cystic disease of the liver and kidney in a pygmy goat. J. Vet. Diagn. Invest., 12(4):374–378, 2000.

Nickel, R. Schummer, A., Seiferle, E. and Sack, W.O.: The Viscera of Domestic Animals. New York, Springer-Verlag, 1973.

O'Brien, T.D., et al.: Hepatic necrosis following halothane anesthesia in goats. J. Am. Vet. Med. Assoc., 189:1591–1595, 1986.

Olsson, K. and Dahlborn, K.: Fluid balance during heat stress in lactating goats. Q. J. Exp. Physiol., 74:645–659, 1989.

Olsson, K., Benlamlih, S., Dahlborn, K., and Orberg, J.: A serial study of fluid balance during pregnancy, lactation, and anestrus in goats. Acta Physiol. Scand., 115:39–45, 1982.

Osweiler, G.D., Carson, T.L., Buck, W.B. and Van Gelder, G.A.: Clinical and Diagnostic Veterinary Toxicology. 3rd Ed. Dubuque, Kendall Hunt Publ. Co., 1985.

Palmer, J.L., Dykes, N.L., Love, K. and Fubini, S.L.: Contrast radiography of the lower urinary tract in the management of obstructive urolithiasis in small ruminants and swine. Vet. Radiol. Ultrasound, 39(3):175–180, 1998.

Pathak, S.K. and Bhowmik, M.K. The chronic toxicity of inorganic mercury in goats: clinical signs, toxicopathological changes and residual concentrations. Vet. Res. Commun., 22(2):131–138, 1998.

Peet, R.L., Dickson, J. and Hare, M.: Kikuyu poisoning in goats and sheep. Aust. Vet. J., 67(6):229–230, 1990.

Petersson, K.H., Warner, R.G., Kallfelz, F.A. and Crosetti, C.F.: Influence of magnesium, water, and sodium chloride on urolithiasis in veal calves. J. Dairy Sci., *71*:3369–3377, 1988.

Pfister, P., et al.: Pollakisuria in a dwarf goat due to pathologic enlargement of the uterus. Vet. Q., 29(3):112–116, 2007.

Pieterse, M.C.: Practice Tip. Wool Wattles, 22(3):11, 1994.

Prakash, P. and Kumar, A.: Surgical significance of preputial muscles and their innervation in goat. Indian J. Vet. Surg., 4:50–54, 1983.

Prasad, G. and Sinha, R.D.: Occurrence of accessory adrenal cortical nodule in the domestic animals. Indian J. Anim. Sci., 50:1060–1063, 1980.

Prasad, G. and Sinha, R.D.: Micrometric observations on the adrenal glands of domestic animals. Indian J. Anim. Sci., 51:1144–1147, 1981.

Prozesky, L. and Du Plessis, J.L.: Heartwater in Angora goats. II. A pathological study of artificially infected, treated and untreated goats. Onderstepoort J. Vet. Res., 52:13–19, 1985.

Qin, S., Zhang, B.X., Liu, B.F. and Zhao, X.J.: Experimental induction of poisoning in goats with natural selenium-containing feeds. Clinical signs and pathology. Acta Vet. Zootech. Sin., 25(4):363–367, 1994.

Radi, Z.A., Thomsen, B.V. and Summers, B.A.: Renal (uremic) encephalopathy in a goat. J. Vet. Med. A, 52:397–400, 2005.

Radostits, O.M., Gay, C.C., Hinchcliff, K.W. and Constable, P.D.: Veterinary Medicine. A textbook of the diseases of cattle, horse, sheep, pigs and goats. 10th Edition, Edinburgh, Saunders Elsevier, 2007.

Rajan, A., Valsala, K.V., Mariamma, K.I. and Nair, M.K.: Pathology of the endocrine glands in Johne's disease in goats. Kerala J. Vet. Sci., 11:166–173, 1980.

Rakestraw, P.C., Fubini, S.L., Gilbert, R.O. and Ward, J.O.: Tube cystostomy for treatment of obstructive urolithiasis in small ruminants. Vet. Surg., 24:498–505, 1995.

Raoofi, A., Mardjanmehr, S.H. and Rahimi, A.: Transitional cell papilloma and leiomyoma of the urinary bladder in two goats. Vet. Rec., 160(2):56–57, 2007.

Rawlings C.A., et al.: Diagnostic quality of percutaneous kidney biopsy specimens obtained with laparoscopy versus ultrasound guidance in dogs. J. Am. Vet. Med. Assoc., 223(3):317–321, 2003.

Richter, W.R.: Adrenal cortical adenomata in the goat. Am. J. Vet. Res., 19:895–901, 1958.

Roperto, F., et al.: Natural caprine herpesvirus 1 (CpHV-1) infection in kids. J. Comp. Pathol. 122(4):298–302, 2000.

Ruhr, L.P., Nicholson, S.S., Confer, A.W. and Blakewood, B. W.: Acute intoxication from a hematinic in calves. J. Am. Vet. Med. Assoc., 182:616–618, 1983.

Saito, J.K., et al.: A new herpesvirus isolate from goats: preliminary report. Am. J. Vet. Res. 35(6):847–848, 1974.

Samarajeewa, U., Arseculeratne, S.N. and Tennekoon, G.E.: Spontaneous and experimental aflatoxicosis in goats. Res. Vet. Sci., 19:269–277, 1975.

Sankarappa, E.V., and Rao, P.R.: Renal lesions in sheep and goats in Andhra Pradesh. Indian Vet. J., 59:705–708, 1982.

Sato, H. and Omori, S.: Incidence of urinary calculi in goats fed a high phosphorus diet. Jpn. J. Vet. Sci., 39,531–537, 1977.

Schmidt, H.: Vitamin A deficiencies in ruminants. Am. J. Vet. Res., 2:373–389, 1941.

Schneider, D.J., Marasas, W.F.O., Collett, M.G. and Van der Westhuizen, G.C.A.: An experimental mycotoxicosis in sheep and goats caused by *Drechslera campanulata*, a fungal pathogen of green oats. Onderstepoort J. Vet. Res., 52:93–100, 1985.

Schöntag, H.: Der artifizielle Penisprolaps bei Hengst, Bulle, Eber, Schaf—und Ziegenbock. Tierärztlichen Fakultät der Universität München, Germany, 1984. (Thesis.)

Shaham, D., et al.: Neural control of renal function in newly rehydrated Bedouin goats. Compar. Biochem. Physiol. A, Compar. Physiol., 107(1):57–61, 1994.

Shelton, M. and Livingston, C.W.: Posthitis in Angora wethers. J. Am. Vet. Med. Assoc., 167:154–155, 1975.

Shokry, M. and Al-Saadi, H.: Retractor penis myotomy for catheterization in sheep and goats. Mod. Vet. Pract., 61:700, 1980.

Silanikove, N.: Renal excretion of urea in response to changes in nitrogen intake in desert (black Bedouin) and non-desert (Swiss Saanen) goats. Comp. Biochem. Physiol., 79A:651–654, 1984.

Singh, K.K., Jha, G.J., Chauhan, V.S. and Singh, P.N.: Pathology of chronic aldrin intoxication in goats. Zbl. Vet. Med. A, 32:437–444, 1985.

Singh, N. and Rajya, B.S.: Pathology of female reproductive system in goats. Indian J. Anim. Sci., 47:22–28, 1977.

Singh, N., Rajya, B.S. and Mohanty, G.C.: Pathology of *Mycoplasma agalactiae* induced granular vulvovaginitis (GVV) in goats. Cornell Vet., 65:363–373, 1975.

Sisson, S.: Ruminant urogenital system. In: The Anatomy of the Domestic Animals. R. Getty, ed. Philadelphia, W.B. Saunders Co., 1975.

Six, A., et al.: Latency and reactivation of bovine herpesvirus a (BHV-1) in goats and of caprine herpesvirus 1 (CapHV-1) in calves. Arch. Virol., 146:1325–1335, 2001.

Stewart, S.R., Emerick, R.J and. Pritchard, R.H.: Effects of dietary ammonium chloride and variations in calcium to phosphorus ratio on silica urolithiasis in sheep. J. Anim. Sci., 69(5):2225–2229, 1991.

Stone, W.C., et al.: Prepubic urethrostomy for relief of urethral obstruction in a sheep and a goat. J. Am. Vet. Med. Assoc., 210(7):939–941, 1997.

Stratton-Phelps, M. and House, J.K.: Effect of a commercial anion dietary supplement on acid-base balance, urine volume, and urinary ion excretion in male goats fed oat or grass hay diets. Am. J. Vet. Res., 65(10):1391–1397, 2004.

Streeter, R.N., Washburn, K.E. and McCauley, C.T.: Percutaneous tube cystostomy and vesicular irrigation for treatment of obstructive urolithiasis in a goat. J. Am. Vet. Med. Assoc., 221(4):546–549, 2002.

Suliman, H.B., Wasfi, I.A. and Adam, S.E.I.: The toxic effects of *Tephrosia apollinea* on goats. J. Comp. Pathol., 92:309–315, 1982.

Suliman, H.B., Wasfi, I.A., Tartour, G., and Adam, S.E.I.: The effects of *Indigofera hochstetteri* on goats. Rev. Élev. Méd. vét. Pays. trop., 36:393–402, 1983.

Tarigan, S., Ladds, P.W. and Foster, R.A.: Genital pathology of feral male goats. Aust. Vet. J., 67:286–290, 1990.

Tarigan, S., Webb, R.F. and Kirkland, D.: Caprine herpesvirus from balanoposthitis. Aust. Vet. J., 64:321, 1987.

Tayal, R., Singh, A.P., Chandna, I.S. and Chawla, S.K.: Contrast cystography in the goat *(Capra hircus).* Vet. Radiol., 25:260–264, 1984.

Tempesta, M., et al.: Natural reactivation of caprine herpesvirus 1 in latently infected goats. Vet. Rec., 143(7):200, 1998.

Tempesta, M. Pratelli, A. Corrente, M. and Buonavoglia, C.: A preliminary study on the pathogenicity of a strain of caprine herpesvirus-1. Comp. Immunol. Microbiol. Infect. Dis., 22(2):137–143, 1999.

Tempesta, M., et al.: Detection of caprine herpesvirus 1 in sacral ganglia of latently infected goats by PCR. J. Clin. Microbiol., 37(5):1598–1599, 1999a.

Tempesta, M., et al.: Experimental intravaginal infection of goats with caprine herpesvirus 1. J. Vet. Med. Series B. 47(3):197–201, 2000.

Tempesta, M., et al.: A classical inactivated vaccine induces protection against caprine herpesvirus 1 infection in goats. Vaccine. 19(28/29):3860–3864, 2001.

Tempesta, M., et al.: Experimental infection of goats at different stages of pregnancy with caprine herpesvirus 1. Comp. Immunol. Microbiol. Infect. Dis., 2004. 27(1): 25–32, 2004.

Tempesta, M. et al.: Analysis of antibody response in goats to caprine herpesvirus 1. Biologicals, 33(4):283–287, 2005.

Tempesta, M. et al.: Cidofovir is effective against caprine herpesvirus 1 infection in goats. Antiviral Res., 74:138–141, 2007.

Tham, V.L. and Bunn, C.M.: Amyloidosis in an Angora goat. Austral. Vet. J., 69(2):40–41, 1992.

Thamsborg, S.M., Jorgensen, R.J. and Brummerstedt, E.: Sawfly poisoning in sheep and goats. Vet. Rec., 121:253–255, 1987.

Thiry, J. et al.: Ruminant alphaherpesviruses related to bovine herpesvirus 1. Vet. Res., 37:169–190, 2006.

Thiry, J. et al.: A live attenuated glycoprotein E negative bovine herpesvirus 1 vaccine induces a partial cross-protection against caprine herpesvirus 1 infection in goats. Vet. Microbiol., 113:303–308, 2006a.

Thiry, J., et al.: Serological evidence of caprine herpesvirus 1 infection in Mediterranean France. Vet. Microbiol., 128(3/4):261–268, 2008.

Thompson, S.W., Bogdon, T.R. and Yost, D.H.: Some histochemical studies of "cloisonné kidney" in the male Angora goat. Am. J. Vet. Res. 22:757–763, 1961.

Thomson, E.M., Forsling, M.L. and Thompson, G.E.: The effect of cold exposure on fluid balance, circulating arginine vasopressin concentration and milk secretion in the goat. Pflug. Arch., 383:241–244, 1980.

Tibary, A. and Van Metre, D.C.: Surgery of the sheep and goat reproductive system and urinary tract. In: Farm Animal Surgery. S.L. Fubini and N.G. Ducharme, eds. St. Louis, Saunders, pp. 527–547, 2004.

Timurkaan, N., Yener, Z. and Yuksel, H.: Leiomyoma of the urinary bladder in a goat. Aust. Vet. J., 79(10):708–709, 2001.

Tiwana, J.S., Singh, N. and Kwatra, M.S.: Isolation of *Mycoplasma* and *Acholeplasma* from vulvovaginitis in goats. Indian J. Comp. Microbiol. Immunol. Infect. Dis., 5:17–19, 1984.

Todhunter P., Baird, A.N. and Wolfe D.F.: Erection failure as a sequela to obstructive urolithiasis in a male goat. J. Am. Vet. Med. Assoc., 209(3):650–652, 1996.

Tomar, D.S.: Studies on the pathology of caprine kidneys. Indian J. Vet. Pathol., 8:73, 1984.

Tontis, A. and Zwahlen, R.: Zur Graviditätstoxikose der kleinen Ruminanten mit besonderer Berucksichtigung der Pathomorphologie. Tierärztl. Prax. 15:25–29, 1987.

Toofanian, F., Aliakbari, S. and Ivoghli, B.: Acute diesel fuel poisoning in goats. Trop. Anim. Health Prod., 11:98–101, 1979.

Twomey, D.F., et al.: Multisystemic necrotising vasculitis in a pygmy goat (*Capra hircus*). Vet. Rec., 158:867–869, 2006.

Unanian, M.D.S. and Silva, A.E.D.F.: Doencas Mais Frequentes Observadas nos Caprinos do Nordeste. Brasilia, EMBRAPA, 1987.

Unanian, M.D.S., Silva, A.E.D.F. and Santa Rosa, J.: Observations on several cases of urolithiasis in goats. Proceedings, Third Internat. Conf. Goat Prod. Dis., Scottsdale, Arizona, Dairy Goat Publ. Co., p 348, 1982.

Unanian, M.M., Santa Rosa, J. and Silva, A.E.D.F.: Urolitiase experimental em caprinos: possiveis causas e profilaxia. Pesq. Agropec. Bras., 20:467–474, 1985.

Uzal, F.A., et al.: Abortion and ulcerative posthitis associated with caprine herpesvirus-1 infection in goats in California. J. Vet. Diagn. Invest., 16:478–484, 2004.

Vagg, M.J. and Payne, J.M.: The effect of ammonium chloride induced acidosis on calcium metabolism in ruminants. Br. Vet. J., 126:531–537, 1970.

Van Metre, D.C. and Fubini, S.L.: Ovine and caprine urolithiasis: another piece of the puzzle. Vet. Surg., 35:413–416, 2006.

Van Metre, D.C., et al.: Obstructive urolithiasis in ruminants: medical treatment and urethral surgery. Compend. Cont. Educ. Pract. Vet., 18(3):317–328, 1996.

Van Metre, D.C., et al.: Obstructive urolithiasis in ruminants: surgical management and prevention. Compend. Cont. Educ. Pract. Vet., 18(10):S275-S289, 1996a.

Van Rensburg, S.J.: Reproductive physiology and endocrinology of normal and aborting Angora goats. Onderstepoort J. Vet. Res. 38(1):1–62, 1971.

van Weeren, P.R., Klein, W.R. and Voorhout, G.: Urolithiasis in small ruminants. II. Cysto-urethrography as a new aid in diagnosis. Vet. Q., 9:79–83, 1987.

van Weeren, R.P., Klein, W.R. and Voorhout, G.: Urolithiasis in small ruminants. I. A retrospective evaluation of urethrostomy. Vet. Q., 9:76–79, 1987a.

Vihan, V.S.: Hexachloroethane toxicity in goats. Indian Vet. J., 64:180–181, 1987.

Visser, I.J.R., van den Hoven, R., Vos, J.H. and van den Ingh, T.S.G.A.M.: *Pieris japonica* (pieris) intoxication in two goats. Tijdschr. Diergeneeskd., 113:185–189, 1988.

Vyas, U.K., Arya, P.L., and Sharma, S.N.: Studies on experimentally produced uremia in sheep and goats. Indian J. Anim. Sci., 48:749–753, 1978.

Wahbi, A.A., El Dirdiri, N., Tageldin, M.H.: Sevin toxicity to Sudanese Nubian goats. Bull. Anim. Health Prod. Afr., 35:53–58, 1987.

Wentzel, D., Morgenthal, J.C. and Van Niekerk, C.H.: The habitually aborting Angora doe. IV. Adrenal function in normal and aborter does. Agroanimalia, 7:27–34, 1975.

Wentzel, D., Viljoen, K.S. and Botha, L.J.J.: Seasonal variation in adrenal and thyroid function of Angora goats. Agroanimalia, 11:1–3, 1979.

Wessels, M.: Chronic arthritis and systemic amyloidosis in three goat kids associated with seroconversion to *Erysipelothrix rhusiopathiae*. Vet. Rec., 152:302–304, 2003.

Whetstone, C.A. and Evermann, J.F.: Characterization of bovine herpesviruses isolated from six sheep and four goats by restriction endonuclease analysis and radioimmunoprecipitation. Am. J. Vet. Res., 49:781–785, 1988.

Widmer, W.R., Biller, D.S. and Adams, L.G.: Ultrasonography of the urinary tract in small animals. J. Am. Vet. Med. Assoc., 225(1):46–54, 2004.

Wilkinson, J.S.: Kidney disease and urine analysis. In: Textbook of Veterinary Clinical Pathology. W. Medway, J.E. Prier and J.S. Wilkinson, eds. Baltimore, Williams and Wilkins Co., 1969.

Williams, N.M., et al.: Multiple abortions associated with caprine herpesvirus infection in a goat herd. J. Am. Vet. Med. Assoc., 211(1):89–91, 1997.

Wisløff, H., Flåøyen, A., Ottesen, N. and Hovig, T.: *Narthecium ossifragum* (L.) Huds. causes kidney damage in goats: morphologic and functional effects. Vet. Pathol., 40:317–327, 2003.

Wittenberg, C., et al.: Effect of dehydration and rapid rehydration on renal function and on plasma renin and aldosterone levels in the black Bedouin goat. Pflug. Archiv, 406:405–408, 1986.

Zahawi, S.: A. Symmetrical cortical siderosis of the kidneys in goats. Am. J. Vet. Res. 18: 861–867, 1957.

13

Reproductive System

It is beyond the scope of this book to consider in detail reproductive physiology, estrus synchronization, artificial insemination, embryo transfer, and other topics more closely related to herd management than to disease. These facets of caprine reproduction have been discussed in various theriogenology textbooks (Morrow 1986; Youngquist and Threlfall 2007) and elsewhere (Evans and Maxwell 1987; Kraemer 1989; Haibel 1990a; Amoah and Gelaye 1990, 1991; Chemineau et al. 1991; Ishwar and Memon 1996; Gordon 1997; Cognie 1999; Bretzlaff and Romano 2001; Rubianes and Menchaca 2003).

Instead, this chapter attempts to provide the basic information needed by the veterinary practitioner.

Guidelines for handling infertility, abortions, and obstetric problems are included. Additional illustrations of many of the conditions discussed in this chapter are available through the Drost Project on the World Wide Web (Drost 2008).

THE DOE

The female goat is called a doe in polite circles or when discussing valuable or cherished animals. A doeling is a young female, often one that has not yet kidded. The term "nanny" should be avoided when there is a chance of offending an owner by its use, although this is the standard terminology for an Angora doe in Texas.

The anatomic features of the reproductive tract of nonpregnant and pregnant goats have been reviewed by Lyngset (1968b, 1968c). The uterus is bicornual and the cervix has approximately five fibrous rings. These rings impede passage of a pipette if the doe is not in estrus. A canine vaginal speculum, caprine artificial insemination speculum, human proctoscope, or glass test tube (22 to 25 mm diameter) with a hole fire-polished in its rounded end permits visualization of the vagina and external cervical os (Haibel 1986b).

The Estrous Cycle

In temperate regions, goats are seasonally polyestrous. Cycling begins under the influence of decreasing day length. After the days begin to lengthen again in winter, cycling gradually ceases. The duration of the period when regular estrous cycles occur varies with the region, breed, and herd. Individual factors also come into play, as high-producing dairy goats are less likely to exhibit estrus shortly after parturition than are healthy animals producing little or no milk. As a rough approximation, August until March in the northern hemisphere, and particularly October until December, encompass the normal breeding season. Some animals in a herd in temperate regions may be capable of cycling year-round, and this is typical in the tropics, where the availability of forage is more important than day length. Owners who desire out-of-season breeding should select as herd replacements the offspring of animals that bred in the traditionally anestrous period.

Macroscopic and histologic changes occurring in the ovarian structures of the goat during the estrous cycle have been reported by Harrison (1948). The estrous cycle, and particularly the ovulation, of research goats (Dukelow et al. 1971) and sheep (Oldham and Lindsay 1980) have been monitored by laparoscopic methods since the early 1970s. Equipment and techniques used for laparoscopic artificial insemination of sheep (Seeger and Klatt 1980; Killen and Caffery 1982; Gourley and Riese 1990) are also suitable for goats.

Transrectal ultrasonography using a probe extender may be useful for monitoring ovarian activity in select cases, if a probe with adequate resolution (at least 7.5 MHz) is available. The ovaries can be visualized to the left and right of the bladder by slow methodical scanning. Normal mature follicles are 9 to 12 mm in diameter (Buergelt 1997). Other ultrasonographic studies in Boer goats (Padilla and Holtz 2000) and Serrana goats (Simoes et al. 2006) have documented three to five waves of follicles per cycle (reviewed by Rubianes and Menchaca 2003), with follicular diameter at ovulation typically 7 to 8 mm. Ovulation can be confirmed by disappearance of one or more large follicles and development of corpora lutea (Baril et al. 1999). A corpus luteum is less echogenic than the surrounding ovarian stroma and may have a central fluid-filled cavity (Kähn 1994). Inactive ovaries and follicles smaller than 4 mm are difficult to identify. Large, cystic follicles could conceivably be found and monitored over time, but this has not been reported.

Cycle Length

The typical length of an estrous cycle for European dairy breeds is twenty-one days. African pygmy goats are more variable (eighteen to twenty-four days). At the beginning and end of the season, cycles of irregular length, not always accompanied by overt estrus, may occur (Phillips et al. 1943; Camp et al. 1983). Short cycles of five to seven days are to be considered normal during the transition periods, especially in kids, but persist throughout the breeding season in certain populations of goats, and more importantly, in certain individual problem breeders and in some goats superovulated for embryo transfer purposes (Armstrong et al. 1983, 1987; Stubbings et al. 1986). In these does, the corpus luteum is short-lived, demonstrated by only a brief increase in progesterone. The problem can be circumvented in embryo transfer donors by administering a progestogen sponge or implant four days after breeding. Pretreatment with a progestogen (45 mg fluorogestone acetate (FGA)-impregnated sponge for seventeen days or a single injection of 5.2 mg FGA) eliminated the occurrence of short-lived corpora lutea associated with introduction of the buck to anestrous does (Chemineau 1985).

Short cycles are also common after prostaglandin-induced abortion and are associated with delayed pre-ovulatory luteinizing hormone surges of reduced magnitude (Bretzlaff et al. 1988). Elevated prostaglandin F2α levels and shortened estrous cycles have been documented in goats in Kenya infected with *Trypanosoma congolense* (Mutayoba et al. 1989). Nymphomania has been observed in mature goats after several years of a copper-deficient diet (Anke et al. 1977). Synthetic corticosteroids (dexamethasone 10 mg twice daily for ten days) extend the cycle length by prolonging luteal function (Alan et al. 1989).

Empirical treatments for short cycles or continuous signs of estrus include gonadotropin releasing hormone (GnRH, one-fourth to one-half a bovine dose), human chorionic gonadotropin (hCG, 1,000 IU), a pregnant mare serum gonadotropin-hCG product for swine (PG600, Intervet, 2 cc) at the time of estrus, or a three-week application of exogenous progesterone (by implant, sponge, or injection as discussed below under control of estrus). In an ultrasonographic study of five goats from Japan, cystic ovaries (defined as persistence of a follicle greater than 10 mm in diameter for ten days or more in the absence of a corpus luteum) was successfully treated with GnRH followed ten days later by prostaglandin. Four of the goats became pregnant to the induced estrus (Medan et al. 2004).

Signs of Estrus

Standing estrus lasts approximately twenty-four hours in doelings but may last two to three days in mature does. It is shortened if service by a buck is permitted (Romano and Benech 1996). The estrous doe is generally easy to identify if a mature and odoriferous buck is nearby; the doe walks restlessly along the perimeter of her enclosure, searching for a way to reach the buck, or remains close to the fence (Figure 13.1). The vulva becomes somewhat swollen and the doe's tail wags vigorously. This tail wag, which can often be observed even in the absence of a buck, presumably has the function of sending pheromones from the doe's reproductive tract into the environs to attract a buck. Other signs of estrus include a plaintive voice, increased frequency of urination, decreased appetite, and decreased milk yield. The doe in estrus normally stands firmly when a buck attempts to mount and may even back up to the buck. Some does, however, find some bucks (for instance, young or descented males) sexually unattractive and will not stand to be bred.

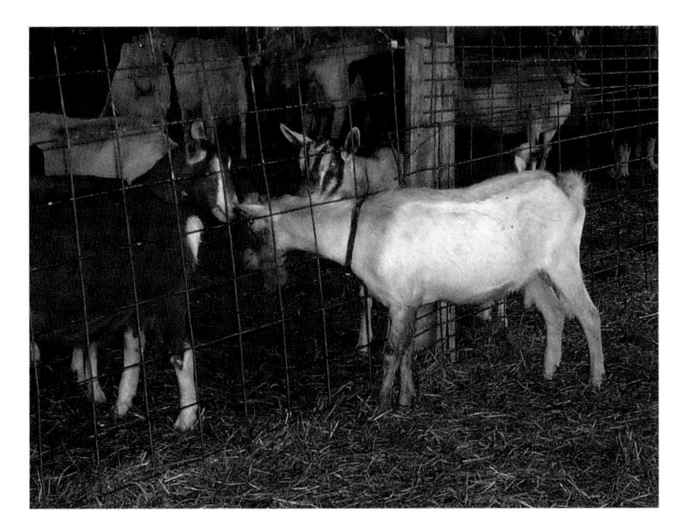

Figure 13.1. This buck in rut is teasing does in estrus through the panel. Note staining of the beard and front legs where he has urinated on himself. (Courtesy Dr. M.C. Smith.)

The vaginal discharge at the beginning of estrus is thin, clear, and colorless. It becomes progressively thicker and whiter toward the end of standing estrus and ovulation (Pretorius 1977). It is important to recognize this aspect of caprine physiology as normal; otherwise practitioners might mistakenly assume that animals with a cloudy white discharge full of neutrophils need antibiotic therapy. Ovulation typically occurs near the end of standing estrus and approximately twenty-four hours after a serum peak in luteinizing hormone (Greyling and van Niekerk 1990).

Vaginal cytology during the estrous cycle has been studied but appears to have limited clinical application. During estrus, superficial keratinized acidophilic cells from the stratum corneum predominate in the vaginal smear. In the case of ovulation there is a sudden influx of leukocytes. Superficial cells and leukocytes are soon replaced by basal and parabasal cells from the stratum germinativum and intermediate cells from the stratum spinosum, which predominate during the corpus luteum phase (Schmidt 1961). Histologic changes of the vaginal mucosa have also been described (Hamilton and Harrison 1951).

Control of Estrus

Although a full discussion of estrus induction and synchronization can be found in other texts, any practitioner dealing with dairy goats will want to be familiar with some of the problems and techniques involved in year-round breeding or synchronization for artificial insemination.

Breeding Season

The methods that can be used successfully vary with the physiologic state of the goat (Smith 1986b). Thus, during the regular breeding season, prostaglandin F 2 alpha (2.5 mg) or cloprostenol (62 mcg) during the luteal phase of the cycle normally induces estrus in approximately 48 hours although some researchers have seen better response with and producers commonly use double these doses (Nuti et al. 1992; Mellado et al. 1994). Even lower doses of prostaglandin F2 alpha (1.25 mg) have been documented to be effective (Bretzlaff et al. 1981). If the doe is not known to be at day five or beyond in the cycle, paired prostaglandin injections ten days apart increase the probability of response to prostaglandin by the time of the second injection.

Although not currently available in the United States, various progestogens can be placed for five to ten days and prostaglandin given at the time of implant or pessary removal. Products that have been used this way include ear implants (3 mg norgestomet, half of a 6 mg Synchro-Mate-B implant), vaginal pessaries (45 mg fluorogestone acetate; FGA, Cronolone, Intervet or 60 mg methyl-acetoxy progesterone; MAP, Upjohn) and controlled internal drug releasers (CIDR-G with 300 mg progesterone). Melengestrol acetate (MGA) can also be fed in some countries. A typical dose is 0.125 mg/head twice a day for ten to fourteen days, followed by a prostaglandin injection. Concerns about unknown meat and milk residues plague the use of most of these products.

Transition

During the transitional period (between the anestrous and breeding seasons), response to prostaglandin alone would be erratic, but either sudden introduction of a buck or application of exogenous progestogens followed by prostaglandin should be effective in inducing cyclicity. Although not currently available in the United States, both vaginal pessaries and subcutaneous progestogen implants work well during the transition period (East and Rowe 1989). Adding gonadotropins such as human chorionic gonadotropin (hCG) combined with equine chorionic gonadotropin (eCG, previously called pregnant mare serum gonadotrophin, PMSG) (PG600, Intervet) to the regimen may be beneficial, as during the anestrous season (Rowe and East 1996).

The buck effect usually synchronizes a group of does to begin cycling within eight days (Shelton 1960; Ott et al. 1980). The buck effect also hastens the onset of puberty in doelings (Amoah and Bryant 1984). If more precise control is needed, the does could be aborted very early in pregnancy and rebred to the buck of choice. Bright security lights in the barnyard might delay the onset of cyclicity in the fall (Bretzlaff 1989).

Anestrous Season

Breeding during the anestrous season is not so easily achieved. Two injections of prostaglandin are ineffective (Greyling and Van Niekerk 1991a), because (except for goats in false pregnancy) there is no corpus luteum available for luteolysis. Some herds, including those in the tropics (Chemineau 1984), may respond to the buck effect. One study in Mexico showed that the buck effect induced ovulation in does that were not otherwise manipulated as long as the bucks used were sexually active. This state was achieved by exposing the bucks to sixteen-hour-long days for two months and then inserting two subcutaneous melatonin implants of 18 mg each when the bucks were returned to ambient day length for a further two months, before being used as teasers (Flores et al. 2000). Based on research done with rams (Pearce and Oldham 1988), it is likely that introduction of a novel buck would be effective in inducing ovulation if does have become habituated to a resident buck by continuous contact.

Photoperiod manipulation of does is a commonly used technique in North America. Herds can be subjected to two months of artificially lengthened days (nineteen to twenty hours of light per day) or to a one- to two-hour "flash" of light beginning sixteen hours after dawn; minimum 200 lux) and then returned to a shorter day length. Cycling begins approximately six weeks later. Some herd owners find the cost of electricity prohibitive. Goats experiencing hydrometra are unlikely to respond but could be identified by ultrasound and treated in advance (see below).

Abrupt introduction of a buck (also light-treated, but held away from the does) six weeks after the end of the long days appears to improve the success rate with photoperiod treatment (BonDurant 1986; Pellicer-Rubio et al. 2007). Improved fertility out of season also seems possible with administration to the does of a melatonin implant at the end of the artificially long days (Chemineau et al. 1986, 1999; Chemineau 1989; du Preez 2001). Melatonin, a hormone normally produced by the pineal gland during hours of darkness, serves as a signal that the nights are now long. These implants are not currently available in the United States.

Finally, the various exogenous progestogen treatments discussed under breeding season can be applied for twenty-one days with good fertility on the induced estrus if equine chorionic gonadotropin (eCG, previously called PMSG) can be given two days before removal of pessary or implant. Fertility is improved if the progestogen treatment is reduced to eleven days and prostaglandin is given simultaneously with the eCG (Corteel et al. 1988). The dose of eCG needed varies with the age and milk production of the goat (400 IU for a nulliparous doeling, 750 IU for a mature doe in early lactation). A generic protocol is then to insert progestogen source on day zero, give prostaglandin and eCG on day nine, remove progestogen on day eleven, and expect estrus thirty-six to forty-eight hours later. In goat herds where eCG is not available, there has been little success with sponges and implants during the anestrous season, although some producers in the United States have successfully used the available swine hCG/eCG product (PG600, Intervet). Adding the buck effect may improve pregnancy rates (Bretzlaff et al. 1991).

PREGNANCY DIAGNOSIS

An excellent general discussion of pregnancy diagnosis has been provided by C.S.F. Williams (1986a)

Table 13.1. Pregnancy diagnosis techniques for goats.

Technique	*Stage of Pregnancy*	*Accuracy %*		*Potential errors*	*Comment*
		Pregnant	*Nonpregnant*		
Estrus detection	18–24 days or until term	Varies with detection method, may stand when pregnant		End of breeding season, buck not "acceptable."	Observe tail wag; use buck, testosterone-treated doe, intersex.
Serum progesterone (Thibier et al. 1982)	19–24 days	87	97	Irregular cycle, false pregnancy, early abortion.	Best used as nonpregnancy test.
Milk progesterone (Pennington et al. 1982; Dionysius 1991)	19–24 days	Varies with each kit/antiserum. 71–98	80–100	False negative unless antiserum detects 5-pregnanedione; false positive may occur during estrus (Holdsworth and Davies 1979; Bretzlaff et al. 1989).	Concentrations more variable and higher than serum progesterone (Murray and Newstead 1988).
Urinary or serum estrone sulfate (Williams 1986a; Sardjana et al. 1988a)	After 50–60 days, some possible by 30 days	About 100	About 100	Testing milk unreliable unless in full production.	Negative in false pregnancy; secretion decreases rapidly if abortion.
PSPB	After 25 days	High	High	False positive if recent fetal death.	
Ballottement	After 100 days			Goat fat or tense.	Swing entire abdomen or push in with fist.
Radiography (Barker and Cawley 1967)	After 70–90 days	About 100	About 100	Diagnosing by uterine enlargement rather than skeleton.	Hold off feed; can count fetuses.
Amplitude depth ultrasound	60 (80)–120 days			False pregnant does positive; late pregnant does may be negative.	Clip hair right side above udder.
Doppler (Lindahl 1969; Fraser et al. 1971; Ott et al. 1981)	>35 days (rectal)	95	25–75	Increased blood flow in false pregnancy.	Fetal heart two times maternal rate.
Real-time ultrasound (Buckrell 1988; Baronet and Vaillancourt 1989)	>25 days (rectal) >35 days (abdominal)	About 100	87	False pregnancy (fluid, no fetus or caruncles); late pregnancy more difficult to visualize.	Transabdominal test earlier in older does.

and updated to include B-mode ultrasonography by Matsas (2007). Table 13.1 outlines many different methods of pregnancy diagnosis and the sensitivity and specificity of the tests for which published information is available. In fact, the apparent accuracy of most of these methods varies from farm to farm, according to the prevalence of infectious abortions, nutritional deficiencies causing early embryonic loss, and hydrometra. Experience of the examiner also affects accuracy.

Diagnostic Techniques

The most accurate tests are those that measure or detect something that is only produced by a viable fetus and that is always present when the goat has reached a certain stage of pregnancy.

Hormonal Assays

Hormones that have been used as predictors of pregnancy include progesterone, estrone sulfate, placental lactogen, and pregnancy associated glyocoproteins.

Progesterone, because it is produced only by the ovaries and not by the placenta, is best used as a nonpregnancy test (Dionysius 1991; Gonzalez et al. 2004), although the probability that a goat with elevated progesterone is actually pregnant is increased during the anestrous season (Fleming et al. 1990). Goats with low progesterone in serum or milk five days or more after breeding are judged to be not pregnant. The exact cut-off varies with test method, and most commercial kits have not been validated for goats. Goats with elevated progesterone at twenty-one days after breeding could be pregnant or could have a different cycle length or be pseudopregnant. One study found that using milk progesterone kits at twenty days after breeding was no more accurate for pregnancy diagnosis than using a buck to detect return to estrus at eighteen to twenty-four days (Engeland et al. 1997).

Estrogens are produced by both the ovaries and placenta, but estrone sulfate is thought to be a product of steroid conjugation by fetal or placental tissues (Refsal et al. 1991). Estrone sulfate in whole milk or whey can be used for pregnancy diagnosis (Chaplin and Holdsworth 1982; McArthur and Geary 1986), and total urinary estrogen has also been used by a commercial laboratory (B.E.T. Reproductive Laboratories, Lexington, KY), beginning at about fifty days of gestation. Occasional false negative results in the B.E.T. test are reported in pregnant does well beyond fifty days of gestation.

Placental lactogen is a hormone produced only by the placenta (Hayden et al. 1980; Byatt et al. 1992). Concentrations in plasma or milk can be assayed after sixty days to diagnose pregnancy. The hormone concentration is also correlated with the total weight of kids produced (Sardjana et al. 1988b). Commercial assays for the caprine hormone are not currently available. Several pregnancy associated glycoproteins (PAGs) are produced by chorionic binucleate cells from the placenta and have been detected as early as twenty-one days of gestation by radioimmunoassay (Gonzalez et al. 1999, 2000, 2004). No PAG is detected if a pseudopregnancy develops early, and sequential tests show a decrease in PAG concentration when one fetus in a litter dies (Zarrouk et al. 1999). Currently, an ELISA test for the closely related pregnancy-specific protein B (PSPB) is available from Bio Tracking (Moscow, ID). This is a placental hormone that has been used as an indicator of pregnancy in goats (Humblot et al. 1990), cattle, and sheep (Ruder et al. 1988). Detection of pregnancy is possible using PSPB by twenty-six days in goats. It is not known how long the test remains positive in a pseudopregnant goat when an embryo reached the stage of hormone production before dying. It is also not yet known if concentrations of placental hormones vary according to previous selection pressures on a given breed for milk or meat production.

Amplitude Depth Ultrasound

The first ultrasound machines on the market detected the interface between a fluid-filled organ (the uterus) and the abdominal viscera. These machines are still commonly used for pregnancy diagnosis in swine and are relatively inexpensive. They are very unsatisfactory for use in dairy goats because of low accuracy. Nonpregnant animals with fluid in the uterus (false pregnancy) are classified as pregnant, thus escaping detection. Also, a false-negative diagnosis is delivered if the ultrasound beam encounters fetus rather than large pockets of fluid.

Doppler

When the limitations of the amplitude depth machines were recognized, interest switched to Doppler techniques. Doppler machines permit the operator to hear the blood flow in maternal and fetal vessels. When used rectally (after thirty-five days), the external iliac vessels are first located by directing the probe laterally within the pelvic canal. When the maternal pulse rate is ascertained, the probe is advanced and directed ventrad to search for a fetal heartbeat or blood flow in the umbilical artery, at approximately twice the maternal rate. The fetal heart rate is negatively correlated with fetal age (Fraser et al. 1971). Loud whooshing sounds at the maternal rate but ventrally located indicate increased blood flow to the uterus; this should not be taken as conclusive evidence of pregnancy because it is also heard in goats with hydrometra and might be detected in does that have recently kidded (Wani et al. 1998). After forty-five days, detection of the fetal heartbeat can be accomplished transabdominally. This technique may also be used to assess fetal viability in goats with pregnancy toxemia. The equipment is more affordable than a real-time ultrasound machine.

Real-time Ultrasound

A real-time ultrasound machine eliminates worries about false positives if the diagnosis is always based on visualizing either fetus or caruncles (Haibel 1990b). False negatives are still possible if later, unrecorded matings have occurred. Administering prostaglandin, then, should generally be delayed until the doe has been rechecked, unless later breedings are absolutely impossible. Accuracy also improves with operator experience (Bretzlaff et al. 1993). Sector scanners generally have superior resolution to linear array systems and make counting fetuses easier, but the equipment is more expensive. Portable generators permit the use of real-time technology even under range conditions. With some machines, it is important not to disconnect the probe or let the generator run out of fuel while the power is on. Smaller battery operated units are now available.

TRANSRECTAL SCANNING. Equine and bovine linear array units with 5-mHz transducers can be used rectally for early diagnosis (twenty to thirty days) or transabdominally later in pregnancy (day thirty-five and beyond) (Buckrell 1988). Withholding food and water for twelve hours improves visualization of the uterus but is usually not necessary and might lead to pregnancy toxemia (Bretzlaff et al. 1993). Taping an insemination rod or a longitudinally split section of plastic pipe to the head and cord of the transducer simplifies manipulations within the rectum. Although more expensive, a human prostate probe also works well. A small amount of lubricant is introduced into the rectum before inserting the lubricated probe. The pregnant uterus is usually located anterior and ventral to the urinary bladder. Elevating the abdomen by placing the goat across a hay bale makes transrectal diagnosis reliable even after thirty-five days (Baronet and Vaillancourt 1989). The earliest that the embryo is reliably detected by transrectal exam is twenty-five or twenty-six days after breeding (Gonzalez et al. 2004). In another small study, at least one embryo of each pregnant doe had a detectable heart beat by day twenty-three (Martinez et al. 1998).

TRANSABDOMINAL SCANNING. For transabdominal examination, does are generally scanned standing, from the right side, and clipping hair immediately lateral and dorsal to the udder improves contact between transducer and skin. Otherwise (show does, for instance), much contact gel (such as methyl-cellulose rectal lubricant), vegetable oil, or alcohol is needed to wet the hair. Examination in dorsal recumbency (in a padded trough) has been used in early research trials (Tainturier et al. 1983), but stresses the doe to an unnecessary degree.

Early in pregnancy (thirty to forty-five days), the ultrasound beam should be directed toward the pelvic inlet. Subsequently, the uterus is usually positioned against the right ventral abdominal wall (Haibel 1986a). Late in pregnancy, the 5-MHz transducer may not penetrate as far as the fetus (caruncles are visible but not well outlined by fluid) or part of a fetus may fill the screen and be overlooked unless bones or beating fetal heart (nonechogenic because of the blood in it) is noted. A 3.5-MHz transducer is preferred but not imperative in late gestation.

A sector scanner is preferred for determining fetal numbers. The best time for counting fetuses is between forty and seventy days of gestation (Lavoir and Taverne 1989; Hesselink and Taverne 1994). The number of triplet litters is underestimated before fifty days (Dawson et al. 1994).

In early pregnancy, numerous fluid-filled cross sections of uterus are visualized. This phenomenon can be explained by circumferential folds of endometrium which protrude into the lumen (Kähn 1994). If a fetus is clearly visualized, its heartbeat can be detected by twenty-five to thirty days. It has been stated that caruncles are routinely found by day thirty (Buckrell et al. 1986; Baronet and Vaillancourt 1989) or day thirty-five (Doizé et al. 1997), but others feel that day forty or fifty is a safer date if a goat is to be called open because caruncles are not visualized. This allows for variations in resolution of the machine and position of the uterus. The caruncles appear to be doughnut- or C-shaped by forty-five to fifty days (Haibel 1986a) and are outlined by fluid (Figure 13.2). There are approximately 120 to 125 caruncles in a goat's uterus, arranged in four rows in each horn (Lyngset 1968c).

FETAL AGE DETERMINATION. With practice, the size of the fetus can be used to estimate stage of gestation. In Saanens and Alpines, the crown-rump length of the fetus is approximately 40 mm at forty-five days, 100 mm at sixty days, and 250 mm at ninety days (Mialot et al. 1991). Fetal age in dairy goats also can be

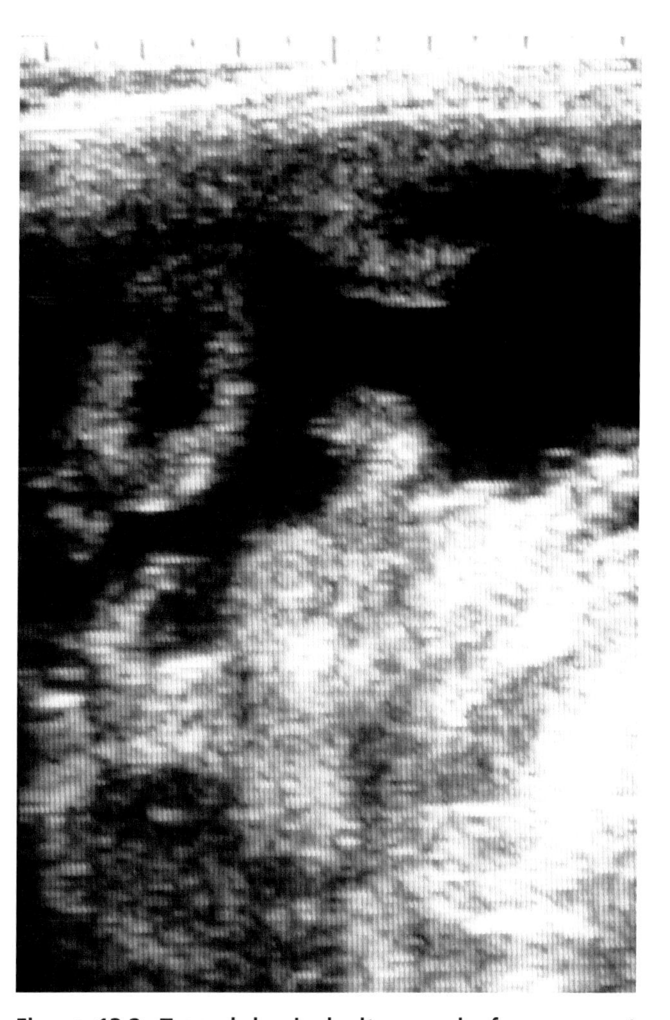

Figure 13.2. Transabdominal ultrasound of a pregnant doe showing a donut-shaped caruncle clearly outlined by black uterine fluid. (Courtesy Dr. M.C. Smith.)

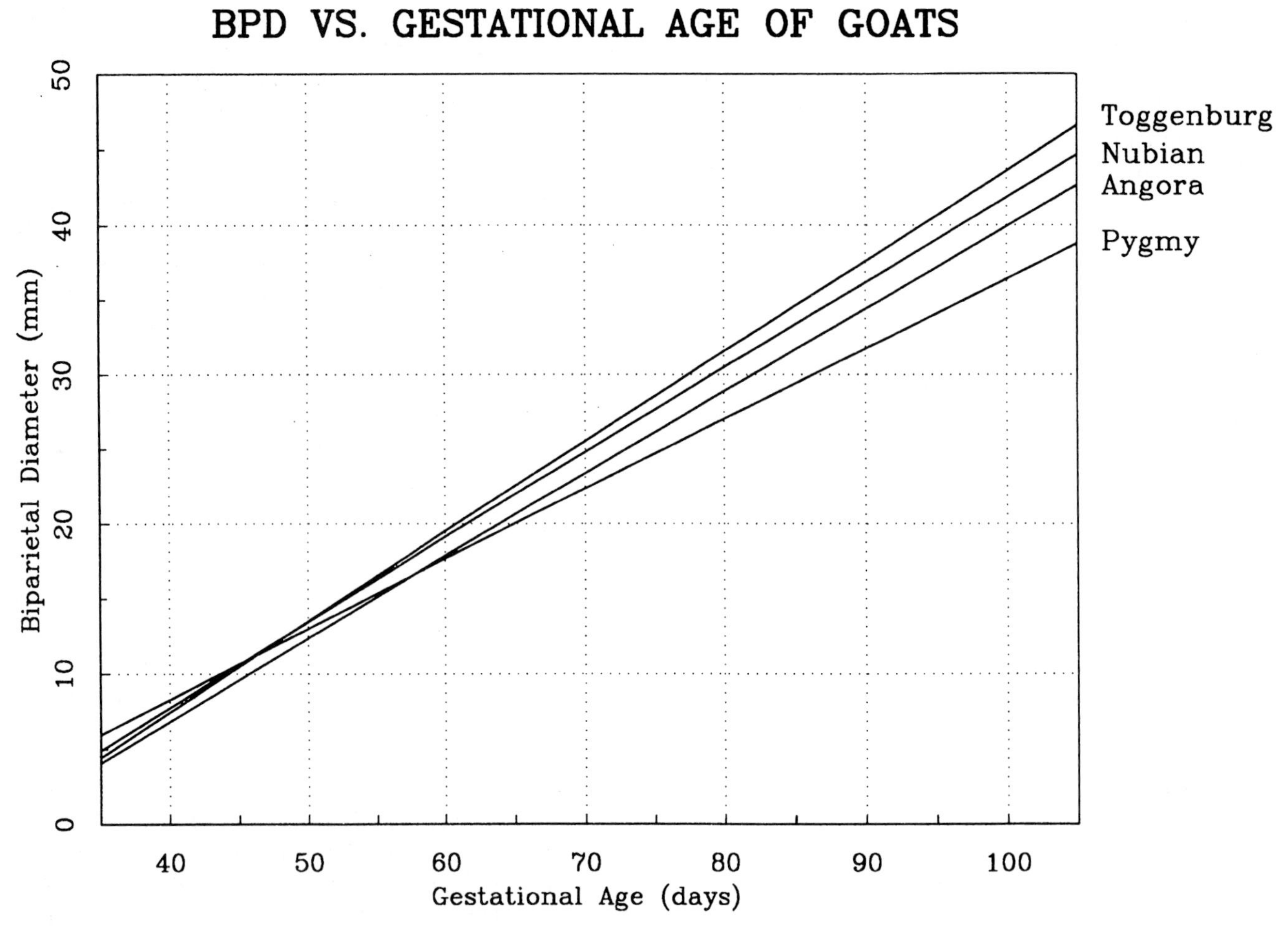

Figure 13.3. Correlation of biparietal diameter and fetal age. (From Haibel, G.K.: Use of ultrasonography in reproductive management of sheep and goat herds. Vet. Clin. N. Am., Food Anim. Prac., 6(3):608, 1990.)

estimated by measuring the width of the fetal head during real-time examination (Figure 13.3). Between forty and one hundred days gestation, the biparietal diameter (measured from a symmetrical, maximum width image) correlates very closely with age (Haibel 1988, Haibel et al. 1989). A similar correlation has been reported for second trimester pygmy goat fetuses (Reichle and Haibel 1991). Later in pregnancy, there is too much difference in size of the fetuses and it is no longer possible to date pregnancies accurately enough to permit safe induction of parturition based on the estimated fetal age.

Caruncular size is also quite variable and not very useful for estimating age, except early in pregnancy. The caruncles increase in size until a maximum is reached at about ninety days of gestation. Before this time the diameter of the caruncles in the uterine body as imaged transrectally can be used as a predictor of stage of pregnancy but less precision might be expected from transabdominal measurements of caruncles in random parts of the uterus (Doizé et al. 1997).

Fetal Sex Determination. Real-time ultrasound permits visualization of the genital tubercle of the developing fetus, an embryologic structure that is initially located between the hind limbs but moves forward to near the umbilicus in males and back toward the tail in females. Transrectal scanning using an adaptor to manipulate the probe gives excellent results for single kids between fifty-five and seventy-five days of gestation, but it is not always possible to visualize the genital tubercle or external genitalia in twins or triplets (Santos et al. 2007). Other authors prefer to use presence of two thin teats between the hind legs and absence of a triangular appearing scrotum in this region to diagnose a female fetus, because the tail may obscure the female genital tubercle (Burstel et al. 2002). The penis/prepuce is located immediately behind the nonechogenic, circular umbilical cord.

Other Techniques

Where Doppler or real-time ultrasound is not available and hormonal assays are prohibitively expensive, other, less sophisticated techniques may be used. For instance, rapid field laparotomy has been used to diagnose pregnancy in goats. Hulet's rod for recto-abdominal palpation has also been used in goats, but American practitioners will probably find this technique less than satisfactory. Goats do not lie quietly on their backs for this examination, as is typical for sheep to do, and rectal lacerations and abortions may occur (Ott et al. 1981). In a relaxed doe in late pregnancy, it may be possible to palpate or ballot a fetus in the right ventral abdomen or to observe fetal movements.

A bimanual technique has been developed for detecting early pregnancy in goats and sheep (Kutty 1999). After overnight fasting of the doe, a gloved index finger is introduced into the rectum of the standing animal and used to evacuate fecal pellets and express the bladder. Then the examiner's right hand is pushed vertically in the caudal abdomen, to displace intestines forward and the uterus caudally into the pelvic canal where it can be palpated by the left index finger. Ovaries could also be trapped between the two index fingers and palpated. A fluid distension of the uterine horns is reported to be palpable at thirty and forty-five days but cannot be distinguished from hydrometra. By ninety days, retroversion of the uterus is no longer possible, but placentomes and softening of the cervix are palpable.

For the answer to the in-passing "do you think she's pregnant?" question, the sacrotuberous ligament and other ligaments near the base of the tail should be evaluated for softening. This is easiest when comparison with a nonpregnant doe is possible. In practiced hands and the second half of pregnancy, this is a free version of the urinary estrone sulfate test. Increased elasticity of the skin around the vulva and pinbones has also been used by laymen as an indicator of pregnancy (DeArmond 1990). Development of an udder, even in yearlings, should not be taken as proof of pregnancy (see inappropriate lactation syndrome, discussed in Chapter 14).

Use of Test Results

Pregnancy diagnosis is performed for a variety of reasons, depending on the management of the goat herd. It may be desirable to cull nonpregnant does after the end of a breeding season or in times of feed shortage. Verifying pregnancy before drying off a dairy doe is becoming routine. It is also very important to monitor the success of out-of-season breeding programs, because of extremely variable results and the relatively high risk of hydrometra in these does.

What one does with the results of a pregnancy test depends on one's faith in the test results. If a goat is thought to be pregnant, usually nothing is done unless mismating has occurred or nutritional resources are so short that only well-grown, pregnant goats can be fed adequately to maintain pregnancy. Animals carrying multiple fetuses might be fed more than those with singles, to decrease the risks of pregnancy toxemia in one group and obesity in the other (see Chapter 19). When the diagnosis is that of nonpregnancy, the owner may choose to restrict feed or continue milking the goat or stop staying up nights, waiting for it to kid. If rebreeding is desired, it is very likely that the use of prostaglandins to induce estrus will come under discussion. At this point, the practitioner must be very certain of his or her diagnosis of "open." Goats with negative progesterone test results twenty-one days after synchronized breeding could be given a new vaginal sponge or ear implant (de Montigny 1988), but even these techniques frequently include prostaglandin in the synchronization protocol.

FALSE PREGNANCY AND HYDROMETRA

Goats occasionally exhibit prolonged luteal function and absence of estrus even though they are not pregnant. Some of these does were bred and may have conceived at the time that the persistent corpus luteum first developed. One study summarized by Chemineau et al. (1999) documented that approximately half of the pseudopregnancies identified by ultrasonography at forty-five days post breeding were preceded by an embryo that lived long enough to produce pregnancy specific protein B. Other affected does have never even been exposed to a buck.

Historical Perspectives and Clinical Signs

Until recent years, it was very difficult to diagnose or study this phenomenon. Results of progesterone analysis (Holdsworth and Davies 1979) and amplitude-depth ultrasound were suggestive of pregnancy. The rectal Doppler examination indicated increased blood flow to the uterus. Radiographic evaluation (absence of fetal skeleton) or laparotomy was required to make the diagnosis. Owners noticed that some apparently pregnant does (no return to estrus, with or without a gradual enlargement of the abdomen) delivered fluid but no placenta or fetus. The lay term "cloud burst" has been applied to the natural termination of a false pregnancy accompanied by discharge of large volumes of fluid. When practitioners examined goats with marked abdominal distension that had not delivered at the calculated due date, hydrometra was sometimes recognized. Surgical drainage of the uterus was soon replaced by treatment with prostaglandin to induce resorption of the corpus luteum followed by voiding of the retained fluid. A few animals that had been included in various reproductive research trials spontaneously developed false pregnancy, thereby providing retrospective hormonal profiles.

Etiology

The etiology of the condition is not yet known. It seems likely that the prevalence is greater in herds trying to delay breeding of some does (for winter milk production) than in those in which all does are bred on the first estrus of the breeding season. Certain infectious diseases—trypanosomosis if controlled with trypanocidal drugs (Llewelyn et al. 1987), toxoplasmosis (Debenedetti et al. 1989), border disease (Løken 1987)—may possibly increase the prevalence of false pregnancy. Involvement of phytoestrogens in the forage has been proposed as contributing to the occurrence of false pregnancies in certain herds (Malher and Ben Younes 1987). Others have suggested that treating short cycles with human chorionic gonadotropin or gonadotropin releasing hormone may predispose the goat to development of false pregnancy (East 1983).

Prolonged luteal function and hydrometra have been recreated experimentally by immunizing goats against prostaglandin F2 alpha (Taverne et al. 1995; Kornalijnslijper et al. 1997). Fluid accumulation is first detectable between days twenty-nine and thirty-eight of the luteal phase. Prolactin does not appear to be involved in the etiology (Hesselink et al. 1995). Possible suppression of testosterone secretion has not been investigated in relation to false pregnancy. Testosterone is usually required for luteolysis in the goat (Cooke 1989). The possibility of a genetic predisposition is supported by a study in which the daughters of goats with hydrometra had a 38% frequency of hydrometra, compared with 9% of the daughters of unaffected goats (Hesselink and Elving 1996). In another study, 20% of 125 daughters of five sires developed pseudopregnancy, as compared with 0% of the 326 daughters of twelve other sires, all in the same herd (Chemineau et al. 1999).

Epidemiology

The prevalence of the condition in privately owned herds is uncertain, but this information should be easy to estimate when pregnancy diagnosis by real-time ultrasound becomes routine. In one French herd studied in 1986, the buck was introduced to 124 adult goats in early April. Ultrasound at day fifty-four revealed that ninety-two goats were pregnant but twenty-one other goats (17%), all of which had experienced a normal gestation the past year, had hydrometra (Malher and Ben Younes 1987). In another study in France (Mialot et al. 1991; Duquesnel et al. 1992), ultrasound was performed more than 5,000 times on sixty-eight farms in 1989 and on seventy-one farms in 1990, and pseudopregnancy was diagnosed in 2.1% and 2.9% of the examinations. In 10% of the herds, the prevalence was more than 5%. The condition was most commonly diagnosed in adult goats after a fall (November to December) kidding without rebreeding or after an out-of-season synchronization program that did not include prostaglandin. A Dutch study found a mean incidence of 9% with the condition being more common in older goats (Hesselink 1993a). In a German study, 143 of 2,434 dairy goats were affected, as diagnosed by ultrasound, with an average incidence of 5.78% (Wittek et al. 1997, 1998).

Diagnosis

With the development of real-time ultrasound, it has become possible to easily differentiate a false from a true pregnancy and to institute early treatment and monitor the success of therapy (Pieterse and Taverne 1986). When a goat with advanced hydrometra is scanned from either flank, large, fluid-filled compartments are seen (Figure 13.4). Thin tissue walls separate the compartments and undulate when the goat moves or succussion of the abdomen is performed. These walls represent sections of curved horn overlapping each other rather than internal trabeculae (Hesselink and Taverne 1994). Fetus and caruncles are absent. White flecks may be seen in the fluid and settle down like snow after succussion. Diagnosis of an early stage of hydrometra is more difficult. Before forty days, when caruncles may not yet be visible by ultrasound, hydrometra is difficult to distinguish from normal pregnancy because it is not always possible to visualize the fetus when scanning an early pregnancy. In these goats, and in those when the breeding date is unknown, re-evaluation several weeks later verifies the existence of hydrometra if fetus or caruncles still cannot be found.

Diagnosis can also be confirmed by laparotomy or necropsy. The volume of fluid in the uterus is quite variable, 1 to 7.2 liters in one study (Mialot et al. 1991), and 0.25 to 8.3 liters in another (Wittek et al. 1997). In the goat that spontaneously voids the fluid (mucoid discharge on tail, decreased abdominal size), the diagnosis is presumptive. Some does that correct spontaneously early in the course of a pseudopregnancy have a bloody discharge. The condition in these animals cannot be distinguished from early embryonic loss (unless the goat was not bred) without a prior ultrasound diagnosis.

Treatment and Prevention

Prostaglandin is the treatment of hydrometra as confirmed by ultrasound or of false pregnancy as suspected in an anestrous doe that cannot possibly have been exposed to a buck. Both natural (5 to 10 mg prostaglandin F2 alpha) and synthetic (125 to 250 mcg clo-

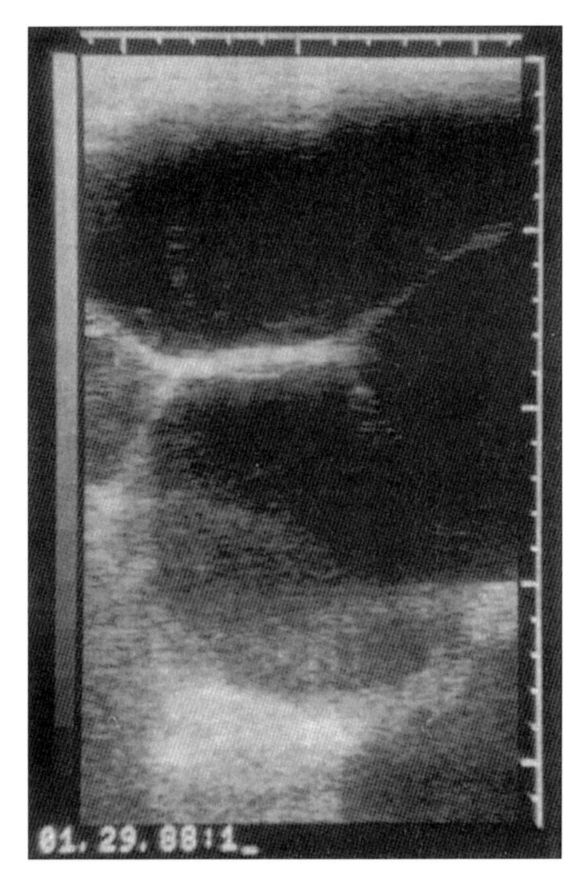

Figure 13.4. Real-time ultrasound image of hydrometra. (Courtesy Dr. M.C. Smith.)

prostenol) hormones cause regression of the corpus luteum and emptying of the uterus. Repeated doses of oxytocin (50 IU twice a day for four days) also induce emptying of the uterus, and might be attempted if scanning several days after prostaglandin therapy indicates continued presence of fluid in the uterus. The rare animal that fails to respond to therapy may have segmental aplasia of the uterus or cervix (Webb 1985; Batista et al. 2006). Many goats return to estrus after treatment and can become pregnant within two months of resolution of the hydrometra (Pieterse and Taverne 1986; Duquesnel et al. 1992). Some of these develop a new pseudopregnancy the following year. Recurrence shortly after treatment has also been observed (Batista et al. 2001), but the risk of this decreases if the goat receives a second dose of prostaglandin twelve days after the initial discharge of fluid (Hesselink 1993b).

In intensively managed herds that practice out-of-season breeding, ultrasound should be performed on all bred does before drying off (Duquesnel et al. 1992). Those that are pseudopregnant should then remain in the milking herd and be treated with prostaglandin, and their milk production will increase. Likewise, goats to be synchronized out of season should be examined by ultrasound first so that affected does that would be expected to have poor fertility at the induced estrus can be treated with prostaglandin and synchronization can be delayed until resolution of the hydrometra is achieved.

Preventing hydrometra in pet goats that will not be bred or even just preventing estrus and associated noisy behavior in these pets can be achieved by ovariectomy. The surgery is done under general anesthesia or heavy sedation and a local block (Mobini et al. 2002). The animal is placed in dorsal recumbency and each ovary is removed after ligation of the pedicle by laparoscopy or via a ventral midline incision just cranial to the udder. Temporary elevation of the rear end of the doe by 25 or 30 degrees simplifies location of the ovaries but prolonged weight of the rumen on the diaphragm is not desirable (Wolfe and Baird 1997). Exposure of the contralateral ovary is difficult from a flank incision, but this approach is preferred for unilateral ovariectomy, as for an ovarian tumor.

A case report of mucometra in a mature West African pygmy goat in Germany documented persistent accumulation of fluid in the uterus in the absence of a functional corpus luteum. This doe did not respond to prostaglandin but was successfully managed by ovariorhystectomy performed from a ventral midline incision caudal to the umbilicus (Trasch et al. 2002).

ABORTION

Abortion by one or more goats in a herd may signal an infectious disease or some other condition that could be controlled by proper management.

Diagnostic Workup for Abortions

Practitioners are often asked to determine the cause of an abortion or to offer an opinion as to the need for diagnostic testing. The owner should be instructed to keep detailed records and accurately identify each aborting animal and the stage of gestation when fetal loss occurred. In addition to crown rump length data, guidelines for estimating the gestational age of tropical breeds in Nigeria have been reported (Sivachelvan et al. 1996) and are summerized as follows.

Week	Developmental characteristic
10–11	Hairs on eyelids
13–14	Hairs on dorsum of neck and entire calvarium hard
14–15	Eyelids separable
16–17	Body sparsely covered with hair
17–20	Body densely covered with hair, teeth buds prominent
At birth	1–3 pair incisors erupted

Similar information exists for West African Dwarf goats (Osuagwuh and Aire 1986) and Norwegian goats (Lyngset 1971).

The serious risk of zoonotic disease and prompt disposal of all fetuses or placentas not submitted for diagnostic workup must be stressed. Uterine discharges are an important source of infection for others in the herd, and thus all aborting does should be isolated at once from the rest of the herd. Pregnant does should be fed from feeders to limit exposure to discharges on the ground. When abortion has occurred outside, the immediate area can be disinfected by burning (straw and diesel fuel). It is also good policy to separate pregnant females of different species because some abortion storms may cross species lines.

After consulting with the regional diagnostic laboratory, fetus, placenta, and paired sera should be collected. If it is not convenient to submit the entire fetus, fetal tissues and fluids (stomach fluid, heart blood) should be harvested for culture and serology tests and submitted along with formalin-fixed tissues (including brain) for histology (see Table 13.2). Impression smears of the cut surface of cotyledons may permit identification of infectious agents by special stains or fluorescent antibody techniques when the placenta itself is too autolysed or contaminated to easily evaluate by culture or routine histology. Exudate from the vagina may be substituted in some tests if placenta is not available. Owners should be alerted to the unsuitability of a mummified fetus for many tests, so that long drives and expenses associated with laboratory submission of a mummy can be avoided. Although not ideal, it is possible to freeze the first aborted fetus and placenta, along with serum from the dam, then await the possible development of a herd problem.

Laboratory procedures for identifying the various causes of abortion have been described in Kirkbride's manual (Kirkbride 1990).

The importance of the placenta cannot be overemphasized. Table 13.3 summarizes the placental changes that may have diagnostic value. Small white amniotic plaques of proliferating epithelial tissue are inconsistent but normal findings (Lyngset 1971). Unfortunately, many does either eat the placenta or retain it, so that this extremely important tissue is not always available. Also, grossly visible placental lesions are not invariably present.

The diagnosis in an abortion storm often is not available for several days. In fact, absence of placentas, autolysis, bacterial contamination, or submission of unrepresentative fetuses (bad luck) may result in no diagnosis being achieved. It is reasonable to begin treatment of remaining pregnant does with tetracycline in case a susceptible infectious agent is involved. One possible protocol is three subcutaneous injections of long-lasting tetracycline (Biomycin 200®, BioCeutic) at 9 mg/lb (20 mg/kg) at three-day intervals. The intramuscular route should be avoided, because it

Table 13.2. Diagnostic samples for abortion testing.

	Fluids in test tube	Tissues		Formalin-fixed histology
		Fresh bacteriology	Fresh virology	
Maternal blood	X			
Fetal heart blood or thoracic fluid	X			
Abomasal fluid	X			
Placenta (note gross lesions); cotyledon and intercotyledonary areas		X	X	X
Kidney		X	X	X
Liver		X	X	X
Lung		X	X	X
Spleen		X	X	X
Brain (note gross lesions)				X
Skeletal muscle				X
Heart				X

Table 13.3. Changes observed in placentas from aborting goats.

Disease	*Placental lesion*
Border disease	Pinpoint grey foci of necrosis in cotyledons.
Brucellosis	No reports, placental edema, necrosis of cotyledons in sheep.
Campylobacteriosis	Placental edema, necrosis of cotyledons.
Chlamydiosis	Thickening and necrosis of cotyledonary and intercotyledonary tissue, brownish exudate.
Listeriosis	No reports in goats. Thickened necrotic leathery cotyledons (sheep).
Q fever	Intercotyledonary and cotyledonary necrosis and mineralization; exudate on surface.
Toxoplasmosis	Small opaque white foci of mineralization in cotyledons. Intercotyledonary areas normal.
Yersiniosis	White foci in cotyledons.

causes severe muscle necrosis. Obvious nutritional deficiencies should also be addressed.

Early Abortion

In the field it is often impossible to differentiate early abortions from simple failure to conceive and false pregnancy. Similarly, when more corpora lutea than embryos are found in slaughterhouse studies, the contribution of fertilization failure cannot be determined (Lyngset 1968a). One possible genetic cause of early embryonic death, the Robertsonian translocation, is discussed later in this chapter.

Veterinarians occasionally prescribe progesterone maintenance therapy for goats that have aborted repeatedly and may have inadequate hormone levels. It may be inappropriate to assist in reproducing reproductive misfits. The presence of a live fetus should also be verified (real-time ultrasound) before progesterone administration is begun. Experimentally, progesterone in oil (25 mg daily) prevented abortion in three ovariectomized goats (Meites et al. 1951).

Drug-induced Malformations

Before attachment of the blastocyst at day fifteen, the uterus contains a fluid of increased pH that accumulates high concentrations of acidic drugs administered to the dam. Even after attachment, drugs may disrupt organogenesis. Specific information related to the goat is lacking, but in general unnecessary drugs, including anthelmintics and anesthetics, should be avoided during the first thirty-five days of pregnancy. Diazepam, xylazine, and acetylpromazine are potentially deleterious drugs, whereas thiopental, thiamylal, ketamine, and the major inhalation anesthetic agents are not believed to be teratogenic (Ludders 1988). In sheep, parbendazole (at doses of 60 mg/kg), cambendazole (at 50 mg/kg), and netobimin (at 20 mg/kg) are teratogenic and cambendazole is also embryotoxic (Szabo 1989; Navarro et al. 1998). Malformations involving vital organs may lead to early loss of embryo or fetus.

Sheep and Goat Hybrids

When flocks of sheep and goats are kept together, breeding usually only occurs between members of the same species. However, if does are housed with a fertile male sheep and no buck is available, interbreeding occurs. An embryo forms but usually does not survive beyond the second month of pregnancy. Fertilization rarely occurs when a ewe is bred by a buck (Kelk et al. 1997).

The goat has sixty chromosomes, all acrocentric. The sheep has fifty-four chromosomes, six of which are metacentric while the rest are acrocentric. The hybrid embryo has fifty-seven chromosomes, three of which are metacentric (Ilbery et al. 1967). Some hybrid embryos fail to attach to the maternal caruncles. Histologically, those that attach show evidence of rejection of the trophoblastic tissue that invades the caruncles (Hancock et al. 1968; Dent et al. 1971). The embryo degenerates and is expelled. Passage of the placenta may astound an owner who had not realized that a pregnancy had been initiated. Occasionally mummification occurs and the fetus is expelled at a later date. Rejection typically occurs in the sixth week of pregnancy (or sooner, in goats carrying a hybrid embryo for the second time). Only very rarely has a hybrid fetus (documented by karyotype) survived to term (Bunch et al. 1976; Denis et al. 1988; Letshwenyo and Kedikilwe 2000; Mine et al. 2000).

Goat-lambs (or "geep") are a different, artificial phenomenon produced by manipulation and combination of a goat embryo and a sheep embryo. The resulting chimera is then implanted in a recipient sheep or goat (Fehilly et al. 1984). If the chimeric embryo is constructed in such a way that the trophectoderm and thus the chorionic epithelium arise entirely from cells of the same species as the recipient, rejection of the embryo is avoided. In chimeras prepared by the blastomere aggregation technique (Ruffing et al. 1993), placentas and binucleate cells of some fetuses surviving to term were also chimeric. The highly publicized reports of these chimeras surviving to birth and beyond inevitably have been misinterpreted by some people as evidence that a viable sheep × goat hybrid can be produced.

Toxoplasmosis

It is reasonable to suspect that infection of a doe with *Toxoplasma gondii* in early gestation might occasionally lead to early embryonic death, rather than overt abortion. Animals affected in this way might return to estrus after an irregular interval or merely be found open when parturition was expected. Early embryonic loss has been documented in experimental infections with *Toxoplasma* (Dubey 1988), but is difficult to confirm in field cases (Calamel and Giauffret 1975; Nurse and Lenghaus 1986). Some early deaths may be the result of the febrile response in the infected doe, rather than of invasion of the placenta and fetus. In a serologic study of sheep from farms where toxoplasmosis had been identified as a cause of abortion, a significantly larger proportion of barren ewes than of lambing ewes had high titers for toxoplasmosis (Johnston 1988).

Nutritional Factors

Deficiencies of several trace minerals have been associated with lowered conception rates and abortions in controlled experiments with goats. These include copper and iodine (Anke et al. 1977). Experimental selenium deficiency leads to a lowered apparent conception rate but not to early abortions (Anke et al. 1989). Conversely, prolonged selenium toxicity (caused by excess selenium in soil and therefore in feeds) has been reported to cause abortion and failure of conception in goats in India (Gupta et al. 1982).

Under adverse field conditions, such as prolonged drought, deficiencies of several nutrients (e.g., protein, magnesium, and copper) have been suspected to cause abortion, based on lowered concentrations in the blood of does aborting early in pregnancy (Unanian and Feliciano-Silva 1984), but the exact cause of the abortions remains unproven.

Studies in Angoras have suggested that simultaneous deficiencies of energy and protein (rather than just one or the other) are required for early embryonic mortality to occur (Van der Westhuysen and Roelofse 1971). Dairy does for which both energy and protein were restricted had a lower ovulation rate and increased embryonic losses when compared with goats on a control, maintenance diet. Circulating progesterone concentrations were not affected (Mani et al. 1992, 1995). A protein and mineral supplement should be offered if reproductive failure coincides with probable nutritional deprivation. Supplementation of a low protein grass diet with leguminous browse has decreased abortion losses in West African dwarf goats (Pamo et al. 2006). Other long-term feeding trials of does have suggested that energy is more critical to successful reproduction in goats than is protein (Sachdeva et al. 1973). This suggests that a supplement that does not improve the digestible nutrients in the ration may not be effective in restoring reproduction.

Prevention of Early Losses by Flushing

Flushing is the technique of increasing energy intake just before breeding to increase ovulation rate. Maintaining the improved nutrition through the first month of gestation is advised to give the embryos ample opportunity to survive this critical period. Flushing is often interpreted as feeding grain. In range or grazing animals, other management options appear to be useful to improve the nutritional balance. These include moving to a better pasture, deworming at this strategic time, or shearing (Angoras). Shearing probably stimulates an increase in feed intake until a protective layer of fleece grows back. A study by Hart et al. (1999) failed to show an increase in conception rate or litter size with increases in either energy or protein fed to Spanish meat goats.

LATE ABORTION: INFECTIOUS CAUSES

In the United States, chlamydiosis, Q fever, and toxoplasmosis appear to be the most frequently identified infectious causes of caprine abortion. Other agents may cause serious losses in individual herds. Additional literature has been reviewed by Lefèvre (1987). The zoonotic potential of most of these agents should not be forgotten.

Akabane Virus

Akabane virus has caused abortions and perinatal mortality of calves, lambs, and kids (Markusfeld and Mayer 1971; Inaba et al. 1975).

Etiology and Epidemiology

Akabane virus is an arbovirus of the bunyavirus group. The virus is arthropod-borne, by gnats and mosquitoes. The disease has been recognized in Japan, Israel, and Australia. It is exotic to the United States. Outbreaks are believed to occur when susceptible females are in early pregnancy during periods of increased vector activity. As many as 50% of kids born on some farms have been affected (Shimshony 1980).

Pathogenesis

The pregnant dam develops viremia. Akabane virus infects lambs transplacentally at thirty to thirty-six days of gestation (Parsonson et al. 1981). The critical time for infection of kids has not been determined, but is probably similar (Kurogi et al. 1977). At this early period, the virus destroys embryonic cells in the cerebral cortex. Fetal muscles undergo neurogenic atrophy, as discussed in Chapter 4. Fetal death and mummification may occur. If the fetus survives, the virus is cleared but precolostral antibodies remain as evidence of the infection.

Clinical Signs

The disease is sometimes referred to as congenital arthrogryposis-hydranencephaly syndrome. Malformations associated with Akabane virus include micrencephaly, hydrocephalus, hydranencephaly, porencephaly, arthrogryposis, and reduced muscle mass (Haughey et al. 1988). Fetuses may be stillborn or die very soon after birth. Arthrogryposis or prepartum death of the fetus may contribute to dystocia. The pregnant dam shows no overt clinical signs at the time of initial infection.

Similarity to Cache Valley Virus

A similar arthropod-borne bunyavirus, the Cache Valley virus, is endemic to parts of North America and has caused epizootics of arthrogryposis with hydrocephalus, hydranencephaly, or cerebellar dysplasia in lambs in Texas, Michigan, and Nebraska (Edwards et al. 1989; Chung et al. 1990b; de la Concha-Bermejillo 2003) and elsewhere. A high prevalence of mummified fetuses, stillbirths, and weak lambs has been observed in infected flocks and reproduced experimentally by inoculation at twenty-seven to fifty-four days of gestation (Chung et al. 1990a). Oligohydroamnion contributes to lack of fetal movement and consequent arthrogryposis. Although case reports are rare, goat fetuses are also susceptible to Cache Valley virus (Edwards et al. 2003).

Diagnosis and Control

Congenital malformations, as described above, are suggestive of Akabane or Cache Valley virus infections. Retrospectively, the first trimester of pregnancy will have occurred during a period of biting insect activity, especially mosquitoes. A warm, humid period after several years of drought results in a large population of insect vectors interacting with a naive population of small ruminants.

Virus isolation may be attempted from placenta, fetal muscle, or fetal brain, but is always unsuccessful in full term fetuses. Demonstration of precolostral or fetal serum antibodies against one of these viruses is evidence of involvement of the virus. Maternal antibodies will probably have peaked by the time parturition occurs, and merely indicate that infection of the dam has occurred (Kalmar et al. 1975). Lack of maternal antibodies rules out the agent as cause of fetal malformation. Control of Akabane disease is discussed in Chapter 4 and elsewhere (Committee on Foreign Animal Diseases 1998).

Chlamydiosis

Chlamydiosis is a well-documented cause of abortion in goats worldwide. It remains the most frequently diagnosed cause of caprine abortion in California (Moeller 2001).

Etiology

The agent responsible for chlamydiosis is *Chlamydophila abortus* (formerly *Chlamydia psittaci*) (Everett 2000), a Gram-negative, intracellular organism that contains both RNA and DNA. The infectious particles that carry the infection to other cells are called elementary bodies. Previous names for the organism include psittacosis-lymphogranuloma venereum-trachoma agent, *Miyagawanella*, and *Bedsonia*. It is not very host-specific, but strain differences are important in determining which disease syndromes occur. Arthritis, keratoconjunctivitis, and respiratory disease caused by chlamydial infections are discussed elsewhere in this text. The abortion disease in sheep and goats is commonly referred to as enzootic or virus abortion.

Epidemiology and Pathogenesis

The intestinal tract is the natural location for chlamydia (Shewen 1980). *Chlamydophila abortus* is an organism that can only replicate in an intracellular location. The organism multiplies (according to strain and host resistance) in epithelial cells of the intestinal or genital tract or conjunctiva and in cells of the reticulo-endothelial system.

Chlamydia gain access to the placenta and fetus after an episode of chlamydemia. Inflammation and necrosis caused by multiplication of the chlamydia prevent normal transfer of nutrients across the placenta, and the fetus dies and is aborted. Other animals become infected by ingestion of placenta or uterine discharges and may abort in their next pregnancy, or (if sufficient time remains for placental damage to occur, approximately forty days) in the current pregnancy (Blewett et al. 1982). Shedding in vaginal secretions has been documented to begin as early as nine days before abortion and to last as long as twelve days after abortion (Rodolakis et al. 1984). Whereas some authors believe that immune does and ewes may remain fecal shedders and sources of infection, others believe that they do not become carriers (Wilsmore et al. 1990). Research documenting that ewes shed the organism when in estrus, even when immunity is adequate to prevent subsequent abortion (Papp et al. 1994), also may be relevant for goats. Chlamydia have been isolated from the semen and genital organs of rams (Pienaar and Schutte 1975), but the possibility that bucks spread the organism during breeding has not been investigated.

Clinical Signs

Chlamydial abortion in goats typically occurs in the last two months of pregnancy and especially the last two weeks (Yalçin and Gane 1970). In an endemic situation, abortion is primarily confined to primiparous does (Faye et al. 1971; East 1983). When the agent is first introduced into a herd, abortions occur in goats of all ages and parities (McCauley and Tieken 1968). Fetuses usually appear fresh. Sometimes infected kids are delivered at term, either stillborn or alive but weak (McCauley and Tieken 1968). The doe is usually not clinically ill, and the placenta is usually not retained (Metcalfe et al. 1968). In experimental reproduction of the disease, delivery of autolysed fetuses, retained placenta, and metritis have occurred in some does (Rodolakis et al. 1984).

Fertility is usually normal in pregnancies subsequent to the abortion, though some feel that immunity decreases after three years and chlamydial abortions may then recur.

Diagnosis

The placenta of the aborting doe is of great diagnostic importance. Lesions resemble those seen in chlamydia-induced ovine abortions (Pienaar and Schutte 1975; Appleyard et al. 1983; Rodolakis et al. 1984). Gross lesions include thickening and necrosis of cotyledons and intercotyledonary tissue. Microscopic lesions include infiltration in the hilar region with neutrophils, lymphocytes, and macrophages. Epithelial and mesenchymal necrosis occur and elementary bodies are present in epithelial cells of the chorionic villi, intercotyledonary chorium, and exudates. The bodies are basophilic (red in acid-fast stains) and measure 250 to 450 nm in diameter (Pienaar and Schutte 1975). Vasculitis is prominent, in contrast with Q fever.

Although abortion is usually the result of placental damage, histologic lesions are occasionally recognized in the fetus. Enlargement and focal necrosis of the liver have been reported in aborted kids (McCauley and Tieken 1968; Shefki 1987).

Many laboratories make a presumptive diagnosis of chlamydial infection based on demonstration of elementary bodies in impression smears or exudates. Stains used include Giemsa, Stamp, Macchiavello's, and modified Ziehl-Neelsen. A cotyledon is transected and the cut surface used to make the impression smear. If placenta is not available, impression smears of vaginal swabs, fetal umbilicus or hair coat, and fetal liver (cut surface) may yield elementary bodies (Bloxham et al. 1977). The same impression smears and swabs may be used for immunohistochemistry testing (Szeredi and Bacsadi 2002) or PCR. Fetal tissues are generally far less satisfactory than placenta for diagnosis by either special stains or immunofluorescence. Rickettsia (Q fever) have a similar appearance in stained smears (Aitken 1986).

Isolation of the organism is usually attempted in embryonated chicken eggs or cell culture. Isolation is followed by demonstration of elementary bodies and group antigen. Recently, enzyme immunoassay tests, such as those developed to detect group antigen of *Chlamydia trachomatis* infection in humans, have been used to detect *C. abortus* in ovine and caprine placental and vaginal swabs (Souriau and Rodolakis 1986; Sanderson and Andersen 1989). Vaginal swabs should be collected within three days after abortion for best results.

The complement fixation (CF) test has been used in the past for screening (Giauffret and Russo 1976). Because the antigen used is group specific, the presence of nonpathogenic intestinal strains may give false-positive tests unless diagnosis is based on an increase in titer. It is helpful to compare titers of aborting and nonaborting goats (Shefki 1987). Animals that have recently aborted because of chlamydiosis generally have a CF titer of at least 1:80. However, infected animals that do not abort may still mount a serologic response (Giauffret and Russo 1976). The CF titers generally are not protective against experimental challenge.

Skin testing has also been used in France and appears to be more sensitive than CF testing (Rodolakis et al. 1977). Cell-mediated immunity, as identified by skin testing, is probably protective (Wilsmore et al. 1986).

Treatment

If chlamydial abortion is confirmed or highly likely to be present, it is common to treat all females remaining at risk of aborting with tetracycline. Suppression of the organism may prevent additional placental damage. Also, reduced shedding of chlamydia by treated does could decrease the number of new infections and thus the number of animals developing a carrier state that will terminate with abortion in the next pregnancy. Large sheep flocks are commonly medicated with oral oxytetracycline or chlortetracycline at 400 to 500 mg per head per day. This is a reasonable approach for fiber-producing does, perhaps at a reduced dosage in view of smaller body size. In dairy herds it is more customary to treat individual nonlactating does by injection rather than to remove all lactating does from the group to be treated so that antibiotics in the feed will not cause milk contamination. Long-acting oxytetracycline preparations given at a dose of 20 mg/kg every ten to fourteen days should decrease the abortion rate during an outbreak (Rodolakis et al. 1980). Others have given the drug every three days.

Tylosin is another antibiotic that has been used in an attempt to control chlamydial abortion outbreaks. A dose of 200 mg/head per day orally in a salt/meal supplement was used with apparent success in a herd of Angoras (Eugster et al. 1977). Chlamydia are also susceptible to rifamicin and chloramphenicol, antibiotics that may be used in some countries but not in the United States.

Prevention

Prevention of chlamydiosis depends on both hygiene and vaccination. Replacement sheep and goats, even unbred kids, should not be purchased from a herd where the disease is endemic. If acquisition of specific genetics from a diseased herd is necessary, embryo transfer into disease-free recipients avoids introduction of the agent, at least in sheep (Williams et al. 1998). If chlamydial abortions occur (introduced animals or endemic infection), all aborted fetuses and placentas should be removed and destroyed if not used for diagnostic testing. Aborting females should be isolated for several weeks until vaginal discharges cease. They should not be used as foster mothers. Animals should not be fed from the ground.

Vaccination of all animals (including bucks) before breeding with a sheep chlamydial vaccine has been helpful in some herds (Polydorou 1981b; Rodolakis and Souriau 1986). Annual revaccination, or, at the very least, vaccination of each year's crop of doelings, should continue indefinitely. Vaccination helps to prevent abortion but it does not eliminate infection. Vaccine availability has been sporadic at best in the United States.

Zoonotic Potential

Chlamydophila abortus is contagious to humans. During kidding or lambing season, pregnant women assisting with parturitions may become infected with the ruminant strain and abort (Johnson et al. 1985; Hyde and Benirschke 1997; Jorgensen 1997; Pospischil et al. 2002). An influenza-like syndrome also has occurred in men assisting lambing in infected flocks (Aitken 1986). People attending normal parturitions, dystocias, or abortions should wear plastic gloves to limit exposure to uterine fluids. The same precautions apply when collecting fetuses or placentas for disposal or diagnostic evaluation. Pregnant women should avoid contact with the herd during the parturition season.

Q Fever

Query or Queensland fever is a zoonotic infection (McQuiston et al. 2002). Signs in humans vary from inapparent infections to flu-like disease, abortion, pneumonia, or heart disease. Except for abortion, clinical signs in ruminants are rare. Human cases are notifiable nationally in the United States since 1999.

Etiology

Q fever is caused by the obligate intracellular rickettsial organism *Coxiella burnetii* that develops inside phagolysosomes. It is pleomorphic (coccoid to short rod), weakly acid-fast, and variably Gram-negative. In nature, *C. burnetii* exists in Phase I, which is virulent and analogous to smooth bacteria. When cultivated in embryonated eggs or cell cultures, the organism mutates irreversibly to a less virulent Phase II form, analogous to rough bacteria (Arricau-Bouvery and Rodolakis 2005).

Epidemiology

Cattle, sheep, goats, and wildlife throughout the world may carry the organism, which is then shed heavily in placentas, birth fluids, colostrum, milk, and feces. Stresses such as overcrowding or poor nutrition probably play an important role in determining if an infected goat will abort (Crowther and Spicer 1976). Abortion outbreaks may occur in well managed naive herds if first exposed during pregnancy. Reproductive failure associated with Q fever usually does not recur in the season following the abortion storm (Berri et al. 2005). The organism is resistant to heat and drying (Arricau-Bouvery and Rodolakis 2005), with the result that animals and humans can be infected by inhaling dust (Polydorou 1981a; Dupuis et al. 1984). Grazing contaminated pastures and tick bites are other modes of transmission.

Shedding of the organism in milk can persist for three months after parturition/abortion but was not detected during the subsequent kidding season in one study (Berri et al. 2005).

Diagnosis

Because *C. burnetii* can be shed heavily at the time of normal kidding, isolation of the organism is not proof of cause of abortion (Miller et al. 1986). Q fever abortion or stillbirth occurs in late pregnancy, but only when placental damage has been severe. Pathologic changes are rarely seen in fetal tissues. Thus, examination of the placenta is necessary for diagnosis (Moeller 2001). Intercotyledonary areas of the placenta are thickened (Waldhalm et al. 1978; Palmer et al. 1983; Copeland et al. 1991) and may be mineralized (Sanford et al. 1994). Abundant exudate is usually present. There is necrosis and neutrophilic infiltration of cotyledonary and intercotyledonary epithelium. Placental vasculitis may be present (Moore et al. 1991). The organism (pleomorphic, acid-fast) is abundant in trophoblastic cells of the chorion. Placental smears that are stained with the Gimenez method show acid-fast rod-like organisms slightly larger than chlamydia. Fluorescent antibody testing, polymerase chain reaction tests (PCR), laboratory animal inoculation, and isolation in embryonated eggs are other possible diagnostic techniques. However, it is still imperative that other causes of abortion be ruled out before the diagnosis is made. Many older reports of Q fever abortion in goats only ruled out brucellosis.

Acute and convalescent sera showing an increase in titer are suggestive, but a titer increase is also observed in late pregnant carrier animals that do not abort. A CF titer greater than or equal to 1:8 is considered positive by some, while others use a cut-off of 1:20. Other serologic tests include enzyme-linked immunoabsorbent assay and micro-agglutination. Even seronegative animals may shed the organism (Arricau-Bouvery and Rodolakis 2005). Serologic evidence of infection in goats is common. For instance, 24% of 1,054 goats and 26% of 234 herds in California were seropositive (Ruppanner et al. 1978). In an Ontario study, 20% (four of twenty) of herds had seroreactors (Lang 1988). Very high titers (>1:4,096) were observed in some goats in a Newfoundland farm experiencing an abortion storm and many human infections (Hatchette et al. 2001).

Treatment and Control

If Q fever is suspected, aborting goats and others in late pregnancy should be treated with tetracycline. Placentas and aborted fetuses should be destroyed, such as by burning. Abortion outbreaks observed after exposure to parturient goats at a fair underscore the need to isolate all aborting animals (Sanford et al. 1994).

Q fever abortion is usually prevented by providing good nutrition and management. This also limits environmental contamination. In private herds, prevention of the zoonotic infection is aided by pasteurization of milk and sanitation (including the use of gloves) at time of abortion or kidding. A tightly fitting particle mask should be worn when removing manure from the barn. The organism is resistant to many disinfectants, including 0.5% hypochlorite, 2% Roccal, 5% Lysol, and 5% formalin, for twenty-four hours but can be inactivated in thirty minutes by 70% ethyl alcohol or at least one quaternary ammonium compound (Scott and Williams 1990). Because the environment can remain infected for a long time and many other species can be carriers, test and cull strategies are not appropriate for infected goat herds.

Control in research herds, where government regulations may be aimed at protecting researchers, animal caretakers, and other staff, presents a special problem. Researchers seeking to assemble seronegative herds of goats on the basis of prepurchase serology find the task daunting and some believe that serologic tests are not useful for determining which animals are a current risk for transmission (McQuiston et al. 2002). Protocols for human protection have been suggested (Ruppaner et al. 1983; Behymer et al. 1985; Singh and Lang 1985) and individual universities may post their recommendations electronically. Human vaccination is routinely used for high-risk groups in Australia.

Vaccine development is progressing. An experimental model of Q fever reliably produces abortion when the goats are infected at ninety days gestation and shedding can be monitored by PCR (Arricau-Bouvery et al. 2003). A commercial vaccine using inactivated phase I *Coxiella* (Coxevac®, CEVA Santé Animal, France) protected against abortion and excretion in milk and vaginal discharges, while an inactivated phase II vaccine did not (Souriau et al. 2003; Arricau-Bouvery et al. 2005). Phase I vaccines are dangerous to produce, so subunit vaccines are being investigated (Arricau-Bouvery and Rodolakis 2005).

Brucellosis

In endemic regions (Corbel 1997) (Mediterranean countries, Middle East, India, China, parts of Latin America), herd infection may first be suspected because of an outbreak of human brucellosis (Malta fever). People become infected by direct contact with infected goats or sheep or by consuming contaminated dairy products.

Etiology

Brucella melitensis is the usual cause of brucellosis in goats, although *Brucella abortus* has been shown to infect goats both naturally and experimentally (Meador and Deyoe 1986). It is a small Gram-negative facultative intracellular coccobacillus.

Pathogenesis and Epidemiology

The organism is excreted in milk, urine, and feces and in fetuses, placenta, and (for two to three months after parturition) vaginal discharges. The organism enters other adult goats by way of the nasopharynx or by direct penetration of the skin (Alton et al. 1984). In resistant animals, macrophages in the nearest lymph node kill the organism, while susceptible animals are unable to control the infection and a bacteremia ensues, with infection of the placenta and udder. Kids born alive to infected does often are infected and capable of shedding the organism. Cows in contact with infected sheep or goats may become infected and shed the organism in milk (Godfroid et al. 2005).

Clinical Signs

When goats in an endemic herd are in a stressful environment and management is not adequate to control nutritional and parasitic diseases, then abortion will occur in the last two months of pregnancy or even earlier. A mid- to late-gestation abortion storm can be expected even in a well-managed herd when the disease is first introduced (Renoux 1957).

Diagnosis

Identification of brucellosis as the cause of abortion is usually made by isolating the organism from fetus, placenta, or vaginal discharges. Selective media are used. Gross placental lesions are not mentioned in reports of natural outbreaks in goats. A polymerase chain reaction test for the organism in milk has been used to detect carrier animals (Gupta et al. 2006).

Various agglutination, precipitation, and complement fixation tests are used to detect carrier goats (Alton et al. 1984; Mikolon et al. 1998). Agglutinins usually appear before precipitins and complement fixing antibodies. In chronic infections, sometimes only the CF test results remain positive (Waghela 1978). An allergic skin test can be used as a screening test to identify infected herds (Alton et al. 1984). The milk ring test gives poor results, even with the addition of cow cream, but a milk ELISA performs better (Mikolon et al. 1998). An agglutination test on whey is possible but not sensitive.

A recently developed indirect ELISA permits monitoring of bulk tank samples, though a maximum group size of fifty goats is suggested, to allow detection of one animal with low antibody concentration (Funk et al. 2005).

False positives occur in most tests for one year or longer after vaccination. Some tests give false-positive results because of cross reactions with antibodies against enterobacteria such as *Yersinia enterocolitica*, but a recently developed competitive serum ELISA avoids this problem (Portanti et al. 2006). Serologic tests are unreliable in young kids.

Control

In countries or regions where the prevalence of infection is very low, slaughtering the entire herd (both goats and sheep) is probably the control measure of choice. This was the method successfully used to eradicate the infection in the most recently reported outbreaks in the United States, in Texas in 1969 (Whiting et al. 1970) and 1999 (AVMA 2000). In other situations, a test and slaughter program is more appropriate (Polydorou 1979, 1984). This does, however, expose personnel testing the herd to a significant risk of contracting brucellosis (Stiles 1950). Testing of dogs in the flock during eradication programs and euthanasia of positive reactors has also been recommended.

Most countries affected with caprine brucellosis control the disease by vaccination, especially in kids and lambs three to six months of age. This procedure not only protects the livestock but also limits the infection of people in contact with the small ruminants. Unfortunately, compliance is often inadequate to achieve regional eradication, even after a vaccination program that lasts for many years (Blasco 1997). Whole herd vaccination during the lactation period may be required, though safety of vaccines in lactating goats and breeding bucks has not been studied. The preferred vaccine is *B. melitensis* Rev 1 (Gaumont et al. 1984; Alton 1987; OIE 2004). This live, attenuated vaccine is usually given subcutaneously, but conjunctival vaccination has also been investigated (Alton 1987). Rev 1 causes bacteremia but does not spread to nonvaccinates. The vaccine causes abortion, and thus is to be avoided in pregnant goats or those within one month before mating. Immunity from a single dose is considered to be lifelong but is not absolute. Conjunctival vaccination still results in abortion and reduced dose vaccination (to avoid abortion) does not provide solid immunity (Blasco 1997). In an infected herd it is also important to decrease natural challenge by appropriate hygiene at kidding and milking time. Placentas and aborted fetuses should be burned or buried deeply. Communal pastures and importation of untested goats should be avoided.

Based on experimental work with both sheep and goats, treatment of particularly valuable animals could be attempted using long-acting oxytetracycline (25 mg/kg intramuscularly every other day for four weeks) combined with streptomycin (20 mg/kg intramuscularly every other day for two weeks). This protocol resulted in bacteriologic cure in thirty-six of thirty-six goats (Radwan 1992).

Campylobacteriosis

Etiology

Although both *Campylobacter fetus* subsp *fetus* (formerly *Vibrio fetus intestinalis*) and *C. jejuni* are common causes of abortion in sheep, campylobacteriosis is reported only rarely as a cause of abortion in goats in North America (Dobbs and McIntyre 1951; Anderson et al. 1983; Gough 1987; Moeller 2001). *Campylobacter jejuni* seems to be more common in goats than *C. fetus*. Zoonotic infections (especially diarrhea) may occur.

Clinical Signs and Diagnosis

In South Africa, where campylobacter abortion appears to be more common, as many as 30% of aborted kids have grossly visible liver necrosis. The placenta is often edematous, with necrosis of cotyledons (Van der Westhuysen et al. 1988; Moeller 2001). In one outbreak in the United States, five of twenty-one late-pregnant goats aborted and two of the does became systemically ill; *C. jejuni* was isolated (Anderson et al. 1983). The organism was later isolated from diarrheic feces in the same herd.

The diagnosis should not be difficult because many laboratories are accustomed to isolating the organism from fetal lamb abomasal contents (microaerophilic conditions required) or demonstrating Gram-negative curved organisms in smears. Thus, the paucity of reports probably indicates that this agent is of minor importance in goats, although of public health significance.

Control

In an undiagnosed abortion storm, administration of tetracycline might be expected to limit the losses if campylobacteriosis were involved, while simultaneously being effective against several other agents. However, antibiotic resistance in *Campylobacter* spp. seems to be an emerging issue (Sahin et al. 2008). In a confirmed outbreak, vaccination of all pregnant does with an ovine bivalent *Campylobacter* bacterin is advisable. Fecal contamination of feed should be prevented and aborting animals should be isolated (Anderson 1986). As with other abortions, placentas and fetuses should be burned or buried deeply.

Leptospirosis

Etiology and Epidemiology

Several serovars of *Leptospira interrogans* have been shown to cause abortion in goats, but the prevalence of losses is unknown. In a California survey, the agent was identified in only one of 211 caprine abortion submissions to the state diagnostic laboratory system (Moeller 2001). Goats probably do not serve as primary reservoirs for leptospirosis, and infection probably occurs from exposure to an environment contaminated by urine of other species (Schollum and Blackmore 1981; Leon-Vizcaino et al. 1987). Goats experimentally infected with *L. interrogans* serovar Pomona, however, remained clinically healthy but shed the organism in their urine (Morse and Langham 1958).

Clinical Signs

L. interrogans serovar Grippotyphosa has caused severe clinical illness in goats in Israel. Signs included anorexia, marked jaundice, hemoglobinuria, abortion, and death of does (Van der Hoeden 1953). The systemic signs of leptospirosis are discussed in Chapter 7. Other does experienced inapparent infections, as determined by increased agglutination titers in the absence of overt disease. *L. interrogans* serovar Hardjo has been implicated as a cause of caprine abortions in several reports that do not present the supporting evidence (McSporran et al. 1985). *L. interrogans* serovar Pomona was identified as the cause of six abortion outbreaks (out of 262 studied) while serovar Sejroe and serovar Icterohaemorrhagiae were each associated with one outbreak in goat herds in Spain (Leon-Vizcaino et al. 1987). From 10% to 43% of pregnant does in these herds aborted. Several animals in one herd also showed fever, jaundice, and anemia.

Diagnosis and Control

The organism is difficult to isolate from contaminated specimens. Dark field microscopy, immunofluorescence testing, and silver stains on fetal fluids and tissues are used to confirm the diagnosis. Microscopic agglutination titers may be static or absent in infected animals (Songer and Thiermann 1988), assuming goats and cattle respond to infection with leptospires in a similar fashion. Paired sera showing an increase in titer after abortion would suggest association with leptospirosis. A single positive serum is of no diagnostic value, because many healthy goats are serologically positive. Vaccination twice a year is a logical prophylactic measure in regions where leptospirosis is prevalent in goats or other ruminants. Other measures recommended include separating animal species, controlling rodents, and maintaining a clean water supply (Lefèvre 1987).

Listeriosis

Listeria monocytogenes causes abortion, septicemia, and encephalitis in goats. The neurologic disease is discussed in Chapter 5.

Etiology and Pathogenesis

The organism is Gram-positive and is not acid-fast. Both short rods and coccoid elements appear in culture (Timoney et al. 1988). Virulent strains are hemolytic. Abortion strains are often serotype 1. The abortion form and the encephalitic form of listeriosis do not usually occur simultaneously in a herd. Experimental intravenous inoculation of the organism has caused a rapid drop in pregnancy-associated glycoprotein normally produced by trophoblastic cells in the placenta as well as a drop in serum progesterone, with abortion typically occurring in nine to eleven days (Engeland et al. 1997; Zarrouk et al. 1999).

Epidemiology

Listeria monocytogenes is a ubiquitous organism that may be found in soil, water, plant litter, ensiled forages, and the digestive tract of ruminants and humans (Timoney et al. 1988). The ability of the organism to multiply at cold temperatures in poor quality silages (pH levels greater than 5.5) is well known and undoubtedly contributes to the occurrence of listeriosis in goats fed silage. Silage feeding also appears to have immunosuppressive effects. Excretion of listeria by healthy animals seems to increase toward the end of gestation, presumably caused by hormonal immunosuppression (Løken et al. 1982; Grønstøl 1984).

Clinical Signs and Diagnosis

Abortion is typically preceded by listerial septicemia. Signs of septicemia may include fever and reduced appetite and milk production (Grønstøl 1984). Clinical signs are minimal or absent in other goats that abort (Sandbu 1956). Some goats recover quickly after aborting while others die. During and after the septicemic stage, goats often excrete listeria in feces and milk. Kids grafted onto the aborting doe may die of listerial septicemia contracted through the umbilicus or the milk (Grønstøl 1984). The diagnosis of septicemia may be confirmed by an increase in serum antibodies by an indirect hemagglutination technique (Løken et al.

1982). Culture of the organism from the fetus confirms a listerial abortion. Ribotyping of the isolate may be helpful in epidemiological investigations (Nightingale et al. 2004).

Prevention and Control

If silages are being fed, check the pH after mixing a sample with a small quantity of distilled water; the pH should be below 5.5. Soil contamination of the feed is another risk factor, and silages should not be made from fields with many molehills, nor should they be fed if the ash content exceeds 70 mg/kg DM (Low and Linklater 1985). Feeding poor quality or spoiled silages should be discontinued if possible. If no other forages are available on the farm, better feed should be purchased. Feeding adequate energy appears to protect somewhat against abortions associated with feeding goats aerobically-deteriorated silage from round bales (Hussain et al. 1996).

Vaccination with an aim of producing cellular immunity has been investigated. Theoretically, live vaccines should be more effective than killed preparations. Two doses of reduced virulence live vaccine before breeding provided significant protection against experimental challenge in pregnant goats (Fensterbank 1987). Administration of live vaccine to late pregnant goats has occasionally been followed by abortion, but this risk would not necessarily rule out vaccination of pregnant goats in the face of an outbreak (Guerrault et al. 1988).

Salmonellosis

Salmonella enterica serovar Abortusovis was first implicated as a cause of abortion in three- to four-month pregnant goats in Cyprus in 1932 (Manley 1932). Aborting goats showed no other symptoms of illness. Abortion with subsequent death of the doe has been produced experimentally by intravenous or oral inoculation during the last month of gestation. In-contact animals became infected and excreted the organism (Tadjebakhche et al. 1974). The organism also has been isolated from goat fetuses and placentas in France. The disease was believed to be transmitted orally to other goats at the time of abortion. Control recommendations made included injecting pregnant does with tetracycline and chloramphenicol and administering two doses of vaccine, followed by an annual booster (Yalçin and Gane 1970).

Specific agglutinins can be demonstrated in the sera of adults in the herd and in aborted fetuses (Mura et al. 1952). Only sheep and goats are affected by *S.* Abortusovis. Salmonellosis as an enteric disease of goats is discussed in Chapter 10. *Salmonella* Typhimurium and *S.* Dublin have both been associated with abortion (Lefèvre 1987). The endotoxin (lipopolysaccharide) produced by *S.* Typhimurium has been documented to cause prostaglandin release and luteolysis, thereby leading to abortion in pregnant goats (Fredriksson et al. 1985).

Toxoplasmosis

Etiology

The protozoan *Toxoplasma gondii* is a very important cause of abortion, mummification, stillbirth, and birth of weak young in goats as it is in sheep.

Epidemiology and pathogenesis

Cats serve as the definitive host for this parasite (Buxton 1998); they become infected by consuming uncooked meat scraps, placentas, and small rodents (Dubey 1986). Recently infected cats then shed oocysts in their feces. Oocyst shedding typically lasts from three to nineteen days, but oocysts may persist in moist and shaded soil for as long as eighteen months (Frenkel 1982).

Goats become infected by eating grass, hay, or grain contaminated by cat feces. After initial invasion of the goat's small intestine and associated lymph nodes, the *Toxoplasma* organisms spread via the bloodstream to other tissues, including muscle, brain, and liver. Here the parasite may remain encysted for months or even the life of the goat. If the goat is pregnant at the time of initial infection, *Toxoplasma* commonly invade the placenta and fetus approximately two weeks after initial infection of the doe. Fetuses infected in the first half of pregnancy are more apt to die than fetuses infected in the second half. Sometimes abortion is repeated in the next gestation (Dubey 1982), but previously infected goats are usually resistant to abortion or other clinical signs when challenged with *T. gondii* (Obendorf et al. 1990).

Diagnosis

Fetal serology is a very specific test for abortive toxoplasmosis (Munday et al. 1987). The ovine fetus (and presumably the caprine fetus) begins to develop immunocompetency at sixty to seventy days of gestation. First immunoglobin M is produced, but by ninety days immunoglobin G is being synthesized. Thus, if the fetus is infected after midgestation, it will usually produce antibody detectable by a variety of immunologic tests (Dubey 1987; Wilson et al. 1990). A modified direct agglutination test (MAT) is considered to be very sensitive and can be used on any species, including goats, because species-specific conjugates are not used (Dubey et al. 1987). The antigen for the MAT, however, is not yet marketed in the United States (as of 2007).

Heart blood or thoracic fluid can be harvested from the fetus. Fetal autolysis does not always preclude identification of toxoplasma antibodies. Absence of antibodies in the fetus does not rule out toxoplasmosis because the fetus may have been infected too young or antibodies may have decomposed. Screening at both high and low dilutions is recommended to avoid false negatives when the antibody concentration is so high as to occupy all binding sites (prozone effect).

Serologic testing of the doe at time of abortion is useful. Absence of antibodies is considered to be conclusive evidence that toxoplasmosis was *not* the cause of abortion (Figure 13.5). An increasing titer would at least indicate recent infection, but a stable, even high titer can persist for months or even years after initial infection of the doe. Thus, a high titer in the dam is not proof of abortion caused by toxoplasmosis (Gunson et al. 1983).

Large surveys of goats in the western United States have revealed a seroprevalence of 20% or more in yearlings or older goats (Dubey and Adams 1990), while fifty-four of ninety-nine does (55%) on nine farms in or near Tennessee were positive by indirect hemagglutination (Patton et al. 1990). In a study in Ontario, Canada, 63% of 399 sera tested positive (1:16 or greater) by the Sabin-Feldman dye test (Tizard et al. 1977). In a serological survey conducted in Turkey, 51% of 170 goats (mostly Angoras) were positive at 1:4 or more in the Sabin-Feldman dye test and 25% were positive at 1:16 or more (Weiland and Dalchow 1970). The Sabin-Feldman dye test uses intact parasites as antigen and requires maintenance of live organisms. Enzyme-linked immunoabsorbent assay tests, which are easily automated and use soluble antigens from disrupted toxoplasma organisms, have become more popular (Denmark and Chessum 1978; Buxton 1998). Other serologic tests currently used include the indirect haemagglutination test, indirect immunofluorescent antibody test, and latex agglutination test (Buxton 1998).

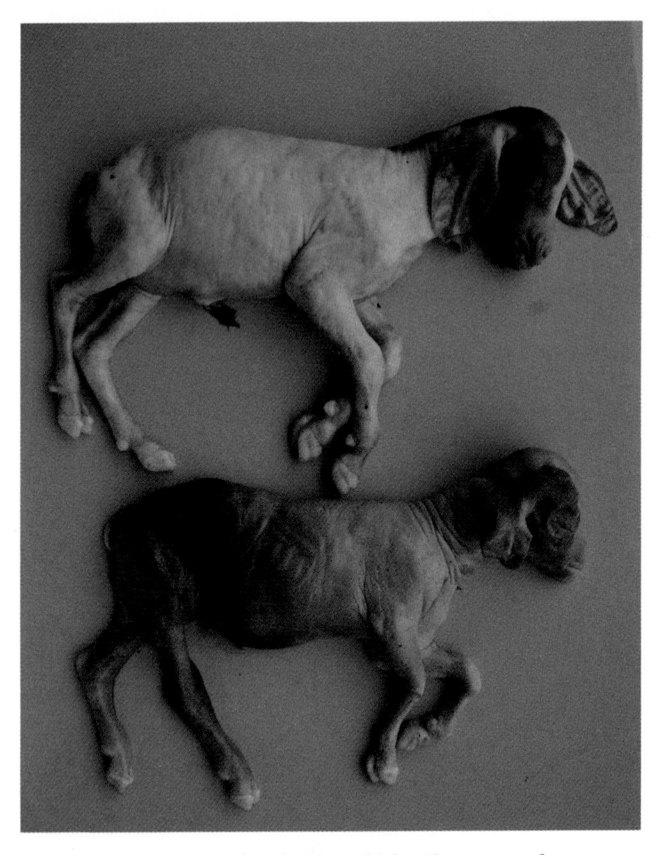

Figure 13.5. Aborted twin Boer kids. The upper fetus was alive at delivery while the lower fetus had been dead long enough to begin to mummify, as demonstrated by the sunken eye sockets. Although these findings were suggestive of toxoplasmosis, the dam was serologically negative, ruling out toxoplasmosis as the cause of abortion. (Courtesy Dr. M.C. Smith.)

If the diagnosis is to be made by histology, it is very important that placenta be submitted. Small yellowish-white foci of mineralization confined to cotyledons are apparent grossly if abortion is delayed until forty-five days or more after infection. Washing the cotyledons thoroughly in isotonic saline solution makes deeper foci easier to visualize. Another useful technique is to compress the cotyledon with a glass microscope slide; the mineralized foci resist squashing. Microscopic foci of necrosis can be identified after thirty days; tachyzooites are sparse in these lesions and difficult to locate (Dubey 1988). Nonsuppurative encephalomyelitis is found more consistently than myocarditis, but even under ideal experimental conditions it is difficult to find *T. gondii* organisms in tissue sections. Very careful histologic examination or immunohistochemistry distinguishes *Toxoplasma* from the far less common *Neospora* infection (Dubey et al. 1992).

Prevention

The control of toxoplasmosis can be approached in several ways. The first is to prevent exposure of susceptible goats to the oocysts in cat feces during the period of danger, which is pregnancy. In particular, grain should be stored in covered containers and the mangers kept clean. Contamination of the hay supply (by cats living in the hay barn) has been implicated in several outbreaks (McSporran et al. 1985; Nurse and Lenghaus 1986). If possible, feed the hay off the top of the stack to the nonpregnant does and young stock. Because exclusion of all cats from a farm is very difficult, it is usually suggested to maintain a stable population of adult neutered cats; kittens younger than six months of age are far more apt to shed oocysts than are adults. A vasectomized tomcat might be helpful in keeping stray cats off the farm, but this technique has not been evaluated. Raw meat should not be fed to cats.

Exposure of doelings to a contaminated environment (buildings where feral cats live or pastures spread with manure from such buildings) before breeding to develop protective immunity might be effective (Buxton 1998). Rubbing their noses with placentas from aborted fetuses has been suggested as one way of infecting doelings (Delahaye 1987), but this is ill-advised if other causes of abortion such as chlamydiosis were active in the herd. In the milking herd this would increase the risk of acute shedding of toxoplasmosis in milk.

A live toxoplasmosis vaccine available for sheep in the UK might be effective in goats (Chartier and Mallereau 2001) but will probably never be licensed in the United States because it is infective to humans. Repeated administration of killed vaccine or vaccination with a related but nonpathogenic organism (*Hammondia*) might be effective in preventing abortion (Dubey 1981; Munday and Dubey 1988) but would certainly be expensive; such vaccines are unlikely to be marketed in the near future. Chemoprophylaxis by feeding ionophores such as monensin during pregnancy, at the normal anticoccidial rate, initially showed promise (Blewett and Trees 1987; Buxton et al. 1988). However, fatal mixing errors may occur with ionophores. Daily decoquinate at 2 mg/kg bodyweight is a safer drug to try and is licensed in the UK for controlling toxoplasmosis in sheep (Buxton 1998).

When abortions caused by toxoplasmosis are diagnosed, emphasis should be put on properly disposing fetuses and placentas, wearing protective gloves when handling these items, and properly pasteurizing milk and cooking meat. Pregnant women should be especially careful.

Miscellaneous Infections

Other infections that induce a febrile response or generalized illness may cause abortion in does. One such agent is foot and mouth disease, as described in Chapter 4. Others that lead to occasional abortions are described below.

Bluetongue

Bluetongue is an infectious, noncontagious disease of ruminants, especially sheep, caused by an orbivirus and transmitted by *Culicoides* midges. The disease occurs in North and South America, Africa, the Middle East, Asia, and recently in northern Europe. Abortion and birth of malformed lambs are common in sheep. Goats are frequently infected in endemic regions, as evidenced by serologic surveys (Lefèvre and Calvez 1986; Flanagan 1995; Ting et al. 2005), but clinical signs are rarely recorded (Van Tonder 1975). Thus, bluetongue is unlikely to be the cause of abortions in goats. See further discussion of bluetongue in Chapter 10.

Border Disease

Border disease of sheep is caused by a pestivirus serologically similar to bovine virus diarrhea (BVD) virus, and BVD strains isolated from cattle can also produce disease in small ruminants. The disease has been under diagnosed in the past because early work concentrated on neurologic and fleece changes in lambs infected in utero. As the pathogenesis of the disease became clearer, in conjunction with important discoveries relating to BVD virus, it was learned that lambs infected in utero often remain persistently infected for life. Some fail to thrive, but others are silent carriers and shedders of the virus and can introduce the disease into other flocks. Infected ewes regularly produce persistently infected lambs. Also, some strains of the virus apparently do not produce neurologic and fleece changes (Bonniwell et al. 1987).

Spontaneous border disease (tremors, no hair coat changes) has been reported only rarely in goats (Løken et al. 1982; Løken 2000). Of three goats in Norway that seroconverted during pregnancy (out of 145 experiencing gestation failure and being sampled twice), one had an apparent false pregnancy while the other two each produced a normal and a weak-born kid (Løken 1990). Additionally, an experimental contagious ecthyma vaccine contaminated with a noncytopathic pestivirus was associated with reproductive failure in 213 of 261 goats vaccinated early in pregnancy (Løken et al. 1991) but no kids with border disease were born. A BVD type 2 virus was isolated from goats in a Korean herd experiencing abortions, stillbirths, and neonatal deaths (Kim et al. 2006). Nonpregnant goats exposed on pasture to calves persistently infected with BVD seroconverted rapidly, with ten of ten positive within six weeks (Broaddus et al. 2007).

Border disease has been experimentally reproduced in goats by inoculation of tissues of affected sheep; abortions and ataxic or shaker kids have been produced (Huck 1973; Barlow et al. 1975). In another study, intramuscular inoculation of a cytopathic bovine strain of BVD virus to does approximately forty days in pregnancy resulted in partial resorption of the fetuses and presence of 1 to 1.5 liters of fluid (hydrometra) in the uterus on slaughter at four months after breeding. Kids were clinically normal when infection occurred at one hundred days (Løken 1987). In a later study comparing a border disease strain and a BVD strain, results were similar in both groups, and all goats inoculated around forty days experienced reproductive failure. At least two viable kids were produced from later inoculations that were persistently infected (Løken and Bjerkås 1991). Some aborted and weak kids had presuckle antibodies. In another study, kids that survived experimental infection during gestation were not persistently infected (Depner et al. 1991).

Placental lesions, including multiple pinpoint foci of necrosis in the cotyledons, resemble those of toxoplasmosis (Barlow et al. 1975; Løken 1987). Birthcoat changes have not been reproduced experimentally in goats (Orr and Barlow 1978).

Caprine Herpesvirus

This agent causes a generalized infection in kids and adult goats, but not in lambs or calves; it is discussed in detail in Chapter 12. A diphasic fever has been observed in adults and may contribute to the occurrence of abortion. Fetuses aborted from experimentally infected does were passed in a very autolytic state three to eight weeks after infection in one study (Berrios et al. 1975). In another study, fetal death occurred by four days after inoculation in one goat and the fetuses were harvested by cesarean section the next day while abortion occurred in the other inoculated doe on day seven without previous ultrasonographic evidence of fetal death. Virus was recovered from the fresh placentas and from one fetal lung, but maternal rather than fetal infection was believed to be the cause of fetal death (Waldvogel et al. 1981). More recently, the caprine herpesvirus has caused cross-placental infection and death of neonates in conjunction with abortion storms. Fetal infection has been confirmed by PCR in aborted fetuses (Keuser et al. 2002; Chénier et al. 2004) and neonates (Roperto et al. 2000), and foci of coagulative necrosis with intranuclear inclusion bodies may be found in numerous tissues, including the liver and thymus (Williams et al. 1997; Chénier et al. 2004; Uzal et al. 2004; McCoy et al. 2007). Viral isolation is difficult if the fetus is autolyzed (Tempesta et al. 2004). A marked increase in serologic titer of the dam to the caprine (not bovine) herpesvirus would be strongly suggestive of the diagnosis.

In one follow-up study of a meat goat herd that experienced a caprine herpesvirus abortion storm, there were no reproductive repercussions the following year. Many does that aborted rebred in the same season, and kids born from these does and from does that were infected but did not abort during the initial outbreak remained seronegative ten months later (McCoy et al. 2007).

Nairobi Sheep Disease

Nairobi sheep disease is a noncontagious tick-transmitted bunyavirus of small ruminants (Terpstra 1990). The virus has been found especially in Kenya but also in other parts of East and Central Africa. Signs are more severe in sheep than goats and include fever, hemorrhagic gastroenteritis, abortion, and increased mortality rates. Histologically, glomerulo-tubular nephritis is present (Mugera and Chema 1967). Tick control and prophylactic vaccination could be recommended but are not warranted for controlling Nairobi sheep disease in enzootic areas, except when susceptible animals are introduced (Davies and Terpstra 2004). The disease is discussed in Chapter 10.

Peste des Petits Ruminants

Peste des petits ruminants is a morbillivirus infection of goats and sheep in Africa, the Middle East, and Asia. Signs include stomatitis, diarrhea, pneumonia, and a fever that persists for five to eight days. Pregnant animals may abort. The disease is discussed in Chapter 10.

Rift Valley Fever

Rift Valley fever is a mosquito-borne bunyavirus disease of ruminants and humans in Africa (Yedloutschnig and Walker 1986; Kasari et al. 2008) and is described in detail in Chapter 11. Abortion may come after fever and viremia in adults (Daubney et al. 1931). Goats are generally more resistant than sheep or cattle (Erasmus and Coetzer 1981) and show a lower abortion rate. Very young kids also may die. Hemorrhages and hepatic necrosis are found at necropsy. Because serious human infection also occurs, abortion samples should be collected carefully. A modified live virus vaccine produces lifelong immunity but must not be given to pregnant sheep or goats, because it produces fetal malformations, especially of the brain (Bath and de Wet 2000).

Wesselsbron Disease

Wesselsbron disease is a mosquito-borne flavivirus disease of sheep, cattle, and goats. It is restricted to sub-Saharan Africa and may cause abortion in pregnant does (Van Tonder 1975; Van der Westhuysen et al. 1988) and ewes and neonatal mortality. Seroconversion of the aborting doe can be used for diagnosis (Mushi et al. 1998). Adult nonpregnant does rarely show any signs except fever. Differentiation from Rift Valley fever is described in Chapter 11. Live virus vaccines against both of these diseases can cause abortion if given during pregnancy. A low incidence of congenital anomalies (i.e., arthrogryposis, porencephaly, hydranencephaly, cerebellar hypoplasia) is reported in sheep infected with Wesselsbron disease but apparently not documented in goats, perhaps because goats are not numerous in the areas of virus activity.

Mycoplasmosis

Numerous *Mycoplasma* species have been isolated from goats and associated with specific clinical syndromes discussed elsewhere in this text (i.e., arthritis, keratoconjunctivitis, mastitis, pneumonia). Abortions occasionally occur during outbreaks of mycoplasma-induced disease but documentation that mycoplasms caused these abortions is often lacking. For instance, an abortion rate of 80% was reported in a pen of fifty goats during an outbreak of mastitis and arthritis caused by *M. putrefaciens* (DaMassa et al. 1987). In another outbreak, however, transplacental infection was documented by the birth of weak kids already demonstrating swollen joints from which *M. mycoides* subsp. *mycoides* was isolated (Bar-Moshe and Rapapport 1981).

Yersiniosis

Yersinia pseudotuberculosis is a zoonotic bacterium commonly carried by wild birds or rodents. Fecal-oral infection of goats can result in establishment of an enteric infection with subsequent bacteremia. Abortions and early neonatal deaths of kids have been reported (Sulochana and Sudharma 1985; Witte et al. 1985; Albert 1988). Opaque white foci were seen in cotyledons, and microscopic lesions included suppurative placentitis and suppurative pneumonia (Witte et al. 1985). Tetracycline may be useful for halting an abortion storm.

Tick-borne Fever

Anaplasma phagocytophilum (formerly *Ehrlichia, Cytoecetes, Rickettsia phagocytophila*) causes a mild to acute, noncontagious disease of sheep, goats, and cattle in the United Kingdom, Europe, Africa, and India (Baas 1986). Although the organism is considered to be a common tick-borne zoonotic agent in the United States, reports of clinical disease in goats in this country are lacking. Natural transmission requires ticks such as *Ixodes ricinus* or *Rhipicephalus haemaphysaloides*, but the disease can be spread by anything that transfers blood. Signs include fever, listlessness, decreased milk production, lameness, and abortion. Secondary infections with *Staphylococcus, Pasteurella, Listeria*, and other organisms occur commonly and may contribute to abortion.

Diagnosis is by demonstration of cytoplasmic inclusions in granulocytes and monocytes in the blood and by complement fixation tests. The inclusions are grayish-blue in Giemsa-stained blood smears, which should be made as soon after abortion as possible. The organism does not invade the fetus, and thus smears of fetal tissue are not helpful (Scott 1983). Tetracycline is used for treatment (Anika et al. 1986). Pregnant animals should not be placed on pastures heavily infested with ticks. Pasture exposure of kids may prevent later economic losses from decreased production of milking goats (Melby 1984).

Anaplasmosis

Anaplasma ovis infection in goats usually causes a subclinical, mild, febrile disease. However, Boer goats in semi-arid regions of South Africa that had to walk long distances for food aborted and aborting does had low hematocrits. Organisms were found in the red blood cells of these goats. Ten of twenty experimentally infected pregnant goats aborted or resorbed their fetuses under conditions that included driving them 800 meters twice a day (Barry and van Niekerk 1990). Goats showed respiratory distress and pulmonary edema when driven. The average peak in body temperature was 2°F (1.1°C) above pre-infection levels and the mean hematocrit dropped from 30% to 22% at the peak of parasitemia, with the lowest recorded hematocrit being 10%. Transplacental infection occurred; *A. ovis* organisms were observed in red blood cells of aborted and live born kids. Means of control of this tick-borne infection, which is usually subclinical, are yet to be determined.

Neosporosis

Neospora caninum is a protozoal parasite similar to *Toxoplasma gondii* that can cause abortion in goats. Cattle are more commonly affected. Whitetail deer may be involved in a sylvatic cycle and dogs and coyotes have been identified as definitive hosts (Gay 2006). Experimental infection of pygmy goats has produced resorption, abortion, and stillbirths (Lindsay et al. 1995). Diagnosis is by isolation from the placenta or by histology and immunohistochemistry, which distinguishes *Neospora* from *Toxoplasma* infection (Dubey et al. 1992). Lesions in the fetal brain include meningoencephalitis with necrosis, gliosis, perivascular cuffs, and protozoal tissue cysts approximately 10 μm in diameter (Dubey et al. 1996). Hydrocephalus and cerebellar atrophy were seen in this case. Diagnosis by PCR is also possible (Eleni et al. 2004). Few serologic surveys have been done, but prevalence of antibodies was only 1% to 2% in dairy goats in western France (Chartier et al. 2000).

Sarcocystosis

Sarcocystis is a genus of cyst-forming protozoa. Cysts are frequently noted as an incidental finding on histological examination of cardiac and skeletal muscle of many species. In a New Zealand study, sarcocysts with mean cross-sectional diameters of 69 × 54 microns were found in 28% of samples from diaphragms of feral goats. When muscle from goat carcasses was fed to dogs and cats, only the dogs shed sporocysts in their feces (Collins and Crawford 1978). Experimental inoculation of goats seventy-five to 105 days pregnant with 10,000 sporocysts from coyote feces and believed to be *Sarcocystis capracanis* resulted in illness and abortions. Because no *Sarcocystis* meronts were found in the placenta or fetuses, the abortions were probably an indirect result of acute sarcocystosis. Naturally occurring abortion caused by sarcocystosis has been reported once in goats (Mackie et al. 1992; Mackie and Dubey 1996).

LATE ABORTION: NONINFECTIOUS CAUSES

Although multiple late abortions suggest the presence of one or more infectious agents in the herd, nutritional, hereditary, and toxic etiologies should not be overlooked. In addition, inadequate nutrition increases the prevalence of abortion caused by infectious agents such as Q fever and others that compromise placental function.

Malnutrition, Stress, and Other Environmental Factors

Stress abortions are common in undernourished Angoras on range and are occasionally seen in other breeds in the United States. When inadequate energy or protein is fed in late gestation, kids may be aborted or stillborn or born alive but small or weak. Colostrum and milk production may be inadequate for survival of the live-born kids. If the major deficiency is one of energy, pregnancy toxemia is likely to occur in does carrying multiple fetuses. If just protein is lacking, the does may not be thin or ketotic. Reduction in the size of the thymus has been proposed to be an indication of a stress abortion.

The underlying cause in a nutritional abortion outbreak may be poor quality (grass) roughage, inadequate feeder space, or very cold weather. Young, undeveloped females should not be bred if feed conditions are unlikely to permit them to complete gestation successfully.

An epidemiologic study of twenty-two dairy goat herds in Norway revealed fetal loss in 11% of the 1,439 goats, with losses in individual herds varying from 3% to 38%. In almost all herds there was no evidence of infectious disease. Decomposed fetuses were typically expelled during the last two months of pregnancy, and mature does (at least three years old) were at greatest risk. Inadequate natural lighting in the barn, more goats per pen, and less floor space per goat were identified as possible risk factors. Progesterone and cortisol were normal before abortion but estrone sulfate was reduced, suggesting placental malfunction (Engeland et al. 1998, 1999).

Inherited Abortion of Angoras

In South Africa, where selection for fine quality mohair has been intense, a genetic habitual abortion problem has been identified in older does (Van Rensburg 1971b; Van Tonder 1975).

Pathogenesis and Clinical Signs

The newborn doe kids destined to become habitual aborters (and the buckling that carries the trait) are above average in weight and have a very fine hair coat. As the animals mature, they produce higher-than-average mohair yields because of decreased adrenal function. The doelings show heat and conceive better in the first breeding season. The apparently desirable offspring of the first few pregnancies are kept for breeding, thus perpetuating the trait in the herd.

Habitual abortion usually does not appear until does reach four or five years of age. Animals with the greatest mohair production relative to body size tend to abort at approximately one hundred days gestation, a time when fetal growth rate increases but placental growth ceases. Adrenal malfunction is involved. Death of the fetus apparently occurs because of placental insufficiency (Van Rensburg 1971a). Luteal function is not impaired, and dead edematous fetuses may be retained for days or weeks. Stresses such as inclement weather, shearing, and dipping promote the expulsion of dead fetuses, causing an apparent abortion storm in the herd.

The older aborter develops both pituitary and adrenal hypertrophy, which are believed to be compensatory for previous adrenal insufficiency. These does have short estrous cycles and a lowered conception rate. A decreased amount of finer mohair is produced. Some of these does show other external evidence of hyperadrenalcorticism, such as muscle wasting and abdominal distension.

Prevention of Habitual Abortion

Mature does that abort or fail to conceive should be removed from the breeding flock. This policy has been shown to decrease the frequency of abortion in Angora herds (Van Heerden 1964). However, under certain nutritional and environmental conditions, progress in decreasing the flock abortion rate is minimal (Van der Westhuysen and Wentzel 1971). The previous offspring of aborters should also be culled. Breeding males in particular should be selected from older does with no history of abortion.

In addition, adequate dietary energy should be supplied for pregnancy maintenance, because both the habitual aborters and "normal" Angoras are more apt to abort if underfed. If a correct diet cannot be supplied, provision of shelter reduces the abortion rate in times of cold weather (Van der Westhuysen and Roelofse 1971). In Mexico, producers associate cold and rainy weather with abortion in dairy goats, often primiparous animals. A greatly increased maternal cortisol level has been documented to precede some of these abortions (Romero-R et al. 1998).

Vitamins and Minerals

A severe vitamin A deficiency (caused by six months on dry pasture without green grass) was implicated as the cause of thirty-two abortions in a goat herd in

Brazil (Caldas 1961). Vitamin A concentrations were undetectable in aborting does.

Selenium deficiency can be a cause of abortions and stillbirths in localities where feedstuffs are low in this mineral. Manganese, iodine, and copper deficiencies have also been shown to cause abortions and weak kids (Anke et al. 1972, 1977; Hennig et al. 1972; Singh et al. 2003). Some aborted fetuses are mummified when does are fed copper-deficient rations. If copper deficiency (or molybdenum or sulfur excess; see Chapter 19) is the cause of abortion or stillbirth in the second to fifth month of pregnancy, some kids in the flock might be expected to be born with weakness or swayback, as described in Chapter 5. Demyelination of white matter in spinal cord and brain has been observed in fetuses aborted due to copper deficiency (Moeller 2001). Liver copper concentrations should be determined to verify the diagnosis. One herd of African dwarf goats experienced 54% loss by two weeks of age until pregnant does were supplemented several times with 10 ml of a 2% solution of copper sulfate (Senf 1974). If iodine deficiency has caused stillbirths, affected kids usually have goiters. Conversely, however, goitrous kids in endemic iodine-deficient areas might be aborted in response to an additional etiologic agent (Wilson 1975).

When goats are kept for several generations under conditions of a trace element deficiency, such as manganese, there is selection for animals that are less susceptible to the deficiency (Hennig et al. 1972). This means that imported goats may show abortions and stillbirths under conditions that permit native goats to reproduce successfully.

Toxic Plants

Several toxic plants have been associated with abortion or birth defects in goats, including *Gutierrezia* spp. (broomweed) (Dollahite and Allen 1959; Dollahite et al. 1962; Gardner et al. 1999), *Astragalus lentiginosus* (Furlan et al. 2007), *Lupinus formosus* (Panter et al. 1992), *Conium maculatum* (Panter et al. 1990), *Nicotiana tabacum* (Panter et al. 1990), and *Veratrum californicum* (Binns et al. 1972) in the United States. Ponderosa pine (*Pinus ponderosa*) does not cause abortion when fed experimentally to goats (Short et al. 1992). The normally nutritious pods of the *Acacia nilotica* tree in South Africa cause abortion and methemoglobinemia when large amounts are consumed (Terblanche et al. 1967; Kellerman et al. 2005). Experimental oral administration of *Claviceps purpurea* sclerotia (ergot) has caused abortion and fetal mummification (Engeland et al. 1998). Additional plants are documented to cause congenital defects in sheep: *Astragalus* (abortions and limb defects), *Lathyrus*, and *Sophora* (limb defects) (Szabo 1989). Akabane virus and Cache Valley virus produce similar malformations.

Drugs

The pharmacokinetics of a few drugs have been studied in pregnant goats (Davis and Koritz 1983). In does pregnant 110 to 115 days, three fetuses were aborted from seven does given 4.4 mg/kg chlorpromazine intravenously. These fetuses showed histologic evidence of major liver damage. When phenylbutazone was given intravenously to six does at 33 mg/kg at the same stage of gestation, two kids had renal insufficiency and histologic kidney lesions after birth.

Anthelmintics, because of their frequent use during pregnancy, and corticosteroids have been implicated as causes of abortion.

Phenothiazine

Abortions have been observed in sheep and goats given phenothiazine as an anthelmintic in the last month of pregnancy (Osweiler et al. 1985). Photosensitization and associated bilateral keratitis may also occur and are well documented to be caused by phenothiazine.

Levamisole

Levamisole (the levo-isomer of tetramisole) is an anthelmintic that has been used extensively in goats, although it is not approved for this purpose in the United States. Word of mouth reports of abortions in goats have led to a general, conservative recommendation that the drug not be used in late pregnancy (Guss 1977). These abortions have not been reproduced experimentally. Likewise, tetramisole did not cause abortion in Angora goats (Philip and Shone 1967). More recently, a possibly genetic polymorphism in the metabolism of levamisole (mediated by hepatic P450 isozymes) has been identified (Babish et al. 1990). The greatly prolonged half-life of levamisole in some goats might contribute to occasional toxicity, or the temporal association of abortion after levamisole administration might be caused by chance alone.

Corticosteroids

Corticosteroids are sometimes administered for an anti-inflammatory effect to goats with infectious disease or with injuries. This should be avoided during the last month of pregnancy. The intentional use of drugs to induce parturition is discussed below.

INDUCED ABORTION OR PARTURITION

Induction of abortion or parturition is easily accomplished in the doe.

Indications

Management errors and eager bucks often result in the natural breeding of goats that the owner did not wish to become pregnant. Sometimes the problem is a buckling that is left with females past puberty or that is incompletely castrated. Frequently, a mature buck gains access to does that are considered too young or have been retained for breeding at a later time or to a different buck. Unless close examination of the buckling reveals that his urethral process is still adhered to the prepuce, effectively preventing intromission, the exposed females are usually treated with prostaglandin (see below) without waiting to confirm that pregnancy has been established.

Owners or veterinarians may desire to induce parturition in goats for a variety of reasons. Disease or injury to the doe may make survival to term and completion of normal parturition unlikely. Pregnancy toxemia appears to fit in this category, but cases must be evaluated carefully. As discussed later, early pregnancy toxemia responds to medical treatment, assuming underlying causes of anorexia can be resolved. Goats with advanced pregnancy toxemia commonly die before the hormonal sequence of events culminating in induced parturition can be completed (often thirty-six to forty-eight hours in a sick doe). These animals require surgical intervention.

Fractures, arthritis, and laminitis may be easier to manage if the goat can be relieved of the weight of fetus, placenta, and associated fluids. If a disease or injury in the late pregnant doe is expected to interfere with feed consumption for several days, (induced) parturition may prevent the otherwise inevitable development of pregnancy toxemia.

Another very important indication is the convenience of predicting the time of parturition. Owners may wish to be present to offer assistance to a primiparous or aged doe. Even more commonly, disease control programs may require rapid removal of the newborn to a clean isolation area so that exposure to disease organisms that the dam might be carrying can be limited. Included here are colostral and milk-borne diseases (CAE, mycoplasmosis), fecally transmitted diseases (paratuberculosis, intestinal parasites), and other conditions that might be contracted while the newborn kid is searching for the udder (caseous lymphadenitis, demodecosis). Hormonal induction of parturition permits the scheduling of most births for daytime or even weekend hours.

Drugs Used

The normal sequence of hormonal events in the initiation of parturition has been described as beginning with an increase in fetal cortisol, which increases placental secretion of estrogen. As maternal estrogen concentrations rise, the uterus produces prostaglandin F2 alpha, which causes luteolysis and a drop in progesterone. High estrogen and low progesterone levels together permit uterine contractions to occur and labor begins (Flint et al. 1978). There is a final surge of prostaglandin in the last few hours before delivery (Umo et al. 1976).

Historically, three classes of drugs have been used to induce parturition.

Corticosteroids

Corticosteroids (e.g., dexamethasone, 20 to 25 mg) act by increasing placental estrogen synthesis. Generally, the fetus and placenta need to have reached a stage of maturity where placental C21-steroid 17alpha-hydroxylase activity can be induced (Flint et al. 1978). This is approximately the same stage of maturity required for survival of the fetus, or roughly 141 days. Younger fetuses may fail to respond, which may be desirable if fetal survival is important, or undesirable if rapid termination of pregnancy is imperative. The average time to parturition in goats receiving corticosteroids has not been well characterized, but is approximately forty-four to forty-eight hours in animals close to term. In one study in which four does received 20 mg dexamethasone ten days before their due date, the average time to delivery was fifty-five hours (Jain and Madan 1982, 1989). By comparison, methylprednisolone acetate (240 to 270 mg) on day 111 or 125 of gestation caused abortion in six days (Van Rensburg 1971b).

Estrogen

The second group of hormones to be used is estrogens (e.g., estradiol 17-beta, 16 mg). The time to parturition is similar to that for corticosteroids, but abortion of nonviable kids can be expected if treatment is attempted too early in gestation. In a study of thirty-six goats each given two doses of estradiol benzoate (15 or 25 mg on days 147 and 148), most of the does kidded on day 149, but five of the does receiving the higher dose did not conceive in the next season (Bosc et al. 1977).

Prostaglandin

Currently, the most popular means of ending pregnancy is prostaglandin. Because the goat depends on progesterone from corpora lutea to maintain pregnancy (the placenta does not produce progesterone), prostaglandins are theoretically effective at all stages of gestation past day five. Thus, if a "buck escape" occurs, all does for which breeding was not desired can be treated with 5 mg prostaglandin F2 alpha seven to ten days later. Attention must be given to adequate buck restraint when many does return to estrus simultaneously two days after prostaglandin treatment. Because the occasional doe is not aborted by this treatment, a second dose of 5 to 10 mg might be given to animals not seen to return to estrus. In a study involving does that were approximately three months pregnant, two doses of 5 mg of prostaglandin F2 alpha twenty-four hours apart resulted in abortion between thirty-four and eighty-one hours after the first injection. Retained placenta occurred in thirty-one of forty-one does thus aborted (Memon et al. 1986b). Thus, abortion in midgestation using prostaglandin appears to take longer than induction of parturition at term. In addition to the increased risk of retained placenta, there are anecdotal reports of difficulties rebreeding in the same breeding season does thus aborted.

The owner who plans to induce parturition (as for CAE control) must faithfully record all breeding dates and prevent later reexposure to a buck. Alternatively, biparietal diameter of the fetuses can be determined by real-time ultrasound, as described above, to date the pregnancy. Injection should not be performed until day 144 of gestation or later because triplets or quadruplets may be so small as to have reduced viability (Williams 1986b). Corticosteroid pretreatment twelve to twenty-four hours in advance may hasten lung maturation and improve viability if early induction is necessary.

There is some question as to the dose of prostaglandin required. Doses of prostaglandin F2 alpha (Lutalyse, Pfizer) as small as 2.5 mg might be expected to work, but several authors have suggested that higher doses (up to 20 mg) narrow the time period when parturition is expected to occur (Bretzlaff and Ott 1983). Reported studies have involved too few goats to justify this conclusion. Many producers use 7.5 to 10 mg, given intramuscularly in the morning, with most parturitions expected the next day, twenty-nine to thirty-six hours later. If the prostaglandin is given in the evening, a similar interval to parturition results, such that the kids are delivered during the night (Romano et al. 2001). An appropriate dose of the synthetic prostaglandin cloprostenol (Estrumate, Haver) is 62.5 to 125 µg (Williams 1986b) or 150 µg (Maule Walker 1983). A Brazilian study documented that 75 µg was an adequate dose, as 100 µg did not improve the response (Santos et al. 1992). Fenprostalene has been used successfully at 0.5 mg subcutaneously, with a mean interval to kidding in eleven does of thirty-two hours (Haibel and Hull 1988).

Retained placenta and sometimes metritis have been reported after prostaglandin-induced parturition (Bosu et al. 1979; Maule Walker 1983), but are not common in the experience of other researchers (McDougall 1990; Romano et al. 2001) or owners who routinely induce parturition in their does. In one report from New Zealand, cloprostenol was administered to 360 pregnant goats. Fourteen of them died with *Clostridium chauvoei* infection and toxemia, though they did not have retained placenta. The authors recommended that clostridial vaccination be given before abortion is induced (Day and Southwell 1979).

Experimental Techniques

In herds in which exact breeding dates are not known, it may still be desirable to have parturitions occur during the day. Observation, assistance in case of dystocia, and proper identification or early removal of kids are all simplified. Other approaches might be applicable when prostaglandin cannot be used to safely modify the time of parturition. Two techniques that have been tried on sheep are controlling the time of feeding and administering a tocolytic drug to delay parturition. Thus, sheep fed once a day tend to lamb during the period from four hours before to eight hours after feeding (Gonyou and Cobb 1986). Clenbuterol (0.2 mg per ewe) delayed parturition for ten hours or more in most ewes judged to be very near to lambing (Plant and Bowler 1988), but use of this drug is forbidden in the United States. Because kidding occurs naturally during the day (Bosc et al. 1988), these techniques have received little attention in goats.

PARTURITION

The average gestation length of the goat is 150 days. There is a tendency for goats bearing triplets to kid slightly earlier (149 days) than goats with single kids (151 days) (Peaker 1978). Doe kids tended to be carried one day longer than male kids in one study (Amoah and Bryant 1983). One Mexican study of 1,468 pregnancies showed breed effects on gestation length as well as advantages to kid survival of a longer gestation, because of increased birthweight (Mellado et al. 2000). The birthweights of twins and triplets are approximately 0.91 and 0.82 of the weight of a single dairy goat kid. Parturition in the doe is termed kidding. Births are concentrated during the daylight period with a maximum at midday and early afternoon in stabled goats (Lickliter 1984/85; Bosc et al. 1988).

Normal Parturition

Signs of impending delivery include relaxation of the pelvic ligaments at the base of the tail, separation from the herd and defense of the area chosen for giving birth, increased restlessness (up and down, pawing), and low pitched vocalizations with closed mouth. For the actual delivery of the kids, the doe lies down next to a vertical surface such as a wall, fence, or feed trough (Lickliter 1984/85). The doe should be left undisturbed and in its natural surroundings, to avoid interfering with normal delivery.

Parturition is traditionally divided into three stages. First stage labor, when the cervix softens and relaxes and uterine contractions force placenta, fetus, and fluids against the cervix to help dilate it, lasts up to twelve hours in primiparous does (Bliss 1988). Multiparous does typically proceed faster. Second-stage labor, which is accompanied by straining (contraction

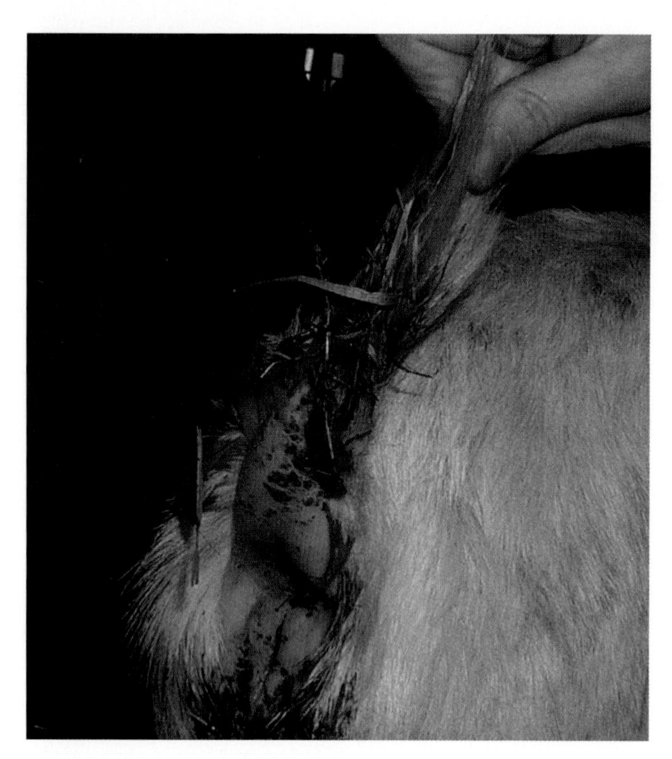

Figure 13.6. Postpartum doe with lochia adhering to the tail. (Courtesy Dr. M.C. Smith.)

of abdominal muscles), typically lasts two hours or less and is completed by expulsion of the last kid. The third stage involves expulsion of the placenta (normally within four hours) and involution of the uterus. Lochia, which should not have a foul odor, is normally discharged for as long as three weeks (Wittek and Elze 2001). Owners may choose to clip or wash the tail to prevent unsightly accumulation of lochia (Figure 13.6). Macroscopic involution of the uterus is complete in approximately four weeks (Greyling and Van Niekerk 1991b).

Evaluation for Dystocia

Most kiddings occur uneventfully and without any human assistance. In one report of records kept by breeders, 95% of does required no help (Engum and Lyngset 1970). Some does experience difficulty delivering their kids because of problems such as fetal malpresentation or oversize or failure of cervical dilation. These animals may or may not be observed to be in active labor (straining) and placenta or fetal parts may or may not be visible. Thus, the question frequently arises of whether or not the goat is in labor or in need of assistance. Certainly, if hard labor produces no kids in one-half to one hour or if placenta has been showing for that long, closer evaluation of the doe is warranted (Yankovich 1990). Yellow staining of the mucus with fetal meconium (Figure 13.7) also indicates that assistance should be provided at once. To limit discomfort

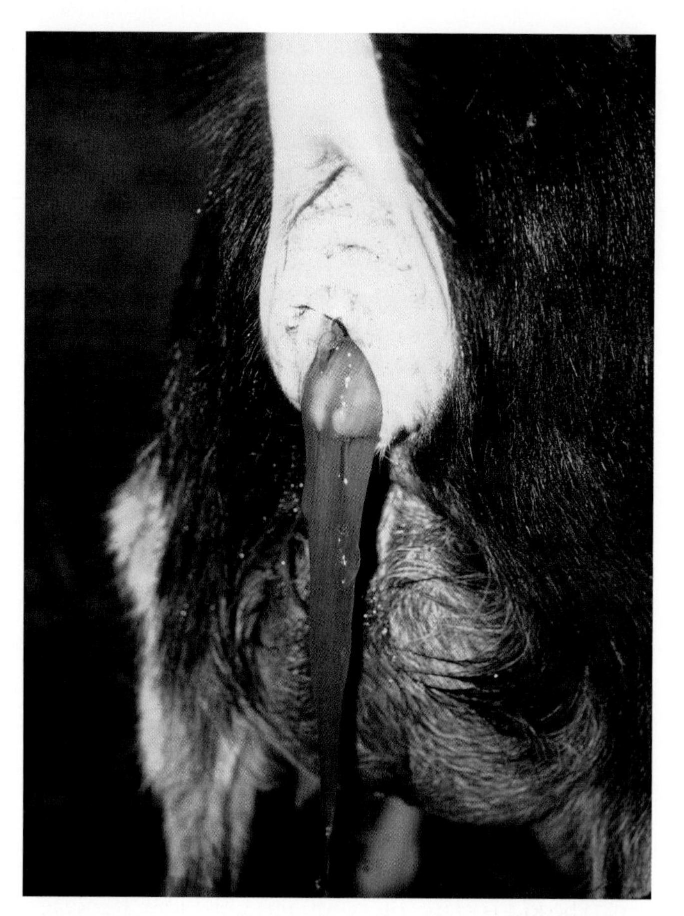

Figure 13.7. Meconium staining of the mucus indicates fetal distress and need for intervention. (Courtesy Dr. M.C. Smith.)

or bruising of the doe and subsequent infection of her reproductive tract, the vulva should be washed with mild soap. Examination should be made with a gloved, well-lubricated, small hand or (less traumatic) glass artificial insemination speculum. In one study of sixty normal parturitions, the fetal forelegs appeared from three to thirty-eight minutes (average twelve minutes) before delivery of the kid was completed (Lickliter 1984/85).

When the main source of concern is merely that the seemingly happy doe is overdue to kid, the calculations of due date (including the possibility of rebreeding) should be checked. Normal does undergo a softening of ligaments around the birth canal before the onset of parturition. If the sacrotuberous ligaments (extending from tailhead to tuber ischiadicum, or pinbone, bilaterally) have softened to the point of disappearing completely, then parturition usually occurs within twelve hours (Yankovich 1989). The doe should be examined carefully if nothing happens within the next twelve to sixteen hours. Progesterone in the blood also drops within twenty-four hours of parturition (Fredriksson et al. 1984). A bovine or canine CITE test value that is low (<2.8 ng/ml) correlates with imminent parturition, while a high value (>5 ng/ml) usually means that parturition is more than a day away (Singer et al. 2004). Induction of parturition, discussed above, shortens the period when close observation is required.

Care of the Newborn Kid

In all kids, whether born naturally or assisted, or delivered by cesarean section, attention should be given to important health measures. Unless special care is given to undersized kids, they are especially susceptible to death from hypothermia and starvation (Bajhau and Kennedy 1990). How feral goats care for their kids is described in Chapter 1.

Respiration

The parturient doe normally licks the kid intensely, beginning with its head and neck. Placental membranes (if present) are torn from the head and fluid is manually removed from the nostrils and mouth if the doe does not attend to these matters. The kid can be stimulated to breathe and fluids cleared from its nose (but not lungs) by swinging it (in a location away from walls and other hard objects). The hind limbs of the kid are held firmly by one hand while the other hand and forearm support the head, neck, and shoulder area. The kid is swung in a 90-degree arc once or twice, then returned to the ground and rubbed briskly with a clean dry towel or straw. Kids that still are not breathing but that have a palpable heartbeat may be given a respiratory stimulant such as doxopram HCl (1 to 1.5 mg/kg intravenously or sublingually). A resuscitation device for lambs has been described (Weaver and Angell-James 1986) that should be equally valuable in establishing respiration in apneic kids. It consists of a mouth piece (milk inflation), one-way valve, flange, and oral tube approximately 9.5 cm long. A lung inflation rate of twenty times per minute is recommended. Owners and veterinarians alike should resist the urge to supply direct mouth-to-mouth respiration when the kid does not respond to swinging and rubbing. Many dystocias and weak kids are the result of *in utero* infection with zoonotic pathogens.

Umbilicus

The umbilical stump should be dipped in iodine. Some authors recommend 7% tincture of iodine, while others consider 2% tincture of iodine or povidone iodine to be preferable. The stronger solution has the advantage of drying the tissues, to prevent later penetration of bacteria. However, availability of 7% tincture of iodine is currently restricted in the United States because of potential misuse for methamphetamine production. Excess length should be trimmed off the cord with clean scissors and the fresh end thoroughly immersed in the iodine. Do not dip the prepuce of the male kid. Using a partially filled plastic film canister or small paper cup avoids contamination of the stock solution. In herds experiencing problems with omphalophlebitis or septicemia, repeated dipping on a daily or twice-daily basis might be advocated. A clean, dry environment is a more effective prophylactic measure.

Housing

In cold weather, careful attention should be given to drying the kid, especially the extremities. Otherwise, the tips of the ears may be lost through frostbite. Folded ears can be straightened out and splinted at this time, using portions of a Styrofoam cup or plastic hair rollers. If the doe is to raise her kid, mother and offspring should be penned together on clean bedding or at least observed closely until a pair bond is established and the kid is nursing and following well. Kids to be raised artificially should be removed to another location where they should not be in contact with kids more than two weeks older than themselves. Heat lamps, with space for the kids to get away if they become overheated, may be used with caution in cold weather. Body socks made of sweatshirt sleeves or wool socks (toe removed, holes cut for the front feet) in place of heat lamps avoid all danger of barn fires.

If kids are chilled at birth, force feeding or rewarming may be necessary for survival. The chilled kid does not suckle. Determining the rectal temperature is helpful when choosing the method of rewarming (Eales et al. 1984). If the temperature is 98°F to 100°F (36.7°C to 37.8°C), it is often adequate to tube feed warm colostrum and place the kid under a heat lamp. Colder kids can be rewarmed in a water bath or with the aid of a hair dryer or space heater aimed into a box or a dog crate. Some producers heat bath towels in the dryer, turn it off, and install the kid into the nest of towels. Continue to monitor the rectal temperature because overheating can easily occur. If the chilled kid is to be raised by its dam, the water bath technique may wash away birth fluids and thereby cause rejection by the mother. This can be avoided by placing the kid's body into a plastic bag before it goes into the water bath.

Colostrum

Nursing kids should be assisted to obtain colostrum. Plugs should be stripped out of each teat by hand and the udder secretion inspected for evidence of mastitis. The fullness of the kid's abdomen should be monitored regularly, because this, rather than time spent sucking on a teat, is what counts. Obviously, a kid with atresia of anus or colon remains distended, even after nursing ceases, but otherwise the plump kids can be assumed to be drinking well. If kids are to be raised artificially or are too weak to suckle, the section of Chapter 19 devoted to feeding newborn kids should be consulted. Dietary deficiencies discussed in Chapter 19 (iodine, selenium, copper, vitamin E) may contribute to a herd problem with weak kids that do not suckle. Heat treatment of colostrum and milk for disease control is discussed under caprine arthritis encephalitis in Chapter 4. Failure of passive transfer of immunity is discussed in Chapter 7.

PERIPARTURIENT PROBLEMS

A variety of serious complications can interfere with normal parturition. Frequent close observation of the doe is the best insurance that difficulties will be recognized in time to save doe and kids.

Pregnancy Toxemia

Does that are carrying multiple fetuses may become anorectic and ketonuric in the last four to six weeks of gestation if feed intake does not match the metabolic needs of both the dam and the fetuses. Possible sequelae include dystocia and stillbirth or even death of the dam. A full discussion of pregnancy toxemia is included in Chapter 19. It is very important to check late pregnant goats for ketonuria if they show any signs of ill health. Treatment of the ketotic state is equally important whether the condition is primary (caused by improper nutrition) or secondary to some other disease or misadventure.

Prolapsed Vagina

Prepartum eversion of part or all of the vagina leads to discomfort and straining by the doe. This results in eversion of more tissue (Figure 13.8). Infection or laceration of the wall of the vagina and loss of the cervical seal (with subsequent entry of infection into the uterus) commonly occur. If the bladder becomes incorporated into the prolapse, kinking of the urethra impedes urination while enlargement of the bladder provokes even more straining. Causes of vaginal prolapse are not well understood in goats but might include heredity, increased intra-abdominal pressure from a large litter or indigestible roughage diet, excess estrogen in the forage, lack of exercise, or previous prolapse (Braun 2007). Unfortunately, failure of cervical dilation often leads to dystocia when labor begins after a vaginal prolapse.

The anatomy, including innervation, of the pelvic outlet of the doe has been reported in detail (Hartman 1975).

Management of Mild Prolapses

A mild prolapse is one that is visible when the doe is lying down but disappears when the animal stands up. Sometimes this condition can be handled by restraining the doe full time in such a way that her front end is lower than her hind end whenever she lies down. Possibilities include tying the doe in a corner where an excavation big enough for her frontquarters has been made in the bedding pack or confining the doe to a narrow pen such as a metabolic cage and then raising the posterior end of the platform on which she stands and sleeps.

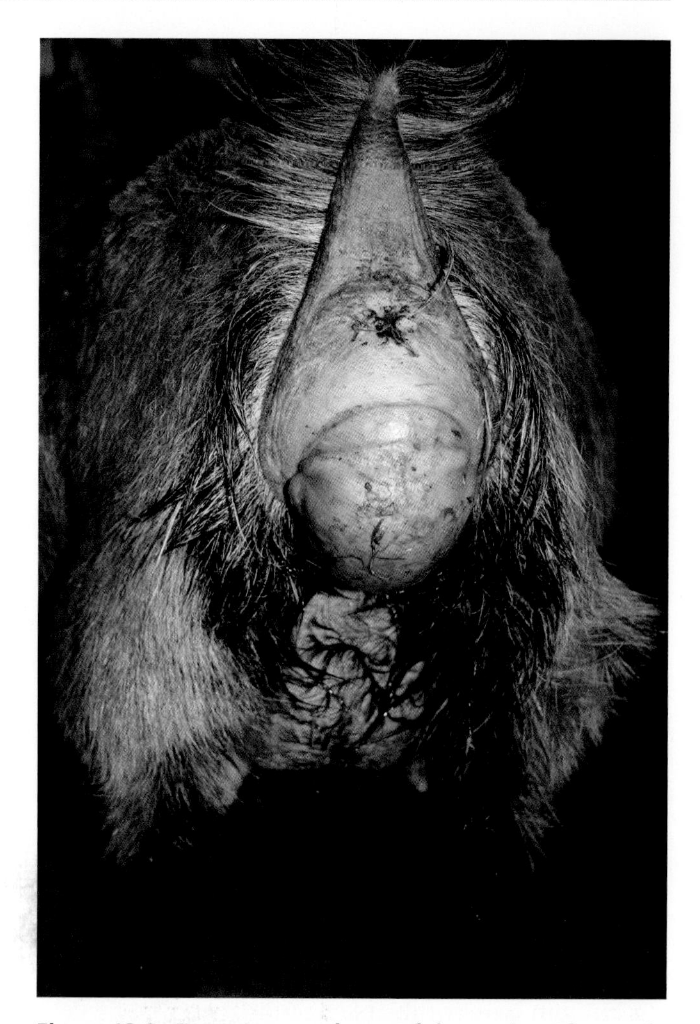

Figure 13.8. Prepartum prolapse of the vagina. The cervix of this pygmy doe failed to dilate when she went into labor, necessitating a cesarean section. (Courtesy Dr. M.C. Smith.)

Retainers and Trusses

A prolapse that does not correct itself when the doe stands up should be cleansed with a nonirritating soap, coated with an emollient or oily antibiotic preparation that includes a topical anesthetic, and manually replaced. If the prolapse appears to be too large to replace, lift up from below to unkink the urethra and permit emptying of the trapped bladder. Then some means must be found to keep the vagina in its normal position until parturition brings a decrease in the dimensions of the vagina and the estrogen-induced relaxation of surrounding tissues. Parturition is usually not possible until the vagina has been replaced. A paddle-shaped plastic bearing retainer is frequently used to treat vaginal prolapses in sheep. The same device can be used in goats, but a way must be found to attach it to the doe. Where a fleece is lacking, a length of umbilical tape can be glued to the doe's hair on each side of the hindquarters, near the point of the hip, and the two ends of the retainer are then tied to these tapes. Alternatively, a loop of suture can be placed in the skin on each side for attachment of the umbilical tapes. Presence of the retainer does not prevent kidding.

A rope truss that puts external pressure on each side of the vulva is also effective in sheep and Angora goats, but it is more difficult to keep the truss properly adjusted on the slippery hair coat of other breeds of goats. Still, the truss has the distinct advantages that it does not provoke straining by the doe and introduces no danger of infection. The center of a long piece of clothesline is placed over the doe's neck. The ends are then crossed under the chest (between the front legs) and crossed again over the back. They are then passed between thigh and udder on each side, continuing up along the vulva and forward to be secured to the rope over the neck. Short pieces of rope are used to connect the two lines above and below the base of the tail and just below the vulva. Alternatively, supporting pressure can be applied to the vulva by means of a stiff rubber, leather, or aluminum rod truss of triangular shape, with loops at the two upper lateral and single ventral corners simplifying attachment to the rope harness (Babin 1981).

Vulvar Sutures

Other methods of retaining a prolapsed vagina include several deep mattress or cruciate sutures across the vulva and a buried pursestring (Rahim and Arthur 1989). The doe must be watched very carefully because the sutures prevent parturition and cause tissue infection. A less invasive technique involves bootlacing across the vulva with a soft strip of cloth or gauze, using small loops of umbilical tape that are placed in rows lateral to each side of the vulva. A single anchoring loop between vulva and anus serves to prevent the lacing from slipping ventrally. The owner can loosen the lacing and check on the progress of parturition without causing further tissue damage or discomfort to the doe.

Sacrocaudal Extradural Anesthesia

Local anesthesia is often desirable, either temporarily for placement of some sort of retaining sutures or with a longer duration to prevent continued straining and repetition of the prolapse. Sacrocaudal extradural anesthesia has been investigated for this purpose in sheep. A dose of 1.5 ml of 2% Hostacaine provided anesthesia for forty-five minutes in sheep averaging 64 kg, whereas 2 to 3 ml resulted in ataxia and inability to rise. An injection of 2 ml of 48% ethyl alcohol created anesthesia of the genital area, croup, and thigh that persisted one to two weeks but did not impair mobility. A 0.80×40 mm needle is directed cranioventrally until it touches the bony floor of the vertebral canal between the last sacral and first (moveable) caudal vertebrae. The needle is then withdrawn slightly and checked to be sure that blood cannot be aspirated. The anesthetic should flow easily if the needle is properly placed (Schwesig 1986).

Milk Fever and Uterine Inertia

Clinical signs of hypocalcemia (inappetence, unsteady gait, weakened uterine contractions, eventual recumbency) are occasionally noted in periparturient goats. Also, a mild hypocalcemia might contribute to prolongation of first stage labor. If milk fever is suspected, calcium borogluconate (60 to 100 ml of a 20% to 25% solution) can be given very slowly intravenously or subcutaneously, split into four sites. Products with phosphorus and dextrose should be avoided subcutaneously because they cause painful abscess formation. Intravenous infusion should be avoided if the animal appears to be toxic. Other explanations for the illness, such as indigestion, pregnancy toxemia, ruptured uterus or uterine artery, metritis, and mastitis, should be ruled out. Milk fever is discussed in detail in Chapter 19.

Failure of Cervical Dilation

"Ringwomb," or incomplete dilation of the cervix, is observed occasionally in goats, as in sheep. In one study in Iraq, ringwomb accounted for 24% of 136 goats presented to a referral clinic for dystocia (Majeed and Taha 1989). The etiology remains unexplained in both species. Primiparous does may be predisposed to the condition. Undoubtedly, some cases diagnosed as incomplete dilation merely represent too early intervention. Others are accompanied by pregnancy toxemia, uterine inertia, or fetal malpresentation (Rahim and Arthur 1982). Sometimes the cervix is actually closing again after failure of parturition to occur at the appropriate time. When the cervix only opens enough for a small sack of placenta to pass and the fetuses are dead or premature, it seems likely that inadequate hormonal preparation for parturition may have been involved, as with diseases involving the placenta. Toxoplasmosis is one disease that has been documented to affect hormone production by the placenta (Engeland et al. 1996).

Possible treatments include careful manual stretching of the cervix (success in two of sixteen cases) (Ghosh et al. 1992), administration of calcium and/or estrogen and waiting a few hours, and cesarean section. Prostaglandin F2 alpha (7.5 mg intramuscularly) has been proposed as an effective treatment, as judged by delivery of kids within four hours (Majeed and Taha 1989). Cloprostenol (500 μg IM) has also been reported to be effective, though the time to delivery was reported to be thirty-nine to fifty-one hours (Ghosh et al. 1992). The possibility that the final preparturient surge of prostaglandin is absent in animals with ringwomb needs to be investigated. It is tempting to ascribe a response to prostaglandin to induction of relaxin, a glycoprotein hormone which softens the cervix in some species (Senger 2005), but relaxin has not yet been studied in the doe. If a true ringwomb is present, manual dilation can easily rupture the cervix or uterus (Engum and Lyngset 1970). Oxytocin also should be avoided. If placenta is visible and other techniques fail, surgery should not be delayed longer than a few hours.

Abnormal Fetal Presentation, Position, or Posture

Both anterior presentation (with head and forelimbs extended) and posterior presentation (with hind limbs extended) are considered to be normal in goats. However, posterior presentation has been reported in only 3% to 9% of kids, is even rarer in single kids, and appears to predispose to dystocia (Engum and Lyngset 1970). Problems occur when multiple kids become tangled in the birth canal or the head or limbs are retained. Careful attention is necessary to distinguish front feet from hind feet and to verify that traction is being applied to the extremities of only one fetus at a time. Normal deliveries and various dystocias in goats have been well illustrated in a French publication (Babin 1981).

Some breeders report increased frequency of dystocia in Pygmy goats and suggest that selection in the show ring for a very short and compact body type is to blame (Brown 1988). Apparently there is not enough room in the doe's abdomen for the kid to present itself properly. A radiographic study of dystocia in thirty West African dwarf goats in Nigeria, with no show ring selection, demonstrated that abnormal fetal posture was more common than a small maternal pelvis as a cause of dystocia (Kene 1991). Pygmy goats were overrepresented in one study of goats undergoing cesarean section in the United States (Brounts et al. 2004).

General Guidelines for Mutation and Delivery

Wild goats are said to stand with their forequarters downhill from the hindquarters to give fetuses the opportunity to rearrange themselves. This gravitational advantage should be remembered when parturition is assisted. If it is necessary to retrieve the head or a limb of a fetus in a recumbent doe, this is easiest if the dam is positioned so that the retained extremity is uppermost. Delivery is usually possible with either one forelimb or one hind limb retained. If there is adequate room for manipulations, the second limb can be properly positioned before extraction begins. If the head is out, it is sometimes possible to deliver the normal sized kid by simple traction, without retrieving either forelimb. If the uterus is contracted around the fetus subsequent to prolonged dystocia, intramuscular epinephrine (1 ml of a 1:1,000 solution to a dairy or meat breed doe) greatly facilitates safe manipulations by relaxing the uterus.

When the kid is properly positioned, it is pulled out and downward in an arc. If a dystocia occurs when head and two forefeet are presenting, the difficulty may be a simple elbow lock; pulling firmly on one limb at a time extends the elbow joint so that the tip of the nose is positioned closer to the carpus rather than directly over the hooves. It is also possible that parts of more than one fetus are represented or that a relative fetal oversize is present.

Deviation of the Head

One should never try to extract a kid in anterior presentation unless the head and neck have either been properly positioned or amputated. Rupture of the uterus is very likely to occur and may already be present before human intervention when the fetal head is retained. A lamb puller (Nasco, Fort Atkinson, WI) makes an excellent head snare. The head typically deviates to the side of the fetus but occasionally drops down between the front limbs. It is usually necessary to repel the fetus by pushing the front limbs inward or elevating the hindquarters of the doe to have space to straighten out the head. Epinephrine, as described above, may also be helpful.

Retention of Forelimbs

Sometimes the head of a kid is delivered but then progress stops because of retention of both forelimbs. Assistance should be provided at once; the neck is followed to a shoulder and then the corresponding limb is retrieved. It may be necessary to repel the head to have room for passing a hand as far as the shoulders. Care must be taken not to push the head around to one side.

If the head of a live kid with retained forelimbs passes beyond the lips of the vulva, compression of the jugular veins results in edema of the head. The head swells to the extent that repulsion becomes impossible yet there is no room to reach inside and straighten a leg. Extensive lubrication may permit delivery of a small kid in this position without additional manipulation. If the kid is dead, there should be no hesitation about amputating the head at the atlanto-occipital joint with a scalpel blade to provide more room for mutation.

Multiple Fetuses or Transverse or Malformed Fetus

When more than one kid is presented simultaneously, it is important to accurately identify the extremities in the birth canal and to trace them back to the body of the fetus. In general, it is preferable to first deliver a kid whose head is in the birth canal rather than risk creating a more difficult dystocia by repelling the head. Otherwise, a kid in posterior presentation is easier to deliver first. If a kid is transversely positioned, it should be moved (with the finger tips) into a posterior, breech position. From this point, retrieval of at least one hind limb usually permits delivery. Epinephrine to relax the uterus, as described above, may be helpful.

A schistosomus reflexus fetus (Buergelt 1997; Gutierrez et al. 1999) could cause dystocia that resembled the simultaneous presentation of twins. If correctly diagnosed by noting abdominal organs outside the fetal body, the dystocia can be relieved by a single cut with a regular fetotome.

Controlling Straining

An epidural injection of lidocaine (with or without xylazine) can be used to decrease straining, as discussed in Chapter 17. The beta-adrenergic compound clenbuterol (Ventipulmin; Boehringer, Ingelheim) is available in some countries as a tocolytic drug to temporarily cause myometrial relaxation. Initial favorable studies in cattle suggest that the drug might also be useful during correction of fetal malposition or exteriorization of the uterus during cesarean section in goats. A possible dose to try is 0.8 µg/kg intramuscularly (Menard and Diaz 1987). The use of this drug in food animals is forbidden in the United States, but epinephrine may be substituted (see above).

Relative Fetal Oversize and Fetotomy

Multiple kids are rarely too large for the birth canal unless the doe is severely stunted or has suffered some injury such as ankylosis of a fractured tail (Engum and Lyngset 1970). On the other hand, a single large kid may be too large for a small first freshener. Owners rarely have the luxury of breeding doelings to a buck of known kidding ease. Addition of lubricant to the birth canal may assist delivery of a large kid, but often the fetus is emphysematous, malformed, or too large to be extracted intact.

Fetal hydrops (anasarca, dropsy) is a specific cause of fetal oversize that warrants discussion. Massive accumulation of fluid in fetal tissues and body cavities may make extraction impossible unless incisions are first made with a finger knife to drain the fluid. Accumulation of fluid within the placenta may be so great that abnormal distension of the dam's abdomen occurs and the subsequent interference with circulation, respiration, and locomotion necessitates a cesarean section or induction of parturition to save the dam. Anasarcous kids may be cotwin to normal, viable kids, and the same doe may produce another affected kid in a subsequent gestation (Elze and Müller 1960; Walser 1963). In one herd, eleven kids with hydrops were produced, all sired by a single buck. The condition may be inherited as a simple recessive character (Ricordeau 1981). Hypothyroidism is another proposed cause (Kumar et al. 1989). Wesselsbron disease (Chapter 11) is also reported to cause hydrops, at least in sheep.

Unless the kid is alive and its value warrants the expense of a cesarean section, consideration should be given to a subcutaneous fetotomy. This procedure is relatively safe for the doe because instruments are not used in the birth canal and the fetal skin protects the friable maternal tissues. An initial skin incision is made with a scalpel just above and all the way around the carpus, and is then extended as far as possible up the medial side of the leg. The skin is then pushed proximally and the front limb is torn loose from the thorax and extracted, an easy process if the fetus is autolyzed. This procedure is repeated with the other front limb. The thorax can be compressed by sliding a hand beneath the kid's skin and manually fracturing the ribs. Rotation of the head and trunk causes the vertebral column to fall apart in the lumbar region. The hind limbs can then be pulled out. A complete subcutaneous fetotomy is rarely necessary (Engum and Lyngset 1970).

Special tools have been described for fetotomy in small ruminants. A long-handled nipper with blunt-tipped jaws bent upward has been used to amputate a front or back limb or the head. Fetal pieces are then extracted with the aid of small tongs (Deckwer 1951).

Hydrops of the Uterus

Rarely, distention of the pregnant uterus with excess amniotic or allantoic fluid occurs. Extreme abdominal distension, discomfort, and difficulty rising may be noted. Presence of caruncles and fetus on ultrasound distinguishes hydrops from hydrometra. Pregnancy toxemia (see Chapter 19) may be concomitant or incorrectly suspected. The normal allantoic fluid volume in sheep and goats has been reported to be between 0.5 and 1.5 liters, while one doe with hydrallantois had approximately 12 liters of fluid at the time of successful treatment by cesarean section (Morin et al. 1994). Hormonal induction of parturition permits slower release of the accumulated fluid but the delivery is also slow and probably requires assistance because of weakness of the myometrium (Jones and Fecteau 1995). It has been proposed that ram × doe hybrid pregnancies are predisposed to the development of hydrops of the uterus (Kelk et al. 1997).

Uterine Torsion

Torsion of the pregnant uterus is occasionally observed in goats (Wyssmann 1945) as in sheep (Smith and Ross 1985). In one report from Kerala, India, torsion was identified as the cause of dystocia in twenty-two of fifty-three goats treated by cesarean section during a five-year period (Philip et al. 1985). The condition is more likely to occur with a single fetus than with bicornual twins. The torsion may involve the vagina, but it also may involve only the cervix or body of the uterus. Thus, when a doe is in dystocia, as evidenced by ineffective straining, it may not be possible to distinguish uterine torsion from incomplete dilation of the cervix. Early cesarean section permits differentiation and correction of both of these conditions. Ultrasound examination may demonstrate marked thickening and edema of the uterine wall near the site of torsion (Wehrend et al. 2002).

If the torsion is recognized at the time of examination for dystocia, correction may be attempted by rolling the doe while weight is applied to the abdomen to prevent rotation of the fetus (Sathiamoorthy and Kathirchelvan 2005). Thus, if the torsion palpable in vagina or cervix is to the left, the doe is placed in left lateral recumbency and rolled over her back to the other side while the uterus is prevented from turning by hand pressure or a weighted plank held across the flank. Suspending the doe by her hind limbs and shaking the doe or manipulating the uterus through the body wall is an older, but sometimes successful approach to repositioning the uterus.

Cesarean Section

When pregnancy toxemia or other misadventure makes immediate termination of pregnancy desirable or when a dystocia cannot otherwise be resolved without sacrificing the life of a kid, surgical delivery of the fetuses is necessary. Ultrasound can be used to assess fetal viability, as immediate slaughter might be the economically correct decision if the fetuses are dead. Research or disease eradication programs requiring gnotobiotic kids may involve elective cesarean section. Because many goats shed the Q fever organism (*Coxiella burnetii*) in birth fluids, all people assisting with the surgery or aftercare of fetuses should wear gloves and tightly fitting masks.

Anesthesia and Surgical Approach

Either general or local anesthesia may be chosen (Benson 1986). Suitable general anesthetic agents (halothane, isoflurane) are rapidly cleared after surgery so that there is minimal respiratory depression of the kids or interference with maternal behavior. Xylazine tranquilization should be kept to a minimum or avoided altogether, unless reversal agents (yohimbine or tolazoline) are available. Intramuscular xylazine at 0.2 mg/kg causes hypoxemia, respiratory acidosis, uterine contractions, and decreased uterine blood flow in the pregnant goat (Sakamoto et al. 1996). Tranquilization with diazepam is preferable to xylazine. An intravenous diazepam dose of 5 mg per goat has been suggested for standing surgery (Snyder 2007). When the doe is toxic or exhausted, local anesthesia (see Chapter 17) alone is adequate. Intravenous fluid therapy should be begun on these patients before surgery commences.

The doe may be tied in right lateral recumbency, with a towel covering the eyes. A vertical incision is made halfway down the left paralumbar fossa. Care should be taken to enter the abdominal cavity rather than the perirenal retroperitoneal space. A ventral midline incision along the linea alba starting at the base of the udder and extending cranially 20 cm is an alternative that requires less suturing to close, but dorsal recumbency increases pressure on major blood vessels and the danger of regurgitation. Using a cuffed endotracheal tube and positive pressure ventilation overcome these disadvantages. A ventral abdominal paramedian approach, between the linea alba and the subcutaneous abdominal vein, is yet another option (Tibary and Van Metre 2004).

Surgical Techniques

When the abdominal cavity has been opened, the greater omentum should be retracted cranially and the abdomen explored to determine the number and location of fetuses. A gravid horn is then exposed and packed off with moistened towels. A single incision along the dorsal curvature of one horn usually permits removal of all fetuses from one site (Wallace 1982). Placentomes should be avoided. Extremities (e.g., hind feet) are grasped and the first kid is gently delivered from the abdomen. Additional kids are milked to the same incision. The umbilical cord is separated by grasping it firmly close to the kid's abdominal wall with one hand and tugging firmly with the other hand that grasps the cord several inches distally. If the cord fails to break, it should be clamped with Carmalt forceps and ligated. The placenta is only removed if it is no longer attached to caruncles. After the surgeon is sure that all fetuses have been removed, the uterus is closed with one or two layers of inverting 0 or 1 chromic catgut or synthetic absorbable sutures. After the surface of the uterus has been lavaged, closure of the abdominal incision is routine (Tibary and Van Metre 2004).

If the doe has a problem that prevents vaginal delivery on subsequent pregnancies but it is to be kept as a pet, ovariectomy should be considered before abdominal closure, as the surest way to prevent rebreeding.

Aftercare

Aftercare of kids is as described for vaginal deliveries. Ideally, an assistant should attend to the kids, because their body temperature can drop dangerously low during the time it takes to finish the surgery. If the doe is to raise the kids, she should be permitted to mother them as soon as possible. Systemic antibiotics (penicillin, ceftiofur, or tetracycline) and tetanus prophylaxis are generally administered to the dam. Oxytocin (5 units) should not be given until suturing of the uterus is completed. Research conducted in ewes suggests that oxytocin doses exceeding 3 or 4 IU intramuscularly cause a prolonged and undesirable spastic contraction of the periparturient uterus (Marnet et al. 1985), but higher (empirical) doses have been recommended in small ruminants. Analgesics such as flunixin meglumine (1.1 mg/kg intramuscularly or intravenously) may be given if needed to control postoperative pain (Vivrette 1986).

The prognosis for life and fertility of the doe is good if the surgery was elective (Brounts et al. 2004), but must be guarded if the fetus was macerated or the doe was seriously ill, as with pregnancy toxemia, before surgery.

Prolapsed Uterus

Eversion of the uterus (typically one horn) occurs occasionally, but is apparently less common when goats are loose-housed than when they are confined to individual stalls (Engum and Lyngset 1970). The prognosis is usually good, even if the prolapse has been present for twenty-four hours. The uterus should be washed with copious water and a mild disinfectant. The hindquarters are then elevated with the hind limbs spread apart. Working through a towel while replacing the uterus protects against accidental perforation. When the uterus is back through the cervix, manipulation with fingers held together is continued until the very tip of the uterine horn is replaced. An antibiotic powder is placed in the uterine cavity and oxytocin (perhaps 5 IU) is given to contract the uterus. Systemic antibiotics may be given for several days. Tetanus prophylaxis should not be neglected. Some authors recommend suturing the vulva, but this should not be necessary if replacement is complete and the doe can get up easily. A truss could be used.

If the prolapse is older than thirty-six hours or is extensively damaged, amputation of the uterus is required. A tight ligature is required, and a stay suture should be placed ahead of the ligature in case the ligature should slip during amputation and retrieval of the cut end should be required (Engum and Lyngset 1970).

Uterine Artery Rupture

Though this condition is not well described in the literature, rupture of the uterine artery occurs occasionally in the postpartum goat. It is conceivable that some does merely experience hematoma formation in the broad ligament, but a problem is usually only diagnosed if fatal hemorrhage occurs. The doe may be found dead or dying; cold skin, muscle tremors, and bloat in the hypovolemic animal may suggest hypocalcemia. Death may occur before the packed cell volume has time to fall. The author has seen goats that bled to death as long as four days post partum.

Retained Placenta and Metritis

The placenta is normally passed within three or four hours. If the placenta has not been expelled within twelve hours after delivery of the last kid, it is then considered to be retained (Franklin 1986). Retained placenta may occur in an infectious abortion (or birth of a live kid from an infected doe) caused by diseases such as toxoplasmosis (Calamel and Giauffret 1975) and chlamydiosis. Practitioners have associated a dietary deficiency of selenium with herd problems of retained placenta in goats, and recommended injectable and oral selenium supplementation for prevention (Cochran 1980). Some delay the injection until ten days before the due date, in light of label warnings against the use in pregnant animals, reasoning that kids might still be viable if treatment induced early parturition. Cesarean section is another risk factor for retained placenta (Brounts et al. 2004).

Metritis associated with retained placenta, retained kids, or trauma and infection of the uterus in the course of dystocia may lead to signs of systemic illness shortly after parturition. Fever, depression, anorexia, and a malodorous vaginal discharge are typical. The occurrence of a retained placenta may be difficult to confirm without a vaginal examination because goats commonly eat all or part of the placenta. In one study of sixty normal parturitions, the placentas were eaten by 38% of the does (Lickliter 1984/85). Transabdominal ultrasound during the first week, at least in sheep, permits identification of hyperechoic placenta in fluid in the uterine lumen, attached to hypoechoic caruncles (Hauser and Bostedt 2002). Peritoneal fluid analysis may suggest peritonitis if a severe metritis or uterine tear is present. If a vaginal examination is performed, intrauterine antibiotics are commonly administered, but manual removal of the placenta should not be attempted. Instead, oxytocin may be administered (5 IU subcutaneously or intramuscularly several times a day) and systemic antibiotics are recommended to prevent development of a life-threatening toxemia or septicemia. It is the author's personal preference to give penicillin prophylactically but to use oxytetracycline if the goat is already systemically ill. Tetanus prophylaxis should be ensured.

Postparturient or genital gas gangrene caused by infection of the uterus with clostridial organisms is common in Angora goats in South Africa that are penned for kidding (Van Tonder 1975). Signs usually develop six to twenty-four hours after kidding. Metritis is accompanied by septicemia and death occurs in untreated animals in twelve to seventy-two hours.

Pyometra appears to be far less common in goats than is mucometra or hydrometra associated with false pregnancy (Hesselink and Taverne 1994). Previous dystocia with cervical damage may predispose to pyometra (Haibel 1986a), as does the presence of parts of a macerated fetus (Lyngset 1968d). The contents of the uterus are more uniformly echogenic when examined by real-time ultrasound than is the fluid in a hydrometra. Fetal bones are sometimes found embedded in the wall of the reproductive tract at necropsy. Treatment is with prostaglandin, systemic antibiotics, and possibly surgical emptying of the uterus.

Vulvovaginitis

Vaginal discharge (other than clear or cloudy heat mucus and lochia) or lesions of the vaginal mucosa in the absence of uterine or urinary tract disease warrant a speculum examination of the vagina. Traumatic lesions and retained vaginal pessaries should be ruled out before investigating the possibility of specific infections localized to the caudal portions of the reproductive tract. Ectopic mammary gland (see Chapter 3) should not be mistaken for inflammatory disease of the vulva.

Caprine Herpesvirus

Postbreeding genital disease (papules, vesicles, and pustules coalescing to form ulcers) associated with caprine herpesvirus-1 has been reported in does in New Zealand (Horner et al. 1982) and Australia (Grewal and Wells 1986). Lesions healed in four to six days and does developed neutralizing antibody. Vaginal lesions have also been produced by experimental infection and reactivated by estrus or corticosteroids (Tempesta et al. 2002). There is no apparent interference with fertility.

Infection can be confirmed by viral isolation from vaginal swabs or by rising serum neutralization titers. The condition is discussed in Chapter 12.

Mycoplasma

A granular vulvovaginitis has been observed in spontaneous cases and reproduced experimentally by inoculation of scarified vulvar mucosa with *Mycoplasma agalactiae* (Singh et al. 1974, 1975). Spontaneously affected goats have a mucopurulent vaginal discharge with multiple, yellowish-white, pinhead-sized elevations, especially near the clitoris. Occasionally the granules are red and ulcerated. Histologically, findings include perivascular cuffing, accumulation of lymphocytes and plasma cells in the lamina propria, and lymphoid follicles in the vulvovaginal region. Numerous other mycoplasmas, including *M. bovigenitalium* and *Acholeplasma laidlawii*, have been isolated from Nigerian goats with clinical vulvovaginitis (Chima et al. 1986). *Acholeplasma laidlawii* is found on all mucosal membranes (Rosendal 1994) and is of questionable pathogenicity, but experimentally has been reported to cause lymphocytic vulvitis and vaginitis in goats (Gupta et al. 1990).

There is no published evidence that this condition interferes with fertility or that its occurrence or duration can be limited by treatment. To avoid additional spread, however, it seems prudent to avoid natural mating until clinical signs disappear.

Leiomyofibromatosis

A prolonged vaginal discharge (purulent or serosanquinous) has been reported from a Saanen goat with multiple firm nodular polyps in the vaginal wall. Based on histology, a diagnosis of vaginal leiomyofibromatosis was made and an association with follicular ovarian cysts was proposed (Haibel et al. 1990). One of the authors (MCS) is aware of a similar case in a goat with bilateral granulosa cell tumors. Because the diagnosis was only considered retrospectively after review of the first report, it seems likely that leiomyofibromatosis also may have been overlooked in other goats. Ovariectomy has been proposed for alleviation of the condition. This option is presumably limited to pet goats unless a unilateral ovarian disease were discovered at laparotomy.

NEOPLASIA OF THE FEMALE REPRODUCTIVE TRACT

Few tumors of the genital system have been reported in does. Select cases might be treated by ovariectomy or hysterectomy.

Ovarian Tumors

A 400 g cystic ovarian tumor histologically resembling a granulosa cell tumor was identified in an Alpine doeling that first underwent a false pregnancy with udder development and lactation and then developed masculine appearance, behavior, and odor. Metastasis to the uterus occurred. Histologically, pituitary, adrenal, and thyroid glands were normal (Dewalque 1963). Another granulosa tumor caused short estrous cycles and masculine behavior in a three-year-old Toggenburg doe (Lofstedt and Williams 1986); its removal allowed establishment of a normal pregnancy. Additional granulosa cell tumors were reported by Cooke and Merrall (1992) and Kutty and Mathew (1995). A dysgerminoma weighing 1,450 g was ballottable through the abdominal wall of an aged doe (Smith 1980). A mucinous adenocarcinoma of the ovary of a six-year-old Nubian doe was associated with accumulation of 30 liters of ascitic fluid in the abdomen (Memon et al. 1995). Ovarian involvement with multicentric lymphosarcoma has also been reported (DiGrassie et al. 1997).

Uterine and Cervical Tumors

The most commonly observed tumor of the tubular genitalia of the doe may be the leiomyosarcoma, which grows by slow invasion and rarely metastasizes. Vaginal bleeding is a common presentation, and Saanens may be predisposed to this tumor. Seven cases were diagnosed over a twenty-year period at a diagnostic laboratory in New York, and five of these were in Saanens, including co-twins affected at twelve and thirteen years of age (Whitney et al. 2000). A seven-year-old Saanen doe with a leiomyosarcoma of the body of the uterus collapsed and died from hemorrhage when the uterus ruptured at the tumor site. The tumor had invaded the broad ligament but had not metastasized to lymph nodes, liver, or lungs (Ryan 1980).

Leiomyomas occur occasionally and may be an incidental finding at necropsy (Ramadan and ElHassan 1975). One reported leiomyoma of the uterus caused dystocia and was removed per vagina after parturition (Kaikini and Deshmukh 1977). Another leiomyoma of the cervix of a nine-year-old Toggenburg invaded the vagina and uterus; it caused a hemorrhagic discharge and severe straining and was diagnosed by vaginal examination (Cockcroft and McInnes 1998). Other reported tumors include a leiomyofibroma of the uterus in a five-year-old goat (Damodaran and Parthasarathy 1972), fibromas of the uterus and vagina and an adenoma of the vagina (Kronberger 1961), a cervical fibroma that protruded from the vulva (Gokak 1988), and a fibroid (Sastry 1959). A twelve-year-old goat in poor body condition that had not become pregnant for many years was found to have a uterine adenocarcinoma that had metastasized extensively to oviduct, ovary, lymph nodes, lung, liver, spleen, and skeletal muscle (Riedel 1964). Lymphosarcoma can also involve the uterus (Whitney et al. 2000).

THE INTERSEX

Although the older literature describes hermaphrodites (ovarian and testicular tissue both present) and pseudohermaphrodites (gonads of one sex but some morphological structures typical of the other sex), the term intersex is currently preferred and can be applied even when the exact nature of the gonads is unknown. An intersex, then, is an animal that shows both male and female characteristics.

The Polled Intersex

Within the breeds originating in western Europe (such as Saanen [Soller 1963], Alpine [Boyajean 1969], and Toggenburg [Eaton 1943]), there is a well known and much studied association between the natural absence of horns and the intersex condition. The condition also occurs in the Damascus or Shami goat (Al-Ani et al. 1998). It is likely that Nubian and Angora goats have a different inheritance of horns (Crepin 1958). The polled intersex condition is not reported in these breeds, although freemartins may occur.

Etiology

The polled condition in the European breeds is determined by an autosomal dominant gene that is the same as or very closely linked to a recessive gene causing infertility. One older theory held that this gene, where homozygous, causes expression of H-Y antigen (Wachtel et al. 1978). The H-Y gene is normally on the Y chromosome. Translocation of a subcritical portion of H-Y genes to an autosome would give rise to a recessive mode of inheritance. H-Y antigen is secreted in hormone-like fashion and binds to cells of the developing ovary (Wachtel 1980). A variable H-Y dosage would explain the extreme variability in phenotype of polled intersex goats (Shalev et al. 1980).

Polled intersex goats have been shown to be negative for SRY, the sex-determining region of the Y chromosome which is one of the major genes responsible for testicular induction (Just et al. 1994). Recently, an 11.7-kb deletion on chromosome 1 of the goat known as the PIS (polled trait related intersex syndrome) deletion has been identified as causing the polled condition (Basrur and Kochhar 2007). The deleted segment of DNA normally has regulatory effects on nearby genes for horn bud development and development of fetal ovaries. Female goats homozygous for the deletion show sex reversal because testis promoting genes in the fetal ovary become active; the intricacies of the sex determination cascade in the developing fetus are detailed by Basrur and Kochhar (2007).

Clinical Signs and Management

Affected animals are genetically female but may exhibit male, female, or mixed external characteristics (Eaton 1943). An enlarged clitoris in a doe-like animal or a decreased ano-genital distance in a more masculine individual is typical. Hypospadias may be present. The gonads (usually testes or ovotestes) may be scrotal, inguinal, or abdominal in location and are smaller than the testes of normal bucks of the same age. In one instance, the uterine tubes attached to the scrotal testes also herniated into the scrotal sac (Ramadan et al. 1991). Testosterone is commonly produced, which accounts for masculine behavior, neck development, erect hair on the neck, and odor (Hamerton 1969; Zlotnik 1973). Sperm are not produced, and thus the intersex can be used as a teaser animal. Gonadectomy is generally required if the animal is to be kept as a pet.

Unless the masculinized intersex goats are counted as females, the sex ratio in European breeds favors males rather than females (Eaton 1945; Soller et al. 1969). Polled does tend to have a larger litter size than horned does (Soller and Kempenich 1964; Constantinou et al. 1981).

Diagnosis

The anatomic variations just described are very suggestive of this condition, if the animal is naturally polled and both parents were polled. In this regard it should be remembered that some breeders disbud every kid at a very young age without paying close attention to hair swirls that would permit differentiation of polled from horned animals (Chapter 18). Thus some polled goats have been "disbudded" and recorded as horned. Likewise, a small horny scur is usually taken as evidence of previous horn removal but conceivably could represent partial growth in a heterozygous animal. If a polled doe is fertile, she is presumed to be heterozygous for the polled gene. Differentiation of a polled intersex from a freemartin requires karyotyping; the polled intersex is a chromosomal female.

Difficulties are encountered in identifying the intersex animal with normal or nearly normal (slight projection of the vulva) external genitalia. Failure to exhibit estrus, development of male odor or behavior during the breeding season, a shortened vagina on speculum examination, or smaller than normal teats may be first signs that the intersex condition is present. At the other end of the spectrum, polled genetic females with male phenotype and hypoplastic testes are difficult to identify without a karyotype until they are old enough that sperm production would be expected (Corteel et al. 1969; Soller et al. 1969). Karyotyping is available from various commercial laboratories, including the Veterinary Genetics Laboratory at the University of California, Davis.

Prevention

The occurrence of intersex goats associated with the polled condition can be avoided by insisting that one goat in each breeding pair have been born with horns and is therefore homozygous for the gene for horns (p). This ensures that no kids are born homozygous for the PIS polled gene mutation/deletion (P) and its associated recessive effects on fertility. A polled buck can be heterozygous or homozygous. A polled doe, on the other hand, must be heterozygous if she is fertile. The potential for obtaining undesirable offspring by mating polled animals is detailed in Figure 13.9.

Freemartins

A freemartin is a female rendered sterile by being co-twin to a male fetus.

Pathogenesis

In cattle, freemartinism is common because the fetal membranes from twin calves generally fuse, thereby permitting exchange of cells and hormones (testosterone and Müllerian inhibiting substance) between male and female fetuses (Padula 2005). Although multiple births are common in goats, freemartins are not. This is presumably because placental fusion does not usually occur, at least not until after differentiation of fetal gonads is completed (Basrur and Kochhar, 2007).

Diagnosis

Caprine freemartins cannot be distinguished on the basis of external or internal genitalia from polled intersexes (Basrur and Kochhar 2007). The gonads may be partially descended testes devoid of germ cells or internal testes or ovotestes. The goat may be polled or horned. A male litter mate must have been present in the uterus early in embryologic development, but might not have persisted to term (the case of the

Homozygous buck		P	P
Doe	P	polled **PP** intersex if female	polled **PP** intersex if female
	p	polled **P**p fertile	polled **P**p fertile

Heterozygous buck		P	p
Doe	P	polled **PP** intersex if female	polled **P**p fertile
	p	polled **P**p fertile	horned pp fertile

Figure 13.9. Results of crossing a polled doe (always heterozygous, Pp) with a homozygous (PP) or heterozygous (Pp) polled buck.

missing womb mate). The diagnosis can be confirmed by demonstrating XX-XY blood chimerism (BonDurant et al. 1980; Ricordeau 1981; Smith and Dunn 1981; Bosu and Basrur 1984). The expense of karyotyping is usually prohibitive. Some laboratories, such as the Veterinary Genetics Laboratory at the University of California, Davis, offer freemartin testing of goats for a lower price than a karyotype, but even this may not be warranted, because clinical management of a freemartin is the same as for a polled intersex.

Other Chromosome Abnormalities

The karyotype of the domestic goat consists of sixty chromosomes; all except the small metacentric Y chromosome are acrocentric. Because the acrosomes appear similar under conventional staining techniques, identifying individual autosomes requires special staining techniques such as G-banding (Cribiu and Matejka 1987a) and R-banding (Cribiu and Matejka 1987b).

If karyotyping is done on infertile goats, very occasional animals are identified that have abnormalities other than the polled XX intersex condition or XX-XY blood chimerism of freemartins. Fusion of embryos and other genetic accidents may be proposed. Goats that are true hermaphrodites are often whole-body chimeras (Basrur and Kochhar 2007). There is a report of a single fertile Saanen × Beetal buck goat with both XY and XXY cell lines in its blood, but the mechanism by which this mosaic was created could not be determined. At least four of the buck's sixteen progeny were culled for breeding problems (Bhatia and Shanker 1992).

Robertsonian Translocation

An inherited centric fusion (Robertsonian translocation) of two acrocentric chromosomes (resulting in a chromosome number of fifty-nine instead of sixty) has been identified in a family of Saanen goats (Soller et al. 1966). Similar Robertsonian translocations involving different chromosomes have been reported in other populations of Saanen or Toggenburg goats (Popescu 1972; Cribiu and Lherm 1986; Burguete et al. 1987). In most instances, no anatomic abnormalities have been identified. In one case, two sterile bucks (with one and two polled parents) were found to have a centric fusion (Ricordeau et al. 1972a). Females carrying this chromosomal abnormality tended to produce fewer kids than did noncarrier sisters (Ricordeau 1972), which suggests increased embryonic mortality rates. Homozygotes with fifty-eight chromosomes were not reported (Ricordeau 1981), again suggesting that the trait was lethal in the homozygous state.

A translocation involving chromosomes five and fifteen in a Saanen buck in Brazil, imported from Switzerland, produced no adverse effects on fertility. Test matings showed that homozygous offspring were viable and produced in the expected frequency (Gonçalves et al. 1994).

THE BUCK

The male goat is called a buck or billy. Many dairy goat owners are offended by the term "billy," and Angora breeders are often confused by "buck" because in many parts of the United States, the ram (male sheep) is referred to as a buck.

The buck is frequently described as half of the breeding herd. Many owners find him the more difficult half to control. Because of his size and strength and his distinctive odor, the buck is often skipped when the does are dewormed, vaccinated, given selenium injections, or foot trimmed. Unless pens are massive and fences both sturdy and high, a resident buck breeds does earlier in the breeding season than desired and leaves no written records of his activities. Owners choosing to raise or purchase a buck for breeding would do well to read lay articles on the subject of buck management (Hicks 1987) before getting into this phase of goat husbandry.

Anatomy

The anatomy of the male goat's reproductive tract has been reviewed elsewhere (Smith 1986c; Garrett 1988; Constantinescu 2001). The scrotum is pendulous and in some animals it is divided to a greater or lesser extent into two sacs. There is little evidence that this trait (bipartite scrotum) is detrimental to fertility in the absence of other anatomic defects.

The testes are present in the scrotum at birth and are positioned with the longitudinal axis vertical. Approximately fifteen to twenty efferent tubules collect spermatozoa from the testis and join the head of the epididymis, which is located on the dorsolateral aspect of the testis. The body of the epididymis is caudal and slightly medial, and the tail of the epididymis, where semen is stored before ejaculation, is ventral. Blood is supplied to the testis by the testicular artery, which is precooled by its proximity to the pampiniform venous plexus in the spermatic cord. The cremaster muscles and smooth muscle in the wall of the scrotum also serve to control the testicular temperature by adjusting the position of the testis relative to the abdomen.

The deferent duct passes dorsally on the medial side of the testis and spermatic cord to the inguinal ring, then passes medial to the ureter and widens to form an ampulla before emptying into the pelvic urethra on the side of the seminal colliculus. The vesicular glands cover the dorsal aspect of the ampullae. Their excretory ducts open at the seminal colliculus, usually through common ejaculatory ducts and orifices that also serve the deferent ducts (Constantinescu 2001). The prostate gland is disseminated in the wall of the pelvic urethra and opens into its lumen by many small ducts. A recess extends caudodorsally from the urethra where the pelvic urethra turns ventrally after leaving the pelvic canal. The bulbourethral glands open into the lumen of the urethral recess, on the fold of mucous membrane that separates the recess from the pelvic urethra.

The bulb of the penis (corpus spongiosum penis) surrounds the penile urethra and is itself covered by the bulbospongiosus muscle ventral to the anus. There are two crura of the penis that are formed by the corpus cavernosum penis surrounded by the heavy tunica albuginea and are covered by the ischiocavernosus muscle, which is important for erection. The hemodynamics of penile erection have been reported by Beckett et al. (1972a, 1972b). Paired retractor penis muscles insert ventrally on the fibroelastic penis just distal to its prominent sigmoid flexure. The penis ends with the glans penis, but the urethra continues as the urethral process, which extends 3 or 4 cm past the glans.

Physiology and Sexual Development of the Male

Breed, age, and nutrition all contribute to the onset of sexual maturity. In Boer goats, spermatogenesis was found to begin as early as eighty-four days of age, with spermatozoa present in the epididymis at 140 days of age (Skinner 1970). In another study of twenty Boer goats, puberty (as defined by presence of spermatozoa in the ejaculate) was reached at 115 to 234 days (Louw and Joubert 1964). Fast-growing, well-fed kids are able to breed sooner than starved males born at the same time. In dairy breeds in the United States, many bucklings are fertile by five months of age, but successful breeding has occurred as early as three months of age. Some other breeds, under other management conditions, mature much later (Elwishy and Elsawaf 1971).

Natural adhesions of the urethral process and glans penis to the prepuce render the immature male incapable of copulation (Figure 13.10). Under the influence of testosterone, the urethral process becomes free, beginning at its tip, and finally the penis separates from the preputial mucosa (Skalet et al. 1988). This separation never occurs in the early-castrated wether.

Serum testosterone concentrations in normal bucks in temperate climates vary with the season; the highest are in the fall breeding season. Increases in testosterone are preceded by increases in luteinizing hormone from the pituitary. Testosterone rises earlier in bucks provided with a high quality diet than in those that are underfed (Walkden-Brown et al. 1994). Mean values in yearling pygmy goats in the fall reach 15 ng/ml (Muduuli et al. 1979). In an Australian study of six Angora bucks, the mean androgen level was approximately ten times more in March (10.25 ng/ml) than in July, at the end of the breeding season (1.05 ng/ml) (Ritar 1991). There is also a diurnal pattern (Bosu and Barker 1982), although this pattern was not consistent throughout the year in another study (Ritar 1991). In Black Bengal goats, higher testosterone concentrations have been reported in two- to three-month-old kids (7 ng/ml) than in three- to five-month-old (3 ng/ml) or mature bucks (5 ng/ml) (Georgie et al. 1985). When samples are taken for analysis, testosterone appears to be stable in the plasma or serum of bucks for at least twenty-four hours (Fahmi et al. 1985).

The buck odor, originating in part from sebaceous glands caudomedial to the horns, contributes to the breeding success of a male. The odor stimulates onset of cyclicity, demonstration of overt estrus, and receptivity in females. Bucks that were descented during disbudding may be ignored or rejected by some choosy does. The glands are testosterone responsive and the odor is most intense during the breeding season (Walkden-Brown et al. 1994).

Sexual behavior and sperm production also vary with season. In a French study, the percentage of bucks that failed to ejaculate increased to as high as 25% in the nonbreeding season, especially May to August. Testicular weight and total spermatozoa in the ejaculate also decreased out of season (Delgadillo et al. 1991). Similar seasonal variations have been seen in semen quality of dairy bucks in England (Ahmad and Noakes 1996b). Photoperiod control, alternating two months of long, sixteen-hour days with two months of short, eight-hour days, largely abolished the seasonality in sexual activity and semen characteristics (Delgadillo et al. 1991). This could be very useful for managing semen production by bucks at artificial insemination centers.

The effect of rearing conditions other than nutrition on the development of sexual activity in bucks has received little attention. In one study, twenty male goats at weaning were raised in individual pens and an additional sixteen male goats were group housed with four females of the same age that had been ovariectomized before puberty. Collection of semen with an artificial vagina was begun between seven and eight months of age. There was no difference in sexual behavior or sperm output between the two groups, but the average semen volume was significantly higher in the group-housed bucks, caused by increased seminal plasma (Orgeur et al. 1984). A "female effect," where exposure of bucks to estrous does stimulates pulsatile release of luteinizing hormone by the buck, with consequent increase in testosterone production, has also been noted (Gordon 1997).

Breeding Soundness Examination

The ability of the buck to be a successful, highly fertile breeder can never be guaranteed, but close evaluation should permit identification of problems that might interfere with fertility. This is ideally done several months before intended onset of breeding, so

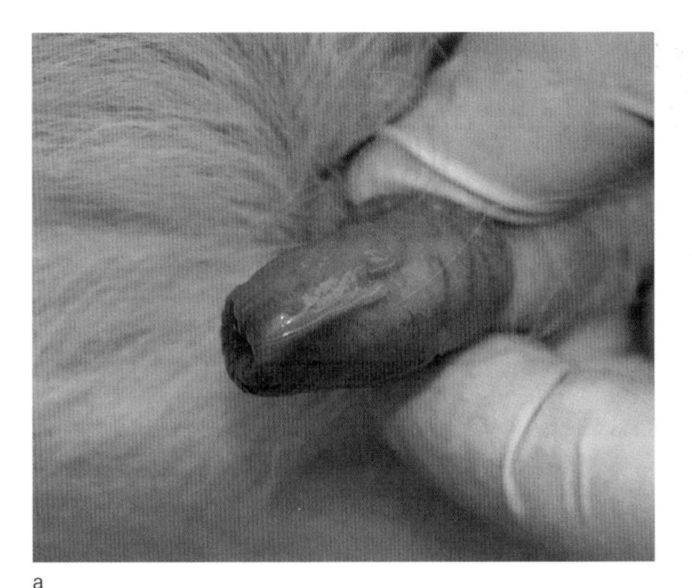

a

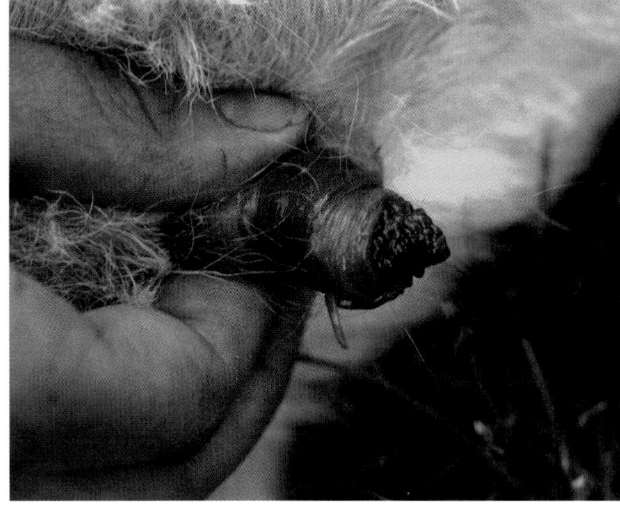

b

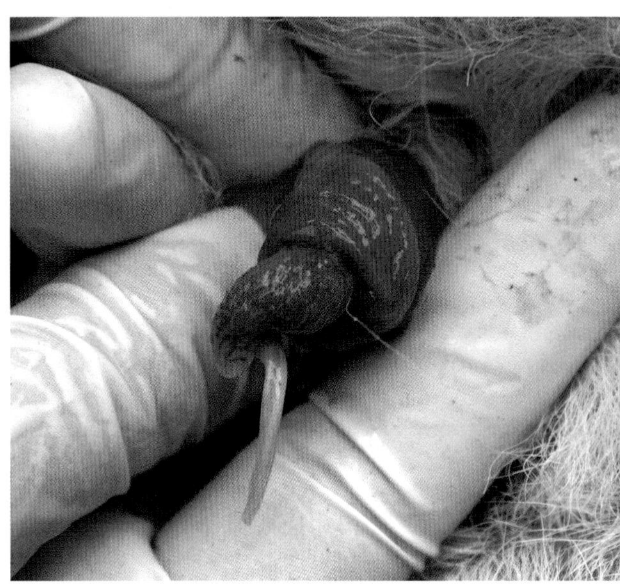

c

Figure 13.10. Normal maturation of the penis. a. The urethral process is completely adhered to the lining of the prepuce; b. separation of the urethral process and glans penis has begun, giving a striking, although normal, red cauliflower-like appearance; c. The urethral process and glans penis are completely separated from the prepuce, and intromission is now possible. (Courtesy Dr. M.C. Smith.)

that the buck can be treated or replaced if found to be "unsound." However, it is more difficult to evaluate libido outside the fall breeding season.

The Society for Theriogenology has developed scoring methods for evaluating the bull and ram. A formal system for the buck has not been widely used, and even the validity of those for the major species has been questioned (Ott 1987). It is inappropriate to assign points for each portion of the examination and then compare the total with an "acceptable" value. Superiority in one aspect of the evaluation does not compensate for poor performance elsewhere.

Physical Examination

The first portion of the breeding soundness examination is a thorough physical examination for general health (Ott 1978; Ott and Memon 1980; Memon et al. 2007). Body condition, color of mucous membranes, and sleekness of hair coat should be evaluated for evidence of parasitism, malnutrition, or chronic infection. Teeth, eyes, feet, and joints should be in good condition so that the buck can continue to eat well and can follow and mount the doe in estrus. The buck should be free of known genetic or possibly hereditary defects such as hernias, jaw malformations, or supernumerary teats. The presence of extra teats apparently has no relationship to the fertility of the buck (Schönherr 1956), but if the trait is passed to the next generation, the buck's offspring may be less suitable for milking. Next, the reproductive organs should be examined. This includes palpating the scrotal contents and inspecting the prepuce and penis for various abnormal conditions described in detail in later sections.

Scrotal Circumference

Although scrotal circumference or testicular diameter charts are lacking for most breeds of goats, it is reasonable to assume that, as for bulls and rams, the male with the larger testicular size at a given age is likely to produce more sperm. The risk that the goat has testicular hypoplasia or an intersex condition (polled intersex or freemartin) is also less when scrotal circumference is larger. It has been suggested that the habitual abortion trait in Angoras is associated with small testicular size (Van Heerden 1964).

Some researchers selecting sheep for accelerated lambing and year-round lambing programs believe that rams that show little seasonal (from October to April) decrease in scrotal circumference sire ewes that have less seasonal breeding tendencies (Ringwall et al. 1990). This possibility should be investigated in commercial goat herds striving for out-of-season breeding. Photoperiod effects appeared to account for a 2-cm difference in scrotal circumference in Alpine and Nubian bucks kept in environmental chambers (Nuti and McWhinney 1987).

The scrotal circumference can be measured with a specially designed metal tape (Lane Manufacturing Inc., Denver, Colorado) or with any other measuring tape or even a cord whose length can be compared with a ruler. The circumference is measured at the widest part of the scrotum with both testes held at the same level; it is important not to distract the testes by grasping the neck of the scrotum (Ott 1986; Memon et al. 2007). When bucks have similar age and bodyweight, those with above average scrotal circumference may be expected to produce offspring with earlier sexual maturity and greater fertility. Older bucks are expected to have larger testes and more sperm, but do not underestimate the potential breeding capacity of a young buck.

As an approximate guideline for dairy goat breeds in the United States, bucks weighing more than 40 kg should have a scrotal circumference of at least 25 cm. Bucks of British breeds had a mean scrotal circumference of 24 cm when they reached sexual maturity at five and a half months, but the value decreased several cm in the following January and February (Ahmad and Noakes 1996a, 1996b). In another study, the scrotal circumference of mature (three- to four-year old) Nubian bucks of proven fertility was 30 to 33 cm (Skalet et al. 1988). In ten young bucks of German breeds, the scrotal circumference was 24 to 28 cm in October, when the bucks were eight months old and weighed 26 to 52 kg. Scrotal circumference decreased a median of 3 cm when poor hay was fed for two months, then increased again by February with improved nutrition (Arbeiter 1963). A study of Creole goats found that nutrition, rather than photoperiod, determined scrotal circumference in this breed as managed locally (de la Vega 2006). Likewise, Australian cashmere bucks on a high-quality diet had markedly higher scrotal circumference than bucks fed a low quality diet. In both groups the testicular weight dropped through the fall breeding season (when voluntary feed intake was low) and reached a low point early in the winter (Walkden-Brown et al. 1994). In Jordan, Damascus goats had the largest scrotal circumference in the spring, when day length was increasing, which is their normal breeding season (Al-Ghalban et al. 2004). In a young, growing buck, a sudden increase in testicular size indicates the onset of spermatogenesis (Skinner 1970; Bongso et al. 1982).

As an alternative to scrotal circumference, scrotal volume can be measured by measuring the amount of water displaced when the scrotum is immersed. In one study of six Angora bucks, the scrotal volume peaked nine weeks after day length began to shorten (Ritar 1991).

Semen Collection

Collecting and evaluating semen (Eaton and Simmons 1952; Chemineau et al. 1991; Memon et al. 2007) comprise the final portion of the breeding soundness examination. The most representative semen samples for laboratory evaluation are obtained by artificial vagina (AV) (Barker 1958; Austin et al. 1968). The technique has been described elsewhere (Refsal 1986; Memon et al. 2007). Most bucks of normal libido in the breeding season try to mount any restrained goat, though a cycling doe treated two days previously with 5 mg of prostaglandin F2 alpha or a doe or wether treated with estrogen (1 mg estradiol administered one or two days previously) may make a more willing mount. Assuming that the temperature of the AV is appropriate (104°F to 113°F; 40°C to 45°C), even untrained dairy bucks can usually be collected without difficulty. The volume of an ejaculate is typically 0.5 to 1.5 ml.

Vocalization by the buck, contraction of voluntary muscles during electroejaculation, and the more dilute semen obtained make electroejaculation less desirable than the use of an AV (Greyling and Grobbelaar 1983; Memon et al. 1986a). It also is impossible to evaluate libido during electroejaculation. This technique, however, may be the only practical way to collect semen from a range buck (O'Brien et al. 1963). One report suggested (but certainly did not prove) that a sine-wave electroejaculator resulted in collection of more sperm with less distress to the buck than a pulse-wave electroejaculator (Carter et al. 1990). The animal is initially set up on its hindquarters to extrude the penis, which can be prevented from retracting by wrapping it in gauze clamped in place with a spring paper clip.

Induction of erection and ejaculation in bucks, rams, and bulls by massage of the glans penis within the sheath has been described (Megale 1968). The animal should be standing unrestrained in a quiet environment. After the penis is extruded from the preputial orifice, ejaculation may occur spontaneously (into a funnel) or semen can be collected with an artificial vagina.

SPERM MORPHOLOGY. Morphology should be carefully evaluated. Previously, sperm abnormalities were designated to be primary if they were thought to have originated in the seminiferous epithelium (i.e., abnormal head shape, abnormal acrosome, midpiece abnormalities, strongly coiled tails) or secondary if they were thought to have occurred in the epididymis (i.e., proximal and distal cytoplasmic droplets, tailless heads, single bent tails). Newer work in bulls favors designation of the various abnormalities as major or minor (Ott 1986). It is not yet known which morphologic abnormalities are of greatest significance relative to buck fertility.

Many veterinarians mix eosin nigrosin stain with a drop of semen on a slide and quickly draw the mixture out with another slide to create a smear. Evaluation of the air-dried smear with a bright-field microscope allows differentiation of live (appearing white) sperm from dead ones (red because of uptake of eosin) as well as visualization of many morphologic defects. The use of formol saline, or glutaraldehyde fixation (without staining) and a phase contrast microscope permits detection of more abnormalities. So will greater experience with semen evaluation. It is best to count at least 200 spermatozoa per sample. The number of each type of abnormality should be recorded. If the first sample yields unsatisfactory spermatozoa, a second sample should be collected on the same day (Schönherr 1956). Repeated semen evaluations during several months may be necessary to establish an accurate prognosis. In particular, a variety of febrile diseases may be followed by poor semen quality that lasts for as long as two months.

A high prevalence of morphologic abnormalities may be associated with either sexual immaturity or degenerative changes. Arbeiter (1964) found 15% abnormal sperm in 144 ejaculates from nine healthy German bucks initially nine months old. In a two-year study of four "yearling" dairy bucks collected multiple times in fall (November) of two successive years, the percent of abnormal acrosomes and of most other sperm abnormalities was decreased the second year (Chandler et al. 1988). In one study involving Nubian bucks, 65% of sperm cells were abnormal at the onset of puberty but only 12% were abnormal by eight months of age (Skalet et al. 1988). Misshapen heads, abnormal midpieces (abaxial, double, coiled, bent, looped) and proximal droplets were common in the young bucks. By eight months of age, only the midpiece abnormalities were common. Dead sperm are more common in the semen of young bucks in spring and summer than in fall and winter (Ahmad and Noakes 1996b).

In older bucks, the season did not influence sperm abnormalities. Likewise, no seasonal effect on sperm morphology was observed in bucks of native breeds in India (Sahni and Roy 1972) although small increases in percentage of abnormal spermatozoa were noted in bucks in Greece in the nonbreeding season (Karagiannidis et al. 2000). However, it has been shown that in hot climates, bucks with a divided scrotum (each testis in a separate scrotal pouch) produce sperm with fewer morphologic abnormalities, presumably because of enhanced cooling. The average percentage of sperm abnormalities was 5.4% for six Moxotó bucks with a divided scrotum and 32.9% for four bucks with no scrotal division collected during the dry season (Nunes et al. 1983). The percentage of live sperm was decreased in the dry season compared with the rainy season, and sperm abnormalities were increased in the dry season (Silva and Nunes 1988).

Few reports are available on the influence of disease on semen quality. Detached heads, tightly coiled tails, and thickened midpieces were prominent in semen samples from an eighteen-month-old infertile LaMancha buck with testicular degeneration (Refsal et al. 1983). Detached heads and acrosomal defects were increased in goat semen after fever was induced by an injection of Freund's complete adjuvant (Yokoki and Akira 1977). Detached heads were also common (70% of the spermatozoa) in the semen of a Nubian buck with seminal vesiculitis diagnosed by histology (Ahmad et al. 1993). Semen changes associated with various infections are described in the discussion of the individual diseases.

SEMEN MOTILITY AND CONCENTRATION. Motility has received much attention in the past. Because it is very difficult to optimally maintain conditions such as temperature, it is common for normal semen (expected motility of 70% to 90%) to have very poor motility when examined under field conditions. Thus, motility is no longer considered to be an important part of the breeding soundness examination. Concentration of spermatozoa in semen of bucks collected by artificial vagina should be estimated. This can be done by hemocytometer techniques or measurement of optical density, after the instrument is calibrated for buck semen. Concentrations of 2.5 to 3 billion/ml are normal (Eaton and Simmons 1952). Concentration decreases somewhat with more frequent electroejaculation (Oyeyemi et al. 2001).

An approximation of concentration can be determined by spinning the semen for ten minutes in a microhematocrit centrifuge (Foote 1958). One spermatocrit point represents approximately 200 × 10^6 sperm/ml (Foote, 1992). Spermatocrits of 25 to 33 in normal bucks have been observed by the author. A commercial Unopette system (Becton-Dickinson, Rutherford, NJ) can also be used to estimate sperm concentration (Memon et al. 2007). The yellow color often seen in the seminal plasma is caused by riboflavin (Mendoza et al. 1989; Ahmad and Noakes 1996b) and does not influence semen quality.

Processing Semen for Artificial Insemination

Undiluted fresh semen can be used for artificial insemination when the buck and does are on the same premises, but usually the semen is extended for short- or long-term storage. Methods of semen preservation and insemination have been described elsewhere (Corteel 1981; Haibel 1986b; Leboeuf et al. 2000; Purdy 2006; Nuti 2007). Skim milk (such as UHT milk) -based extenders are often used. High concentrations of egg yolk should not be used in an extender for unwashed semen because a lipase enzyme secreted by the bulbourethral glands (Chemineau et al. 1999) hydrolyzes egg yolk lecithins to products that are toxic to sperm. When semen is to be kept frozen for many months, washing the spermatozoa to remove most of the seminal plasma before freezing has sometimes improved fertility, especially with breeds or seasons when the original ejaculate volume was small (Corteel 1981; Corteel et al. 1984). Nonbreeding season seminal plasma is more detrimental to post-thaw motility than breeding season seminal plasma (Leboeuf et al. 2000). Photoperiod treatment (alternating two months of long days with two months of short days) alleviates adverse effects of the nonbreeding season on post-thaw semen quality (Chemineau et al. 1999).

Although fertility was low, cryopreserved epididymal sperm collected from postpubertal bucks at necropsy has been successful in producing a pregnancy (Blash et al. 2000).

TESTICULAR AND EPIDIDYMAL ABNORMALITIES

Except for changes induced by fever or malnutrition, most abnormalities are not amenable to treatment.

Procedures for Evaluating Testis and Epididymis

In addition to judging the testicular volume by scrotal circumference or the diameter of each testis by the use of calipers, the consistency of the testes should be evaluated. Normal testicular tissue should feel resilient and approximately as firm as muscle. Its ultrasonographic appearance is uniformly homogeneous with a central hyperechoic line representing the mediastinum testis. The testicular tunics and testicular capsule are also distinct hyperechoic lines, whereas fluid around the testis (hydrocele) is hypoechoic (Eilts et al. 1989). The tail of the epididymis is more heterogeneous and less echogenic than the testis (Ahmad et al. 1991). The use of ultrasonography for evaluating testicular lesions has also been described for bulls (Pechman and Eilts 1987; Powe et al. 1988).

Testicular biopsy is not routinely used in goats. In bulls, biopsy procedures have led to decreased semen quality. It is important to avoid highly vascular areas and to suture the incision in the tunica albuginea, or else hemorrhage and infarction may occur (McEntee 1990).

Testicular Atrophy or Degeneration

A common cause of testicular degeneration is debility from malnutrition or parasitism (Memon 1983). The chronically recumbent buck might also experience testicular atrophy because of impaired thermoregulation in the scrotum. Sperm granulomas (see below) cause progressive testicular degeneration. Testicular atrophy of unknown etiology but accompanied by abnormal spermatozoa appears to be common in some goat populations. The testes often are more elongated and smaller than normal. The head of the epididymis may undergo a palpable loss in lobulation (Fraser 1971). Multiple foci of calcinosis are grossly visible on cut surfaces of the testis. Histologically, granuloma formation occurs where masses of dead sperm have accumulated in collecting ducts (Fraser and Wilson 1966).

Foci of testicular necrosis or mineralization are hyperechoic during ultrasonographic examination but only the echogenicity of the near-field testis should be assessed, because of attenuation of the far-field ultrasound beam. Firm, mineralized parenchyma, detectable by ultrasound, has been observed in elderly or infertile bucks (Buckrell 1988). These changes are irreversible. Testicular neoplasia, although rare in goats, should also be detectable by ultrasonography.

Atrophy and degeneration of the seminiferous tubules have been reported in goats in the Sudan experimentally fed *Acanthospermum hispidum*, which also causes hepatic necrosis and fibrosis (Ali and Adam 1978). Likewise, the feeding of *Leucaena leucocephala* is reported to cause mild degeneration of the testes. (Rajan et al. 1991), possibly secondary to hypothyroidism. Experimental hypothyroidism in goats (achieved by feeding thiouracil) was associated with a relative decrease in the weight of the testis and epididymis, a reduction in spermatogenesis, and degenerative changes in the testis and accessory sex glands. There was loss of libido, decreased ejaculate volume, and decreased sperm concentration, motility, and viability, and an increase in abnormal spermatozoa. These changes were reversible (Sreekumaran and Rajan 1978;

Reddi and Rajan 1985, 1986). Thyroidectomy in young male goats also results in smaller than normal testes (Reineke et al. 1941). Detrimental effects of naturally occurring hypothyroidism on testicular function in adult goats have not been documented. Additional discussion of thyroid function and goiter is provided in Chapter 3.

Testicular Hypoplasia

Abnormally small testes most commonly occur with severe malnutrition (Neathery et al. 1973) or in animals that are actually intersexes (i.e., polled intersexes or freemartins). Hypoplasia is often difficult to distinguish from atrophy, but with either condition, testicular size and function should improve with proper feeding if malnutrition is responsible. Intersexes and freemartins do not produce any sperm at all, even in the breeding season, and generally are less odoriferous than normal bucks. Their testes do not undergo the increase in size that normally occurs at puberty, or else the testes may atrophy at that time.

One case of testicular hypoplasia has been reported in a horned buck with chromosomal mosaicism (XXY and XY) (Jorge and Takebayasi 1987). Two sterile polled bucks with a Robertsonian translocation were found to have normal seminiferous tubules interspersed with tubules devoid of germinal cells (Ricordeau 1972). Histologically, similar findings have been reported in polled bucks with sperm granulomas obstructing the epididymis but with normal karyotype (Corteel et al. 1969).

Bucks with severe experimental zinc deficiency compounded by reduced feed intake and control bucks with just reduced feed intake in the same trial showed normal tubules adjacent to tubules containing only spermatogonia (Neathery et al. 1973). A secondary zinc deficiency, caused by excessive fertilization of fields, resulted in atrophy of the seminiferous tubules, hyperplasia of the germinal epithelium, and thickening of the walls of blood vessels in the testes of young Black Bengal bucks (Ray et al. 1997).

Unilateral testicular hypoplasia (in males producing sperm) has been reported in two goats in India (Mathew and Raja 1978b) and in a polled Saanen XY buck in the United States (Sponenberg et al. 1983). In the Indian bucks, spermatogenesis only progressed to the formation of spermatocytes, while in the latter case, some seminiferous tubules in the affected testis were devoid of sperm cells while others were normal. Three additional bucks (horned feral animals) in Australia with unilateral hypoplasia had small seminiferous tubules lined by Sertoli cells (Tarigan et al. 1990). A unilateral segmental tubular hypoplasia in a testis of normal size but with discrete pale areas on section also has been observed in two animals in this Australian slaughterhouse survey of 1,000 bucks.

Cryptorchidism

Intersex animals, as discussed previously, may exhibit retained testes or ovotestes. The gonad may be abdominal or inguinal in location. The animals are usually genetic females or freemartins. No sperm are produced.

Failure of one testis to descend into the scrotum has been reported frequently in Angora goats. Bilateral cryptorchidism appears to be rare in this breed. The cryptorchid goat is sometimes referred to as a "ridgling."

Etiology

Cryptorchidism is hereditary in Angora goats but is not related to the polled intersex condition, which does not occur in this breed. Affected Angoras are genetic males (Skinner et al. 1972). The cryptorchid trait is recessive but controlled by a few pairs of genes (Warwick 1961). In other breeds, cryptorchidism in XY males occurs occasionally, and although less is known about the etiology, a genetic explanation is probable.

Clinical Signs and Surgical or Necropsy Findings

The testes normally descend into the scrotum by twelve to thirteen weeks of gestation (Sivalchelvan et al. 1996). Cryptorchidism is detectable at birth. If the condition is bilateral, no scrotum is present. In Texas Angoras (Lush et al. 1930) and in Indian goats of unspecified breed (Mathew and Raja 1978a), the right testis was retained, whereas in South African Angoras, the left testis was retained (Skinner et al. 1972). In one research farm in India, six of eighty-nine Tellicherry bucks born during a four-year period were unilaterally cryptorchid. In five of these the right testis was retained (Murali et al. 2005). In a slaughterhouse study in Ethiopia, twenty-two of 404 (5.5%) horned native breed bucks were cryptorchid; eighteen of these were unilateral and ten involved the right testis (Regassa et al. 2003). The unilaterally affected buck is generally fertile, although semen volume and sperm concentration are reduced. Mohair quality in cryptorchid Angoras is normal.

In the unilateral cryptorchid, the retained testis is often located near the kidney. In two Anglo-Nubian bucks in Brazil with unilateral cryptorchidism, the retained testis (one left, one right) was located at the entrance to the inguinal canal (Vinha and Humenhuk 1976). If castration is required, as for a pet animal, the location of the testis can be confirmed before surgery by ultrasound. The tunica albuginea of the retained testis is echogenic and clearly demarcates it from surrounding tissue (Kaulfuss 2006). This testis is generally smaller than the scrotal testis.

The cryptorchid testis resembles a prepuberal testis histologically. Sertoli cell degeneration has been described in the cryptorchid testis in West African dwarf goats (Ezeasor and Singh 1987), whereas tubular degeneration and Sertoli cell hyperplasia have been reported in two cryptorchid feral goats in Australia (Tarigan et al. 1990).

Prevention

The prevalence of the condition in a flock varies with the selection pressure against it, often approximately 2% but as much as 10% in commercial herds and more than 60% when cryptorchids are intentionally bred. Breeders wishing to sell bucks realize that a unilateral cryptorchid is of little commercial value. To decrease the prevalence of the condition, cryptorchid bucks should not be used for breeding and their sires and dams should also be culled. Even stricter selection involves culling all offspring of known carriers (Warwick 1961).

Persistent Müllerian Duct Syndrome

A single male (60, XY) Nubian goat with bilateral cryptorchidism and persistent Müllerian duct syndrome has been described (Haibel and Rojko 1990). Hypoplastic testes, rudimentary epididymides, and a bicornuate uterus were present. Vesicular glands, bulbourethral glands, and penis resembled those of a normal male. Similar syndromes are seen in Miniature Schnauzers and human males and are thought to be associated with a lack of either secretion of or receptors for Müllerian inhibiting substance, normally of fetal Sertoli cell origin.

Infectious Diseases Causing Orchitis and Epididymitis

Bacterial orchitis and epididymitis are far less common in goats than in sheep. Expected clinical findings include swelling, increased heat, and pain on palpation of the testis. The semen may contain pus and the percentage of live spermatozoa drops. In one case report, transrectal ultrasonography also demonstrated changes in the echogenicity of the seminal vesicles (Santiago Moreno et al. 1996).

Coliform bacteria and *Pseudomonas* have been cultured from ejaculates of young bucks. Coliforms have caused both orchitis and epididymitis when injected into the testis (Löliger 1956, 1957). *Actinobacillus seminis* was isolated from four of forty Angora bucks examined in South Africa, but details as to clinical presentation were not supplied (Van Tonder 1975). When pathologic changes are not palpable, they might be suspected based on the presence of increased leukocytes in the semen. The major differential diagnosis is the nonsuppurative sperm granuloma originating from a malformation of the epididymis.

In one five-year-old buck, unilateral testicular enlargement progressed to five times the normal size. The animal was inappetent and walked with a stiff, straddling gait. The affected testis was firm and fixed in the scrotum. *Staphylococcus pyogenes* was isolated from a purulent epididymitis at time of unilateral castration. Involvement of the second testis was obvious within three weeks (Jackson and White 1982). In another report, *Corynebacterium pseudotuberculosis* was associated with epididymitis and orchitis in two bucks in Brazil (Alves et al. 2004). *Burkholderia (Pseudomonas) pseudomallei* caused orchitis and peri-orchitis in a buck (Fatimah et al. 1984). The buck was inappetent and the swollen testes developed pyogranulomas. There was no response to antibiotic therapy.

Mycoplasma putrefaciens was isolated from the testes of a buck that died during a severe herd outbreak of contagious agalactia with concomitant infection with *M. agalactiae* and *M. putrefaciens*. Spermatozoa were absent in seminiferous tubules and there was calcification and loss of germinative epithelium, with only Sertoli cells remaining (Gil et al. 2003).

Brucellosis

Brucella ovis is an important cause of epididymitis and orchitis in sheep. Stamps stain can be used to demonstrate the organism in semen smears, and white blood cells and detached heads are commonly found in the semen. This organism is not recognized as a cause of natural infections in goats. Experimental infection of bucks by conjunctival or intrapreputial inoculation of this organism has led to clinical and histological epididymitis, transient infection, and serologic response (García-Carrillo et al. 1974). In a subsequent trial, the organism was isolated from the semen of one of fifteen goats (García-Carrillo et al. 1977). In another experiment, inoculation of *B. ovis* onto the preputial epithelium (two yearling goats) and nasal mucosa (two goats) led to an antibody response best detected by enzyme-linked immunoabsorbent assay but also (in three animals) by CF testing. One intranasally inoculated buck persistently shed *B. ovis* and white cells in semen. The experiment was concluded at ninety-eight days, when chronic epididymitis and seminal vesiculitis were demonstrated only in the goat that had excreted organisms (Burgess et al. 1985). Thus, if bucks engage in homosexual activity with infected rams there is some potential for transmission to occur.

Brucella melitensis occasionally causes orchitis in bucks (Dubois 1911). The Rev 1 vaccine strain has also caused orchitis in a buck kid vaccinated at five months of age (Tolari and Salvi 1980). In South Africa, where the Rev 1 *melitensis* vaccine has been used to control *Brucella ovis* in sheep, orchitis and epididymitis have developed in Angora bucks soon after vaccination (Vermeulen et al. 1988). The authors failed to create clinical disease in bucks by experimental infection with *Brucella ovis* and concluded that bucks should not be vaccinated unless *B. ovis* has been confirmed on the farm or *B. melitensis* is causing abortions in the herd.

Trypanosomosis

Trypanosoma brucei and *T. vivax* have been associated with inflammatory and degenerative changes in the testis and epididymis of sheep and goats in Africa. After experimental infection with *T. brucei* (in rams), persistent scrotal edema and a nonsuppurative granulomatous periorchitis developed associated with tissue invasion by the parasite. Trypanosomes were readily detected in fluid from the scrotal sac. Secondary degenerative changes in the testis included atrophy and calcification of seminiferous tubules and intertubular sclerosis (Isoun and Anosa 1974; Ikede 1979). In bucks experimentally infected with *T. vivax*, organisms were not seen outside blood vessels in the testes and it was postulated that testicular degeneration occurred because of recurrent fever (Anosa and Isoun 1980). Affected animals are expected to have low fertility until some time after the infection has cleared.

Experimental infection of bucks with *Trypanosoma evansi* also caused microthrombi in testicular blood vessels, severe mononuclear cell infiltration in the epididymis and testicular interstitium, and subsequent dystrophic mineralization. The number of abnormal and dead sperm increased greatly, and bucks with clinical orchitis became aspermic (Ngeranwa et al. 1991). A later experimental infection of bucks with an equine isolate of the same organism caused scrotal edema in 20%, degeneration of spermatogonia and Sertoli cells, and infiltration of the testes with macrophages and lymphoid cells (Dargantes et al. 2005). Experimental infection of bucks with *Trypanosoma congolense*, a plasma parasite that does not invade tissue, also has caused testicular degeneration with marked shrinking of seminiferous tubules and epididymides, but the pathogenesis is unknown (Kaaya and Oduor-Okelo 1980). Trypanosomosis is described in Chapter 7.

Besnoitiosis

There is one report of a buck in Africa with masses of *Besnoitia* cysts in the wall and lumen of veins and arteries of the pampiniform plexus; parasitic cysts were also present in the epididymis and testis. Thrombosis of vessels, absence of sperm production, and extensive testicular fibrosis were believed to be caused by the parasite (Bwangamoi et al. 1989). Encrustation of the scrotum and presence of numerous *Besnoitia* cysts in the tunica vaginalis, tunica albuginea, and interstitium of the epididymis were reported from two male wild goats in Iran (Cheema and Toofanian 1979). The existence of a distinct species, *Besnoitia caprae*, has been proposed in Kenya, where cattle housed with infected goats do not develop besnoitiosis (Njenga, J.M., et al. 1993).

Sperm Granulomas

Obstruction of the head of the epididymis is a common cause of infertility in polled male (XY genotype) goats (Hamerton et al. 1969). Bucks of the Damascus breed in Jordan have higher reproductive capabilities when horned rather than polled (Al-Ghalban et al. 2004), but sperm granulomas have not been documented in this breed.

Etiology and Pathogenesis

This condition is believed to be hereditary and recessive, with incomplete penetrance (estimated in one study as 0.55) (Ricordeau et al. 1972a). An early theory that the problem was caused by excessive nutrient intake by the young buck came about because better nutrition leads to earlier puberty and thus earlier expression of the problem. Other early theories included psychological factors and abnormal thyroid function (Schönherr 1956).

The normal head of the epididymis forms from the union of approximately sixteen to nineteen efferent ductules (Hemeida et al. 1978). The direct cause of the obstruction is believed to be one or more of these ductules that end blindly (Machens 1937). The ducts become distended with inspissated sperm until rupture occurs and sperm are released into the stroma of the epididymis (Figure 13.11). A severe inflammatory reaction with lymphocytes and giant cells occurs in response to the sperm cells and eventually a granuloma forms. The granuloma may calcify. Epididymal ducts that were previously patent may become obstructed by the

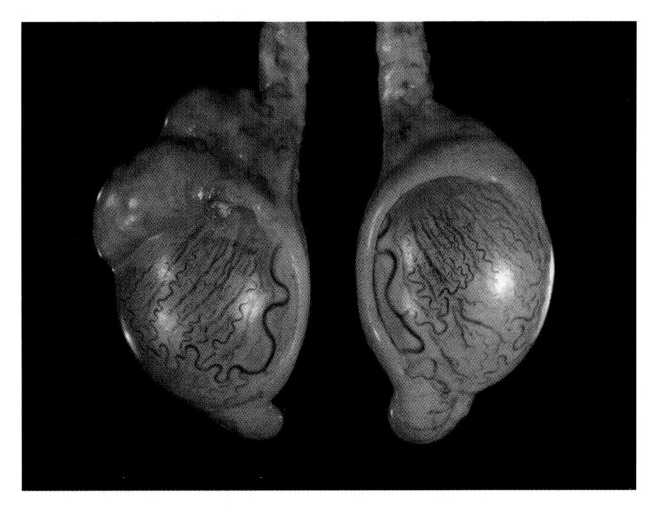

Figure 13.11. Sperm granuloma in the head of the epididymis of the testis on the left, from a polled buck. (Courtesy Dr. M.C. Smith.)

granuloma (by compression or fibrosis) (Machens 1937). Back pressure eventually leads to degeneration and even mineralization of the testicular stroma (Corteel et al. 1969; Soller et al. 1969).

A partially split scrotum has been associated with increased frequency of sperm granulomas in Germany (Schönherr 1956), but appears to be a desirable trait in breeds native to very hot climates, where cooling of the testes is facilitated.

Clinical Signs and Diagnosis

Some animals are sterile from the beginning because all of the efferent ducts are affected. Others are initially fertile but become infertile if bilateral granulomas form. Normal libido persists.

By the end stage, both the firm granuloma (lentil- to egg-sized) in the head of the epididymis and the reduced size of the testis are palpable. Less commonly, granulomas form in the body or tail of the epididymis. Normal epididymis is clearly softer than normal testis (München 1951). In ultrasonographic evaluations, appearance of sperm granulomas (in a ram) has been described as fluid-filled structures within a ring of echogenic tissue (Buckrell 1988). Ultrasound examination is also useful for demonstrating testicular mineralization, the end stage of degeneration induced by back pressure.

Correction of this defect is not possible. The diagnosis can be confirmed by gross and histological examination after castration or slaughter.

Prevention

Because sperm granulomas are very strongly correlated with the homozygous polled condition, breeders can avoid the expense of raising animals that will be (or become) sterile because of this defect by culling all young bucks that are by phenotype homozygous for the polled gene. These bucks have very smooth, well-separated protuberances on the poll. Heterozygous bucks, in contrast, typically have bean-shaped protuberances that converge anteriorly and many have irregular horny bosses that become evident by three to six months of age (Ricordeau et al. 1972b). If polled bucks are kept for breeding, their potential fertility should be monitored regularly by palpation and semen evaluation.

Segmental Aplasia of the Epididymis

In a slaughterhouse study of one hundred bucks in Brazil, three were found to have segmental aplasia of the body of the epididymis. One buck was affected bilaterally. Two bucks were horned and one (Moxotó breed) was polled. The head of the epididymis was distended, the body could not be palpated, and the tail was reduced in size (Humenhuk and Vinha 1976).

Scrotal Hernia

Scrotal and inguinal hernias have not been described in goats, but are seen in sheep and generally presumed to be hereditary in that species. Clinical signs include distension of one side of the scrotum with a freely movable, fluctuant loop of intestine. If a hernia is identified in a buck and surgical correction is desired, the buck should be castrated bilaterally.

Other Scrotal Lesions

Wounds (shearing cuts, dog bites, vasectomy) involving the scrotum may result in establishment of a purulent orchitis or periorchitis. Fly strike and grass awn migration might also occur, although these conditions are better described in rams. Some breeders in Texas believe that a split scrotum increases the risk of injury to the scrotum by burrs or brambles (Drummond 1988). Other causes of scrotal dermatitis include mange (Kambarage 1992), bacterial infections, zinc deficiency, and frostbite; the reader is referred to Chapter 2.

Elastosis and fibroblastic proliferation of the intima of the testicular artery have been observed in goats, as has calcification of the wall of the testicular artery and veins (Panebianco et al. 1985). Possible effects of these vascular lesions on fertility are unclear. Varicocele does not seem to have been reported in goats.

PENILE AND PREPUTIAL ABNORMALITIES

Examination of the penis is most easily performed with the buck positioned on his rump. Tranquilization may be helpful, because goats rarely rest quietly in the sitting position. The shaft of the penis is pushed anteriorly with one hand while the prepuce is pushed posteriorly with the other hand. The young buck kid is held in a sitting position in the examiner's lap, with legs pointing away from the person, to facilitate exteriorization and examination of the penis.

Malformations

Most congenital malformations (i.e., hypospadias [Al-Ani et al. 1998], shortened penis of some intersexes) are easily detected by physical examination. Congenital diverticula in the urethra were associated with swelling of the ventral sheath and continuous dribbling of urine in eleven goat kids two to six months of age in India. Ten of these animals also had a completely divided scrotum. The animals recovered after surgical excision of the diverticula (Gahlot et al. 1982).

Maturation of the Penis

When the sexual maturity of a male is questioned (e.g., during a breeding soundness exam or when he has inadvertently gained access to females that were not to be bred), the penis should be carefully examined. As long as the urethral process and glans penis are adhered to the prepuce, successful copulation is unlikely to occur. These adhesions, normal in the immature buck, break down with testosterone, time, and good nutrition.

Injuries

Traumatic hematoma of the penis is rare in small ruminants; a single case report describes successful surgical treatment in a buck with return to normal breeding (Bani Ismail and Ababneh 2007). The presence of a hair ring (accumulation of loosely matted hairs) around the shaft of the penis may be accompanied by irritation (Tarigan et al. 1990). Grass awns in the prepuce can also cause irritation.

Loss of the urethral process is a common shearing accident in Angoras. If the urethral process is absent but the glans penis is intact and normal, no direct adverse effect on fertility is expected (Ott 1978). In other goat breeds, a previous bout of urolithiasis is usually responsible for loss of the urethral process. Re-obstruction at a later date may endanger the buck's life or fertility. There also might be an increased risk of contamination of the semen by urine, caused by damage to sphincter muscles during obstruction. There is a single report of erection failure in a Nubian buck after urolithiasis, secondary to a vascular obstruction in the corpus cavernosum penis (Todhunter et al. 1996). Urolithiasis is discussed in Chapter 12.

Posthitis

Posthitis, the inflammatory condition of the prepuce also termed "pizzle rot," often results from overgrowth of urea-splitting bacteria in the prepuce of males consuming excessive dietary protein. Free ammonia scalds the preputial and penile mucosa. Wethers appear to be more susceptible than intact males (Shelton and Livingston 1975). This condition is discussed in Chapter 12.

Pustules and ulcers on the prepuce and penis of bucks have been ascribed to caprine herpesvirus-1, which is associated with abortion and with vulvovaginitis in does (Tarigan et al. 1987; Uzal et al. 2004). The gross appearance varies with the extent of secondary bacterial infection. Histologically, findings of acidophilic intranuclear inclusion bodies and chromatin margination in epithelial cells adjacent to the ulcers are considered highly suggestive of the herpesvirus infection (Tarigan et al. 1990). It is also reported that bucks that spread the infection to does during mating may remain free of clinical signs (Grewal and Wells 1986). This condition is discussed further in Chapter 12.

Trichomoniasis

Trichomonad protozoa have been observed in large numbers in the semen of Alpine and Saanen bucks in France and Sardinia and in Angoras in South Africa. The parasite, which is approximately the size of a sperm head, infests the sheath and urethra. Quantity and quality of ejaculates are decreased, as is libido. The infections have been treated successfully with dimetridazole (3 or 5 g, divided into three intravenous doses at twenty-four-hour intervals), but use of this drug is currently illegal in goats in the United States. Routine treatment of all bucks in the artificial insemination centers in France each summer, before the season of semen collection, has been proposed as an alternative to repeated testing of each buck (Corteel 1991). Effects of this organism on the doe have not been elucidated and recent reports of the condition are lacking.

OTHER PROBLEMS AFFECTING THE BUCK

Poor Libido

Mounting and thrusting behavior, sniffing of the anogenital region, and flehmen are well established as common behaviors of normal goat kids of both sexes before the age of one month (Sambraus 1971). Normal libido, then, although necessary for fertility, is clearly not sufficient.

In the anestrous season it may be difficult to obtain an ejaculate by artificial vagina or the buck may be very slow to serve a doe in heat. The buck may rest his head on the doe's hindquarters but fail to align himself with the longitudinal axis of the doe. Proper alignment is gradually approached as the breeding season nears (Fraser 1964). If heat detection is all that is needed, a doe or wether can be treated with testosterone propionate (100 mg every three days) until male behavior is observed. Testosterone is a controlled substance in the United States. Additionally, extralabel drug use for production purposes is not permitted.

Testosterone should not be given to the breeding buck because of its negative feedback effect on sperm production. Instead, the buck to be used out of season should be prepared in advance by a light treatment at the same time the does are exposed to a nineteen- to twenty-hour photoperiod. Daily training with a doe treated with estrogen may increase libido as the planned breeding time approaches (Van der Westhuysen et al. 1988), or else eCG (500 IU once) (Skinner and Hofmeyr 1969) or GnRH (40 µg every eight hours for four days) (Minnia et al. 1987) may be administered to the buck.

Gynecomastia

Development of mammary glands in bucks is occasionally observed (Heidrich and Renk 1967). The best description of the condition comes from the German literature.

Etiology and Pathogenesis

One documented case involved a polled one-and-a-half-year-old fertile male Fawn German goat (Deutsche bunte Edelziege) that yielded 20 ml of milk daily. The animal was determined to be a chromosomal mosaic with variable deletions of the Y chromosome (XO/XY) (Rieck et al. 1975). The authors suggested that gynecomastia might be an early sign of feminization, analogous to the XO/XY condition in humans. Another buck that yielded 250 to 300 ml of milk per day had drum sticks in 45% of neutrophil nuclei, suggesting a genetic intersex, but karyotyping was not performed (Panchadevi and Pandit 1979).

Earlier reports of gynecomastia in bucks do not include karyotype (Harms 1937; Ullner 1961; Hamori 1983). Presumably, a variety of conditions disturbing the endocrine balances in a goat (i.e., hypophyseal, testicular, or adrenal abnormalities, administration of exogenous hormones) could be accompanied by gynecomastia. For example, a six-year-old Toggenburg wether of normal (60, XY) karyotype developed gynecomastia that was traced to estradiol 17 beta production from an adrenal adenoma (Lofstedt et al. 1994). Another fertile Toggenburg buck with normal karyotype had normal plasma testosterone and estradiol concentrations but prolactin was markedly elevated (Janett et al. 1996). A fertile Nubian buck with gynecomastia associated with hyperplasia of acidophilic cells in the pituitary has also been reported (Buergelt 1997). Some case reports lack hormonal studies (Al Jassim and Khamas 1997).

In England, mammary gland development is seen in bucks from high producing lines of British Saanens (Matthews 1991). The phenomenon is usually observed in the summer and fertility is unaffected. This suggests a genetic basis and perhaps an increased production of hormones or an increased sensitivity of mammary tissue to normal hormones.

Clinical Signs

Polled intersex goats (genetic females) that have a masculine phenotype are best excluded from this discussion. Thus, if a given "male" animal has no history of being fertile, the discussion of intersexes should be consulted. Unfortunately, early writers considered gynecomastia to be just another expression of the intersex problem. In affected fertile bucks, the teats are enlarged and the mammary gland is developed to a variable, often asymmetrical, degree (Figure 13.12). There is true glandular development rather than just local fat deposition. These signs generally appear after sexual maturity is reached. Analysis of the milk has disclosed no major differences from milk of does. There appear to be seasonal variations in milk production as production is lower during the breeding season.

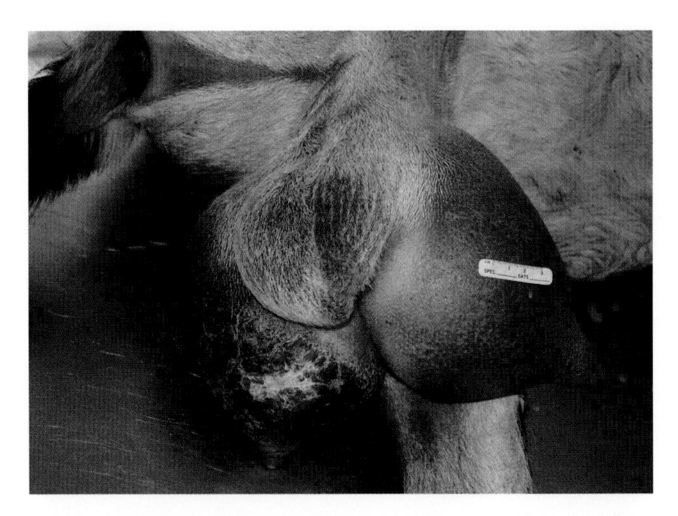

Figure 13.12. Gynecomastia in a five-year-old Nubian buck. Although initially fertile, severe chronic mastitis led to weight loss and testicular degeneration. (Courtesy Dr. M.C. Smith.)

Several animals that have been followed closely showed a progressive decline in libido and semen quality (Ullner 1961). At time of slaughter, mineralization of the testicular parenchyma has been identified. The authors were unable to determine if the testicular lesions preceded (and might have caused) the gynecomastia. In another study, milk secretion by four mature bucks could not be associated with reduced fertility (Schönherr 1956).

Treatment and Control

Reducing the protein and energy levels in the feed during the summer has been suggested for managing gynecomastia in bucks from high producing lines. This may reduce the risk of mastitis (Matthews 1991). Apparently the superior milk production of the daughters of these bucks discourages culling, though gynecomastia occurs in the male offspring.

No specific treatment has been suggested that might not be detrimental to fertility. Amputation of the glands may be attempted if nonresponsive mastitis (Dafalla et al. 1990) or neoplasia (Wooldridge et al. 1999) develops. Semen quality should be monitored so that the buck may be culled if infertility develops, but there is insufficient evidence at this time to justify automatic culling of the fertile animal. Researchers might choose to karyotype these animals.

Neoplasms of the Male Reproductive Tract

Reports of testicular tumors in goats are very scarce. One seminoma has been reported (Pamukcu 1954). A single case of hemangiosarcoma of the bulbourethral gland was also found in a slaughterhouse survey (Tarigan et al. 1990). Adrenal cortical adenomas are a relatively common but incidental finding in castrated male goats. Fifteen percent of wethers examined in one study (Altman et al. 1969) and 26% of wethers in another study (Richter 1958) were affected. Most of these animals were Angoras, the breed of goats in which wethers are most commonly allowed to live to an old age. Lack of testicular negative feedback on release of pituitary gonadotrophins may be involved in the pathogenesis of these tumors. Hyperplastic adrenal cortical nodules (subcapsular, intracapsular, or extracapsular) are also common. They have been found in the head of the epididymis of intersexes (three of ten) and of polled (six of twenty-seven) and horned (one of eight) bucks (Widmaier 1959).

Arthritis and the Breeding Buck

In the United States, one of the most common reasons for a buck to come to the end of his breeding career is arthritis. Painful hips, stifles, or hocks cause a reluctance or inability to mount. The occasional very willing doe manages to get into a compatible position for breeding, but most service attempts fail. If several bucks are run together with the does, the arthritic male may interfere with and prevent breeding by another, normal buck. The lame buck also tends to lose body condition because it does not get up to eat as much as it should.

The decision regarding how to handle the arthritic buck deserves careful thought. In particular, it is important to know the etiology of the lameness. If arthritis involves one limb and is the result of a known traumatic event, then continued breeding with semen from the buck is a reasonable goal, assuming his progeny are of adequate quality. If the buck has clinical caprine arthritis encephalitis (CAE), then the breeder should consider retiring the buck from breeding. Clinical disease is more common in some families than others, suggesting an inherited susceptibility to the effects of the virus. Also, research has shown that clinical CAE is associated with certain histocompatibility antigens, again suggesting a hereditary component (Ruff and Lazary 1989). A herd with a goal of eradicating the CAE virus should not be propagating inherently disease-susceptible animals. That means that the practice of freezing as much semen as possible from a crippled buck must be questioned. Transmission of CAE infection by natural breeding appears to occur infrequently (Adams et al. 1983), although virus has been detected in the seminal fluid and non-sperm cellular fraction of semen from infected bucks (Travassos et al. 1999; Martinez-Rodriguez et al. 2005). Handmating (to decrease contact with other secretions of the infected buck) or washing and extending the semen would presumably reduce the risk of venereal transmission of CAEV.

Similarly, if the buck's lameness is caused by degenerative arthritis, in turn caused by congenitally poor conformation or anatomy, he should not be used for breeding. The veterinarian needs only to think of the increased incidence of stifle injuries in certain breeds of dogs to imagine the long-term results of indiscriminate propagation of such traits.

If the buck has no genetic faults or the owner refuses to consider these arguments as valid, then semen is collected with an artificial vagina or (less commonly) by electroejaculation. The semen can then be frozen or used fresh. Many bucks are willing to serve an AV while standing behind the doe in heat. The undiluted semen can be used to breed that doe, or semen can be diluted in heat-treated milk if several does are in estrus simultaneously. As the buck's condition worsens, an owner may choose to collect as much semen as possible for freezing, then euthanatize the buck. Custom freezers of goat semen have reported poor semen quality and freezability when semen is processed from bucks with severe CAE that have received phenylbutazone. This might be because of direct effects of the virus on testicular function, prolonged recumbency, or decreasing body condition as the disease advances rather than a toxic effect of the anti-inflammatory drugs. No detrimental effects of phenylbutazone on semen quality of artificial insemination stud bulls have been demonstrated.

Diseases Transmissible by Semen or Embryos

When it is desirable to transfer genetic material between herds or even between countries, the risks of introducing an infectious agent must be considered. Our knowledge concerning the transmission of diseases via semen is still fragmentary (Hare 1985; Philpott 1993). Agents known to be transmitted this way in small ruminants include foot and mouth disease virus, bluetongue virus, leptospires, mycoplasma, *Mycobacterium paratuberculosis* (Eppleston and Whittington 2001), and *Toxoplasma gondii* (Dubey and Sharma 1980). Probably transmitted agents include peste des petits ruminants and *Brucella melitensis*. Most infectious agents survive the freezing process. This means that a single ejaculate can potentially infect does in several herds or seasons. On the other hand, extended semen may have less than the minimum infective dose of an organism present. Also, if bucks are kept in artificial insemination centers, they can be routinely screened for many diseases.

When evaluating the risks from embryo transfer, it should be noted that infection could come from the ovum, the sperm, uterine fluids, or infection of the embryo by the dam after fertilization. In general, if embryos are deep frozen after collection, there will be time to complete laboratory tests on the donor dam and collection fluid from the donor before embryos are transported to the recipient herd. Protocols to decrease the risk of disease transfer by embryos to near zero include requiring an intact zona pellucida and ten consecutive washings at 1:100 dilution with use of a new sterile pipette for each washing.

Almost no research with goat embryos has been reported to date. Preliminary work suggests that bluetongue virus (Chemineau et al. 1986) and caprine arthritis encephalitis virus (Wolfe et al. 1987) are not transmitted by embryos. Also, scrapie is apparently not transmitted by either artificial insemination or embryo transfer (Foote et al. 1986). However, the International Embryo Transfer Society (Givens et al. 2007; OIE 2007) still places bluetongue and scrapie in goats into category 4, indicating that either no conclusions are possible or else there is evidence for a nonnegligible risk of disease transfer by embryo transfer.

SURGERY OF THE MALE REPRODUCTIVE TRACT

Preparation of Teaser Bucks

There are many situations in which the presence of a teaser animal is desirable. A teaser can be used to stimulate the onset of cyclicity at the beginning of the breeding season or in the off season (male effect). If the teaser is incapable of inseminating his does, breeding can be intentionally postponed until the second estrus, when there is an increased ovulation rate.

A teaser animal may also be more efficient than a human caretaker at eliciting or observing signs of estrus, including tail wag, buck-seeking behavior, and willingness to stand. The teaser, then, generally simplifies protocols involving superovulation, artificial insemination, or breeding to a distant buck. It can also be used to detect returns to estrus when rebreeding must be to the same distant buck or buck in a straw. One study showed a decrease in the duration of estrus and an increase in fertility to artificial insemination (from 59% to 74%) when a vasectomized buck serviced the does before AI was performed (Romano et al. 2000). Finally, the owner can be more sure of the last possible due date, as for induction of parturition, if there was no post-breeding exposure to a fertile buck.

Angora goats are reported to be inactive outside the normal breeding season, and selection and preparation of a less seasonal goat such as the Boer has been recommended for use as an early season teaser in South Africa (Van der Westhuysen et al. 1988).

Nonsurgical Teasers

There is a teaser to fit almost every situation. If a small herd has only one buck, that animal can be fitted with an apron to ensure that copulation does not occur. If no bucks are present, other animals can be substituted. One of the simplest teasers is the intersex goat. This infertile animal usually has no idea that it is a genetic female. Where year-round masculine behavior is not desired or the expense of maintaining an otherwise nonproductive animal is too great, a temporary teaser can be created with hormones. A wether or a doe that will not be bred for several months is chosen. The animal is then given testosterone by injection to develop adequate libido. One protocol involves using 100 mg of testosterone propionate every third day (Barker and Bosu 1980; Bosu and Barker 1982). Another uses 150 mg repositol testosterone weekly, beginning three weeks before intended use and continuing until the teasing job is done for the year (Herndon 1989). Intravaginal sponges impregnated with 100 mg testosterone have also been used (Gordon 1997). Practitioners in the United States should note that testosterone is currently regulated as a schedule III drug under the Controlled Substance Act (Parkhie 1991).

Penile Translocation

The owner of a large herd may want one or more surgically prepared teasers. A penile translocation (deviation) is the surgery of choice if later breeding to the selected buck might be desirable (Barker 1977). The buck should be held off feed and water twelve hours before surgery because he will be positioned in dorsal recumbency. If surgery is done under general anesthesia, a cuffed endotracheal tube should be used. If the buck is only tranquilized and analgesia is provided with local injection of 1% lidocaine, the head should be positioned lower than the neck. The abdomen is clipped and scrubbed and a new location, above the fold of the flank and on an angle from the base of the scrotum that is 45 degrees off midline, is chosen for the preputial opening. The right flank is preferred if a right handed person is trying to collect semen from the buck with an artificial vagina at a later date. A circle of skin and cutaneous trunci muscle (4 to 5 cm in diameter, lower edge 1 cm above the fold of the flank) is removed and discarded (Ames 1988; Mobini et al. 2002). Next, a circumferential skin incision approximately the same size as that of the target hole (5 cm diameter) is made around the preputial orifice and extended along the midline, over the shaft of the penis, from the preputial incision two-thirds of the way to the base of the scrotum (Figure 13.13). The prepuce and penis are dissected free of the body wall. A reference suture is placed to mark the most cranial aspect of the skin of the prepuce (Mobini et al. 2002), and the finger of a sterile glove is slipped over the prepuce to prevent tissue contamination as the penis is pulled through a subcutaneous tunnel to the flank incision with the aid of long forceps. Finally, the prepuce is sutured into its new location with two layers of interrupted absorbable sutures, being careful to locate the reference suture dorsally. The midline incision is closed except for the most cranial aspect, which is left open for drainage (Mobini et al. 2002). Postoperative penicillin and tetanus

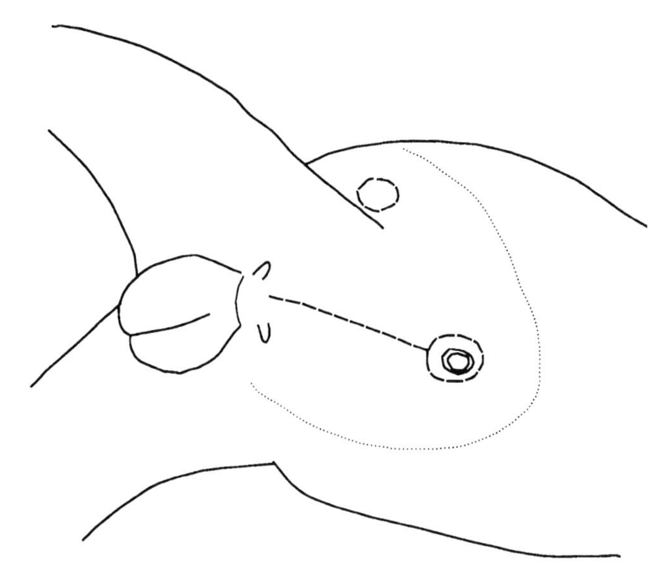

Figure 13.13. Location of incisions for penile deviation. —— = incision lines; ..... = line for infiltration or local anesthetic.

prophylaxis are warranted. Hot-packing or anti-inflammatory drugs may be needed for several days to control swelling at the preputial orifice. The buck thus prepared can still breed an artificial vagina. He can also breed a cooperative doe, given adequate time for maneuvering, and he should not be allowed to run loose with the does unless aproned or sterilized with a further surgery.

Vasectomy

If no additional breeding with the animal is planned, a vasectomy can be used to create a permanent teaser. Possibilities for anesthesia (see Chapter 17) include sedation and local infiltration, epidural anesthesia, or general anesthesia. The procedure is as for rams and has been well described elsewhere (Copland 1986). Briefly, the neck of the scrotum is prepared for surgery. An incision can be made anteriorly, laterally, or posteriorly, according to the surgeon's preference. It is also possible to perform a bilateral vasectomy through a single cranial midscrotal incision (Lofstedt 1982). The firm, cord-like ductus deferens is located and ligated twice and a section 2 to 3 cm long is removed between the ligatures. Both pieces of excised ductus should be examined to verify that an artery was not removed by mistake. An impression smear can be made to look for sperm in the ductus of a mature male. The center of the ductus of an immature male appears as a red dot. Under a dissecting scope, however, the lining has a stellate appearance. The tissue should be preserved in formalin in case histologic verification of the vasectomy should be required. The vaginal tunics need not be sutured; skin can be closed with absorbable or nonabsorbable suture or with wound clips. The vasectomized buck should be permanently identified (e.g., by tattoo) to prevent later confusion, and it should not be used for at least two weeks after surgery. Some authors suggest a minimum of thirty days before the animal should be used as a teaser (Mobini et al. 2001), but numbers are greatly decreased and 95% of the sperm in the ejaculate are already dead by one week (Batista et al. 2002a).

Inflammatory and degenerative changes have been reported after vasectomy. Palpable granulomas, anechogenic on ultrasound and consisting of dead sperm, develop in the firm and enlarged tail of the epididymis. Efferent ductules may rupture, causing extravasation of spermatozoa into the tissues and evoking an immune response with multinucleated giant cells (Batista et al. 2002b). Some bucks showed degeneration of seminiferous tubules by four months after vasectomy. In another report, anechoic granulomas developed in the deferent duct of six bucks and in the head of the epididymis of a seventh. Only in the latter animal, with obstruction of the epididymis occurring close to the testis, were ultrasonographic changes visible in the parenchyma of the testis by five months after vasectomy (Ahmad and Noakes 1995).

Epididymal Surgery

An alternative to vasectomy is destruction or removal of the tail of the epididymis. Tranquilization or infiltration of a local analgesic may be used, although neither is mentioned in the original descriptions. As always, tetanus prophylaxis should be ensured.

One technique involves simply incising through skin and tunics over the tail of the epididymis and then amputating it with scissors. Heat cautery or ligation of the exposed stumps of epididymal tissue is recommended to hinder recanalization (Van Rensburg et al. 1963; Shelton and Klindt 1974; Mobini et al. 2001), which otherwise frequently occurs. The skin should be sutured to avoid infection, unless the surgery was not aseptic. Another technique involves injecting a sclerosing agent such as 1 ml of 10% calcium chloride into the tail of each epididymis (Smith 1986a).

Castration

Castration is commonly performed to avoid undesirable odors and aggressive sexual behavior in male goats kept as pets and to prevent breeding by bucks deemed to be of inferior genetic quality. The flavor of the meat of males raised past puberty is also affected by castration, although in some societies, especially where meat is served with plenty of spices, the rank buck remains quite acceptable. An intact male is preferred for some religious feasts (Muslim), so producers should plan according to their intended markets.

Numerous methods of castration are covered in standard surgery and medicine textbooks (for one example, see Mobini et al. 2001). The procedure is usually performed by an experienced producer; the veterinarian is asked to castrate the maturing pet or the buck with a scrotal lesion (abscess, hernia). Tetanus prophylaxis is advised for all techniques. (See discussion in Chapter 18.) Small goats are restrained on their rumps with front and hind limbs held together on each side by an assistant. Larger (tranquilized) goats are held in a standing or laterally recumbent position.

When a goat is to be kept as a pet wether, delaying castration until puberty permits separation of urethral process and glans penis from the prepuce, thus simplifying manipulations to examine or catheterize the goat if urolithiasis develops. Delaying castration also may lead to some additional increase in diameter of the urethra (Kumar et al. 1982). In general, anyone willing to plan this far ahead to prevent deaths caused by urolithiasis should be encouraged to choose a doe kid as a pet instead. Ejaculatory behavior may be retained for months after castration of adult bucks (Hart and Jones 1975).

Surgical Castration

Young kids (less than one month old) are often castrated by producers by the knife method, without anesthesia. By the time the well-fed kid is several months old, surgical removal of the testes is the preferred technique unless environmental conditions make an open wound unacceptable. By this age the desirability of anesthesia is also evident; older bucks sometimes die very quickly after being subjected to the stress and pain of castration.

Large bucks are tranquilized lightly. Diluted (0.5% to 1%) lidocaine can be injected with a fine needle to avoid provoking as much reaction from the injections as castration itself would have engendered. One to 2 ml, depending on the size of the goat, is deposited in each of four sites: high in the cord and at the distal end of the scrotal sac bilaterally. Alternatively (and especially in larger animals), an intratesticular injection can be made, placing 2 to 10 ml of 1% local anesthetic into each side with most of this being injected into the testis and the remainder being deposited subcutaneously in the bottom of the scrotum (Hall and Clarke 1983).

A U-shaped skin incision is made over each testis or the distal third of the scrotum is cut off. Testes, still within their tunics, are expressed and removed by scraping the cords with a sterile knife or (for larger bucks) by an emasculator with a crushing blade. Caprine testicular size approaches that of a stallion, and a good, well used equine emasculator is appropriate. If such an instrument is not available, the cords of a mature buck should be transfix ligated with absorbable suture. An alternative technique for bloodless castration of a large buck is use of a Henderson Castrating Instrument (Stone Manufacturing, Kansas City, Missouri). This device is clamped across tunic and cord above the testis and rotated with a variable speed drill until tissue separation occurs. General anesthesia (see Chapter 17) in addition to the local anesthetic seems ideal.

If very young kids are castrated by simply pulling on the testis until the cord snaps, a finger should be placed at the inguinal ring to avoid enlarging it while traction is being applied, with subsequent risk of herniation. In warm weather, a fly repellant is needed and the kid should ideally be kept on clean grass rather than in a dirty pen or on sawdust. Hands and equipment should be disinfected between animals.

Rubber Rings and Banding

Very young kids are commonly castrated with elastrator rings, very heavy rubber rings that are first soaked in alcohol or iodine to disinfect them and then placed around the neck of the scrotum with a special applicator. The scrotal sac and whatever has been trapped within it (hopefully both testes and none of the penis) become ischemic and eventually drop off several weeks later. There is no hemorrhage and no open wound, but there is an increased risk of tetanus relative to several of the other techniques, and blowflies may be attracted to the gangrenous scrotum in hot weather (Van der Westhuysen et al. 1988). Rubber bands also evoke more prolonged signs of pain in older animals than does surgical castration (Shutt et al. 1988) but this might be attenuated by intratesticular lidocaine in advance of application. On humane grounds, it seems preferable to restrict the use of rubber rings to kids younger than three weeks of age. There is a very real danger of an incomplete castration if the operator is not careful to verify the entrapment of both testes in the scrotum below the band. While fertility is probably decreased because of the elevated temperature of a testis forced into an inguinal position, testosterone production (and thus male behavior and odor) will continue. Some unwanted pregnancies might occur if the improperly castrated male is allowed to run with females.

Special instruments have been produced to tightly stretch solid rubber tubing around the neck of the scrotum of bulls. These same devices, such as the Callicrate bander® (No-Bull Enterprises, St. Francis, Kansas) can be used to castrate mature bucks. The band is applied close to the dorsal aspect of the testes, because higher placement results in a larger skin defect when the scrotum sloughs. The animal should receive two doses of tetanus toxoid in advance. With the aid of light tranquilization, 7 to 10 ml of 1% lidocaine is infiltrated into the skin of the neck of the scrotum and into the spermatic cords before the band is applied. The scrotum should be amputated about 1 inch (2.5 cm) distal to the band three days later and the stump sprayed with a fly repellant. This technique is especially useful for avoiding hemorrhage or when the animal must be bedded on shavings which would otherwise contaminate an open castration wound.

Burdizzo

The small Burdizzo emasculatome can be used to crush the contents of the cord above each testis (Ames 1988). Each cord in turn is held tightly against the lateral aspect of the scrotum with one hand while the instrument is applied twice on each side. The crushes are made approximately 1 to 2 cm apart, both above the testis, and should not cross the midline of the scrotum (to avoid sloughing skin) or include the penis. The testis is manipulated vigorously while the instrument is in place in an attempt to snap the cord. The kid should be evaluated one month or longer afterward to ensure that both testes have atrophied. Improper technique or a sprung instrument (as from using it to dock tails) gives the Burdizzo method a bad reputation. If castration is delayed until the testes enlarge with spermatogenesis, too much tissue will be present to be completely resorbed. The infarcted testis (often with a viable epididymis, see Figure 13.14) remains as a palpable mass in the scrotum, engendering uncertainty in the owner's mind as to the sterility of the wether.

The chief advantages of this technique are the absence of hemorrhage and open wounds and the decreased risk of tetanus. Anesthesia is usually not used, except when the buckling is dehorned at the same time. A small (to avoid toxicity) quantity of lidocaine can be injected into the cords before crushing. Disadvantages include swelling or sloughing of the scrotum or survival of a testis if the clamp is not applied properly.

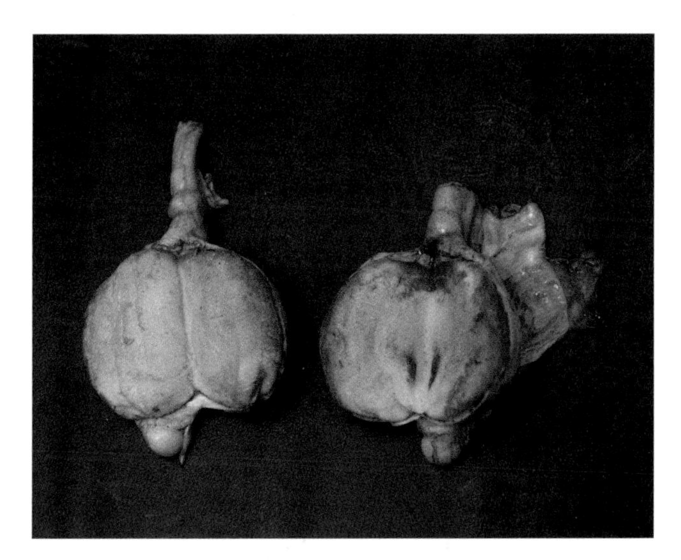

Figure 13.14. Necrotic testicular parenchyma and crimp lines on the cords above the testes following Burdizzo castration. The testes were too large when the procedure was performed to be resorbed. (Courtesy Dr. M.C. Smith.)

Similar results might be obtained using a pinhole castration technique recently described for calves (Ponvijay 2007). Under local anesthesia, the spermatic cord is forced laterally, and an 18-gauge needle is used as a guide to pass absorbable suture through the scrotum. The needle is then withdrawn, the cord forced medially, and the needle reinserted through the same holes, to permit passage of the suture to now completely encircle the cord. After ligation to constrict the cord within the neck of the scrotum, the knot is trimmed short and becomes subcutaneous.

Manipulation of the Testes into the Inguinal Ring

It has been reported that in Venezuela, producers twist each testis around the spermatic cord and push it back into the inguinal canal (Gall 1981). This takes manual dexterity and must be done at an early age. The animal is rendered sterile without risk of hemorrhage, infection, or tetanus and without the need for any specialized equipment. The more rapid growth characteristics and carcass composition of the buck kid are retained. The results of a short scrotum castration (elastrator band intentionally applied below the testes) would have similar effects on growth, although the potential for partial fertility has not been studied in bucks.

Chemical Castration

In the United States, an 88% solution of lactic acid was briefly marketed for castration of calves (Chemcast®, Bio-Ceutic Labs Inc., St. Joseph, Missouri). This product was used on lambs and kids also. A 20-gauge or smaller needle (to avoid leakage from the injection site) was inserted from above, downward into the center of each testis. A small quantity (0.3 to 0.5 ml) of solution was deposited; larger amounts leaked back and caused adhesions between testis and scrotum or draining tracts (Blackburn 1985). Although this method was praised by the manufacturer as being superior to the Burdizzo technique, verification of castration before "wethers" are allowed to run with females of breeding age should be mandatory. Other sclerosing chemicals such as cadmium chloride (200 μg/kg) (Kar 1962) have also been injected to destroy testicular tissue, without consideration of possible meat contamination. More recently, injectable zinc gluconate has been licensed for castrating dogs (Levy et al. 2008), but evaluation of efficacy in goats has not been reported.

REFERENCES

Adams, D.S., et al.: Observations on caprine arthritis-encephalitis in Kenya. Vet. Rec., 112:227–228, 1983.

Ahmad, N. and Noakes, D.E.: A clinical and ultrasonographic study of the testes and related structures of goats and rams after unilateral vasectomy. Vet. Rec., 137:112–117, 1995.

Ahmad, N. and Noakes, D.E.: Sexual maturity in British breeds of goat kids. Br. Vet. J., 152:93–103, 1996a.

Ahmad, N. and Noakes, D.E.: Seasonal variations in the semen quality of young British goats. Br. Vet. J., 152:225–236, 1996b.

Ahmad, N., Noakes, D.E. and Middleton, D.J.: Seminal vesiculitis and epididymitis in an Anglo-Nubian buck. Vet. Rec., 133:322–323, 1993.

Ahmad, N., Noakes, D.E. and Subandrio, A.L.: B-mode real time ultrasonographic imaging of the testis and epididymis of sheep and goats. Vet. Rec., 128:491–496, 1991.

Aitken, I.: Chlamydial abortion in sheep. In Practice, 8:236–237, 1986.

Al-Ani, F.K., et al.: Occurrence of congenital anomalies in Shami breed goats: 211 cases investigated in 19 herds. Small Rumin. Res., 28:225–232, 1998.

Al-Ghalban, A.M., Tabbaa, M.J. and Kridli, R.T.: Factors affecting semen characteristics and scrotal circumference in Damascus bucks. Small Rumin. Res., 53:141–149, 2004.

Al Jassim, R. and Khamas, W.A.: Gynaecomastia and galactorrhea in a goat buck. Aust. Vet. J., 75:669–670, 1997.

Alan, M.G.S., Ahmed, J.U. and Jahan, S.: Effect of dexamethasone on the estrous cycle length in Black Bengal goats (*Capra hircus*). Theriogenology, 31:935–941, 1989.

Albert, K.: Verlammen und Todesfälle durch enzootisches Auftreten von *Yersinia pseudotuberculosis* in einer Ziegenherde. (Abortion and mortality due to *Yersinia pseudotuberculosis* in a herd of goats.) Tierärtzl. Umschau, 43:718–720, 1988.

Ali, B. and Adam, S.E.I.: Effects of *Acanthospermum hispidum* on goats. J. Comp. Pathol., 88:533–544, 1978.

Altman, N.H., Streett, C.S. and Terner, J.Y.: Castration and its relationship to tumors of the adrenal gland in the goat. Am. J. Vet. Res., 30:583–589, 1969.

Alton, G.G.: Control of *Brucella melitensis* in sheep and goats: a review. Trop. Anim. Health Prod., 19:65–74, 1987.

Alton, G.G., Fensterbank, R., Plommet, M. and Verger, J.M.: La brucellose de la chèvre. In: Les Maladies de la Chèvre, Niort, France, 9–11 pp. 69–91, Octobre 1984.

Alves, F.S.F., et al.: Orchitis-epididymitis caused by *Corynebacterium pseudotuberculosis* in goats. Rev. Bras. Med. Vet., 26(1): 11–16, 2004.

Ames, N.K.: The male genital system. Sheep and goat. In: Textbook of Large Animal Surgery. 2nd Ed. F.W. Oehme, ed. Baltimore, Williams and Wilkins, pp. 544–548, 1988.

Amoah, E.A. and Bryant, M.J.: Gestation period, litter size and birth weight in the goat. Anim. Prod., 36:105–110, 1983.

Amoah, E.A. and Bryant, M.J.: A note on the effect of contact with male goats on occurrence of puberty in female goat kids. Anim. Prod., 38:141–144, 1984.

Amoah, E.A. and Gelaye, S.: Superovulation, synchronization and breeding of does. Small Rumin. Res., 3:63–72, 1990.

Amoah, E.A. and Gelaye, S.: Embryo recovery, evaluation, storage and transfer in goats. Small Rumin. Res., 6:119–129, 1991.

Anderson, K.L.: Campylobacteriosis (formerly vibriosis). In: Current Therapy in Theriogenology 2. D.A. Morrow, ed. Philadelphia, W.B. Saunders Co., pp. 605–606, 1986.

Anderson, K.L., et al.: Isolation of *Campylobacter jejuni* from an aborted caprine fetus. J. Am. Vet. Med. Assoc., 183:90–92, 1983.

Anika, S.M., et al.: Chemotherapy and pharmacokinetics of some antimicrobial agents in healthy dwarf goats and those infected with *Ehrlichia phagocytophilia* (tickborne-fever). Res. Vet. Sci., 41:386–390, 1986.

Anke, M., Groppel, B. and Lüdke, H.: Kupfermangel bei Wiederkäuern in der DDR. Tierzucht, 26:56–58, 1972.

Anke, M., et al.: Der Einfluss des Mangan-, Zink-, Kupfer-, Jod-, Selen-, Molybdän- und Nickelmangels auf die Fortpflanzungsleistung des Wiederkäuers. Wissenschaftliche Zeitschrift Karl-Marx-Universität Leipzig, Mathematisch-Naturwissenschaftliche Reihe, 26:283–292, 1977.

Anke, M., et al.: The effect of selenium deficiency on reproduction and milk performance of goats. Arch. Anim. Nutr. Berl., 39:483–490, 1989.

Anosa, V.O. and Isoun, T.T.: Further observations on the testicular pathology in *Trypanosoma vivax* infection of sheep and goats. Res.Vet. Sci., 151–160, 1980.

Appleyard, W.T., Aitken, I.D. and Anderson, I.: Outbreak of chlamydial abortion in goats. Vet. Rec., 113:63, 1983.

Arbeiter, E.: Beitrag zur Spermien-Morphologie der Ziegenböcke. Dtsche. Tierärztl. Wochenschr., 71:60–62, 1964.

Arbeiter, K.: Untersuchungen über den Einfluss verschiedener Heuqualitäten auf die biologische Samenbeschaffenheit von Ziegenböcken. Zuchthyg., 7:349–362, 1963.

Armstrong, D.T., Kiehm, D.J., Warnes, G.M. and Seamark, R.F.: Corpus luteum (CL) failure and embryonic loss in superovulated goats. Theriogenology, 27:207, 1987. (Abstract.)

Armstrong, D.T., Pfitzner, A.P., Warnes, G.M. and Seamark, R.F.: Superovulation treatments and embryo transfer in Angora goats. J. Reprod. Fert., 67:403–410, 1983.

Arricau-Bouvery, N. and Rodolakis, A.: Is Q fever an emerging or re-emerging zoonosis? Vet. Res., 36:327–349, 2005.

Arricau-Bouvery, N., et al.: Excretion of *Coxiella burnetii* during an experimental infection of pregnant goats with an abortive goat strain CbC1. Ann. N.Y. Acad. Sci., 990:524–526, 2003.

Arricau-Bouvery, N., et al.: Effect of vaccination with phase I and phase II *Coxiella burnetii* vaccines in pregnant goats. Vaccine, 23:4392–4402, 2005.

Austin, J.W., Leidy, R.B., Krise, G.M. and Hupp, E.W.: Normal values for semen collected from Spanish goats by two methods. J. Appl. Physiol., 24:369–372, 1968.

AVMA: *Brucella melitensis* infection discovered in cattle for first time, goats also infected. J. Am. Vet. Med. Assoc., 216:648, 2000. (News)

Baas, E.J.: Tick-borne fever. In: Current Veterinary Therapy Food Animal Practice 2. J.L. Howard, ed. Philadelphia, W.B. Saunders Co., pp. 645–646, 1986.

Babin, M., et al.: Élevage des Jeunes Caprins. 2nd Ed. Paris, Institut Technique de l'Élevage Ovin et Caprin, 1981.

Babish, J.G., et al.: Toxicity and tissue residue depletion of levamisole hydrochloride in young goats. Am. J. Vet. Res., 51:1126–1130, 1990.

Bajhau, H.S. and Kennedy, J.P.: Influence of pre- and post-partum nutrition on growth of goat kids. Small Rumin. Res., 3:227–236, 1990.

Bani Ismail, Z.A. and Ababneh, M.: Penile hematoma in a Shami buck. Can. Vet. J. 48:433–434, 2007.

Bar-Moshe, B. and Rapapport, E.: Observations on *Mycoplasma mycoides* subsp. *mycoides* infection in Saanen goats. Isr. J. Med. Sci., 17:537–539, 1981.

Baril, G., et al.: [Use of transrectal ultrasonography to follow ovarian activity in goats.] Rev. Méd. Vét, 150:261–264, 1999.

Barker, C.A.V.: The collection of semen from bulls, rams and bucks by electro-ejaculator. Can. J. Comp. Med., 22:3–8, 1958.

Barker, C.A.V.: Penile deviation. Teaser bucks—a new development for dairy goat A/I. Dairy Goat J., 55(11):65 and 69, 1977.

Barker, C.A.V. and Bosu, W.T.K.: Studies on experimentally androgenized females: goats. Dairy Goat J., 58:944–945 and 948, 1980.

Barker, C.A.V. and Cawley, A.J.: Radiographic detection of fetal numbers in goats. Can. Vet. J., 8:59–61, 1967.

Barlow, R.M., et al.: Experiments in border disease VII. The disease in goats. J. Comp. Pathol., 85:291–297, 1975.

Baronet, D. and Vaillancourt, D.: Pregnancy diagnosis in goat with linear array real-time ultrasound scanning. Méd. Vét. Quebec, 19(2):67–73, 1989.

Barry, D.M. and van Niekerk, C.H.: Anaplasmosis in improved Boer goats in South Africa artificially infected with *Anaplasma ovis*. Small Rumin. Res., 3:191–197, 1990.

Basrur, P.K. and Kochhar, H.S.: Inherited sex abnormalities in goats. In: Current Therapy in Large Animal Theriogenology 2. R.S. Youngquist and W.R. Threlfall, eds. St. Louis, Saunders Elsevier, pp. 590–594, 2007.

Bath, G. and de Wet, J.: Sheep and Goat Diseases. Capetown, Tafelberg, 2000.

Batista, M., et al.: Incidence and treatment of hydrometra in Canary Island goats. Vet. Rec., 149:329–330, 2001.

Batista, M., et al.: Semen characteristics and plasma levels of testosterone after bilateral vasectomy in bucks. Reprod. Domest. Anim., 37:375–378, 2002a.

Batista, M., et al.: Structural changes in the testes and epididymides of bucks 16 weeks after bilateral vasectomy. Vet. Rec., 151:740–741, 2002b.

Batista, M., et al.: Segmental aplasia of the uterus associated with hydrometra in a goat. Vet. Rec., 159:597–598, 2006.

Beckett, S.D., Reynolds, T.M., Hudson, R.S. and Holley, R.S.: Serial angiography of the crus penis of the goat during erection. Biol. Reprod., 7:365–369, 1972b.

Beckett, S.D., et al.: Corpus cavernosum penis pressure and external penile muscle activity during erection in the goat. Biol. Reprod., 7:359–364, 1972a.

Behymer, D.E., et al.: Enzyme immunoassay for surveillance of Q fever. Am. J. Vet. Res., 46:2413–2417, 1985.

Benson, G.J.: Anesthetic management of ruminants and swine with selected pathophysiologic alterations. Vet. Clin. N. Am. Food Anim. Pract., 2:677–691, 1986.

Berri, M., et al.: Progression of Q fever and *Coxiella burnetii* shedding in milk after an outbreak of enzootic abortion in a goat herd. Vet. Rec., 156:548–549, 2005.

Berrios, P.E., McKercher, D.G. and Knight, H.D.: Pathogenicity of a caprine herpesvirus. Am. J. Vet. Res., 36:1763–1769, 1975.

Bhatia, S. and Shanker, V.: First report of a XX/XXY fertile goat buck. Vet. Rec., 130:271–272, 1992.

Binns, W., Keeler, R.F. and Balls, L.D.: Congenital deformities in lambs, calves, and goats resulting from maternal ingestion of *Veratrum californicum*: hare lip, cleft palate, ataxia, and hypoplasia of metacarpal and metatarsal bones. Clin. Toxicol. 5:245–261, 1972.

Blackburn, L.: Castration. Pygmy Goat Memo, 10(2):12–13, 1985.

Blasco, J.M.: A review of the use of *B. melitensis* Rev1 vaccine in adult sheep and goats. Prev. Vet. Med., 31:275–283, 1997.

Blash, S., Melican, D. and Gavin, W.: Cryopreservation of epididymal sperm obtained at necropsy from goats. Theriogenology, 54:899–905, 2000.

Blewett, D.A. and Trees, A.J.: The epidemiology of ovine toxoplasmosis with especial respect to control. Br. Vet. J., 143:128–135, 1987.

Blewett, D.A., et al.: Ovine enzootic abortion: the acquisition of infection and consequent abortion within a single lambing season. Vet. Rec., 111:499–501, 1982.

Bliss, E.L.: Obstetrics and neonatal care in goats. Proceedings, Society for Theriogenology, Orlando, FL, pp. 283–284, Sept. 16–17, 1988.

Bloxham, P.A., Davis, G.W. and Charlesworth, A.: Ovine enzootic abortion diagnosis. Vet. Rec., 100:371–372, 1977.

BonDurant, R.H.: Induction of estrus in does by introduction of buck or photoperiod manipulation. In: Current Therapy in Theriogenology 2. D.A. Morrow, ed. Philadelphia, W.B. Saunders Co., pp. 579–581, 1986.

BonDurant, R.H., McDonald, M.C. and Trommershausen-Bowling, A.: Probable freemartinism in a goat. J. Am. Vet. Med. Assoc., 177:1024–1025, 1980.

Bongso, T.A., Jainudeen, M.R. and Zahrah, A.S.: Relationship of scrotal circumference to age, body weight and onset of spermatogenesis in goats. Theriogenology, 18:513–524, 1982.

Bonniwell, M.A., et al.: Border disease without nervous signs or fleece changes. Vet. Rec., 120:246–249, 1987.

Bosc, M.J., Delouis, C. and Terqui, M.: Control of the time of parturition of sheep and goat. In: Management of Reproduction in Sheep and Goats. Symposium, Univ. of Wisconsin, Madison, WI, July 24–25, pp. 89–100, 1977.

Bosc, M., et al.: Hourly distribution of time of parturition in the domestic goat. Theriogenology 30:23–33, 1988.

Bosu, W.T.K. and Barker, C.A.V.: Steroid levels after intramuscular injection of testosterone propionate in the caprine. Can. J. Comp. Med., 46:390–394, 1982.

Bosu, W.T.K. and Basrur, P.K: Morphological and hormonal features of an ovine and a caprine intersex. Can. J. Comp. Med., 48:402–409, 1984.

Bosu, W.T.K., Garibay, J.A.S. and Barker, C.A.V.: Peripheral plasma levels of progesterone in pregnant goats and in pregnant goats treated with prostaglandin F2α. Theriogenology, 11:131–148, 1979.

Boyajean, D.: Intersexualité associée à l'absence de cornes chez la chèvre d'origine alpine. Ann. Génét. Sél. Anim., 1:447–463, 1969.

Braun, W., Jr: Periparturient infections and structural abnormalities. In: Current Therapy in Large Animal Theriogenology 2. R.S. Youngquist and W.R. Threlfall, eds. St. Louis, Saunders Elsevier, 2007, pp. 572–574.

Bretzlaff, K.: Reproduction problems in goats. In: Proceedings, Symposium on Diseases of Small Ruminants. American Association of Small Ruminant Practitioners, pp. 13–16 Boise, Idaho, June 1–3, 1989.

Bretzlaff, K.N., Elmore, R.G. and Nuti, L.C.: Use of an enzyme immunoassay to determine concentrations of progesterone in caprine plasma and milk. J. Am. Vet. Med. Assoc., 194:664–668, 1989.

Bretzlaff, K.N. and Ott, R.S.: Doses of prostaglandin F2-alpha effective for induction of parturition in goats. Theriogenology, 19:849–853, 1983.

Bretzlaff, K.N. and Romano, J.E.: Advanced reproductive techniques in goats. Vet. Clin. N. Am. Food Anim. Pract., 17:421–434, 2001.

Bretzlaff, K.N., et al.: Doses of prostaglandin F2 alpha effective for induction of estrus in goats. Theriogenology, 16:587–591, 1981.

Bretzlaff, K.N., et al.: Plasma luteinizing hormone and progesterone concentrations in goats with estrous cycles of normal or short duration after prostaglandin F2α administration during diestrus or pregnancy. Am. J. Vet. Res., 49:939–943, 1988.

Bretzlaff, K.N., et al.: Luteinizing hormone and progesterone concentrations and induction of estrus after use of norgestomet ear implants or constant infusion of gonadotropin-releasing hormone in anestrous, nonlactating dairy goats. Am. J. Vet. Res., 52:1423–1426, 1991.

Bretzlaff, K., et al.: Ultrasonographic determination of pregnancy in small ruminants. Vet. Med., 88:12–24, 1993.

Broaddus, C.C., et al.: Transmission of bovine viral diarrhea virus to adult goats from persistently infected cattle. J. Vet. Diagn. Invest., 19:545–548, 2007.

Brounts, S.H., et al.: Outcome and subsequent fertility of sheep and goats undergoing cesarean section because of dystocia: 110 cases (1981–2001). J. Am. Vet. Med. Assoc., 224:275–279, 2004.

Brown, N.: Ribbons and dollar bills vs. the health and welfare of the Pygmy goat. Pygmy Goat Memo., 13(2):16–17, 1988.

Buckrell, B.C.: Applications of ultrasonography in reproduction in sheep and goats. Theriogenology, 29:71–84, 1988.

Buckrell, B.C., Bonnett, B.N. and Johnson, W.H.: The use of real-time ultrasound rectally for early pregnancy diagnosis in sheep. Theriogenology, 25:665–673, 1986.

Buergelt, C.D.: Color Atlas of Reproductive Pathology of Domestic Animals. St. Louis, Mosby, 1997.

Bunch, T.D., Foote, W.C. and Spillett, J.J.: Sheep-goat hybrid karyotypes. Theriogenology, 6:379–385, 1976.

Burgess, G.W., Spencer, T.L. and Norris, M.J.: Experimental infection of goats with *Brucella ovis*. Aust. Vet. J., 62:262–264, 1985.

Burguete, I., et al.: Cytogenetic observations on a Robertsonian translocation in Saanen goats. Génét. Sél. Evol., 19:391–398, 1987.

Burstel, D., Meinecke-Tillman, S. and Meinecke, B.: Ultrasonographic diagnosis of fetal sex in small ruminants bearing multiple fetuses. Vet. Rec., 151:635–636, 2002.

Buxton, D.: Protozoan infections (*Toxoplasma gondii*, *Neospora caninum* and *Sarcocystis* spp.) in sheep and goats: recent advances. Vet. Res., 29:289–310, 1998.

Buxton, D., et al.: Further studies on the use of monensin in the control of experimental ovine toxoplasmosis. J. Comp. Pathol., 98:225–236, 1988.

Bwangamoi, O., Carles, A.B. and Wandera, J.G.: An epidemic of besnoitiosis in goats in Kenya. Vet. Rec., 125:461, 1989.

Byatt, J.C., et al.: Ruminant placental lactogens: structure and biology. J. Anim. Sci., 70:2911–2923, 1992.

Calamel, M.M. and Giauffret, A.: Une enzootie de toxoplasmose caprine abortive. Acad. Vét. Fr. Bull., 48:41–45, 1975.

Caldas, A.D.: Avitaminose A espontânea em caprinos (Spontaneous avitaminosis A in goats.) O Biológico, 27:266–270, 1961.

Camp, J.C., et al.: Ovarian activity during normal and abnormal length estrous cycles in the goat. Biol. Reprod., 28:673–681, 1983.

Carter, P.D., Hamilton, P.A. and Dufty, J.H.: Electroejaculation in goats. Aust. Vet. J., 67:91–93, 1990.

Chandler, J.E., et al.: Semen quality characteristics of dairy goats. J. Dairy Sci., 71:1638–1646, 1988.

Chaplin, V.M. and Holdsworth, R.J.: Oestrone sulphate in goats' milk. Vet. Rec., 111:224, 1982.

Chartier, C. and Mallereau, M.P.: (Vaccinal efficacy of *Toxoplasma gondii* S48 strain tested in an experimental trial in goats.) Ann. Méd. Vét., 145:202–209, 2001.

Chartier, C., et al.: Neosporosis in goats: results of two serological surveys in western France. Point Vet., 31(209): 65–69, 2000.

Cheema, A.H. and Toofanian, F.: Besnoitiosis in wild and domestic goats in Iran. Cornell Vet., 69:159–168, 1979.

Chemineau, P.: "Buck effect" in tropical goats. In: The Male in Farm Animal Reproduction. M. Courot, ed. Boston, Martinus Nijhoff Publishers, pp. 310–315, 1984.

Chemineau, P.: Effects of a progestagen on buck-induced short ovarian cycles in the Creole meat goat. Anim. Reprod. Sci., 9:87–94, 1985.

Chemineau, P.: Le désaisonnement des chèvres par la lumière et la mélatonine. La Chèvre 171:18–22, 1989.

Chemineau, P., Normant, E., Ravault, J.P. and Thimonier, J.: Induction and persistence of pituitary and ovarian activity in the out-of-season lactating dairy goat after a treatment combining a skeleton photoperiod, melatonin and the male effect. J. Reprod. Fert., 78:497–504, 1986.

Chemineau, P., et al.: Production, freezing and transfer of embryos from a bluetongue-infected goat herd without bluetongue transmission. Theriogenology, 26:279–290, 1986.

Chemineau, P., et al.: Training Manual on Artificial Insemination in Sheep and Goats. Rome, Food and Agricultural Organization of the United Nations, FAO Animal Production and Health Paper 83, 1991.

Chemineau, P., et al.: Implications of recent advances in reproductive physiology for reproductive management of goats. J. Reprod. Fert. Suppl., 54:129–142, 1999.

Chénier, S., Montpetit, C. and Hélie, P.: Caprine herpesvirus-1 abortion storm in a goat herd in Quebec. Can. Vet. J., 45:241–243, 2004.

Chima, J.C., Ernø, H. and Ojo, M.O.: Characterization and identification of caprine genital mycoplasmas. Acta Vet. Scand., 27:531–539, 1986.

Chung, S.I., et al.: Congenital malformations in sheep resulting from in utero inoculation of Cache Valley virus. Am. J. Vet. Res., 51:1645–1648, 1990a.

Chung, S.I., et al.: Evidence that Cache Valley virus induces congenital malformations in sheep. Vet. Microbiol., 21:297–307, 1990b.

Cochran, D.E.: Clinical selenium-tocopherol deficiency (STD) in dairy goats. Dairy Goat J., 58:48–51, 1980.

Cockcroft, P.D. and McInnes, E.F.: Abdominal straining in a goat with a leiomyoma of the cervix. Vet. Rec., 142:171, 1998.

Cognie, Y.: State of the art in sheep—goat embryo transfer. Theriogenology, 51:105–116, 1999.

Committee on Foreign Animal Diseases: Foreign Animal Diseases. Richmond, VA, United States Animal Health Association. Revised, 1998.

Constantinescu, G.M.: Guide to Regional Ruminant Anatomy Based on the Dissection of the Goat. Ames, IA, Iowa State Univ. Press, 2001.

Constantinou, A., Louca, A. and Mavrogenis, A.P.: The effect of the gene for polledness on conception rate and litter size in the Damascus goat. Ann. Génét. Sél. Anim., 13:111–118, 1981.

Cooke, M.M. and Merrall, M.: Mammary adenocarcinoma and granulosa cell tumour in an aged Toggenberg goat. N. Z. Vet. J., 40:31–33, 1992.

Cooke, R.G.: Testosterone secretion during early pregnancy in the goat. Theriogenology, 32:331–334, 1989.

Copland, M.D.: Surgical procedures of the reproductive tract of sheep. In: Current Therapy in Theriogenology 2. D.A. Morrow, ed. Philadelphia, W.B. Saunders Co., pp. 890–893, 1986.

Copeland, S., Chirino-Trejo, M., Bourque, P. and Biernacki, A.: Abortion due to *Coxiella burnetii* in a goat. Can. Vet. J., 32:245, 1991.

Corbel, M.: Brucellosis: an overview. Emerg. Infect. Dis., 3(2), 1997. http://www.cdc.gov/ncidod/EID/vol3no2/corbel.htm.

Corteel, J.M.: Collection, processing and artificial insemination of goat semen. In: Goat Production. C. Gall, ed. New York, Academic Press, pp. 171–191, 1981.

Corteel, J.M., Nouzilly, France, personal communication, 1991.

Corteel, J.M., Baril, G., Leboeuf, B. and Nunès, J.F.: Goat semen technology. In: The Male in Farm Animal Reproduction. Edited by M. Courot. Boston, MA, Martinus Nijhoff Publishers, pp. 237–256, 1984.

Corteel, J.M., Leboeuf, B. and Baril, G.: Artificial breeding of adult goats and kids induced with hormones to ovulate outside the breeding season. Small Rumin. Res., 1:19–35, 1988.

Corteel, J.-M., et al.: Examens morphologiques, caryologiques, physiologiques et pathologiques de boucs stériles sans cornes. Ann. Génét. Sél. Anim., 1:341–348, 1969.

Crepin, P.: Les cornes dans l'espèce caprine. (Horns in the goat.) Mouton, 13:79, 1958. Anim. Breed. Abstr., 26(2017):412, 1958.

Cribiu, E.P. and Lherm, C.: Caryotype normal et anomalies chromosomiques de la chèvre domestique (*Capra hircus*). Rec. Méd. Vét., 162:163–167, 1986.

Cribiu, E.P. and Matejka, M.: Idiogram and standardized G-band karyotype of the goat (*Capra hircus*). Zuchthyg., 22:1–7, 1987a.

Cribiu, E.P. and Matejka, M.: Standardized R-band karyotype of the goat (*Capra hircus*). Zuchthyg., 22:260–266, 1987b.

Crowther, R.W. and Spicer, A.J.: Abortion in sheep and goats in Cyprus caused by *Coxiella burneti* (sic). Vet. Rec., 99:29–30, 1976.

Dafalla, E.A., et al.: A functioning udder in a male goat. J. Vet. Med. Ser. A., 37:686–691, 1990.

DaMassa, A.J., Brooks, D.L., Holmberg, C.A. and Moe, A.I.: Caprine mycoplasmosis: An outbreak of mastitis and arthritis requiring destruction of 700 goats. Vet. Rec., 120:409–413, 1987.

Damodaran, S. and Parthasarathy, K.R.: Neoplasms of goats and sheep. Indian Vet. J., 49:649–652, 1972.

Dargantes, A.P., et al.: Experimental *Trypanosoma evansi* infection in the goat. II. Pathology. J. Comp. Pathol., 133:267–276, 2005.

Daubney, R., Hudson, J.R. and Garnham, P.C.: Enzootic hepatitis or Rift Valley fever. An undescribed virus disease of sheep, cattle and man from East Africa. J. Pathol. Bacteriol., 34:545–579, 1931.

Davies, F.G. and Terpstra, C.: Nairobi sheep disease. In: Infectious Diseases of Livestock, Volume Two, 2nd Ed. J. A.W. Coetzer and R.C. Tustin, eds. Oxford Univ. Press, Oxford, pp. 1071–1076, 2004.

Davis, L.E. and Koritz, G.D.: Placental transfer of drugs in ruminant animals. In: Veterinary Pharmacology and Toxicology. Y. Ruckebusch, P.L. Toutain and G.D. Koritz, eds. Westport, CT, AVI Publ. Co., Inc, pp. 23–37, 1983.

Dawson, L.J., et al.: Determination of fetal numbers in Alpine does by real-time ultrasonography. Small Rumin. Res., 14:225–231, 1994.

Day, A.M. and Southwell, S.R.G.: Termination of pregnancy in goats using cloprostenol. N. Z. Vet. J., 27:207–208, 1979.

de la Concha-Bermejillo, A.: Cache Valley virus is a cause of fetal malformation and pregnancy loss in sheep. Small Rumin. Res., 49:1–9, 2003.

de la Vega, A.C., et al.: Annual variation of scrotal circumference in male Creole goats. Arch. Zootec., 55:113–116, 2006.

de Montigny, G.: Le "DG" par la progesterone. La Chèvre, 168:18–19, 1988.

DeArmond, D.: No-cost no-fault pregnancy test. Dairy Goat J., 68(1):7 and 62, 1990.

Debenedetti, A., Malfatti, A., Moretti, A. and Lucaroni, A.: Anomalies précoces de la gestation et toxoplasmose chez la chèvre. Goat Diseases and Productions, Second International Colloquium in Niort, France, June 26–29 1989. Abstracts p. 91.

Deckwer, N.: Embryotomien bei Schafen und Ziegen mit neuen Instrumenten. Berl. Münch. Tierärztl. Wochenschr, (64):150–153, 1951.

Delahaye, J.: Gare aux avortements. La Chèvre, 161:8, 1987.

Delgadillo, J.A., Leboef, B. and Chemineau, P.: Decrease in the seasonality of sexual behavior and sperm production in bucks by exposure to short photoperiodic cycles. Theriogenology, 36:755–770, 1991.

Denis, B., et al.: Chabin: L'hybride chèvre × mouton. La Chèvre, 168:24–25, Sept-Oct 1988.

Denmark, J.R. and Chessum, B.S.: Standardization of enzyme-linked immunosorbent assay (ELISA) and the detection of *Toxoplasma* antibody. Med. Lab. Sci., 35:227–232, 1978.

Dent, J., McGovern, P.T. and Hancock, J.L.: Immunological implications of ultrastructural studies of goat × sheep hybrid placentae. Nature, 231:116–117, 1971.

Depner, K., Hubschle, O.J.B. and Liess, B.: BVD-virus infection in goats–experimental studies on transplacental transmissibility of the virus and its effect on reproduction. Arch. Virol., Suppl. 3:253–256, 1991.

Dewalque, J.: Tumeur ovarienne et masculinisation chez une chèvre chamoisée des Alpes. Ann. Méd. Vét., 107:322–328, 1963.

DiGrassie, W.A., Wallace, M.A. and Sponenberg, D.P.: Multicentric lymphosarcoma with ovarian involvement in a Nubian goat. Can. Vet. J., 38:383–384, 1997.

Dionysius, D.A.: Pregnancy diagnosis in dairy goats and cows using progesterone assay kits. Aust. Vet. J., 68:14–16, 1991.

Dobbs, E.M. and McIntyre, R.W.: A case of vibrionic abortion in a goat herd. Calif. Vet., 4(4):19, 1951.

Doizé, F., et al.: Determination of gestational age in sheep and goats using transrectal ultrasonographic measurement of placentomes. Theriogenology, 48:449–460, 1997.

Dollahite, J.W. and Allen, T.J.: Feeding perennial broomweed to cattle, swine, sheep, goats, rabbits, guinea pigs and chickens. Tex. Agric. Exp. Stat. Prog. Rep., 2105, 1959.

Dollahite, J.W., Shaver, T. and Camp, B.J.: Injected saponins as abortifacients. Am. J. Vet. Res., 23:1261–1263, 1962.

Drost, M.: The Drost project. Visual Guide to Caprine Reproduction. 2008. http://www.drostproject.vetmed.ufl.edu/drost_guides.html.

Drummond, S.B.: Angora Goats the Northern Way. 2nd Ed. Freeport, MI, Stony Lonesome Farm, 1988.

du Preez, E.R., et al.: Out-of-season breeding of milk goats—the effect of light treatment, melatonin and breed. J. S. Afr. Vet. Assoc., 72:228–231, 2001.

Dubey, J.P.: Prevention of abortion and neonatal death due to toxoplasmosis by vaccination of goats with the non-pathogenic coccidium *Hammondia hammondi*. Am. J. Vet. Res., 42:2155–2157, 1981.

Dubey, J.P.: Repeat transplacental transfer of *Toxoplasma gondii* in goats. J. Am. Vet. Med. Assoc., 180:1220–1221, 1982.

Dubey, J.P.: Transplacental toxoplasmosis in goats. In: Current Therapy in Theriogenology 2. Edited by D.A. Morrow. Philadelphia, W.B. Saunders Co., 1986, pp. 606–607.

Dubey, J.P.: Toxoplasmosis in goats. Agri-Practice, 8:43–52, 1987.

Dubey, J.P.: Lesions in transplacentally induced toxoplasmosis in goats. Am. J. Vet. Res., 49:905–909, 1988.

Dubey, J.P., Acland, H.M. and Hamir, A.N.: *Neospora caninum* (Apicomplexa) in a stillborn goat. J. Parasitol., 78:532–534, 1992.

Dubey, J.P. and Adams, D.S.: Prevalence of *Toxoplasma gondii* antibodies in dairy goats from 1982 to 1984. J. Am. Vet. Med. Assoc., 196:295–296, 1990.

Dubey, J.P. and Sharma, S.P.: Prolonged excretion of *Toxoplasma gondii* in semen of goats. Am. J. Vet. Res., 41:794–795, 1980.

Dubey, J.P., et al.: Serodiagnosis of postnatally and prenatally induced toxoplasmosis in sheep. Am. J. Vet. Res., 48:1239–1243, 1987.

Dubey, J.P., et al.: Neosporosis-associated abortion in a dairy goat. J. Am. Vet. Med. Assoc., 208:263–265, 1996.

Dubois, C.: La fièvre de Malte chez les animaux domestiques. Rev. Vét. [Toulouse], 68:129–140, 199–212, 269–281, 1911.

Dukelow, W.R., Jarosz, S.J., Jewett, D.A. and Harrison, R.M.: Laparoscopic examination of the ovaries in goats and primates. Lab. Anim. Sci., 21:594–597, 1971.

Dupuis, G., et al.: Q fever outbreak–Switzerland. Morb. Mort. Wkly. Rep., 33:355–356 and 361, 1984.

Duquesnel, R., et al.: La pseudogestation chez la chèvre. Ann. Zootech. 41:407–415, 1992.

Eales, F.A. et al.: Effectiveness in commercial practice of a new system for detecting and treating hypothermia in newborn lambs. Vet. Rec., 114:469–471, 1984.

East, N.E.: Pregnancy toxemia, abortions, and periparturient diseases. Vet. Clin. N. Am. Large Anim. Pract., 5:601–618, 1983.

East, N.E. and Rowe, J.D.: Subcutaneous progestin implants versus intravaginal sponges for dairy goat estrus synchronization during the transitional period. Theriogenology, 32:921–928, 1989.

Eaton, O.N.: An anatomical study of hermaphrodism in goats. Am. J. Vet. Res., 4:333–343, 1943.

Eaton, O.N.: The relation between polled and hermaphroditic characters in dairy goats. Genetics, 30:51–61, 1945.

Eaton, O.N. and Simmons, V.L.: A semen study of goats. Am. J. Vet. Res., 13:537–544, 1952.

Edwards, J.F., Angulo, A.B. and Pannill, E.C.: Theriogenology question of the month. J. Am. Vet. Med. Assoc., 222:1361–1362, 2003.

Edwards, J.F., et al.: Ovine arthrogryposis and central nervous system malformations associated with in utero Cache Valley virus infection: Spontaneous disease. Vet. Pathol., 26:33–39, 1989.

Eilts, B.E., Pechman, R.D., Taylor, H.W. and Usenik, E.A.: Ultrasonographic evaluation of induced testicular lesions in male goats. Am. J. Vet. Res., 50:1361–1364, 1989.

Eleni, C., et al.: Detection of *Neospora caninum* in an aborted goat fetus. Vet. Parasitol. 123:271–274, 2004.

Elwishy, A.B. and Elsawaf, S.A.: Development of sexual activity in male Damascus goats. Indian J. Anim. Sci., 41:350–356, 1971.

Elze, K. and Müller, H.: Ein Beitrag zum Hydrops universalis congenitus (Anasarka) beim Kalb und Ziegenlamm. Monatsheft f. Veterinärmed., 15:373–376, 1960.

Engeland, I.V., et al.: Effect of *Toxoplasma gondii* infection on the development of pregnancy and on endocrine foetal-placental function in the goat. Vet. Parasitol., 67:61–74, 1996.

Engeland, I.V., et al.: Effect of experimental infection with *Listeria monocytogenes* on the development of pregnancy and on concentrations of progesterone, oestrone sulphate and 15-ketodihydro-PGF-2alpha in the goat. Anim. Reprod. Sci., 45:311–327, 1997.

Engeland, I.V., et al.: Pregnancy diagnosis in dairy goats using progesterone assay kits and oestrous observation. Anim. Reprod. Sci., 47:237–243, 1997.

Engeland, I.V., et al.: Effect of fungal alkaloids on the development of pregnancy and endocrine foetal-placental function in the goat. Anim. Reprod. Sci., 52:289–302, 1998.

Engeland, I.V., et al.: Foetal loss in dairy goats: An epidemiological study in 22 herds. Small Rumin. Res., 30:37–48, 1998.

Engeland, I.V., et al.: Foetal loss in dairy goats: function of the adrenal glands, corpus luteum and the foetal-placental unit. Anim. Reprod. Sci., 55:205–222, 1999.

Engum, J. and Lyngset, O.: Gynecology and obstetrics in the goat. Iowa State Univ. Vet., 32:120–124, 1970.

Eppleston, J. and Whittington, R.J.: Isolation of *Mycobacterium avium* subsp *paratuberculosis* from the semen of rams with clinical Johne's disease. Aust. Vet. J., 79:776–777, 2001.

Erasmus, B.J. and Coetzer, J.A.W.: The symptomatology and pathology of Rift Valley fever in domestic animals. In: Contributions to Epidemiology and Biostatistics. 3. Rift Valley Fever. Basel, Karger, 1981, pp. 77–82.

Eugster, A.K., Jones, L.P. and Gayle, L.G.: Epizootics of chlamydial abortions and keratoconjunctivitis in goats. Ann. Proc. Am. Assoc. Vet. Lab. Diagnost., 20:69–78, 1977.

Evans, G. and Maxwell, W.M.C.: Salamon's Artificial Insemination of Sheep and Goats. Sydney, Butterworths, 1987.

Everett, K.D.E.: *Chlamydia* and *Chlamydiales*: more than meets the eye. Vet. Microbiol., 75:109–126, 2000.

Ezeasor, D.N. and Singh, A.: Morphologic features of Sertoli cells in the intra-abdominal testes of cryptorchid dwarf goats. Am. J. Vet. Res., 48:1736–1745, 1987.

Fahmi, H.A., et al.: The influence of some sample handling factors on progesterone and testosterone analysis in goats. Theriogenology, 24:227–234, 1985.

Fatimah, I., Ikede, B.O. and Mutalib, R.A.: Granulomatous orchitis and periorchitis caused by *Pseudomonas pseudomallei* in a goat. Vet. Rec., 114:67–68, 1984.

Faye, P., et al.: Avortement enzootique <<à virus>> (*Rakeia*) de la chèvre. Bull. Acad. Vét., 44:61–64, 1971.

Fehilly, C.R., Willadsen, S.M. and Tucker, E.M.: Interspecific chimaerism between sheep and goat. Nature, 307:634–636, 1984.

Fensterbank, R.: Vaccination with a *Listeria* strain of reduced virulence against experimental *Listeria* abortion in goats. Ann. Rech. Vét., 18:415–419, 1987.

Flanagan, M., Dashorst, M.E., Ward, M.P. and Morris, C.M.: Antibodies to bluetongue and related orbiviruses in sheep and goats in bluetongue virus-endemic areas of northern and central Queensland. Aust. Vet. J., 72:31–32, 1995.

Fleming, S.A., et al.: Serum progesterone determination as an aid for pregnancy diagnosis in goats bred out of season. Can. Vet. J., 31:104–107, 1990.

Flint, A.P.F., Kingston, E.J., Robinson, J.S. and Thorburn, G.D.: Initiation of parturition in the goat: Evidence for control by foetal glucocorticoid through activation of placental C21-steroid 17α-hydroxylase. J. Endocrinol., 78:367–378, 1978.

Flores, J.A., et al.: Male reproductive condition is the limiting factor of efficiency in the male effect during seasonal anestrus in female goats. Biol. Reprod., 62:1409–1414, 2000.

Foote, R.H.: Estimation of bull sperm concentration by packed cell volume. J. Dairy Sci., 41:1109–1110, 1958.

Foote, Robert H.: Ithaca, NY, personal communication 1992.

Foote, W.C., Call, J.W., Bunch, T.D. and Pitcher, J.R.: Embryo transfer in the control of transmission of scrapie in sheep and goats. Proceedings, U.S. Animal Health Assoc., 413–416, 1986.

Franklin, J.S.: Retained placenta, metritis and pyometra. In: Current Therapy in Theriogenology 2. D.A. Morrow, ed. Philadelphia, W.B. Saunders Co., p. 595, 1986.

Fraser, A.F.: Observations on the pre-coital behaviour of the male goat. Anim. Behav., 12:31–33, 1964.

Fraser, A.F.: Infertility in goats related to testicular atrophy. Trop. Anim. Health Prod., 3:173–182, 1971.

Fraser, A.F., Nagaratnam, V. and Callicott, R.B.: The comprehensive use of Doppler ultra-sound in farm animal reproduction. Vet. Rec., 88:202–205, 1971.

Fraser, A.F. and Wilson, J.C.: Testicular calcinosis in domestic ruminants. Nature (London), 210:547, 1966.

Fredriksson, G., Kindahl, H. and Edqvist, L-E.: Periparturient release of prostaglandin F-2alpha in the goat. Zbl. Vet. Med. A, 31:386–392, 1984.

Fredriksson, G., Kindahl, H. and Edqvist, L-E.: Endotoxin-induced prostaglandin release and corpus luteum function in goats. Anim. Reprod. Sci., 8:109–121, 1985.

Frenkel, J.K.: Common questions on toxoplasmosis: veterinary, medical, and public health considerations. Vet. Med., 77:1188–1196, 1982.

Funk, N.D., et al.: Indirect enzyme-linked immunosorbent assay for detection of *Brucella melitensis*-specific antibodies in goat milk. J. Clin. Microbiol., 43:721–725, 2005.

Furlan, S., et al.: Fetotoxic effects of locoweed (*Astragalus lentiginosus*) in pregnant goats. In: Poisonous Plants: Global Research and Solutions. K.E. Panter, et al., eds. Cambridge, MA, CABI Publ., pp. 130–135, 2007.

Gahlot, T.K., Ranka, A.K., Chouhan, D.S. and Choudhary, R.J.: Congenital urethral deverticulum (sic) in male goat (*Capra hircus*)–surgical management. Indian J. Vet. Surg., 3(2):95–97, 1982.

Gall, C.: Husbandry. In: Goat Production. C. Gall, ed. New York, Academic Press, p. 429, 1981.

García-Carrillo, C., Cuba-Caparó, A. and Myers, D.M.: Susceptibilidad comparada de cabritos y carneros a la infección causada por *Brucella ovis*: estudios serológicos, bacteriológicos y patológicos. Gaceta Vet., 36:355–374, 1974.

García-Carrillo, C., et al.: (Experimental infection of male goats with *Brucella ovis*. Bacteriological, serological and histopathological study.) Revista Asoc. Argentina Microbiol., 9(3):101–108, 1977. Abstract 5259 in Vet. Bull., 48:755, 1978.

Gardner, D.R., et al.: Ponderosa pine and broom snakeweed: Poisonous plants that affect livestock. J. Nat. Toxicol., 1999; 8:27–34, 1999.

Garrett, P.D.: Guide to Ruminant Anatomy Based on the Dissection of the Goat. Ames, IA, Iowa State Univ. Press, 1988.

Gaumont, R., Trap, D. and Dhennin, L.: Immunisation de la chèvre primipare contre l'infection expérimentale à *Brucella melitensis*. Comparison des vaccins Rev. 1 et H.38. In: Les Maladies de la Chèvre, Niort, France, 9–11, pp. 111–120, Octobre 1984.

Gay, J.M.: Neosporosis in dairy cattle: an update from an epidemiological perspective. Theriogenology, 66:629–632, 2006.

Georgie, G.C., et al.: Peripheral plasma testosterone levels in two Indian breeds of goats and their reciprocal crosses. Anim. Reprod. Sci., 9:95–98, 1985.

Ghosh, A., Yeasmin, F. and Alam, M.G.S.: Studies of ringwomb in Black Bengal goats (*Capra hircus*). Theriogenology, 37:527–532, 1992.

Giauffret, A. and Russo, P.: Enquête sérologique sur la chlamydiose des petits ruminants. Rec. Méd. Vét., 152:535–541, 1976.

Gil, M.C., et al.: Genital lesions in an outbreak of caprine contagious agalactia caused by *Mycoplasma agalactiae* and *Mycoplasma putrefaciens*. J. Vet. Med. Ser. B, 50:484–487. 2003.

Givens, M.D., Gard, J.A. and Stringfellow, D.A.: Relative risks and approaches to biosecurity in the use of embryo technologies in livestock. Theriogenology, 68:298–307, 2007.

Godfroid, J., et al.: From the discovery of the Malta fever's agent to the discovery of a marine mammal reservoir, brucellosis has continuously been a re-emerging zoonosis. Vet. Res., 36:313–326, 2005.

Gokak, A.G.: A case report of fibroma of the cervix in a female goat. Indian Vet. J., 65:834, 1998.

Gonçalves, H.C., et al.: Chromosomal constitution in rob (5/15) goat progeny. Small Rumin. Res., 15:73–76, 1994.

Gonyou, H.W. and Cobb, A.R.: The influence of time of feeding on the time of parturition in ewes. J. Anim. Sci., 66:569–574, 1986.

Gonzalez, F., et al.: Early pregnancy diagnosis in goats by determination of pregnancy-associated glycoprotein concentrations in plasma samples. Theriogenology, 52:717–725, 1999.

Gonzalez, F., et al.: The pregnancy associated glycoproteins (Pags) in the caprine species: fundamental and clinical approach. Proceedings, 7th International Conference on Goats, Tours, France, Vol 1, pp 413–415, May 2000.

Gonzalez, F., et al.: A comparison of diagnosis of pregnancy in the goat via transrectal ultrasound scanning, progesterone, and pregnancy-associated glycoprotein assays. Theriogenology, 62:1108–1115, 2004.

Gordon, I.: Controlled Reproduction in Sheep and Goats. Oxon UK, CAB International, 1997.

Gough, J.F.: *Campylobacter jejuni* isolated from an aborted caprine fetus in Ontario. Can. Vet. J., 28:670, 1987.

Gourley, D.D. and Riese, R.L.: Laparoscopic artificial insemination in sheep. Vet. Clin. N. Am. Food Anim. Pract., 6:615–633, 1990.

Grewal, A.S. and Wells, R.: Vulvovaginitis of goats due to a herpesvirus. Aust. Vet. J., 63:79–82, 1986.

Greyling, J.P.C. and Grobbelaar, J.A.N.: Seasonal variation in semen quality of Boer and Angora goat rams using different collection techniques. S. Afr. J. Anim. Sci., 13:250–252, 1983.

Greyling, J.P.C. and van Niekerk, C.H.: Ovulation in the Boer goat doe. Small Rumin. Res., 3:457–464, 1990.

Greyling, J.P.C. and Van Niekerk, C.H.: Different synchronization techniques in Boer goat does outside the normal breeding season. Small Rumin. Res., 5:233–243, 1991a.

Greyling, J.P.C. and Van Niekerk, C.H.: Macroscopic uterine involution in the postpartum Boer goat. Small Rumin. Res., 4:277–283, 1991b.

Grønstøl, H.: Listeriosis in goats. In: Les Maladies de la Chèvre, Niort, France, pp. 189–192, 9–11 Octobre 1984.

Guerrault, P., Perrin, G. and Fensterbank, R.: Essai de vaccination des caprins contre la listériose. Bull. Soc. Vét. Prat. Fr., 72:223–229, 1988.

Gunson, D.E., Acland, H.M., Gillette, D.M. and Pearson, J.E.: Abortion and stillbirth associated with *Chlamydia psittaci* var *ovis* in dairy goats with high titers to *Toxoplasma gondii*. J. Am. Vet. Med. Assoc., 183:1447–1450, 1983.

Gupta, P.P., et al.: Pathology of the genital tract of goats experimentally infected with *Acholeplasma laidlawii*. Indian Vet. J., 67:871–872, 1990.

Gupta, R.C., Kwatra, M.S. and Singh, N.: Chronic selenium toxicity as a cause of hoof and horn deformities in buffalo, cattle and goat. Indian Vet. J., 59:738–740, 1982.

Gupta, V.K., et al.: Polymerase chain reaction (PCR) for detection of *Brucella melitensis* in goat milk. Small Rumin. Res., 65:79–84, 2006.

Guss, S.B.: Management and Diseases of Dairy Goats. Scottsdale, AZ, Dairy Goat Journal Publ. Co., 1977.

Gutierrez, C., et al.: Two cases of schistosomus reflexus and two of omphalocele in the Canarian goat. J. Appl. Anim. Res., 15:93–96, 1999.

Haibel, G.K.: Real-time ultrasound assessment of the uterus and fetus in small ruminants. Proceedings, Annual Meeting, Society for Theriogenology, Rochester, New York, pp. 275–277, Sept. 17–19, 1986a.

Haibel, G.K.: Semen freezing and artificial insemination. In: Current Therapy in Theriogenology 2. D.A. Morrow, ed. Philadelphia, W.B. Saunders Co., pp. 624–626, 1986b.

Haibel, G.K.: Real-time ultrasonic fetal head measurement and gestational age in dairy goats. Theriogenology, 30: 1053–1057, 1988.

Haibel, G.K.: Out-of-season breeding in goats. Vet. Clin. N. Am. Food Anim. Pract., 6:577–583, 1990a.

Haibel, G.K.: Use of ultrasonography in reproductive management of sheep and goat herds. Vet. Clin. N. Am. Food Anim. Pract., 6:597–613, 1990b.

Haibel, G.K., Constable, P.D. and Rojko, J.L.: Vaginal leiomyofibromatosis and goiter in a goat. J. Am. Vet. Med. Assoc., 196:627–629, 1990.

Haibel, G.K. and Hull, B.L.: Induction of parturition in goats with fenprostalene. Theriogenology, 30:901–903, 1988.

Haibel, G.K., Perkins, N.R. and Lidl, G.M.: Breed differences in biparietal diameters of second trimester Toggenburg, Nubian and Angora goat fetuses. Theriogenology, 32:827–834, 1989.

Haibel, G.K. and Rojko, J.L.: Persistent Müllerian duct syndrome in a goat. Vet. Pathol., 27:135–137, 1990.

Hall, L.W. and Clarke, K.W.: Veterinary Anaesthesia. 8th Ed. London, Baillière Tindall, 1983.

Hamerton, J.L., et al.: Genetic intersexuality in goats. J. Reprod. Fert. Suppl. 7:25–51, 1969.

Hamilton, W.J. and Harrison, R.J.: Cyclical changes in the uterine mucosa and vagina of the goat. J. Anat., 85:316–324, 1951.

Hamori, D.: Constitutional Disorders and Hereditary Diseases in Domestic Animals. Developments in Animal and Veterinary Sciences 11. New York, Elsevier Scientific Publ. Co., 1983.

Hancock, J.L., McGovern, P.T. and Stamp, J.T.: Failure of gestation of goat × sheep hybrids in goats and sheep. J. Reprod. Fert. Suppl., 3:29–36, 1968.

Hare, W.C.D.: Diseases transmissible by semen and embryo transfer techniques. Office International des Epizooties, Paris, Technical Series No. 4, 1985.

Harms, J.W.: Zuchtfähige Ziegenböcke mit funktionierenden Milchdrüsen. Zool. Anz., 119(5/6):113–123, 1937.

Harrison, R.J.: The changes occurring in the ovary of the goat during the estrous cycle and in early pregnancy. J. Anat., 82:21–48, 1948.

Hart, B.L. and Jones, T.O.A.C.: Effects of castration on sexual behavior of tropical male goats. Horm. Behav., 6:247–258, 1975.

Hart, S. et al.: Nutritional flushing to increase ovulation and kidding rate in Spanish meat goats. J. Anim. Sci., 77(Suppl 1):265, 1999.

Hartman, W.: The anatomy and embryology of the pelvic outlet in female goats. Anat. Histol. Embryol., 4:127–148, 1975.

Hatchette, T.F., et al.: Goat-associated Q fever: a new disease in Newfoundland. Emerg. Infect. Dis., 7:413–419, 2001.

Haughey, K.G., Hartley, W.J., Della-Porta, A.J. and Murray, M.D.: Akabane disease in sheep. Aust. Vet. J., 65:136–140, 1988.

Hauser, B. and Bostedt, H.: Ultrasonographic observations of the uterine regression in the ewe under different obstetrical conditions. J. Vet. Med. A, 49:511–516, 2002.

Hayden, T.J., Thomas, C.R., Smith, S.V. and Forsyth, I.A.: Placental lactogen in the goat in relation to stage of gestation, number of fetuses, metabolites, progesterone and time of day. J. Endocrinol., 86:279–290, 1980.

Heidrich, H.J. and Renk, W.: Diseases of the Mammary Glands of Domestic Animals. Translated by L.W. van den Heever. Philadelphia, W.B. Saunders Co., 1967.

Hemeida, N.A., Sack, W.O. and McEntee, K.: Ductuli efferentes in the epididymis of boar, goat, ram, bull, and stallion. Am. J. Vet. Res., 39:1892–1900, 1978.

Hennig, A., et al.: Manganmangel beim Wiederkäuer, 1: Der Einfluss des Manganmangels auf die Lebenmassentwicklung. Arch. Tierernährung, 22:601–614, 1972.

Herndon, E.: Uvalde, TX, personal communication, 1989.

Hesselink, J.W.: Incidence of hydrometra in dairy goats. Vet. Rec., 132:110–112, 1993a.

Hesselink, J.W.: Hydrometra in dairy goats: reproductive performance after treatment with prostaglandins. Vet. Rec., 133:186–187, 1993b.

Hesselink, J.W. and Elving, L.: Pedigree analysis in a herd of dairy goats with respect to the incidence of hydrometra. Vet. Q., 18:24–25, 1996.

Hesselink, J.W. and Taverne, M.A.M.: Ultrasonography of the uterus of the goat. Vet. Q., 16:41–45, 1994.

Hesselink, J.W., et al.: Serum prolactin concentration in pseudopregnant and normally reproducing goats. Vet. Rec. 137:166–168, 1995.

Hicks, M.: Bucks will be bucks; management of the herd sire. Dairy Goat J., 65(8):494 and 504, 1987.

Holdsworth, R.J. and Davies, J.: Measurement of progesterone in goat's milk: An early pregnancy test. Vet. Rec., 105:535, 1979.

Horner, G.W., Hunter, R. and Day, A.M.: An outbreak of vulvovaginitis in goats caused by a caprine herpesvirus. N. Z. Vet. J., 30:150–152, 1982.

Huck, R.A.: Transmission of Border disease in goats. Vet. Rec., 92:151, 1973.

Humblot, P., et al.: Pregnancy-specific protein B and progesterone concentrations in French Alpine goats throughout gestation. J. Reprod. Fert., 89:205–212, 1990.

Humenhuk, R.A. and Vinha, N.A.: [Preliminary observations on the pathology of the testicle and epididymis in goats. III-Segmental aplasia of the mesonephric duct.] Arq. Escola Vet. Univ. Fed. Minas Gerais, 28:325–328, 1976.

Hussain, Q., et al.: Effect of type of roughage and energy level on reproductive performance of pregnant goats. Small Rumin. Res., 21:97–103, 1996.

Hyde, S.R. and Benirschke, K.: Gestational psittacosis: Case report and literature review. Mod. Pathol., 10:602–607, 1997.

Ikede, B.O.: Genital lesions in experimental chronic *Trypanosoma brucei* infection in rams. Res. Vet. Sci., 26:145–151, 1979.

Ilbery, P.L.T., Alexander, G. and Williams, D.: The chromosomes of sheep × goat hybrids. Aust. J. Biol. Sci., 20:1245–1247, 1967.

Inaba, Y., Kurogi, H. and Omori, T.: Akabane disease: epizootic abortion, premature birth, stillbirth and congenital arthrogryposis-hydranencephaly in cattle, sheep and goats caused by Akabane virus. Aust. Vet. J., 51:584–585, 1975.

Ishwar, A.K. and Memon, M.A.: Embryo transfer in sheep and goats: a review. Small Rumin. Res., 19:35–43, 1996.

Isoun, T.T. and Anosa, V.O.: Lesions in the reproductive organs of sheep and goats experimentally infected with *Trypanosoma vivax*. Tropenmed. Parasitol., 25:469–476, 1974.

Jackson, P.G.G. and White, R.A.S.: Epididymitis in a goat. Vet. Rec., 111:81–82, 1982.

Jain, G.C. and Madan, M.L.: Effect of prostin F2 alpha and dexamethasone on prostaglandin F and estradiol-17 beta level during induced parturition in goats. Proceedings, Third International Conference on Goat Production and Disease. Tucson, Arizona, p. 313, 1982.

Jain, G.C. and Madan, M.L.: Plasma prostaglandin F, oestradiol-17β, cortisol and progesterone in induced parturient goats. Int. J. Anim. Sci., 4:152–156, 1989.

Janett, F., et al.: Gynecomastia in a goat buck. Schweiz. Arch. Tierheilkunde, 138:241–244, 1996.

Johnson, F.W.A., et al.: Abortion due to infection with *Chlamydia psittaci* in a sheep farmer's wife. Br. Med. J., 290:592–594, 1985.

Johnston, W.S.: An investigation into toxoplasmosis as a cause of barrenness in ewes. Vet. Rec., 122:283–284, 1988.

Jones, S.L. and Fecteau, G.: Hydrops uteri in a caprine doe pregnant with goat-sheep hybrid fetuses. J. Am. Vet. Med. Assoc., 206:1920–1922, 1995.

Jorge, W. and Takebayasi, S.: Chromosomal mosaicism associated with testicular hypoplasia in goats. In: Proceedings, IVth International Conference on Goats, Brasilia, Brazil, 1987, EMBRAPA, Vol. II, abstr. 52, p. 1339.

Jorgensen, D.M.: Gestational psittacosis in a Montana sheep rancher. Emerg. Infect. Dis., 3:191–194, 1997.

Just, W., et al.: The male pseudohermaphrodite XX polled goat is Zfy and Sry negative. Hereditas, 120:71–75, 1994.

Kaaya, G.P. and Oduor-Okelo, D.: The effects of *Trypanosoma congolense* infection on the testis and epididymis of the goat. Bull. Anim. Health Prod. Afr., 28:1–5, 1980.

Kähn, W.: Veterinary Reproductive Ultrasonography. London, Mosby-Wolfe, 1994.

Kaikini, A.S. and Deshmukh, V.B.: Uterine leiomyoma in a goat (*Capra hircus* L). Indian Vet. J., 54:583+ plate, 1977.

Kasari, T.R., et al.: Evaluation of pathways for release of Rift Valley fever virus into domestic ruminant livestock, ruminant wildlife, and human populations in the continental United States. J. Am. Vet. Med. Assoc., 232:514–529, 2008.

Kalmar, E., Peleg, B.A. and Savir, D.: Arthrogryposis-hydranencephaly syndrome in newborn cattle, sheep and goats—Serological survey for antibodies against the Akabane virus. Refuah Vet., 32:47–54, 1975.

Kambarage, D.M.: Sarcoptic mange infestation in goats. Bull. Anim. Health Prod. Afr., 40:239–244, 1992.

Kar, A.B.: Chemical sterilization of male goats. Indian J. Vet. Sci., 32:70–73, 1962.

Karagiannidis, A., Varsakeli, S. and Karatzas, G.: Characteristics and seasonal variations in the semen of Alpine, Saanen and Damascus goat bucks born and raised in Greece. Theriogenology, 53:1285–1293, 2000.

Kaulfuss, K.-H.: [Case report: Diagnosis of cryptorchid male lambs and of ovine and caprine intersex by real-time ultrasound.] Tierärztl. Umschau, 61:86–90, 2006.

Kelk, D.A., et al.: The interbreeding of sheep and goats. Can. Vet. J., 38:235–237, 1997.

Kellerman, T.S., et al.: Plant Poisonings and Mycotoxicoses of Livestock in Southern Africa. 2nd edition. Oxford, Oxford Univ. Press, 2005.

Kene, R.O.C.: Radiographic investigation of dystocia in the West African dwarf goat. Br. Vet. J., 147:283–289, 1991.

Keuser, V., Gogev, S., Schynts, F. and Thiry, E.: Demonstration of generalized infection with caprine herpesvirus 1 diagnosed in an aborted caprine fetus by PCR. Vet. Res. Commun., 26:221–226, 2002.

Killen, I.D. and Caffery, G.J.: Uterine insemination of ewes with the aid of a laparoscope. Aust. Vet. J., 59:95, 1982.

Kim, I., et al.: Identification of bovine viral diarrhea virus type 2 in Korean native goat (*Capra hircus*). Virus Res., 121:103–106, 2006.

Kirkbride, C.A. (ed): Laboratory Diagnosis of Livestock Abortion. 3rd Ed. Ames, IA, Iowa State University Press, 1990.

Kornalijnslijper, J.E., et al.: Induction of hydrometra in goats by means of active immunization against prostaglandin $F_{2\alpha}$. Anim. Reprod. Sci., 46:109–122, 1997.

Kraemer, D.C.: Embryo collection and transfer in small ruminants. Theriogenology, 31:141–148, 1989.

Kronberger, H.: Kritische Sichtung des dem Institute in den Jahren 1917–1959 eingesandten Geschwulst-materials von Haussäugetieren. Monatshefte f. Veterinärmed, 16:296–302, 1961.

Kumar, R., Sharma, A.K. and Prasad, M.C.: Foetal hydrops in a goat. Goat Vet. Soc. J., 10(1):52, 1989.

Kumar, R., et al.: Effect of castration on urethra and accessory sex glands in goats. Indian Vet. J., 59:304–308, 1982.

Kurogi, H., et al.: Experimental infection of pregnant goats with Akabane virus. Natl. Inst. Anim. Health Q. (Tokyo), 17:1–9, 1977.

Kutty, C.I.: Gynecological examination and pregnancy diagnosis in small ruminants using bimanual palpation technique: a review. Theriogenology, 51:1555–1564, 1999.

Kutty, C.I. and Mathew, S.: Granulosa cell tumour in a goat. J. Vet. Anim. Sci., 26:127–128, 1995.

Lang, G.H.: Serosurvey of *Coxiella burnetii* infection in dairy goat herds in Ontario. A comparison of two methods of enzyme-linked immunosorbent assay. Can. J. Vet. Res., 52:37–41, 1988.

Lavoir, M.C. and Taverne, M.A.M.: The diagnosis of pregnancy and pseudopregnancy, and the determination of foetal numbers of goats, by means of real-time ultrasound scanning. In: Diagnostic Ultrasound and Animal Reproduction. M.A.M. Taverne and A.H. Willesme, eds. Dordrecht, Kluwer Acad. Publ., 1989.

Leboeuf, B., Restall, B. and Salamon, S.: Production and storage of goat semen for artificial insemination. Anim. Reprod. Sci., 62:113–141, 2000.

Lefèvre, P.C.: In utero infections causing abortions and weak kids. In: Proceedings, Fourth International Conference on Goats, Brasilia, Brazil, EMBRAPA, Volume I, pp. 355–371 March 8–13, 1987.

Lefèvre, P.C. and Calvez, D.: La fièvre catarrhale du mouton (bluetongue) en Afrique intertropicale: influence des facteurs écologiques sur la prévalence de l'infection. Rev. Élev. Méd. Vét. Pays Trop., 39:263–268, 1986.

Leon-Vizcaino, L., Hermoso de Mendoza, M. and Garrido, F.: Incidence of abortions caused by leptospirosis in sheep and goats in Spain. Comp. Immunol. Microbiol. Infect. Dis., 10:149–153, 1987.

Letshwenyo, M. and Kedikilwe, K.: Goat-sheep hybrid born under natural conditions in Botswana. Vet. Rec., 146:732–734, 2000.

Levy, J.K., et al.: Comparison of intratesticular injection of zinc gluconate versus surgical castration to sterilize male dogs. Am. J. Vet. Res., 69:140–143, 2008.

Lickliter, R.E.: Behavior associated with parturition in the domestic goat. Appl. Anim. Behav. Sci., 13:335–345, 1984/85.

Lindahl, I.L.: Pregnancy diagnosis in dairy goats using ultrasonic Doppler instruments. J. Dairy Sci., 52:529–530, 1969.

Lindsay, D.S., et al.: Abortions, fetal death, and stillbirths in pregnant pygmy goats inoculated with tachyzoites of *Neospora caninum*. Am. J. Vet. Res., 56:1176–1180, 1995.

Llewelyn, C.A., Luckins, A.G., Munro, C.D. and Perrie, J.: The effect of *Trypanosoma congolense* infection on the oestrous cycle of the goat. Br. Vet. J., 143:423–431, 1987.

Lofstedt. R.M.: Vasectomy in ruminants: A cranial midscrotal approach. J. Am. Vet. Med. Assoc., 181:373–375, 1982.

Lofstedt, R.M., Laarveld, B. and Ihle, S.L.: Adrenal neoplasia causing lactation in a castrated male goat. J. Vet. Int. Med., 8:382–384, 1994.

Lofstedt, R.M. and Williams, R.J.: Granulosa cell tumor in a goat. J. Am. Vet. Med. Assoc., 189:206–208, 1986.
Løken, T.: Experimentally-induced border disease in goats. J. Comp. Pathol., 97:85–89, 1987.
Løken, T.: Pestivirus infections in Norway. Epidemiological studies in goats. J. Comp. Pathol., 103:1–10, 1990.
Løken, T., Aspøy, E. and Grønstøl, H.: *Listeria monocytogenes* excretion and humoral immunity in goats in a herd with outbreaks of listeriosis and in a healthy herd. Acta Vet. Scand., 23:392–399, 1982.
Løken, T.: Border disease in goats. In: Recent Advances in Goat Diseases. M. Tempesta, ed. Accessed online at <http://www.ivis.org/advances/Disease_Tempesta/Loken/chapter.asp>. November 23, 2000.
Løken, T. and Bjerkås, I.: Experimental pestivirus infections in pregnant goats. J. Comp. Pathol., 105:123–140, 1991.
Løken, T, Bjerkås, I. and Hyllseth, B.: Border disease in goats in Norway. Res. Vet. Sci., 33:130–131, 1982.
Løken, T., Krogsrud, J. and Bjerkås, I.: Outbreaks of border disease in goats induced by a pestivirus-contaminated orf vaccine, with virus transmission to sheep and cattle. J. Comp. Pathol., 104:195–209, 1991.
Löliger, H.-C.: Experimentelle Coli-Orchitis beim Ziegenbock. Arch. Exp. Vet., 10:582–590, 1956.
Löliger, H.-C.: Die Pathogenese der sog. Samenstauung im Nebenhoden der Ziegenböcke. Zentralblatt f. Veterinärmed., 4:892–906, 1957.
Louw, D.F.J. and Joubert, D.M.: Puberty in the male Dorper sheep and Boer goat. So. Afr. J. Agr. Sci., 7:509–520, 1964.
Low, C. and Linklater, K.: Listeriosis in sheep. In Practice, 7:66–67, 1985.
Ludders, J.W.: Anesthesia for the pregnant patient. Soc. Theriogenology Proc Ann. Meeting, Orlando, Florida, pp. 36–54, September 16–17, 1988.
Lush, J.L., Jones, J.M. and Dameron, W.H.: The inheritance of cryptorchidism in goats. Tex. Agric. Exp. Stn. Bull. No. 407, 1930.
Lyngset, O.: Embryonic mortality in the goat. VIe Congr. Intern. Reprod. Anim. Insem. Artif., Paris., 1:439–441, 1968a.
Lyngset, O.: Studies on reproduction in the goat, I. The normal genital organs of the nonpregnant goat. Acta Vet. Scand., 9:208–222, 1968b.
Lyngset, O.: Studies on reproduction in the goat, II. The genital organs of the pregnant goat. Acta Vet. Scand., 9:242–252, 1968c.
Lyngset, O.: Studies on reproduction in the goat. V. Pathological conditions and malformations of the genital organs of the goat. Acta Vet. Scand., 9:364–375, 1968d.
Lyngset, O.: Studies on reproduction in the goat. VII. Pregnancy and the development of the foetus and the foetal accessories of the goat. Acta Vet. Scand., 12:185–201, 1971.
Machens, A.: Beobachtungen über die Samenstauung der Ziegenböcke. Dtsch. Tierärztl. Wochenschr., 45:123–125, 1937.
Mackie, J.T., Rahaley, R.S. and Nugent, R.: Suspected *Sarcocystis* encephalitis in a stillborn kid. Aust. Vet. J., 69:114–115, 1992.
Mackie, J.T. and Dubey, J.P.: Congenital sarcocystosis in a Saanen goat. J. Parasitol., 82:350–351, 1996.
Majeed, A.F. and Taha, M.B.: Preliminary study on treatment of ringwomb in Iraqi goats. Anim. Reprod. Sci., 18:199–203, 1989.
Malher, X. and Ben Younes, A.: Les facteurs zootechniques de l'infécondité dans l'espèce caprine. Rec. Méd. Vét., 163:831–838, 1987.
Mani, A.U., McKelvey, W.A.C. and Watson, E.D.: The effects of low level of feeding on response to synchronization of estrus, ovulation rate and embryo loss in goats. Theriogenology, 38:1013–1022, 1992.
Mani, A.U., Watson, E.D. and McKelvey, W.A.C.: Effect of undernutrition on progesterone concentration during the early luteal phase and mid-gestation in goats. Vet. Rec., 136:518–519, 1995.
Manley, F.H.: Contagious abortion of sheep and goats in Cyprus. J. Comp. Pathol. Ther., 45:293–300, 1932.
Markusfeld, O. and Mayer, E.: An arthrogryposis and hydranencephaly syndrome in calves in Israel, 1969/70—Epidemiological and clinical aspects. Refuah Vet., 28:51–61, 1971.
Marnet, P.G., Laurentie, M.P., Garcia-Villar, R. and Toutain, P.L.: Effets de doses excessives d'ocytocine sur la contractilité utérine chez la brebis. Rev. Méd. Vét., 136:315–320, 1985.
Martinez, M.F., Bosch, P. and Bosch, R.A.: Determination of early pregnancy and embryonic growth in goats by transrectal ultrasound scanning. Theriogenology, 49:1555–1565, 1998.
Martinez-Rodriguez, H.A., et al.: Effect of the caprine arthritis encephalitis virus in the reproductive system of male goats. Vet. Mex., 36:159–176, 2005.
Mathew, J. and Raja, C.K.S.V.: Investigation on the incidence of cryptorchidism in goats. Kerala J. Vet. Sci., 9(1):47–52, 1978a.
Mathew, J. and Raja, C.K.S.V.: Studies on testicular hypoplasia in goats. Kerala J. Vet. Sci., 9:24–30, 1978b.
Matsas, D.: Pregnancy diagnosis in goats. In: Current Therapy in Large Animal Theriogenology 2. R.S. Youngquist and W.R. Threlfall, eds. St. Louis, Saunders Elsevier, pp. 547–554, 2007.
Matthews, J.G.: Outline of Clinical Diagnosis in the Goat. London, Wright, 1991.
Maule Walker, F.M.: Lactation and fertility in goats after the induction of parturition with an analogue of prostaglandin F2α, cloprostenol. Res. Vet. Sci., 34:280–286, 1983.
McArthur, C.P. and Geary, A.: Field evaluation of a pregnancy immunoassay for the detection of oestrone sulphate in goats. J. Endocrinol. 110:133–136, 1986.
McCauley, E.H. and Tieken, E.L.: Psittacosis-lymphogranuloma venereum agent isolated during an abortion epizootic in goats. J. Am. Vet. Med. Assoc., 152:1758–1765, 1968.
McCoy, M.H., et al.: Serologic and reproductive findings after a herpesvirus-1 abortion storm in goats. J. Am. Vet. Med. Assoc., 231:1236–1239, 2007.
McDougall, S.: Induction of parturition in milking goats. Aust. Vet. J., 67:465–466, 1990.
McEntee, K.: Reproductive Pathology of Domestic Mammals. New York, Academic Press, 1990.
McQuiston, J.H., Childs, J.E. and Thompson, H.A.: Q fever. J. Am. Vet. Med. Assoc., 221:796–799, 2002.

McSporran, K.D., McCaughan, C. and Demsteegt, A.: Toxoplasmosis in goats. N. Z. Vet. J., 33:39–40, 1985.

Meador, V.P. and Deyoe, B.L.: Experimentally induced *Brucella abortus* infection in pregnant goats. Am. J. Vet. Res., 47:2337–2342, 1986.

Medan, M.S., Watanabe, G., Sasaki, K. and Taya, K.: Transrectal ultrasonic diagnosis of ovarian follicular cysts in goats and treatment with GnRH. Domestic Anim. Endocrinol., 27:115–124, 2004.

Megale, F.: Induction of erection and ejaculation in the bull by local massage. Cornell Vet., 58:88–89, 1968.

Meites, J., et al.: Effects of corpora lutea removal and replacement with progesterone on pregnancy in goats. J. Anim. Sci., 10:411–416, 1951.

Melby, H.P.: Sjodogg (Tick-borne fever) hos geit. Norsk Veterinaertidsskrift, 96:87–90, 1984.

Mellado, M., et al.: Effect of prostaglandin F2α dosage and route of administration on estrus response in Criollo goats under range conditions. Small Rumin. Res., 14:205–208, 1994.

Mellado, M., et al.: Factors affecting gestation length in goats and the effect of gestation period on kid survival. J. Agric. Sci., 135:85–89, 2000.

Memon, M.A.: Male infertility. Vet. Clin. N. Am. Large Anim. Pract., 5:619–635, 1983.

Memon, M.A., Bretzlaff, K.N. and Ott, R.S.: Comparison of semen collection techniques in goats. Theriogenology, 26:823–827, 1986a.

Memon, M.A., et al.: Observations on the use of prostaglandin F-2-alpha as an abortifacient and effect of gonadotropin-releasing hormone on ovarian activity after induced abortion during the breeding season in goats. Theriogenology, 25:653–658, 1986b.

Memon, M.A., Mickelsen, W.D. and Goyal, H.O.: Examination of the reproductive tract and evaluation of potential breeding soundness in the buck. In: Current Therapy in Large Animal Theriogenology 2. R.S. Youngquist and W. R. Threlfall, eds. St. Louis, Saunders Elsevier, pp. 515–518, 2007.

Memon, M.A., Schelling, S.C. and Sherman, D.M.: Mucinous adenocarcinoma of the ovary as a cause of ascites in a goat. J. Am. Vet. Med. Assoc., 206:362–264, 1995.

Menard, L. and Diaz, C.S.: The use of clenbuterol for the management of large animal dystocias: surgical corrections in the cow and ewe. Can. Vet. J., 28:585–590, 1987.

Mendoza, G., White, I.G. and Chow, P.: Studies on chemical components of Angora goat seminal plasma. Theriogenology, 32:455–466, 1989.

Metcalfe, J., et al.: The pygmy goat as an experimental animal. In: Symposium on Animal Models for Biomedical Research. Natl. Acad. Sci. Publ., 1594:55–63, 1968.

Mialot, J.-P., Lévy, I., and Emery, P.: Echographie et gestion des troupeaux caprins. Rec. Méd. Vét., 168:399–406, 1991.

Mialot, J.P., et al.: La pseudogestation chez la chèvre: observations préliminaires. (Pseudo-pregnancy in goats: preliminary observations.) Rec. Méd. Vét., 167:383–390, 1991.

Mikolon, A.B., et al.: Evaluation of North American antibody detection tests for diagnosis of brucellosis in goats. J. Clin. Microbiol., 36:1716–1722, 1998.

Miller, R.B., Palmer, N.C. and Kierstad, M.: *Coxiella burnetii* infection in goats. In: Current Therapy in Theriogenology, 2: Edited by D.A. Morrow. Philadelphia, W.B. Saunders Co., pp. 607–609, 1986.

Mine, O.M., et al.: Sheep-goat hybrid born under natural conditions. Small Rumin. Res., 37:141–145, 2000.

Minnia, P., Lacalandra, G.M., Lattanzi, M. and Bufano, G.: Reproductive management of anestrus goats with Gn-RH or "male effect." Proceedings, Fourth International Conference on Goats, Brasilia, Brazil (Abstract.) EMBRAPA Vol. 2, p. 1497, 1987.

Mobini, S., Heath, A.M. and Pugh, D.G.: Theriogenology of sheep and goats. In: Sheep and Goat Medicine. D.G. Pugh, ed. Philadelphia, W.B. Saunders, pp. 129–186, 2002.

Moeller, Jr., R.B.: Causes of caprine abortion: diagnostic assessment of 211 cases (1991–1998). J. Vet. Diagn. Invest., 13:265–270, 2001.

Moore, J.D., et al.: Pathology and diagnosis of *Coxiella burnetii* infection in a goat herd. Vet. Pathol., 28:81–84, 1991.

Morin, D.E., et al.: Hydrallantois in a caprine doe. J. Am. Vet. Med. Assoc., 204:108–111, 1994.

Morrow, D.A. (ed.): Current Therapy in Theriogenology 2. Philadelphia, W.B. Saunders Co, 1986.

Morse, E.V. and Langham, R.F.: Experimental leptospirosis, III. Caprine *Leptospira pomona* infections. Am. J. Vet. Res., 19:139–144, 1958.

Muduuli, D.S., Sanford, L.M., Palmer, W.M. and Howland, B.E.: Secretory patterns and circadian and seasonal changes in luteinizing hormone, follicle stimulating hormone, prolactin and testosterone in the male pygmy goat. J. Anim. Sci., 49:543–553, 1979.

Mugera, G.M. and Chema, S.: Nairobi sheep disease: a study of its pathogenesis in sheep, goats and suckling mice. Bull. Epizoot. Dis. Afr., 15:337–354, 1967.

München, W.K.: Die Diagnose der Sterilität bei Ziegen. Tierärztl. Umschau., 6:153–155, 1951.

Munday, B.L. and Dubey, J.P.: Prevention of *Toxoplasma gondii* abortion in goats by vaccination with oocysts of *Hammondia hammondi*. Aust. Vet. J., 65:150–153, 1988.

Munday, B.L., Obendorf, D.L., Handlinger, J.H. and Mason, R.W.: Diagnosis of congenital toxoplasmosis in ovine fetuses. Aust. Vet. J., 64:292, 1987.

Mura, D., Altieri, M. and Contini, A.: (*Salmonella abortus-ovis* infection in sheep and goats.) Atti Soc. Ital. Sci. Vet. Sanremo, 6:673–676, 1952. Abstract in Vet. Bull., 24:294 (abstr. 1797), 1954.

Murali, N., Jagatheesan, P.N.R. and Kumar, V.R.S.: Unilateral cryptorchidism in Tellicherry bucks. Indian Vet. J., 82:1122–1123, 2005.

Murray, R.D. and Newstead, R.: Determination of steroid hormones in goats' milk and plasma as an aid to pregnancy diagnosis using an ELISA. Vet. Rec., 122:158–161, 1988.

Mushi, E.Z., Binta, M.G. and Raborokgwe, M.: Wesselsbron disease virus associated with abortions in goats in Botswana. J. Vet. Diagn. Invest., 10:191, 1998.

Mutayoba, B.M., Meyer, H.H.D., Osaso, J. and Gombe, S.: Trypanosome-induced increase in prostaglandin F2α and its relationship with corpus luteum function in the goat. Theriogenology, 32:545–555, 1989.

Navarro, M., et al.: Anthelmintic induced congenital malformations in sheep embryos using netobimin. Vet. Rec., 142:86–90, 1998.

Neathery, M.W., et al.: Effects of long term zinc deficiency on feed utilization, reproductive characteristics, and hair growth in the sexually mature male goat. J. Dairy Sci., 56:98–105, 1973.

Ngeranwa, J.J.N., et al.: The effects of experimental *Trypanosoma* (*Trypanozoon*) (*brucei*) *evansi* infection on the fertility of male goats. Vet. Res. Commun., 15:301–308, 1991.

Nightingale, K.K., et al.: Ecology and transmission of *Listeria monocytogenes* infecting ruminants and in the farm environment. Appl. Environ. Microbiol., 70:4458–4467, 2004.

Njenga, J.M., et al.: Preliminary findings from an experimental study of caprine besnoitiosis in Kenya. Vet. Res. Commun., 17:203–208, 1993.

Nunes, J.F., et al.: Preliminary report on observed differences in goat sperm characteristics based on scrotal morphology. In: Reproduction des Ruminants en Zone Tropicale. Pointe-à-Pitre, INRA Publ., 1984 (Les Colloques de l'INRA, no. 20) pp. 251–264, June 8–10, 1983.

Nurse, G.H. and Lenghaus, C.: An outbreak of *Toxoplasma gondii* abortion, mummification and perinatal death in goats. Aust. Vet. J., 63:27–29, 1986.

Nuti, L.: Techniques for artificial insemination of goats. In: Current Therapy in Large Animal Theriogenology 2. R.S. Youngquist and W.R. Threlfall, eds. St. Louis, Saunders Elsevier, pp.529–534, 2007.

Nuti, L.C. and McWhinney, D.R.: Photoperiod effects on reproductive parameters in two breeds of dairy goat bucks (*Capra hircus*). Proceedings, Fourth International Conference on Goats, Brasilia, Brazil, Vol. 2, (Abstract.), pp. 1508–1509, 1987.

Nuti, L.C., et al.: Synchronization of estrus in dairy goats treated with prostaglandin F at various stages of the estrous cycle. Am. J. Vet. Res., 53:935–937, 1992.

Obendorf, D.L., Statham, P. and Munday, B.L.: Resistance to *Toxoplasma* abortion in female goats previously exposed to *Toxoplasma* infection. Aust. Vet. J., 67:233–234, 1990.

O'Brien, C., Szabuniewicz, M. and Sorensen, A.M., Jr.: Simplified method for semen collection from rams and billies. Southwest. Vet., 17:32–33, 1963.

OIE: Manual of Diagnostic Tests and Vaccines for Terrestrial Animals, Vol. 2, 5th Ed. Office International des Épizooties (OIE), Paris, 2004.

OIE: Terrestrial Animal Health Code 2007. Appendix 3.3.5. Categorisation of diseases and pathogenic agents by the International Embryo Transfer Society. http://www.oie.int/eng/normes/mcode/en_chapitre_3.3.5.htm (Accessed 2 Feb 2008.)

Oldham, C.M. and Lindsay, D.R.: Laparoscopy in the ewe: a photographic record of the ovarian activity of ewes experiencing normal or abnormal oestrous cycles. Anim. Reprod. Sci., 3:119–124, 1980.

Orgeur, P., Signoret, J.P. and Leboeuf, B.: Effects of rearing conditions upon the development of sexual activity and semen production in young male goats. In: The Male in Farm Animal Reproduction. M. Courot, ed. Boston, MA, Martinus Nijhoff Publishers, pp. 135–140, 1984.

Orr, M.B. and Barlow, R.M.: Experiments in Border disease. X. The postnatal skin lesion in sheep and goats. J. Comp. Pathol., 88:295–302, 1978.

Osuagwuh, A.I.A. and Aire, T.A.: Studies on the estimation of the developmental age of the caprine foetus. 1. External measurements and appearance. Trop. Vet., 4:39–51, 1986.

Osweiler, G.D., Carson, T.L., Buck, W.B. and Van Gelder, G.A.: Clinical and Diagnostic Veterinary Toxicology, 3rd Ed. Dubuque, Iowa, Kendall/Hunt Publ. Co., 1985.

Ott, R.S.: Examination of bucks for breeding soundness. Vet. Med. Small Anim. Clin., 73:1561–1563, 1978.

Ott, R.S.: Breeding soundness examination of bulls. In: Current Therapy in Theriogenology 2. D.A. Morrow, ed. Philadelphia, W.B. Saunders Co. pp. 125–136, 1986.

Ott, R.S.: Current thinking on breeding soundness examination of bulls. Proceedings, Society for Theriogenology Annual Meeting, Austin, Texas, pp. 14–31, 1987.

Ott, R.S. and Memon, M.A.: Breeding soundness examination of rams and bucks: A review. Theriogenology, 13:155–164, 1980.

Ott, R.S., Nelson, D.R. and Hixon, J.E.: Effect of presence of the male on initiation of estrous cycle activity of goats. Theriogenology, 13:183–190, 1980.

Ott, R.S., et al.: A comparison of intrarectal Doppler and rectal abdominal palpation for pregnancy testing in goats. J. Am. Vet. Med. Assoc., 178:730–731, 1981.

Oyeyemi, M.O., Akusu, M.O. and Ola-Davies, O.E.: Effect of successive ejaculation on the spermiogram of West African Dwarf goats. Israel J. Vet. Med., 56:151–153, 2001.

Padilla, G. and Holtz, W.: Follicular dynamics in cycling Boer goats. Proceedings, 7th International Conference on Goats, Tours, France, Vol. 1, p 479 May 2000.

Padula, A.M.: The freemartin syndrome: an update. Anim. Reprod. Sci., 87:93–109, 2005.

Palmer, N.C., et al.: Placentitis and abortion in goats and sheep in Ontario caused by *Coxiella burnetii*. Can. Vet. J., 24:60–61, 1983.

Pamo, E.T., et al.: Influence of supplementary feeding with multipurpose leguminous tree leaves on kid growth and milk production in the West African dwarf goat. Small Rum. Res., 63:142–149, 2006.

Pamukcu, A.M.: Seminoma of the testicles in an Ankara goat. Ankara Univ. Vet. Fak. Dergisi, 1:42–46, 1954.

Panchadevi, S.M. and Pandit, R.V.: Milking males—two case studies. Indian Vet. J., 56:590–592, 1979.

Panebianco, A., Zanghi, A. and Catone, G.: Su alcune vasculopatie del cordone testicolare in ovini e caprini. [Some angiopathies of spermatic cord in sheep and goat.] Clin. Vet., 108:441–449, 1985.

Panter, K.E., James, L.F., Keeler, R.F. and Bunch, T.D.: Radio-ultrasound observations of poisonous plant-induced fetotoxicity in livestock. In: Poisonous Plants. Proceedings of the Third International Symposium. L.F. James, et al., eds. Ames, IA, Iowa State Univ. Press, pp. 481–488, 1992.

Panter, K.E., Keeler, R.F., Bunch, T.D. and Callan, R.J.: Congenital skeletal malformations and cleft palate induced in goats by ingestion of *Lupinus*, *Conium* and *Nicotiana* species. Toxicon (Oxford), 28:1377–1385, 1990.

Papp, J.R., Shewen, P.E. and Gartley, C.J.: Abortion and subsequent excretion of chlamydiae from the reproductive tract of sheep during estrus. Infect. Immun., 62:3786–3792, 1994.

Parkhie, M.R.: Abuse of anabolic steroids. J. Am. Vet. Med. Assoc., 199:11–12, 1991.

Parsonson, I.M., Della-Porta, A.J. and Snowdon, W.A.: Akabane virus infection in the pregnant ewe, 2: Pathology of the foetus. Vet. Microbiol., 6:209–224, 1981.
Patton, S., Johnson, S.S. and Puckett, K.: Prevalence of *Toxoplasma gondii* antibodies in nine populations of dairy goats: compared titers using modified direct agglutination and indirect hemaglutination. J. Parasitol., 76:74–77, 1990.
Peaker, M.: Gestation period and litter size in the goat. Br. Vet. J., 134:379–383, 1978.
Pearce, G.P. and Oldham, C.M.: Importance of non-olfactory ram stimuli in mediating ram-induced ovulation in the ewe. J. Reprod. Fert., 88:333–339, 1988.
Pechman, R.D. and Eilts, B.E.: B-mode ultrasonography of the bull testicle. Theriogenology, 27:431–441, 1987.
Pellicer-Rubio, M.T., et al.: Highly synchronous and fertile reproductive activity induced by the male effect during deep anoestrus in lactating goats subjected to treatment with artificially long days followed by a natural photoperiod. Anim. Reprod. Sci., 98:241–258, 2007.
Pennington, J.A., et al.: Milk progesterone for pregnancy diagnosis in dairy goats. J. Dairy Sci., 65:2011–2014, 1982.
Philip, J.R. and Shone, D.K.: Anthelmintic and toxicity studies with tetramisole. II Toxicity studies in sheep and goats. J. S. Afr. Vet. Med. Assoc., 38:287–292, 1967.
Philip, P.J., et al.: Caesarean section in goats: A clinical study. Indian J. Vet. Surg., 6(1):41–43, 1985.
Phillips, R.W., Simmons, V.L. and Schott, R.G.: Observations on the normal estrous cycle and breeding season in goats and possibilities of modification of the breeding season with gonadotrophic hormones. Am. J. Vet. Res., 4:360–367, 1943.
Philpott, M.: The dangers of disease transmission by artificial insemination and embryo transfer. Br. Vet. J., 149:339–369, 1993.
Pienaar, J.G. and Schutte, A.P.: The occurrence and pathology of chlamydiosis in domestic and laboratory animals: a review. Onderstepoort J. Vet. Res., 42(3):77–90, 1975.
Pieterse, M.C. and Taverne, M.A.M.: Hydrometra in goats: diagnosis with real-time ultrasound and treatment with prostaglandins or oxytocin. Theriogenology, 26:813–821, 1986.
Plant, J.W. and Bowler, J.K.: Controlled parturition in sheep using clenbuterol hydrochloride. Aust. Vet. J., 65:91–93, 1988.
Polydorou, K.: Brucellosis in sheep and goats in Cyprus. Comp. Immunol. Microbiol. Infect. Dis., 2:99–106, 1979.
Polydorou, K.: Q fever in Cyprus: a short review. Br. Vet. J., 137:470–477, 1981a.
Polydorou, K.: The control of enzootic abortion in sheep and goats in Cyprus. Br. Vet. J., 137:411–415, 1981b.
Polydorou, K.: Caprine brucellosis in Cyprus. In: Les Maladies de la Chèvre, Niort, France, pp. 93–99, 9–11 Octobre 1984.
Ponvijay, K.S.: Pinhole castration: a novel minimally invasive technique for in situ spermatic cord ligation. Vet. Surg., 36:74–79, 2007.
Popescu, C.P.: Mode de transmission d'une fusion centrique dans la descendance d'un bouc (*Capra hircus* L.) hétérozygote. Ann. Génét. Sél. Anim., 4:355–361, 1972.
Portanti, O., et al.: Development and validation of a competitive ELISA kit for the serological diagnosis of ovine, caprine and bovine brucellosis. J. Vet. Med. Ser. B, 53:494–498, 2006.
Pospischil, A., et al.: Abortion in humans by *Chlamydophila abortus* (*Chlamydia psittaci* serovar 1). Schweiz. Arch. Tierheilkunde, 144:463–466, 2002.
Powe, T.A., et al.: B-mode ultrasonography of testicular pathology in the bull. Agri-Practice, 9(5):43–45, 1988.
Pretorius, P.S.: Vaginal cytological changes in the cycling and anoestrous Angora goat doe. J. S. Afr. Vet. Assoc., 48:169–171, 1977.
Purdy, P.H.: A review on goat sperm cryopreservation. Small Rumin. Res., 63:215–225, 2006.
Radwan, A.I., Bekairi, S.I. and Mukayel, A.A.: Treatment of *Brucella melitensis* infection in sheep and goats with oxytetracycline combined with streptomycin. Rev. Sci. Tech. Off. Int. Epiz., 11:845–857, 1992.
Rahim, A.T.A. and Arthur, G.H.: Obstetrical conditions in goats. Cornell Vet., 72:279–284, 1982.
Rajan, A., et al.: An assessment of the goitrogenic effect of *Leucaena leucocephala*. Indian Vet. J., 68:413–417, 1991.
Ramadan, R.O. and El Hassan, A.M.: Leiomyoma in the cervix and hyperplastic ectopic mammary tissue in a goat. Aust. Vet. J., 51:362, 1975.
Ramadan, R.O., et al.: Bilateral scrotal hysterocele in an intersex goat. J. Vet. Med. A, 38:441–444, 1991.
Ray, S.K., et al.: Studies on "zinc deficiency syndrome" in Black Bengal goats (*Capra hircus*) fed with fodder (*Andropogon gayanus*) grown on soil treated with an excess of calcium and phosphorus fertilizer. Vet. Res. Commun., 21:541–546, 1997.
Reddi, N.M. and Rajan, A.: Pathology of the reproductive organs in experimental hypothyroidism in male goats. Indian Vet. J., 62:837–842, 1985.
Reddi, N.M. and Rajan, A.: Reproductive behaviour and semen characteristics in experimental hypothyroidism in goats. Theriogenology, 25:263–274, 1986.
Refsal, K.R.: Collection and evaluation of caprine semen. In: Current Therapy in Theriogenology 2. D.A. Morrow, ed. Philadelphia, W.B. Saunders Co. pp. 619–621, 1986.
Refsal, K.R., et al.: Concentrations of estrone sulfate in peripheral serum of pregnant goats: relationships with gestation length, fetal number and the occurrence of fetal death *in utero*. Theriogenology, 36:449–461, 1991.
Refsal, K.R., Simpson, D.A. and Gunther, J.D.: Testicular degeneration in a male goat: A case report. Theriogenology, 19:685–691, 1983.
Regassa, F., Terefe, F. and Bekana, M.: Abnormalities of the testes and epididymis in bucks and rams slaughtered at Debre Zeit abattoir, Ethiopia. Trop. Anim. Health Prod., 35:541–549, 2003.
Reichle, J.K. and Haibel, G.K.: Ultrasonic biparietal diameter of second trimester pygmy goat foetuses. Theriogenology 35:689–694, 1991.
Reineke, E.P., Bergman, A.J. and Turner, C.W.: Effect of thyroidectomy of young male goats upon certain AP hormones. Endocrinology, 29:306–312, 1941.
Renoux, G.: Brucellosis in goats and sheep. In: Advances in Veterinary Science 3. C.A. Brandly and E.L. Jungherr, eds. New York and London, Academic Press, 1957, pp. 241–273.

Richter, W.R.: Adrenal cortical adenomata in the goat. Am. J. Vet. Res., 19:895–901, 1958.

Ricordeau, G.: Observations sur les caractères de reproduction des produits mâles et femelles issus d'un bouc porteur d'une "fusion centrique." Ann. Génét. Sél. Anim., 4:593–598, 1972.

Ricordeau, G.: Genetics: breeding plans. In: Goat Production. C. Gall, ed. New York, Academic Press, 1981.

Ricordeau, G., Bouillon, J. and Hulot, F.: Pénétrance de l'effet de stérilité totale lié au gène sans cornes P, chez les boucs. Ann. Génét. Sél. Anim., 4:537–542, 1972a.

Ricordeau, G., et al.: Distinction phénotypique des caprins homo- et hétérozygotes sans cornes. Ann. Génét. Sél. Anim., 4:469–475, 1972b.

Rieck, G.W., et al.: Gynäkomastie bei einem Ziegenbock. II. Zytogenetische Befunde: XO/XY-Mosaik mit variablen Deletionen des Y-Chromosoms. Zuchthyg., 10:159–168, 1975.

Riedel, W.: Ein metastasierendes Uteruskarzinom einer Ziege. Berl. Münch. Tierärztl. Wochenschr., 77:395–398, 1964.

Ringwall, K.A., Wettemann, R.P. and Whiteman, J.V.: Seasonal reproduction in rams: May-June reproductive performance of mature F2 Finnish Landrace × Dorset rams selected for extreme or slight seasonal changes in scrotal circumference. SID Sheep Res. J., 6(1):1–4, 1990.

Ritar, A.J.: Seasonal changes in LH, androgens and testes in the male Angora goat. Theriogenology, 36:959–972, 1991.

Rodolakis, A., Boullet, C. and Souriau, A.: *Chlamydia psittaci* experimental abortion in goats. Am. J. Vet. Res., 45:2086–2089, 1984.

Rodolakis, A., Dufrenoy, J. and Souriau, A.: Diagnostic allergique de la chlamydiose abortive de la chèvre. Ann. Rech. Vét., 8:213–219, 1977.

Rodolakis, A. and Souriau, A.: Response of goats to vaccination with temperature-sensitive mutants of *Chlamydia psittaci* obtained by nitrosoguandidine mutagenesis. Am. J. Vet. Res., 47:2627–2631, 1986.

Rodolakis, A., Souriau, A., Raynaud, J.-P. and Brunault, G.: Efficacy of a long-acting oxytetracycline against chlamydial ovine abortion. Ann. Rech. Vét., 11:437–444, 1980.

Romano, J.E. and Benech, A.: Effect of service and vaginal-cervical anesthesia on estrus duration in dairy goats. Theriogenology, 45:691–696, 1996.

Romano, J.E., Crabo, B.G. and Christians, C.J.: Effect of sterile service on estrus duration, fertility and prolificacy in artificially inseminated dairy goats. Theriogenology, 53:1345–1353, 2000.

Romano, J.E., Rodas, E. and Ferreira, A.: Timing of prostaglandin F2alpha administration for induction of parturition in dairy goats. Small Rumin. Res., 42:199–202, 2001.

Romero-R, C.M., Lopez, G. and Luna-M, M.: Abortion in goats associated with increased maternal cortisol. Small Rumin. Res., 30:7–12, 1998.

Roperto, F., et al.: Natural caprine herpesvirus 1 (CpHV-1) infection in kids. J. Comp. Pathol., 122:298–302, 2000.

Rosendal, S.: Ovine and caprine mycoplasmas. In: Mycoplasmosis in Animals: Laboratory Diagnosis. Ames, Iowa, Iowa State University Press, pp. 84–96, 1994.

Rowe, J.D. and East, N.B.: Comparison of two sources of gonadotropin for estrus synchronization in does. Theriogenology, 45:1569–1575, 1996.

Rubianes, E. and Menchaca, A.: The pattern and manipulation of ovarian follicular growth in goats. Anim. Reprod. Sci., 78:271–287, 2003.

Ruder, C.A., Stellflug, J.N., Dahmen, J.J. and Sasser, R.G.: Detection of pregnancy in sheep by radioimmunoassay of sera for pregnancy-specific protein B. Theriogenology, 29:905–912, 1988.

Ruff, G. and Lazary, S.: Possible influence of the caprine leucocyte antigen (CLA) system on development of caprine arthritis encephalitis (CAE) in family and population studies. Goat Diseases and Productions, 2nd International Colloquium in Niort, France, Abstracts p. 7, June 26–29, 1989.

Ruffing, N.A., et al.: Effects of chimerism in sheep-goat concepti that developed from blastomere-aggregation embryos. Biol. Reprod., 48:889–904, 1993.

Ruppanner, R., et al.: Prevalence of *Coxiella burnetii* (Q fever) and *Toxoplasma gondii* among dairy goats in California. Am. J. Vet. Res., 39:867–870, 1978.

Ruppanner, R., et al.: Q fever hazards from sheep and goats used in research. Arch. Environ. Hlth., 37:103–110, 1982.

Ryan, M.J.: Leiomyosarcoma of the uterus in a goat. Vet. Pathol., 17:389–390, 1980.

Sachdeva, K.K., Sengar, O.P.S., Singh, S.N. and Lindahl, I.L.: Studies on goats, 1: Effect of plane of nutrition on the reproductive performance of does. J. Agric. Sci. Cambr., 80:375–379, 1973.

Sahin, O., et al.: Emergence of a tetracycline-resistant *Campylobacter jejuni* clone associated with outbreaks of ovine abortion in the United States. J. Clin. Microbiol., 46:1663–1671, 2008.

Sahni, K.L. and Roy, A.: A note on seasonal variation in the occurrence of abnormal spermatozoa in different breeds of sheep and goat under tropical conditions. Indian J. Anim. Sci., 42:501–504, 1972.

Sakamoto, H., et al.: The effects of xylazine on intrauterine pressure, uterine blood flow, maternal and fetal cardiovascular and pulmonary function in pregnant goats. J. Vet. Med. Sci., 58:211–217, 1996.

Sambraus, H.H.: Ontogenese des Sexualverhaltens von Ziegen. Zuchthyg., 1:15–19, 1971.

Sandbu, H.: *Listeria monocytogenes* som abortårsak hos geit. Nord. Vet. Med., 8:585–594, 1956.

Sanderson, T.P. and Andersen, A.A.: Evaluation of an enzyme immunoassay for detection of *Chlamydia psittaci* in vaginal secretions, placentas, and fetal tissues from aborting ewes. J. Vet. Diag. Inv., 1:309–315, 1989.

Sanford, S.E., Josephson, G.K.A. and MacDonald, A.: *Coxiella burnetii* (Q fever) abortion storms in goat herds after attendance at an annual fair. Can. Vet. J., 35:376–378, 1994.

Santiago Moreno, J., Cortes, S. and Gonzalez de Bulnes, A.: Ultrasound diagnosis of orchitis and seminal vesiculitis in a goat. Med. Vet., 13:49–54, 1996.

Santos, D.O., Simplicio, A.A. and Machado, R.: Induction of parturition in goats through intramuscular injection of cloprostenol. Rev. Bras. Reprod. Anim., 16:41–54, 1992.

Santos, M.H.B., et al.: Early fetal sexing of Saanen goats by use of transrectal ultrasonography to identify the genital tubercle and external genitalia. Am. J. Vet. Res., 68:561–563, 2007.

Sardjana, I.K.W., Tainturier, D. and André, F.: Étude du sulfate d'oestrone dans le plasma et dans le lait au cours de la gestation et le post-partum chez la chèvre. (Application au diagnostic tardif de gestation). Rev. Méd. Vét., 139:827–835, 1988a.

Sardjana, I.K.W., Tainturier, D. and Djiane, J.: Étude de l'hormone chorionique somatomammotrophique dans le plasma et le lactoserum au cours de la gestation et du post-partum chez la chèvre (application au diagnostic tardif de gestation). Rev. Méd. Vét., 139:1045–1052, 1988b.

Sastry, G.A.: Neoplasms of animals in India. Vet. Med., 54:428–430, 1959.

Sathiamoorthy, T. and Kathirchelvan, M.: Uterine torsion in a goat. Indian Vet. J., 82:984, 2005.

Schmidt, V.: Der Scheidenzyklus der Ziege (vergleichende zytologische und klinische Untersuchungen). [The vaginal cycle of the goat (comparative cytological and clinical examinations.)] Wissenschaftliche Zeitschrift der Humboldt-Universität zu Berlin, 10:551–562+ plates, 1961.

Schollum, L.M. and Blackmore, D.K.: The serological and cultural prevalence of leptospirosis in a sample of feral goats. N. Z. Vet. J., 29:104–106, 1981.

Schönherr, S.: Die Unfruchtbarkeit der Ziegenböcke, ihre Verbreitung, frühzeitige Erkennung und Bekämpfung. Z. Tierz. Zuchtsbiol., 66:209–234 and 381–416, 1956.

Schwesig, K.-P.: Die sakrokokzygeale Extraduralanästhesie in der Therapie und Prophylaxe des Prolapsus vaginae sive uteri bei Schafmüttern. Hannover, Germany, 1986. Thesis.

Scott, G.R.: Tick-associated infections. In: Disease of Sheep. W.B. Martin, ed. Oxford, Blackwell Scientific Publ., pp. 209–213, 1983.

Scott, G.H. and Williams, J.C.: Susceptibility of *Coxiella burnetii* to chemical disinfectants. In: Rickettsiology: Current Issues and Perspectives. Ann. N.Y. Acad. Sci., 590:291–296, 1990.

Seeger, K.H. and Klatt, P.R.: Laparoscopy in the sheep and goat. In: Animal Laparoscopy. R.M. Harrison and D.E. Wildt, eds. Baltimore, Williams and Wilkins, 1980.

Senf, W.: Beitrag zur Kupfermangelerkrankung—Swayback-bei Afrikanischen Zwergziegen und anderen Zootieren. XVI Internationalen Symposiums über die Erkrankungen der Zootiere, pp. 239–243, 1974.

Senger, P.L.: Pathways to Pregnancy and Parturition. 2nd Rev. Ed. Pullman WA, Current Conceptions Inc, 2005.

Shalev, A., Short, R.V. and Hamerton, J.L.: Immunogenetics of sex determination in the polled goat. Cytogenet. Cell Genet., 28:195–202, 1980.

Shefki, M.D.: Enzootic abortion in goats. Br. Vet. J., 119:430–433, 1963, 1987.

Shelton, M.: Influence of the presence of a male goat on the initiation of estrous cycling and ovulation of Angora does. J. Anim. Sci., 19:368–375, 1960.

Shelton, M. and Klindt, J.M.: A simple method of male sterilization for use with sheep and goats. Texas Agric. Expt. Stat. Research Reports. Sheep and Goat, Wool and Mohair, PR-3286, pp. 10–11, 1974.

Shelton, M. and Livingston, C.W. Jr.: Posthitis in Angora wethers. J. Am. Vet. Med. Assoc., 167:154–155, 1975.

Shewen, P.E.: Chlamydial infection in animals: a review. Can. Vet. J., 21:2–11, 1980.

Shimshony, S.: An epizootic of Akabane disease in bovines, ovines and caprines in Israel, 1969–70: Epidemiologic assessment. Acta Morph. Acad. Sci. Hung., 28(1–2):197–199, 1980.

Short, R.E., et al.: Effects of feeding ponderosa pine needles during pregnancy: comparative studies with bison, cattle, goats, and sheep. J. Anim. Sci., 70:3498–3504, 1992.

Shutt, D.A., Fell, L.R., Connell, R. and Bell, A.K.: Stress responses in lambs docked and castrated surgically or by the application of rubber rings. Aust. Vet. J., 65:5–7, 1988.

Silva, A.E.D.F. and Nunes, J.F.: Comportamento sexual do macho caprino da raça Moxotó às variaçøs estacionais no Nordeste do Brasil, EMBRAPA-CNPC, Boletim de Pesquisa, (17 pp.) Número 6, 1988.

Simoes, J., et al.: Follicular dynamics in Serrana goats. Anim. Reprod. Sci., 95:16–26, 2006.

Singer, L.A., et al.: Predicting the onset of parturition in the goat by determining progesterone levels by enzyme immunoassay. Small Rumin. Res., 52:203–209, 2004.

Singh, J.L., et al.: Clinico-biochemical profile and therapeutic management of congenital goitre in kids. Indian J. Vet. Med., 23:83–87, 2003.

Singh, N., Rajya, B.S. and Mohanty, G.C.: Granular vulvovaginitis (GVV) in goats associated with *Mycoplasma agalactiae*. Cornell Vet., 64:435–442, 1974.

Singh, N., Rajya, B.S. and Mohanty, G.C.: Pathology of *Mycoplasma agalactiae* induced granular vulvovaginitis (GVV) in goats. Cornell Vet., 65:363–373, 1975.

Singh, S.B. and Lang, C.M.: Q fever serologic surveillance program for sheep and goats at a research animal facility. Am. J. Vet. Res., 46:321–325, 1985.

Sivachelvan, M.N., Ghali Ali, M. and Chibuzo, G.A.: Foetal age estimation in sheep and goats. Small Rumin. Res., 19:69–76, 1996.

Skalet, L.H., et al.: Effects of age and season on the type and occurrence of sperm abnormalities in Nubian bucks. Am. J. Vet. Res., 49:1284–1289, 1988.

Skinner, J.D.: Post-natal development of the reproductive tract of the male Boer goat. Agroanimalia, 2:177–180, 1970.

Skinner, J.D. and Hofmeyr, H.S.: Effect of the male goat and of progesterone and PMSG treatment on the incidence of oestrus in the anoestrous Boer goat doe. Proc. S. Afr. Soc. Anim. Prod., 8:155–156, 1969.

Skinner, J.D., van Heerden, J.A.H. and Goris, E.J.: A note on cryptorchidism in Angora goats. S. Afr. J. Anim. Sci., 2:93–95, 1972.

Smith, M.C.: Caprine reproduction. In: Current Therapy in Theriogenology. D.A. Morrow, ed. Philadelphia, W.B. Saunders Co., pp. 971–1004, 1980.

Smith, M.C.: Castration and preparation of teasers. In: Current Therapy in Theriogenology 2. D.A. Morrow, ed. Philadelphia, W.B. Saunders Co., pp. 627–628, 1986a.

Smith, M.C.: Synchronization of estrus and the use of implants and vaginal sponges. In: Current Therapy in Theriogenology 2. D.A. Morrow, ed. Philadelphia, W.B. Saunders Co., pp. 582–583, 1986b.

Smith, M.C.: The reproductive anatomy and physiology of the male goat. In: Current Therapy in Theriogenology 2. D.A. Morrow, ed. Philadelphia, W.B. Saunders Co., pp. 616–618, 1986c.

Smith, M.C. and Dunn, H.O.: Freemartin condition in a goat. J. Am. Vet. Med. Assoc., 178:736–737, 1981.

Smith, M.C. and Ross, M.: Uterine torsion in three ewes. Comp. Cont. Educ. Pract. Vet., 7(5):S303-S306, 1985.

Snyder, J.H.: Anesthesia and analgesia. Minor surgeries in small ruminants. AABP Proceedings, 40:183–187, 2007.

Soller, M. and Kempenich, O.: Polledness and litter size in Saanen goats. J. Hered., 55:301–304, 1964.

Soller, M., Padeh, B., Wysoki, M. and Ayalon, N.: Cytogenetics of Saanen goats showing abnormal development of the reproductive tract associated with the dominant gene for polledness. Cytogenetics, 8:51–67, 1969.

Soller, M., Wysoki, M. and Padeh, B.: A chromosomal abnormality in phenotypically normal Saanen goats. Cytogenetics, 5:88–93, 1966.

Soller, M., et al.: Polledness and infertility in male Saanen goats. J. Hered., 54:237–240, 1963.

Songer, J.G. and Thiermann, A.B.: Leptospirosis. J. Am. Vet. Med. Assoc., 193:1250–1254, 1988.

Souriau, A. and Rodolakis, A.: Rapid detection of *Chlamydia psittaci* in vaginal swabs of aborted ewes and goats by enzyme linked immunosorbent assay (ELISA). Vet. Microbiol., 11:251–259, 1986.

Souriau, A., et al.: Comparison of the efficacy of Q fever vaccines against *Coxiella burnetii* experimental challenge in pregnant goats. Annals N.Y. Acad. Sci., 990:521–523, 2003.

Sponenberg, D.P., Smith, M.C. and Johnson, R.J.: Unilateral testicular hypoplasia in a goat. Vet. Pathol., 20:503–506, 1983.

Sreekumaran, T. and Rajan, A.: Pathology of gonads in experimental hypothyroidism in goats. Kerala J. Vet. Sci., 9(1):92–100, 1978.

Stiles, G.W.: Controlling brucellosis in Colorado goats. Proceedings, Third Interamerican Congress on Brucellosis, Washington, D.C., pp. 226–237, November 6–10, 1950.

Stubbings, R.B., Bosu, W.T.K., Barker, C.A.V. and King, G.J.: Serum progesterone concentrations associated with superovulation and premature corpus luteum failure in dairy goats. Can. J. Vet. Res., 50:369–373, 1986.

Sulochana, S. and Sudharma, D.: Isolation of *Yersinia pseudotuberculosis* from cases of abortion in goats. Kerala J. Vet. Sci., 16(2):139–142, 1985.

Szabo, K.T.: Congenital Malformations in Laboratory and Farm Animals. New York, Academic Press, Inc., 1989.

Szeredi, L. and Bacsadi, A.: Detection of *Chlamydophila* (*Chlamydia*) *abortus* and *Toxoplasma gondii* in smears from cases of ovine and caprine abortion by the streptavidin-biotin method. J. Comp. Pathol., 127:257–263, 2002.

Tadjebakhche, H., Hosseinioun, M. and Nadalian, M.: Infection expérimentale due à *Salmonella abortus ovis* chez la chèvre. Rev. Méd. Vét., 125:711–718, 1974.

Tainturier, D., et al.: Diagnostic de la gestation chez la chèvre par échotomographie. Rev. Méd. Vét., 134(3):597–599, 1983.

Tarigan, S., Ladds, P.W. and Foster, R.A.: Genital pathology of feral male goats. Aust. Vet. J., 67:286–290, 1990.

Tarigan, S., Webb, R.F. and Kirkland, D.: Caprine herpesvirus from balanoposthitis. Aust. Vet. J., 64:321, 1987.

Taverne, M.A.M., et al.: Aetiology and endocrinology of pseudopregnancy in the goat. Reprod. Dom. Anim., 30:228–230, 1995.

Tempesta, M., et al.: Reactivation of caprine herpesvirus 1 in experimentally infected goats. Vet. Rec., 150:116–117, 2002.

Tempesta, M., et al.: Experimental infection of goats at different stages of pregnancy with caprine herpesvirus 1. Comp. Immunol. Microbiol. Infect. Dis., 27:25–32, 2004.

Terblanche, M., et al.: *Acacia nilotica* (L.) Del. subsp. *kraussiana* (Benth.)Brenan, as a poisonous plant in South Africa. J. S. Afr. Vet. Med. Assoc., 38:57–62, 1967.

Terpstra, C.: Nairobi sheep disease virus. In: Virus Infections of Vertebrates. Vol. 3. Virus Infections of Ruminants. Z. Dinter and B. Morein, eds. New York, Elsevier Science Publ., pp. 495–500, 1990.

Thibier, M., Jeanguyot, N. and de Montigny, G.: Accuracy of early pregnancy diagnosis in goats based on plasma and milk progesterone concentrations. Int. Goat Sheep Res., 2(1):1–6, 1982.

Tibary, A. and Van Metre, D.: Surgery of the sheep and goat reproductive system and urinary tract. In: Farm Animal Surgery. S.L. Fubini and N.G. Ducharme, eds. St Louis, Saunders, pp. 527–547, 2004.

Timoney, J.F., Gillespie, J.H., Scott, F.W. and Barlough, J.E.: Hagan and Bruner's Microbiology and Infectious Diseases of Domestic Animals. 8th Ed. Ithaca, NY, Comstock Publ. Assoc., 1988.

Ting, L.J., et al.: Identification of bluetongue virus in goats in Taiwan. Vet. Rec., 156:52, 2005.

Tizard, I.R., Carrington, M. and Lai, C.H.: Toxoplasmosis in goats in southern Ontario—a public health hazard? Can. Vet. J., 18:274–277, 1977.

Todhunter, P., Baird, A.N. and Wolfe, D.F.: Erection failure as a sequela to obstructive urolithiasis in a male goat. J. Am. Vet. Med. Assoc., 209:650–652, 1996.

Tolari, F. and Salvi, G.: Bilateral orchitis in a kid after vaccination with Rev 1. Ann. Fac. Med. Vet. Pisa 33:87–91, 1980.

Trasch, K., Wehrend, A. and Bostedt, H.: [Ovariohysterectomy in a goat with progesterone-independent hydrometra.] Tierärztl. Prax., 30(G):234–239, 2002.

Travassos, C.E., et al.: Caprine arthritis-encephalitis virus in semen of naturally infected bucks. Small Rum. Res., 32:101–106, 1999.

Ullner, W.: Über 2 Fälle von Gynäkomastie bei Ziegenböken. Tierärztl. Umschau, 16:146–151, 1961.

Umo, I., Fitzpatrick, R.J. and Ward, W.R.: Parturition in the goat: Plasma concentrations of prostaglandin F and steroid hormones and uterine activity during late pregnancy and parturtion. J. Endocrinol., 68:383–389, 1976.

Unanian, M.D.S. and Feliciano-Silva, A.E.D.: Trace elements deficiency: Association with early abortion in goats. Int. Goat Sheep Res., 2:129–134, 1984.

Uzal, F.A., et al.: Abortion and ulcerative posthitis associated with caprine herpesvirus-1 infection in goats in California. J. Vet. Diagn. Invest., 16:478–484, 2004.

Van der Hoeden, J.: Leptospirosis among goats in Israel. J. Comp. Pathol., 63:101–111, 1953.

Van der Westhuysen, J.M. and Roelofse, C.S.M.B.: Effect of shelter and different levels of dietary energy and protein on reproductive performance in Angora goats with special reference to the habitual aborter. Agroanimalia, 3:129–132, 1971.

Van der Westhuysen, J.M. and Wentzel, D.: Progress through selection against the aborting Angora goat. S. Afr. J. Anim. Sci., 1:101–102, 1971.

Van der Westhuysen, J.M., Wentzl, D. and Grobler, M.C.: Angora Goats and Mohair in South Africa. 3rd Ed. Port Elizabeth, South Africa, NMB Printers, 1988.

Van Heerden, K.M.: The effect of culling aborting ewes, on the abortion rate in Angora ewes. J. S. Afr. Vet. Med. Assoc., 35(1):19–20, 1964.

Van Rensburg, S.J.: Malnutrition of the foetus as a cause of abortion. J. S. Afr. Vet. Med. Assoc., 42:305–308, 1971a.

Van Rensburg, S.J.: Reproductive physiology and endocrinology of normal and habitually aborting Angora does. Onderstepoort J. Vet. Res., 38:1–62, 1971b.

Van Rensburg, S.J., McFarlane, I.S. and van Rensburg, S.W.J.: Sterilization of teaser male ruminants—The reliability of surgical methods. S. Afr. Vet. Med. Assoc. J., 34:249–253, 1963.

Van Tonder, E.M.: Notes on some disease problems in Angora goats in South Africa. Vet. Med. Rev., 1/2:109–138, 1975.

Vermeulen, S.O., et al.: *Brucella ovis* as a possible cause of epididymitis in an Angora goat. J. S. Afr. Vet. Assoc., 59:177–179, 1988.

Vinha, N.A. and Humenhuk, R.A.: (Preliminary observations on the pathology of the testicle and epididymis in goats. I. Cryptorchidism.) Arq. Escola Vet. Univ. Fed. Minas Ger., 28:249–253, 1976.

Vivrette, S.: Cesarean section in goats. In: Current Therapy in Theriogenology 2. D.A. Morrow, ed. Philadelphia, W.B. Saunders Co., pp. 592–593, 1986.

Wachtel, S.S.: The dysgenetic gonad: aberrant testicular differentiation. Biol. Reprod., 22:1–8, 1980.

Wachtel, S.S., Basrur, P. and Koo, G.C.: Recessive male-determining genes. Cell, 15:279–281, 1978.

Waghela, S.: Serological response of adult goats infected with live *Brucella melitensis*. Br. Vet. J., 134:565–571, 1978.

Waldhalm, D.G., Stoenner, H.G., Simmons, R.E. and Thomas, L.A.: Abortion associated with *Coxiella burnetii* infection in dairy goats. J. Am. Vet. Med. Assoc., 173:1580–1581, 1978.

Waldvogel, A., et al.: Caprine herpesvirus infection in Switzerland: some aspects of its pathogenicity. Zbl. Vet. Med. B., 28:612–623, 1981.

Walkden-Brown, S.W., et al.: Effect of nutrition on seasonal patterns of LH, FSH and testosterone concentration, testicular mass, sebaceous gland volume and odour in Australian cashmere goats. J. Reprod. Fert., 102:351–360, 1994.

Wallace, C.E.: A technique for performing cesarean section in goats. Vet. Med. Small Anim. Clin., 77:791–793, 1982.

Walser, K.: Wiederholte hydropische Gravidität bei einer Ziege. Berl. Münch. Tierärztl. Wochenschr., 76:206–208, 1963.

Wani, N.A., et al.: Ultrasonic pregnancy diagnosis in Gaddi goats. Small Rum. Res., 29:239–240, 1998.

Warwick, B.L.: Selection against cryptorchidism in Angora goats. J. Anim. Sci., 20:10–14, 1961.

Weaver, B.M.Q. and Angell-James, J.: A simple device for respiratory resuscitation of newborn calves and lambs. Vet. Rec., 119:86–88, 1986.

Webb, P.: Segmental aplasia and hydrometra in a goat. Vet. Rec., 117:13, 1985.

Wehrend, A., Bostedt, H. and Burkhardt, E.: The use of trans-abdominal B mode ultrasonography to diagnose intra-partum uterine torsion in the ewe. Vet. J., 164:69–70, 2002.

Weiland, G. and Dalchow, W.: *Toxoplasma*-Infektionen bei Haustieren in der Türkei (Serologische Untersuchungen im Sabin-Feldman-Test). Berl. Münch. Tierärztl. Wochenschr., 83:65–68, 1970.

Whiting, R.D., White, B.M. and Stiles, F.C. Jr.: An epizootic of *Brucella melitensis* infection in Texas. J. Am. Vet. Med. Assoc., 157:1860–1863, 1970.

Whitney, K.M., Valentine, B.A. and Schlafer, D.H.: Caprine genital leiomyosarcoma. Vet. Pathol., 37:89–94, 2000.

Widmaier, R.: Nebennierenrindenknötchen in Nebenhodenkopf bei Ziegenböckchen. Zbl. Vet. Med., 6:368–379, 1959.

Williams, A.F.J., Beck, N.F.G. and Williams, S.P.: The production of EAE-free lambs from infected dams using multiple ovulation and embryo transfer. Vet. J., 155:79–84, 1998.

Williams, C.S.F.: Pregnancy diagnosis. In: Current Therapy in Theriogenology 2. D.A. Morrow, ed. Philadelphia, W.B. Saunders Co., pp. 587–588, 1986a.

Williams, C.S.F.: Practical management of induced parturition. In: Current Therapy in Theriogenology 2. D.A. Morrow, ed. Philadelphia, W.B. Saunders Co., pp. 588–589, 1986b.

Williams, N.M., et al.: Multiple abortions associated with caprine herpesvirus infection in a goat herd. J. Am. Vet. Med. Assoc., 211:89–91, 1997.

Wilsmore, A.J., Dawson, M., Arthur, M.J. and Davies, D.C.: The use of a delayed hypersensitivity test and long-acting oxytetracycline in a flock affected with ovine enzootic abortion. Br. Vet. J., 142:557–561, 1986.

Wilsmore, A.J., Izzard, K.A., Wilsmore, B.C. and Dagnall, G.J.R.: Breeding performance of sheep infected with *Chlamydia psittaci* (*ovis*) during their preceding pregnancy. Vet. Rec., 126:40–41, 1990.

Wilson, J.G.: Hypothyroidism in ruminants with special reference to foetal goitre. Vet. Rec., 97:161–164, 1975.

Wilson, M., Ware, D.A. and Juranek, D.D.: Serologic aspects of toxoplasmosis. J. Am. Vet. Med. Assoc., 196:277–281, 1990.

Witte, S.T., Sponenberg, D.P. and Collins, T.C.: Abortion and early neonatal death of kids attributed to intrauterine *Yersinia pseudotuberculosis* infection. J. Am. Vet. Med. Assoc., 187:834, 1985.

Wittek, T. and Elze, K.: [A contribution to the clinical puerperium and different parameters of blood serum in dairy goats during early puerperium.] Tierärztl. Umschau, 56:369–375, 2001.

Wittek, T., Erices, J. and Elze, K.: Histology of the endometrium, clinical-chemical parameters of the uterine fluid and blood plasma concentrations of progesterone, estradiol-17beta and prolactin during hydrometra in goats. Small Rumin. Res., 30:105–112, 1998.

Wittek, T., et al.: [Hydrometra in goats: incidence, diagnosis, therapy and following fertility performance.] Tierärztl. Prax., 25:576–582, 1997.

Wolfe, D.F. and Baird, A.N.: Urogenital surgery in goats. In: Current Therapy in Large Animal Theriogenology. R.S. Youngquist, ed. Philadelphia, W.B. Saunders, pp. 494–498, 1997.

Wolfe, D.F. et al.: Embryo transfer from goats seropositive for caprine arthritis-encephalitis virus. Theriogenology, 28:307–316, 1987.

Wooldridge, A.A., et al.: Gynecomastia and mammary gland adenocarcinoma in a Nubian buck. Can. Vet. J., 40:663–665, 1999.

Wyssmann, E.: Statistische Erhebungen uber Schwergeburten bei Ziegen. Schweiz. Arch. Tierheilkunde, 87:57–65, 83–90, 1945.

Yalçin, N. and Gane, P.: Les avortements salmonellique et néorickettsien des chèvres. Rec. Méd. Vét., 146:705–709, 1970.

Yankovich, L.: You're kidding. Dairy Goat J., 67:798–799, 1989.

Yankovich, L.I.: You're not kidding! Dairy Goat J., 68:31–32, 1990.

Yedloutschnig, R.J. and Walker, J.S.: Rift Valley fever in sheep and goats. In: Current Veterinary Therapy Food Animal Practice 2. J.L. Howard, ed. Philadelphia, W.B. Saunders Co., p. 526, 1986.

Yokoki, Y. and Akira, O.: Effects of hyperthermia on semen production in goats. Jpn. J. Anim. Reprod., 23(3):93–98 + plate, 1977.

Youngquist, R.S. and Threlfall, W.R. (eds.): Current Therapy in Large Animal Theriogenology 2. St. Louis, Saunders Elsevier, 2007.

Zarrouk, A., et al.: Determination of pregnancy-associated glycoprotein concentrations in goats (*Capra hircus*) with unsuccessful pregnancies: a retrospective study. Theriogenology, 51:1321–1331, 1999.

Zarrouk, A., et al.: Pregnancy-associated glycoprotein levels in pregnant goats inoculated with *Toxoplasma gondii* or *Listeria monocytogenes*: a retrospective study. Theriogenology, 52:1095–1104, 1999.

Zlotnik, G.: Testosterone levels in intersex goats. J. Reprod. Fert., 32:287–290, 1973. Supplement.

14

Mammary Gland and Milk Production

ANATOMY OF THE UDDER AND MALFORMATIONS

The goat's udder is composed of two glands, called halves or sides. In the male, teats are present but the glands usually remain rudimentary.

Normal Anatomy

Each gland has a single large teat. Six to nine large milk ducts join to form the gland cistern. The gland cistern blends with the teat cistern, which ends at a single streak canal and a single teat opening (Turner 1952; Heidrich and Renk 1967). The major blood supply is provided by the external pudendal artery. Venous return is via the external pudendal vein and the subcutaneous abdominal vein. The genitofemoral nerve, which passes through the inguinal ring with the external pudendal vessels, supplies most of the udder. Some skin innervation is also supplied by the lumbar cutaneous nerves cranially and the mammary branch of the pudendal nerve caudally.

The glands are separated by a median suspensory ligament. The lateral laminae of the suspensory apparatus are lateral to the external pudendal vessels and attach to the symphysial tendon caudally and the tunica flava abdominis cranially. The mammary (superficial inguinal) lymph nodes are located deep to the lateral laminae and caudal to the external pudendal arteries (Garrett 1988; Constantinescu 2001).

The ultrasonographic anatomy of the bovine teat and udder has been well described (Trostle and O'Brien 1998) and the images supplied should be applicable to the goat udder as well. A 5-MHz rectal probe can be used but a 7.5-MHz probe gives better resolution. Isopropyl alcohol or coupling gel is applied to achieve good contact with the skin, and the teat is scanned in longitudinal and transverse planes. The gain of the machine is adjusted until the normal milk appears anechoic. Using a commercial standoff device or a saline-filled examination glove between probe and skin improves the image of superficial tissues. The near teat wall can be used as a convenient standoff for imaging lesions of the far teat wall.

Supernumerary Teats

Small supernumerary teats, completely separate from and usually cranial to the main teats, are occasionally observed in goats. Almost 12% of Barbari goats in one study had supernumerary teats (Bhat 1988), as did 30% of West African dwarf goats in Ghana (Oppong and Gumedze 1982), while goats with supernumerary teats predominated in a population of native goats in Japan (Nozawa 1970). These teats represent remnants of the embryologic mammary line that extends to the vulva, where ectopic milk secreting tissue also may be located. The distinct supernumerary teats are commonly amputated with scissors while the doe kid is still young. Tetanus prophylaxis (such as 200 to 300 IU antitoxin) is recommended (Smith and Roguinsky 1977).

Rarely, the extra teats are of a size comparable to the normal teats, resulting in an udder divided into four equal glands (Balasurbramanian et al. 1994).

Double or Fused Teats

It is relatively common for goats, especially of breeds that have not been selected for dairy purposes, such as Pygmy and meat goats, to have double teats on one or both sides of the udder. The abnormal teats may be fused to the tip but have two orifices (including fishtail teats). Forked teats (Figure 14.1), where both ends are of similar size, and small spurs protruding from the side of larger teats are other variations. Double teats are probably inherited in a complex way (Cunningham 1931–1932).

Kids (both does and bucks) of dairy breeds should be examined at birth, and all those with teat malformations other than simple, discrete, supernumerary teats should be marked for culling. Breed associations vary in the importance they place on abnormal teats. The American Veterinary Medical Association has determined that removing an extra teat that would have interfered with milking is not ethical in an animal to be shown, bred, or sold (AVMA 1976). Owners who are unconcerned about the possible genetic basis for these malformations occasionally choose to cut off part of a double teat. Sometimes the wrong guess is made and the doe freshens with a small spur off a separate, larger gland that no longer has a teat orifice. Infections may also become established in the remaining gland at time of spur removal.

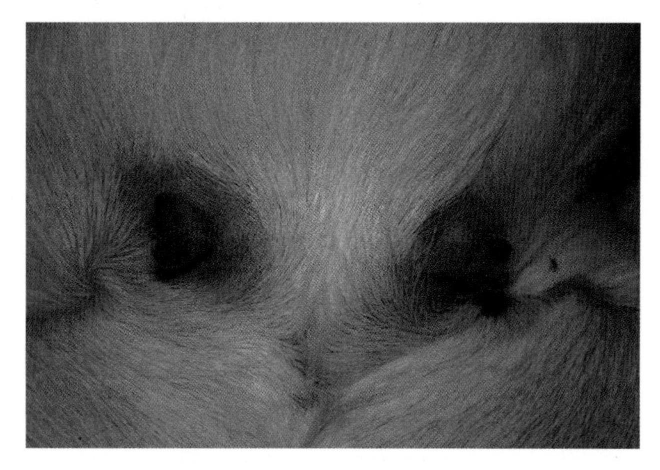

Figure 14.1. Bilateral forked teats in a Boer kid. (Courtesy Dr. M.C. Smith.)

Weeping Teats and Teat Wall Cysts

Some goats have milk secreting tissue in the wall of the teat, especially near its base. If this tissue communicates through one or more pores in the skin to the outside, milk oozes out. The condition is noticed when the hand of the milker becomes wet. Cauterization of the opening(s) with silver nitrate sticks after each milking may solve the problem. If the glandular tissue does not communicate with the outside or to the teat cistern, a cyst may form in the wall of the teat and interfere with milking. Real-time ultrasound clearly demonstrates a fluid-filled cavity. If the cyst is large, it may need to be drained occasionally using aseptic techniques.

An extreme version of this condition, possibly hereditary, has been reported in Israel, where nineteen of 324 lactating mixed-breed goats in one herd had multiple cysts 3 to 8 mm in diameter in the wall of the teat near its base. Most of these cysts contained clear rather than milky fluid (Yeruham et al. 2005).

Blind Udder Halves

A presumably congenital abnormality has been described in a single Saanen goat in which the primary milk ducts ended blindly instead of joining the gland cistern. The mammary gland was capable of secretion, but no milk could be obtained from either teat (Turner and Berousek 1942). Absence of leukocytic infiltration in the udder tissue made a bacterial or retroviral etiology unlikely. Blind teats are common in artificially reared calves that suck on each other, and presumably scar tissue in the teat end could cause a similar problem in goats.

Poor Udder Suspension

The various suspensory ligaments of the udder should be strong and broad so that the udder is held tightly against the body with the floor of the udder above hock level (Considine and Trimberger 1978). Low-slung udders are prone to injury and are also bruised by alternately wrapping around one hind leg and then the other as the goat runs. Affected does and their offspring should not be allowed to contribute more to the gene pool in the herd. The heritability of the medial suspensory ligament as scored by the American Dairy Goat Association linear appraisal program has been estimated at 0.33 (Wiggans and Hubbard 2001). An enlarged, pendulous udder may also be the result, rather than the cause, of mastitis (Addo et al. 1980).

Neoplasia and Fibrocystic Disease

Neoplasms of the parenchyma of the udder are rarely reported in goats. In one Indian slaughterhouse study of 2,000 female goats four years of age or older, multiple gray-white dots seen grossly in three udders were identified as intraductal carcinomas. The tumors were multicentric, with diffuse intraluminal proliferation of cells. Metastasis to the supramammary lymph node had occurred in one animal (Singh and Iyer 1972). In another study of more than 4,000 mature goats, two more multicentric intraductal carcinomas were identified (Sharma and Iyer 1974). Diffuse involvement of both glands with a mammary adenocarcinoma was observed in a seven-year-old doe that had not kidded or lactated for five years. Tumor metastases were found in the bronchial lymph node (Miller 1992). An aged Toggenburg doe with a chronic history of mastitis was found at necropsy to have a locally infiltrative adenocarcinoma in the udder and a granulosa cell tumor on one ovary, suggesting that high estrogen concentrations might be a risk factor for mammary cancer (Cooke and Merrall 1992)

Slaughterhouse studies from India report a condition termed fibrocystic disease or cystic hyperplasia (Singh and Iyer 1973; Sharma and Iyer 1974; Tripathi et al. 1989; Upadhyaya and Rao 1994). Affected goat udders are enlarged and very firm/indurated, with multiple pea- to grape-sized nodules containing straw-colored fluid. Periductal and perilobular fibrosis with mononuclear cell infiltration surrounds dilated ducts filled with proteinaceous material. A predisposition of fibrocystic disease to the development of intraductal carcinomas has been proposed (Tripathi et al. 1989). A unilateral fibroepithelial hyperplasia of the udder of a nulliparous goat has also been reported and compared to mammary fibroepithelial hyperplasia in young, sexually intact cats (Andreasen et al. 1993). Because the histologic findings in biopsies from the udders of goats with inappropriate lactation syndrome (see below) are often suggestive of neoplasia, these various syndromes may be related.

MILK PRODUCTION BY KIDS AND UNBRED GOATS

Udder development and even milk production are relatively common in unbred doelings of dairy breeds. Gynecomastia in bucks is discussed in Chapter 13.

Witch's Milk

Occasionally kids have enough udder development at birth that the glands are tense and conical. Milk sometimes can be expressed from the teats, but this is not desirable because of the risk of mastitis once the teat seal is broken. The condition occurs in other species, including human infants (Nelson 1964). It is presumed to occur in response to increased levels of hormones (estrogen, prolactin, placental lactogen) in utero. No treatment is necessary.

Inappropriate Lactation Syndrome

Unbred goats frequently develop a large "precocious" udder. In some animals, the udder enlargement is mainly because of deposition of adipose tissue. In others, milk is actually produced from one or both glands without a preceding parturition (Figure 14.2). Precocious milking may be a hereditary trait (Campbell 1961). It has been said that doelings who lactate precociously, also termed "maiden milkers," generally come from genetic stock with high production potential (Baxendell 1984a; Matthews 1999). It should be noted, however, that some intersex animals lactate (Hamerton et al. 1969).

Neither the etiologic basis nor the ideal treatment for such inappropriate lactation has been determined. Two affected does have been reported to have increased prolactin from an acidophilic pituitary adenoma (Miller et al. 1997), but this is a rare explanation for a common clinical condition. One theory is that some goats are very sensitive to either prolonged progesterone exposure from a persistent corpus luteum or to elevated prolactin levels in the spring.

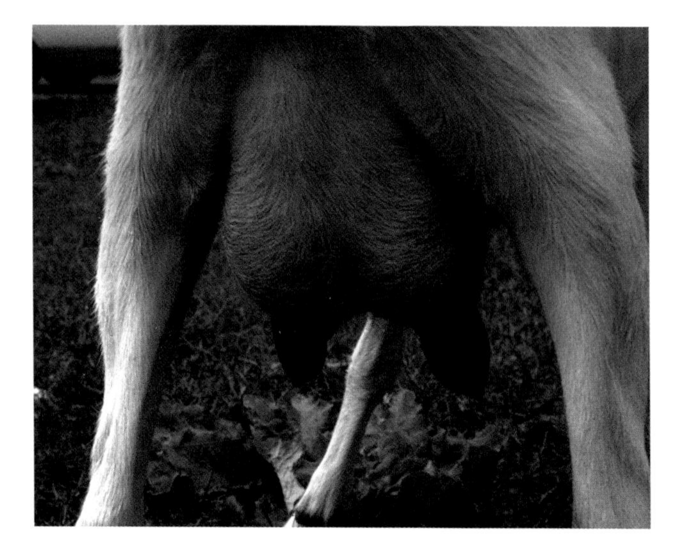

Figure 14.2. Precocious udder in a doe that was never bred. The udder produced one cup of normal milk per day. (Courtesy Dr. M.C. Smith.)

A possible treatment if false pregnancy is suspected is a luteolytic dose of prostaglandin (2.5 to 5 mg prostaglandin F2 alpha), although withdrawal of progesterone by natural termination of the false pregnancy may have already occurred before the udder developed. Progesterone and estrogens should stimulate additional mammary gland development, and are therefore contra-indicated. Feeds with estrogenic action, such as moldy corn or subterranean clover, should be eliminated from the diet. Temporarily eliminating the grain ration and feeding dry hay should discourage milk production, but water deprivation is not warranted. Milking the goat is not desirable because disrupting the seal in the teat predisposes to mastitis if the goat is not milked regularly. If the udder becomes painfully engorged so that milking is necessary or if the owner has milked the goat before seeking advice, a milk culture should be taken to check for mastitis and a bovine dry period treatment infused into the udder after it has been emptied completely.

If this regimen fails to stop lactation, the goat can be milked daily for several months and dry-off can be attempted again, preferably in the fall, the season when production naturally decreases. An expensive and as of yet inadequately tested alternative is the administration of an antiprolactin drug such as bromocryptine (5 mg bromocryptine mesylate [Parlodel, Sandoz]/day for fourteen days orally). A similar empirical treatment is cabergoline, 5 µg/kg orally for four to six days (Galostop, Boerhringer) (Matthews 1999), but owners report that this treatment has not worked. Also, the bromocryptine-induced decrease in milk production is only temporary in normal goats (Forsyth and Lee 1993).

There are anecdotal reports of destroying the secretory tissue by infusing a destructive substance such as ether or 2% chlorhexidine solution (5 to 10 ml only) into the affected gland. Occasionally the precocious udder develops severe chronic mastitis or becomes so pendulous that udder amputation is advisable. In summary, milking, mating, or mastectomy seem to be the most reliable options for treating persistent maiden milkers (John Matthews, personal communication 2007).

Self-sucking

Because the simple act of trying to extract milk from a teat on a regular basis stimulates development of milk-secreting tissue, the possibility that another goat has been nursing the doeling with a developed udder or that she is a self-sucker should be investigated. The first possibility can be handled by separating the animals involved or by fitting the animal engaged in illicit sucking with a halter that holds a wooden bit in the mouth (Gall 1981). Self-sucking, on the other hand, is a difficult habit to break. Many goats like the flavor of milk and drink their own regularly when they have learned the trick. The behavior has been observed in a feral goat (O'Brien 1982) and theorized to have begun as an attempt to relieve discomfort from a turgid udder.

Treatments that have been tried with variable success include applying teat tape (as for preventing suckling in CAE control programs), painting the teats with a solution distasteful to the goat, and fitting the goat with an Elizabethan collar or a bra-like udder bag. A side brace constructed of aluminum rod is another possibility; the side extensions of a padded neck ring are taped to the forward-directed ends of a padded arch that goes over the lumbar area. A strap made of tape joins the two sides of the brace underneath the abdomen.

Hormonal Induction of Lactation

Lactation physiologists have made extensive use of goats in their study of hormonal treatments (e.g., estrogen, progesterone, prolactin, and corticosteroids) that will induce udder development and lactation in non-pregnant animals (Erb 1977). Space does not permit review of this information here. A successful protocol for inducing lactation in the field was developed in France but was not pursued because of regulatory constraints on sale of milk from treated goats. It consisted of 17β-estradiol (0.25 mg/kg bw twice daily) and progesterone (0.625 mg/kg twice daily) in alcohol, given subcutaneously for seven days. Machine milking and hydrocortisone (25 mg/goat intramuscularly twice daily for three to five days) were begun on day twenty-one after initiation of treatment (Delouis 1975) or else the hydrocortisone was given before milking began, on days eighteen, nineteen, and twenty (Lerondelle et al. 1989). Recently, the addition of reserpine as a prolactin-releasing agent has been found to be beneficial (Salama et al. 2007). The technique is useful for goats that aborted or were found to be nonpregnant after having been dried off. However, milk production will be low, subsequent reproduction may be adversely affected (Salama et al. 2007), and extralabel use of drugs for production purposes in the United States is illegal. Hormonal induction of lactation of both immature does and bucks has been used to permit early expression of recombinant proteins in the milk of transgenic goats (Cammuso et al. 2000).

SKIN DISEASES AND INJURIES OF THE UDDER

Skin diseases that are frequently localized to the udder include bacterial folliculitis and contagious ecthyma (sore mouth). Readers should refer to Chapter 2 when additional information is desired or when symptoms are more general (e.g., capripox infection, bluetongue).

Contagious Ecthyma

Parapoxvirus infection may be limited to the teats or present elsewhere on the body. In regions where capripox virus also occurs, both viruses cause similar lesions on the udder and teats of lactating goats (Okoh and Obasaju 1983).

Pathogenesis and Clinical Signs

Contagious ecthyma lesions predispose to mastitis by interfering with the function of the streak canal while simultaneously harboring many pathogenic bacteria. A kid with sore mouth lesions can pass the infection to a doe's teats during suckling. Milking equipment and bedding contaminated by other infected does are other possible sources. The lesions are proliferative and crusty. Often they are secondarily infected with staphylococci.

Treatment and Prevention

Affected goats should be milked last, and an antiseptic udder salve may be applied to keep the scabs pliable and control bacterial proliferation until self-healing occurs. The arguments for and against herd vaccination are discussed in Chapter 2. The zoonotic potential of the virus must not be forgotten.

Staphylococcal Dermatitis

Lesions of the udder caused by staphylococcal infection include folliculitis, moist dermatitis in the intramammary sulcus, and deep furuncles.

Etiology

Staphylococcus aureus is the most important cause of folliculitis and furunculosis of the teats and udder skin of goats, but other staphylococci and streptococci may be involved.

Clinical Signs and Diagnosis

Pinhead- to pea-sized pustules typically develop on the skin on the back of the udder, base of the teat, or intramammary sulcus (Figure 14.3). Lesions are usually not painful. When a deeper furuncle develops, there is a reddened, warm, and tender swollen area that develops into an abscess (Fontanelli and Caparrini 1955; Heidrich and Renk 1967).

Cultures are rarely performed unless the condition is unresponsive to conventional therapy or spreads to other parts of the goat. Important differentials include contagious ecthyma, capripox, and warts when lesions are superficial; furuncles can be differentiated from milk cysts by careful palpation and, if necessary, aspiration. Enlarged or abscessed supramammary lymph nodes are located more dorsally than furuncles.

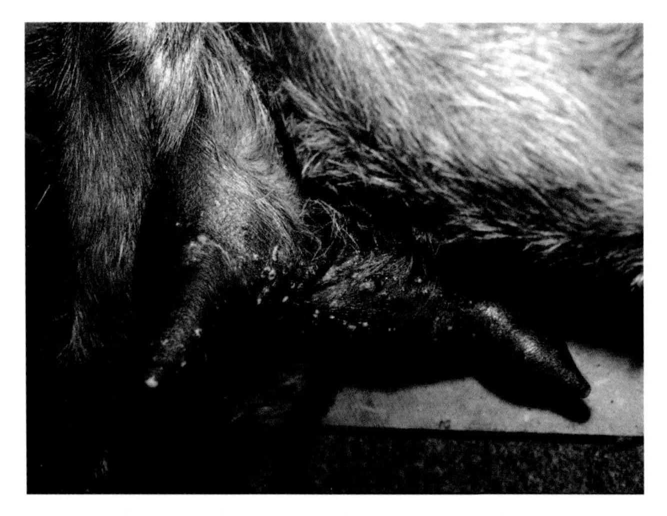

Figure 14.3. Pustules on the skin of the udder and moist dermatitis between the udder halves caused by *Staphylococcus aureus* infection. The doe later developed gangrenous mastitis. (Courtesy Dr. M.C. Smith.)

Therapy and Prevention

Lesions should be washed with a mild disinfectant and dried with single service towels. Disinfectant ointment or spray is applied after milking. Affected animals are to be milked last, and the milker should wear gloves or wash hands to avoid spread to other goats. Furuncles can be encouraged to point with ointments containing iodine or ichthyol. The abscess is then lanced and flushed. Autogenous *Staphylococcus aureus* vaccine (two doses) has appeared to limit the course and spread of the disease in some goat herds (Heidrich and Renk 1967).

Caseous Lymphadenitis

In herds in which *Corynebacterium pseudotuberculosis* is endemic, wounds to the teats or udder permit penetration of the organism. Infection of the wound may be noted, but more commonly, the problem first becomes obvious when an abscess develops in a supramammary lymph node (Figure 14.4). This abscess may break and drain pus down the back of the udder, or additional enlarged nodes may appear in a chain that extends upward toward the vulva. Caseous lymphadenitis is discussed in detail in Chapter 3.

Dermatomycosis

Flat, slightly thickened, circular, nonpainful skin lesions on the udders of goats in Florida have been diagnosed as tinea versicolor, a dermatomycosis of humans resulting from *Melassezia furfur* (Bliss 1984). Lesions on dark skin appear depigmented, whereas on lightly pigmented skin they are lightly colored. Biopsy specimens contained basophilic, PAS (periodic acid-Schiff stain) -positive filamentous organisms and oval,

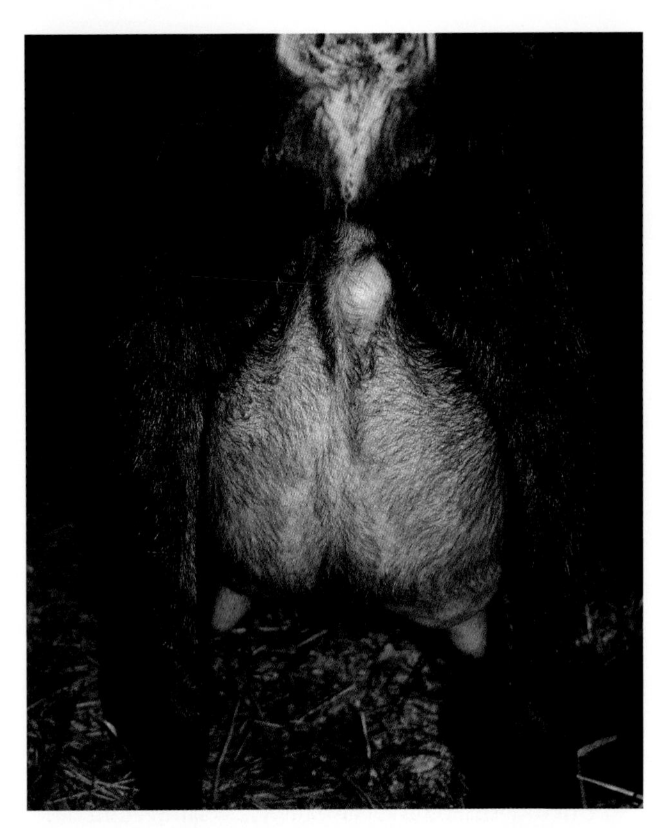

Figure 14.4. Abscess in the supramammary lymph node of a doe in a herd with endemic caseous lymphadenitis. (Courtesy Dr. M.C. Smith.)

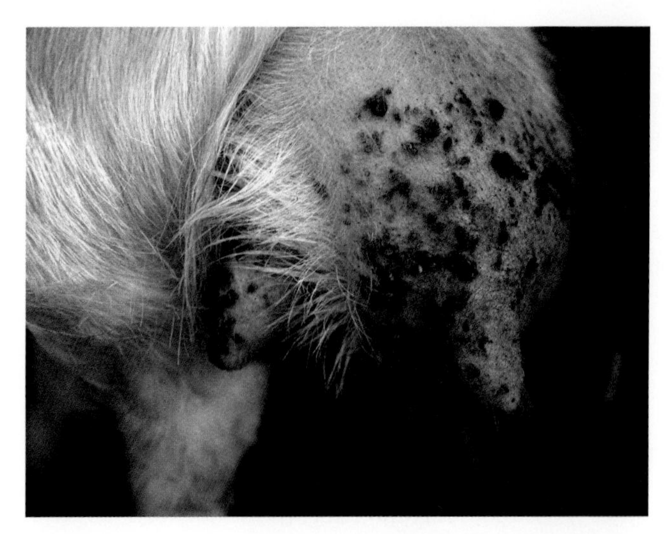

Figure 14.5. Udder warts on a Saanen doe. (Courtesy Dr. M.C. Smith.)

thick-walled cells (nicknamed "spaghetti and meatballs") in the stratum corneum. No treatment has been attempted.

Frostbite

If the teats are wet from inadequate drying after udder preparation for milking or from confinement in a wet environment, frostbite may occur when the goat is exposed to extreme cold and wind. Pendulous or edematous udders are especially vulnerable. Mildly chapped teats may be treated with protective ointments. If the full thickness of a teat is frozen, thawing in warm water 106°F to 111°F (41°C to 44°C) and protecting from refreezing are advised (Scott 1988). Sloughing of skin on the teat and secondary bacterial mastitis are to be expected. Powder teat dips are available for dipping in cold weather after milking.

Sunburn

Does with light-colored udder and teat skin are subject to sunburn when first turned out in the spring, even with cloud cover. The best means of avoiding a painful burn is to initially permit only very brief grazing, then drive the animal back into the barn. With succeeding days the exposure to sunlight is gradually lengthened. This protocol also avoids indigestion in goats changing from dry hay to green grass. Many owners lack time, patience, or both. Their animals can be protected by application of colored teat dip or a sunscreen sold for human use. All such material must be washed off before the next milking to avoid contamination of the milk.

Saanen does that have pale pink udders at the end of the housing season often have large black spots akin to freckles on the udder after a summer on pasture. This condition is not pathological and requires no treatment.

Warts and Squamous Cell Carcinomas

Papillomas (warts) of the udder of white goats are a very serious problem, especially in areas with abundant sunshine (Moulton 1954; Ficken et al. 1983; Theilen et al. 1985).

Etiology and Epidemiology

Most attempts to demonstrate virus in these lesions have failed. Recently, papillomavirus-like sequences have been detected in wart-like lesions by DNA hybridization, even though no virions were found by electron microscopy (Manni et al. 1998). An epidemiologic survey (Ficken et al. 1983) revealed that appearance of udder warts in the herd often begins three to six months after introduction of an affected goat. Exposure to sunlight appears to be involved.

Pathogenesis and Clinical Signs

The warts are multiple and initially may be flat and scaly (Figure 14.5) or prolonged into cutaneous horns. Some flake off the teat or bleed during milking. In some animals the warts regress completely during the nonlactation period. In other goats, the warts partially or totally regress but recur the next spring and summer (during lactation). The animals with persistent lesions may develop squamous cell carcinomas in subsequent years. The carcinomas have a flat base and often an ulcerated surface. They occasionally metastasize to the supramammary node. Much more serious is their propensity to eventually erode through the wall of the teat. This leads to mastitis and loss of the udder half, as may penetration of the streak canal by bacteria harbored in tumors located near the teat orifice. Myiasis may also occur.

Treatment and Prevention

No effective treatment is known. Neither have vaccines been of any value. The recently affected goat could be housed in the hopes that permanent regression will occur. Certain carcinomas may be surgically removed; cryosurgery has the advantage of minimizing hemorrhage. Prevention involves excluding affected goats from the herd and selecting for other breeds or at least for pigmentation of the skin of the udder in white breeds. The prevalence of udder warts in Saanens in Queensland, Australia, has been greatly decreased by selecting for tan skin on the udder (Baxendell 1984a). In South Africa, providing adequate shade for milking Saanens has prevented the development of squamous cell carcinomas (Donkin and Boyazoglu 2004).

Teat Obstruction and Stenosis

A doe at kidding may have a temporary teat obstruction caused by a plug blocking the streak canal. This material can be manually expressed from the teat, and afterward the doe milks easily. When kids are allowed to suckle the doe, it is important to remove a squirt or two of colostrum from each half of the udder. Not only does this allow inspection of the secretion for evidence of clinical mastitis, but it avoids starvation of the kid that is too weak to suck out the teat seal on its own. Even a strong kid prefers to suckle the side that yields milk for less effort. The unmilked side then becomes distended and painful, and the doe no longer permits nursing on that teat. Stripping out milk from the enlarged gland as soon as the udder is noticed to be lopsided is necessary if both glands are to remain productive in the current lactation.

If difficulty in milking persists after removal of the initial teat plug, an experienced person should evaluate the teats of the goat in question. People who are just learning to hand-milk goats may have difficulties because of lack of proper technique. If a teat sphincter is too tight for milking, it is important to determine if scar tissue from a previous injury is responsible. If no scar tissue is detected, the doe and its offspring should not be kept for breeding purposes. In such an animal and in goats that previously milked normally, a stenotic teat opening sometimes can be corrected by removing a core of tissue with a disposable 18-gauge needle (Nigam and Tyagi 1973) after previous infusion or spraying of local anesthetic. Consideration should be given to antibiotic therapy after such manipulation because the protective keratin lining of the streak canal will undoubtedly be damaged. In large teats with scar tissue or an excessively tight sphincter, several cuts (on opposite sides, with care to avoid incising skin) with a teat bistoury may be tried; milk should drip from the teat end immediately after surgery, as some contraction is to be expected during healing.

If the udder of a multiparous doe appears to be distended but no milk reaches the teat cistern, the problem may be scar tissue at the base of the teat. This develops as the result of chewing behavior by hungry nursing kids when milk production is inadequate. The obstruction may not be recognized until the subsequent lactation. An important differential is hard udder, in which interstitial mastitis caused by the caprine arthritis encephalitis virus (see below) prevents milk from reaching the teat end.

Milkstones, lactoliths, or "peas," small, hard concretions floating in the teat cistern, may occasionally work as a ball valve and interfere with milking. An association with incomplete milkout has been proposed (Guss 1980). Stones that cannot be forcibly expressed from the teat or crushed with alligator forceps could be removed surgically.

Udder and Teat Wounds

Udders with poor suspensory ligaments or long teats can be injured during grazing activities. Barbed wire, dog attacks, and horn punctures can also tear the skin of the teats or udder. Repair of the wound follows general surgical principles but has been described in some detail by Anderson et al. (2002). After cleansing and debriding to bleeding tissue, the fascial layer of the udder or the inner teat lining (depending on the location of the wound) is closed with a fine (4-0) absorbable suture material. Nonabsorbable sutures or wound clips can be placed in the skin. The goat is given systemic antibiotics (penicillin) and the gland is infused with a bovine intramammary antibiotic product. Tetanus prophylaxis must not be neglected. Aftercare involves frequent gentle milking or drainage with a sterile teat cannula to prevent back pressure, leakage, and formation of a permanent fistula.

In fiber-producing goats, teats are occasionally cut off accidentally during shearing. Does with only one teat remaining may not be able to raise a kid under range conditions.

Teat biting is an abnormal behavior which has been observed in dairy goats at the time of estrus if the group is being reserved for later breeding. The teat may be scratched or bruised or bitten completely off. Often the goat that is biting the teats of other animals is not identified, but sometimes it is a frustrated buck, sticking his head through a fence to a waiting doe. The use of a sexually active vasectomized buck has been recommended to prevent this problem (Coleshaw 2004).

Udder Edema

Periparturient udder edema, characterized by excessive accumulation of fluid in the interstitial spaces and pitting on digital pressure of the skin of the udder, has been reported in goats but has received little scientific attention. The goat may be uncomfortable and difficult to milk. Does kidding for the first time are frequently affected. Differential diagnosis includes mastitis, hard udder caused by caprine arthritis encephalitis, hematoma, and rupture of the prepubic tendon (Al-Ani and Vestweber 1983). Treatment with exercise, massage, and a diuretic (e.g., 50 to 100 mg furosemide, although a goat dosage has not been established) can be tried, but the edema often resolves within a few days after parturition without any treatment except milking. Vitamin D_3 has been suggested to aid resolution of udder edema by counteracting hypocalcemic effects of hypomagnesemia (Mills 1983a, 1983b). Some owners start milking a week before parturition as a means of controlling edema (Baxendell 1984b); the first milking colostrum should be heat treated and frozen for later feeding to the kids. Draining the fluid with one or more 3-cm incisions in the skin caudal to the teat has been reported to be effective and innocuous in goats (Rebesko et al. 1974), but is not presently recommended. Because the pathogenesis of udder edema remains unclear, even in cattle (Al-Ani and Vestweber 1986; Goff 2006), one can only speculate on how to prevent the condition in goats. Limiting salt before parturition is reasonable, but limiting grain, as commonly recommended, might cause pregnancy toxemia.

MASTITIS

Mastitis, or inflammation of the mammary gland, is a broad diagnosis that may be based on changes in the physical characteristics of the udder or its secretion. Mastitis usually results from an infectious agent, although consuming avocado leaves also causes marked inflammation (Craigmill et al. 1992). Several reviews of caprine mastitis have been published (Smith and Roguinsky 1977; Lewter et al. 1984; Menzies and Ramanoon 2001; Bergonier et al. 2003; Contreras et al. 2007).

DIAGNOSIS OF MASTITIS

Physical examination for changes in the milk or signs of inflammation and culture of the mammary secretion are the most commonly used techniques for identifying clinical or subclinical mastitis. Various other laboratory tests, especially those relating to cell enumeration, have been investigated as possible indicators of mastitis. Tests currently available other than culture are unsatisfactory in goats, in the author's opinion. Monthly somatic cell determinations on all herd members are valuable for keeping track of increased cell counts (and satisfying government regulations) but are rarely worth the expense regarding mastitis control.

Clinical Examination

Early indications of clinical mastitis include a decrease in milk production by one gland or a lameness on the affected side as the goat attempts to avoid contact of the hind limb with the tender half of the udder. Nursing kids may appear to be hungry, and mastitis is associated with increased kid mortality rates (Addo et al. 1980). Visual inspection of the udder from behind and from the sides may reveal asymmetry whereby the affected gland is swollen (acute) or atrophied (long-term inflammation). Predisposing teat end lesions (Kapur and Singh 1978) (wounds, contagious ecthyma, warts) also may be identified. Palpation may disclose the presence of heat, tenderness and swelling (acute), induration or atrophy (chronic mastitis), or even multiple abscesses. Regarding acute mastitis, the goat may be systemically ill, with signs of fever, anorexia, and depression. If the teat is cold and edematous or the secretion red and watery, gangrenous mastitis should be suspected. This severest clinical form is discussed in detail below.

Culture

Culture of an aseptically obtained milk sample is necessary to identify the etiologic agent of bacterial mastitis. The ideal sampling technique begins with brushing off any loose debris and discarding several streams of milk. The teats are then predipped in an approved bovine product and the predip is allowed thirty seconds of contact time before being wiped off with an individual paper towel. Finally, the teat end should be carefully disinfected with a cotton ball moistened with 70% ethyl or isopropyl alcohol before a milk sample is collected in a sterile vial (National Mastitis Council 1999). Refrigerate the samples promptly, or freeze if culture will be delayed more than forty-eight hours. Freezing results in a minimal decrease in recovery of organisms from goat milk samples (McDougall 2000; Sanchez et al. 2003). Sensitivity testing using routine techniques sometimes assists in selecting antibiotic therapy.

Some researchers require positive cultures from two consecutive milk samples from the same gland before a culture result can be interpreted as positive (Contreras et al. 1997b). Two or more consecutive negative culture test results are often presumed to indicate absence of infection.

Practitioners who wish to perform in-house mastitis cultures find that most mastitis isolates grow on blood agar at 95°F to 98.6°F (35°C to 37°C) and can be identified on the basis of a few simple tests such as colony characteristics and hemolysis on blood agar, Gram stain, and catalase tests. A standard reference book that includes color photographs of culture plates is extremely helpful (National Mastitis Council 1999). A simplified flow chart for identifying common pathogens adapted from this reference is provided in Figure 14.6. An organism is catalase positive if bubbles are produced when a colony is emulsified in 3% hydrogen peroxide. The oxidase test requires special discs and should not be performed on colonies grown on selective media such as MacConkey agar (National Mastitis Council 1999).

Various multipartite culture plates are also available commercially that include selective media for Gram-negative or Gram-positive organisms, staphylococci, or streptococci. An example is the Bi-plate from the University of Minnesota Laboratory for Udder Health, St. Paul, Minnesota, which includes Factor medium (Gram-positive growth, *S. aureus* shows hemolysis) and MacConkey medium (Gram-negative growth).

Mycoplasma are more difficult to grow in the laboratory. *Mycoplasma mycoides* subsp. *mycoides* (large colony type) grows on blood agar plates supplemented with ovine blood; "fried egg" colonies 1 mm in diameter and beta hemolysis are detectable after one week (DaMassa et al. 1983). Isolating the other species usually requires special mycoplasma medium and a moist 10% CO_2 incubator (National Mastitis Council 1999). Plates are observed under 20 to 50× magnification for seven to ten days before being termed

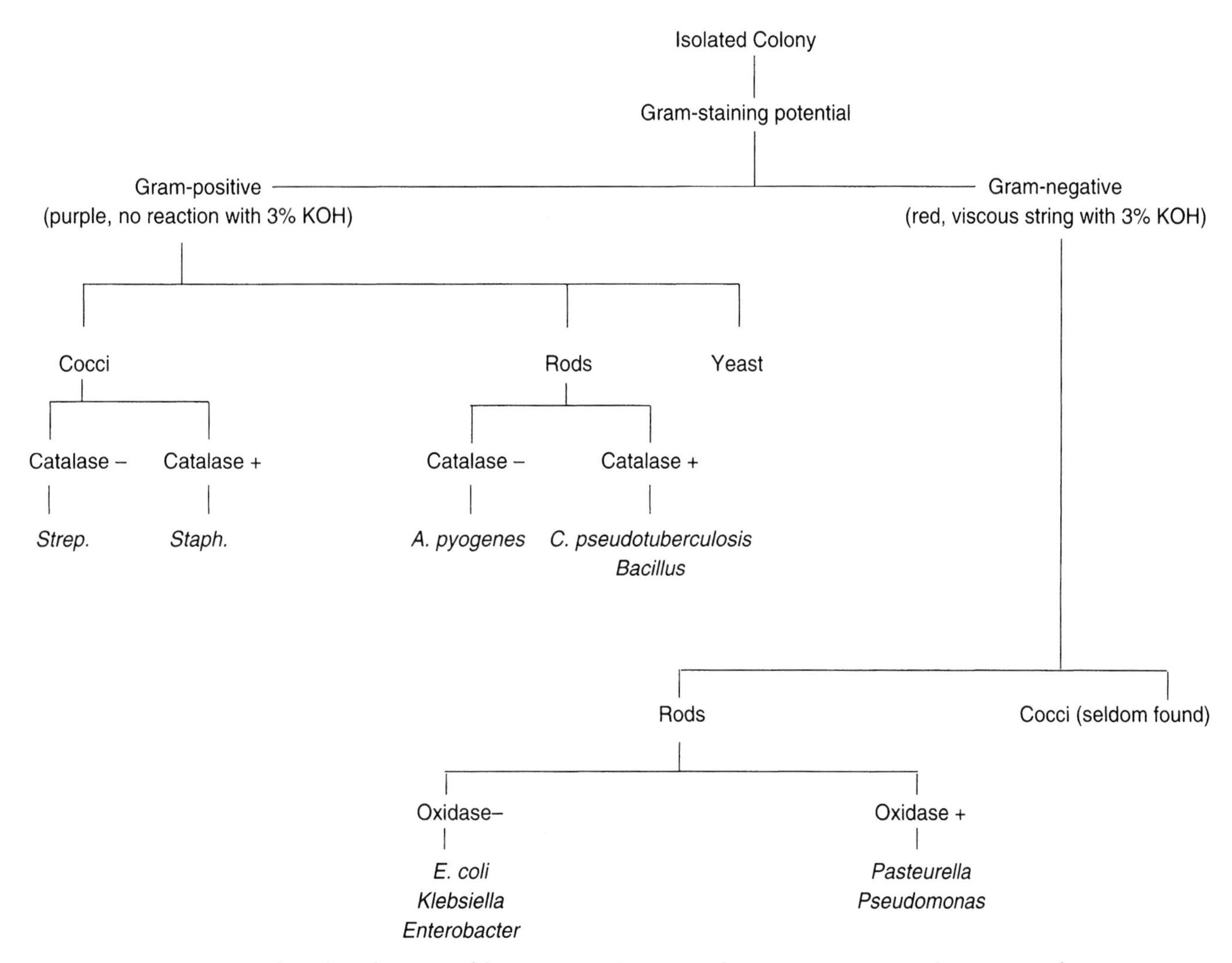

Figure 14.6. Flow chart for identification of bacteria causing mastitis.—represents negative test result, + represents positive test result.

negative. Most colonies have a fried egg appearance. Exact identification of an isolate is difficult, and typing is performed by only a few laboratories.

Cell Enumeration

An increase in the number of somatic cells in milk has been used as an indication of mastitis, including subclinical mastitis, in cows. Application to dairy goats of tests and regulations developed for cattle frequently has led to panic in the commercial producer who interprets "high" cell counts as evidence of a serious mastitis problem or who is threatened by the inspector with loss of a milk market. Currently the legal limit for somatic cell count (SCC) in goat milk in the United States is 1 million cells/ml. In a survey of seventy-one commercial U.S. herds in November and December, only 35% could achieve this low a count (Droke et al. 1993). A legal limit has not yet been set in the European Union (Paape et al. 2007). Numerous factors affecting cell count in goat milk have been reviewed recently (Haenlein 2002; Paape et al. 2007).

Cytoplasmic Particles and Epithelial Cells

In discussions of bovine mastitis, the number of somatic cells per ml of milk is generally assumed to correlate directly with the severity of mastitis or the degree of irritation to the mammary gland. The relationship of somatic cell count (SCC) to caprine mastitis is limited, unless tests appropriate to caprine milk are used. This is partly because goat milk differs from cow milk due to the presence of cytoplasmic particles and epithelial cells. The caprine mammary gland produces milk by a process called apocrine secretion (Wooding et al. 1970). Portions of the cytoplasm of the epithelial cells are pinched off and appear in the milk as DNA-free particles similar in size to leukocytes (Dulin et al. 1982). By contrast, ewes produce milk with approximately 10% of the number of cytoplasmic particles found in goat milk (Paape et al. 2001). Also present in variable numbers in goat milk are intact epithelial cells sloughed from acini and ducts.

Interpretation of Reports and Counting Methods

Very careful attention must be paid to the counting technique when comparing or contrasting various reports or when attempting to estimate the prevalence of mastitis in a goat herd. Another inadequacy of much of the literature is in the realm of determining mean SCC. Most older studies have not used a log transformation such as the linear score (also called somatic cell score) developed for bovine SCC where linear score $= 3 + \log_2 (X/100)$ for a somatic cell count of $X \times 10^3$ cells/ml. Somatic cell scores and equivalent SCC are: 1 = 25,000; 2 = 50,000; 3 = 100,000; 4 = 200,000; 5 = 400,000; 6 = 800,000; 7 = 1.6 million; 8 = 3.2 million/ml.

The direct microscopic somatic cell count, using a stain appropriate for goat milk, is the standard against which other counting methods should be judged.

Direct Microscopic Somatic Cell Count

The confirmatory test for somatic cell numbers in bovine milk is usually a direct microscopic examination of 0.01 ml of milk on a slide within an area of 1 cm^2. The Levovitz-Weber modification of the Newman-Lampert stain is commonly used to stain somatic cells for counting (Schalm et al. 1971). This stain is inappropriate for goat milk because staining is similar for cytoplasmic particles and cells (Dulin et al. 1982). A research technician might be able to recognize the difference between particles and cells, but over counting would be expected in a commercial laboratory.

Currently, the stain preferred for determining SCC in goat milk in the United States is the pyronin Y-methyl green stain (Dulin et al. 1982; Paape et al. 2001), often referred to simply as the green stain. Methyl green is specific for DNA and pyronin Y is specific for RNA. Chromosomes, then, stain blue-lavender while cytoplasmic particles and the cytoplasm of epithelial cells stain red. Neutrophils do not contain pyronin Y-positive material (Paape et al. 1963). Unfortunately, this staining is difficult to do and the reagents are potentially toxic to laboratory workers. Neutrophils are the predominant cell type in goat milk from both infected and uninfected glands, whereas the macrophage is the predominant cell in milk from uninfected sheep and cows (Sierra et al. 1999; Paape et al. 2001).

Leukocytes and epithelial cells in goat milk have also been differentiated by a modified Wright's stain technique (Hinckley and Williams 1981). Others have reported that many leukocytes are masked by the background in smears prepared with Wright's stain (Paape et al. 1963).

California Mastitis Test (CMT) and Teepol Test

The CMT is a simple, semiquantitative test for determining the number of nucleated cells (both neutrophils and epithelial cells) in milk (Schalm and Noorlander 1957). Equal quantities (typically 2 ml) of milk and the commercial reagent (Nasco, Inc., Fort Atkinson, WI, and others), which contains 3% alkyl arylsulfonate and bromcresol purple as a pH level indicator, are combined in the cup on a white paddle and swirled. Different scoring schemes are used in different parts of the world. As described originally, there is no change with a negative reaction, while a T (trace) reaction consists of a slight thickening of the milk. Scores of 1, 2, and 3 are given with increasing gel formation and deepening of color. A score of 3 means that a gel has formed that pulls away from the edge and collects in

Table 14.1. CMT scores on goat milk (after Schalm 1971).

CMT score	Scand. system	Samples	Neutrophil leukocytes/ml	
			Range	Median
0	1	46	0–480,000	60,000
trace	2	43	0–640,000	270,000
1	3	29	240,000–1,440,000	660,000
2	4	16	1,080,000–5,850,000	2,400,000
3	5	6	>10,000,000	—

the center of the cup. It is potentially confusing that some workers designate the same five categories as scores of 1 to 5 (Scandinavian system).

The reaction detects the presence of DNA, which is released when the detergent ruptures somatic cells. The approximate numbers of leukocytes for each score for goat milk (Schalm et al. 1971) are indicated in Table 14.1. In a Norwegian study, the total numbers of leukocytes and epithelial cells were 690, 800, 820, 1,230, and $4{,}520 \times 10^3$/ml for the five CMT scores from 1,966 goat milk samples (Pettersen 1981). A French study of midlactation samples that categorized any reaction greater than a trace as positive concluded that a positive CMT result had a sensitivity of 88% and a specificity of 93% for detecting SCC by Fossomatic methods greater than 750,000 cells/ml (Perrin et al. 1997). It is generally believed that scores of T or 1 (up to 1 million cells/ml) are usually no reason for concern.

In France, the equivalent to the CMT is called the Teepol test, after a European brand of neutral liquid detergent. The commercial detergent is diluted 1:10 and then used as the reagent (Lefrileux 2002). It reacts with both epithelial cells and neutrophils. Test results with goat milk have been graded and interpreted as follows (Roguinsky et al. 1971):

1. No or fine precipitation (as many as 500,000 cells/ml): normal
2. Granular precipitate (200,000 to 1 million cells): mild irritation, as by improper milking
3. Filamentous precipitate (500,000 to 2 million cells/ml): weakly pathogenic organism such as nonhemolytic staphylococcus
4. Viscous precipitate (more than 1.5 million cells/ml): suggests presence of *Staph. aureus*

The CMT is more useful for ruling out than for diagnosing mastitis in goats (Contreras et al. 1996). In a Norwegian study of 1,161 milk samples, 331 of 422 samples with CMT values of 1 to 3 in the American system yielded no bacterial growth; 732 of 739 with a negative or trace CMT score yielded no growth (Nesbakken 1978b). High scores at the end of lactation (Maisi 1990) or in systemically ill goats with drastically reduced milk production occur in the absence of mastitis. A sick goat with a negative or trace CMT reaction is probably not sick because of mastitis. If there is a marked difference between the scores of two halves of a goat's udder, mastitis is very likely. The usefulness of the CMT (or any other test) for diagnosing subclinical mastitis depends on the prevalence of mastitis in a herd. In a well-managed herd, the predictive value of a positive test is unacceptably low (Hueston et al. 1986).

Wisconsin Mastitis Test (WMT)

The Wisconsin Mastitis Test uses diluted CMT reagent. It is more objective than the CMT because the viscosity of the milk-reagent mixture is estimated from the volume remaining in a special tube after draining through a standard-sized hole for fifteen seconds (Schalm et al. 1971). The WMT is considered to be DNA-specific. Results obtained using standard conversion factors for cow milk are similar to counts obtained by the Fossomatic method (Dulin et al. 1982).

That the test results accurately predict the etiologic agent of mastitis has not been adequately documented.

Fossomatic and DeLaval Cell Counters

The Fossomatic method (Foss-O-Matic, Foss Electric, Hillerod, Denmark) of determining SCC is an automated fluorescent technique that uses a dye that specifically binds to the DNA of cell nuclei. With Fossomatic equipment currently used by dairy herd improvement associations in the United States, both epithelial cells and leukocytes are counted, but counts are not confounded by cytoplasmic particles. There is good correlation between Fossomatic counts and those obtained by direct microscopic exam using the pyronin Y-methyl green stain (Droke et al. 1993).

Test temperature (104°F versus 140°F; 40°C versus 60°C), use of bronopol preservative, and sample storage time (one to four days) have little effect on SCC results (Sierra et al. 2006). Counts are slightly lower when azidiol is used as the preservative (Sanchez et al. 2005). If the Fossomatic machine is calibrated according to the manufacturer's directions using goat milk standards, the SCC is 27% lower than when cow standards are used (Zeng 1996).

The DeLaval counter (DeLaval International AB, Tumba, Sweden) is a newer device that is portable and can be used on the farm. A single-use cassette is employed for each milk sample and the technique is DNA-specific. Fluorescence of cell nuclei is detected as a digital image. There is a high correlation (95%) with cell counts obtained with the more laborious direct microscopic method using the pyronin Y-methyl green stain on goat milk (Berry and Broughan 2007). Early, mid, and late lactation goats were included in this study.

Coulter Counter

The Coulter counter enumerates particles as milk flows past an electronic eye. Because cytoplasmic particles are similar in size to leukocytes, they too are counted in goat milk. Certain counters with channels that permit categorizing cells by cell diameter may improve differentiation of mastitic from nonmastitic samples (Smith and Roguinsky 1977). Coulter counter cell counts tend to be approximately double the counts in goat milk determined by Fossomatic equipment (Poutrel and Lerondelle 1983; Lerondelle 1984).

One study involving 483 half samples from goats in Scotland found that SCC by Coulter counter is neither specific nor sensitive for diagnosing caprine mastitis. Approximately one-third of noninfected samples or those yielding coagulase-negative staphylococci gave counts more than 2 million, whereas 73% of samples yielding *Staphylococcus aureus* had SCC more than 2 million (Hunter 1984). The stage of lactation and yield were not specified for these goats. In a longitudinal study in Greece, the SCC by Coulter counter increased as lactation progressed in uninfected goats, varied with the breed of goat, and was higher is goats infected with *S. aureus* than in animals with coagulase-negative staphylococci, which in turn were higher than the count from goats with no infection (Boscos et al. 1996), demonstrating the same relationships seen by others with Fossomatic counts.

Cell Counts in the Course of a Normal Lactation

The number of cells and distribution of cell types are not constant throughout lactation. Epithelial cells are most numerous in late lactation. In a study that did not distinguish stage of lactation and did count cytoplasmic particles, epithelial cells accounted for 5.6% of the total cells plus particles (Sierra et al. 1999). Macrophages are also increased in late lactation and may have a foamy cytoplasm due to phagocytized fat globules. They are extremely difficult to differentiate from epithelial cells. In the fall, when many goats in the herd are "stressed" by estrus, the percentage of neutrophils in the milk increases (Atherton 1992) as does the overall SCC (Haenlein 2002). An association has also been proposed between herd events such as vaccination or nutritional problems leading to acidosis and increased cell counts (Lerondelle et al. 1992). Cytoplasmic particle numbers change little with stage of lactation (Dulin et al. 1983).

The proportion of polymorphonuclear cells in the milk increases as days in milk increases (Rota et al. 1993). A differential count of cells from uninfected goat milk in late lactation has revealed that approximately 80% of the cells are polymorphonuclear cells. This is due to the presence of chemotactic factors different from those found in mastitic milk (Manlongat et al. 1998). These cells may participate in the involution of the udder and protect from new infections. In one study, increased SCC was clearly linked to advancing lactation and decreased production. Goats producing less than one pound (454 g) of milk per day all had counts more than 5 million/ml (using a DNA-specific method) (Perez and Schultz 1979). Other studies have also shown SCC above 1 million/ml in uninfected goats in late lactation (Zeng and Escobar 1995). In a seasonal dairy goat herd, then, where most animals are in late lactation simultaneously, cell counts determined by whatever method often exceed regulatory standards for cow milk even with low prevalence of mastitis. It has been proposed that the regulatory threshold should be adjusted according to herd average days in milk (Haenlein 2002), but implementation might be easier if month of the year were considered instead, in regions where seasonal breeding is the norm. The cell count may also vary with time of day, as one study found higher SCC for afternoon than morning milk samples (Randy et al. 1988).

The arithmetic mean cell count by Coulter counter at drying off is approximately three times the cell count in midlactation in halves infected with nonhemolytic staphylococci or in halves with negative bacterial cultures. Thus, in noninfected halves, the Coulter counter cell count mean in one study was 1.54×10^6 cells/ml (n = 1061) in lactation versus 4.31×10^6 cells/ml (n = 617) at drying off (Lerondelle and Poutrel 1984). In another study, the sum of cytoplasmic particle count and mononuclear (epithelial) cell count exceeded 10 million/ml in several goats in very early and very late lactation, although it was not clear if they were actually free of mastitis (Hinckley 1983).

Cell Counts in Mastitis

It is very difficult to establish a threshold cell count for the diagnosis of mastitis. Many authors have attempted to do so, but their results cannot be combined because different techniques for cell enumeration were used. Marked herd differences in SCC of milk from uninfected goats have been reported in several studies. Also, the specificity of a given threshold as an indicator of mastitis is greatly decreased at or near drying off (Lerondelle and Poutrel 1984). In other words, goats with a high SCC in midlactation are more likely to be infected than are late lactation goats with elevated counts. A threshold of 1 million cells/ml has been proposed for detecting major pathogens in early and midlactation (Poutrel and Lerondelle 1983).

The presence of more than 3 million cells/ml in one or both of the first two monthly tests in lactation has been used in France to diagnose infection with *S. aureus*, with a sensitivity of 82% and a specificity of 95% (Baudry et al. 1999). In another French study of

5,905 samples from 1,060 goats in eight herds, the geometric mean cell count per ml (by Fossomatic) was 272,000 for uninfected glands, 932,000 for coagulase-negative staphylococci, and 2,443,000 for glands infected with major pathogens (Poutrel et al. 1996). In an eight-year survey of herds in Rhode Island and Connecticut, 2,911 milk samples were evaluated. Of these, 466 had SCC above the 1×10^6 threshold but were culture negative, representing 44% of all samples classified as mastitic by SCC (White and Hinckley 1999). A marked difference in the cell count (by whatever test) between halves is a very good indicator of infection in the gland with the higher cell count.

Whatever the cell counting technique and threshold used, it is also very important to realize that the prevalence of infection affects the predictive value of a positive test. Thus, using sensitivity and specificity determined in a Fossomatic study at forty days of lactation, the predictive value of an SCC above 1 million was 0.21 at an infection prevalence of 5%, 0.57 at a prevalence of 20%, and 0.84 at a prevalence of 50%. The corresponding predictive values with a 3 million threshold were 0.39, 0.76, and 0.93 (McDougall et al. 2001). One study concluded that approximately 90% of the difference in goat somatic cell counts cannot be explained by infection, and that a better test for milk quality is needed (Wilson et al. 1995).

Most (but not all) goats with subclinical *Staph. aureus* infection show an elevated cell count (Lerondelle and Poutrel 1984). The nucleated cell count in the milk from a half chronically infected with *Staphylococcus aureus* can fluctuate widely from week to week (Nesbakken 1978a). The SCC in the half infected with *Staph. aureus* is higher than the SCC of the goat's other gland if it is uninfected (Moroni et al. 2005b). A decrease from 10 million to 1 million per ml cannot be used as evidence of elimination of the infection.

Most studies show increased SCC in goats infected with coagulase-negative staphylococci as compared with noninfected herdmates, while others show no or minimal difference (Sheldrake et al. 1981; Hunter 1984; Manser 1986; Paape et al. 2001; Moroni et al. 2005d; Schaeren and Maurer 2006). In one study, the proportion of cells that were neutrophils was increased (approximately 75% compared with approximately 50%) in milk from goats with coagulase-negative staphylococci when compared with milk from goats with negative culture test results (Dulin et al. 1983). It has been proposed that strain differences in pathogenicity are responsible for variation in inflammatory response in different herds. Contreras et al. (1999) reported that *S. epidermidis* was associated with a higher SCC than other coagulase-negative staphylococci in the same herd. Hemolytic strains of coagulase-negative staphylococci induce a higher SCC response than nonhemolytic strains (Bergonier et al. 2003). However, one recent study failed to find a difference in SCC according to species of coagulase negative staphylococci (Leitner et al. 2004b).

Infections with coliforms or other bacteria producing endotoxin can result in increased nucleated cell counts, and specifically neutrophils, in goats as in cattle. Several workers have demonstrated this by infusing endotoxin into the udder (Dhondt et al. 1977; Jarman and Caruolo 1984). Various species of *Mycoplasma* have also been associated with increased leukocyte counts in goat milk (Prasad et al. 1985).

Some researchers feel that caprine arthritis encephalitis (CAE) virus infection leads to higher cell counts in goats and accounts for part of the difference between SCC of "normal" goats and cows. French workers have noted an increase in the proportion of mononuclear cells in milk from goats with interstitial mastitis caused by CAE (Lerondelle 1988; Lerondelle et al. 1989, 1992). In one study, goats serologically positive for CAE had increased cell counts but also had more subclinical infections with staphylococci than did CAE-negative herdmates (Smith and Cutlip 1988). A similar study from Italy found significantly higher SSC and lower protein and lactose in seropositive doelings but did not determine bacteriologic status (Turin et al. 2005). A Norwegian study of 1,799 goats from sixty-six herds found increased SCC but no statistical differences in production of milk, fat, protein, or lactose in seropositive goats (Nord and Adnoy 1997). Several studies of goats free of bacterial infection have reported increased SCC in milk of CAE positive animals (Ryan et al. 1993; Sánchez et al. 2001). Some researchers have found no effect of CAE status on SCC (Luengo et al. 2004).

The feeding of avocado leaves (*Persea americana*) of the Guatemalan but not Mexican variety to goats has caused a marked drop in milk production, udder edema, grossly curdled milk, and somatic cell counts that were markedly increased (mean more than 7 million/ml; technique not reported but probably Fossomatic) (Craigmill et al. 1984, 1989). There is an apparent injury to the microcirculation of the gland followed by coagulative and lytic necrosis of acinar epithelium (Craigmill et al. 1992). Doses of 20 g fresh leaves/kg body weight cause mastitis while higher doses cause a cardiomyopathy.

Finally, some intramammary infusion products cause a marked increase in SCC; swelling and tenderness of the udder and flakes or clots in the milk occur when given to healthy goats. Oxytetracyline increased the SCC by an average of forty-two times twelve hours after infusion, erythromycin by an average of twenty-three times, and penicillin and cephapirin by six times pretreatment cell counts (Ziv 1984). In a more recent study using bovine mastitis infusion tubes available in South Africa after three consecutive milkings, a cefuroxime product caused no irritation, whereas an ampicillin/cloxicillin product caused a significant (but unspecified) increase in SCC and the irritation caused by a cephalexin/neomycin/prednisolone treatment was less marked (Karzis et al 2007).

Cell Counts and Cheese Yield

Work with cow milk has shown a small decrease in cheese yield from milk with high SCC. It is believed that proteolytic enzymes from neutrophils break down milk solids into smaller fragments that are then lost in the whey. Lipolysis, which results in off-flavor and decreased yield, also increases, apparently caused by increased susceptibility of the milk fat to lipolysis when mastitis is present (Murphy et al. 1989). Preliminary work with goat milk has failed to show any abnormal protein composition related to increased neutrophil production (Atherton 1992). However, a goat study that compared the milk of uninfected halves with halves infected with coagulase-negative staphylococci demonstrated higher somatic cell counts, lower lactose concentration, and decreased cheese curd yield from the infected glands (Silanikove et al. 2005). Another study found that cheese yield increased in late lactation and was negatively correlated with CMT but that there was no correlation with SCC by Fossomatic (Galina et al. 1996).

Other Tests Correlated with Mastitis

Various constituents and properties of normal goat milk have been reviewed by Jenness (1980). The chloride content of goat milk is greater than in cow milk, with means in various studies ranging from 121 to 204 mg/100 ml.

Bacterial infections in the udder alter cell wall permeability and permit an increased flow of sodium and chloride into the milk. Lactose and potassium concentrations decrease (Linzell and Peaker 1972), but these substances have not been used to diagnose caprine mastitis.

Electrical Conductivity

Subclinical infections by minor pathogens that do not damage mammary epithelium may be of little or no concern to udder health or milk production. With this in mind, researchers have tried to use electrical conductivity of the milk as an indicator of the severity of a mastitis infection (Linzell and Peaker 1975; Fernando et al. 1982; Sheldrake et al. 1983; Norberg et al. 2004). A convincing increase in accuracy of detecting bovine mastitis, relative to somatic cell counting, has not been demonstrated.

Preliminary work has not shown electrical conductivity to be useful in screening for subclinical mastitis in goats. One group failed to find a correlation between SCC (Fossomatic) and electrical conductivity (Park and Nuti 1985; Park 1991). They noted little variation between conductivity of foremilk and strippings of the same goat but demonstrated a negative correlation between electrical conductivity and butterfat percentage. Another study showed no correlation of electrical conductivity with SCC, a positive correlation with butterfat, and an increase in electrical conductivity as lactation progressed (Das and Singh 2000). Another study showed that electrical conductivity of goat milk was a poor predictor of infection status and less accurate than somatic cell count (McDougall et al. 2001).

NAGase

N-acetyl-β-D-glucosaminidase (NAGase) has received attention as a possible marker for inflammation in both bovine and caprine milk. Because this enzyme is present in the cytoplasm of epithelial cells of the mammary gland and in sloughed-off cytoplasmic particles, and because NAGase is increased in the colostrum and late lactation milk of goats free of bacterial mastitis (Maisi 1990), it suffers from the same problems relative to interpretation as do cell counting techniques.

Several studies have confirmed that NAGase is elevated in milk from halves with major pathogens and with coagulase negative staphylococci (Timms and Schultz 1985; Maisi and Riipinen 1988; Vihan 1989; Maisi and Riipinen 1991; Leitner et al. 2004a, 2004b). Increased NAGase has also been demonstrated in milk from CAE positive goats free of bacterial infection, when compared with CAE negative, bacteria negative goats (Ryan et al. 1993). The test has been reported to be less sensitive than CMT for detecting infection and there is no significant difference between NAGase levels in the infected and uninfected halves of the same goat according to one study (Maisi 1990). Others have concluded that NAGase is superior to cell counting techniques for diagnosing subclinical mastitis in goats (Vihan 1989, 1996).

INFECTIOUS CAUSES OF MASTITIS

Numerous bacterial and mycoplasmal agents have long been associated with caprine mastitis. More recently, retroviral infections have been recognized as an important cause of udder inflammation.

Retroviral Mastitis (Hard Udder)

Goat owners in the United States and Australia have been frustrated for many years by a condition known as "hard udder." More recently a milder form of the condition has been recognized in many countries.

Etiology and Epidemiology

Undoubtedly, the diagnostic characteristics of a firm udder at parturition with scanty milk flow are not specific enough to limit "hard udder" to a single etiology. However, it has become clear since the discovery of CAE (caprine arthritis encephalitis) that the condition as a herd problem tends to disappear when CAE is eradicated from the farm (Kapture 1983). Interstitial mastitis has been recognized in two goats experimentally infected with CAE virus (Cork and Narayan 1980). A similar hard udder syndrome has been recognized in sheep infected with the closely related ovine progressive pneumonia and maedi-visna viruses (Cutlip et al. 1985; van der Molen and Houwers 1987). A recent histologic study of sixty-two agar gel immunodiffusion (AGID) positive native goats in Japan found nonsuppurative mastitis in 80% of the animals (Konishi et al. 2006). Infection is readily spread and histologic lesions created by introducing infected cells into the udder (Lerondelle et al. 1995). There is one report of another as of yet unidentified virus smaller than CAEV in the cytoplasm of inflammatory cells in the udder of a goat with typical hard udder (Post et al. 1984)

It is not clear if CAE is involved in the etiology of cystic hyperplasia of the caprine mammary gland described in the older literature from India (Singh and Iyer 1973; Sharma and Iyer 1974). Periductal and perilobular fibrosis infiltrated by lymphocytes was associated with dilated ducts in the cystic lesions. "Udder edema" accompanied by decreased milk flow is another poorly described condition that might be related to CAEV (Sedgman 1982). When true udder edema is present (as described earlier in this chapter), the skin pits on pressure.

There is a recent suggestion that the scrapie agent could be excreted in the milk of sheep with retroviral interstitial mastitis (Ligios et al. 2005). Scrapie is not common in goats (see Chapter 5), but the possibility of horizontal spread of scrapie via milk of CAE infected goats is intriguing.

Clinical Signs

When the acute form of retroviral mastitis appears at parturition, the udder is very firm, almost like a rock, but the overlying skin is loose and free of edema. Heat and erythema are also absent. Almost no milk can be obtained, even with the aid of oxytocin and warm compresses. What milk is obtained appears normal but has an elevated cell count (Lerondelle 1988). Signs of systemic illness are absent. Some affected goats come gradually to milk over a period of several weeks, which has allowed numerous medical or herbal treatments to appear to be effective. In other animals, palpable induration of the udder or udder half persists (Zwahlen et al. 1983). Supramammary lymph nodes are enlarged. Clinical signs may be less severe and cell counts lower in subsequent lactations (Le Guillou 1989; Lerondelle 1989).

Careful udder palpation reveals increased firmness in additional does that appear to be milking normally. A Swiss study based on palpation of the udder of 1,517 animals found palpable changes (diffuse or focal induration of the parenchyma) in 23% of ELISA seropositive goats, 19% of suspicious goats, and only 7% of seronegative animals (Krieg and Peterhans 1990). Bacteriologic cultures were not undertaken.

Diagnosis

Diagnostic evaluation should include a physical examination to detect other problems such as metritis, udder edema, and teat obstructions. Udder biopsy might be performed but microscopic examination is more commonly performed at necropsy. Histological changes reported for retroviral mastitis in goats and sheep include accumulation of mononuclear cells (lymphocytes, macrophages, and plasmacytes) in the parenchyma and around ducts in the udder (Zwahlen 1983). These mononuclear cells are sometimes organized into lymphoid follicles, a histologic change that has been seen in a three-month-old doeling infected naturally with CAE and in adults (Kennedy-Stoskopf et al. 1985). These cellular infiltrations may externally compress ducts or protrude into ducts, preventing the passage of milk (Post et al. 1986). Lobular atrophy and prominent corpora amylacea are also reported in CAE-affected udders.

Bacterial and mycoplasmal cultures and herd testing for CAE are performed if the owner or veterinarian is unsure of the diagnosis. Not every animal infected with the CAE virus has detectable serum antibody, especially at parturition when circulating antibody has passed into the colostrum. Demonstration of virus by isolation or immunofluorescence testing could be attempted on milk or udder tissue from serologically negative goats. Many goats with CAE infection (including many shedding virus in their milk) do not develop a hard udder. Thus, serology is inconclusive at best. However, if the entire herd is free of evidence of the virus, the diagnosis becomes very unlikely.

Treatment and Control

No cure for the interstitial mastitis has been identified, and culling is indicated. Cortisone administered two days before expected parturition has been reported to cause regression of clinical signs in some goats (Lerondelle 1988). Control is through a CAE eradication program, as discussed in Chapter 4. Kids should be removed from the affected doe and fed virus-free colostrum and milk. Infected animals, if left in the herd, should be separated and milked last, and milk or whey should not be fed back to any goats in the herd without proper heat treatment.

Mycoplasma Mastitis

When repeated efforts to isolate bacteria from udders affected with clinical mastitis yield no growth or only non-hemolytic staphylococci, the possibility of mycoplasmal involvement should be investigated. The simultaneous presence of mastitis with other clinical signs such as arthritis, pneumonia, or conjunctivitis also warrants consideration of mycoplasma.

Etiology

Numerous species of mycoplasma have been isolated from the milk of goats (DaMassa et al. 1992; Bergonier and Poumarat 1996), sometimes with more than one species present in the same animal (Gil et al. 1999a) or the same herd (Kinde et al. 1994). Others have been infused experimentally into goat udders to test pathogenicity. The various organisms cannot be distinguished on clinical grounds.

MYCOPLASMA AGALACTIAE. Contagious agalactia of sheep and goats is a specific disease common in Mediterranean countries, much of Europe, the Middle East, and South Africa. The causative agent is classically *Mycoplasma agalactiae*, although some authors now use the term contagious agalactia for almost any mycoplasmal mastitis of small ruminants (OIE 2004; Corrales et al. 2007). As discussed in Chapter 4, *M. agalactiae*, *M. capricolum* subsp. *capricolum*, *M. putrefaciens*, and *M. mycoides* subsp. *mycoides* large colony (LC) type are recognized by the World Organization for Animal Health (OIE) as causes of contagious agalactia for regulatory purposes. *M. agalactiae* is generally considered to be exotic to the United States, although it has been isolated from goats in California (DaMassa 1983; Kinde et al. 1994). In many regions, this condition must be reported to regulatory authorities.

Septicemia occurs in infected animals, and the organism may then localize in the udder, joints, or eyes. *Mycoplasma agalactiae* is shed for months via milk, urine, feces, and ocular and nasal discharges. Infection can be by either ingestion or inhalation. The environment becomes contaminated, and infections may spread via communal browsing areas or driving routes (Dhanda et al. 1959; Corrales et al. 2007).

MYCOPLASMA MYCOIDES SUBSP. MYCOIDES (LARGE COLONY). California goat dairies have experienced mastitis outbreaks and polyarthritis in kids due to *Mycoplasma mycoides* subsp. *mycoides* (large colony type) (East et al. 1983). Its role in respiratory disease is discussed in Chapter 9. This same organism is isolated frequently enough in Europe that recent authors classify it as one of the causes of contagious agalactia (Corrales et al. 2007). In Israel, udder inflammation and agalactia in does and conjunctivitis and polyarthritis in kids have been reported to be caused by *Mycoplasma mycoides* subsp. *mycoides* (ovine/caprine) serogroup 8 (Bar-Moshe and Rapapport 1978, 1981), which is possibly the same organism.

MYCOPLASMA PUTREFACIENS. *Mycoplasma putrefaciens* has caused an outbreak of mastitis, agalactia, abortion, and arthritis in a large California dairy (DaMassa et al. 1987) and in Europe (Gaillard-Perrin et al 1986; Mercier et al. 2000) and the Middle East. Subclinical mastitis can occur also. Some goats infected with *M. putrefaciens* have no visible changes in the milk nor palpable inflammation or fibrosis (although milk leukocyte percentages are increased). Even when agalactia develops, fibrosis is absent (Adler et al. 1980). The organism does not seem to induce a febrile response (DaMassa et al. 1992).

OTHER MYCOPLASMAS. *Mycoplasma mycoides* subsp. *capri* (normally a cause of pleuropneumonia) and *M. capricolum* subsp. *capricolum* have been isolated from goats with mastitis in France (Perreau 1972; Perreau and Breard 1979; Picavet et al. 1983). Intramammary inoculation of several *M. capricolum* strains produced severe mastitis (thick yellowish secretion, increased cell count, agalactia, enlargement of the supramammary nodes) in does, and pneumonia, polyarthritis, and keratoconjunctivitis in nursing kids (Taoudi et al. 1988). In India, *M. mycoides* subsp. *capri* has produced a purulent mastitis after experimental inoculation (Misri et al. 1988). *Mycoplasma capricolum* has also been isolated from California goats.

Mycoplasma arginini has produced natural cases of purulent mastitis in goats in India (Prasad et al. 1984), and the condition has been reproduced experimentally (Prasad et al. 1985). Leukocyte counts were markedly increased and agalactia developed. In contrast, Jones (1985) was unable to demonstrate pathogenicity of *M. arginini* to the goat udder. The organism is usually considered to be nonpathogenic (DaMassa et al. 1992).

Experimental inoculation of goat udders with *Acholeplasma laidlawii* has produced mastitis leading to agalactia and marked fibrosis (Singh et al. 1990). The goat udder has also been used to test other strains of mycoplasmas isolated from other species or body systems for potential pathogenicity (Pal et al. 1983; Jones 1985).

Clinical Signs

Contagious agalactia (*M. agalactiae*) often appears in a herd in the spring, soon after lactation begins. An incubation period of seven to fifty-six days has been reported. Early signs (during the septicemic stage) include inappetence, depression or malaise, and an unwillingness to follow the herd (U.S. Animal Health Assoc. 1998). A purulent mastitis and agalactia then develop. The secretion is initially watery but later turns thick or lumpy. Keratoconjunctivitis or arthritis may occur in the same goats or in kids drinking unpasteurized milk. Mortality of untreated animals can approach 20%. Some herds have animals infected with and shedding *M. agalactiae* in milk without clinical mastitis or elevation in the bulk tank somatic cell count (Corrales et al. 2004).

Clinical signs with other mycoplasma infections are variable. The classic mastitic mycoplasma milk sample is one that separates into a granular sediment and a greenish-yellow watery supernatant. The milk is said to have a putrefactive odor when *M. putrefaciens* is the cause of the mastitis. In acute, severe cases both mammary gland and supramammary lymph node are enlarged. Both halves of the udder are often but not always affected, and there is no response to treatment. Milk production ceases quickly, with does essentially agalactic in two to three days. The udder atrophies but may be completely functional after the next parturition. Some does die during the acute stage of the disease (East et al. 1983; Gil et al. 1999b). Some mycoplasmas also may be associated with respiratory disease or abortion.

Diagnosis

Mycoplasma should be suspected if blood agar cultures of milk samples from a herd outbreak of mastitis are negative. Appropriate cultures for mycoplasma (for instance on Hayflick's medium) should then be initiated. In herds with *M. mycoides* subsp. *mycoides* LC, it has been noted that most milking does are asymptomatic with normal appearance to the milk, though large numbers of mycoplasma are present. This species is somewhat unique in that it can be isolated on sheep or calf blood agar, where colonies resemble alpha-hemolytic streptococci but no bacteria are seen on Gram stain (Rosendal 1994). When contagious agalactia is suspected, other samples from septicemic animals can also be positive by culture, including ocular swabs, ear swabs, joint fluid, blood, liver, spleen, feces, and urine. As with respiratory disease, the identification of the species of mycoplasma involved in a mastitis outbreak can be hastened and simplified by using appropriate polymerase chain reaction tests (Nicholas 2002; Corrales et al. 2007). Serologic testing using ELISA can also be helpful if vaccination is not part of the control strategy (Corrales et al. 2007). Commercial ELISA kits for *M. agalactiae* are available in Europe (OIE 2004).

Histopathologic examination of the mammary gland reveals marked interstitial infiltration with mononuclear leukocytes, especially around acini and ducts. Mononuclear cells and desquamated epithelial cells are seen in ducts. Giemsa stain can be used to demonstrate the mycoplasma (Dhanda et al. 1959), but immunochemistry is more specific and preferred (Corrales et al. 2007).

Treatment

Treatment is generally ineffective. Improvement in systemic signs is usually noted with drugs generally used against mycoplasma (such as tetracycline, tylosin, erythromycin, spiramycin, lincomycin, tiamulin, florfenicol, or fluoroquinolones where legal), but the goat is apt to become an inapparent carrier (Perreau 1974; Bergonier and Poumarat 1996; Nicholas 2002). Thus, slaughter of all infected goats is recommended unless the herd is in an endemic region. Practitioners should particularly avoid infusion into the udder of preparations of tylosin or erythromycin meant for systemic administration. The irritating nature of these drugs often ensures destruction of milk secreting tissue, even if the infection can be eliminated. It has been reported that tiamulin at 10 mg/kg intramuscularly can maintain concentrations in the udder inhibitory for *M. agalactiae* for twelve hours (Ziv et al. 1983). Spectinomycin penetrates the udder poorly. In endemic herds, using an antimycoplasma treatment for all animals at dry off has been recommended (Corrales et al. 2007).

Control

Because mycoplasma mastitis is usually introduced into the herd by a carrier goat or sheep (Ruhnke et al. 1983), it is very important to investigate the health status of the herd of origin before buying or boarding an animal. Serologic tests have been undertaken in some countries with an aim of eradicating infection from herds and preventing re-introduction. The variety of species possibly involved complicates this approach. Serology using enzyme-linked immunoabsorbent assay tests for *M. agalactiae* and *M. mycoides* subsp. *mycoides* LC has shown promise for identifying individual carrier goats (Davidson et al. 1989). Culture tests of bulk tank samples appear to be a starting point in regions where the problem occurs. An outbreak of mastitis may be delayed until several months or years after introduction of carrier animals (Picavet et al. 1983). Stress, as is associated with parturition or with transport and adjustment to a new herd, appears to trigger shedding of the organism.

As with all cases of mastitis, affected animals should be milked last and hands or milking machines disinfected before milking other goats. Common udder towels should be avoided. In dairy herds undertaking an eradication program for *M. mycoides* subsp. *mycoides* LC, one approach is to cull all positive animals to slaughter based on an initial herd culture. Then colostrum is cultured from each doe at freshening. The eradication efforts are monitored by frequent culturing of tank milk from each milking string (East et al. 1983). Because feeding of raw colostrum and milk can be the source of serious joint and lung infections, a pasteurizer should be used if goat milk is to be fed to kids.

Mycoplasma agalactiae organisms are shed in urine and feces, making the environment an important source of infection to other sheep and goats. Stalls should be disinfected and litter removed. Mycoplasma are inactivated by many routine disinfectants, including sodium hypochlorite (30 ml of household bleach in

1 gallon or 4 liters of water), cresol, 1% formalin, and ionic and nonionic detergents (U.S. Animal Health Association 1998). A variety of vaccines against *M. agalactiae*, both killed and attenuated, have been evaluated. Although some provide protection from clinical disease and are thus very useful in endemic areas, carrier states may still develop (Foggie et al. 1970, 1971; Arisoy 1973; U.S. Animal Health Assoc. 1998). In regions where vaccination is routine, leaving a small population of unvaccinated sentinel animals in the herd permits monitoring of disease activity by serologic screening (Corrales et al. 2007). Goats previously inoculated with *M. putrefaciens* showed resistance to subsequent challenge for at least one year (Brooks et al. 1981), suggesting that a vaccine might also help to control this organism.

Bacterial Mastitis

Bacteria causing caprine mastitis, with a few exceptions, usually enter the udder through the teat end. Clinical cases occur most commonly in early lactation (Moroni et al. 2005c). Control is achieved by udder hygiene during and between milkings.

Organisms and Clinical Syndromes

The clinician cannot expect to identify the organism by the nature of the secretion but can often make a tentative diagnosis based on herd history (prior probability). Culturing the etiologic agent from the milk or udder tissue is necessary to identify the cause of mastitis. In turn, identifying the organism involved assists the veterinarian and owner in designing future control programs. Organisms are discussed in alphabetical order because prevalence and importance vary between herds and regions.

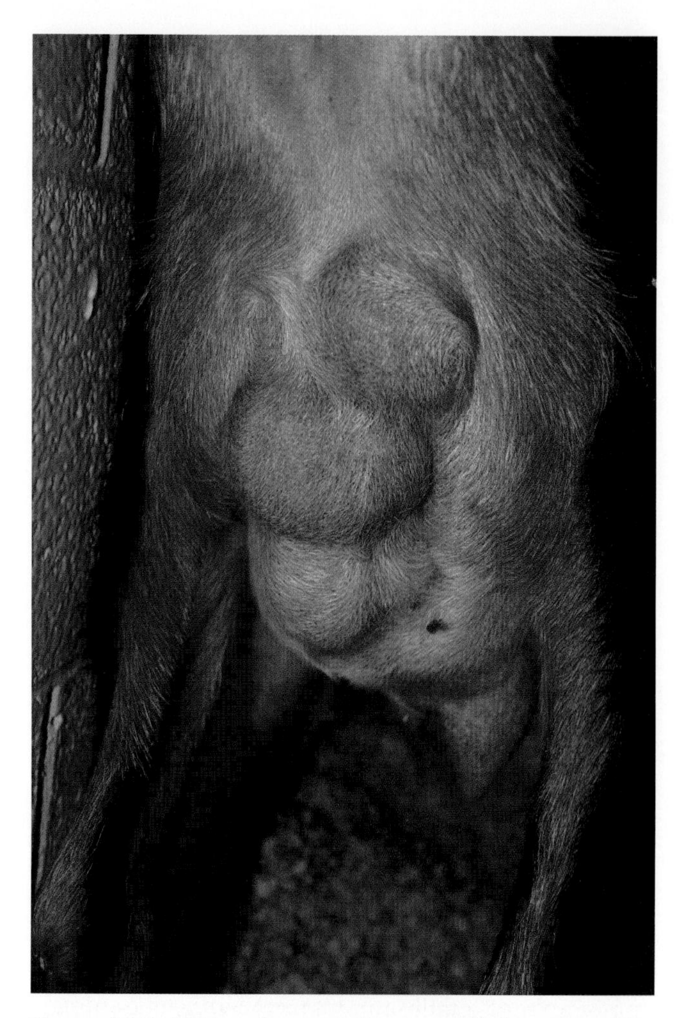

Figure 14.7. Udder abscesses in an aged doe caused by *Arcanobacterium pyogenes*. The animal was managed by udder amputation. (Courtesy Dr. M.C. Smith.)

Arcanobacterium (Actinomyces, Corynebacterium) pyogenes. This organism is frequently isolated from udders containing multiple abscesses (Figure 14.7). Teat or udder wounds predispose to the entry and establishment of the infection in the udder. In experimental infections, nonlactating glands are more severely affected than lactating glands (Jain and Sharma 1964). In the chronic stage, culling is advisable, although teat (Sasshofer et al. 1987) and udder amputation return the goat to systemic good health if localization in other organs has not occurred. The organism grows slowly on blood agar. Colonies are tiny at forty-eight hours but made visible by a narrow zone of clear hemolysis. The organism is a small Gram-positive rod and is catalase-negative.

Brucellosis. *Brucella melitensis* and *Br. abortus* can cause a subclinical interstitial lymphoplasmacytic mastitis (Heidrich and Renk 1967). The organism is carried by macrophages to the udder and then to the supramammary lymph node, which may be enlarged (Meador et al. 1989). The number of organisms in the milk and the degree of inflammation in the gland are increased by milk stasis, as when milking or nursing does not occur (Meador and Deyoe 1991). The presence of these organisms is often first suspected when brucellosis is diagnosed as a cause of abortion in the herd (see Chapter 13) or if humans consuming raw milk products develop undulant or Malta fever (Stiles 1950). Serologic testing of the goats is then undertaken, because the milk ring test is not accurate in goat milk (see Chapter 13). Sometimes a clinical mastitis occurs with palpable nodules in the udder parenchyma and flakes in the secretion (Dubois 1911). The mastitis resolves spontaneously, but the goat should be slaughtered to avoid human infections.

Coliforms. Coliforms, including *Escherichia coli* and *Klebsiella* spp, occasionally cause clinical mastitis in goats (Adinarayanan and Singh 1968; Lewter et al. 1984). The organisms are Gram-negative, KOH-positive, oxidase-negative rods. Colonies are large, gray or yellow, and moist. *E. coli* gives off a fecal odor.

Infection appears to be more common in periparturient does. Clinical signs in acute cases include anorexia, fever, and a yellowish or reddish watery secretion with an increased somatic cell count. The affected gland is warm, swollen, and painful. These signs have been reproduced experimentally by intramammary infusion of *E. coli* endotoxin (Dhondt et al. 1977). Occasionally signs progress to gangrene (Ameh et al. 1994).

These organisms represent "environmental" mastitis. Thus, control involves keeping sleeping areas clean and dry, drying teats thoroughly before milking, and avoiding teat-end injuries. Using post-milking teat dipping does not aid much in controlling coliform infections, because these are initiated between milkings, except when wet udders are milked.

Corynebacterium pseudotuberculosis. Though caseous lymphadenitis is very common in goats, mastitis caused by this disease is relatively rare. Infection of skin wounds on the udder may cause abscessation of the supramammary lymph node with no involvement of mammary gland tissue. Occasionally, goats develop mastitis or abscesses in the parenchyma of the udder (Addo et al. 1980; Burrell 1981; Schreuder et al. 1990). Positive catalase test results distinguish *C. pseudotuberculosis* from *A. pyogenes*.

Listeria. It has been suggested that *Listeria monocytogenes* can cause a subclinical interstitial mastitis, with diagnosis based on isolation of the organism from milk (Sasshofer et al. 1987). A chronic inflammatory lesion with lymphocyte infiltration, alveolar destruction, and fibrosis has been seen in the udder of sheep shedding listeria in the milk after natural or experimental infection (Tzora et al. 1999). Documentation of an inflammatory lesion in the goat udder is lacking, but listeria are commonly shed in the milk of clinically normal goats during herd outbreaks of listeriosis or immediately after parturition (Løken et al. 1982). Shedding of *L. monocytogenes* in the milk of goats correlates well with the presence of antibodies against the organism in the milk as detected by an ELISA (Bourry et al. 1997). *Listeria ivanovii* has been isolated from a mastitic goat in India (Elezebeth et al. 2007). *Listeria* are more important from a food safety perspective (Pearson and Marth 1990) than as a cause of mastitis in goats.

Mannheimia. Mannheimia (Pasteurella) haemolytica has been isolated only occasionally from goat milk (Schröter 1954; Bagadi and Razig 1976; Manser 1986; Donkin and Boyazoglu 2004), although it is a well-recognized cause of mastitis (including gangrene) of sheep. In an Italian study of 720 goats over an entire lactation, it was responsible for 16% of clinical cases (Moroni et al. 2005c). In Angoras in South Africa, *M. haemolytica* is reported to be a more frequent cause of acute mastitis than *Staphylococcus aureus*, typically occurring four to six weeks after parturition and seldom being accompanied by gangrenous color changes (Van Tonder 1975). The infection is most likely acquired from suckling kids, since it is a common inhabitant of the upper respiratory tract. The organism is a Gram-negative, oxidase-positive, bipolar rod. Colonies are medium, gray, transparent, and hemolytic on blood agar plates.

Mycobacterium Infections (Tuberculosis). Mycobacterium bovis, M. tuberculosis, and *M. avium* can all be associated with tubercular mastitis in goats (Murray et al. 1921; Davies 1947; Sasshofer et al. 1987). In regions where bovine tuberculosis is common, cows infect goats by the respiratory or alimentary routes (Heidrich and Renk 1967). The udder becomes involved during generalization of the infection to other organs such as lungs, liver, and spleen. Often, the source is infected humans.

The infection is subacute to chronic and manifests itself by slight swelling of the udder and development of firm, caseous or calcified, nodules in the parenchyma (Davies 1947; Soliman et al. 1953). Supramammary lymph node enlargement occurs. Antemortem diagnosis is by tuberculin test. Culture requires special media. Affected goats are slaughtered because of the risk they pose to human health.

Pseudomonas. Like *Mannheimia*, *Pseudomonas* species are oxidase-positive, Gram-negative rods, but colonies are usually granular and dry and may be a variety of colors. The source is usually contaminated water or teat dips, old pitted inflations, or wet bedding. If the water system is contaminated, flushing with heavily chlorinated hot water (160°F; 71°C or hotter) should kill the *Pseudomonas*, which are otherwise protected by a biofilm. Cleaning directions for pipeline systems (Dairy Practices Council 2000) are applicable. Paracetic acid can also be used to flush hoses and the water system in the parlor (Yeruham et al. 2005).

In one natural outbreak, systemic signs of illness were so severe that gangrenous staphylococcal mastitis was originally suspected. Only when appropriate antibiotics (based on a sensitivity test) were administered did affected goats survive (Petgen and Martain 1977). In another herd outbreak, 18% of 450 goats were infected and 12.5% developed clinical mastitis due to *Pseudomonas aeruginosa*. These does were depressed, inappetent, and febrile and the udders were firm, swollen, and painful. Many of these animals developed gangrenous mastitis and twenty-five died while the other fifty-seven infected goats were culled because they did not respond to treatment (Yeruham et al. 2005). In some herds, prolonged infections develop and clinical signs occur periodically.

Goats have been experimentally infected, but inoculation of the udder with large numbers of *Pseudomonas aeruginosa* was required; clinical signs varied from mild mastitis to severe, hemorrhagic mastitis with terminal septicemia (Lepper and Matthews 1966).

Burkholderia (*Pseudomonas*) *pseudomallei*, the causative agent of melioidosis, is a soil saprophyte found in parts of Australia and tropical Asia. Mastitis sometimes occurs, although abscesses are most common in lymph nodes, spleen, and lungs. This may take the form of udder swelling with pus in the milk (Thomas et al. 1988; van der Lugt and Henton 1995). Abscesses in the udder that repeatedly break and drain to the outside also have been observed (Olds and Lewis 1954). The organism has been isolated from macroscopically normal goat milk. Treatment (with tetracycline) is often unsuccessful, and affected goats are usually destroyed because of public health concerns.

Staphylococcus Aureus. Coagulase-positive (usually hemolytic) staphylococci are a common major pathogen of the goat's udder. In regions free of mycoplasmal mastitis, these organisms are often the most prevalent cause of clinical mastitis in dairy goats. *Staphylococcus aureus* isolates from caprine mastitis have been shown to resemble bovine mastitis strains in that most contain surface protein A (that binds to immunoglobin G) and fibronectin binding protein (involved in bacterial adherence and colonization) (Jarp et al. 1989). Most strains produce both alpha hemolysin and beta hemolysin (Roguinsky and Grandemy 1978). Colonies are large on blood agar media and usually surrounded by a zone of incomplete hemolysis or more than 2 mm of complete hemolysis (Figure 14.8). The organisms are Gram-positive cocci in pairs or clumps and are catalase-positive. Although the coagulase test is commonly used to identify *S. aureus*, *S. intermedius*, and *S. hyicus* can also be coagulase-positive (National Mastitis Council 1999) and are occasionally isolated from goat milk (Kalogridou-Vassiliadou 1991; Kyozaire et al. 2005) when full speciation is performed.

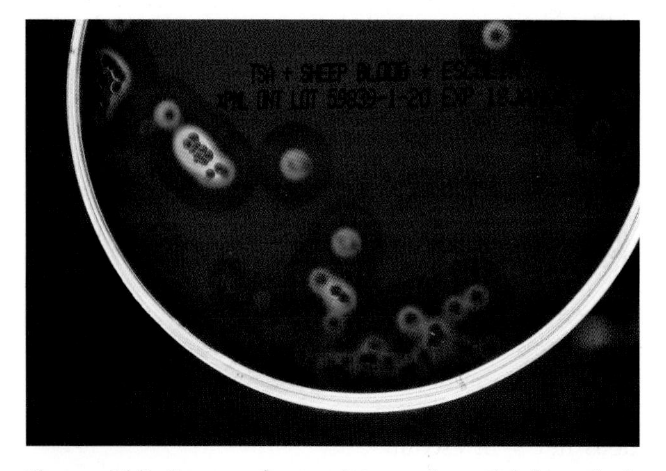

Figure 14.8. Zones of complete and partial hemolysis around colonies of *Staphylococcus aureus* growing on blood agar. (Courtesy Dr. M.C. Smith.)

The infection can be subclinical (identified by culture during herd survey), chronic (decreased production accompanied by induration and abscess formation), or acute (swollen, hot, painful half of the udder, accompanied by systemic illness). The most severe, acute form is gangrenous mastitis, which is described in detail below. These same forms have been reproduced by experimental inoculation of *S. aureus* into goat udders (Derbyshire 1958a).

As is the case with cows, the organism resides in microabscesses in chronically infected goats and infections are very difficult to cure (Derbyshire 1958b). Transmission to other goats occurs during milking. Animals that are culture positive for *S. aureus* should be culled to slaughter or milked last. In larger herds with machine milking, a "staph" unit can be identified and used to milk only *S. aureus* infected goats. If these animals are retained in the herd, they should certainly be dry treated and then should remain in the "staph string" (the group of infected goats) into the beginning of the next lactation. Intermittent shedding is common, and a single negative culture of a previously infected goat is not proof of a cure. If cultures are repeatedly negative and somatic cell counts remain low, the animal could be returned to the main herd.

Ideally, the milk of infected does should be pasteurized before it is fed to kids. Diarrhea, pneumonia, and death of nursing kids, with isolation of *S. aureus* from heart blood and abomasal and intestinal contents, have been reported (Paliwal et al. 1977).

Gangrenous Mastitis. Gangrenous mastitis in goats is most frequently due to *Staphylococcus aureus* in animals lacking adequate concentrations of antitoxin against the necrotizing alpha-toxin produced by the organism. Clostridial infections have also been implicated, as have coliforms (Renk 1957, Petris 1963).

The condition usually is restricted to the period of lactation. However, sometimes gangrenous mastitis occurs during the last week of pregnancy, when it often causes loss of the fetuses and death of the doe from toxemia (Petris 1963). Affected goats have poor appetite and a transient fever. In early cases, the skin of the teat or udder floor becomes cool and edematous, and the goat appears lame. A reddish (Figure 14.9), then bluish discoloration of the skin is noted next. The secretion becomes watery and red; gas bubbles may be present and produce a squeaking sound when the teat is stripped. Death may occur within twenty-four hours. In animals that survive the acute phase, a clear line of demarcation forms on the udder and the gangrenous portions are sloughed after several days or weeks.

Histologically, there is venous thrombosis, and the initial inflammatory changes are replaced by necrosis and sloughing of epithelial cells (Derbyshire 1958b). This thrombosis is probably responsible for edema of the mammary gland and ventral abdominal wall. The

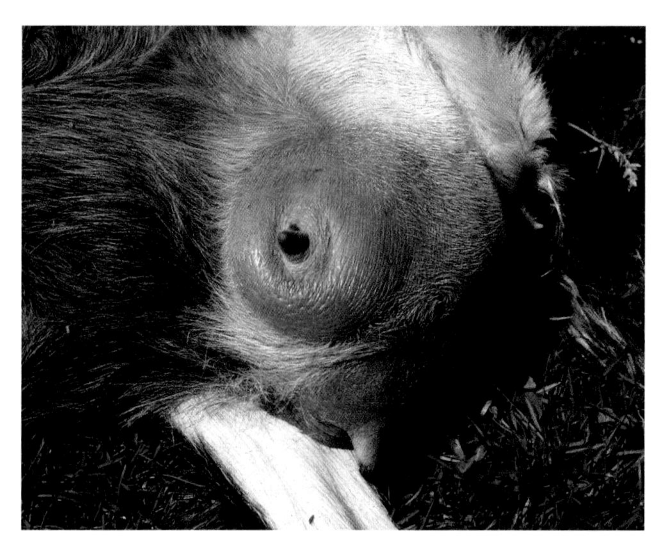

Figure 14.9. Early gangrenous mastitis with edema and erythema of the udder. *Staphylococcus aureus* was isolated from the milk and a portion of the gland sloughed. (Courtesy Dr. M.C. Smith.)

supramammary lymph node is enlarged, edematous, and hemorrhagic.

Because of its dramatic presentation and associated great economic loss, gangrenous mastitis caused by *S. aureus* is often the most prevalent form of mastitis recognized in herds free of mycoplasmal infections. In one report from Cyprus in 1961, almost 9% of 8,000 goats were affected with gangrene (Petris 1963). The average case fatality rate in this study was 40%.

COAGULASE-NEGATIVE STAPHYLOCOCCI. In many herd surveys, the most commonly isolated organisms are staphylococci other than *S. aureus*. As many as 71% of udder halves in a herd have been found to be infected (Sheldrake et al. 1981; Poutrel 1984). In a large California survey (sixteen herds, 2,522 lactating does), coagulase-negative *Staphylococcus* spp. were isolated from 17.5% of does (East et al. 1987). In four commercial herds in Australia, the prevalence was 13.3% of 896 halves tested (Ryan and Greenwood 1990). In a study in Italy that sampled 305 goats monthly throughout the lactation, 1,474 of 4,571 udder half samples cultured coagulase negative staphylococci (Moroni et al. 2005b). Numerous staphylococcal species have been identified, including *Staphylococcus epidermidis*, *S. intermedius*, *S. caprae*, and *S. hyicus* (Poutrel 1984; Maisi and Riipinen 1988; Maisi 1990; Kalogridou-Vassiliadou 1991). Many studies have been summarized by Contreras et al. (2003). Because different staphylococcal test systems often result in different species assignments, reported species prevalences in the literature may not be comparable (Burriel and Scott, 1998). These infections tend to persist throughout much of the lactation and are more common in older goats (Contreras et al. 1997b; Sanchez et al. 1999) and later lactation. Bilateral infections are common (Moroni et al. 2005b). The organisms commonly reside on the skin or in the environment (Valle et al. 1991; National Mastitis Council 1999).

Some authors regard the coagulase-negative organisms as major pathogens (Dulin et al. 1983), while others see them as minor pathogens or incidental infections (Moroni et al. 2005d). In a study comparing milk production of the udder halves of twenty-five unilaterally infected goats (Leitner et al. 2004a), production was significantly higher (0.98 kg/milking) in the uninfected halves, as compared with the infected halves (0.69 kg/milking). Some authors define an increased cell count to be equivalent to a serious mastitis and then conclude that because some goat milk samples with an increased cell count yield the organism, it must therefore have caused serious mastitis (Hinckley et al. 1985). The economic importance of coagulase-negative staphylococci remains unclear. Generally, the practitioner should look further to explain serious illness or marked loss in production because the coagulase-negative staphylococci are unlikely to be the cause. However, a high prevalence of these bacteria may suggest suboptimal milking procedures that should be addressed (Contreras et al. 2003).

STREPTOCOCCUS AGALACTIAE. Infection with *Streptococcus agalactiae* has been reported in goats in sporadic or epizootic forms, but occurs less frequently than in cattle. Most reports are in the older literature (Heidrich and Renk 1967) or from India (Mukherjee and Das 1957), New Zealand (McDougall and Anniss 2005), or Brazil (Langoni et al. 2006). The organism does not appear to be a problem in goats in the United States (White and Hinckley 1999).

The goat is not systemically ill, but induration of the udder and loss of secretory tissue may occur. *Streptococcus agalactiae* has been associated with severe stromal proliferation and fibrosis in goat udders (Addo 1984). The lesions have been reproduced experimentally (Pattison 1951). Abscess formation does not occur. The disease is transmitted from cow to goat or goat to goat, by milk on the inflations or the hands of the milker. Introduction of the disease to the herd can be avoided by screening bulk tank milk from the herd of origin or culturing the milk of the individual purchased doe before it joins the milking herd. Most isolates are sensitive to penicillin.

Colonies are not sufficiently characteristic in blood agar cultures to permit differentiation from other streptococci (see below), because *Streptococcus agalactiae* may be accompanied by greening of the medium, beta hemolysis, or no hemolysis. *Streptococcus agalactia* does not split esculin. The CAMP test is frequently used to make a presumptive diagnosis of *Streptococcus agalactiae* (Schalm et al. 1971). Erythrocytes sensitized by beta hemolysin from a nearby streak of *Staph. aureus* are completely hemolyzed by a factor diffusing into the agar from the *S. agalactiae*.

Other Streptococci. Streptococci other than *S. agalactiae* are occasionally the cause of sporadic cases of mastitis of environmental origin (Mallikeswaran and Padmanaban 1991). In one study that followed 720 machine milked goats over a complete lactation, 16% of the clinical cases of mastitis were ascribed to *Streptococcus* species, as compared with 74% due to *Staphylococcus aureus* (Moroni et al. 2005c). A herd outbreak of mastitis caused by *Streptococcus zooepidemicus* (twenty-eight of fifty animals with chronic mastitis) was ascribed to poor hygiene. Clinical signs included udder atrophy, induration, and abscessation (Nesbakken 1975). Outbreaks of *Streptococcus zooepidemicus* in three herds in Spain resembled contagious agalactia due to mycoplasma, including the occurrence of septic arthritis, and were controlled with an autogenous vaccine (Ruiz Santa Quiteria et al. 1991). Somatic cell counts are elevated, even in subclinically infected goats (Hall and Rycroft 2007). Provision of a clean, dry environment for the goats and assuring that the udder is clean and dry at milking should help to prevent new infections.

Streptococcal species form colonies on blood agar that are smaller than staphylococci, and the bacteria are catalase-negative. Many streptococci of environmental origin are esculin-negative (National Mastitis Council 1999).

Miscellaneous Bacterial and Fungal Organisms. It is conceivable that any pathogenic bacterium introduced into the udder might cause mastitis. For instance, isolation of the environmental organism *Serratia* is occasionally reported on herd surveys. Based on experience with cattle, antibiotic therapy is not helpful, but hygiene of the barn and teat dip should be investigated (National Mastitis Council 1999). If treatment has preceded isolation of an uncommon agent, the possibility of iatrogenic inoculation of the udder cannot be discounted. Miscellaneous organisms isolated from mastitic goat milk include *Yersinia pseudotuberculosis* (Cappucci et al. 1978; Jones 1982), *Nocardia* (Dafaalla and Gharib 1958; Bassam and Hasso 1997; Rozear et al. 1998), *Cryptococcus neoformans* (Pal and Randhawa 1976; Aljaburi and Kalra 1983), and numerous other fungi (Lepper 1964; Pal 1982; Jensen et al. 1996). Fungal mastitis has also been produced experimentally in goats using numerous *Candida* species and *Rhodotorula glutinis*. Antibiotic treatment prolonged the disease (Jand and Dhillon 1975). *Corynebacterium* spp. (Schaeren and Maurer 2006; Hall and Rycroft 2007) and yeasts (McDougall 2000) have been isolated from clinically normal goats. The isolation of *Corynebacterium bovis* from dairy cows is usually interpreted as evidence for inadequate teat dipping (National Mastitis Council 1999).

Treatment of Bacterial Mastitis

Although the owner of a valuable or pet goat expects and desires treatment for the doe with mastitis, culling of affected animals is often an economically sound alternative. Culling serves to decrease exposure of other does to contagious organisms and to increase selection pressure for genetic resistance to infection. Culling is also a logical choice when abscesses are found in the udder of a fiber-producing or meat goat during weaning or when selection for rebreeding occurs.

Lactation Treatment with Antibiotics. If treatment is elected, it should begin as soon as clinical signs are noted. Otherwise, additional destruction of milk secreting tissue may occur or the mastitis may turn gangrenous (*Staphylococcus aureus*). Lactational treatment of subclinical mastitis detected by culture or somatic cell determination usually is not economically profitable, except possibly for *Streptococcus agalactiae*, which is uncommon in goats. Milking such animals last is desirable.

Choice of Antibiotics. The range of antibiotics available for either intramammary or parenteral treatment of mastitis varies from country to country. Practitioners should evaluate the antibiotic sensitivity of isolates relative to drugs that are available, legal, and not prohibitively expensive. Because *Staphylococcus aureus* is the most frequent cause of clinical mastitis in many herds, initial treatment (in the absence of sensitivity results) should ideally be with a drug this organism is normally sensitive to; tetracycline and cephapirin are frequently effective *in vitro*. Resistance to penicillin is common, while ampicillin and amoxicillin have a broader spectrum of efficacy. Some studies have not shown beta lactamase production by goat isolates (Moroni et al. 2005a). Unless the animal is systemically ill, treatment is often limited to intramammary infusion with a full bovine tube administered two or three times at twelve- or twenty-four-hour intervals.

When extensive swelling or tissue penetration by bacteria such as *S. aureus* has occurred, parenteral administration of an antibiotic with good bio-availability for five to seven days is recommended (Ziv 1980). Because of pharmacokinetic considerations, some drugs that are administered parenterally do not achieve adequate concentrations in the udder (Ziv and Soback 1989). Gentamicin penetrates the udder poorly, and cephalosporins also do not pass readily from blood to milk. Oxytetracyline and potentiated sulfonamides are broad-spectrum and nontoxic but also have limited or variable penetration. Chloramphenicol has excellent properties for parenteral treatment of mastitis but is forbidden in many countries. Slow-release formulations (penicillin, tetracycline) are not usually effective in maintaining adequate milk concentrations.

Infusion of the udder on a prescription basis with gentamicin or trimethoprim/sulfadiazine has been recommended for confirmed coliform mastitis (Lewter et al. 1984). Research in cows suggests that gentamicin therapy does not affect severity or duration of *E. coli* mastitis, and clearance of gentamicin from kidney tissue requires many months (Erskine et al. 1991). The use of this antibiotic, then, is best avoided. Furthermore, infusion of any antibiotic solution other than a commercial mastitis tube is undesirable because of sterility, safety, and residue issues.

The antibacterial and udder penetration properties of several newer agents have been summarized by Ziv and Soback (1989). Florfenicol, enrofloxacin, norfloxacin nicotinate, tiamulin, and doxycycline afford good or excellent udder penetration after parenteral administration. The use of enrofloxacin and other fluoroquinolones in goats is expressly forbidden in the United States.

Infusion Techniques. Most commercial bovine infusion tubes have an applicator tip that is too large to be inserted into an average goat's teat. It is currently recognized that full insertion, even in a cow, damages the lining of the streak canal. In addition, bacteria that colonize the keratin lining are forced upward into the teat cistern, thereby predisposing to new infections. Thus, even in the case of a large teat opening, the applicator tip should be inserted only far enough to prevent leakage of the product during infusion. A specially designed 3.5-mm (one-eighth-inch) syringe tip (Opti-Sert, Ft. Dodge Labs, Ft. Dodge IA) should make partial insertion easier. When the teat sphincter is too tight or the doe too uncooperative, a sterile tom cat catheter may be used to infuse the mastitis medicine into the teat. Some authors recommend treating both halves even if only one is clinically affected (Sasshofer et al. 1987).

Teat dipping with a disinfectant before and after infusion is advisable, as is cleansing of the teat end with alcohol. Owners may need instruction in the importance of clean hands (or gloves) and sanitary techniques.

Antibiotic Residue Avoidance. The owner or veterinarian who has treated the lactating goat with antibiotics is left with the question of when the milk will be free of antibiotic residues. In one study using commercial lactating cow infusion tubes in the United States, erythromycin, oxytetracycline, penicillin, and cephapirin were administered according to label directions to ten goats. Antibiotic residues were not detected after the labeled discard periods (thirty-six, ninety-six, sixty, and ninety-six hours, respectively) except for one goat that still had detectable penicillin after seventy-two hours (Long et al. 1984). Another study found that oxytetracycline (426 mg) was still detectable at 108 hours and cloxacillin (200 mg) at 156 hours after last treatment (Hill et al. 1984). A commercial combination product (200 mg amoxicillin trihydrate, 50 mg potassium clavulanate, and 10 mg prednisolone) labeled with a forty-eight-hour withdrawal in dairy cows required 112 hours withholding time to achieve acceptable amoxicillin concentrations in goat milk (Buswell et al. 1989). It seems prudent to at least double the recommended bovine withdrawal period when treating goats. European regulations specify a seven-day withdrawal period for extralabel intramammary treatment of lactating small ruminants (Bergonier et al. 2003).

Duration of antibiotic residues in healthy goats after intramammary treatment (thirty-five commercially available infusion products) or parenteral treatment (twenty-seven injectable products) has been reported by Ziv (1984). Ceftiofur is labeled for systemic use in goats in the United States with zero milk withdrawal but does not penetrate the udder well. Systemic oxytetracycline is expected to be cleared from goat milk as fast as or faster than cows clear the antibiotic, but a milk discard period of six days has been suggested after high or prolonged dosage (Martin-Jimenez et al. 1997). Duration of penicillin residues in goat milk is variable, especially if given by the subcutaneous route, and testing of the milk is advised (Payne et al. 2006).

As the sensitivity of assays in use increases, it can be expected that the prudent withdrawal period will lengthen. Several residue tests have been shown to detect antibiotic concentrations in goat milk below the tolerance limit set for cow milk in the United States (Zeng et al. 1998); typically no confirmatory testing is done and the producer is presumed to be guilty of supplying milk with an illegal residue. It is also important to remember that detectable concentrations of antibiotics appear in milk from the untreated half (Hill et al. 1984). Even when residue levels are too low to endanger any except the most allergic human consumers, a cultured cheese may fail because of antibiotics in the milk. Ideally, milk from treated does should be tested at a milk plant or laboratory with the most sensitive antibiotic test available; milk with positive test results should not be used for human consumption.

False-positive Inhibitor Tests. Normal goat milk appears to have some antibacterial action. In one study, 24% of pre-antibiotic treatment milk samples from seventy-five healthy goats showed false-positive Delvotest results, and in 11% of the seventy-five animals the natural inhibitors were heat stable (140°F or 60°C for twenty minutes) (Ziv 1984). Small zones of inhibition (halos) are sometimes noted with the *Bacillus stearothermophilus* disc assay, especially late in lactation, and this naturally attracts the attention of regulatory officials (Hinckley 1991). Iron-binding protein (lactoferrin) in goat milk has been shown to be bacteriostatic for *B. stearothermophilus* (Oram and Reiter 1968). Both the bacteriostatic effect and the lactoferrin concentration are increased in dry secretion. Rancidity (lipolysis) is also increased in late lactation, and heat treatment does not affect bacterial inhibition due to fatty acids (Hinckley 1991; Atherton 1992). The *B. stearothermophilus* test may be inappropriate for goat milk (Klima 1980). The Delvotest P® culture medium version of the *B. stearothermophilus* assay has been shown to produce false positive results when compared with the disc assay (Zeng et al. 1996). The Penzyme® test for beta lactam residues has been reported to be sensitive and specific when used on goat milk containing penicillin or cephapirin (Zeng et al. 1996). Another study using eight different test kits and milk from clinically normal goats found all kits, including Penzyme®, to be suitable for screening goat milk when performed according to the manufacturer's directions because specificity was at least 0.99 (Contreras et al. 1997a).

Incubating bovine milk samples at warm temperatures, with resulting increase in bacterial numbers and decrease in pH levels, has been shown to cause inhibitory zones in disc assays. Some of these inhibitory zones, like those caused by antibiotics, persisted after raw milk had been heated to 180°F (82.2°C) for five minutes (Kosikowski 1963). Thus, improper handling of milk samples may contribute to false-positive residue test reactions.

Non-antibiotic inhibitors in milk may have an importance that transcends regulatory considerations. Residues of disinfectant in milk or iodine originating from excessive dietary levels may interfere with bacterial acidification necessary for cultured products (Le Jaouen 1987).

Supportive Therapy for Mastitis

Frequent stripping, which serves to remove both bacteria and toxins, is beneficial. Oxytocin (5 to 10 units) and hot compresses assist in achieving milk letdown from a painful gland. Infection or starvation of kids and spread to other does are potential risks if kids are left on the doe to aid in removal of secretions from the udder.

Anti-inflammatory agents such as intravenous or oral flunixin meglumine (1 mg/kg once or twice daily) or corticosteroids (dexamethasone 0.44 mg/kg single dose) are frequently administered to animals with signs of discomfort or toxemia. In an experimental intramammary *E. coli* challenge, goats treated with anti-inflammatory agents showed some improvement in clinical signs without any adverse effects on bacterial clearance (Anderson et al. 1991). In a clinical trial, intramuscular flunixin meglumine at approximately 2.5 mg/kg once daily for two treatments resulted in more rapid resolution of clinical signs compared with control goats receiving the same intramammary antibiotic but no anti-inflammatory drug (Mavrogianni et al. 2004). Phenylbutazone should be avoided in goats to be used for meat or milk and is explicitly forbidden in some countries. Intravenous fluids may be indicated in systemically ill animals. If the goat is still ambulatory, oral fluids, such as commercial electrolyte products, can be substituted and are less expensive. Systemic antibiotics are commonly administered when the mastitis is severe or chronic.

Treatment of Gangrenous Mastitis

When a reddish udder secretion is accompanied by blue discoloration and coolness of the udder skin, the severity of the mastitis warrants intensive therapy and, usually, a poor prognosis for return to function.

Medical Management. In the early stages, when the affected gland is warmer than normal and painful and the secretion is blood tinged, successful medical treatment has been reported. Even when signs of gangrene were unequivocal (i.e., coolness, pitting edema, loss of skin sensation, and a watery red secretion), complete recovery was reported in 91% of eighty-one goats in the Sudan (Abu-Samra et al. 1988). Oxytetracycline systemically (5 mg/kg intravenously) and intramammary (426 mg daily) for five days was used in the Sudanese study, but cephapirin also seems to be a rational choice. The secretion was drained with a sterile teat cannula. In addition, a diuretic (40 mg furosemide) daily for five days and topical treatment of the udder with an antiseptic cream were used.

Most authors do not claim such successful results with less intensive medical treatment. For instance, in a study from Cyprus in which 9% of 8,000 goats suffered from gangrenous mastitis, in no case was there complete recovery of the udder (Petris 1963).

Mastectomy. Surgical removal of one half or of the entire udder is sometimes performed.

- **Indications and reservations**. Amputation of the udder can be a life-saving procedure if the goat is very toxic with gangrenous mastitis. Udder amputation avoids the unhygienic and unpleasant process of sloughing of necrotic tissue (Abu-Samra et al. 1988). Another candidate for the surgery is the goat that has chronic abscesses in the udder and is in poor body condition; udder amputation may result in a return to good health (Cable et al. 2004).

  The reason for saving the goat's life should be discussed with the owner in advance. Is it a pet or a commercial animal? Salvaging an animal for later slaughter in societies where meat from sick animals is not consumed is justification for udder amputation and also for use of inexpensive surgery techniques. Salvaging the goat for continued breeding is hard to justify unless the mastitis was clearly the result of an injury and cannot be attributed to a decreased genetic resistance. In herds participating in a Swedish mastitis control program, goats with milk cultures that were positive for *Staphylococcus aureus* are slaughtered because of the poor prognosis for microbiologic cure and the danger to people consuming unpasteurized goat milk products. Therefore, mastitis has become relatively rare in these herds (Danielsson et al. 1980). Owners become more careful and goats are selected for genetic resistance.

- **Anesthesia.** A variety of anesthetic regimens have been used successfully. The choice depends on the previous experience of the veterinarian and the drugs and facilities available. In the United States, gas anesthesia or a ketamine/xylazine combination is commonly selected. Intravenous barbiturates and lumbosacral spinal anesthesia are other possibilities. These methods are discussed in detail in Chapter 17. Antibiotic therapy (penicillin or ceftiofur) should be begun before surgery commences and intravenous fluids should be administered during surgery.
- **Surgical techniques** (Otte 1958; Kerr and Wallace 1978; Matthews 1999; Anderson et al. 2002; Cable et al. 2004). The animal should be fasted for twenty-four hours before surgery if possible. The goat is placed in lateral recumbency with the upper hind limb pulled caudally or in dorsal recumbency, depending on whether one or both glands are to be removed. A clamp attached to the teat simplifies manipulation of the udder during surgery. After skin preparation, an elliptical incision is made around the base of the teat or udder, leaving as much skin as possible to provide for closure. Blunt dissection is used to separate the gland from the skin and, if only half is to be removed, from the median suspensory ligament. The supramammary lymph node (caudal and dorsal to the gland) should also be removed. Major vessels that need to be ligated include first the external pudendal artery at the inguinal ring (double ligate), and then the external pudendal vein, the subcutaneous abdominal vein, and the perineal vein (Figure 14.10). Dead space is closed with subcutaneous sutures and drains are placed if deemed necessary. A potential blood donor and equipment for obtaining a blood transfusion should be located before the surgery is undertaken.
- **Other alternatives to udder amputation.** Amputation of the teat under tranquilization and local anesthesia has been used in goats to improve drainage of purulent or gangrenous infections of the udder. The base of the teat is clamped and the teat is amputated in its proximal one-third, distal to the large vessels. Hemostasis is achieved with cautery or ligation after removing the clamp (Sasshofer et al. 1987).

In selected cases, when surgery is not an option, the gangrenous gland can be infused once with 60 ml of 5% to 10% formalin (normally used for fixation of pathological specimens). The formalin kills organisms and binds toxins produced by

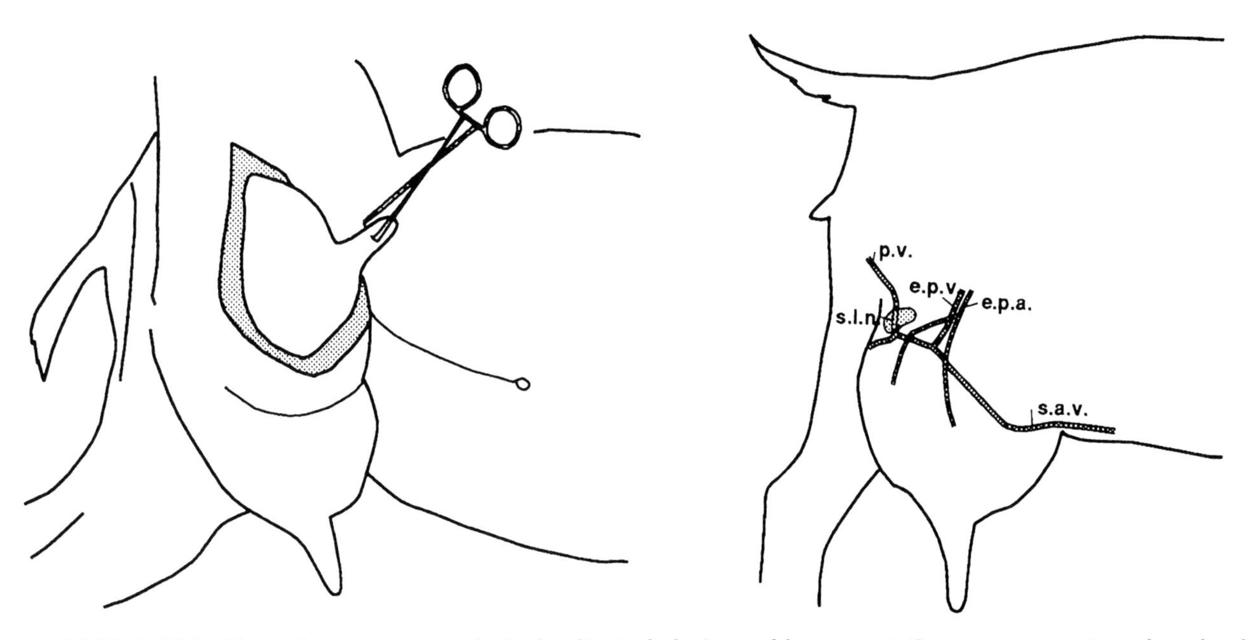

Figure 14.10. Initial skin incision and vessels to be ligated during udder amputation. e.p.a. = external pudendal (mammary) artery; e.p.v. = external pudendal vein; s.a.v. = subcutaneous abdominal vein; p.v. = perineal vein; s.l.n. = supramammary lymph node.

either the infectious agent or the necrosis of tissue. The gland thus treated does not return to production, but the doe's life may be preserved. In cattle, both 2% chlorhexidine and 5% povidone iodine have been used to cause cessation of lactation in chronically infected glands (Smith et al. 2005); a dose of 10 ml might be appropriate for goats.

Dry-off Procedures and Dry Period Therapy

Dairy goats are commonly allowed a two- to three-month nonlactating ("dry") period before the next parturition occurs. Provision of this rest period increases milk production in the next lactation. It also permits production of colostrum for protection of neonates; colostrum from goats with a fifty-six-day dry period had an IgG concentration of 42.4 mg/ml, as compared with 5.6 mg/ml in goats not given a dry period (Caja et al. 2006). It is possible to milk a goat daily for several years with reasonable milk yield if production of kids is not desired or the doe fails to conceive.

When does are milking heavily at the time of weaning or dry-off, it is helpful to restrict feed to a poor quality roughage and (if climate permits) to limit water for several days. During this time, animals should be kept clean and dry and observed for inordinate udder swelling. In commercial dairy herds, careful infusion of a dry period mastitis preparation is recommended. Udders that become severely distended should be milked out and retreated five to seven days later. It is very important to clearly mark the animal that has been dry treated, because it is likely to try to return to the milking group if it is put into a different pen, and antibiotic residues will follow.

In one survey, 76% of udder half infections caused by major pathogens (*Staph. aureus* or streptococci) and 55% of infections caused by coagulase-negative staphylococci persisted through the dry period to the next lactation (Lerondelle and Poutrel 1984). Infusions of an appropriate long-lasting dry cow preparation (one tube per half) at the time of drying off should increase the cure rate during the dry period while simultaneously preventing some new infections during this period. In one report, approximately two-thirds of infections were eliminated in goats receiving dry treatment (Plommet 1974). A study using a cattle cephapirin benzathine product found a 79% cure rate of infections, most of which were coagulase negative staphylococci (Fox et al. 1992). In a study from New Zealand, a dry treatment licensed for goats containing 300 mg procaine penicillin, 100 mg dihydrostreptomycin, and 100 mg of nafcillin resulted in a 92% cure rate, compared with 31% cure of untreated glands. *Staphylococcus aureus* did not respond as well as other organisms. At the same time, new infections were reduced from 9% to 2% (McDougall and Anniss 2005), although most authors have not shown an effect on new infections. A 66% to 78% cure rate was found in another study using the same antibiotics (Poutrel et al.1997) with no antibiotic residues detected seven days after parturition. Cloxacillin has also been shown to be efficacious (Paape et al. 2001). There are anecdotal reports of severe systemic reactions in goats treated with erythromycin dry cow preparations, so this drug should probably be avoided.

It has been suggested that herds with more than 30% or 40% subclinical mastitis should treat all goats at dry-off, while herds with lower infection rates should treat selectively those animals that are infected (Paape et al. 2001). In herds free of mycoplasma infection, two or more monthly cell counts greater than 2 million/ml have been shown to be indicative of *S. aureus* infection with a sensitivity of 100% and a specificity of 74%, thus aiding in the selection of goats to be dry treated (Baudry et al. 1999). Teat dipping before and after infusion and partial insertion of the tube are recommended.

Prevention of Bacterial Mastitis

Management decisions that decrease the risk of injury to the udder or teat (such as selecting for improved udder attachment) or that control skin lesions on the teats (including contagious ecthyma, staphylococcal infections, or warts; see Chapter 2) should decrease the risk of mastitis. Genetic aspects of udder conformation also affect risk of mastitis via ease of machine milking (Barillet 2007). Attention to sanitation, proper milking procedures, teat dipping, and dry period antibiotic therapy are also beneficial. Less is known regarding the value of nutritional adjustments or vaccination programs in preventing mastitis in goats.

Environmental Considerations. Dry, clean surroundings are especially important at freshening and at dry-off. When goats are housed and fed dry hay, the dry consistency of their fecal pellets combined with their tendency to bed themselves on wasted hay usually ensures acceptable conditions. Otherwise, slatted floors or elevated sleeping platforms may help to keep conditions sanitary. Teat end injuries predispose to mastitis and thus should be prevented as much as possible (Ameh and Tari 2000).

Milking Procedures. The method of udder preparation for milking is very important in determining the incidence of new cases of mastitis in goats, as it is in cows. For example, herds in which individual towels were used to wash and dry the udder had a decreased prevalence of intramammary infections compared with herds in which common towels were used (East et al. 1987). Hands and udders should be clean and dry. Disposable nitrile gloves are recommended. Goat udders are usually cleaner than cow udders. If washing is required, only the teats should be washed. It is better not to wash at all than to leave the udder and teats wet. Sanitizer solution for washing teats should be delivered from a hose or spray bottle, rather than from an open bucket. Animals with mastitis or with skin lesions on the teats should be milked last, with appropriate sanitation of hands between affected animals. Careful attention to unit placement to prevent liner slip and teat end impacts (causing reverse flow of milk into the udder) is important to prevent introduction of bacteria, mycoplasma, and the CAE virus into the gland during milking.

Goats should be milked gently and in quiet surroundings to encourage oxytocin release and milk letdown. The physiology of these events has been reviewed elsewhere (Martinet and Richard 1974). The biological half-life of oxytocin has been calculated to be approximately twenty-two minutes in goats (Homeida and Cooke 1984). The premilking stimulation afforded by udder washing is not necessary for goats to milk out completely. Research, then, has demonstrated no effect of udder washing on milking time or milk yield (Ricordeau and Labussière 1970). This is because the goat holds nearly 80% of its milk in the cistern rather than in the alveoli and means that the machine can be attached immediately if the teats are clean (Ohnstad 2006). The satisfied goat often ruminates while being milked. Vigorous stripping, by hand or machine, should be avoided. Overmilking of late lactation does may contribute to the risk of mastitis (East et al. 1987). Restraining goats during milking by pulling on the teats has been proposed as one reason for a high incidence of gangrenous staphylococcal mastitis in Cyprus (Petris 1963). When machine milking, it is important to use a vacuum cut-off valve before removing the teat cups, to avoid teat end impacts (Bergonier et al. 2003).

Milking should occur at regular times, but equal twelve-hour intervals are not necessary. The goat has a relatively large gland cistern for holding milk. One study found no difference in yield with milk intervals of 16:8 hours and 12:12 hours (Henderson et al. 1983). Yield is increased by milking three times a day. French workers have also investigated the effects of omitting the Sunday evening milking and have found a reduced milk yield of 4.5% if this practice is begun one month into the lactation, and only 1.2% if begun after five months. An increase in mastitis has not been noted, and on some farms the savings in labor costs more than offset the decrease in yield (Le Du 1987).

Preliminary research in France suggests that the speed of milking is under genetic control, with the goats homozygous for the recessive gene "hd" having the most rapid milk flow (Bouillon 1990). How this gene might affect the incidence of mastitis remains to be investigated.

Milking Parlor Design. A raised platform is the most basic equipment for milking goats, and most owners of small herds use individual milking stands. When herd size justifies construction of a parlor, several different designs are satisfactory and have been described (Le Du1987; Mottram et al. 1991). These include a side-by-side parlor with milking from behind, herringbone parlor with milking from the side, inverted herringbone with milking from the front, and tunnel parlor with milking from the side. To additionally increase throughput, the goats, stalls, and milking units can be mounted on a rotating platform.

Milking Machine Function. When a commercial goat dairy installs or modifies a machine milking system, attention should be given to choosing an efficient system that milks goats under low vacuum with minimal vacuum fluctuation. Low-line systems, in which the milk line is just below the edge of the pit or elevated milking platform, are generally preferred. Vacuum levels of 11.5 to 12 inches Hg are adequate for low-line systems, but higher vacuum is needed for high-line systems. Machines available for milking goats in France are operated at comparable vacuum levels (gauge pressures) of 30 to 38 cm Hg (Darracq 1974). Yet another vacuum unit in use in the literature is the Pascal, which equals 10 dyne/cm^2 or 7.5×10^{-3} mm Hg; a kPa equals 0.75 cm Hg.

The vacuum pump should have a capacity of 30 cubic feet per minute (CFM) (ASME standard) for the pipeline system, 1.5 CFM per unit, and 3 to 4 CFM reserve air flow. Bucket milker systems require 10 CFM reserve and 1 CFM per unit (East and Birnie 1983; Spencer 1984).

Pulsation rates of 70 to 100 per minute and pulsation ratios of 50:50 to 70:30 (milk: rest) have been recommended for goats (Le Du 1987). In a study that attempted to optimize milking rate and somatic cell counts, a pulsation ratio of 60:40, a pulsation rate of 90 per minute, and a vacuum level of 45 to 52 kPa were judged to be optimal (Lu et al. 1991). Another recommendation is for a vacuum of 37 to 38 kPa, a pulsation rate of 90 to 120 per minute, and a 50:50 pulsation ratio (Ohnstad 2006).

Inflations should be replaced before they become worn and cracked. Some authors propose changing inflations on the same schedule used for cows (every 1,000 to 1,500 milkings for molded liners) (East and Birnie 1983). In Europe, allowances are apparently made for the very short milking time (one to two minutes) per goat. One producers' guide from France recommends changing inflations twice a year (Cardoen and Delahaye 1977). Because liners tend to deteriorate with time, washing, and use, they should not be used for longer than sixty days.

Teat Dips. Although few studies have been conducted in goats, it is generally accepted that teat dipping or spraying with a properly mixed and uncontaminated solution is of economical benefit via prevention of bacterial mastitis (Plommet 1974; Bergonier et al. 2003; Contreras et al. 2007). One French study documented a 62% decrease in new infections in early lactation and a 41% decrease over the entire lactation when the right teat was dipped but the left teat was an undipped control (Baudry et al. 2000). Some studies have found a beneficial effect on somatic cell counts (Paape et al. 2001) while others have not (Poutrel et al. 1997). Products with evidence of efficacy for preventing mastitis in dairy cows (e.g., 0.5% iodine or 0.5% chlorhexidine) are commonly used. Nisin, a bacteriocin protein synthesized by the bacterium *Lactococcus lactis* subspecies *lactis* and long used as a food grade preservative in dairy products, has also been shown to be effective in goats (Paape et al. 2001). Recently concerns have been raised that use of teat dips increases selection for bacteria that are resistant to disinfectants, which might impact human health (Contreras et al. 2007).

In small herds, purchasing large quantities of teat dip at one time should be discouraged because settling of the product may occur and cause teat irritation. Even a newly purchased supply may cause problems because of past freezing or prolonged storage. When concentrates are used, they should be mixed with clean water; some pathogens such as *Pseudomonas* or even the common saprophyte *Serratia* can survive and even multiply in the teat dip (Van Damme 1982). Owners should also empty and sanitize the dipper after every milking. Hand pumps or aerosol sprays (e.g., chlorhexidine; Fightbac-SmithKline Animal Health Products, West Chester, Pennsylvania) help to avoid contamination of the teat dip, but the milker must take the time to ensure that the teat ends are adequately covered. Teat dipping for one week after dry off or before kidding probably is of no value.

Dry Period Therapy. Infusion of an antibiotic into the udder at time of dry-off, as discussed previously, helps to prevent new cases of mastitis in addition to curing some pre-existing infections.

Vaccination. Staphylococcal toxoid vaccinations have been used in herds experiencing clinical mastitis caused by *Staph. aureus* (Petris 1963; Lerondelle and Poutrel 1984). An adjuvanted cell-toxoid vaccine (formolized cells and toxoid adjuvanted with aluminum hydroxide gel) has been used in studies using goats as a model for cows (Derbyshire 1960). These vaccines do not lower the prevalence of infection but do decrease severity. In contrast, a polyvalent somatic antigen vaccine did not prevent mastitis or decrease severity of clinical signs (Lepper 1967). Field experiments with sheep vaccinated twice with oil adjuvanted alpha and beta staphylococcal toxoids demonstrated a reduced rate of clinical mastitis when compared with unvaccinated control sheep (Plommet and Bézard 1974). Recent studies on vaccination of goats for this organism or its toxins are lacking. An attempt to increase resistance by gene therapy, causing expression of lysostaphin in the goat udder, failed because of adverse immune reactions to the molecule (Fan et al. 2004).

Although *E. coli* mastitis is relatively rare in goats and vaccination as a substitute for hygiene is not justified, goats have been proposed as a model for coliform vaccination research in cattle. A J5 vaccine moderated the clinical signs and decreased shedding in the milk after experimental challenge (Aslam et al. 1995).

Nutrition. Although it seems reasonable that nutritional deficiencies should increase an animal's susceptibility to mastitis and other infectious diseases, few studies in goats are available. However, it has been shown that selenium deficiency is associated with reduced neutrophil function in goats (Aziz et al 1984; Aziz and Klesius 1986). Also, somatic cell count (by Fossomatic) was decreased and milk production increased in Finngoats with a high glutathione peroxidase activity when compared with goats with decreased selenium status judged by this enzyme's activity (Atroshi et al. 1985). This study did not include cultures of milk samples. In a selenium-deficient region in Spain, an injection of slow release barium selenate before mating to half of the goats in four herds was associated with a significant decrease in somatic cell counts and the incidence of clinical mastitis in the subsequent lactation of the supplemented goats. There were ten clinically affected goats out of 260 treated animals, compared with forty clinical mastitis cases in the 260 controls (Sánchez et al. 2007). Improved bactericidal activity of neutrophils in selenium-supplemented cows is believed to moderate the severity of *E. coli* mastitis in that species (Erskine et al. 1989). Vitamin E status is probably important for resistance to mastitis as well.

NONMASTITIC ALTERATIONS IN GOAT MILK

The presence of blood or unpleasant flavors in goat milk decreases the desirability of milk and cheese for human consumption. Decreased butterfat is another common but serious problem for commercial producers of fluid milk or cheese.

Bloody Milk

Sometimes goat milk is slightly pink or a red sediment collects on the bottom of the milk container in the refrigerator because of ruptured blood vessels in the udder. The skin over the udder is not cold or blue, and the goat is not systemically ill (in the absence of other disease conditions). The need to distinguish bloody milk from gangrenous mastitis often prompts performance of a milk culture. One author advises telling the owner to call for results in five days, because by then the blood has usually disappeared from the milk (Baxendell 1984a). The irrelevancy of a coagulase-negative staph species to the condition should be discussed in advance if the owner is to obtain maximum assurance from the culture test results.

If the goat has kidded recently, the possibility of hypocalcemia could be investigated. Some veterinarians administer vitamin K or other blood coagulant therapy. The results have not been compared with the self-cure rate. The environment should be examined for sources of trauma to the udder, including high door sills and rough milkers, be they hands, machines, or butting kids.

Off-flavored Milk

Off flavors or milk taint problems must be considered in relationship to the intended use for the goat milk. In Scandinavia, the aim is to produce certain cheeses with a characteristic "goaty" flavor. To achieve this flavor, producers may feed more dry hay or store the milk for as long as forty-two hours before processing into cheese. They also can use genetic selection, as the hereditability coefficient for goat flavor in Norwegian goats has been calculated to be 0.25 (Trodahl et al. 1981). In America or Australia, where a relatively larger proportion of the milk is consumed in the fluid form, goaty flavors are only tolerated by owners who have become so accustomed to the taste as not to notice it. Otherwise, good goat milk should taste like good cow milk. Some of the possible causes for undesirable flavors in milk from the entire herd or from individual goats are outlined in the box titled "Causes of Abnormal Flavors in Goat Milk."

Causes of Abnormal Flavors in Goat Milk

Herd Problem

a) *Hygiene:* Buckets should be chemically sanitized or scalded to avoid introduction of psychrophils that multiply in refrigerated milk. Stainless steel, glass, and enamel are preferred over other materials because of ease of cleaning. Clean, well-ventilated barns avoid inhalation of ammonia and other malodorous agents.

b) *Milk Handling Procedures:* Milk should be rapidly cooled and stored in covered containers in the refrigerator. Exposure of milk or cheese to copper or iron metal, sunlight, or fluorescent light results in oxidized flavors that are variously described as "cardboardy," "metallic," or "oily." Copper tubing should be avoided in the milkhouse, especially if water pH is less than 7.0. Airborne taints may be absorbed if the milk container is not properly sealed. Violent agitation of milk (as from air leaks in pipeline milkers) may rupture the lipid membrane around fat globules. Mixing warm raw milk with cold or pasteurized milk allows active lipase to attack damaged fat globules, which also leads to lipolysis and rancid flavors.

c) *Nutritional Considerations:*
   1) Cobalt deficiency: Expect a response within a few days after providing a mineral block containing cobalt or after injecting vitamin B_{12}.
   2) Vitamin B_{12} deficiency secondary to helminthiasis has been proposed as a frequent cause of tainted milk (Mews 1987).
   3) Vitamin E deficiency: Without vitamin E's antioxidant effects (e.g., winter feeding), oxidized flavors may develop. Based on recommendations for cattle of daily supplementation with 1,000 to 7,000 IU of vitamin E, feeding an additional 400 IU vitamin E/day/goat for one to two weeks could be tried (Ishler and Roberts 2002).
   4) Unsaturated fatty acids in milk are more susceptible to oxidation and may be limited by decreasing fat (full-fat soybeans, whole cottonseed, added fats) in the diet and by increasing the forage to concentrate ratio.
   5) Inadequate dietary protein may lead to weakened fat globule membranes and thus to rancidity (Ishler and Roberts 2002).
   6) Feed or weed flavors: Plants incriminated include silage, cabbage, turnip, fresh alfalfa, ragweed, goldenrod, honeysuckle, buttercups, blackberry, and grape leaves (Lovegrove 1990).
   7) Garlic preparations used for possible anthelmintic effect.
   8) Drugs such as anthelmintics that are secreted into milk.

d) *Buck Odor:* Housing the buck with the does usually has not caused flavor problems unless the milk is not properly handled.

Individual Goat Problem

a) *Genetic Flavor:* The reverse of the Scandinavian approach suggests selecting for does with a good flavor to their milk.

b) *Spontaneous Lipolysis:* Abnormal flavor develops under refrigeration.

c) *Ketosis.*

d) *Mastitis.*

e) *Feed Flavors:* Strong-flavored feeds should be fed after milking, not within the four hours preceding milking.

Table 14.2. Zoonotic diseases potentially transmitted by raw goat milk.

Causative agent secreted in milk	*Fecal contaminants in milk*
Brucellosis	Campylobacteriosis
Caseous lymphadenitis	Cryptosporidiosis
Cryptococcosis	*Escherichia coli*
Leptospirosis	Listeriosis
Listeriosis	Salmonellosis
Louping-ill	Yersiniosis
Melioidosis	
Q Fever	
Staphylococcal food poisoning	
Toxoplasmosis	
Tuberculosis	

Evaluating Off-flavored Milk

While investigating a milk flavor problem, the owner needs to determine if the flavor is present at milking or if it develops with storage. Is the milk tainted from one half (suggestive of mastitis) or from both halves of one goat? Is the milk from certain pairs of goats incompatible, such that mixing produces the problem? Are many goats involved? If the owner has not yet evaluated the flavor from each half of each goat separately, immediately after milking, the veterinarian should at least suggest pasteurization to avoid any danger of the zoonotic diseases listed in Table 14.2. If a single goat is involved and if mastitis can be ruled out, the goat can then be kept in a stall and fed only weed-free hay for several days. If the abnormal taste disappears, it was probably caused by feed. The goat is then introduced again to one feed at a time and then one pasture at a time until the source of the offending feed or weed is identified (Baxendell 1984c). See also an investigation scheme by Matthews (1999).

Milk Lipase and its Effects

Goat milk contains an intrinsic milk lipase (e.g., lipoprotein lipase, LPL) that is capable of causing enzymatic hydrolysis of milk fat and an increase in free fatty acid content of the milk. Approximately 46% of the lipoprotein lipase is to be found in the cream portion of goat milk. The enzyme is responsible for both "spontaneous lipolysis" (initiated by cooling fresh milk) and "induced lipolysis" (initiated by mechanical or thermal treatment of milk). The LPL activity is correlated with the degree of spontaneous lipolysis that occurs in the milk sample, with an r-value ranging from 0.65 to 0.80 (Chilliard et al. 1984).

There are great differences between goats in LPL activities and in milk lipolysis. In one study (Chilliard et al. 1984), the most susceptible sample released twenty-six times more free fatty acids in twenty-four hours than did the least active sample. In France, the level of lipolysis is approximately four times greater in milk collected during the summer months (midlactation) than in the winter (LeMens 1987). Evening goat milk has relatively more LPL than morning milk. Other activators and inhibitors that might be involved in the process have not yet been identified. Dairy processing plants can determine acid degree values (ADV) as an objective determination of rancidity. At least for cow milk, a soapy-bitter rancid flavor is expected if the ADV is more than 1.0 (Ishler and Roberts 2002).

When an individual goat's milk is subject to spontaneous lipolysis, the milk initially tastes normal but deteriorates rapidly with storage in the refrigerator. The problem can be controlled by heating the milk to 135°F (57°C) immediately after collection to partially inactivate the enzyme. This process is called heat treatment to avoid upsetting owners who have a strong aversion to anything suggestive of pasteurization. Unless the milk will be made into an aged cheese (more than sixty days), pasteurization is still advised. Pasteurization, and even boiling, do not completely inactivate lipase in goat milk (Jandal 1995).

Low Butterfat

The normal butterfat concentration of most European dairy goat breeds under temperate conditions is approximately 3.8%, whereas Nubians and Pygmy goats traditionally give a richer milk (Jenness 1980; Haenlein and Caccese 1984). Goat milk fat is higher in medium chain triglycerides than that of cow milk (Sanz Sampelayo et al. 2007). The same authors review the effects of diet on the fatty acid profile of goat milk. Genetic selection for high volume secretion of milk without consideration of solids composition gradually causes decreased butterfat concentrations. As butterfat levels decrease, there is a decrease in cheese yield. Also, the milk may no longer achieve legal standards for marketing.

Dietary Roughage versus Concentrates and Dietary Fat

One of the most common causes of low butterfat is a ratio of dietary concentrates to roughages of more than 2:1. This typically occurs in herds striving for increased milk production. A concentrate mixture that contains more than 35% heat-treated starchy grains such as corn, milo, and barley has also been incriminated (Adams 1986). Normal milk fat production requires maintaining cellulose-digesting, acetate-producing microbes in the rumen. Rapid digestion of concentrates and decreased saliva flow result in a decrease in rumen pH to a level unfavorable for the bacteria producing acetate. In general, dietary concentrates do not have a detrimental effect on butterfat if limited to 50% or less of the total diet (Morand-Fehr et al. 2000).

How the concentrates are distributed to the goat also affects rumen acidosis and butterfat production. Thus, roughage should be fed before grain in the morning. Dividing the concentrate portion of the diet into more than two meals per day is also helpful. Long alfalfa hay supports higher butterfat concentration than a chopped dehydrated product (Morand-Fehr et al. 1999). Additional discussion is provided in Chapter 19.

Excessive dietary fat can decrease butterfat production by coating rumen fiber and interfering with its digestion. However, rumen protected fats at up to 8% of the diet increase butterfat without detrimental effects on milk protein production (Morand-Fehr et al. 2000). Contrary to what occurs in cows, supplementation of the goat's diet with vegetable oils rich in polyunsaturated fatty acids does not decrease butterfat production (Sanz Sampelayo et al. 2007).

Use of Buffers

Roughage is more effective than sodium bicarbonate in elevating ruminal pH and acetate molar fraction (Hadjipanayiotou 1982). However, supplementing a low roughage diet with $NaHCO_3$ (at 4% of the concentrates) significantly increases milk fat production. The improvement is noticeable two to three weeks after incorporating the buffer into the diet (Hadjipanayiotou 1988). Supplementing the low fiber diet with bicarbonate at 1% to 1.5% of total dry matter intake tends to increase butterfat and adding probiotics may also be beneficial (Morand-Fehr et al. 2000).

Environmental Temperature

High environmental temperatures contribute to low butterfat through their effect on roughage consumption (Devendra 1982). The heat-stressed goat eats less roughage or preferentially selects the more digestible portions of the roughage available. This decreases the heat of digestion liberated in the rumen but also decreases acetate production, and thereby butterfat synthesis. Providing good ventilation, plentiful water, and multiple smaller meals helps to alleviate the effects of environmental temperature.

Other Techniques for Increasing Butterfat

Feeding larger quantities of dried brewer's grains has resulted in increased butterfat production (Sauvant et al. 1987). More complete milk out also increases the butterfat percentage (Morand-Fehr et al. 1999).

When all else has failed, or often long before appropriate changes in management have been made, a producer may purchase several Nubian goats to raise the herd butterfat concentration to exceed the minimum legal limit in the state or country.

RAW MILK AND OTHER SAFETY ISSUES

Few topics elicit such heated discussion among goat owners as the raw versus pasteurized milk controversy. People who have drunk raw milk all their lives or whose babies returned to good health after being switched from cow to goat milk find it hard to believe that such a "natural" food should be anything but healthful. People who have for centuries prepared certain types of cheeses from raw milk complain that the result is not the same if pasteurized milk is used. Also, pasteurization destroys the stability and keeping qualities of milk, which is critical where refrigeration is not available.

Zoonotic Diseases

Many industrialized countries have regulations requiring pasteurization of milk to be sold unless very stringent sanitary requirements are adhered to. These laws were generally formulated in an attempt to prevent human infection with brucellosis or tuberculosis. In regions where those two diseases have been eradicated, the laws seem, to the layman, quite antiquated. In the meantime, however, an ever-growing number of additional infectious agents have been isolated from goat milk (Pritchard 1987; Klinger and Rosenthal 1997). These are listed in Table 14.2.

Supporting references for acquiring these conditions from goat milk products include: brucellosis (Stiles 1950; Renoux 1957; Young and Suvannoparrat 1975; Wallach et al. 1994; Vogt and Hasler 1999; Wyatt 2005; Gupta et al. 2006), caseous lymphadenitis (Goldberger et al. 1981; Schreuder et al. 1990), listeriosis (Løken et al. 1982; Tham 1988; Azadian et al. 1989; Eilertz et al. 1993; Abou Eleinin et al. 2000), louping-ill (Reid et al. 1984) and other tick-borne encephalitis diseases (Heinz and Kunz 2004), melioidosis (Olds and Lewis 1954), Q fever (Caminopetros 1948a, 1948b; Ruppaner et al. 1978; Fishbein and Raoult 1992; Hatchette et al. 2001; Berri et al. 2005), staphylococcal food poisoning (Geringer 1983; Gross et al. 1988; Hahn et al. 1992), *Streptococcus zooepidemicus* (Kuusi et al. 2006), toxoplasmosis (Riemann et al. 1975; Sacks et al. 1982; Chiari and Neves 1985; Skinner et al. 1990), campylobacteriosis (Jackson 1985; Jelley 1985; Harris et al. 1987), *E. coli* (McIntyre et al. 2002), salmonellosis (Jensen and Hughes 1980; Galbraith et al. 1982; Desenclos 1996), and yersiniosis (Hughes and Jensen 1981; Walker and Gilmour 1986).

Many of these diseases are not serious in immunecompetent, healthy people. Chronically ill babies, old people, pregnant women, people receiving cancer therapy, and those infected with the AIDS (acquired immune deficiency syndrome) virus are less able to withstand infection with these agents. Goat owners wishing to avoid legal or moral responsibility for illness in their milk-drinking customers should continue to pasteurize or at the very least explain the need for and method of pasteurization of the milk they sell. The American Veterinary Medical Association has taken a stand against the use of raw milk (Summers and New 1985).

In the UK, 47% of one hundred samples of raw goat milk offered for sale did not meet the regulatory dairy product standards (Little and de Louvois 1999). When raw milk is to be used for cheese production, standard coliform screening detects lapses in proper milk hygiene and thus an increased likelihood of potentially dangerous fecal contaminants.

Home Pasteurization

Several types of commercial home pasteurizers are available to simplify making goat milk safe for human consumption. They are also very convenient for implementing programs to control milk-borne diseases of goats such as CAE and mycoplasmosis. A variety of time and temperature combinations are suitable for controlling zoonotic agents. These include heating the milk to 145°F (63°C) for thirty minutes or 161°F (72°C) for fifteen seconds. For home pasteurization, longer times are often recommended to ensure that all of the milk reaches the desired temperature (e.g., 150°F to 155°F [65.5°C to 68.3°C] for thirty minutes, 165°F to 170°F [73.8°C to 76.6°C] for thirty seconds) (Vasavada 1986). The pasteurized milk must then be cooled rapidly and transferred carefully to a sterile container for storage in the refrigerator. Post-pasteurization contamination of milk is a very real risk, both in the home and in the large scale dairy plant.

When a pasteurizer is not available, the milk can be treated in a similar way in a double boiler or in glass jars placed in a heated water bath. A cooking thermometer and frequent stirring and heat adjustment are necessary. Alternatively, once the milk has been heated to the desired temperature, it can be poured into a thermos that was preheated with boiling water. The milk must be checked at the end of the holding period to verify that it remained at or above the target temperature. Finally, although testing with *Listeria* and *Coxiella* has not been performed, the home microwave oven has been shown capable of greatly reducing bacterial counts and increasing shelf life of goat milk. Heating to 149°F (65°C) for thirty minutes is recommended, using a temperature probe with "temperature hold" feature (Thompson and Thompson 1990).

Alkaline phosphatase activity is reported to be low in goat milk relative to cow milk, and the activity in sheep milk is ten to twenty times higher than in goat milk (Raynal-Ljutovac et al. 2007). Bovine standards for phosphatase activity as evidence of proper pasteurization may not be applicable to goat milk (Klinger and Rosenthal 1997; Vamvakaki et al. 2006) and psychrotrophic bacteria multiplying in the refrigerator may produce alkaline phosphatase resistant to destruction by proper pasteurization (Raynal-Ljutovac et al. 2007).

Toxins Excreted in Milk

The possible presence of toxins of feed or iatrogenic origin is not limited to raw milk or necessarily affected by pasteurization. However, home produced goat milk is more likely than commercially marketed milk to cause human illness because the protective effects of toxin dilution by admixture with normal milk are often lost. It should be noted that pasteurization does not destroy preformed staphylococcal enterotoxins, which may be present in the milk of goats with either *Staphylococcus aureus* or coagulase negative staphyloccal infections (Valle et al. 1990). The potential for contamination of milk by natural plant toxins has been reviewed (Panter and James 1990). Numerous other chemicals, including pesticides, have the potential to be excreted in milk and are unlikely to be affected by pasteurization. Research performed with cattle should be largely applicable to goat milk. Neonates, because of incompletely developed detoxification pathways, may be especially susceptible.

Pyrrolizidine Alkaloids

Plants of the genera *Senecio*, *Crotalaria*, *Heliotropium*, *Echium*, *Amsinckia*, *Symphytum*, *Cynoglossum*, and *Festuca* contain pyrrolizidine alkaloids that cause hepatotoxic and veno-occlusive disease and may be carcinogenic. These toxins may be excreted in goat milk (Dickinson and King 1978; Deinzer et al. 1982; Goeger et al. 1982). Of special concern is *Symphytum* (comfrey), because some goat owners intentionally feed this plant to their livestock.

Tremetol

Ageratina altissima (white snakeroot, synonym *Eupatorium rugosum*) and *Haplopappus* (*Aplopappus*) sp. (rayless goldenrod, synonym *Isocoma wrightii* [McGinty 1987]) both contain tremetol, a higher alcohol that is excreted in milk and not destroyed by pasteurization. A syndrome called milk sickness (weakness, prostration, nausea) occurs in people ingesting milk from animals grazing the plants. Goat kids may also develop muscular tremors and recumbency from consuming the toxin in milk.

Other Plant Toxins and Mycotoxins

There is a single report of skeletal abnormalities and red cell aplasia in a child in California whose mother drank goat milk from goats grazing lupine (*Lupinus latifolius*) (Ortega and Lazerson 1987). Puppies from a dog fed the same goat milk were also malformed, as were several aborted goat kids. Quinolizidine alkaloids such as anagyrine were thought to be responsible for this outbreak, which resembled crooked calf disease. Anagyrine appeared in the milk of a goat experimentally fed lupine seeds (Kilgore et al. 1981).

Milk collected from cows and ewes consuming *Astragalus lentiginosus* contains a toxin (probably swainsonine) that causes foamy cytoplasmic vacuolation when the milk is fed to the animals (James and Hartley 1977). Swainsonine inhibits α-mannosidase, causing a lysosomal storage disease.

At least of theoretic concern is the occurrence of carcinogenic, toxic, and mutagenic compounds (ptaquiloside) in the milk of cows grazing bracken fern (*Pteridium aquilinum*) (Hopkins 1990). Also of note is the goitrogenic effect of milk from goats fed goitrogenic plants (White and Cheeke 1983). Thiocyanate has been shown to transfer from dams administered potassium cyanide (KCN) daily to suckling kids via the milk (Soto-Blanco and Górniak 2004).

Aflatoxins, and especially aflatoxin M1, are excreted in the milk of dairy cows consuming moldy feeds (Osweiler et al. 1985). The potential for contamination of goat milk should not be ignored, because this has been demonstrated experimentally (Smith et al. 1994). Aflatoxin-producing fungi can also contaminate cheese.

Antibiotics and Anthelmintics

Antibiotic contamination from intramammary or systemic medication of the goat or from consumption of "medicated" feeds may lead to allergic reactions in sensitive people, interference with cultured products, or regulatory action against the producer. As noted before, the commonly used *B. stearothermophilus* assay may be inappropriate for goat milk. Because withdrawal periods have rarely been established for goat milk, especially for sick animals, veterinarians should advise exaggerated withdrawals (longer than for dairy cattle) to allow for different rates of metabolism or excretion. If goats kid less than two months after receiving a dry period intramammary treatment, a withdrawal of fourteen days has been recommended (Bergonier et al. 2003). Toxic parasiticides that have not been approved for dairy cows should not be used for dairy goats either.

Thiabendazole has antifungal properties that inhibit *Penicillium* while enhancing several undesirable mold species. Thus, thiabendazole at 200 mg/kg clearly interfered with proper curing of goat cheese while 50 or 100 mg/kg sometimes did so, especially in milk from animals with low production (Toussaint et al. 1976). By contrast, pyrantel (25 mg/kg), morantel (10 mg/kg), or double these doses did not perturb the fabrication, appearance, or taste of the cheese. In another study, a taste panel detected a decrease in quality of a soft cheese made from milk of goats treated with netobimin (20 mg/kg twelve hours before) or albendazole (8 mg/kg twenty-four hours before). Morantel tartrate (10 mg/kg), pyrantel tartrate (20 mg/kg), oxfendazole (5 mg/kg), and diamfenetide (240 mg/kg) had no effect, while the deleterious effect of tetramisole (12 mg/kg twenty-four hours before) was judged to be not significant (Cabaret et al. 1987). Even if the chemical cannot be tasted in the finished product and the consumer is not allergic, the sale of milk or cheese containing these compounds is illegal.

REFERENCES

Abou Eleinin, A.A.M., et al.: Incidence and seasonal variation of *Listeria* species in bulk tank goat's milk. J. Food Prot., 63:1208–1213, 2000.

Abu-Samra, M.T., et al.: Studies on gangrenous mastitis in goats. Cornell Vet., 78:281–300, 1988.

Adams, R.S.: Dietary management in goats. In: Current Veterinary Therapy Food Animal Practice 2. J.L. Howard, ed. Philadelphia, W.B. Saunders Co., pp. 266–271, 1986.

Addo, P.B.: Chronic caprine mastitis: clinical, microbiological and pathological findings in spontaneously occurring cases in Nigerian goats. Int. Goat Sheep Res., 2:266–273, 1984.

Addo, P.B., Chineme, C.N. and Eid, F.I.A.: Incidence and importance of chronic mastitis in Nigerian goats. Bull. Anim. Health Prod. Afr., 28:225–231, 1980.

Adinarayanan, N. and Singh, S.B.: Caprine mastitis due to *Klebsiella pneumoniae*. Indian Vet. J., 45:373–377, 1968.

Adler, H.E., DaMassa, A.J. and Brooks, D.L.: Caprine mycoplasmosis: *Mycoplasma putrefaciens*, a new cause of mastitis in goats. Am. J. Vet. Res., 41:1677–1681, 1980.

Al-Ani, F.K. and Vestweber, J.G.E.: Udder edema in goats. Dairy Goat J., 61:1126–1127, 1983.

Al-Ani, F.K. and Vestweber, J.G.E.: Udder edema: an updated review. Vet. Bull., 56:763–769, 1986.

Aljaburi, A.M.I. and Kalra, D.S.: Cryptococcal mastitis in a goat—a case report. Haryana Vet., 22:120–121, 1983. Abstract 5620, Vet. Bull., 55:690, 1985.

Ameh, J.A. and Tari, I.S.: Observations on the prevalence of caprine mastitis in relation to predisposing factors in Maiduguri. Small Rumin. Res., 35:1–5, 2000.

Ameh, J.A., et al.: Gangrenous caprine coliform mastitis. Small Rumin. Res., 13:307–309, 1994.

Anderson, D.E., Hull, B.L. and Pugh, D.G.: Diseases of the mammary gland. In: Sheep and Goat Medicine. D.G. Pugh, ed. Philadelphia, W.B. Saunders, pp. 341–358, 2002.

Anderson, K.L., Hunt, E. and Davis, B.J.: The influence of anti-inflammatory therapy on bacterial clearance following intramammary *Escherichia coli* challenge in goats. Vet. Res. Commun., 15:147–161, 1991.

Andreasen, C.B., Huber, M.J. and Mattoon, J.S.: Unilateral fibroepithelial hyperplasia of the mammary gland in a goat. J. Am. Vet. Med. Assoc., 202:1279–1280, 1993.

Arisoy, F.: Large scale field trials on sheep and goats using living and dead agalactia vaccines in Turkey. In: Symposium sur la Traite Mécanique des Petits Ruminants. Millau, pp. 113–115, 1973.

Aslam, M., Whitemore, H.L. and Kakoma, I.: Effect of *E. coli* J5 vaccine and intramammary challenge with live *Escherichia coli* in lactating dairy goats. Small Rumin. Res., 17:275–281, 1995.

Atherton, H.V.: Using somatic cells and antibiotic tests for determining the quality of goat milk. Proceedings, National Symposium on Dairy Goat Production and Marketing, Oklahoma City, U.S., pp. 128–135, 1992.

Atroshi, F., Sankari, S. and Lindström, U.B.: Glutathione peroxidase activity in dairy goat erythrocytes in relation to somatic cell counts and milk production. Arch. Exp. Veterinärmed., 39:520–524, 1985.

AVMA, American Veterinary Medical Association: Unacceptable surgical procedures applicable to domestic animals. J. Am. Vet. Med. Assoc., 168:947–953, 1976.

Azadian, B.S., Finnerty, G.T. and Pearson, A.D.: Cheeseborne *Listeria* meningitis in immunocompetent patient. Lancet, 1(8633):322–323, 1989.

Aziz, E. and Klesius, P.H.: Effect of selenium deficiency on caprine polymorphonuclear leukocyte production of leukotriene B4 and its neutrophil chemotactic activity. Am. J. Vet. Res., 47:426–428, 1986.

Aziz, E.S., Klesius, P.H. and Frandsen, J.C.: Effects of selenium on polymorphonuclear leukocyte function in goats. Am. J. Vet. Res., 45:1715–1718, 1984.

Bagadi, H.O. and Razig, S.E.: Caprine mastitis caused by *Pasteurella mastitidis* (*P. haemolytica*). Vet. Rec., 99:13, 1976.

Balasurbramanian, S., Thilagar, S. and Rameshkumar, B.: Four functional mammary glands in a goat. Vet. Rec., 135:532, 1994.

Bar-Moshe, B. and Rapapport, E.: A contagious agalactia-like disease in goats caused by *Mycoplasma mycoides* subsp *mycoides* (ovine/caprine) serogroup 8. Refuah Vet., 35:75–77, 1978.

Bar-Moshe, B. and Rapapport, E.: Observations on *Mycoplasma mycoides* subsp. *mycoides* infection in Saanen goats. Isr. J. Med. Sci., 17:537–539, 1981.

Barillet, F.: Genetic improvement for dairy production in sheep and goats. Small Rumin. Res., 70:60–75, 2007.

Bassam, L.S. and Hasso, S.A.: Mastitis in goats caused by *Nocardia asteroides*. Small Rumin. Res., 26:287–290, 1997.

Baudry, C., et al.: Utilisation des numérations cellulaires individuelles pour la détection des infections mammaires subcliniques de la chèvre: définition de seuils. In: Milking and Milk Production of Dairy Sheep and Goats. EAAP Publication no. 95. Wageningen Pers, Wageningen, pp. 119–123, 1999.

Baudry, C., et al.: Evaluation of postmilking efficacy in goat. Rev. Méd. Vét., 151:1035–1040, 2000.

Baxendell, S.A.: Caprine udder conditions. In: Refresher Course for Veterinarians, Proceedings No. 73, Goats, The University of Sydney, The Post-Graduate Committee in Veterinary Science, Sydney, N.S.W., Australia, pp. 241–246, 1984a.

Baxendell, S.A.: Other udder conditions of goats. In: Refresher Course for Veterinarians, Proceedings No. 73, Goats. The University of Sydney, The Post-Graduate Committee in Veterinary Science, Sydney, N.S.W., Australia, pp. 484–489, 1984b.

Baxendell, S.A.: Goat milk taints. In: Refresher Course for Veterinarians, Proceedings No. 73, Goats, The University of Sydney, The Post-Graduate Committee in Veterinary Science, Sydney, N.S.W., Australia, pp. 493–494, 1984c.

Bergonier, D, and Poumarat, F.: Agalactie contagieuse des petits ruminants: épidémiologie, diagnostic et contrôle. Rev. Sci. Tech. Off. Int. Epiz., 15:1431–1475, 1996.

Bergonier, D., et al.: Mastitis of dairy small ruminants. Vet. Res., 34:689–716, 2003.

Berri, M., et al.: Progression of Q fever and *Coxiella burnetii* shedding in milk after an outbreak of enzootic abortion in a goat herd. Vet. Rec., 156:548–549, 2005.

Berry, E. and Broughan, J.: Use of the DeLaval cell counter (DCC) on goats' milk. J. Dairy Res., 74:345–358, 2007.

Bhat, P.P.: Inheritance of external traits in Barbari goats. Indian J. Anim. Sci., 58:448–455, 1988.

Bliss, E.L.: *Tinea versicolor* dermatomycosis in the goat. J. Am. Vet. Med. Assoc., 184:1512–1513, 1984.

Boscos, C., et al.: Prevalence of subclinical mastitis and influence of breed, parity, stage of lactation and mammary bacteriological status on Coulter Counter Counts and California Mastitis Test in the milk of Saanen and autochthonous Greek goats. Small Rumin. Res., 21:139–147, 1996.

Bouillon, J.: Rapidité de traite: un critère de sélection à prendre en compte? La Chèvre 180:16–18, 1990.

Bourry, A., Cochard, T. and Poutrel, B.: Serological diagnosis of bovine, caprine, and ovine mastitis caused by *Listeria monocytogenes* by using an enzyme-linked immunosorbent assay. J. Clin. Microbiol., 35:1606–1608, 1997.

Brooks, D.L., DaMassa, A.J. and Adler, H.E.: Caprine mycoplasmosis: Immune response in goats to *Mycoplasma putrefaciens* after intramammary inoculation. Am. J. Vet. Res., 42:1898–1900, 1981.

Burrell, D.H.: Caseous lymphadenitis in goats. Aust. Vet. J., 57:105–110, 1981.

Burriel, A.R. and Scott, M.: A comparison of methods used in species identification of coagulase-negative staphylococci isolated from the milk of sheep. Vet. J., 155:183–188, 1998.

Buswell, J.F., Knight, C.H. and Barber, D.M.L.: Antibiotic persistence and tolerance in the lactating goat following intramammary therapy. Vet. Rec., 125:301–303, 1989.

Cabaret, J., Devillard, J.P. and Richard, S.: Traitements anthelminthiques et qualité des fromages de chèvres fermiers. (Anthelmintic treatments and the quality of farm goat cheese.) Bull. Group. Tech. Vét., 4:88–90, 1987.

Cable, C.S., Peery, K. and Fubini, S.L.: Radical mastectomy in 20 ruminants. Vet. Surg., 33:263–266, 2004.

Caminopetros, J.P.: La "Q" fever en Grèce: le lait source de l'infection pour l'homme et les animaux. Ann. Parasitol. Hum. Comp., 23:107–118, 1948a.

Caminopetros, J.P.: Q fever, a respiratory human epidemic disease in the Mediterranean area, determined a milk-borne infection from goats and sheep. Fourth International Congress on Tropical Medicine and Malaria, Washington D.C., Dept. of State, 1948b, pp. 441–449.

Cammuso, C., et al.: Hormonal induced lactation in transgenic goats. Anim. Biotechnol., 11:1–17, 2000.

Campbell, A.: How to handle precocious milkers. Dairy Goat J., 39(5):5, 1961.
Cappucci, D.T., et al.: Caprine mastitis associated with *Yersinia pseudotuberculosis*. J. Am. Vet. Med. Assoc., 173:1589–1590, 1978.
Cardoen, J.-M. and Delahaye, J.: Comment lutter contre les mammites de la chèvre. Paris, SPEOC, 1977.
Caja, G., Salama, A.A.K. and Such, X.: Omitting the dry-off period negatively affects colostrum and milk yield in dairy goats. J. Dairy Sci., 89:4220–4228, 2006.
Chiari, c. de A. and Neves, D.P.: (Human toxoplasmosis acquired through drinking goats milk.) Mem. Inst. Oswaldo Cruz 79:337–340, 1984. Abstract 2881, Vet. Bull. 55:355, 1985.
Chilliard, Y., et al.: Characteristics of lipolytic system in goat milk. J. Dairy Sci., 67:2216–2223, 1984.
Coleshaw, P.: Teat biting in goats. Goat Vet. Soc. J., 20:8, 2004.
Considine, H. and Trimberger, G.W.: Dairy Goat Judging Techniques. Scottsdale, Arizona, Dairy Goat Journal Publishing Corp., 1978.
Constantinescu, G.M.: Guide to Regional Ruminant Anatomy Based on the Dissection of the Goat. Ames, IA, Iowa State Univ. Press, 2001.
Contreras, A., Paape, M.J. and Miller, R.H.: Prevalence of subclinical intramammary infection caused by *Staphylococcus epidermidis* in a commercial dairy goat herd. Small Rumin. Res., 31:203–208, 1999.
Contreras, A., et al.: Physiological threshold of somatic cell count and California Mastitis Test for diagnosis of caprine subclinical mastitis. Small Rumin. Res., 21:259–264, 1996.
Contreras, A., et al.: Evaluation of selected antibiotic residue screening tests for milk from individual goats. J. Dairy Sci., 80:1113–1118, 1997a.
Contreras, A., et al.: Persistence of subclinical intramammary pathogens in goats throughout lactation. J. Dairy Sci., 80:2815–2819, 1997b.
Contreras, A., et al.: The role of intramammary pathogens in dairy goats. Livestock Prod. Sci., 79:273–283, 2003.
Contreras, A., et al.: Mastitis in small ruminants. Small Rumin. Res., 68:145–153, 2007.
Cooke, M.M. and Merrall, M.: Mammary adenocarcinoma and granulosa cell tumour in an aged Toggenberg goat. N. Z. Vet. J., 40:31–33, 1992.
Cork, L.C. and Narayan, O.: The pathogenesis of viral leukoencephalomyelitis-arthritis of goats. I. Persistent viral infection with progressive pathologic changes. Lab. Invest., 42:596–602, 1980.
Corrales, J.C., et al.: Effect of clinical contagious agalactia on the bulk tank milk somatic cell count in Murcia-Granada goat herds. J. Dairy Sci., 87:3165–3171, 2004.
Corrales, J.C., et al.: Contagious agalactia in small ruminants. Small Rumin. Res., 68:154–166, 2007.
Craigmill, A.L., et al.: Pathological changes in the mammary gland and biochemical changes in milk of the goat following oral dosage with leaf of the avocado (*Persea americana*). Aust. Vet. J., 66:206–211, 1989.
Craigmill, A.L., et al.: Toxicity of avocado (*Persea americana* (Guatemalan var)) leaves: review and preliminary report. Vet. Hum. Toxicol., 26:381–383, 1984.
Craigmill, A.L., et al.: The toxicity of avocado (*Persea americana*) leaves for the lactating mammary gland of the goat. In: Poisonous Plants, Proceedings of the Third International Symposium. L.F. James et al., eds. Ames, IA, Iowa State Univ. Press, pp. 623–625, 1992.
Cunningham, O.C.: Milk goat improvement. Agricultural Experiment Station of the New Mexico College of Agriculture and Mechanic Arts, Annual Report 43:55, 1931–1932.
Cutlip, R.C., et al.: Mastitis associated with ovine progressive pneumonia virus infection in sheep. Am. J. Vet. Res., 46:326–328, 1985.
Dafaalla, E.N. and Gharib, H.M.: A study of mastitis in a goat caused by *Nocardia asteroides*. Br. Vet. J., 114:143–145, 1958.
Dairy Practices Council: Guidelines for the design, installation, and cleaning of small ruminant milking systems. Publication DPC 70, Barre, VT, 29 pp. 2000.
DaMassa, A.J.: Recovery of *Mycoplasma agalactiae* from mastitic goat milk. J. Am. Vet. Med. Assoc., 183:548–549, 1983.
DaMassa, A.J., Brooks, D.L. and Adler, H.E.: Caprine mycoplasmosis: widespread infection in goats with *Mycoplasma mycoides* subsp *mycoides* (large-colony type). Am. J. Vet. Res., 44:322–325, 1983.
DaMassa, A.J., et al.: Caprine mycoplasmosis: An outbreak of mastitis and arthritis requiring destruction of 700 goats. Vet. Rec., 120:409–413, 1987.
DaMassa, A.J., Wakenell, P.S. and Brooks, D.L.: Mycoplasmas of goats and sheep. J. Vet. Diagn. Invest., 4:101–113, 1992.
Danielsson, M.-L., Hammarberg, K.-H. and Wittander, G.: Getostens bakteriologi och hygien. Vår Föda 32 Suppl. 3, 1980.
Darracq, J.: Caractéristiques des machines à traire les chèvres et les brebis et leur contrôle dans les fermes. In: Symposium sur la Traite Mécanique des Petits Ruminants. Millau, 1973, INRA, pp. 217–220, 1974.
Das, M. and Singh, M.: Variation in blood leukocytes, somatic cell count, yield and composition of milk of crossbred goats. Small Rumin. Res., 35:169–174, 2000.
Davidson, I., et al.: Use of an ELISA test for *Mycoplasma agalactiae* and M. *mycoides* var *mycoides* (LC) to detect mycoplasma-infected goats under field conditions. Fourth International. Symp. Machine Milking Small Ruminants. Israel, p. 523, 1989.
Davies, A.A.: Generalized tuberculosis in a goat. J. Am. Vet. Med. Assoc., 110:322, 1947.
Deinzer, M.L., et al.: Gas chromatographic determination of pyrrolizidine alkaloids in goat milk. Anal. Chem., 54:1811–1814, 1982.
Delouis, C.: Induction hormonale de la lactation chez la chèvre. 1ieres Journées de la Recherche Ovine et Caprine. Tome 1: Espèce Caprine. Paris, I.N.R.A., pp. 64–72, 1975.
Derbyshire, J.B.: The experimental production of staphylococcal mastitis in the goat. J. Comp. Pathol., 68:232–241, 1958a.
Derbyshire, J.B.: The pathology of experimental staphylococcal mastitis in the goat. J. Comp. Pathol., 68:449–454 and plates, 1958b.
Derbyshire, J.B.: Studies in immunity to experimental staphylococcal mastitis in the goat and cow. J. Comp. Pathol., 70:222–231, 1960.

Desenclos, J.C., et al.: Large outbreak of *Salmonella enterica* serotype paratyphi B infection caused by a goats' milk cheese, France, 1993: a case finding and epidemiological study. Br. Med. J., 312:91–94, 1996.

Devendra, C.: Goat; dietary factors affecting milk secretion and composition. Int. Goat Sheep Res., 2(1):61–76, 1982.

Dhanda, M.R., Sharma, G.L. and Bhalla, N.P.: Contagious agalactia in goats and sheep. Indian J. Vet. Sci., 29 (2 and 3):62–68, 1959.

Dhondt, G., Burvenich, C. and Peeters, G.: Mammary blood flow during experimental *Escherichia coli* endotoxin induced mastitis in goats and cows. J. Dairy Res., 44:433–440, 1977.

Dickinson, J.O. and King, R.R.: The transfer of pyrrolizidine alkaloids from *Senecio jacobaea* into the milk of lactating cows and goats. In: Effects of Poisonous Plants on Livestock. R.F. Keeler, K.R. Van Kampen, and L.F. James, eds. New York, Academic Press, pp. 201–208, 1978.

Donkin, E.F. and Boyazoglu, P.A.: Diseases and mortality of adult goats in a South African milk goat herd. S. Afr. J. Anim. Sci., 34(Suppl. 1):254–257, 2004.

Droke, E.A., Paape, M.J. and Di Carlo, A.L.: Prevalence of high somatic cell counts in bulk tank goat milk. J. Dairy Sci., 76:1035–1039, 1993.

Dubois, C.: La fièvre de Malte chez les animaux domestiques. Rev. Vét. (Toulouse, France), 68:129–140, 1911.

Dulin, A.M., et al.: Effect of parity, stage of lactation, and intramammary infection on concentration of somatic cells and cytoplasmic particles in goat milk. J. Dairy Sci., 66:2426–2433, 1983.

Dulin, A.M., Paape, M.J. and Wergin, W.P.: Differentiation and enumeration of somatic cell counts in goat milk. J. Food Prot., 45:435–439, 1982.

East, N.E. and Birnie, E.F.: Diseases of the udder. Vet. Clin. N. Am. Large Anim. Pract., 5(3):591–600, 1983.

East, N.E., Birnie, E.F. and Farver, T.B.: Risk factors associated with mastitis in dairy goats. Am. J. Vet. Res., 48:776–779, 1987.

East, N.E., et al.: Milkborne outbreak of *Mycoplasma mycoides* subspecies *mycoides* infection in a commercial goat dairy. J. Am. Vet. Med. Assoc., 182:1338–1341, 1983.

Eilertz, I., et al.: Isolation of *Listeria monocytogenes* from goat cheese associated with a case of listeriosis in goat. Acta Vet. Scand., 34:145–149, 1993.

Elezebeth, G., et al.: The occurrence of *Listeria* species and antibodies against listeriolysin-O in naturally infected goats. Small Rumin. Res., 67:173–178, 2007.

Erb, R.E.: Hormonal control of mammogenesis and onset of lactation in cows: A review. J. Dairy Sci., 60:155–169, 1977.

Erskine, R.J., et al.: Induction of *Escherichia coli* mastitis in cows fed selenium-deficient or selenium-supplemented diets. Am. J. Vet. Res., 50:2093–2100, 1989.

Erskine, R.J., et al.: Theory, use, and realities of efficacy and food safety of antimicrobial treatment of acute coliform mastitis. J. Am. Vet. Med. Assoc., 198:980–984, 1991.

Fan, W., et al.: Persistency of adenoviral-mediated lysostaphin expression in goat mammary glands. J. Dairy Sci., 87:602–608, 2004.

Fernando, R.S., Rindsig, R.B. and Spahr, S.L.: Electrical conductivity of milk for detection of mastitis. J. Dairy Sci., 65:659–664, 1982.

Ficken, M.D., Andrews, J.J. and Engeltes, I.: Papilloma-squamous cell carcinoma of the udder of a Saanen goat. J. Am. Vet. Med. Assoc., 183:467, 1983.

Fishbein, D.B. and Raoult, D.: A cluster of *Coxiella burnetii* infections associated with exposure to vaccinated goats and their unpasteurized dairy products.: Am. J. Trop. Med. Hyg., 47:35–40, 1992.

Foggie, A., et al.: Contagious agalactia of sheep and goats. J. Comp. Pathol., 80:345–358, 1970.

Foggie, A., et al.: Contagious agalactia of sheep and goats, studies on live and dead vaccines in lactating sheep. J. Comp. Pathol., 81:165–172, 1971.

Fontanelli, E. and Caparrini, W.: La dermatite pustulosa mammaria delle pecore e delle capre nella provincia di Viterbo. Zooprofilassi 10:603–608, 1955.

Forsyth, I.A. and Lee, P.D.: Bromocriptine treatment of periparturient goats: long-term suppression of prolactin and lack of effect on lactation. J. Dairy Res., 60:307–317, 1993.

Fox, L.K., Hancock, D.D. and Horner, S.D.: Selective intramammary antibiotic therapy during the nonlactating period in goats. Small Rumin. Res., 9:313–318, 1992.

Gaillard-Perrin, G., Picavet, D.P. and Perrin, G.: Isolation of *Mycoplasma putrefaciens* in two herds of goats showing symptoms of agalactia. Rev. Méd. Vét., 137:67–70, 1986.

Galbraith, N.S., Forbes, P. and Clifford, C.: Communicable disease associated with milk and dairy products in England and Wales 1951–80. Br. Med. J., 284:1761–1765, 1982.

Galina, M.A., et al.: Effect of somatic cell count on lactation and soft cheese yield by dairy goats. Small Rumin. Res., 21:251–257, 1996.

Gall, C.: Husbandry. In: Goat Production. C. Gall, ed. New York, Academic Press, 1981.

Garrett, P.D.: Guide to Ruminant Anatomy Based on the Dissection of the Goat. Ames, IA, Iowa State Univ. Press, 1988.

Geringer, M.: Untersuchungen zum Vorkommen pathogener und enterotoxogener Staphylokokken in Ziegenmilch. (Investigations on the presence of pathogenic and enterotoxigenic staphlylococci in goat milk.) Tierärztl. Umschau., 38:109–110, 1983.

Gil, M.C., et al.: Aetiology of caprine contagious agalactia syndrome in Extremadura, Spain. Vet. Rec., 144:24–25, 1999a.

Gil, M.C., et al.: Mastitis caused by *Mycoplasma mycoides* subspecies *mycoides* (large colony type) in goat flocks in Spain. J. Vet. Med. Ser. B, 46:741–743, 1999b.

Goeger, D.E., et al.: Effect of feeding milk from goats fed tansy ragwort (*Senecio jacobaea*) to rats and calves. Am. J. Vet. Res., 43:1631–1633, 1982.

Goff, J.P.: Major advances in our understanding of nutritional influences on bovine health. J. Dairy Sci., 89:1292–1301, 2006.

Goldberger, A.C., Lipsky, B.A. and Plorde, J.J.: Suppurative granulomatous lymphadenitis caused by *Corynebacterium ovis* (*pseudotuberculosis*). Am. J. Clin. Pathol., 76:486–490, 1981.

Gross, E.M., et al.: Milkborne gastroenteritis due to *Staphylococcus aureus* enterotoxin B from a goat with mastitis. Am. J. Trop. Med. Hyg., 39:103–104, 1988.

Gupta et al.: Polymerase chain reaction (PCR) for detection of *Brucella melitensis* in goat milk. Small Rumin. Res., 65:79–84, 2006.

Guss, S.B.: Veterinary column. Dairy Goat J., 58(6):10,1980.
Hadjipanayiotou, M.: Effect of sodium bicarbonate and of roughage on milk yield and milk composition of goats and on rumen fermentation of sheep. J. Dairy Sci., 65:59–64, 1982.
Hadjipanayiotou, M.: Effect of sodium bicarbonate on milk yield and milk composition of goats and on rumen fermentation of kids. Small Rumin. Res., 1:37–47, 1988.
Haenlein, G.F.W.: Relationship of somatic cell counts in goat milk to mastitis and productivity. Small Rumin. Res., 45:163–178, 2002.
Haenlein, G.F.W. and Caccese, R.: Goat milk versus cow milk. Goat Extension Handbook Factsheet E-1:1, 1984.
Hahn, G., et al.: Bakteriologische Befunde und deren Bewertung in Milch und Milchprodukten von Ziegen und Schafen. Arch. f. Lebensmittelhygiene. 1992; 43:89–93, 1992.
Hall, S.M. and Rycroft, A.N.: Causative organisms and somatic cell counts in subclinical intramammary infections in milking goats in the UK. Vet Rec. 2007 160:19–22, 2007.
Hamerton, J.L., et al.: Genetic intersexuality in goats. J. Reprod. Fert. Suppl., 7:25–51, 1969.
Harris, N.V., et al.: *Campylobacter jejuni* enteritis is associated with raw goat milk. Am. J. Epidemiol., 126:179–186, 1987.
Hatchette et al.: Goat-associated Q fever: a new disease in Newfoundland. Emerg. Infect. Dis., 7:413–419, 2001.
Heidrich, H.J. and Renk, W.: Diseases of the Mammary Glands of Domestic Animals. Translated by L.W. van den Heever. Philadelphia, W.B. Saunders, 1967.
Heinz, F.X. and Kunz, C.: Tick-borne encephalitis and the impact of vaccination. Arch. Virol. Suppl., 18:201–205, 2004.
Henderson, A.J., Blatchford, D.R. and Peaker, M.: The effects of milking thrice instead of twice daily on milk secretion in the goat. Q. J. Exp. Physiol., 68:645–652, 1983.
Hill, B.M., et al.: Antibiotic residues in goat milk following intramammary treatment. N.Z. Vet. J., 32:130–131, 1984.
Hinckley, L.S.: Somatic cell count in relation to caprine mastitis. Vet. Med. Small Anim. Clin., 78:1267–1271, 1983.
Hinckley, L.S.: Quality standards for goat milk. Dairy Food Environ. Sanit., 11:511–512, 1991.
Hinckley, L.S., Post, J.E. and Duval, M.C.: The role of nonhemolytic staphylococci in caprine mastitis. Vet. Med., 80:76–80, 1985.
Hinckley, L.S. and Williams, L.F.: Diagnosis of mastitis in goats. Vet. Med. Small Anim. Clin., 76:711–712, 1981.
Homeida, A.M. and Cooke, R.G.: Biological half-life of oxytocin in the goat. Res. Vet. Sci., 37:364–365, 1984.
Hopkins, A.: Bracken (*Pteridium aquilinum*): Its distribution and animal health implications. Br. Vet. J., 146:316–326, 1990.
Hueston, W.D., Hartwig, N.R. and Judy, J.K.: Detection of ovine intramammary infection with the California mastitis test. J. Am. Vet. Med. Assoc., 188:522–524, 1986.
Hughes, D. and Jensen, N.: *Yersinia enterocolitica* in raw goat's milk.: Appl. Environ. Microbiol., 41:309–310, 1981.
Hunter, A.C.: Microflora and somatic cell content of goat milk. Vet. Rec., 114:318–320, 1984.
Ishler, V. and Roberts, B.: Troubleshooting milk flavor problems. Cooperative Extension Service, Pennsylvania State Univ. Publication DAS-02-39, University Park, PA, 2002.
Jackson, B.: *Campylobacter* in goats. Goat Vet. Soc. J., 6(1):7–9, 1985.
Jain, N.C. and Sharma, G.L.: Studies on *Corynebacterium pyogenes* mastitis in goats. 1. The effect of live organisms on the udder. Indian Vet. J., 41:379–385, 1964.
James, L.F. and Hartley, W.J.: Effects of milk from animals fed locoweed on kittens, calves and lambs. Am. J. Vet. Res., 38:1263–1265, 1977.
Jand, S.K. and Dhillon, S.S.: Mycotic mastitis produced experimentally in goats. Mykosen 18:363–366, 1975.
Jandal, J.M.: Some factors affecting lipase activity in goat milk. Small Rumin. Res., 16:87–91, 1995.
Jarman, R.F. and Caruolo, E.V.: The response of body and mammary temperature, milk somatic cell concentration to mammary infusion of endotoxin in lactating goats. J. Dairy Sci., 67(Suppl. 1):235, 1984. (Abstract.)
Jarp, J., Mamo, W. and Johne, B.: Surface properties of *Staphylococcus aureus* isolated from caprine mastitis. Acta Vet. Scand., 30:335–339, 1989.
Jelley, W.C.N.: Goats—an unusual case of *Campylobacter* enteritis. Environ. Health, 93:154, 1985.
Jenness, R.: Composition and characteristics of goat milk: review 1968–1979. J. Dairy Sci., 63:1605–1630, 1980.
Jensen, H.E., Espinosa de los Monteros, A. and Carrasco, L.: Caprine mastitis due to aspergillosis and zygomycosis: a pathological and immunohistochemical study. J. Comp. Pathol., 114:183–191, 1996.
Jensen, N. and Hughes, D.: Public health aspects of raw goat's milk produced throughout New South Wales. Food Technol. Aust., 32:336–341, 1980.
Jones, G.E.: The pathogenicity of some ovine or caprine mycoplasmas in the lactating mammary gland of sheep and goats. J. Comp. Pathol., 95:305–318, 1985.
Jones, T.O.: Caprine mastitis associated with *Yersinia pseudotuberculosis* infection. Vet. Rec., 110:231, 1982.
Kalogridou-Vassiliadou, D.: Mastitis-related pathogens in goat milk. Small Rumin. Res., 4:203–212, 1991.
Kapur, M.P. and Singh, R.P.: Studies on clinical cases of mastitis in cows, buffaloes and goats in Haryana State. Indian Vet. J., 55:803–806, 1978.
Karzis, J., Donkin, E.F. and Petzer, I.M.: The influence of intramammary antibiotic treatment, presence of bacteria, stage of lactation and parity in dairy goats as measured by the California Milk Cell Test and somatic cell counts. Onderstepoort J. Vet. Res., 74:161–167, 2007.
Kennedy-Stoskopf, S., Narayan, O. and Strandberg, J.D.: The mammary gland as a target organ for infection with caprine arthritis-encephalitis virus. J. Comp. Pathol., 95:609–617, 1985.
Kerr, H.J. and Wallace, C.E.: Mastectomy in a goat (a case report). Vet. Med. Small Anim. Clin., 73:1177–1181, 1978.
Kilgore, W.W., et al.: Toxic plants as possible human teratogens. Calif. Agric., 35:6, 1981.
Kinde, H., et al.: Mycoplasma infection in a commercial goat dairy caused by *Mycoplasma agalactiae* and *Mycoplasma mycoides* subsp. *mycoides* (caprine biotype). J. Vet. Diagn. Invest., 6:423–427, 1994.
Klima, H.: Positiver Hemmstofftest in Ziegenmilchproben mit *B. stearothermophilus*. Arch. Lebensmittelhygiene 31:111, 1980.

Klinger, I. and Rosenthal, I.: Public health and the safety of milk and milk products from sheep and goats. Rev. Sci. Tech. Off. Int. Epiz., 16:482–488, 1997.

Konishi, M., et al.: Epidemiological survey and pathological studies on caprine arthritis-encephalitis (CAE) in Japan. Bull. Natl. Inst. Anim. Health, (113):23–30, 2006.

Kosikowski, F.V.: Induced and natural inhibitor behavior of milk and significance to antibiotic disc assay testing. J. Dairy Sci., 46:95–101, 1963.

Krieg, A. and Peterhans, E.: Caprine arthritis-encephalitis in Switzerland: epidemiological and clinical studies. Schweiz. Archiv Tierheilkd., 132:345–352, 1990.

Kuusi, M., et al.: An outbreak of *Streptococcus equi* subspecies *zooepidemicus* associated with consumption of fresh goat cheese. BMC Infect. Dis., 6(36), 2006. http://www.biomedcentral.com/content/pdf/1471-2334-6-36.pdf.

Kyozaire, J.K., et al.: Microbiological quality of goat's milk obtained under different production systems. J. South Afr. Vet. Assoc., 76:69–73, 2005.

Langoni, H., Domingues, P.F. and Baldini, S.: Goat mastitis: their agents and susceptibility face to the antimicrobial. [Mastite caprina: seus agentes e sensibilidade frente a antimicrobianos.] Rev. Bras. Sci. Vet., 13:51–54, 2006.

Le Du, J.F.: Facilities and equipment for hand and machine milking of goats. Proceedings, Fourth International Conference on Goats, Brasilia, Brazil, EMBRAPA, Volume 1, pp. 269–281, 1987.

Le Jaouen, J.-C.: Défauts du lait: Les inhibiteurs de fermentation. La Chèvre 163:30–31, 1987.

Le Guillou, S.: Pathologie mammaire et production laitière. La Chèvre 174:27–32, 1989.

Lefrileux, Y.: [The Teepol test: the CMT works.] Chèvre (248):24–25, 2002.

Leitner, G., Merin, U. and Silanikove, N.: Changes in milk composition as affected by subclinical mastitis in goats. J. Dairy Sci., 87:1719–1726, 2004a.

Leitner, G., et al.: Effect of subclinical intramammary infection on somatic cell counts, NAGase activity and gross composition of goats' milk. J. Dairy Res., 71:311–315, 2004b.

LeMens, P.: Composition du lait: de nouveaux éléments. La Chèvre 161:10–12, 1987.

Lepper, A.W.D.: Mycotic mastitis in a dairy goat. Vet Rec., 76:1469–1472, 1964.

Lepper, A.W.D.: A trial in goats of an inactivated staphylococcal polyvalent somatic antigen vaccine against mastitis. Br. Vet. J., 123:183–191, 1967.

Lepper, A.W.D. and Matthews, P.R.J.: Experimental mastitis produced by *Pseudomonas aeruginosa* in goats. Res. Vet. Sci., 7:151–160, 1966.

Lerondelle, C.: Dénombrement cellulaire dans le lait de demi-mamelles de chèvre. In: Les Maladies de la Chèvre, (Les Colloques de l'INRA, no. 28) Niort, France, 1984, pp. 225–232.

Lerondelle, C.: L'infection de la mamelle par le virus de l'arthrite et de l'encephalite de la chèvre (CAEV). Sci. Vet. Med. Comp., 90:139–143, 1988.

Lerondelle, C.: L'infection de la mamelle par le virus de l'arthrite et de l'encéphalite caprine. Fourth International Symp. Machine Milking Small Ruminants. Israel, 1989, pp. 381–387.

Lerondelle, C., Fleury, C. and Vialard, J.: La glande mammaire: organe cible de l'infection par le virus de l'arthrite et de l'encéphalite caprine. Ann. Rec. Vét., 20:5764, 1989.

Lerondelle, C. and Poutrel, B.: Characteristics of nonclinical mammary infections of goats. Ann. Rec. Vet., 15:105–112, 1984.

Lerondelle, C., Richard, Y. and Isartial, J.: Factors affecting somatic cell counts in goat milk. Small Rumin. Res., 8:129–139, 1992.

Lerondelle, C., et al.: Infection of lactating goats by mammary instillation of cell-borne caprine arthritis-encephalitis virus. J. Dairy Sci., 78:850–855, 1995.

Lewter, M.M., Mullowney, P.C., Baldwin, E.W. and Walker, R.D.: Mastitis in goats. Compend. Contin. Educ. Pract. Vet., 6(7):S417-S425, 1984.

Ligios, C., et al.: PrP^{Sc} in mammary glands of sheep affected by scrapie and mastitis. Nature Med., 11:1137–1138, 2005.

Linzell, J.L. and Peaker, M.: Day-to-day variations in milk composition in the goat and cow as a guide to the detection of subclinical mastitis. Br. Vet. J., 128:284–295, 1972.

Linzell, J.L. and Peaker, M.: Efficacy of the measurement of the electrical conductivity of milk for the detection of subclinical mastitis in cows: detection of infected cows at a single visit. Br. Vet. J., 131:447–461, 1975.

Little, C.L. and de Louvois, J.: Health risks associated with unpasteurized goats' and ewes' milk on retail sale in England and Wales. Epidemiol. Infect. 122:403–408, 1999.

Løken, T., Aspøy, E. and Grønstøl, H.: *Listeria monocytogenes* excretion and humoral immunity in goats in a herd with outbreaks of listeriosis and in a healthy herd. Acta Vet. Scand., 23:392–399, 1982.

Long, P.E., Heavner, J.E., Ziv, G. and Geleta, J.N.: Depletion of antibiotics from the mammary gland of goats. J. Dairy Sci., 67:707–712, 1984.

Lovegrove, S.: Off-flavors in goat milk: Cause for concern. Dairy Goat J., 68:440, 442, 1990.

Lu, C.D., Potchoiba, M.J. and Loetz, E.R.: Influence of vacuum level, pulsation ratio and rate on milking performance and udder health in dairy goats. Small Rumin. Res., 5:1–8, 1991.

Luengo, C., et al.: Influence of intramammary infection and non-infection factors on somatic cell counts in dairy goats. J. Dairy Res., 71:169–174, 2004.

Maisi, P.: Analysis of physiological changes in caprine milk with CMT, NAGase and antitrypsin. Small Rumin. Res., 3:485–492, 1990.

Maisi, P.: Milk NAGase, CMT and antitrypsin as indicators of caprine subclinical mastitis infections. Small Rumin. Res., 3:493–501, 1990.

Maisi, P. and Riipinen, I.: Use of California mastitis test, N-acetyl-β-glucosaminidase, and antitrypsin to diagnose caprine subclinical mastitis. J. Dairy Res., 55:309–314, 1988.

Maisi, P. and Riipinen, I.: Pathogenicity of different species of staphylococci in caprine udder. Br. Vet. J., 147:126–132, 1991.

Mallikeswaran, K. and Padmanaban, V.D.: Microbial flora of milk of goats affected with clinical mastitis. Indian Vet. J., 68:152–154, 1991.

Manlongat, N., et al.: Physiologic-chemoattractant-induced migration of polymorphonuclear leukocytes in milk. Clin. Diagn. Lab. Immunol., 5:375–381, 1998.

Manni, V., et al.: Presence of papillomavirus-like DNA sequences in cutaneous fibropapillomas of the goat udder. Vet. Microbiol., 61:1–6, 1998.

Manser, P.A.: Prevalence, causes and laboratory diagnosis of subclinical mastitis in the goat. Vet. Rec., 118:552–554, 1986.

Martin-Jimenez, T., Craigmill, A.L. and Riviere, J.E.: Extralabel use of oxytetracycline. J. Am. Vet. Med. Assoc., 211:42–44, 1997.

Martinet, J. and Richard, P.: La réflexe d'éjection du lait chez la brebis et chez la chèvre. In: Symposium sur la Traite Mécanique des Petits Ruminants. Millau, 1973, INRA, pp. 29–49, 1974.

Matthews, J.: Diseases of the Goat. 2nd Ed. Oxford, Blackwell Science, 1999.

Mavrogianni, V.S., Alexopoulos, C. and Fthenakis, G.C.: Field evaluation of flunixin meglumine in the supportive treatment of caprine mastitis. J. Vet. Pharmacol. Ther., 27:373–375, 2004.

McDougall, S.: Recovery of bacteria from goats' milk following freezing and the prevalence of bacterial infection in milk from goats with an elevated somatic cell count. N. Z. Vet. J., 48:27–29, 2000.

McDougall, S. and Anniss, F.: Efficacy of antibiotic treatment at drying-off in curing existing infections and preventing new infections in dairy goats. In: Mastitis in Dairy Production: Current Knowledge and Future Solutions. H. Hogeveen, ed. Wageningen, Netherlands, Wageningen Academic Publishers, pp. 523–528, 2005.

McDougall, S., et al.: Relationships among somatic cell count, California mastitis test, impedance and bacteriological status of milk in goats and sheep in early lactation. Small Rumin. Res., 40:245–254, 2001.

McGinty, A.: Toxic Plant Handbook for Pecos County. Fort Stockton, Texas, Texas Agricultural Service, 1987.

McIntyre, L., et al.: *Escherichia coli* O157 outbreak associated with the ingestion of unpasteurized goat's milk in British Columbia, 2001. Can. Commun. Dis. Rep., 28:6–8, 2002.

Meador, V.P. and Deyoe, B.L.: Effect of milk stasis on *Brucella abortus* infection of the mammary gland in goats. Am. J. Vet. Res., 52:886–890, 1991.

Meador, V.P., Deyoe, B.L. and Cheville, N.F.: Pathogenesis of *Brucella abortus* infection of the mammary gland and supramammary lymph node of the goat. Vet. Pathol., 26:357–368, 1989.

Menzies, P.I. and Ramanoon, S.Z.: Mastitis of sheep and goats. Vet. Clin. N. Am. Food Anim. Pract., 17:333–358, 2001.

Mercier, P., et al.: Agalactia caused by *Mycoplasma putrefaciens* in a goat herd. Point Vét., 31:345–348, 2000.

Mews. A.: Goat milk taints. Goat Vet. Soc. J., 8:29–31, 1987.

Miller, C.C., et al.: Lactation associated with acidophilic pituitary adenoma, pheochromocytoma, and cystic endometrial hyperplasia in two goats. J. Am. Vet. Med. Assoc., 210:378–381, 1997.

Miller, S.: Mammary carcinoma in a goat. Wool Wattles 20(1):11, 1992.

Mills, J.A.: Treatment of afebrile postparturient udder edema in goats. Can. Vet. J., 24:62, 1983a.

Mills, J.A.: Treatment of atypical postparturient udder edema in goats. Can. Vet. J., 24:324, 1983b.

Misri, J., Gupta, P.P. and Sood, N.: Experimental *Mycoplasma capri* mastitis in goats. Aust. Vet. J., 65:33–35, 1988.

Morand-Fehr, P., et al.: Conditions d'apparition des inversions de taux du lait de chèvre et effet des conditions de traite. In: Milking and Milk Production of Dairy Sheep and Goats. EAAP Publication no. 95. Wageningen Pers, Wageningen, pp. 489–494, 1999.

Morand-Fehr, P., et al.: Effect of feeding on the quality of goat milk and cheeses. Proceedings, 7th International Conference on Goats, Tours, France, Vol 1, pp 53–58, May 2000.

Moroni, P., et al.: Characterization of *Staphylococcus aureus* isolated from chronically infected dairy goats. J. Dairy Sci., 88:3500–3509, 2005a.

Moroni, P., et al.: Risk factors for intramammary infections and relationship with somatic-cell counts in Italian dairy goats. Prevent. Vet. Med., 69:163–173, 2005b.

Moroni, P., et al.: Study of intramammary infections in dairy goats from mountainous regions in Italy. N.Z. Vet. J., 53:375–376, 2005c.

Moroni, P., et al.: Subclinical mastitis and antimicrobial susceptibility of *Staphylococcus caprae* and *Staphylococcus epidermidis* isolated from two Italian goat herds. J. Dairy Sci., 88:1694–1704, 2005d.

Mottram, T.T., Smith, D.L.O. and Godwin, R.J.: Analysis of parlour design parameters for goat milking. Small Rumin. Res., 6:1–13, 1991.

Moulton, J.E.: Cutaneous papillomas on the udders of milk goats. N. Am. Vet., 35:29–33, 1954.

Mukherjee, A. and Das, M.S.: Etiology of clinical forms of goat mastitis in West Bengal. Indian Vet. J., 34:339–341, 1957.

Murphy, S.C., et al.: Influence of bovine mastitis on lipolysis and proteolysis in milk. J. Dairy Sci., 72:620–626, 1989.

Murray, C., McNutt, S.H. and Purwin, P.: Tuberculosis of goats. J. Am. Vet. Med. Assoc., 59:82–84, 1921.

National Mastitis Council, Inc.: Laboratory and Field Handbook on Bovine Mastitis. Revised ed. Fort Atkinson, WI, National Mastitis Council, 1999.

Nelson, W.E. (ed.): Textbook of Pediatrics. 8th Ed. Philadelphia, W.B. Saunders Co., 1964.

Nesbakken, T.: Kronisk mastitis forårsaket av *Streptococcus zooepidemicus* som problem i en geitebesetning. Norsk Veterinaertidsskrift 87:188–191, 1975.

Nesbakken, T.: A case of mastitis in a goat. Cytological and bacteriological examinations of milk samples throughout the entire lactation period. Nord. Vet. Med., 30:18–20, 1978a.

Nesbakken, T.: The cell count in milk of goats and the diagnosis of mastitis in goats. Nord. Vet. Med., 30:21–23, 1978b.

Nicholas, R.A.J.: Improvements in the diagnosis and control of diseases of small ruminants caused by mycoplasmas. Small Rumin. Res., 45:145–149, 2002.

Nigam, J.M. and Tyagi, R.P.S.: Caprine teat surgery. Indian Vet. J., 50:588–592, 1973.

Norberg, E., et al.: Electrical conductivity of milk: ability to predict mastitis status. J. Dairy Sci., 87:1099–1107, 2004.

Nord, K. and Adnoy, T.: Effects of infection by caprine arthritis-encephalitis virus on milk production of goats. J. Dairy Sci., 80:2391–2397, 1997.

Nozawa, K.: Population genetics of farm animals. II. Statistical analyses on the polymorphic populations of goats in southwestern islands of Japan. Jpn. J. Genet., 45:45–57, 1970.

O'Brien, P.H.: Self-suckling behaviour by a feral goat. Appl. Anim. Ethol., 8:189–190, 1982.

Ohnstad, I.: Milking machine maintenance for dairy goats. Goat Vet. Soc. J., 22:43–44, 2006.

OIE: Manual of Diagnostic Tests and Vaccines for Terrestrial Animals, Vol. 2, 5th Ed. Office International des Épizooties (OIE), Paris, 2004.

Okoh, A.E.J. and Obasaju, M.F.: A disease simulating goat-specific pox in Kano, Nigeria. Trop. Anim. Health Prod., 15:226, 1983.

Olds, R.J. and Lewis, F.A.: Melioidosis in goats. Aust. Vet. J., 30:253–261, 1954.

Oppong, E.N. and Gumedze, J.S.E.: Supernumerary teats in Ghanaian livestock. I. Sheep and goats. Beitr. Trop. Landwirtschaft Veterinärmed., 20:63–67, 1982.

Oram, J.D. and Reiter, B.: Inhibition of bacteria by lactoferrin and other iron-chelating agents. Biochem. Biophys. Acta, 170:351–365, 1968.

Ortega, J.A. and Lazerson, J.: Anagyrine-induced red cell aplasia, vascular anomaly, and skeletal dysplasia. J. Pediatr., 111:87–89, 1987.

Osweiler, G.D., et al.: Clinical and Diagnostic Veterinary Toxicology. 3rd Ed. Dubuque, Iowa, Kendall/Hunt Publ. Co., 1985.

Otte, E.: Euteramputation bei Schaf und Ziege. Berl. Münch. Tierärtzld. Wochenschr., 71:473–474, 1958.

Paape, M.J., Hafs, H.D. and Snyder, W.W.: Variation of estimated numbers of milk somatic cells stained with Wright's stain or pyronin Y-methyl green stain. J. Dairy Sci., 46:1211–1216, 1963.

Paape, M.J., et al. Milk somatic cells and lactation in small ruminants. J. Dairy Sci., 84(E. Suppl.)E237-E244, 2001.

Paape, M.J., et al.: Monitoring goat and sheep milk somatic cell counts. Small Rumin. Res., 68:114–125, 2007.

Pal, M.: Association of fungi with caprine mastitis. Proceedings, Third Int. Conf. Goat Prod. Dis. Tucson, Arizona, p. 564, 1982.

Pal, M. and Randhawa, H.S.: Caprine mastitis due to *Cryptococcus neoformans*. Sabouraudia 14:261–263, 1976.

Pal, B.C., Singh, P.P. and Pathak, R.C.: *Mycoplasma bovigenitalum* pathogenicity for caprine udder. Indian J. Comp. Microbiol. Immunol. Infect. Dis., 4:262–263, 1983.

Paliwal, O.P., Kulshrestha, S.B. and Krishna, L.: A note on mortality in suckling kids due to *Staphylococcus aureus*. Indian J. Anim. Sci., 47:430–431, 1977.

Panter, K.E. and James, L.F.: Natural plant toxicants in milk: a review. J. Anim. Sci., 68:892–904, 1990.

Park, Y.W.: Interrelationships between somatic cell counts, electrical conductivity, bacteria counts, percent fat and protein in goat milk. Small Rumin. Res., 5:367–375, 1991.

Park, Y.W. and Nuti, L.C.: Electrical conductivity of goat milk in evaluating subclinical mastitis. Proceedings, Third Asian-Australasian Assoc. of Animal Production Animal Science Congress, Seoul, Korea Republic, 2:1272–1274, 1985.

Pattison, I.H.: Studies on experimental streptococcal mastitis. V. Histological findings in experimental streptococcal mastitis in the goat. J. Comp. Pathol., 61:71–87, 1951.

Payne, M.A., et al.: Extralabel use of penicillin in food animals. J. Am. Vet. Med. Assoc., 229:1401–1403, 2006.

Pearson, L.J. and Marth, E.H.: *Listeria* monocytogenes—threat to a safe food supply: A review. J. Dairy Sci., 73:912–928, 1990.

Perez, M. and Schultz, L.H.: Somatic cells in goat milk. Proceedings, Eighteenth Annual Meeting National Mastitis Council, Inc. Louisville, KY, pp. 44–49, 1979.

Perreau, P.: Syndrome d'agalaxie contagieuse à *Mycoplasma mycoides* subsp *capri*. Nouvelles observations. Bull. Acad. Vét. Fr. 47:179–188, 1974.

Perreau, P. and Breard, A.: La mycoplasmose caprine à *M. capricolum*. Comp. Immunol. Microbiol. Infect. Dis., 2:87–97, 1979.

Perreau, P., Cuong, T. and Vallée, A.: Isolement d'un mycoplasme du groupe *Mycoplasma mycoides* var. *capri* à partir d'un lait de mammite chez la chèvre. Bull. Acad. Vét. Fr. 45:109–116, 1972.

Perrin, G.G., et al.: Relationships between California mastitis test (CMT) and somatic cell counts in dairy goats. Small Rumin. Res., 26:167–170, 1997.

Petgen, A. and Martain, L.: Importance du diagnostic en laboratoire des mammites de la chèvre à haute production laitière. Choix du traitement spécifique d'une mammite à *Pseudomonas aeruginosa*. Soc. Vét. Prat. Fr. Bull. Mens., 61:397–398, 400–401, 1977.

Petris, M.A.: Ovine and caprine mastitis in Cyprus. A report on the naturally occurring disease. Bull. Off. Int. Epiz., 60:989–1007, 1963.

Pettersen, K.-E.: Cell content in goat's milk. Acta Vet. Scand., 22:226–237, 1981.

Picavet, D.P., et al.: A propos de quelques foyers d'agalactie contagieuse de la chèvre dans le Sud-Ouest de la France. Rev. Sci. Tech. Off. Int. Epiz 2:489–497, 1983.

Plommet, M.: Mammites et traite mécanique. (Mastitis and mechanical milking.) In: Symposium sur la Traite Mécanique des Petits Ruminants. Millau, 1973, INRA, pp. 87–95, 1974.

Plommet, M. and Bézard, G.: Immunisation anti-staphylococcique de la brebis par anatoxines et adjuvants. Ann. Rec. Vét., 5:29–39, 1974.

Post, J.E., Duval, M.C. and Hinckley, L.S.: Association of caprine arthritis encephalitis virus (CAEV) with mastitis in goats. Bull. Int. Dairy Fed., 202:90–92, 1986.

Post, J.E., Hinckley, L. and Duval, M.: Udder infections with CAE virus in goats. Proc. U.S. Anim. Health Assoc., 88:262–263, 1984.

Poutrel, B.: Udder infection of goats by coagulase-negative staphylococci. Vet. Microbiol., 9:131–137, 1984.

Poutrel, B. and Lerondelle, C.: Cell content of goat milk: California mastitis test, Coulter counter, and Fossomatic for predicting half infection. J. Dairy Sci., 66:2575–2579, 1983.

Poutrel, B., et al.: Relations entre statut infectieux des mamelles et numérations cellulaires du lait de chèvre. In: Somatic Cells and Milk of Small Ruminants. EAAP Publication no. 77. Wageningen Pers, Wageningen, pp. 61–64, 1996.

Poutrel, B., et al.: Control of intramammary infections in goats: Impact on somatic cell counts. J. Anim. Sci., 75:566–570, 1997.

Prasad, L.N., Gupta, P.P. and Singh, N.: Isolation of mycoplasmas from goat mastitis. Indian J. Anim. Sci., 54:1172–1175, 1984.

Prasad, L.N., Gupta, P.P. and Singh, N.: Experimental *Mycoplasma arginini* mastitis in goats. Aust. Vet., J., 62:341–342, 1985.

Pritchard, C.G.: Goats and public health. State Vet. J. (United Kingdom) 41:3–12, 1987.

Randy, H.A., et al.: Effect of age and time of milking on day-to-day variation in milk yield, milk constituents, and somatic cell counts. Small Rumin. Res., 1:151–155, 1988.

Raynal-Ljutovac, K., et al.: Heat stability and enzymatic modifications of goat and sheep milk. Small Rumin. Res., 68:207–220, 2007.

Rebesko, B., Aswad, A. and Fahri, R.: Edemi govedeg i kozjeg vimena (Oedemas in the udder of cows and goats). Vet. Glasnik 28:875–882, 1974.

Reid, H.W., et al.: Transmission of louping-ill virus in goat milk. Vet. Rec., 114:163–165, 1984.

Renk, W.: Beiträge zur Diagnose und Pathogenese der akuten Mastitiden. Zentralblatt f. Veterinärmedizin 4:325–340, 1957.

Renoux, G.: Brucellosis in goats and sheep. In: Advances in Veterinary Science, Vol. 3. C.A. Brandly and E.L. Jungherr, eds. New York and London, Academic Press, pp. 241–273, 1957.

Ricordeau, G. and Labussière, J.: Traite à la machine des chèvres. Ann. Zootech., 19:37–43, 1970.

Riemann, H.P., et al.: Toxoplasmosis in an infant fed unpasteurized goat milk. J. Pediatr., 84:573–575, 1975.

Roguinsky, M., et al.: Causes et diagnostic des mammites de la chèvre. La Chèvre 68:4–5, 1971.

Roguinsky, M. and Grandemy, T.: Caractères des staphylocoques des mammites caprines. La Chèvre 108:25–26, 1978.

Rosendal, S.: Ovine and caprine mycoplasmas. In: Mycoplasmosis in Animals: Laboratory Diagnosis. H.W. Whitford et al., eds. Iowa State Univ. Press, Ames, pp. 84–96, 1994.

Rota, A.M., et al.: Somatic cell types in goats' milk in relation to total cell count, stage and number of lactation. Small Rumin. Res., 12:89–98, 1993.

Rozear, L., Love, N.E. and van Camp, S.L.: Radiographic diagnosis: pulmonary lymphosarcoma in a goat. Vet. Radiol. Ultrasound, 39:528–531, 1998.

Ruhnke, H.L., Rosendal, S., Goltz, J. and Blackwell, T.E.: Isolation of *Mycoplasma mycoides* subspecies *mycoides* from polyarthritis and mastitis of goats in Canada. Can. Vet. J., 24:54–56, 1983.

Ruiz Santa Quiteria, J.A., et al.: [Outbreaks of mastitis in goats caused by group C streptococci.] Advances Aliment. Mejora Anim., 31:27–28, 1991. Vet. Bull. Abst. 2334, 1992.

Ruppanner, R., et al.: Prevalence of *Coxiella burnetii* (Q fever) and *Toxoplasma gondii* among dairy goats in California. Am. J. Vet. Res., 39:867–870, 1978.

Ryan, D.P. and Greenwood, P.L.: Prevalence of udder bacteria in milk samples from four dairy goat herds. Aust. Vet. J., 67:362–363, 1990.

Ryan, D.P., Greenwood, P.L. and Nicholls, P.J.: Effect of caprine arthritis-encephalitis virus infection on milk cell count and N-acetyl-beta-glucosaminidase activity in dairy goats. J. Dairy Res., 60:299–306, 1993.

Sacks, J.J., Roberto, R.R. and Brooks, N.F.: Toxoplasmosis infection associated with raw goat's milk. J. Am. Med. Assoc., 248:1728–1732, 1982.

Salama, A.A.K., et al.: Mammogenesis and induced lactation with or without reserpine in nulliparous dairy goats. J. Dairy Sci., 90:3751–3757, 2007.

Sanchez, A., Contreras, A. and Corrales, J.C.: Parity as a risk factor for caprine subclinical intramammary infection. Small Rumin. Res., 31:197–201, 1999.

Sanchez, A., et al.: Relationships between infection with caprine arthritis encephalitis virus, intramammary bacterial infection and somatic cell counts in dairy goats. Vet. Rec., 148:711–714, 2001.

Sanchez, A., et al.: Effect of freezing goat milk samples on recovery of intramammary bacterial pathogens. Vet. Microbiol., 94:71–77, 2003.

Sanchez, A., et al.: Influence of storage and preservation on fossomatic cell count and composition of goat milk. J. Dairy Sci., 88:3095–3100, 2005.

Sánchez, J., et al.: Prevention of clinical mastitis with barium selenate in dairy goats from a selenium-deficient area. J. Dairy Sci., 90:2350–2354, 2007.

Sanz Sampelayo, M.R., et al.: Influence of type of diet on the fat constituents of goat and sheep milk. Small Rumin. Res., 68:42–63, 2007.

Sasshofer, K., Loibl, A. and Kessler, O.: Erkrankungen bei Schaf und Ziege. 7. Euterentzündungen. Wien. Tierärztl. Monatsschr., 74:125–135, 1987.

Sauvant, D., et al.: Brewer's grain feeding value for dairy goats. Proc. Fourth International Conference on Goats, Brasilia, Brazil, EMBRAPA, p. 1423, 1987.

Schaeren, W. and Maurer, J.: [Prevalence of subclinical udder infections and individual somatic cell counts in three dairy goat herds during a full lactation.] Schweiz. Archiv Tierheilkd., 148:641–648, 2006.

Schalm, O.W., Carroll, E.J. and Jain, N.C.: Bovine Mastitis. Philadelphia, Lea and Febiger, 1971.

Schalm, O.W. and Noorlander, D.O.: Experiments and observations leading to development of the California mastitis test. J. Am. Vet. Med. Assoc., 130:199–204, 1957.

Schreuder, B.E.C. et al.: *Corynebacterium pseudotuberculosis* in milk of CL affected goats. Vet. Rec., 127:387, 1990.

Schröter, A.: Über das Vorkommen von *Bakterium ovium* (Dammann-Freese) bei Ziegen. Berl. Münch. Tierärztl. Wochenschr., 67:3–5, 1954.

Scott, D.W.: Large Animal Dermatology. Philadelphia, W.B. Saunders Co., 1988.

Sedgman, D.K.: How does parenteral phosphorus and vitamin D_3 correct afebrile postparturient udder edema in goats? Can. Vet. J., 23:275, 1982.

Sharma, S.P. and Iyer, P.K.R.: Pathology of chronic lesions in the mammary glands of goats (*Capra hircus*). 2: Fibrocystic disease and intraductal carcinomas. Indian J. Anim. Sci., 44:474–479, 1974.

Sheldrake, R.F., Hoare, R.J.T. and Woodhouse, V.E.: Relationship of somatic cell count and cell volume analysis of goat's milk to intramammary infection with coagulase-negative staphylococci. J. Dairy Res., 48:393–403, 1981.

Sheldrake, R.F., McGregor, G.D. and Hoare, R.J.T.: Somatic cell count, electrical conductivity, and serum albumen

concentration for detecting bovine mastitis. J. Dairy Sci., 66:548–555, 1983.
Sierra, D., et al.: Differential cell counts in goat's milk. In: Milking and Milk Production of Dairy Sheep and Goats. EAAP Publication no. 95. Wageningen Pers, Wageningen, pp. 178–180, 1999.
Sierra, D., et al.: Temperature effects on Fossomatic cell counts in goats milk. Int. Dairy J., 16:385–387, 2006.
Silanikove, N., et al.: Subclinical mastitis affects the plasmin system, milk composition and curd yield in sheep and goats: comparative aspects. In: Mastitis in Dairy Production: Current Knowledge and Future Solutions. H. Hogeveen, ed. Wageningen, Netherlands, Wageningen Academic Publishers, pp. 511–516, 2005.
Singh, A.N.O.O.P., Gupta, P.P. and Banga, H.S.: Pathogenicity of *Acholeplasma laidlawii* for the goat udder. Aust. Vet. J., 67:155–156, 1990.
Singh, B. and Iyer, P.K.R.: Mammary intraductal carcinoma in goats (*Capra hircus*). Vet. Pathol., 9:441–446, 1972.
Singh, B. and Iyer, P.K.R.: A note on fibrocystic disease (cystic hyperplasia) in the mammary glands of goats (*Capra hircus*). Indian J. Anim. Sci., 43:83–85, 1973.
Skinner, L.J., et al.: Simultaneous diagnosis of toxoplasmosis in goats and goatowner's family. Scand. J. Infect. Dis., 22:359–361, 1990.
Smith, E.E., et al.: Dietary hydrated sodium calcium aluminosilicate reduction of aflatoxin M1 residue in dairy goat milk and effects on milk production and components. J. Anim. Sci., 72:677–682, 1994.
Smith, G.W., et al.: Extralabel intramammary use of drugs in dairy cattle. J. Amer. Vet. Med. Assoc., 226:1994–1996, 2005.
Smith, M.C. and Cutlip, R.: Effects of infection with caprine arthritis-encephalitis virus on milk production in goats. J. Am. Vet. Med. Assoc., 193:63–67, 1988.
Smith, M.C. and Roguinsky, M.: Mastitis and other diseases of the goat's udder. J. Am. Vet. Med. Assoc., 171:1241–1248, 1977.
Soliman, K.N., et al.: An outbreak of naturally acquired tuberculosis in goats. Vet. Rec., 65:421–425, 1953.
Soto-Blanco, B. and Górniak, S.L.: Transfer of cyanide and its main metabolite thiocyanate in milk: Study of cyanogenic plants ingestion during lactation in goats. In: Poisonous Plants and Related Toxins. T. Acamovic et al., eds. Cambridge, MA, CABI Publishing, pp. 552–557, 2004.
Spencer, S.B.: Machine milking systems. Goat Extension Handbook Factsheet E-2:1–5, 1984.
Stiles, G.W.: Controlling brucellosis in Colorado goats. Third Interamerican Congress on Brucellosis. Washington, D.C., pp. 226–237, 1950.
Summers, J. and New, J.C.: When doing good can help in doing well—a case study. J. Am. Vet. Med. Assoc., 187:902–905, 1985.
Taoudi, A., et al.: Comparaison du pouvoir pathogène de trois souches de *Mycoplasma capricolum* pour la chèvre et le chevreau nouveau-né. Rev. Élev. Méd Vét. Pays Trop., 41:353–358, 1988.
Tham, W.: Survival of *Listeria monocytogenes* in cheese made of unpasteurized goat milk. Acta Vet. Scand., 29:165–172, 1988.
Theilen, G., et al.: Goat papillomatosis. Am. J. Vet. Res., 46:2519–2525, 1985.
Thomas, A.D., et al.: Clinical and pathological observations on goats experimentally infected with *Pseudomonas pseudomallei*. Aust. Vet. J., 65:43–46, 1988.
Timms, L.L. and Schultz, L.H.: N-acetyl-β-d-glucosaminidase activity and somatic cells in goat milk. J. Dairy Sci., 68:3363–3366, 1985.
Thompson, J.S. and Thompson, A.: In-home pasteurization of raw goat's milk by microwave treatment. Int. J. Food Microbiol., 10:59–64, 1990.
Toussaint, G., et al.: Pertubation éventuelle de la fabrication, de l'apparence et du goût des fromages après administration aux chèvres laitières d'anthelminthiques des familles benzimidazole ou tetrahydropyrimidine. Rev. Méd. Vét., 127:259–288, 1976.
Tripathi, B.N., Chattopadhyay, S.K. and Iyer, P.K.R.: Fibrocystic disease and intraductal carcinoma in mammary glands of sheep and goats. Indian J. Anim. Sci., 59:404–409, 1989.
Trodahl, S., Skjevdal, T. and Steine, T.A.: Goats in cold and temperate climates. In: Goat Production. C. Gall, ed. New York, Academic Press, pp. 489–513, 1981.
Trostle, S.S. and O'Brien, R.T.: Ultrasonography of the bovine mammary gland. Compend. Contin. Educ. Pract. Vet., 20: S64-S71, 1998.
Turin, L., et al.: Correlation between milk parameters in CAEV seropositive and negative primiparous goats during an eradication program in Italian farm. Small Rumin. Res., 57:73–79, 2005.
Turner, C.W.: The Mammary Gland, 1: Anatomy of the Udder of Cattle and Domestic Animals. Columbia, MO, Lucas Bros., 1952.
Turner, C.W. and Berousek, E.R.: Blind halves in a goat's udder. J. Dairy Sci., 25:549–555, 1942.
Tzora, A., Fthenakis, G.C. and Linde, K.: Naturally occurring or experimentally induced subclinical ovine mastitis associated with *Listeria monocytogenes*. In: Milking and Milk Production of Dairy Sheep and Goats. EAAP Publication no. 95. Wageningen Pers, Wageningen, pp. 144–150, 1999.
U.S. Animal Health Assoc., Committee on Foreign Animal Diseases: Foreign Animal Diseases. Richmond, VA, U.S.A.H.A., Revised 1998.
Upadhyaya, T.N. and Rao, A.T.: Pathology of spontaneous mammary lesions in goats. Indian Vet. J., 71:19–22, 1994.
Valle, J, et al.: Enterotoxin production by staphylococci isolated from healthy goats. Appl. Environ. Microbiol., 56:1323–1326, 1990.
Valle, J., et al.: Staphylococci isolated from healthy goats. J. Vet. Med. B, 38:81–89, 1991.
Vamvakaki, A.N., et al.: Residual alkaline phosphatase activity after heat treatment of ovine and caprine milk. Small Rumin. Res., 65:237–241, 2006.
Van Damme, D.M.: Mastitis caused by contaminated teat dip and dipping cup. Vet. Med. Small Anim. Clin., 77:541–544, 1982.
van der Lugt, J.J. and Henton, M.M.: Melioidosis in a goat. J. S. Afr. Vet. Assoc., 66:71–73, 1995.
van der Molen, E.J. and Houwers, D.J.: Indurative lymphocytic mastitis in sheep after experimental infection with maedi-visna virus. Vet. Q., 9:193–202, 1987.
Van Tonder, E.M.: Notes on some disease problems in Angora goats in South Africa. Vet. Med. Rev., 1/2:109–138, 1975.

Vasavada, P.C.: Public health aspects of raw goat milk. Dairy Goat J., 64 226–227 and 262, 1986.

Vihan, V.S.: Determination of NA-Gase activity in milk for diagnosis of subclinical caprine mastitis. Small Rumin. Res., 2:359–366, 1989.

Vihan, V.S.: Determination of lysosomal enzyme activity, somatic cells, percent fat and protein in sub-clinical caprine mastitis. In: Somatic Cells and Milk of Small Ruminants. EAAP Publication no. 77. Wageningen Pers, Wageningen, pp. 31–34, 1996.

Vogt, T. and Hasler, P.: A woman with panic attacks and double vision who liked cheese. Lancet, 354:300, 1999.

Walker, S.J. and Gilmour, A.: The incidence of *Yersinia enterocolitica* and *Yersinia enterocolitica*-like bacteria in goat milk in Northern Ireland. Lett. Appl. Microbiol. 3:49–52, 1986.

Wallach, J.C., et al.: Urban outbreak of a *Brucella melitensis* infection in an Argentine family: clinical and diagnostic aspects. FEMS Immunol. Med. Microbiol., 8:49–56, 1994.

White, E.C. and Hinckley, L.S.: Prevalence of mastitis pathogens in goat milk. Small Rum. Res., 33:117–121, 1999.

White, R.D. and Cheeke, P.R.: Meadowfoam (*Limnanthes alba*) meal as a feedstuff for dairy goats and toxicologic activity of the milk. Can. J. Anim. Sci., 63:391–398, 1983.

Wiggans, G.R. and Hubbard, S.M.: Genetic evaluation of yield and type traits of dairy goats in the United States. J. Dairy Sci., 84 (Elect. Suppl.): E69-E73, 2001.

Wilson, D.J., Stewart, K.N. and Sears, P.M.: Effects of stage of lactation, production, parity and season on somatic cell counts in infected and uninfected dairy goats. Small Rumin. Res., 16:165–169, 1995.

Wooding, F.B.P., Peaker, M. and Linzell, J.L.: Theories of milk secretion: evidence from the electron microscopic examination of milk. Nature 226:762–764, 1970.

Wyatt, H.V.: How Themistocles Zammit found Malta Fever (brucellosis) to be transmitted by the milk of goats. J. R. Soc. Med., 98:451–454, 2005.

Yeruham, I., et al.: Cystic dilation of the teat sinuses in doe goats. Vet. Rec., 156:844, 2005.

Yeruham, I., et al.: Investigation and control of mastitis outbreaks caused by *Pseudomonas aeruginosa* in a sheep flock and a goat herd. Berl. Münch. Tierärztl. Wochenschr., 118:220–223, 2005.

Young, E.J. and Suvannoparrat, U.: Brucellosis outbreak attributed to ingestion of unpasteurized goat cheese. Arch. Intern. Med., 135:240–243, 1975.

Zeng, S.S.: Comparison of goat milk standards and cow milk standards for analyses of somatic cell count, fat and protein in goat milk. Small Rumin. Res., 21:221–225, 1996.

Zeng, S.S. and Escobar, E.N.: Effect of parity and milk production on somatic cell count, standard plate count and composition of goat milk. Small Rumin. Res., 17:269–274, 1995.

Zeng, S.S., Escobar, E.N. and Brown-Crowder, I.: Evaluation of screening tests for detection of antibiotic residues in goat milk. Small Rumin. Res., 21:155–160, 1996.

Zeng, S.S., et al.: Validation of antibiotic residue tests for dairy goats. J. Food Protect., 61:344–349, 1998.

Ziv, G.: Practical pharmacokinetic aspects of mastitis therapy-2: practical and therapeutic applications. Vet. Med. Small Anim. Clin., 75:469–474, 1980.

Ziv, G.: Concentrations and residues of antibiotics in the milk of goats after parenteral and intramammary administration, III. Int. Symp. Machine Milking Small Rum., Valladolid, Spain, pp. 513–527, 1983, 1984.

Ziv, G. and Soback, S.: Pharmacotherapeutics of newer antibacterial agents in lactating ewes and goats: A review. 4th Int. Symp. Machine Milking Small Ruminants, Israel, pp. 408–423, 1989.

Ziv, G., et al.: Clinical pharmacology of tiamulin in ruminants. J. Vet. Pharmacol. Ther., 6:23–32, 1983.

Zwahlen, R., et al.: Lentivirusinfektionen bei Ziegen mit Carpitis und interstitieller Mastitis. Schweiz. Arch. Tierheilkd. 125:281–299, 1983.

15

Wasting Diseases

The loss of weight without other obvious signs of disease, also known as wasting or ill thrift, is a common clinical presentation in goats (Figure 15.1). While any given goat may present with weight loss for individual reasons, the abnormally thin goat is often a sentinel of serious herd problems of infectious, parasitic, or management origin. If thin goats are noticed during a farm visit, the veterinarian should ask to examine them even if they were not the reason for the call.

Ill thrift in mature animals is taken to mean that a loss of weight in individual goats has occurred and the goat has become abnormally thin. In growing animals it can also mean that the animal has lost weight, or alternately, that the rate of weight gain is less than expected from past experience, known breed standards, or in comparison with other animals on the premises. Some conditions discussed in this chapter may cause either actual weight loss or a failure to gain weight in growing animals.

CLINICAL EXAMINATION FOR DIAGNOSIS OF WEIGHT LOSS

Clinical examination of the goat is covered in detail in Chapter 1. Aspects relevant to the problem of ill thrift are briefly reviewed here.

History Taking

A number of the causes of weight loss are infectious diseases with chronic, subclinical, or carrier forms, notably caprine arthritis encephalitis, caseous lymphadenitis, and paratuberculosis. Therefore, it is important to establish how long the herd or flock has been in existence, whether or not the owner knows the original sources of animals in the herd, the disease status of those herds of origin, and whether any pre-purchase testing for these or other diseases was performed on animals brought into the herd.

Determine if and when there have been any previous cases of weight loss. If similar cases occurred in previous years, it suggests an endemic condition. Any patterns of occurrence within a certain age group or with regard to season, housing, pasturing, feeding, or other management conditions should be evaluated. Questions regarding current cases should include information about the possibility of recent stressful situations such as parturition, purchase and introduction into the herd, transport and attendance at sales or shows, or episodes of acute disease, since such stresses can trigger latent paratuberculosis or expose the animal to new infections. Evaluation of parasite control programs is important. Determine that control efforts are directed at all important types of internal and external parasites. Establish that the anthelmintics employed are appropriate and effective and determine how available pastures are used for grazing, including information about rotation and stocking rates.

The history related to feeding may be critical in many cases. Solicit information on the basic ration fed to the group or groups showing weight loss and any recent changes in feedstuffs, feeding methods, feeder space, feeder design, or number of animals fed per group. Be sure that feeding programs are appropriate for the level and type of production being called for in each group. Nutrient requirements for different levels and types of production are given in Chapter 19.

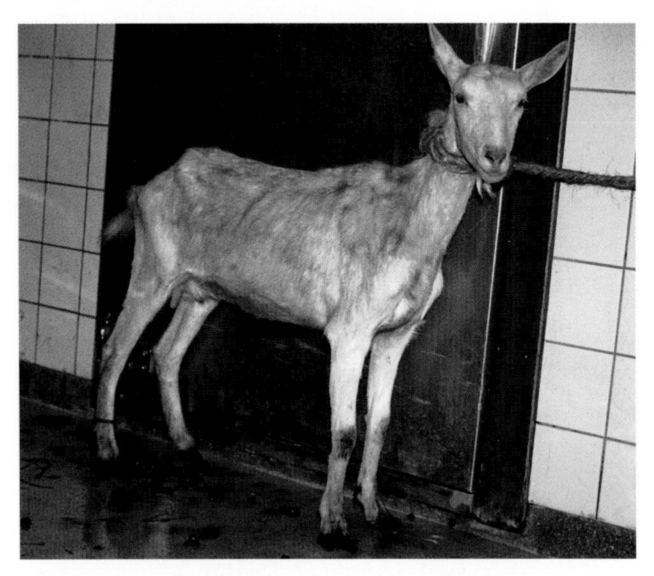

Figure 15.1. Wasting goats such as this one, with no other localizing signs, present a diagnostic challenge for the veterinary practitioner. This particular doe was ultimately diagnosed with paratuberculosis. (Courtesy Dr. Daan Dercksen.)

Physical Examination

All animals in contact with the thin animal should be examined at least from a distance to detect any clinical signs, such as coughing or diarrhea, which might represent conditions that could manifest in a chronic form as weight loss. An assessment of body condition in herd mates by digital palpation of the back, ribs, and sternum is essential to establish the body condition perceived as normal by the owner and to determine the prevalence of thin goats in the group. This is particularly important in Angora goats, in which the fleece may hide body condition. For veterinarians more familiar with dairy breeds, the normal Angora goat feels thin because these animals are more slightly built by nature.

On direct examination, weakness, dullness, lack of appetite, and a rough hair coat are all nonspecific signs associated with ill thrift that may accompany weight loss. Careful physical examination may reveal additional abnormalities undetected by the owner that can help in diagnosis. Some specific points to consider are as follows.

Examine the skin for lice, keds, or fleas by carefully parting the hair on the face, body, and limbs and look in the ears and under the tail for ticks.

A thorough oral examination may reveal brachygnathism, tooth loss, gum or alveolar abscesses, painful sores, or other abnormalities that might interfere with normal prehension, mastication, or swallowing. Evaluate the gums and other mucous membranes for anemia or icterus suggestive of chronic helminthiasis or liver fluke infestation. Check for nasal discharges that could indicate lung disease or nasal adenocarcinomas.

Routine palpation of all superficial lymph nodes is essential because several causes of weight loss may cause lymph node enlargement. These include caseous lymphadenitis, melioidosis, tuberculosis, trypanosomosis, and lymphosarcoma. In thin goats, however, be aware that lymph nodes may be more readily palpable, giving a false impression of enlargement. In this case, asymmetrically sized nodes are of greater significance. Careful auscultation of the lungs may reveal abnormalities consistent with chronic pneumonia. Displacement of the heart by a mediastinal mass may alter normal heart sounds. Because congenital heart disease may occasionally occur and lead to ill thrift, cardiac murmurs should be noted when present.

Establish the presence of normal rumination and gut motility. Assess the animal for ascites or rumen impaction by ballotment or observation of the abdominal contour.

Foot and joint problems should not be overlooked as a cause of inefficient grazing that can result in weight loss. Check the interdigital space for foot scald and pare out the feet to assess for foot rot. Palpate all joints carefully. Forced exercise may help identify signs of limb problems, chronic pneumonia, or anemia.

Environmental Examination

The level of general sanitation is important in confinement operations. Manure buildup contributes to the spread of coccidiosis, paratuberculosis, and chronic mastitis. Overcrowding can facilitate transmission of lice and pneumonia and predispose to herd outbreaks of enteric diseases, some of which can assume chronic forms. Poorly drained paddocks and barns can contribute to foot problems and coccidiosis.

All components of the ration should be inspected for spoilage, molds, and palatability. Look for fouled or frozen water supplies, which can reduce water and feed intake. Chronic weight loss can be related to the way animals are fed. If young animals can climb or defecate in feeders, then fecal contamination promotes the spread of coccidiosis. Keyhole-type feeders common in goat dairies may facilitate the rupture of lymph node abscesses on the head and neck during feeding, causing contamination of feed and spread of caseous lymphadenitis. Inadequate feeder space in either keyhole-type or trough-type feeding systems may deprive individual animals, low in the social pecking order, of adequate feed intake.

In range systems the stocking rate; availability and quality of forage, water, and supplemental feeds; and current weather conditions must be considered when thin animals are observed. Angora goats have specialized needs for supplemental protein and energy at different times in their fiber production and reproductive cycles and these requirements can be heightened by harsh weather.

Laboratory Diagnosis and Necropsy

Despite thorough clinical examination and knowledge of the likely causes, the definitive diagnosis of chronic weight loss may remain elusive. Hematology and clinical chemistry are often unrewarding, merely confirming the presence of undifferentiated chronic disease. Serology, however, can be helpful in the diagnosis of some infectious causes of weight loss, especially CAE and paratuberculosis. Fecal examination can assist in the diagnosis of various endoparasitisms.

When multiple animals are affected in commercial herds or flocks, sacrifice of an individual animal for post mortem examination is justifiable on economic grounds. The animal should be checked thoroughly for evidence of gastrointestinal, pulmonary, and hepatic parasites and for internal abscesses. The degree of rumen fill and the general body condition should be noted. Emaciated goats with obvious loss of muscle mass and perirenal fat, paradoxically, may still have noticeable fat deposits in the mesentery. This should not be interpreted as evidence of good body condition because goats preferentially store whatever fat they have intra-abdominally rather than subcutaneously.

For field necropsy, tissues submitted for histopathological examination in addition to any gross lesions should include kidney, carpal synovial tissue, and ileocecal lymph node and valve for diagnosis of amyloidosis, CAEV infection, and paratuberculosis, respectively, because these conditions may not be evident from gross findings.

CAUSES OF WASTING DISEASE

In this section, likely causes of weight loss in goats are given by etiologic category. The main intent is to provide a list for differential diagnosis, including only that information that may help to determine its relevance to the case at hand. Additional information about the diagnosis, treatment, and prevention of each disease is provided elsewhere in this volume along with references. In general, nutritional deficiencies, parasitisms, and dental disease are the conditions most amenable to treatment.

Nutrition-related Causes

Nutrition-related causes of chronic weight loss fit in either of two categories: primary cases resulting from the unavailability of appropriate feed or specific nutrients, or secondary cases caused by the inability of animals to obtain or use feed when available.

Primary Nutritional Problems

In extensive systems, feed availability can be curtailed by sustained, severe weather conditions such as drought or heavy snow cover, and also by overgrazing, overstocking, or failure to provide supplemental feed when nutrition requirements are not being met. Weight loss, emaciation, or even outright starvation may occur under these circumstances. In confinement systems, inadequate feeder space can lead to weight loss. This should become apparent if animals are observed during feeding. In any management system, specific nutritional deficiencies may be caused by inappropriate feedstuffs, unexpected feed shortages, unbalanced rations, inexperience with livestock feeding, and occasionally, neglect.

Regarding specific deficiencies, inadequate energy and protein levels are most commonly involved in cases of primary nutritional weight loss. Feed analysis may be necessary to establish the availability of protein and energy in the overall ration. The results of such analyses must be compared with established nutrient requirements for goats in the relevant type and stage of production and climatic region.

Cobalt deficiency may be a specific cause of progressive emaciation with no localizing signs in goats. In the United States, portions of New England, the upper midwest, and the southeast have cobalt-deficient soils, as do parts of New Zealand, Australia, the UK, Germany, the Netherlands, and Kenya. Goats grazing cobalt-deficient pastures show loss of appetite, rough hair coat, weakness, muscle wasting, and anemia, and may die after several weeks to months. In pastured animals, cobalt deficiency must be differentiated from gastrointestinal helminthiasis, which produces similar signs. Diagnosis of cobalt deficiency can be established by response to parenteral vitamin B_{12} administration or oral cobalt chloride. Appetite returns within a few days of treatment.

Copper deficiency can cause inadequate weight gains in growing goats. Diagnosis may be aided by the presence of other clinical signs including anemia, pigmentation defects in the hair coat, conjunctivitis, prolonged diarrhea, and incoordination in newborn (swayback) and young goats (enzootic ataxia). Copper deficiency can also increase susceptibility to gastrointestinal parasitism and adult goats with copper deficiency and parasites may be emaciated, anemic, and hypoproteinemic.

Where forage quality is extremely poor, with little or no fresh green forage available, hypovitaminosis A may contribute to progressive emaciation. Other signs of vitamin A deficiency may include night blindness, corneal cloudiness, ocular discharge, and neurologic signs including convulsive seizures.

Secondary Nutritional Problems

A variety of possibilities must be considered which could limit the animal's ability to obtain or use feed. These include the following:

Behavioral Problems. Even when feeder space is adequate, goats with a low social standing in the herd hierarchy may have their attempts to eat thwarted by more dominant goats who drive them away from feeders. This can be determined by observation at feeding time. Regrouping animals or feeding affected individuals separately may resolve the problem.

During the breeding season, bucks, though otherwise healthy, often become quite thin, presumably because of less time spent eating and more time and energy spent in amorous pursuits. It is imperative that bucks enter the breeding season in good health and good body condition because a certain amount of weight loss is inevitable.

Oral Problems. Goats with marked brachygnathism may be unable to prehend and masticate efficiently and not do well under extensive management. In confinement feeding systems, affected animals are usually able to consume adequate feed.

The excessive wear or loss of teeth, a common cause of thin ewe syndrome, can also occur in goats, though it is less frequent. This is because goats are more likely than sheep to browse in range and pasture and therefore less likely to wear away teeth by grazing low to the ground on abrasive soils. Nevertheless, thin does, particularly older does, should be checked for tooth loss. Tooth wear may be aggravated by inadequate dietary calcium or calcium/phosphorus imbalance resulting in softer teeth, or by fluoride toxicity. When cutting and grinding surfaces of teeth are excessively worn, prehension and mastication become inefficient and feed intake and utilization decrease. Water intake can also diminish because worn teeth are more sensitive to cold temperatures. Animals with dental attrition become progressively weaker and emaciated and can succumb to secondary disease processes, particularly pneumonia and pregnancy toxemia.

Periodontal disease can be an additional cause of tooth loss. Coarse feeds or awns of certain plants may pack between gums and teeth, initiating a progressive cycle of infection, tooth loosening, tooth socket deterioration, and additional impaction of foreign material until teeth are dramatically loosened or expelled. Osteomyelitis of the jawbones may also result.

Signs of molar loss include pouching of the cheeks from feed impaction in empty molar sockets, dribbling of fluid from the mouth, excessive staining of the lips and teeth, and a necrotic or stale feed odor to the breath. When a molar is missing, the normally apposing molar grows excessively long because of a lack of occlusal wear, causing trauma to soft tissues in the mouth.

Animals with severe dental attrition or periodontal disease should be culled. The productive life of animals with moderate dental disease can be prolonged by placing them on lusher pasture, feeding processed feeds in confinement, and floating sharp teeth with a flat file. Supplementing calcium and balancing it with phosphorus are indicated as preventive and therapeutic measures in herds in which the diet was previously inadequate.

Soft Tissue Infections. Contagious ecthyma is common in goats worldwide and can produce painful, scabby lesions on the lips that persist from three to six weeks or longer if secondary bacterial infections occur. These lesions can impair feed intake and lead to weight loss. Less common or geographically restricted causes of stomatitis that can cause dysphagia, inappetence, and weight loss are discussed in Chapter 10. Peste des petits ruminants causes severe stomatitis, affecting the gums, tongue, lips, and palate. These lesions may be slow to heal in nonfatal cases, leading to prolonged reduction in feed intake and weight loss. Foot and mouth disease can also affect goats, but foot lesions tend to be more common and severe than oral lesions.

Blindness. Animals fed in confinement can readily adapt to sudden blindness if surroundings are unchanged. Grazing animals on sparse rangelands, however, probably depend heavily on sight for adequate feed intake. Angora goats with excessive hair covering of the face, an inherited trait, graze inefficiently because of impaired vision. They may become thin and often succumb to secondary disease problems.

Blindness in goats may be caused by gid, hypovitaminosis A, permanent corneal damage after outbreaks of infectious keratoconjunctivitis, or as a sequel to polioencephalomalacia.

Locomotor Problems. Foot and leg problems can interfere with efficient grazing or produce sufficient pain to keep animals recumbent instead of standing at the feeders. Weight loss associated with a reluctance of ambulate and eat may precede outward signs of lameness.

Numerous conditions can lead to impaired locomotion. Foot rot, foot scald, and foot abscesses occur in goats. Chronic bacterial polyarthritis can occur in very young kids after navel infection. *Mycoplasma* spp. are an important cause of arthritis in goats worldwide and the caprine arthritis encephalitis (CAE) virus has been recognized as a major cause of arthritis and lameness since 1980. Where it occurs, foot and mouth disease can affect goats and produce lameness with impaired locomotion. Noninfectious conditions that cause impaired mobility and reduced intake include fractures, other traumatic limb injuries, peripheral nerve damage, or rickets secondary to mineral imbalances.

Viral and Prion Causes of Chronic Weight Loss

Caprine Arthritis Encephalitis Virus (CAEV)

It is the arthritic form of CAEV infection which is generally associated with weight loss. This form most often appears clinically between one and two years of age, with great variability in the progression and severity of signs. The first sign of CAE may be unexplained weight loss, followed by stiffness and reluctance to move. Periods of recumbency increase, food intake diminishes, and weight loss becomes more pronounced. Some goats become severely crippled within a few months while others may show only intermittent lameness or stiffness for years, and remain that way indefinitely.

Far less commonly, a pneumonic form of CAE occurs in mature goats that produces long-term interstitial pneumonia with intermittent secondary bacterial pneumonia, exercise intolerance, and weight loss.

Weight loss may occur independently of arthritic or pneumonic signs in goats that are infected with the virus as demonstrated by serology. Because CAEV infection is a chronic infection, wasting may be an effect of endogenous cytokine release, and may not depend only on decreased ambulation and feed intake. Because many serologically positive goats never show any signs of disease, however, other possible causes for weight loss must also be considered in thin, otherwise normal goats with positive CAE serologic tests.

Other Viral and Prion Diseases

Contagious ecthyma is discussed above under oral problems. Foot and mouth disease usually produces mild clinical signs in goats, but lameness and oral lesions may impair feed intake sufficiently to cause weight loss.

Scrapie, a prion infection of small ruminants, is less common in goats as compared to sheep, but a case with weight loss as the principal sign of scrapie in a goat has been reported from Britain. An affected herd mate showed the more typical scrapie signs of progressive incoordination and intense pruritus, while the goat in question showed only progressive weight loss, listlessness, and a premature cessation of milk production. Diagnosis was confirmed by histopathologic examination of the brain.

Peste des petits ruminants can cause pronounced weight loss and debilitation in goats during the prolonged convalescent periods that may follow recovery from the acute diarrheal and respiratory phase of the disease. As mentioned above, severe stomatitis in the acute phase may also contribute to decreased feed intake.

Pulmonary adenomatosis, or jaagsiekte, is a neoplastic transformation of the lung caused by a retrovirus distinct from CAEV. It is primarily a sheep disease but has been reported in goats. The disease produces a syndrome of progressive dyspnea and weight loss with pronounced nasal discharge over a period of several months. Moist lung sounds are audible and considerable fluid drains from the lungs if the animal is held vertically with the head hanging down. Diagnosis is by histopathologic examination of the lungs.

Bacterial Causes of Chronic Weight Loss

Paratuberculosis (Johne's Disease)

It is very likely that paratuberculosis is a frequent but undiagnosed cause of progressive weight loss in adult goats. Failure to diagnose this condition usually results from three factors. First, chronic diarrhea, the cardinal sign of paratuberculosis in cattle, is rarely observed in goats, so veterinarians familiar with the cattle disease may not consider paratuberculosis when confronted with a thin goat. Second, rapid, reliable laboratory tests have not been readily available as aids to clinical diagnosis. Last, gross post mortem lesions of intestinal thickening, common in cattle, are uncommonly seen in affected goats. In most cases, histopathologic examination of intestinal tissue with acid-fast staining and/or mycobacterial culture of feces or intestine must be performed to establish paratuberculosis as the cause of chronic weight loss. Such examinations are warranted in unexplained caprine wasting disease because of the relative importance of paratuberculosis as a cause of weight loss that is commonly overlooked in goats.

Caseous Lymphadenitis

This important chronic infectious disease of goats caused by *Corynebacterium pseudotuberculosis (C. ovis)* is best known by the superficial lymphadenopathy it produces. However, abscesses of internal lymph nodes and viscera also occur, though less commonly. While the impact of superficial lymph node abscesses on general health in goats is not remarkable, a stronger association exists between progressive emaciation and internal abscesses.

Antemortem diagnosis of internal abscesses can be difficult. Goats with internal abscesses often do not have concurrent superficial abscesses. Physical exam rarely establishes proof of an internal lymph node abscess, although large abscesses in the chest may alter normal heart and lung sounds and large abdominal abscesses are sometimes palpable. Radiography or ultrasonography may be helpful if large or focally calcified abscesses are present. Neutrophilia and hypergammaglobulinemia may support the diagnosis but are not pathognomonic. At necropsy, thoracic and abdominal organs should be examined and abscesses cultured because other pyogenic organisms may be involved. Tuberculosis may present similarly.

Tuberculosis

Tuberculosis is uncommon in goats but sporadic cases continue to be reported. *Mycobacterium bovis* is the most common cause, but *M. avium* and *M. tuberculosis* also occur, and the zoonotic potential of the disease should be respected. Tuberculous goats often are commingled with cattle. The presentation of weight loss is variable. It may precede other clinical signs, accompany them, or not occur at all. Clinical tuberculosis most often manifests as chronic pneumonia with a moist, persistent, productive cough. Intestinal tuberculosis also occurs with diarrhea as a presenting sign. Antemortem diagnosis is by intradermal skin test. At post mortem examination, obvious caseated, sometimes calcified, parenchymal or lymph node granulomas are present. Tuberculosis coincident with paratuberculosis in goats has been reported from Spain. In such cases, definitive diagnosis depends on mycobacterial culture of granulomatous lesions.

Melioidosis

This infection caused by a soil saprophyte, *Burkholderia (Pseudomonas) pseudomallei*, is reported from tropical regions, primarily southeast Asia and Australia. It may be endemic in some regions and outbreaks are associated with flooding of pastures. Acute and chronic forms are seen in goats. Clinical manifestations are varied and include high fever, nasal discharge, pneumonia, lymphadenopathy, mastitis, orchitis, polyarthritis, and frequently neurologic signs including ataxia, head tilt, nystagmus, or circling. Acute deaths may occur within twenty-four to forty-eight hours after fever, weakness, and recumbency. Animals that survive may have any of the signs noted in addition to pronounced weight loss. Asymptomatic infections can also occur in the herd. The organism may be transmitted in goat milk and the disease is zoonotic.

Ante mortem diagnosis may be accomplished by bacterial culture of milk, nasal discharges, or aspirates of swollen lymph nodes; skin testing with meliodin; or serologic methods, including complement fixation and indirect hemagglutination assays. Necropsy usually reveals multiple abscesses in numerous organs, especially spleen, liver, and lungs. These abscesses should be cultured (see Chapter 3).

Chronic Bacterial Infection

Any prolonged infection may contribute to a process of progressive debilitation and wasting, referred to as cachexia, which in and of itself can contribute to an adverse patient outcome. The mechanisms of cachexia are multifactorial and not fully understood. Alterations in carbohydrate, protein, and lipid metabolism all contribute to the loss of tissue and body mass. It is believed that these metabolic changes are driven by an inflammatory response and are mediated in part by dysregulated production of proinflammatory cytokines such as interleukin 1, interleukin 6, and tissue necrosis factor. Current knowledge on the mechanisms of cachexia have been recently reviewed (Delano and Moldawer 2006). The mechanisms of cachexia have not been studied directly in the goat, but the process is certainly at play in chronic caprine infections such as paratuberculosis, tuberculosis, and melioidosis, as discussed above. Other chronic bacterial infections likely to be associated with weight loss in goats are as follows:

Pasteurella and *Mannheimia* pneumonias of goats are common and often become chronic due to failure of early detection coupled with inadequate therapy. Chronic pasteurellosis is often complicated by secondary lung abscessation due to *Arcanobacterium pyogenes.* Careful auscultation and radiology may confirm the presence of chronic pneumonia and abscessation.

Chronic mastitis cases are generally culled from commercial goat dairies in a timely fashion. Hobbyists, however, may show a marked reluctance to cull mastitic does. Typically, affected does with chronic mastitis appear thin and depressed, and have a pendulous udder containing extensive fibrotic areas and multiple large firm abscesses, often caused by *Arcanobacterium pyogenes* (Figure 15.2).

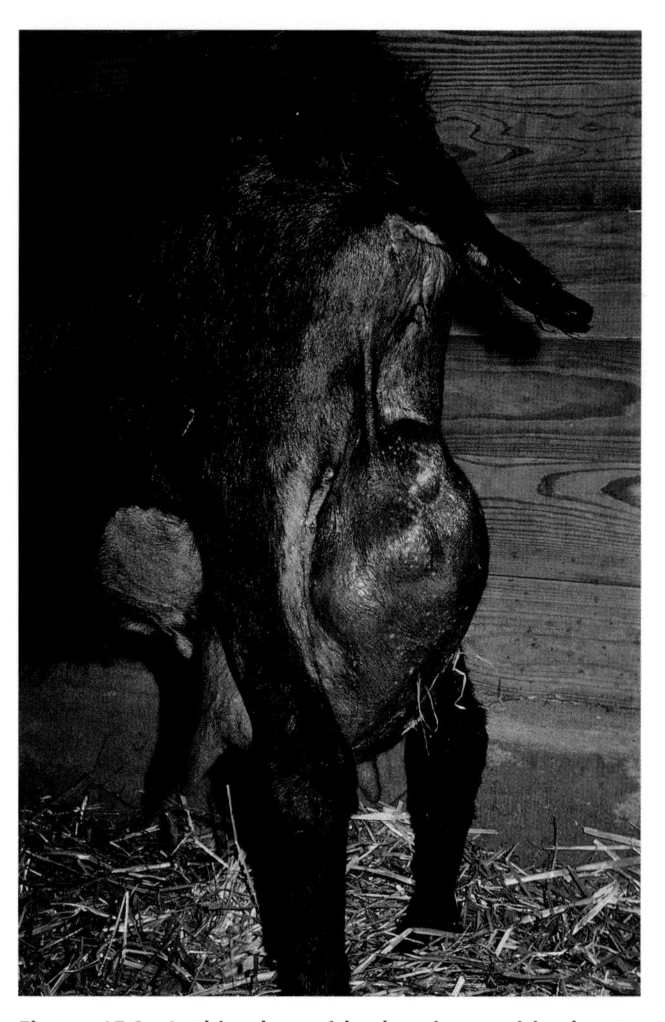

Figure 15.2. A thin doe with chronic mastitis due to *Arcanobacterium pyogenes*. Note the characteristic, large, nodular, multiple abscesses in the udder. (Courtesy Dr. David M. Sherman.)

Peritonitis can occur secondary to a number of conditions. These include rumenitis resulting from grain overload, migration of liver flukes through abdominal organs, administration of irritating drugs intraperitoneally, the rupture of internal abscesses, and as sequelae to abdominal surgery or septicemia. Abscesses, adhesions, and bowel stenosis can occur as a result. Diagnosis is based on history of predisposing conditions, evidence of fever and abdominal pain, digestive dysfunction, an inflammatory blood picture, and supportive abdominocentesis findings. Thin animals with evidence of peritonitis should be culled.

Salmonellosis and enterotoxemia present most often as causes of acute, frequently fatal, enteritis or toxemia. Chronic forms of both diseases, however, occasionally occur in adult goats, and their clinical presentations are quite similar. Both conditions are characterized by periodic intermittent diarrhea accompanied by fever, loss of appetite, and depression. Sporadic recurrences may be observed over several months, accompanied by progressive weight loss. Notably, the chronic form of enterotoxemia can occur even in animals with a strong vaccination history against *Clostridium perfringens* type D. Definitive diagnosis depends on isolation of *Salmonella* spp. during episodes of active diarrhea or, in the case of enterotoxemia, identification of epsilon toxin in diarrheic feces or gut content.

Parasitic Causes of Chronic Weight Loss

Both ectoparasites and endoparasites can contribute significantly to progressive weight loss in goats, either primarily or in association with malnutrition or concurrent disease.

Gastrointestinal Parasitism

Coccidiosis. Coccidiosis is easily diagnosed as a cause of diarrhea, dysentery, dehydration, and often death in young kids. However, less obvious is the fact that animals that survive clinical coccidiosis often suffer sufficient damage to the intestinal mucosa that normal growth and development are permanently impaired, presumably due to occurrence of intestinal malabsorption. Specific diagnosis of this condition is difficult. A history of coccidiosis on the farm and exclusion of other likely causes of poor growth or inadequate weight gain may lead to a presumptive diagnosis of chronic intestinal damage secondary to coccidiosis.

Nematodiasis. Nematodiasis is the most important parasitism contributing to ill thrift. Young animals between two and twenty-four months of age are most often affected, but age-related resistance to parasitism is not as strong in goats as it is in cattle, and clinical parasitism is not uncommon in older animals, particularly when concurrent disease or poor nutrition is present. Clinical evidence of gastrointestinal parasitism includes pale mucous membranes, fluid accumulation between the jaws (bottle jaw), weakness, decreased growth rate or milk production, rough hair coat, and progressive weight loss or emaciation. Diarrhea is not a consistent finding.

Cestodiasis. Tapeworms occur in goats worldwide. Their contributory role in the development of weight loss is controversial, but in general they are not considered to be clinically important unless heavy infestations are found in animals younger than six months of age, in which case they may contribute to poor growth. An inordinate amount of importance is placed on tapeworm infestation by goat owners because they can readily observe tapeworm segments (proglottids) in goat feces.

The goat can serve as an intermediate host for tapeworms of the genera *Taenia* and *Echinococcus*, resulting in cysticercosis and hydatidosis, respectively. These conditions usually remain subclinical, producing no signs other than poor weight gain in young animals. Sometimes they produce peritonitis with accompanying fever, depression, and weakness. Diagnosis is usually accomplished at slaughter or necropsy when numerous, large, larval cysts are found in abdominal viscera, mesentery, and lungs.

Trematodiasis. Four species of liver flukes affect goats: *Fasciola hepatica*, *F. gigantica*, *Fascioloides magna*, and *Dicrocoelium dendriticum*. While acute and chronic forms of liver fluke disease occur, it is the chronic form caused by *Fasciola* spp. that is associated with weight loss. This results from localization and persistence of adult flukes in the bile ducts, where they consume blood and produce bile duct irritation with resultant liver dysfunction. The clinical syndrome produced may be indistinguishable from gastrointestinal nematodiasis, although icterus is sometimes seen. Ova may be found in feces using sedimentation techniques, but diagnosis is easiest at necropsy, where adult flukes and their excretions are found in the bile ducts. Note that *Fascioloides magna* infestation can cause weight loss and death without the appearance of eggs in the feces.

Pancreatic flukes of the genus *Eurytrema* can also produce emaciation in goats. The condition is discussed further in Chapter 11.

Schistosomosis can produce ill thrift in goats in Asia, Africa, the Middle East, South and Central America, and the Mediterranean region. The disease occurs where livestock are exposed to aquatic snails, the intermediate parasite hosts. In the nasal form, weight loss is accompanied by snoring, sneezing, and dyspnea, and in the intestinal form, by diarrhea and anemia. This form may be clinically indistinguishable from gastrointestinal nematodiasis. Diagnosis is based on identifying parasite eggs in feces, urine, liver biopsy specimens, or nasal discharges.

Lungworm Infestations

Three species of lungworms affect goats in the United States. *Dictyocaulus filaria* has a direct life cycle and is considered the most pathogenic. *Protostrongylus rufescens* and *Muellerius capillaris* both have snail intermediate hosts and are considered less pathogenic. All are likely to occur in cool, wet, autumnal weather when younger stock on lowland or irrigated pastures ingest infective larvae or snails. While adult *Dictyocaulus* and *Protostrongylus* cause obvious coughing in affected goats by irritating airways, adult forms of *Muellerius capillaris* do not because they do not reach the airways. They reside in the alveoli, producing small, gray-green nodules visible at necropsy on the surface of the diaphragmatic lobes. Weight loss may accompany respiratory signs in *Dictyocaulus* infection, but may be the only clinical sign of severe *Muellerius* infection.

External Parasites

Ectoparasites can contribute to ill thrift when infestations are severe and concurrent diseases are present. Biting lice such as *Damalina caprae* may cause irritation to affected hosts, leading to reduced feeding efficiency. The blue louse of goats, *Linognathus stenopsis*, feeds on host blood using piercing mouth parts and causes anemia and weight loss. Lice are more common in winter months and are promoted by confinement and overcrowding. Parasites are visible when the hair is parted and the skin carefully observed.

Among the mange mites affecting goats, *Sarcoptes*, and to a lesser extent, *Chorioptes*, can produce intense pruritus which torments the host and results in decreased feeding activity and weight loss. Generalized crusting and flaking of the skin with alopecia are apparent and skin scrapings should confirm the diagnosis. The sheep ked, *Melophagus ovinus*, also affects goats and can produce intense pruritus, particularly in winter. A period of ill thrift has been observed in goats with demodectic mange and also in association with heavy ear mite infestation.

In tropical regions, heavy infestations of goats with fleas of the genus *Ctenocephalides* can cause anorexia, anemia, weight loss, and even death. Kid goats are most severely affected.

Hemoparasites

Trypanosomosis affects goats in the tsetse fly regions of Africa. Acute, subacute, and chronic forms occur. Severe emaciation is associated with chronic disease. Additional clinical signs may include anemia, depression, anorexia, lack of rumen motility, and peripheral lymphadenopathy. Diagnosis is by identifying the hemoparasite on stained blood smears.

Rarely, eperythrozoonosis may be a cause of anemia and ill thrift in goats. Infection is usually subclinical. Caprine infection is reported in Pakistan, South Africa, Australia, and Cuba.

Miscellaneous Causes of Chronic Weight Loss

Plant Toxicities

A wide variety of poisonous plants may affect goats on pasture or range. Most plant intoxications produce sudden death or an acute disease syndrome which does not involve weight loss. One important exception is toxicity due to locoweed (*Astragalus* spp.), a chronic intoxication characterized by mild nervous signs, muscular incoordination, fetal abnormality or abortion, and chronic, progressive weight loss. Locoism is seen most commonly in the western United States. Goats are susceptible, though the disease is seen more often in sheep. Lupinosis, a common cause of weight loss, anorexia, depression, and jaundice in sheep in Europe, Australia, New Zealand, and South Africa, is not reported to occur in goats. In Germany, Austria, and Switzerland (Braun et al. 2000), a syndrome of vitamin D toxicity causing progressive weight loss, lameness, decreased milk production, and calcification of soft tissues has been observed in goats consuming yellow oat grass (*Trisetum flavescens*), which contains 1,25 dihdroxycholecalciferol. This golden oat grass intoxication may also cause cardiovascular abnormalities and is discussed further in Chapter 8.

Gastrointestinal Foreign Bodies

In South Africa, phytobezoars consisting of seed hairs of karoo bushes can cause abomasal impaction in grazing goats. Progressive weight loss accompanied by progressive abdominal distension suggests this diagnosis. Recently, anorexia and progressive weight loss of six weeks duration was reported in three Angora goats, subsequently confirmed by necropsy of two and rumenotomy of the third to have multiple hair balls (trichobezoars) in their rumens (Baillie and Anzuino 2006).

Consumption of plastic trash bags is common where rubbish disposal is uncontrolled and where goats forage in urban areas, as is common in Africa, the Middle East, and South Asia (Figure 15.3). Baling twine can be ingested when confined goats are fed baled hay. These foreign bodies can lead to partial gastrointestinal obstructions, chronic indigestion, abdominal distension, and weight loss. In a study from Jordan, 4.5% of 722 adult goat cases presented at a veterinary teaching hospital over a 3.75-year period were diagnosed with soft foreign bodies (plastic) in their rumens and reticuli (Hailat et al. 1998).

Neoplasia

In general, tumors are an uncommon finding in goats and therefore are a relatively infrequent cause of progressive emaciation. However, neoplasia still should be considered in a differential diagnosis of chronic weight loss, especially in older goats kept as pets, because they are often kept to very advanced ages, with a concurrent increase in the likelihood of neoplasia. Sporadic cases of neoplasia, including intestinal adenocarcinomas, have been diagnosed at necropsy in adult goats after a prolonged course of ill thrift. More consistently, enzootic intranasal tumors of goats have been reported, primarily in Europe. Affected goats show persistent, profuse, often unilateral, serous nasal discharge; progressive dyspnea; and chronic weight loss. It has been demonstrated by transmission studies that these nasal adenocarcinomas are caused by a retrovirus (De las Heras et al. 1995). The disease is discussed further in Chapter 9.

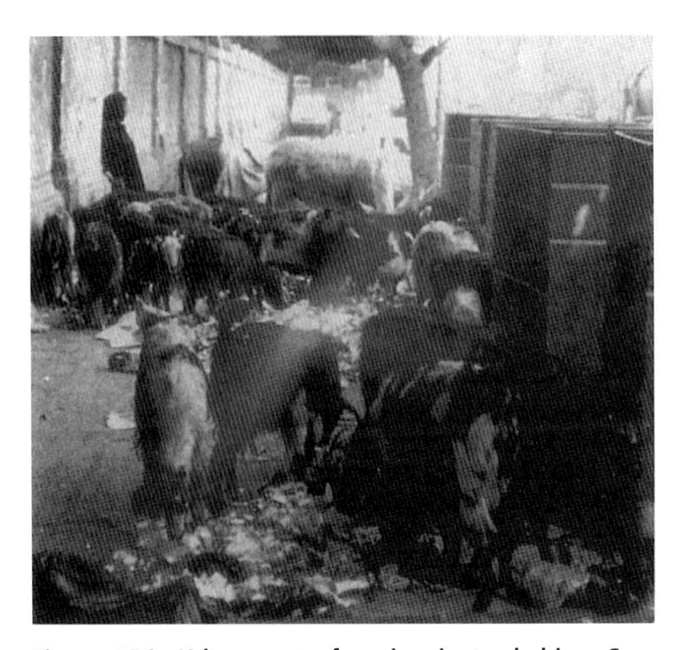

Figure 15.3. Urban goats foraging in trash bins. Consumption of plastic bags can lead to blockage of the reticulo-omasal orifice, resulting in chronic indigestion and weight loss. (Courtesy Dr. Laurie C. Miller.)

Amyloidosis

Goats are used extensively in research and industry to produce antibodies for commerce or research. Repeated immune stimulation in these animals with adjuvanted antigens can stimulate the production and deposition of renal amyloid. Renal amyloidosis manifests clinically as progressive emaciation with weakness, anorexia, depression, and possible edema and ascites caused by hypoproteinemia subsequent to proteinuria. Diarrhea may also be present, caused by hypoproteinemia or concurrent intestinal amyloidosis. Diagnosis is aided by urinalysis and kidney biopsy. There is no treatment for the condition. Although amyloidosis is an unlikely cause of chronic weight loss in the general goat population, it may occur frequently in this specialized group of antibody-producing goats.

Other Sporadic Causes

Though an uncommon occurrence, congenital ventricular septal defect results in poor growth in young, affected goats. Stunted growth may also result from chronic aspiration pneumonia associated with cleft palate or other causes (Figure 15.4). In Nubian goats,

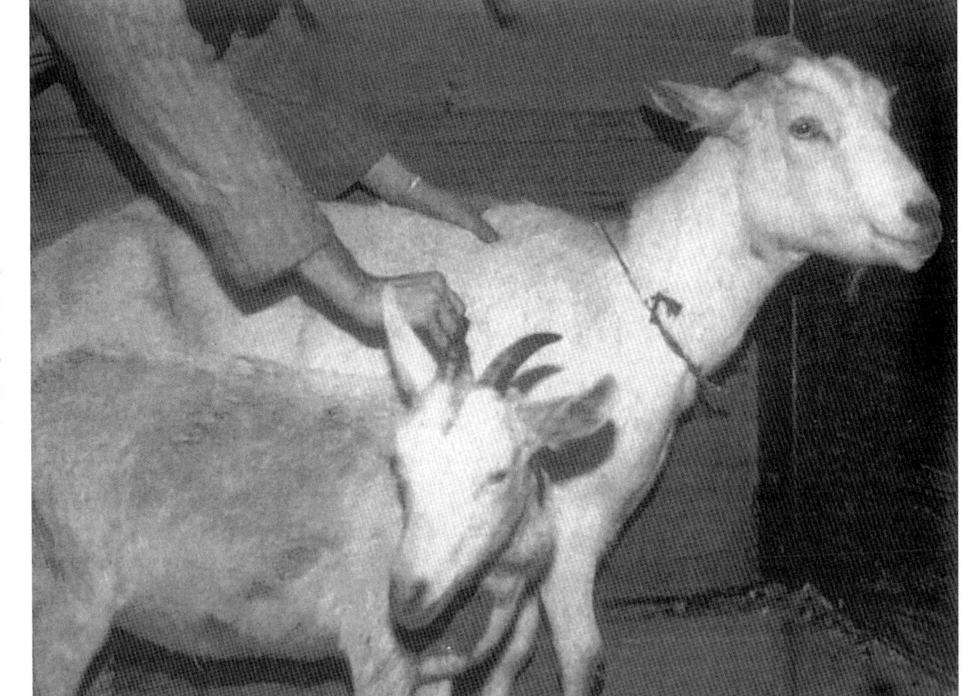

Figure 15.4. Two seven-month-old Saanen doeling sisters. The stunted goat in the foreground was diagnosed at presentation with a cleft palate. (Courtesy Dr. David M. Sherman.)

the inherited lysosomal storage disease mucopolysaccharidosis IIID can cause muscle wasting in homozygous, affected individuals, resulting in weakness and ill-thrift. The condition is discussed further in Chapter 5.

REFERENCES

Baillie, S. and Anzuino, K.: Hairballs as a cause of anorexia in Angora goats. Goat Vet. Soc. J., 22:53–55, 2006.

Braun, U., et al.: Enzootic calcinosis in goats caused by golden oat grass (*Trisetum flavescens*). Vet. Rec., 146:161–162, 2000.

Delano, M.J. and Moldawer, L.L.: The origins of cachexia in acute and chronic inflammatory diseases. Nutr. Clin. Pract., 21(1):68–81, 2006.

De las Heras, M. et al.: Experimental transmission of enzootic intranasal tumors of goats. Vet. Pathol. 32(1):19–23, 1995.

Hailat, N., et al.: Pathology of the rumen in goats caused by plastic foreign bodies with reference to its prevalence in Jordan. Small Rumin. Res., 30(2):77–83, 1998.

16

Sudden Death

The goat that is healthy one night and found dead the next morning poses a particular problem for the owner and the veterinarian. If an explanation for the death cannot be found, appropriate steps cannot be taken to prevent additional losses. On the other hand, a full necropsy by a diagnostic pathologist may be expensive. Not all owners are eager to pay much to get a diagnosis if the condition seems to be sporadic, and if the rest of the herd is not at risk. Note that in Germany, and possibly other countries, on-farm necropsies by owners or private veterinarians are forbidden by law, to avoid potential contamination of the environment with body fluids laden with infectious organisms. Thus, local regulations supercede the advice presented in this chapter.

PRELIMINARY DECISIONS

As a guide for deciding what course to follow, the answers to these questions should be reviewed.

1. Was the animal really healthy when last observed, or did it show some signs, albeit vague, such as poor appetite, weight loss, or lassitude? Is the body emaciated? The goat may have had a prolonged or chronic infection or parasitism, and others in the herd may also be affected.
2. Was the animal larger than, (tending to eat more), smaller than (with tendency for chronic disease, social hierarchy problems), older than, or younger than the others in its group? Was it persistently harassed by other animals or children?
3. Is any information to be gathered from the position of the carcass? Was a pygmy goat or obese animal stuck on its back where it died of bloat? Is the bedding disturbed, as by convulsions? Has the goat been strangled by a collar? Was lightning strike or electrocution possible?
4. Is this the first death, or is a pattern developing?
5. Has there been any change in feed? This includes different amounts or new feeds, even new batches of what is thought to be the same feed. Has the goat recently foraged where it does not usually go: in the garden, a cultivated field, or the grain room? Have children been hand-feeding it bread or other treats? Have irregularities occurred in availability of feed or water?
6. Was the animal recently treated with any anthelminthic, injectable selenium, or other medication?
7. What was the vaccination status of the animal?

Now what? The first decision must be made rapidly. If the body is not to be examined, then it should be disposed of at once, by burning, deep burial, or composting (Koebel et al. 2003), according to local regulations. Rendering companies in the United States usually do not accept carcasses of small ruminants because of the perceived risk of scrapie transmission. The body should not be left for domestic or wild animals to tear apart and drag all over the farm, thereby possibly spreading infectious disease (including hydatidosis) to animals and man; neither should it be buried near a water supply or left as a breeding ground for flies.

Almost every sudden death warrants some degree of investigation. This even includes the aborted fetus in a herd that has had no previous abortions. Because placenta or fetus may not be available from later cases, the first observed abortion becomes very important. The reader should refer to Chapter 13 for a detailed discussion of abortion diagnosis and zoonotic concerns.

The presence of unclotted blood at body orifices raises the specter of anthrax (Okoh 1981; de Vos and Turnbull 2004), and this possibility radically changes the options available. The body should not be opened, because exposure to air promotes sporulation of the causative bacteria. Instead, a veterinarian should take a blood sample in an evacuated tube from the jugular vein to be examined for the anthrax bacillus. Alternatively, an impression smear of ear blood can be used; an ear is grasped with a gloved hand, severed, and sealed in the everted glove for transport. Technicians or other laboratory personnel receiving or handling the specimen should be cautioned regarding possible danger. Anthrax is discussed in Chapter 7.

Examination by the Owner

The level of examination to be chosen varies with the knowledge of the owner and the availability and cost of the services of a veterinarian or diagnostic laboratory. It may also be influenced by the time of day, day of the week, and ambient temperature. It is often better for an owner to do what he can rather than wait for expert evaluation until the next day in hot weather or until two days later in a cold climate. If death is suspected to be caused by dog attack, local laws may permit indemnity payment if the proper authorities are notified before the necropsy is begun.

The practitioner on emergency duty should be prepared to relay instructions if there is no time to personally perform a necropsy. If the owner routinely does home slaughtering, it is often possible for him or her to recognize something in an organ as being different, even if the exact problem cannot be diagnosed. Digital photographs are helpful for documenting these findings. Also, when the examination is guided by the veterinarian, the normality of some organs can be established and recorded to help rule out certain conditions. If the owner does the initial or only examination, then it is exceedingly important that dogs be tied up and that protective, waterproof gloves be worn. Pregnant women should be dissuaded from performing necropsies without full protective garb, including a face mask. Organs or tissues with suspected lesions can be placed in waterproof containers and refrigerated until a veterinarian can examine them. If possible, they should be delivered immediately to the veterinarian's office rather than being stored in a home refrigerator where contamination of food might occur. An insulated box and several plastic jugs of ice provide a temporary cooler.

Necropsy Technique

Every veterinarian has had some instruction in field necropsies, but some may have forgotten important details. The first is to wear protective gloves and to plan ahead for safe disposal of carcass remnants. The next involves writing down the findings, including history, identification (tags and tattoos, color), weight, and age. The owner's statement of age should be compared with the teeth and tattoo.

The color of mucous membranes should be noted relative to possible anemia or icterus. Are the hindquarters soiled with feces (diarrhea) or are formed fecal pellets present in the rectum? Discharges from body orifices should be noted. Anthrax has already been mentioned as a cause of bloody discharges, but it should be noted that a bloody froth is commonly present at the nostrils of animals dead for a myriad of reasons, especially in warm weather.

The body should always be placed in the same position relative to the prosector (e.g., on its left side, head directed to the examiner's right [King 1983]). The necropsy should be performed in a routine and complete manner (Hindson and Winter 2002; King et al. 2005). A sharp post mortem knife is a great asset, but if necessary, the goat can be dissected with a disposable scalpel blade and a pair of foot trimming shears. Begin with a skin incision in the right axilla and cut through muscles beneath the scapula until the front limb can be folded back out of the way. Next, make an incision into the right hip joint and surrounding muscles, to fold back the hind limb. Connect the first two incisions by cutting the skin from the inside out and peeling it back off the thorax and abdomen. Carefully enter the abdominal cavity along the costal arch and reflect the abdominal wall. Observe the amount of omental fat and the position of the viscera. Animals lacking omental fat are in very poor body condition (Figure 16.1). If omental fat is present, verify that there is muscle and fat present over the lumbar vertebrae. The animal that began its illness with copious internal fat may give the false appearance of good body condition, even though it actually has severe muscle wasting.

Next, puncture the diaphragm and listen for the normal inrush of air as the lungs collapse. Cut the diaphragm off the rib cage. Foot trimmers permit cutting of the ribs at the costochondral junction, even in adults. The rib cage of a kid is folded back as one section. In an old goat, it may be necessary to use heavy tree branch loppers or to cut between the ribs and break one at a time near the spinal column. Examine the viscera in the thorax and abdomen systematically and note any fluid accumulations.

The brain of a young kid can be exposed by cutting the calvarium with heavy scissors, but a saw is needed when removing the brain of an adult. Remove skin from the top of the skull and make a first transverse saw cut just caudal to the zygomatic process of the frontal bone. Then make sagittal cuts on each side from just medial to the occipital condyle to join the first cut

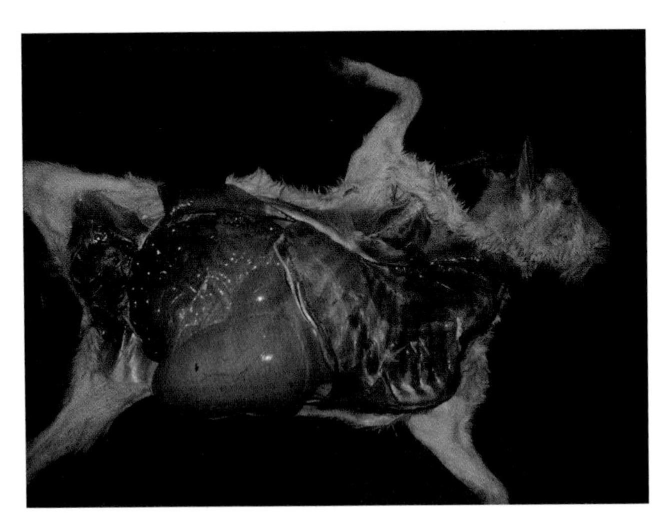

Figure 16.1. Emaciated goat lacking omental fat. The intestines should not be easily seen until the omentum has been removed. (Courtesy Dr. M.C. Smith.)

(King et al. 2005). Alternatively, four saw cuts can be made in a diamond pattern, with the anterior point of the diamond on the midline between the eyes. If the goat has large horns, the first transverse cut is made on the forehead anterior to the horns and angled caudally. The sagittal cuts are slanted toward the midline, and the skull cap with horns can then be lifted off, as illustrated in Figure 16.2.

Heart blood, urine (50 ml if possible), and cerebrospinal fluid (at the atlanto-occipital space) can be aspirated in a clean fashion and set aside for later examination. For instance, glucose is usually present in the urine of a goat that dies of enterotoxemia. Unfortunately, information regarding sensitivity and specificity of various findings in specified reference populations (for example, the percentage of goats dying in New York State with enterotoxemia that have glucosuria [equals sensitivity] or the percentage dying of something other than enterotoxemia that do not have glucosuria [equals specificity] is rarely available). Until the published literature provides such information, practitioners should tabulate their own records as to gross necropsy findings, simple test results, and final diagnosis. This permits later estimation of sensitivity, specificity, and even prior probability in a given practice setting.

Appropriate tissues or swabs (for example, abnormal lung, mammary gland, abscesses, or tied-off section of intestine) should be taken for bacteriologic and virologic testing. The laboratory to receive the specimens should be consulted relative to transport media, packaging, and shipping instructions. Sections should be taken for histologic study from the major organs (i.e., lung, liver, kidney, heart, mesenteric lymph node, brain stem, cerebellum, and cerebrum) and from

Figure 16.2. Opening the cranial cavity of a horned goat. (Courtesy Dr. M.C. Smith; Mr. Patrick Burke, prosector.)

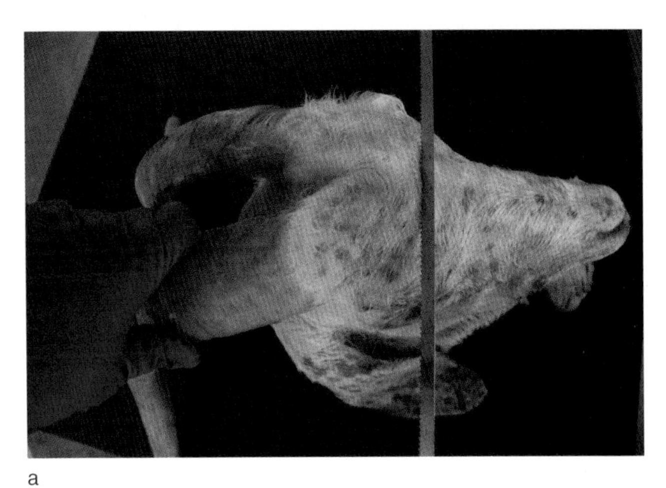

a

Figure 16.2a. The initial transverse saw cut is made on the forehead in front of the horns.

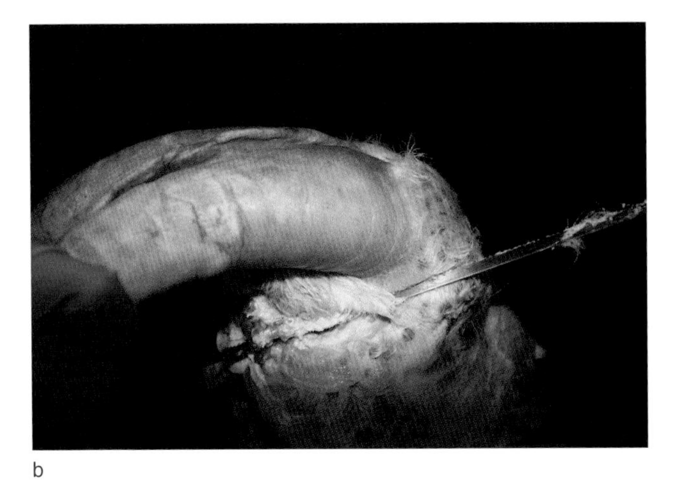

b

Figure 16.2b. The sagittal cuts are almost horizontal.

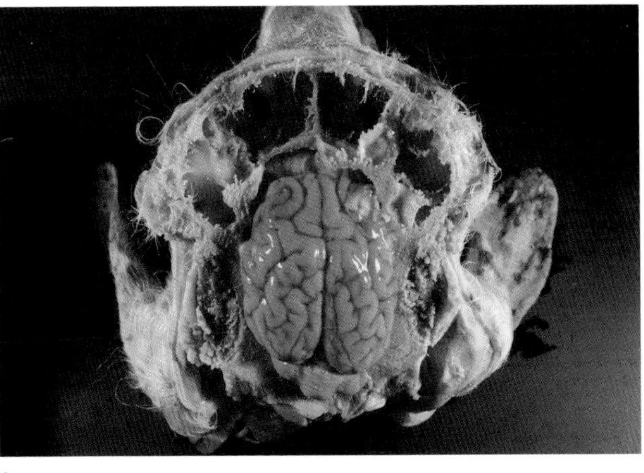

c

Figure 16.2c. The horns and top of the calvarium have been lifted off to expose the brain and frontal sinus.

all suspected lesions. The kidney section should include cortex, medulla, and pelvic epithelium. Whenever possible, some normal tissue at the edge of a lesion should be included. Slices must be thin (no more than 5 mm) and the tissues should be preserved in at least ten times their volume of 10% formalin. A history should accompany the samples to the laboratory. Saving tissues preserved in formalin is advisable, even if the owner does not currently wish to pay for histologic examination.

The gastrointestinal tract should not be opened until the rest of the necropsy is finished, to avoid contamination. At the appropriate time, rumen contents should be examined for pH level, color, smell, and identifiable roughages or grain. A sample of at least 200 g should be labeled and frozen for later reference if toxicity has not yet been ruled out. At the same time, large pieces (at least 100 g each) of liver and kidney should be frozen (King 1983). Liver also may be useful for monitoring trace mineral status of the herd. Plant fragments requiring identification should be dried between layers of newspaper. The abomasum and small intestine should be examined closely for parasites; this serves a herd-monitoring function, even if parasitism did not directly kill the goat (Figure 16.3). A quantitative fecal examination may be warranted. Peyer's patches and mesenteric, bronchial, and mediastinal lymph nodes deserve special attention, and the presence or absence of white foci in the wall of the intestine (coccidiosis) should be determined. Impression smears of intestinal mucosa may be helpful for diagnosis of coccidiosis, cryptosporidiosis, paratuberculosis, and (if the necropsy is done less than four hours after death) enterotoxemia.

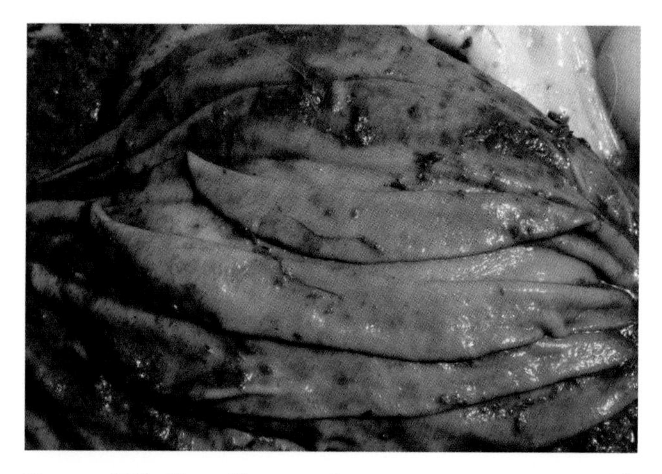

Figure 16.3. Two *Haemonchus contortus* worms with barberpole appearance are present on the abomasal folds. (Courtesy Dr. M.C. Smith.)

INTERPRETATION OF THE FINDINGS

Table 16.1 is an incomplete listing of conditions causing sudden death. A more complete list can be found in the Internet resource Consultant (White 2008). If the carcass is emaciated, refer first to the chapter on wasting diseases. Death may have been sudden, but a long-term problem often exists as the cause of death or predisposition to some terminal accident or infection.

Most of these conditions are discussed elsewhere in this book and will not be repeated here. The situation of the kid found dead shortly after delivery deserves special comment. It is important to determine whether the kid was born alive and whether it breathed; if so, its lung tissue is inflated and floats. If the kid was stillborn, more consideration should be given to the long list of diseases causing abortion. It is critical to know whether the kid ever nursed (milk in the abomasum) as opposed to being too weak at birth to get up and nurse (because of in utero infection, swayback, congenital defects, prematurity, or nutritional muscular dystrophy) or having a dam with malnutrition, udder problems, or poor maternal behavior so that no milk could be obtained. Death from exposure is more common if the abomasum is empty, whereas other explanations should be sought if the kid has a full stomach. One should also evaluate body fat deposits on the pericardial sac and around the kidneys. These fat stores are normally light tan and extensive at birth but quickly become dark red and reduced in volume with starvation. An ileal impression smear is helpful in diagnosing the cause of death of kids that lived long enough to die of enterotoxigenic *E. coli* (packets of Gram-negative rods in microcolonies) or clostridial enterotoxemia (many large Gram-positive rods).

A complete necropsy can provide other information of use in the management of the herd, even if it does not directly pertain to the sudden death of the goat at hand. A record of whether a doe is pregnant and the number of fetuses in the uterus is important for the differential diagnosis of pregnancy toxemia, but it is also needed for monitoring the reproductive efficiency of the herd. Joint diseases are not expected to cause sudden death, but necropsy is an excellent way to verify the presence of arthritis due to caprine arthritis encephalitis virus or mycoplasma infection. Soft bones and a rachitic rosary on the ribs suggest a mineral imbalance in the ration that should be corrected. They may also remind the prosector to examine the vertebral column more closely for a pathologic fracture as cause of the sudden death.

The practitioner should never underestimate how fast a dead goat can rot, even in the winter. A heavy Angora fleece or a body cavity full of fat makes many conditions difficult to diagnose after as little as four

Table 16.1. Conditions causing sudden death in goats.

Diagnosis	*Comments*
All ages	
Trauma, including predation	Subcutaneous hemorrhage, broken bones, ruptured internal viscus. If the eyes are absent, post mortem damage to the carcass by birds is likely.
Exposure	Cold stress caused by exposure to rain and wind after shearing.
Lightning strike, electrical shock	Subcutaneous hemorrhage, singe marks, often no lesions.
Snake bite	Fang marks in localized edematous swelling.
Anesthesia overdose, idiosyncratic reaction	Verify dose actually given.
Anaphylaxis	Death immediately after administration of penicillin, tetanus antitoxin, autogenous bacterins.
Anthrax	Petechiae and echhymoses throughout, large hemorrhagic lymph nodes; may lack bloody discharges from orifices or greatly enlarged pulpy spleen.
Clostridial wound infections	Crepitant (*C. chauvoei*) or edematous (*C. septicum*) tissues with odor of rancid butter (King et al. 2005); confirm by culture or fluorescent antibody.
Enterotoxemia	Fluid and fibrin in pericardial sac, glucosuria; kidneys rot quickly; fresh ileal impression smear shows many Gram-positive rods.
Polioencephalomalacia	Fluorescence of cerebral cortex under Wood's lamp suggestive but may be absent if acute course.
Encephalitis or meningitis	Impression smear of meninges if cloudy, to look for neutrophils or bacteria; evaluation and culture of CSF.
Tetanus	Limbs extended; diagnosis probably not possible if no clinical signs observed; history may include recent dehorning, dystocia, or other wound for entry of the organism.
Pseudorabies	Fluorescent antibody test on liver and brain stem, viral isolation; history of exposure to pigs or syringe contaminated with live virus vaccine.
Poisonous plants (see Table 19.7)	Examine rumen contents carefully; venous blood bright red with cyanide, dark with nitrates.
Chemical poisoning, including insecticides and anthelmintics	Check history, package label. The antibiotic tilmicosin has caused sudden death of goats (U.S. FDA 2006).
Rumensin toxicity	Histologic myocardial damage; may not be visible grossly in acute case; access to improperly mixed feeds or cattle pellets.
Urea toxicity	Rumen pH >7.5; access to improperly mixed feeds, de-icing products, or fertilizer.
Rumen acidosis	Rumen fluid milky, pH <5.5 if rapid death but returns to normal range as saliva enters rumen; sloughing of mucosa also occurs with simple autolysis.
Bloat	Bloat line in esophagus; edema of hindquarters.
Choke	Bolus of food at larynx.
Intestinal volvulus	Dark discoloration of only the involved portion of intestine.
Cecal or abomasal torsion	Rare in goats.
Haemonchosis (not in neonates)	Muscles and other tissues very pale; "barber pole" worms may be numerous in abomasum or absent (King 1983); may have submandibular edema.
Fascioliasis and fascioloidosis	Extensive necrosis and hemorrhage from fluke migration in liver; sometimes live rupture or *Clostridium novyi* infection (black disease).
Inhalation pneumonia	History of force feeding kids or of drenching goats of any age; nutritional muscular dystrophy or neurologic disease can result in inhalation.
Mannheimia and *Pasteurella* pneumonia	Cranioventral lung lobes firm, red; grossly similar to inhalation pneumonia but less septic.
Pulmonary edema	Red watery fluid in lung parenchyma, froth in airways; may have cardiac malformation or history of dog attack.
Heartwater (*Ehrlichia ruminantium*)	Tick-borne disease common in Africa and Caribbean; if noticed ill, history of fever, neurologic signs; look for edema of thoracic contents.

Table 16.1. *Continued*

Diagnosis	*Comments*
More common in kids	
Exposure of neonate to heat or cold, starvation	No milk in abomasum or intestine if kid did not nurse.
Congenital cardiac malformation	Heart may appear globular.
Brain damage from disbudding	Open calvarium to check surface of brain.
Cryptosporidiosis	Demonstrate organisms with acid-fast or other stain, but may be incidental finding.
Coccidiosis	White foci in wall of intestine. Some kids bleed out into intestine acutely.
Ruptured abomasum	Edges of rupture have curled if this happened antemortem.
Nutritional muscular dystrophy of heart	Not always grossly visible; liver edges may be rounded; excess fluid may be present in abdomen or thorax. Gossypol toxicity, from cottonseed, similar.
Ionophore toxicity	Myocardial necrosis; foot and mouth disease can affect kids similarly.
Septicemia	Splenomegaly, possibly polyarthritis; culture the spleen if fresh necropsy; use impression smear to demonstrate *Streptococcus pneumoniae* (Buddle et al. 1986; Vaissaire et al. 1989).
Anemia from sucking lice	Lice macroscopic; Angoras especially susceptible.
More common in adults	
Gangrenous or toxic mastitis	Cut surface of udder changes color; skin may be blue, secretion red.
Listeriosis	Gross lesions seldom visible in acute case; histology of brain stem is indicated if cause of death not evident after gross examination.
Ruptured aneurysm	Blood in body cavity.
Pregnancy toxemia	At least two well-developed kids in uterus, fatty liver, ketones in urine.
Rupture of uterus	Fetus often in anterior presentation with head back.
Rupture of uterine artery	May occur as long as several days after kidding.
Hypocalcemia	Sudden dietary changes or periparturient condition predisposes.
Vegetative endocarditis	Look for predisposing chronic infection, arthritis, or cardiac malformation; common where researchers use indwelling jugular catheters.

hours. Recognition of typical changes resulting from autolysis helps to avoid misdiagnoses. These include greenish or black discoloration of tissues adjacent to the intestine, and pale, even bubbly foci in the liver. A partial list of agonal and postmortem changes (Roth and King 1982; King et al. 2005) follows.

Pseudolesions Resulting from Agonal Death or Autolysis

- **Livor mortis**: Settling of blood to dependent parts of the body.
- Rumen contents in oral or nasal discharge.
- Ingesta in lungs without evidence of inflammation.
- **Rectal or vaginal prolapse**: Caused by post mortem bloat.
- **Pulpy kidney**: Not significant if rest of body also autolytic, otherwise suggestive of enterotoxemia.
- **Tracheal froth**: Agonal. May be significant if signs of pulmonary edema also present.
- **Endocardial, myocardial, epicardial hemorrhages**: Agonal.
- **Rumen mucosal sloughing**: Often an early autolytic change.
- **Post mortem abomasal rupture**: Along greater curvature, but lacks fibrin, hemorrhage.
- **Tiger striping in large intestine**: Terminal tenesmus.
- **Pseudomelanosis**: Blackening of tissues, especially adjacent to autolytic intestine.
- **Melanosis**: Normal black pigment in various organs.

REFERENCES

Buddle, B.M., Herceg, M., Tisdall, C.J. and Tisdall, D.J.: *Streptococcus pneumoniae* septicaemia in an Angora goat kid. N. Z. Vet. J., 34:156–157, 1986.

de Vos, V. and Turnbull, P.C.B: Anthrax. In: Infectious Diseases of Livestock, 2nd Ed., Vol. 3. J.A.W. Coetzer and R. C. Tustin, eds. Capetown, Oxford Univ. Press Southern Africa, pp. 1262–1289, 2004.

Hindson, J.C. and Winter, A.C.: Manual of Sheep Disease, 2nd Ed. Oxford, UK, Blackwell Science, 2002.

King, J.M.: Sudden death in sheep and goats. Vet. Clin. N. Am. Large Anim. Pract., 5:701–710, 1983.

King, J.M., Roth-Johnson, L., Dodd, D.C. and Newson, M.E.: The Necropsy Book, 4th Ed. Gurnee, IL, Charles Louis Davis, DVM. Foundation Publisher, 2005.

Koebel, G., Rafail, A. and Morris, J.: On-farm composting of livestock and poultry mortalities. Ontario Ministry of Agriculture, Food and Rural Affairs Factsheet ISSN 1198-712X, 2003. <http://www.omafra.gov.on.ca/english/livestock/deadstock/facts/03-083.htm>.

Okoh, A.E.J.: An epizootic of anthrax in goats and sheep in Danbatta Nigeria. Bull. Anim. Health Prod. Afr., 29:355–359, 1981.

Roth, L. and King, J.M.: Nonlesions and lesions of no significance. Comp. Cont. Educ. Pract. Vet., 4:S451–S456, 1982.

U.S. Food and Drug Administration: Cumulative veterinary adverse drug experience (ADE) reports. Accessed on-line 10 December 2006 at <http://www.fda.gov/cvm/ade_cum.htm>.

Vaissaire, J., et al.: *Streptococcus pneumoniae* septicaemia in different animal species (cattle, goat, rodents). Demonstration in France. Bull. Mens. Soc. Vet. Pract. Fr., 72:211–213, 216–221, 1988.

White, M.E.: Consultant [database on the Internet]. Ithaca, NY, Cornell University. c2008. http://www.vet.cornell.edu/consultant/consult.asp.

17

Anesthesia

Goats are obviously sensitive to pain and vocalize loudly, sometimes even before being hurt. Most hobby goat owners prefer paying for tranquilization or anesthesia to observing the distress of a loved animal. In addition, goats seem to be prone to shock or perhaps to catecholamine-induced ventricular fibrillation (Gray and McDonell 1986a). Some die quickly after a surgical experience, and these losses can usually be prevented with adequate analgesia. Finally, in some countries humane laws dictate analgesia for surgical operations.

Consideration must be given to withdrawal times when tranquilizers or general anesthetics are given to meat or dairy animals. Because none of the drugs discussed in this chapter is approved for use in goats in the United States, withdrawals should be based on information supplied by the Food Animal Residue Avoidance Databank (FARAD) if available. In most instances, recommendations published for cattle are appropriate for goats, but a twenty-four-hour withdrawal period is recommended to meet the extended withdrawal required for extralabel drug use under AMDUCA, the Animal Medicinal Drug Use Clarification Act, if the cattle withdrawal is zero (Craigmill et al. 1997). See Table 17.1 for some FARAD guidelines for withdrawals in goats.

FARAD specifically declined to provide a withdrawal recommendation for tiletamine hydrochloride and zolazepam (Craigmill et al. 1997) or acepromazine (Haskell et al. 2003). Recommendations are also lacking for medetomidine, bupivacaine, morphine, and butorphanol, although FARAD personnel tend to suggest thirty days for such drugs when scientific data are not available.

Intravenous injections are given easily in the jugular vein (Figure 1.1) of goats. One person can restrain an adult dairy goat by straddling its neck and holding the head to one side with an elbow, leaving both hands free to distend the jugular vein and manipulate a needle and syringe. The presence of both horns and mohair on Angoras makes venipuncture more difficult and an assistant may be welcome. If a goat is short and squirmy, the operator may choose to lift the animal's front quarters off the ground and hold them clamped between the knees for better restraint during venipuncture. The cephalic vein and the recurrent tarsal vein are suitable for placement of butterfly catheters, and some may find 19- or 21-gauge butterfly catheters

Table 17.1. FARAD recommended withdrawal (WD) intervals for tranquilizers and general anesthetics in goats (Craigmill et al. 1997; Haskell et al. 2003).

Drug	*Dose (mg/kg)*	*Meat WD (d)*	*Milk WD (h)*
Acepromazine (Canada)	Up to 0.13 IV; up to 0.44 IM	7	48
Atropine	Adjunct to anesthesia	7	24
Detomidine	Up to 0.08 IM or IV	3	72
Guaifenesin	Up to 100 IV	3	48
Ketamine	Up to 2 IV, 10 IM	3	48
Lidocaine with epinenephrine	Infiltration, epidural	1	24
Tolazoline (cattle)	2 to 4 IV	8	48
Ultra-short acting barbiturates	Thiamylal (up to 5.5) Thialbarbitone (up to 9.4)	1	24
Xylazine	Up to 0.1 IV, 0.3 IM	5	72
Xylazine (cattle)	Up to 0.3 IM	4	24
Yohimbine	Up to 0.3 IV	7	72

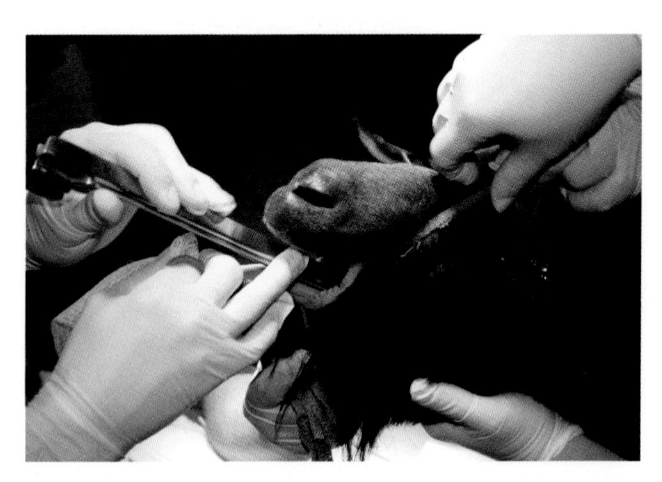

Figure 17.1. Visualizing the larynx with a long laryngoscope blade. Gauze loops hold the goat's mouth open. (Courtesy Dr. M.C. Smith.)

convenient for rapid administration of drugs via the jugular vein.

LOCAL AND REGIONAL ANALGESIA

Local analgesia is commonly used for procedures such as dehorning, castration, cyst removal, and wound repair. Lidocaine is probably the local analgesic agent most commonly used for goats in the United States; other agents include 2% procaine, 2% mepivacaine, and 0.25% to 0.5% bupivacaine solutions. Mixtures of lidocaine and bupivacaine are used to provide immediate analgesia and prolonged duration of pain relief, though meat and milk withdrawals have not been established for bupivacaine. An estimated maximum dose for bupivacaine is 2 mg/kg (Snyder 2007) and it has a greater margin of safety than lidocaine (Skarda and Tranquilli 2007). The use of lidocaine is prohibited in food-producing animals in the UK, where the only licensed product is 5% procaine with epinephrine (Hodgkinson and Dawson 2007).

Lidocaine

Lidocaine has a historical reputation of being toxic to goats. This can be easily demonstrated if small kids are injected without consideration of the total drug dosage being administered per unit bodyweight. In most species the convulsive threshold dose of lidocaine hydrochloride is 10 mg/kg intramuscularly (Gray and McDonell 1986a). For a kid that weighs 3 kg, a 10 mg/kg dose would be equivalent to 1.5 ml of 2% lidocaine. In general, a dosage of 5 mg/kg should be safe. Dilution of the lidocaine to 1% or even 0.5% with saline permits use of a larger volume of analgesic before the toxic level is approached (Skarda and Tranquilli 2007). This is especially helpful if the local blocks (a total of four injections) are to be used when disbudding newborn kids or a line block is used for a large abdominal incision.

Drowsiness, nystagmus, and convulsions are early signs of lidocaine toxicity (Covino and Vassallo 1976). Hypotension, respiratory arrest, and circulatory arrest occur at about five to six times the convulsive dose (Gray and McDonald 1986a). Goats suffering from slight overdoses recover spontaneously, whereas severely affected animals should receive oxygen therapy (if available) and 0.5 mg/kg diazepam intravenously or a short-acting barbiturate to control convulsions. When P_{CO_2} is increased, the convulsive threshold is lowered (Covino and Vassallo 1976).

In human medicine, and less frequently in veterinary medicine, lidocaine has been buffered with sodium bicarbonate to reduce pain associated with intradermal or subdermal injection. A mixture of commercial 2% lidocaine is diluted 5:1 or 10:1 with 8.4% sodium bicarbonate. The resulting solution has a more physiologic pH (7.3 rather than the 6.2 of the straight lidocaine) but the exact mechanism of pain relief is not known (Palmon et al. 1998). No trials have been published concerning efficacy of buffered lidocaine for controlling injection pain in goats.

Paravertebral Block

A line block or an inverted L-block 2 to 3 cm cranial and dorsal to the proposed incision site provides good analgesia for celiotomies. The distal paravertebral block is an alternative, although it requires a better remembrance of anatomy. The thirteenth thoracic and first two or three lumbar nerves are blocked; up to 5 ml of analgesic is injected into each nerve, mostly below the intertransverse ligament but with some above the ligament (Hall et al. 2001) in a fan-shaped pattern near the anterior aspect of the tip of the transverse processes of L1 to L4. The most caudal palpable transverse process is L5, and this is used as a landmark for counting forward to locate L1, which is shortened and often difficult to palpate on an obese animal (Hodgkinson and Dawson 2007). Respect a maximum total lidocaine dose of 6 mg/kg to avoid toxicity.

Alternative injection sites, closer to the midline (proximal paravertebral), have also been described (Gray and McDonell 1986a; Hodgkinson and Dawson 2007; Skarda and Tranquilli 2007). In an adult dairy goat, the transverse processes of L1 and L3 are located and a point marked over the center of each approximately 3 cm (1.25 inches) from the midline. A small subcutaneous bleb of analgesic may be placed at these two spots. Then a 20-gauge, 6-cm spinal needle is introduced through the skin at the point over L1, directed straight down onto the transverse process, and walked off the anterior edge of the bone. When the needle pops through the intertransverse ligament, aspiration is performed to assure no venous injection, and 3 to 5 ml of 1% lidocaine or a lidocaine-bupivacaine mixture is deposited just ventral to the ligament. The needle is then withdrawn slightly and an additional 2 ml deposited above the ligament to block the dorsal branch of the nerve. Next, the needle is walked off the caudal aspect of the transverse process of L1, where 5 ml is deposited below and 2 ml above the intertransverse ligament. The spinal needle is then moved to L3, where the injections are repeated anterior to the transverse process only, unless analgesia of L4 is also desired. In this case, the injections are also repeated caudal to the transverse process of L3. Analgesia persists for approximately one hour.

Intravenous Regional Analgesia

The distal limb of a goat can be anesthetized easily by injecting a local anesthetic into a superficial vein of the limb distal to a tourniquet (Babalola and Oke 1983). This is most desirable when treating serious wounds of the extremity or when amputating a digit. The tourniquet (such as an Esmarch rubber bandage) is applied above the elbow or hock to raise the cephalic vein (crosses the anterior aspect of the middle third of the forearm) or the recurrent tarsal vein (in front of the gastrocnemius tendon laterally). A volume of 3 to 4 ml of 2% lidocaine solution delivered intravenously distal to the tourniquet has been recommended for pygmy goats. Five to 7 ml is appropriate for larger goats (Gray and McDonell 1986a). For a distal lesion, the tourniquet may be applied in the midmetacarpal or midmetatarsal region, a superficial vein located, and a smaller volume of analgesic injected intravenously if this is deemed desirable. The likelihood of hematoma formation can be reduced by draining off some blood before injection, using a fine gauge needle, and applying pressure over the injection site post injection. Analgesia is complete within ten minutes and lasts until the tourniquet is removed. To avoid potential lidocaine toxicity, do not remove the tourniquet for at least fifteen to twenty minutes after the injection (Taylor 1991). The tourniquet should remain on the limb for no longer than forty-five or fifty minutes to avoid postsurgical or delayed ligamentous and neuropathic pain.

Caudal Epidural Block

The most cranial moveable joint of the tail is usually between the first and second caudal vertebrae. Either the sacrocaudal or the first intercaudal (intercoccygeal) space is suitable for caudal epidural injection (Skarda and Tranquilli 2007). Lidocaine, procaine, or mepivacaine (all 2% solutions) can be used. A standard dose to anesthetize the perineum and vagina of an adult without interfering with motor function of the hind limbs is 2 to 4 ml. A 19- or 20-gauge needle is appropriate. If the needle is properly placed, an air bubble in the syringe will not be compressed during injection (Hodgkinson and Dawson 2007).

A longer duration of local anesthesia and a block that extends forward to provide adequate anesthesia after forty to fifty minutes for flank laparotomy or caesarean section can be achieved by adding xylazine at 0.07 mg/kg to the lidocaine (Scott 2000). Although this technique was originally developed for sheep, it also appears to work for goats. Mild ataxia may develop and persist for several hours. Analgesia of perineal tissues appears to last for more than twenty-four hours.

Anterior Epidural Anesthesia

Mammary gland surgery, vasectomy, laparotomy, embryo transfer, prolapse repair, and treatment of hind limb fractures are among the procedures that may be performed under spinal anesthesia. The anterior epidural block is performed at the lumbosacral junction, using a 1.5- to 3-inch 20-gauge spinal needle with stylet. The site is a palpable depression between the tuber coxae; it should be clipped widely and the skin prepared as for surgery. If the animal is restrained in lateral recumbency with the lumbosacral spine flexed, the opening between vertebrae at the lumbosacral junction is effectively larger. The skin may be desensitized with 1 to 2 ml of local anesthetic and an initial skin puncture made with a large bore needle. The finer spinal needle is then directed straight into the space between vertebrae. Appearance of spinal fluid at the hub of the needle usually occurs when the subarachnoid space had been entered. Approximately 1 ml of anesthetic, such as a 2% lidocaine or 2% mepivacaine solution, is injected slowly into the subarachnoid space for each 10 kg of bodyweight.

Loss of sensation to the rear limbs is delayed (five to ten minutes) if the anesthetic is placed epidurally (Riese 1987). Some authors prefer to always give the injection in the epidural location, using 1 ml of 2% lidocaine solution with epinephrine/5 kg (Nelson et al. 1979; Gray and McDonell 1986a), and to routinely give intravenous fluids and a vasopressor drug such as methoxamine at 5 to 10 mg/kg or phenylephrine at perhaps 0.005 to 0.01 mg/kg if hypotension occurs (Hall et al. 2001). After epidural injection, the animal is rolled immediately onto its back if bilateral diffusion of the anesthetic is desired or maintained in lateral recumbency with the side to be desensitized undermost for unilateral analgesia. Paralysis lasts approximately three hours, at least in animals that have been sedated with xylazine (0.1 mg/kg intramuscularly). Recovery is delayed (often longer than eleven hours) when 0.75% bupivacaine is used for epidural anesthesia (Trim 1989). Linzell (1964) recommends performing an epidural injection while the goat is standing and using a lumbar epidural block (5 ml of 1.5% lidocaine plus epinephrine between L1 and L2) to anesthetize the abdominal wall without paralyzing the limbs.

Extradural anesthesia using xylazine at 0.07 mg/kg diluted in sterile water to a volume of 2.5 ml provides adequate anesthesia for a flank incision for caesarean section of ewes forty to fifty minutes later, whether the xylazine is given at the lumbosacral or the previously discussed sacrocaudal site (Scott and Gessert 1997). Medetomidine (0.020 mg/kg in 5 ml of sterile water) administered epidurally at the lumbosacaral site provides adequate anesthesia for flank surgery of goats within five to ten minutes (Mpanduji et al. 2000), although the observed effect may actually represent systemic absorption. Analgesia extends forward to the thorax, front limbs, and neck. Intravenous atipamezole at 0.08 mg/kg rapidly reverses the analgesia and the cardiopulmonary depression effects induced by the medetomidine (Mpanduji et al. 2001). Lumbosacral epidural xylazine at 0.025 mg/kg combined with ketamine at 2.5 mg/kg has been used to produce surgical anesthesia of the perineal region of normal and uremic goats (Singh et al. 2007).

Lumbosacral subarachnoid administration of xylazine at 0.05 mg/kg and of medetomidine at 0.01 mg/kg have been used to provide flank, hind limb, and perineal anesthesia in goats (Kinjavdekar et al. 2000). Doses of 0.001 to 0.002 mg/kg medetomidine may be adequate. Use of subarachnoid ketamine at 3 mg/kg and of subarachnoid xylazine at 0.1 mg/kg has also been reported (DeRossi et al. 2003).

Sacral Paravertebral Alcohol Block

Long-term (four to six weeks) control of straining associated with rectal or vaginal prolapses can be achieved by injecting isopropyl alcohol (70%) where the sacral nerves exit from the spinal column (Eness 1987; Skarda and Tranquilli 2007). A caudal epidural injection of lidocaine simplifies the procedure. A right-handed person inserts the left index finger into the rectum to locate the small bony indentations which mark the junction between two vertebrae. Six injections of 0.25 to 0.5 ml each are made. The first injections are made bilaterally at sacral spinal nerve S5, directly lateral to the sacrococcygeal junction. An 18-gauge 1 to 1.5-inch needle is directed down, about 1 cm from the midline, until the point of the needle can barely be felt with the finger positioned in the rectum. The procedure is repeated at S4 and S3 bilaterally. The S3 injections are omitted for males because prolapse of the prepuce might otherwise occur. If the goat has a problem requiring culling, it should be adequately identified; otherwise complete recovery from the current prolapse will tempt the owner to forget genetic predispositions.

SINGLE AND COMBINATION AGENTS FOR GENERAL ANESTHESIA

A variety of injectable and inhalant anesthetic agents have been used successfully in goats to achieve chemical restraint or general anesthesia. Electrical current and acupuncture stimulation have also been used.

Short-acting Barbiturates

Thiopental sodium (15 to 20 mg/kg in a 2.5% solution given rapidly intravenously) can be used for induction of anesthesia. It produces thirty to fifty seconds of apnea; intubation is easiest to perform during this period, as long as a stylet is used to stiffen the tube. Thiamylal sodium (Surital®, Parke-Davis) has similar effects at 10 mg/kg (Gray and McDonell 1986b). Methohexital sodium (Brevital®) at 4 mg/kg intravenously is said to provide five to seven minutes of anesthesia (Hall et al. 2001). Excitement during recovery can be avoided by premedication with midazolam, diazepam, medetomidine, or xylazine, and the latter two permit use of a lower barbiturate dose for induction. When xylazine has been used, recovery time to standing is shortened by reversal with intravenous yohimbine at 0.125 mg/kg (Mora et al. 1993).

Other Barbiturates

The intravenous dose of pentobarbital for adult goats is 30 mg/kg (Linzell 1964). The animal regains its feet in twenty to sixty minutes unless additional doses to total 6 to 36 mg/kg per hour are administered. Animals vary in their response to this drug, and recovery may be prolonged (Hall et al. 2001). Commercial solutions of pentobarbital often contain propylene glycol, which causes hemolysis and hematuria in goats and sheep (Linzell 1964). Instead, a solution may be prepared by dissolving powdered pentobarbitone in 10% ethyl alcohol in a saline solution.

Laryngospasm sometimes occurs shortly after the administration of barbiturates, especially pentobarbital, and especially during anesthesia of young goats (Bryant 1969). The animal exhibits gasping, ineffective ventilation, and dilated pupils. The emergency requires forceful intubation (or an emergency tracheostomy). Spraying a local anesthetic on the larynx simplifies intubation in this instance.

Xylazine

Xylazine is an excellent drug for sedating goats, although it is not approved for this purpose in the United States. For many minor procedures such as oral and ocular exams, 0.03 to 0.04 mg/kg intravenously provides a brief (ten minutes) period of complacency. For painful procedures, it is safest to use a modest dose (0.05 mg/kg intravenously or 0.10 mg/kg intramuscularly) in combination with local analgesia (Gray and McDonell 1986a). Dosages should be calculated carefully; a 20 mg/ml solution and a tuberculin syringe make it easier to draw up the correct quantity, but beware of extra xylazine in the hub of the needle when the injection is given intravenously. Male goats and those with central nervous system diseases such a listeriosis seem to be especially susceptible to overdosing (M.C. Smith, personal observations). Salivation, bloat, and hyperglycemia are expected complications whenever xylazine is used. The drug has been shown to cause increased myometrial activity, depression of maternal and fetal heart rates, and marked depression of maternal and fetal arterial oxygen partial pressure (PaO_2) when given to late pregnant Rambouillet cross ewes at a dosage of 10 mg intramuscularly. The fetuses recovered within sixty minutes (Jansen et al. 1984). Conservative doses of xylazine are not contra-indicated in healthy pregnant goats and are preferable to the stress associated with physically restraining an excited or painful goat.

Doses of xylazine more than 0.15 mg/kg intravenously are not recommended for sheep and goats because these doses may cause severe cardiovascular and respiratory depression (Gray and McDonell 1986b). Even at the 0.15 mg/kg dosage, clinically important respiratory depression and hypoxemia have been reported in sheep (Doherty et al. 1986), though less consistently in goats (Kutter et al. 2006). PaO_2 decreases by approximately half, and a paradoxical respiratory rhythm has been observed where the thoracic cage collapses on inspiration. The sheep become cyanotic. Later research in sheep has explained how the hypoxemia develops by demonstrating that xylazine at 0.15 mg/kg intravenously causes damage to the capillary endothelium, intra-alveolar hemorrhage, and interstitial and alveolar edema, changes that clear within twelve hours (Celly et al. 1999).

The adverse effects of xylazine can be partially reversed by the α_2-adrenergic receptor antagonists yohimbine at 0.125 mg/kg or tolazoline at 1.5 mg/kg intravenously and administration of oxygen. Yohimbine produces a more rapid and persistent reversal of xylazine than does doxapram (0.4 mg/kg intravenously). Tolazoline may be more effective than yohimbine in ruminants (Gross and Tranquilli 1989). Yohimbine at 0.25 mg/kg in combination with 4-aminopyridine at 0.4 mg/kg, both given intravenously, is more effective than either drug alone (Ndeereh et al. 2001).

Ketamine, Ketamine plus Diazepam

Ketamine alone may be used for anesthetic procedures where muscle relaxation is not important (Kellar and Bauman 1978). A dose of 11 mg/kg intramuscularly or 6 mg/kg intravenously (Hall et al. 2001) supplies fifteen to thirty minutes of adequate anesthesia to adult goats. Larger doses have been recommended for young kids or longer surgery. The eyes remain open (use a lubricating ointment) and nystagmus may occur, as may involuntary limb movements. The animal retains the ability to eructate, cough, and swallow. This is desirable if intubation is not possible but does not guarantee that aspiration will not occur. Diazepam at 0.25 mg/kg combined in the same syringe with ketamine at 5 to 7.5 mg intravenously has been recommended for ten to fifteen minutes of anesthesia (Hall et al. 2001); a similar duration has been reported for diazepam at 0.11 mg/kg plus ketamine at 4.4 mg/kg (Riebold et al. 1995).

Xylazine and Ketamine

Xylazine and ketamine are frequently combined for general anesthesia in goats when inhalation anesthesia is not available. The period of analgesia is prolonged, but so is the recovery time relative to ketamine alone. A frequently quoted regimen is 0.22 mg/kg xylazine followed by 11 mg/kg ketamine ten minutes later; both drugs are given intramuscularly (Kumar et al 1976; Thurmon 1986). Also possible is a single-intramuscular injection of 0.22 mg/kg xylazine and 11 mg/kg ketamine, although the time until immobilization occurs is increased. Anesthesia lasts approximately forty-five minutes and recovery to standing occurs in approximately one and a half hours (Kumar et al. 1983). Increments of 6 mg/kg ketamine are given intramuscularly if prolongation of anesthesia is necessary. Decreased dosage rates (0.10 mg/kg xylazine followed by 5 mg/kg ketamine) are more appropriate for procedures that require fifteen to twenty minutes of anesthesia (Gray and McDonell 1986b).

A xylazine/ketamine/atropine combination has been recommended for disbudding of kids (Pieterse and van Dieten 1995). The dosages are 0.04 mg/kg xylazine, 10 mg/kg ketamine, and 0.1 mg/kg atropine all in one intramuscular injection providing onset of surgical anesthesia in an average of twelve minutes. Note that the combination of xylazine and atropine has been found to cause hypertension and infarction in small animal species. Another intramuscular combination is created by adding 1 ml = 10 mg of butorphanol and 1 ml = 100 mg equine xylazine to a 10-ml vial of 100 mg/ml ketamine. The dose of the cocktail is 1 ml/100 pounds IV or 1 ml/50 pounds IM. Create a new controlled substance recording form for this vial, to simplify required paperwork.

Time to standing (but not to eating) is shortened by intravenous administration of 0.25 mg/kg yohimbine and 0.6 mg/kg 4-aminopyridine (Kruse-Elliott et al. 1987). Intravenous tolazoline at 2.1 mg/kg also significantly shortens the period of recumbency in goats anesthetized with xylazine-ketamine (Dew 1988).

Xylazine Congeners

Clonidine, medetomidine, dexmedetomidine, and detomidine are alpha-2 adrenergic agonists similar in action to xylazine. Intravenous clonidine doses of 0.2 to 7 µg/kg in goats cause dose-dependent sedation ranging from quiet behavior with maintenance of appetite to a sleep-like state (Eriksson and Tuomisto 1983). Intravenous medetomidine at 5 µg/kg causes deep clinical sedation, metabolic alkalosis, and hyperglycemia (Raekallio et al. 1994). Intramuscular medetomidine at 15 µg/kg results in sedation and lateral recumbency, beginning at approximately ten minutes, and lasting approximately one hour. Side effects include bradycardia, hypothermia, rumen stasis, bloating, frequent urination, salivation, and dyspnea, but disappear within two hours after return to standing (Mohammad et al. 1991). Dexmedetomidine (the active d- enantiomer of medetomidine) at 2 ug/kg has recently been shown to severely decrease PaO_2 in goats (Kutter et al. 2006). Detomidine causes mild to moderate sedation and analgesia approximately fifteen minutes after intramuscular injection at 10 to 20 ug/kg (Clark et al. 1993).

Intramuscular medetomidine at 15 ug/kg (fifteen minutes after 0.1 mg/kg atropine) provides sedation that begins approximately seven minutes after injection and lasts approximately forty minutes. When the same doses of medetomidine are followed ten minutes later with 5 mg/kg ketamine intramuscularly, anesthesia onset is rapid and lasts approximately forty-five minutes. Salivation and diuresis are marked. When atipamezole is given intravenously at 15 ug/kg as a reversal agent thirty minutes after medetomidine, the goats are able to walk normally in two to three minutes (Tiwari et al. 1997). Similarly, when an intravenous medetomidine dose of 20 ug/kg was reversed twenty-five minutes later with intravenous atipamezole at 100 ug/kg, the goats stood up an average of one and a half minutes later but were agitated and vocalized (Carroll et al. 2005).

Tiletamine and Zolazepam

Telazol® (Fort Dodge Animal Health) is a nonnarcotic, nonbarbiturate anesthetic agent approved in the United States for intramuscular injection in dogs and cats. It is a combination of a ketamine-like drug, tiletamine (50 mg/ml), and the tranquilizer zolazepam (50 mg/ml). It produces cataleptoid or dissociative anesthesia. Few reports are published on its use in small ruminants, but the drug is effective in sheep and goats. Intramuscular injection of a dosage of 7.5 to 10 mg/kg provides anesthesia within ten minutes and lasting fifteen to thirty-five minutes (Clark et al. 1995). A dosage of 8 to 16 mg/kg was used intravenously to anesthetize eighty laboratory sheep for various surgeries, including celiotomies. The average duration of surgical anesthesia was two and a half hours, and the average time from injection to recovery was 5.6 hours (Conner et al. 1974). A 5.5 mg/kg dosage intravenously provides rapid induction of goats, and additional doses of 0.5 to 1 mg/kg can be used to prolong the surgical anesthesia as needed. Adding butorphanol at 0.1 mg/kg intravenously is not beneficial (Carroll et al. 1997).

Premedication with atropine decreases salivation but is not necessary because the swallowing reflex is preserved. Intubation or at the very least positioning the head low is advised in case regurgitation of rumen contents occurs. An oxygen source and means of assisted ventilation are also desirable (Carroll et al. 1997). Initial screening suggested that doxapram HCl (Dopram-V, A.H. Robins) is useful for arousing dogs that have been overdosed with Telazol® (Hatch et al. 1988). An approximate dose is 5 mg/kg intravenously. There are no reports available of similar testing in goats.

Althesin

Althesin (Saffan®, Schering-Plough) was previously approved as an anesthetic for sheep and goats in New Zealand. This agent contained 9 mg of alphaxalone and 3 mg of alphadolone per ml. The drug is no longer marketed in the United States or New Zealand. The dosage for healthy adult sheep and goats is 2.2 to 3 mg/kg given intravenously to produce ten minutes of surgical anesthesia. Recovery to standing occurs about twenty minutes after injection. An increased dose (6 mg/kg) has been used for disbudding kids (McKeating and Pilsworth 1984; Williams 1985). Althesin causes depression of myocardial contractility in goats (Foëx and Prys-Roberts 1972) and has been reported to cause anaphylaxis in dogs and cats due to the castor oil based vehicle.

Propofol

Propofol is another injectable induction agent with rapid onset of anesthesia, short duration of action, and smooth recovery. In a dose titration study, 5.1 mg/kg given rapidly intravenously was the median effective dose required for induction of anesthesia adequate for intubation in unpremedicated goats (Pablo et al. 1997). The mean induction time was twenty-three seconds, and twenty-seven of twenty-eight goats experienced apnea (mean duration seventy-three seconds). Another study found a dose of 4 mg/kg adequate for induction with only one of five goats experiencing apnea (Reid et al. 1993). Additional doses of propofol should be available if needed to complete induction, and ventilation should be supported if apnea persists. The dose of propofol can be reduced in sedated animals (Branson and Gross 1994). One such protocol uses intramuscular detomidine at 10 μg/kg combined with butorphanol at 0.1 mg/kg before induction with 3 to 4 mg/kg propofol IV (Carroll et al. 1998). Anesthesia can be maintained with intermittent boluses of propofol. An alternative protocol reported is induction with intravenous ketamine (3 mg/kg) and propofol (1 mg/kg) followed by infusion of ketamine (0.03 mg/kg/min) and propofol (0.3 mg/kg/min) and 100% inspired oxygen for maintenance of anesthesia (Larenza et al. 2005).

Opioid Immobilization

Etorphine and carfentanil, more commonly used for capture or immobilization of exotic species, have been evaluated in domestic goats at 5 to 40 μg/kg. Intramuscular carfentanil provides faster catatonic immobilization (five minutes or less) than does etorphine (five to ten minutes; transient struggling occurs attributed to injection site pain). Recovery is slower after carfentanil, as the goat remains recumbent for more than two hours. Blood pressure increases while heart rate decreases (Heard et al. 1996). Oral administration of carfentanil combined with detomidine results in an undesirable prolonged induction time and excitement phase (Sheeman et al. 1997).

Halothane

Halothane has been largely supplanted by newer agents but was once a popular nonexplosive anesthetic among practitioners owning a gas anesthesia machine. Halothane takes effect quickly enough that a small goat can be induced through a mask, though more often an injectable drug such as xylazine or thiamylal sodium is used in older animals (Dhindsa et al. 1970). Recovery from the effects of the gas anesthesia is rapid, and fetal depression is minimal. In light of this, halothane could be used for cesarean section when general anesthesia is desired, although isoflurane is a safer choice.

During mask induction, 4% halothane solution is administered. This takes three to four minutes with a tightly fitting face mask. A canine face mask is suitable, or a mask can be fashioned by cutting the bottom out of a 500-ml plastic bottle and padding the edges with cotton and tape. After intubation, the goat is maintained on a 1% to 2% halothane vaporizer setting at a flow rate of 1 liter of oxygen per minute. Semiclosed circuits require a greater oxygen flow rate than do completely closed circuits.

Occasionally, an acute, massive liver necrosis occurs after halothane anesthesia of seemingly healthy goats (Fetcher 1983; O'Brien et al. 1986). Signs usually occur within twenty-four hours and include depression, inappetence, salivation, teeth grinding, head pressing, and icterus. Serum levels of aspartate aminotransferase (AST), bilirubin, alkaline phosphatase, creatinine, and blood urea nitrogen levels are increased. Death typically occurs within four days. Necropsy reveals centrilobular or massive liver necrosis. In some cases, there is necrosis of the proximal renal tubules, abomasal ulceration, and hepatic encephalopathy. It has been postulated that hypotension and liver hypoxia encourage reductive metabolism of halothane, leading to production of toxic, free radicals. Although unproven, use of xylazine in conjunction with halothane may be a contributing factor because of depressive effects on the circulatory system. Prolonged anesthesia is also a risk factor. Halothane administered for forty-five to 125 minutes did not cause liver injury in young healthy goats premedicated with xylazine at 0.1 mg/kg IM (McEwen et al. 2000).

Methoxyflurane

Methoxyflurane has no advantage over halothane unless the practitioner owns only a Metophane machine. Induction and recovery are slower than with halothane. Methoxyflurane can be used to supplement nitrous oxide (4 l/minute) and oxygen (2 l/minute) in a nonrebreathing system.

Isoflurane and Other Inhalants

Depending on availability and personal preferences of the anesthetist, other agents may be used in goats. These include enflurane (Antognini and Eisele 1993), isoflurane (Ewing 1990), and sevoflurane (Larenza et al. 2005). Mask induction can be done with 3% to 4% isoflurane, with or without nitrous oxide at 50% of the total gas flow (Riebold et al. 1995). Nitrous oxide should be discontinued after induction, to avoid accumulation in the rumen. Anesthesia is maintained with a lower concentration, such as 1% to 2% isoflurane in oxygen. The concentration of isoflurane needed can be further reduced by intravenous morphine at 2 mg/kg (Doherty et al. 2004). Because these agents cause some respiratory depression, controlled ventilation is preferable to spontaneous breathing (Antognini and Eisele 1993). Portable tabletop isoflurane anesthesia units are now available and appropriate for field anesthesia situations.

Ether is undesirable because it produces profuse salivation and a prolonged, unpleasant induction and is highly flammable.

Electroanesthesia

There are several reports of the use of an alternating electric current to anesthetize goats. For instance, a 700 cycle/second alternating sine wave current of 25 milliamps and 10 volts was used for bone plating in one pregnant doe (Vijaykumar and Ramakrishna 1983). It has been suggested that electroimmobilization is unpleasant to ruminants (they show aversion in behavior trials) and also that the technique is inhumane if surgery is performed without additional local analgesia (Thurmon 1986; Trim 1987).

Acupuncture Analgesia

Beginning in the 1970s, acupuncture stimulation has been used in Western countries in both small animal and human medicine to decrease the amount of anesthetic needed or to control postoperative pain. Complex mechanisms of action have been proposed (Janssens 1988), and release of endorphins and encephalins is involved. Because acupuncture lacks sedative effects, goats with a quiet temperament or those extremely depressed because of illness presumably are most suitable for acupuncture analgesia. Otherwise, mild sedation, as with xylazine, should be considered. Few specific reports of the use of either bodypoint or earpoint acupuncture for surgery in goats have been published. Practitioners, then, should fall back on their experience with other species.

PREANESTHETIC CONSIDERATIONS AND TRANQUILIZATION

Anemia from endoparasitism is relatively common in goats. The color of the mucous membranes, specifically the conjunctiva, should be evaluated as part of the preanesthesia physical examination. Determination of a packed cell volume aids in detecting anemia if there is doubt, and it may be prudent to postpone elective surgery until after anthelmintics and good nutrition have corrected the anemia.

Preoperative starvation reduces the volume of digesta in the rumen. The activity of the microfloral population is also reduced; gas production (bloat) during surgery is then reduced. An undesirable effect of starvation is that it makes the digesta more fluid, increasing the risk of regurgitation. Lactation decreases, and there is a risk of pregnancy toxemia in late pregnancy. In general, adults should not be held off feed longer than twelve to twenty-four hours, and four hours is adequate for unweaned kids. Longer periods without food slow the recovery of ruminal activity and appetite of adults and predispose kids to hypoglycemia and hypothermia. Neonatal kids should not be fasted (Riebold et al. 1995).

Premedication with atropine is generally considered unnecessary. A dose small enough to avoid undesirable tachycardia and pupil dilation does not prevent salivation, but merely makes the saliva more viscid and more difficult to clear from the airways (Hall et al. 2001). Some anesthetists use glycopyrrolate as an antisialogogue. Rarely, therapeutic use of atropine at 0.02 mg/kg intravenously has been recommended if bradycardia develops during anesthesia (Trim 1987).

Preanesthetic sedation with acepromazine maleate (0.05 to 0.10 mg/kg intravenously), midazolam (0.4 mg/kg intravenously), or diazepam (0.50 mg/kg intravenously) has been recommended to simplify restraint and reduce the dose of drugs needed to achieve induction (Gray and McDonell 1986b; Larenza et al. 2005). These drugs are considered to cause less cardiopulmonary depression than xylazine. A chlorpromazine dosage of 2 to 2.5 mg/kg intravenously has been suggested for preanesthetic tranquilization of goats (Nawaz 1981). At decreased doses, both diazepam (0.04 mg/kg intravenously) and chlorpromazine (0.5 mg/kg intravenously) have been used to stimulate appetite in goats (Anika 1985). The positive effect on feeding lasts approximately thirty minutes.

INTUBATION

Endotracheal intubation with a cuffed tube is advisable whenever general anesthesia is induced in an adult goat to prevent inhalation of saliva and regurgitated rumen contents (Taylor 1991). A variety of rapidly acting drugs may be used to facilitate intubation. These include short-acting barbiturates, ketamine, xylazine, and halothane or isoflurane (by mask). Intramuscular administration of midazolam at 0.4 mg/kg followed by ketamine at 4 mg/kg intravenously is adequate for

Table 17.2. Endotracheal tube sizes for goats.

Weight of goat	*Tube size*
15 kg	5–6 mm
25 kg	7–8 mm
30–40 kg	9–10 mm
Adult dairy goat	11–12 mm

intubation (Stegmann 1998). Another option is propofol (Waterman 1988) at 3 to 4 mg/kg slowly intravenously (Taylor 1991).

Laryngospasm has been reported, especially during intubation of young goats. This potentially fatal complication can be prevented by spraying the larynx with a local anesthetic at least thirty seconds before attempting intubation (Taylor 1991). Lidocaine is preferred to benzocaine, to avoid methemoglobinemia (Reibold et al. 1995). The endotracheal tube should be left in place until coughing and swallowing reflexes are regained.

Endotracheal Tube Size

The recommendations given in Table 17.2 aid selection of an appropriate tube (Linzell 1964; Gray and McDonell 1986b). A 35-cm long tube is appropriate for an adult goat. Cuffs should be inflated for at least five minutes before induction to detect any slow leaks. It is helpful to stiffen the tube with a wire stylet, which is withdrawn when the tube is in the trachea. Alternatively, a human endotracheal tube exchanger can be preplaced and the endotracheal tube advanced over it (Bush 1996). After intubation, a wooden bite bar can be taped in place to protect the tube.

Intubation Under Visual Observation

Direct observation with a laryngoscope is considered ideal for intubation. The anesthetized goat is left in sternal recumbency, and the head is directed toward the ceiling or the goat is placed on its back with its head and neck fully extended. The latter procedure theoretically increases the risk of regurgitation occurring before intubation can be completed. An assistant holds the tongue out of the mouth using a gauze sponge for a better grip. Gauze loops also allow an assistant to hold the jaws open without being in the way (Figure 17.1). The lower gauze loop could go over the tongue. The anesthetist passes a laryngoscope with a long blade (8 to 11 inches, 20 to 27.5 cm) to behind the base of the tongue, then lifts the blade to expose the larynx and vocal cords. If a long laryngoscope blade is not available, one can be prepared by welding an extension on a shorter blade to achieve a total length of 257 mm or longer (Tillman and Brooks 1983). It is also possible to pass a lubricated endotracheal tube via the inferior nasal meatus, although the tube diameter must be smaller than is listed in Table 17.2 and intubation forceps may be needed (Hall et al. 2001).

Blind Intubation

Blind intubation is worth learning, not only because laryngoscopes are expensive, but also because the batteries lose their charge. The goat is placed in lateral recumbency with the head in slight extension, in line with the thoracic spine. The thumb and first finger of one hand hold the tongue and lower jaw, while the other fingers of the hand press against the hard palate to hold the mouth open. The endotracheal tube is held with the other hand and passed into the pharynx with its concave side against the tongue until its tip is felt to touch the larynx. The tube is then twisted and advanced until the characteristic feel of its passage over the tracheal rings is detected (Hecker 1974).

Others prefer to advance the tube into the pharynx with its convex surface against the tongue, then rotate the tube 180 degrees to ensure that the tip of the tube is not trapped beneath the epiglottis. With this technique, which has been well illustrated by radiographic studies, the larynx is pushed upward with one hand to occlude the esophagus while the other advances the tube (Gray and McDonell 1986b).

PRECAUTIONS DURING ANESTHESIA

Judging the depth of general anesthesia requires assessment of several reflexes and, more importantly, response to surgical manipulations (Gray and McDonell 1986b). Some jaw tone persists under deep anesthesia, but swallowing motions usually mean that the anesthetic depth is lightening. Palpebral reflexes are usually lost during surgical anesthesia, but the corneal reflex is maintained at all levels. The pupils dilate during light anesthesia or when cerebral hypoxia occurs during deep anesthesia. Some authors report that the globe does not rotate in response to depth of anesthesia of the goat (Riebold et al. 1995; Riebold 2007), while others claim that it does (Hall et al. 2001).

Arterial blood pressure can be monitored as an indicator of circulatory adequacy during anesthesia (Wagner and Brodbelt 1997). The normal mean arterial pressure during anesthesia is 75 to 100 mm Hg (Riebold et al. 1995). Hypotension (defined as mean arterial pressure less than 60 mm of Hg) results in underperfusion of the brain and kidneys. An over-the-needle teflon catheter is inserted into an auricular, saphenous, or common digital artery for direct blood pressure measurement, or an ultrasonic flow detector can be placed over a limb artery (Wagner and Brodbelt 1997; Hall et al. 2001; Riebold 2007). Administering intravenous fluids and decreasing the depth of anesthesia usually improve blood pressure. When available, a pulse oximeter attached to tongue, ear, interdigital skin, teat, rectum, or tail permits monitoring of pulse rate and hemoglobin saturation (Haskins 1996; Hodgkinson and Dawson 2007; Snyder 2007).

When anesthesia is apt to be prolonged, lateral recumbency is preferred to dorsal recumbency. Left lateral recumbency reduces the risk or regurgitation, compared with positioning on the other side (Trim 1987). While the animal is in dorsal recumbency, the weight of the rumen and intestinal contents (and the pregnant uterus) compresses the aorta and posterior vena cava and restricts movement of the diaphragm. The function of the lungs is also markedly impaired in lateral recumbency, so efficiency during surgery becomes important to the survival of the goat. Intermittent positive pressure ventilation via use of an Ambu bag and oxygen supply is helpful for correcting respiratory acidosis when general anesthesia is prolonged.

If an endotracheal tube is not used (e.g., when abdominal surgery is performed under tranquilization and local anesthesia), the goat should then be placed on a slanted surface so that the abdomen is below the thorax. This reduces the pressure of abdominal viscera on the lungs. Rumen fluid is less likely to rise to the mouth and be inhaled. At the same time, the head should be placed lower than the neck to permit saliva to drain from the mouth. Ruminal tympany can be controlled by passing a stomach tube or by centesis of the rumen with a 14-gauge needle or trocar. After surgery is complete, the goat should be propped in sternal recumbency to facilitate eructation.

During prolonged general anesthesia (longer than two hours) the goat may lose a large quantity of saliva (up to 500 ml/hour). This leads to acidosis unless intravenous replacement fluids containing sodium bicarbonate are supplied. It is also possible to collect the saliva in a bucket and return it to the goat via stomach tube after surgery (Linzell 1964). Barbiturate anesthesia is associated with a greater loss of saliva and hence of bicarbonate than is inhalant anesthesia with halothane or methoxyflurane (Edjtehadi and Howard 1978). Hypothermia is another serious problem associated with general anesthesia, especially in neonates or if the animal has been held off feed. When surgery is performed on the farm, the goat should be kept in a heated building or supplied with a heating pad, heating blanket, or lamp, or with hot water bottles until it is up and actively feeding again.

If the goat is pregnant, care should be taken to minimize the risk to the fetus (Ludders 1988). This means reducing the dosage of preanesthetics and anesthetics to the minimum necessary for the procedure, avoiding hypoxemia and hypovolemia of the dam, using increased oxygen flow and intra-operative intravenous fluid administration, and keeping the patient warm to speed recovery. If good placental perfusion and oxygenation are not maintained, the fetus may be aborted after the anesthetic episode.

POSTSURGICAL PAIN RELIEF

It is difficult to assess pain in goats, especially if the animals are not habituated to contact with people. Goats are famous for screaming when subjected to nothing more than manual restraint, and yet do not always vocalize or show restless behavior or struggling after surgery that might be expected to cause pain. Inappetence and depression are possible indicators of pain (Hendrickson et al. 1996), as are trembling and bruxism. Analgesics are most effective if administered before pain actually develops (preemptive analgesia).

Morphine has been used as an epidural for pain relief after abdominal or limb surgery (Pablo 1993; Hall et al. 2001). Morphine binds to opiate receptors in the central and peripheral nervous system and inhibits release of pain-related neurotransmitters. Preservative free morphine is diluted in saline and administered at 0.1 mg/kg in the lumbosacral space, using aseptic technique and a spinal needle. Duration of action may be as long as twenty-four hours. Epidural bupivacaine at 1.5 mg/kg affords some pain relief but causes prolonged recumbency (Hendrickson et al. 1996). Lesser doses of bupivacaine are mixed with morphine to provide surgical analgesia and postoperative pain relief.

Intramuscular opioids have also been used, including butorphanol at 0.2 mg/kg and pethidine at 2 to 4 mg/kg (Hall et al. 2001) and morphine at 0.1 mg/kg. Buprenorphine (at 0.02 mg/kg intramuscular or intravenous) does not appear to be suitable for postsurgical pain relief, because it causes agitation and inhibits rumination (Ingvast-Larsson et al. 2007).

Fentanyl is a synthetic opioid agonist that has a short duration of action when given intravenously (Kyles 1998; Carroll et al. 1999). Transdermal fentanyl can be administered via a commercially available patch to provide more prolonged blood concentrations. Hair is clipped on the side of the neck and a 50-μg/hour patch is applied to the skin of an adult goat, under a protective bandage. The patch should be placed twelve to twenty-four hours before surgery for best effect. Because goats show variable and inconsistent absorption of fentanyl from the patch (Carroll et al. 1999), they need to be monitored closely in case additional analgesia is required.

A variety of nonsteroidal anti-inflammatory drugs have been administered to goats, often extrapolating from pharmacokinetic and pharmacodynamic data collected for other species (Lees et al. 2004) and with the assumption that pain relief is also supplied. Salicylates are poorly absorbed from the rumen (Davis and Westfall 1972) and thus aspirin is unlikely to be very effective, even at doses as high as 100 mg/kg. Oral ibuprofen is well absorbed and an appropriate caprine dose may be similar to human doses on a mg/kg basis (DeGraves et al. 1993); however, this drug is not approved for food producing animals in the United States. Flunixin meglumine is an irritating drug that is best given intravenously but is also well absorbed orally (Königsson et al. 2003) and has frequently been given by the subcutaneous route. This is the preferred nonsteroidal drug for use in goats in the United States, because it is approved for other food animals (cattle and swine). A typical dose is 1.1 to 2.2 mg/kg once or twice a day. The extralabel use of nonsteroidal anti-inflammatory drugs in cattle in the United States has been reviewed recently (Smith et al. 2008) and the same decision-making processes for drug selection are applicable for goats.

In other countries, preference might be given to intravenous or intramuscular ketoprofen at 3 mg/kg daily (Arifah et al. 2003) or oral carprofen. The extralabel withdrawal times suggested by FARAD when ketoprofen is given to goats are twenty-four hours for milk and seven days for meat (Damian et al. 1997). Carprofen has been used in England at an anecdotal dose of 50 mg once daily for dairy goats, with a seven-day milk withholding time, and at 20 mg daily for pygmy goats (Matthews 2005). Another suggested carprofen dose is 1.4 mg/kg subcutaneously or intravenously (Hodgkinson and Dawson 2007). Very preliminary studies for meloxicam in goats suggest a dose of 0.5 mg/kg intravenously repeated perhaps every twelve hours, because goats clear the drug rapidly (Hodgkinson and Dawson 2007; Shukla et al. 2007).

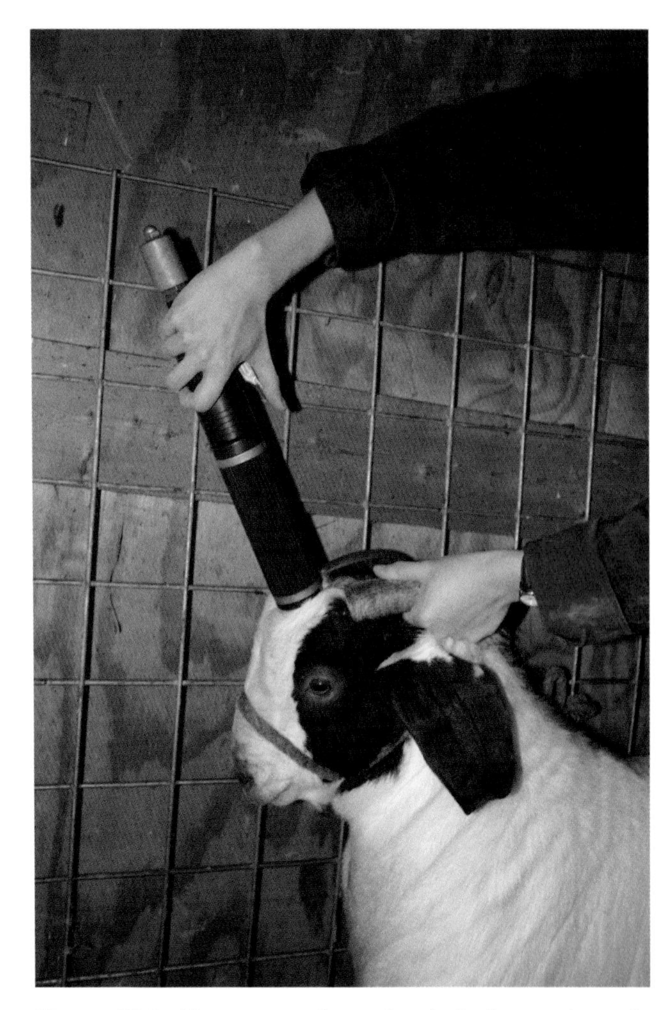

Figure 17.2. Placement of captive bolt for euthanasia from the top of the head, directed toward the spine. (Courtesy Dr. M.C. Smith.)

EUTHANASIA AND SLAUGHTER

When euthanasia of a pet or hospitalized patient is required, overdose of an intravenous barbiturate is usually most appropriate. If an intravenous catheter is not already in place, use of a 19-gauge butterfly catheter reduces the risk of perivascular drug deposition. For commercial animals or for salvage slaughter on the farm, gunshot or penetrating captive bolt to the head is a humane alternative (AVMA 2001), as long as the operator is aware of the landmarks and the brain is not needed for rabies testing or other diagnostic evaluation. The animal is restrained with a halter and offered food if able to eat. The captive bolt gun or firearm is aimed from the top of the skull down toward the spine (Figure 17.2) or from the back of the skull, between the base of the horns, toward the mouth (Figure 17.3) (Longair et al. 1991; Grandin 1994).

Goats are commonly killed by Muslim or Jewish ritual slaughter. A very sharp knife is used to cut the carotid arteries near the jaw, thereby causing rapid exsanguination, without first stunning the animal. Although ritual slaughter is exempt from humane slaughter laws in the United States (Grandin 1994), the animal should not be unduly stressed by inhumane restraint (such as shackling and hoisting upside down from a chain) before slaughter. Welfare during halal or kosher slaughter can be improved by restraining the goat in an upright position with its head and neck extended (Thonney 2007).

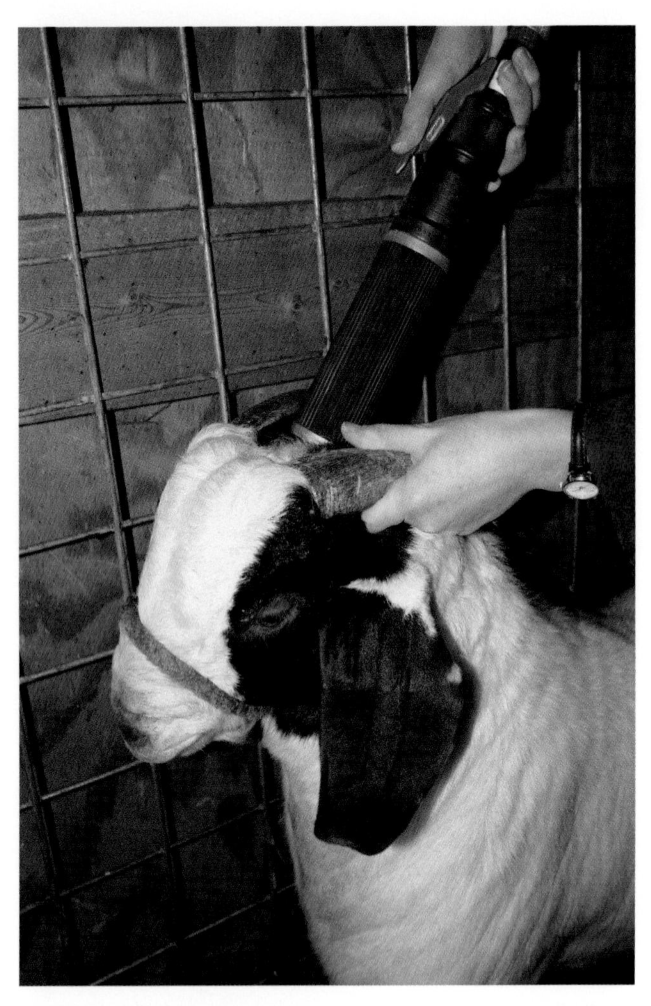

Figure 17.3. Placement of captive bolt for euthanasia between the horns, directed toward the mouth. (Courtesy Dr. M.C. Smith.)

REFERENCES

Anika, S.M.: Diazepam and chlorpromazine stimulate feeding in dwarf goats. Vet. Res. Comm., 9:309–312, 1985.

Antognini, J.F. and Eisele, P.H.: Anesthetic potency and cardiopulmonary effects of enflurane, halothane, and isoflurane in goats. Lab. Anim. Sci., 43:607–610, 1993.

Arifah, A.K., Landoni, M.F. and Lees, P.: Pharmacodynamics, chiral pharmacokinetics and PK-PD modelling of ketoprofen in the goat. J. Vet. Pharmacol. Ther., 26:139–150, 2003.

AVMA: 2000 Report of the AVMA panel on euthanasia. J. Am. Vet. Med. Assoc., 218:669–696, 2001.

Babalola, G.O. and Oke, B.O.: Intravenous regional analgesia for surgery of the limbs in goats. Vet. Q., 5:186–189, 1983.

Branson, K.R. and Gross, M.E.: Propofol in veterinary medicine. J. Am. Vet. Med. Assoc., 204:1888–1890, 1994.

Bryant, S.H.: General anesthesia in the goat. Fed. Proc., 28:1553–1556, 1969.

Bush, M.: A technique for endotracheal intubation of nondomestic bovids and cervids. J. Zoo Wildl. Med., 27:378–381, 1996.

Carroll, G.L., Hartsfield, S.M. and Hambleton, R.: Anesthetic effects of tiletamine-zolazepam, alone or in combination with butorphanol, in goats. J. Am. Vet. Med. Assoc., 211:593–597, 1997.

Carroll, G.L., et al.: Detomidine-butorphanol-propofol for carotid artery translocation and castration or ovariectomy in goats. Vet. Surg., 27:75–82, 1998.

Carroll, G.L., et al.: Pharmacokinetics of fentanyl after intravenous and transdermal administration in goats. Am. J. Vet. Res., 60:986–991, 1999.

Carroll, G.L., et al.: Effect of medetomidine and its antagonism with atipamezole on stress-related hormones, metabolites, physiologic responses, sedation, and mechanical threshold in goats. Vet. Anaesth. Analg., 32:147–157, 2005.

Celly, C.S., et al.: Histopathologic alterations induced in the lungs of sheep by use of α_2-adrenergic receptor agonists. Am. J. Vet. Res., 60:154–161, 1999.

Clark, T.P., Purohit, R.C. and Wilson, R.C.: Evaluation of sedative and analgesic properties of detomidine in goats. Agri-Practice, 14(4):29–33, 1993.

Clark, T.P., Purohit, R.C. and Wilson, R.C.: Evaluation of tiletamine-zolazepam anesthesia in goats. Agri-Practice, 16(6):24–27, 1995.

Conner, G.H., Coppock, R.W. and Beck, C.C.: Laboratory use of CI-744, a cataleptoid anesthetic, in sheep. Vet. Med. Small Anim. Clin., 69:479–482, 1974.

Covino, B.G. and Vassallo, H.G.: Local Anesthetics: Mechanisms of Action and Clinical Use. New York, Grune and Stratton, 1976.

Craigmill, A.L., et al.: Extralabel use of tranquilizers and general anesthetics. J. Am. Vet. Med. Assoc., 211:302–304, 1997.

Damian, P., Craigmill, A.L. and Riviere, J.E.: Extralabel use of nonsteroidal anti-inflammatory drugs. J. Am. Vet. Med. Assoc., 211:860–861, 1997.

Davis, L.E. and Westfall, B.A.: Species differences in biotransformation and excretion of salicylate. Am. J. Vet. Res., 33:1253–1262, 1972.

DeGraves, F.J., Anderson, K.L. and Aucoin, D.P.: Pharmacokinetics of ibuprofen in lactating dairy goats. Am. J. Vet. Res., 54:434–437, 1993.

DeRossi, R., Junqueira, A.L. and Beretta, M.P.: Analgesic and systemic effects of ketamine, xylazine, and lidocaine after subarachnoid administration in goats. Am. J. Vet. Res., 64:51–56, 2003.

Dew, T.L.: Use of tolazoline hydrochloride to reverse multiple anesthetic episodes induced with xylazine hydrochloride and ketamine hydrochloride in white-tailed deer and goats. J. Zoo Anim. Med., 19(1–2):8–13, 1988.

Dhindsa, D.S., Hoversland, A.S. and Kluempke, R.: Halothane semiclosed-circuit anesthesia in pygmy and large goats. Am. J. Vet. Res., 31:1897–1899, 1970.

Doherty, T.J., et al..: Cardiopulmonary effects of xylazine and yohimbine in laterally recumbent sheep. Am. J. Vet. Res., 50:517–521, 1986.

Doherty, T.J., et al.: Effect of morphine and flunixin meglumine on isoflurane minimum alveolar concentration in goats. Vet. Anaesth. Anal., 31:97–101, 2004.

Edjtehadi, M. and Howard, B.R.: The effect of thiopental sodium, methoxyflurane and halothane on the acid-base status of sheep. Can. J. Comp. Med., 42:364–367, 1978.

Eness, P.G.: Alcohol block using the caudal paravertebral procedure. Presented at the AASGP Regional Symposium, Des Moines, IA, 1987.

Eriksson, L. and Tuomisto, L.: Effect of naloxone on the hypotensive action of clonidine in the conscious, normotensive goat. Acta Pharmacol. Toxicol., 52:241–245, 1983.

Ewing, K.K.: Anesthesia techniques in sheep and goats. Vet. Clin. N. Am. Food Anim. Pract., 6:759–778, 1990.

Fetcher, A.: Liver diseases of sheep and goats. Vet. Clin. N. Am. Large Anim. Pract., 5:525–538, 1983.

Foéx, P. and Prys-Roberts, C.: Pulmonary haemodynamics and myocardial effects of Althesin (CT1341) in the goat. Postgrad. Med. J., 48:24–31, 1972.

Grandin, T.: Euthanasia and slaughter of livestock. J. Am. Vet. Med. Assoc., 204:1354–1360, 1994.

Gray, P.R. and McDonell, W.N.: Anesthesia in goats and sheep, Part I: Local analgesia. Compend. Contin. Educ. Pract. Vet., 8:S33–S39, 1986a.

Gray, P.R. and McDonell, W.N.: Anesthesia in goats and sheep, Part II: General anesthesia. Comp. Contin. Educ. Pract. Vet., 8:S127–S135, 1986b.

Gross, M.E. and Tranquilli, W.J.: Use of α_2-adrenergic receptor antagonists. J. Am. Vet. Med. Assoc., 195:378–381, 1989.

Hall, L.W., Clarke, K.W. and Trim, C.M.: Veterinary Anaesthesia. 10th Ed. London and New York, W.B. Saunders, 2001.

Haskell, S.R.R., et al.: Update on FARAD food animal drug withholding recommendations. J. Am. Vet. Med. Assoc., 223:1277–1278, 2003.

Haskins, S.C.: Monitoring the anesthetized patient. In: Lumb and Jones' Veterinary Anesthesia. 3rd Ed. J.C. Thurmon et al., eds. Philadelphia, Lippincott Williams and Wilkins, pp. 409–424, 1996.

Hatch, R.C., et al.: Searching for a safe, effective antagonist to Telazol overdose. Vet. Med., 83:112–117, 1988.

Heard, D.J., et al.: Comparative cardiopulmonary effects of intramuscularly administered etorphine and carfentanil in goats. Am. J. Vet. Res., 57:87–96, 1996.

Hecker, J.F.: Experimental Surgery on Small Ruminants. London, Butterworth and Co., 1974.

Hendrickson, D.A., Kruse-Elliott, K.T. and Broadstone, R.V.: A comparison of epidural saline, morphine, and bupivacaine for pain relief after abdominal surgery in goats. Vet. Surg., 25:83–87, 1996.

Hodgkinson, O. and Dawson, L.: Practical anaesthesia and analgesia in sheep, goats and calves. In Practice, 29:596–603, 2007.

Ingvast-Larsson, C., et al.: Clinical pharmacology of buprenorphine in healthy, lactating goats. J. Vet. Pharmacol. Ther., 30:249–256, 2007.

Jansen, C.A.M., Lowe, K.C. and Nathanielsz, P.W.: The effects of xylazine on uterine activity, fetal and maternal oxygenation, cardiovascular function, and fetal breathing. Am. J. Obst. Gynecol., 148:386–390, 1984.

Janssens, L.A.A., Rogers, P.A.M. and Schoen, A.M.: Acupuncture analgesia: a review. Vet. Rec., 122:355–358, 1988.

Kellar, G.L. and Bauman, D.H.: Ketamine and xylazine anesthesia in the goat. Vet. Med. Small Anim. Clin., 73:443–444, 1978.

Kinjavdekar, P., et al.: Physiologic and biochemical effects of subarachnoidally administered xylazine and medetomidine in goats. Small Rumin. Res., 38:217–228, 2000.

Königsson, K., et al.: Pharmacokinetics and pharmacodynamic effects of flunixin after intravenous, intramuscular and oral administration in dairy goats. Acta Vet. Scand., 44:153–159, 2003.

Kruse-Elliott, K.T., Riebold, T.W. and Swanson, C.R.: Reversal of xylazine-ketamine anesthesia in goats. Vet. Surg., 16:321–322, 1987. (Abstract.)

Kumar, A., Thurmon, J.C. and Hardenbrook, H.J.: Clinical studies of ketamine HCl and xylazine HCl in domestic goats. Vet. Med. Small Anim. Clin., 71:1707–1713, 1976.

Kumar, A., et al.: Response of goats to ketamine hydrochloride with and without premedication of atropine, acetylpromazine, diazepam, or xylazine. Vet. Med. Small Anim. Clin., 78:955–960, 1983.

Kutter, A.P.N., et al.: Cardiopulmonary effects of dexmedetomidine in goats and sheep anaesthetised with sevoflurane. Vet. Rec., 159:624–629, 2006.

Kyles, A.E.: Transdermal fentanyl. Compend. Contin. Educ. Pract. Vet., 20:721–726, 1998.

Larenza, M.P., et al.: Comparison of the cardiopulmonary effects of anesthesia maintained by continuous infusion of ketamine and propofol with anesthesia maintained by inhalation of sevoflurane in goats undergoing magnetic resonance imaging. Am. J. Vet. Res., 66:2135–2141, 2005.

Lees, P., et al.: PK-PD integration and PK-PD modelling of nonsteroidal anti-inflammatory drugs: principles and applications in veterinary pharmacology. J. Vet. Pharmacol. Ther., 27:491–502, 2004.

Linzell, J.L.: Some observations on general and regional anaesthesia in goats. In: Small Animal Anaesthesia. O. Graham-Jones, ed. New York, MacMillan Co., 1964.

Longair, J., et al.: Guidelines for euthanasia of domestic animals by firearms. Can. Vet. J., 32:724–726, 1991.

Ludders, J.W.: Anesthesia for the pregnant patient. Society for Theriogenology, Proceedings of the Annual Meeting, Orlando, FL, pp. 36–54, 1988.

Matthews, J.: Longterm NSAIDS in pet goat. Message posted to AASRP-L discussion list March 12, 2005.

McEwen, M-M. et al.: Hepatic effects of halothane and isoflurane anesthesia in goats. J. Am. Vet. Med. Assoc., 217:1697–1700, 2000.

McKeating, F.J. and Pilsworth, R.C.: 'Disbudding' of kids. Vet. Rec., 115:419, 1984.

Mohammad, F.K., Zangana, I.K. and Al-Kassim, N.A.: Clinical observations in Shami goat kids sedated with medetomidine. Small Rumin. Res., 5:149–153, 1991.

Mora, G., Messen, J. and Cox, J.F.: Effect of yohimbine on xylazine-thiopental anaesthetized Creole goats. Small Rumin. Res., 11:163–169, 1993.

Mpanduji, D.G., et al.: Analgesic, behavioural and cardiopulmonary effects of epidurally injected medetomidine (Domitor®) in goats. J. Vet. Med. Ser. A, 47:65–72, 2000.

Mpanduji, D.G., et al.: Comparison of the effects of atipamezole and tolazoline on analgesia, cardiopulmonary and rectal temperature changes induced by lumbosacral epidural injection of medetomidine in goats. Small Rumin. Res., 40:117–122, 2001.

Nawaz, M.: Pharmacokinetics and dosage of chlorpromazine in goats. J. Vet. Pharmacol. Ther., 4:157–163, 1981.

Ndeereh, D.R., Mbithi, P.M.F. and Kihurani, D.O.: The reversal of xylazine hydrochloride by yohimbine and 4-aminopyridine in goats. J. S. Afr. Vet. Assoc., 72:64–67, 2001.

Nelson, D.R., et al.: Spinal analgesia and sedation of goats with lignocaine and xylazine. Vet. Rec., 105:278–280, 1979.

O'Brien, T.D., et al: Hepatic necrosis following halothane anesthesia in goats. J. Am. Vet. Med. Assoc., 189:1591–1595, 1986.

Pablo, L.S.: Epidural morphine in goats after hindlimb orthopedic surgery. Vet. Surg., 22:307–310, 1993.

Pablo, L.S., Bailey, J.E. and Ko, J.C.H.: Median effective dose of propofol required for induction of anesthesia in goats. J. Am. Vet. Med. Assoc., 211:86–88, 1997.

Palmon, S.C., Lloyd, A.T. and Kirsch, J.R.: The effect of needle gauge and lidocaine pH on pain during intradermal injection. Anesth. Analg., 86:379–81, 1998.

Pieterse, M.C. and van Dieten, J.S.M.M.: [The dehorning of goats and kids.] Tijdschrift v. Diergeneeskunde, 120:36–38, 1995.

Raekallio, M., Hackzell, M. and Eriksson, L.: Influence of medetomidine on acid-base balance and urine excretion in goats. Acta Vet. Scand., 35:283–288, 1994.

Reid, J., Nolan, A.M. and Welsh, E.: Propofol as an induction agent in the goat: a pharmacokinetic study. J. Vet. Pharmacol. Ther., 16:488–493, 1993.

Riebold, T.W., Geiser, D.R. and Goble, D.O.: Large Animal Anesthesia Principles and Techniques. 2nd Ed. Ames, Iowa State Univ. Press, 1995.

Riebold, T.W.: Ruminants. In: Lumb and Jones' Veterinary Anesthesia and Analgesia. 4th Ed. W.J. Tranquilli et al., eds. Ames, IA, Blackwell Publishing, pp. 731–746, 2007.

Riese, R.L.: Epidural and spinal anesthesia in sheep and goats. Presented at the AASGP Regional Symposium, Des Moines, IA, 1987.

Scott, P.R.: Extradural analgesia for field surgery in sheep. Compend. Contin. Educ. Pract. Vet., 22:S68–S75, 2000.

Sheeman, J.M., et al.: Immobilization of domestic goats (*Capra hircus*) using orally administered carfentanil citrate and detomidine hydrochloride. J. Zoo Wildl. Med., 28:158–165, 1997.

Shukla, M., et al.: Comparative plasma pharmacokinetics of meloxicam in sheep and goats following intravenous administration. Comp. Biochem. Physiol. C Toxicol. Pharmacol., 145:528–532, 2007.

Singh, K., et al.: Effects of epidural ketamine-xylazine combination on the clinicophysiological and haematobiochemical parameters of uraemic and healthy goats. Vet. Res. Commun., 31:133–142, 2007.

Skarda, R.T. and Tranquilli, W.J.: Local and regional anesthetic and analgesic techniques: Ruminants and swine. In: Lumb and Jones' Veterinary Anesthesia and Analgesia. 4th Ed. W.J. Tranquilli et al., eds. Ames, IA, Blackwell Publishing, pp. 643–681, 2007.

Smith, G.W., et al.: Extralabel use of nonsteroidal anti-inflammatory drugs in cattle. J. Am. Vet. Med. Assoc., 232:697–701, 2008.

Snyder, J.H.: Anesthesia and analgesia. Minor surgeries in small ruminants. AABP Proc., 40:183–187, 2007.

Stegmann, G.F.: Observations on the use of midazolam for sedation, and induction of anaesthesia with midazolam in combination with ketamine in the goat. J. S. Afr. Vet. Assoc., 69:89–92, 1998.

Taylor, P.M.: Anaesthesia in sheep and goats. In Practice 13:31–36, 1991.

Thonney, M.L.: Halal-Kosher restraining device. On-line presentation at http://sheepgoatmarketing.info/education/restrainer/slideshow/index.html, accessed July 1, 2007.

Thurmon, J.C.: Injectable anesthetic agents and techniques in ruminants and swine. Vet. Clin. N. Am. Food Anim. Pract., 2:567–591, 1986.

Tillman, P.C. and Brooks, D.L.: A rapid method for devocalizing goats. Lab. Anim. Sci., 33:98–100, 1983.

Tiwari, S.K., Kumar, A. and Papikh, P.V.: Effects of medetomidine with and without ketamine, and its reversal with atipamezole in goats. Indian J. Anim. Sci., 67:849–851, 1997.

Trim, C.M.: Special anesthesia considerations in the ruminant. In: Principles and Practice of Veterinary Anesthesia. C.E. Short, ed. Baltimore, Williams and Wilkins, 1987.

Trim, C.M.: Epidural analgesia with 0.75% bupivacaine for laparotomy in goats. J. Am. Vet. Med. Assoc., 194:1292–1296, 1989.

Vijaykumar, D.S. and Ramakrishna, O.: Electroanesthesia for fracture repair in a pregnant doe. Vet. Med. Small Anim. Clin., 78:1111–1112, 1983.

Wagner, A.E. and Brodbelt, D.C.: Arterial blood pressure monitoring in anesthetized animals. J. Am. Vet. Med. Assoc., 210:1279–1285, 1997.

Waterman, A.E.: Use of propofol in sheep. Vet. Rec., 122:26, 1988.

Williams, B.M.: Disbudding kids. Vet. Rec., 116:480, 1985.

18

Dehorning and Descenting

DEHORNING

Horns have evolved in goats, as in other species, because of the protection they afford against predators and the improved social status they impart within a herd. Goats joust frequently to establish and verify social rank. The goat rears up on its hindquarters, twists its head down and to one side, and crashes against the opponent's horns. Ridges on the anterior surface of the horns help to prevent a sudden slipping or shearing motion, and neck muscles are well developed, so that fractured cervical vertebrae are avoided (Reed and Schaffer 1972). In many confrontations (e.g., when food is involved), the abrupt presentation of horns is enough to drive off a subordinate goat; however, when adults are put together for the first time or after even a brief separation, actual contact occurs.

The number of horns is variable: none (polled condition) or two horns are generally present. Goats with more than two horns (as many as eight) have been reported, and the polycerate condition is believed to be inherited (Lush 1926).

The basic anatomy of goat horns resembles that of cattle horns. Each horn is composed of closely packed tubules which are produced by corium and germinal epithelium. The corium in turn is attached to the periosteum of the cornual process of the frontal bone. The cornual diverticulum of the frontal sinus forms a cavity within the horn. The cornual artery, a branch of the superficial temporal, supplies the horn. The nervous supply is described here under disbudding.

Reasons For and Against Dehorning Goats

What is appropriate for wild goats may be undesirable in large herds or for animals in close confinement. If one goat does not acknowledge another's dominance, severe crushing injuries or lacerations may occur. Young kids may be killed by a buck or a dominant doe because they are too slow to take evasive action. If none of the goats in a herd has horns, then fewer serious injuries occur during social interactions. The total absence of horns, however, does not greatly alter social behavior. Goats still rear up and crash down toward each other, sometimes missing by the distance equivalent to two sets of horns. Young kids and subordinate does are still kept away from the feed trough, although biting of ears may be the threat used to enforce territorial rights.

One of the major reasons for dehorning goats, then, is to limit injuries inflicted on herd mates. By the same token, injuries to children and adult goat keepers can be minimized by removing the goats' natural weapons. Destruction of fences and pen partitions is slowed, and the annoying tendency of goats to stick a head through a fence, then yank back and get caught, can be almost totally eliminated. This prevents deaths by hanging and also avoids complaints from passers-by. A final reason for dehorning goats is that, in the United States, dairy goats cannot be registered or shown if they have horns. Horns are permitted in pygmy and pygora goats. It is common for meat goat shows to require that horns be tipped (blunted) if present.

A goat should not be dehorned without due consideration given to the dangers associated with the operation. A placid adult kept as a pet or family goat should not be subjected to the surgery if no children or small animals are nearby to be inadvertently injured. An animal that is destined to live its life on a tether should probably be left with horns so that it can defend itself against marauding dogs. Angora goats also usually need their horns for protection. Large bucks can be led by the horns. Removing the horns from a breeding buck may make it less able to compete with other bucks for females. The dehorned buck may also be perceived as less "macho" in some human societies and may therefore not be chosen for breeding. Finally, the stresses associated with the surgery and adverse sequelae may interfere with milk or sperm production or even cause death of the goat.

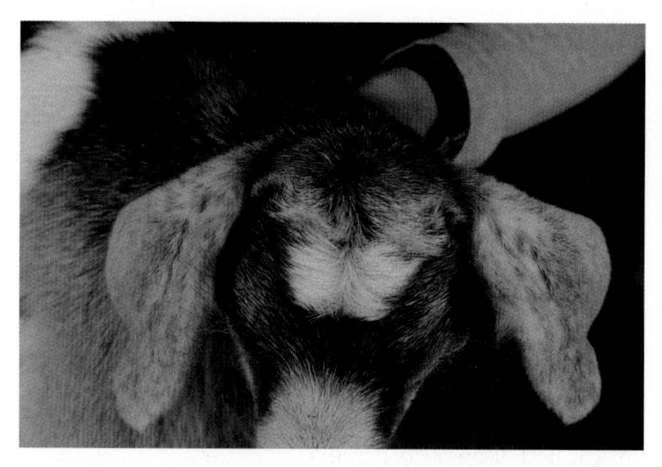

Figure 18.1. Horned kid with twist of hair over each bud. (Courtesy Dr. M.C. Smith.)

The Polled Goat Alternative

It seems logical to avoid all the problems and dangers of dehorning by simply selecting for the absence of horns. Although this works in some breeds, the U.S. dairy goats of European extraction (i.e., Saanen, Alpine, Toggenburg) unfortunately have a serious genetic reproductive disorder linked to the polled condition. In these breeds, the presence of horns is determined by a recessive gene. The polled trait is dominant but is linked to a recessive gene for infertility. A female goat that is homozygous for the polled gene develops into a sterile intersex. The homozygous polled male has an increased risk of developing sperm granulomas in the head of the epididymis. These problems are discussed in Chapter 13. Polled goats of normal reproductive potential can be obtained if one member of each breeding pair is polled and one is naturally horned; eliminating all horned goats from the breeding program results in the production of many infertile goats.

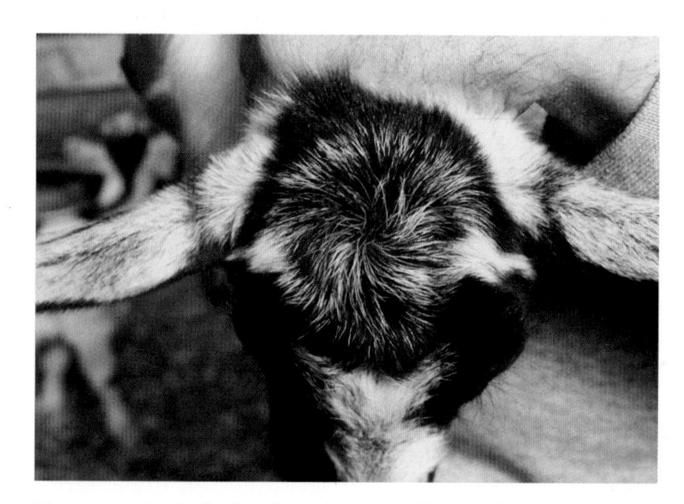

Figure 18.2. Polled kid with central hair whorl. (Courtesy Dr. M.C. Smith.)

Disbudding Kids

If either parent was polled, then the kid may be naturally polled and thus not require disbudding. Some owners ignore this possibility and simply destroy skin in the place where horns would normally be while descenting the kid. For future breeding plans (to avoid intersexes), however, it is important to know whether the kid was polled. Horned kids have a twist of hair over each horn bud (Mackenzie 1975; Ricordeau and Bouillon 1969) (Figure 18.1). The skin of the horn bud is tightly affixed to the underlying bone. Polled kids have just a central whorl of hair on top of the head (Figure 18.2).

Age for Disbudding

For doe kids of European breeds, five to seven days is an ideal age for disbudding. Buck kids have larger horn buds than doe kids of the same age; therefore, disbudding at three to five days of age is preferable for bucks. Disbudding of kids that were very small at birth and of most female Nubians and pygmy goats can usually be delayed until two weeks, as long as the operation is performed carefully (Williams 1990).

Methods

The secret to successful disbudding is to destroy all of the corium from which horn is destined to grow. Although options include surgical removal of a circle of skin, heat cautery, and cryosurgery, only heat cautery will be discussed in detail.

Dehorning paste should be avoided; it can injure the eyes of the kid or eat holes elsewhere in the skin of the kid or other animals in contact with it. These risks can be controlled to some degree by clipping hair, applying a peripheral ring of vaseline to limit spread of the paste, and restraining the kid for thirty minutes. The pain associated with paste dehorning persists longer than does pain from heat cautery. Occasionally, the paste even destroys the calvarium underlying the horn bud, thereby permitting penetration of bacteria to the brain.

Heat cautery is the most commonly used technique in most parts of the world. An electric dehorning iron with a tip of 3/4 to 1 inch diameter is convenient, as long as it becomes and remains hot enough (cherry red) to destroy the skin rapidly. A Rhinehart® dehorner with a half-inch tip (Hoegger Supply, Fayetteville, GA) is more appropriate for pygmy and Nigerian dwarf doe kids. Less expensive, low-wattage dehorners must be applied longer to achieve the same results, with more risk of overheating the brain. Thus, a dehorner producing 200 Watts is applied for five to ten seconds while a 125-Watt dehorner may require twenty seconds of burning (Anonymous 1988). Long extension cords decrease the heat of the iron. Clipping hair from the head improves visibility, decreases burning time, and limits smoke inhalation. When the horn bud is very small, a dehorning tip with a sharp edge can be applied with enough pressure that a ring is burned through the full thickness of the skin. The isolated central circle of skin containing the horn bud can then be lifted off (Figure 18.3). Where electricity is not available, a butane-heated calf dehorner (Portasol®, Nasco, Fort Atkinson, WI) also works well on young goats. Alternatively, a length of metal pipe of the appropriate diameter can be heated in a fire or with a blow torch until cherry red. A 25-mm steel nut can be welded onto a branding iron and heated in the same way (Baxendell 1984).

Some kids, especially bucks, are presented for disbudding when the entire horn bud no longer fits within the dehorner tip. The hot dehorner is applied with less pressure and slid around to burn a larger circle than is required for does. Operators should not aim for a fixed time, but instead, should check each horn bud to determine that the full thickness of skin has been destroyed. This is the case when the skin has turned copper-colored and that color cannot be scraped off with a fingernail. All of the horn corium must be within the final copper ring; the author prefers to burn the center of the ring until it, too, turns copper-colored. On buck kids, an additional crescent toward the front is also burned. If the initial burn is not adequate, then that side of the head should be allowed to cool and the dehorner allowed to reheat before continuing.

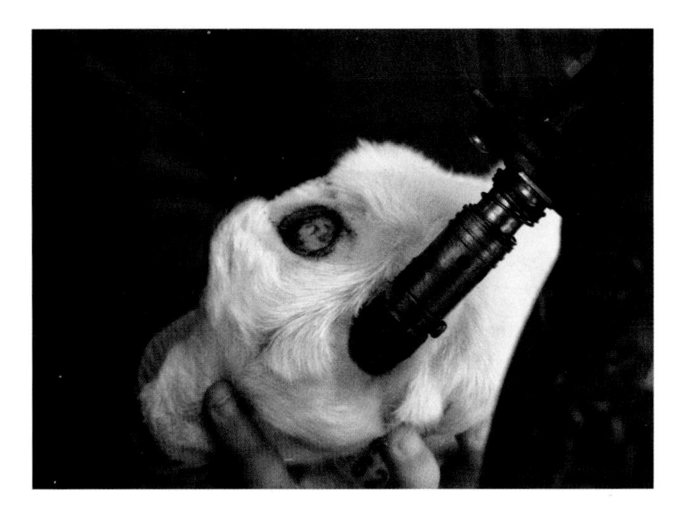

Figure 18.3. Removing horn bud with butane heated dehorner. (Courtesy Dr. M.C. Smith.)

Many other variants exist. Some practitioners without a dehorning iron excise a circle of skin with a scalpel blade. Spark gap electrodesiccation with a Hyfrecator® electrosurgery instrument (previously Birtcher Corp., now CONMED Corp., Utica, New York) has produced good results for some (Koger and McNiece 1982) but regrowth of deformed horns for others (Wright 1983). Disbudding of two-day-old kids with cryosurgery has been reported to be successful and problem-free (Anonymous 1977).

Restraint and Sedation

Restraint for disbudding is done in as many different ways as the surgery itself. In the United States and Australia, disbudding is commonly done without anesthesia, whereas in Great Britain, anesthesia is required by law. In defense of the many who simply hold the kid flat on its side while kneeling on the ground or wrapped in a towel or placed in a narrow wooden box from which only its head protrudes (Williams 1990), it should be noted that all signs of discomfort disappear as soon as the hot iron is removed and the kid is released. The kid immediately resumes nursing, playing, or even sucking on the fingers of the person who held it.

If available, halothane or isoflurane administered through a face mask is an easy way to supply general anesthesia, as long as the oxygen mask is taken away before a hot iron is applied (Buttle et al. 1986). An intramuscular cocktail of injectable drugs is commonly used, such as xylazine, ketamine, and atropine (Pieterse and van Dieten 1995) or xylazine, ketamine, and butorphanol, as described in Chapter 17. Xylazine alone, at doses large enough to produce several hours of somnolence, often does not prevent vocalization during disbudding.

Nerve Block for Disbudding

Local nerve blocks can be used for anesthesia when disbudding young kids, as long as care is taken to avoid a toxic dose of the local anesthetic agent (see Chapter 17). Two nerves supply each horn (Vitums 1954; Elmore 1981). The cornual branch of the lacrimal nerve passes along the temporal line behind

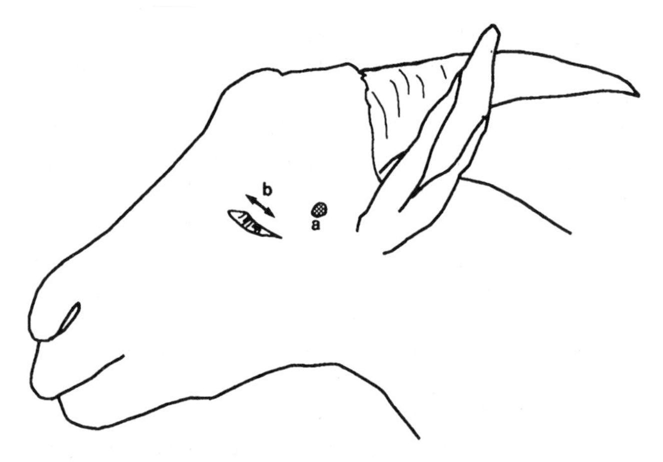

Figure 18.4. Injection sites for the cornual branches of the lacrimal (a) and infratrochlear (b) nerves.

the supraorbital process, between the lateral canthus of the eye and the posterior aspect of the horn. The cornual branch of the infratrochlear nerve passes over the dorsomedial rim of the orbit before it divides into cornual and frontal branches. It can be anesthetized with a line block along the rim of the orbit dorsomedially (Skarda 1986). See Figure 18.4 for location of the nerve blocks. It is the author's preference to dilute 1 ml of 2% lidocaine with epinephrine to 0.5% lidocaine by adding 3 ml of sterile water or saline. This permits the injection of 1 ml over each of the four nerves of a young kid weighing approximately 3 kg. Dilution is not necessary if 0.25 ml of 2% lidocaine can be accurately placed over each nerve. A 1% solution of lidocaine (1 ml per nerve) can be used in older, larger kids and works better.

Dehorning Older Kids

By the time a kid is a few weeks old, a distinct nubbin of horn already extends above the surface of the skull. This horn prevents most dehorner tips from reaching the skin. Heat cautery can still be successful, but first the tip of the horn bud must be removed with a pen knife, hoof trimmer, or shears. A small Barnes calf dehorner can also be used for this purpose as long as it is opened just far enough to remove the protruding bud; a wide enough cut to remove all the skin from which horn might grow could easily go deep enough to expose the goat's brain. Next, the cautery tip is applied to the edges of the wound to achieve a full thickness burn. The tip is slid around to cover a larger area, with particular attention paid to destroying skin over the anterior ridge of the horn.

As the kid grows older, the horn enlarges and both bone and frontal sinus develop within the horn. By the time the kid is six or eight weeks old, it is often simplest to treat it as a small-scale adult and dehorn with scalpel and obstetrical wire or saw.

Dehorning Adults

When facilities are available, general anesthesia makes dehorning of the adult goat more pleasant for the surgeon. However, under field conditions when no one but the owner is available through recovery from anesthesia, sedation with xylazine or diazepam combined with local nerve blocks is an acceptable alternative. Depending on the size of the goat, 2 to 3 ml of 1% or 2% lidocaine is injected for each nerve block, as described under disbudding. There is no anesthesia to the mucous membrane and periosteum lining the horn, however, and supplemental sedation is advisable with older goats (Skarda 1987). The author finds a dose of 0.06 mg/kg xylazine intravenously suitable. Larger doses of xylazine (up to 0.1 mg/kg) have been recommended by others (Bowen 1977; Hague and Hooper 1997), but the associated risks are greater. Recovery is delayed, and supplemental heat may be necessary to avoid hypothermia in cold barns in the winter.

Hair is then clipped widely from around and between the horns, using a razor blade between the horns if necessary. It is helpful to outline the desired skin incisions with an indelible felt-tipped marker before scrubbing and disinfecting the skin. This ensures that the two incisions made will have the same proportions. Except that a narrow strip of skin should be left intact between the horns to speed healing, at least 1 cm of skin should be removed all the way around (Bowen 1977; Turner and McIlwraith 1982). Even more skin must be removed rostrally; the entire base of the ridge that rises to the rostral-medial corner of the horn should be included.

A scalpel blade is used to cut quickly full-thickness through the skin all the way around the horn and to undermine the caudal flap of skin. The person sawing is positioned in front of the goat. An assistant now holds head and horn firmly while obstetrical wire is slipped around the horn and seated in the incision on each side of the horn and under the flap (Figure 18.5). If the horn is not held back during sawing, the frontal bone may splinter. If sedation is not deep enough or too much time has elapsed since xylazine administration, the goat may vocalize or try to rise as the wire passes through the center of the horn. A flat-backed dehorning or miter saw can be used in place of obstetrical wire to remove the horn (Baker 1981). When the first horn is off, the major artery (superficial temporal) situated laterally should be pulled, ligated, or cauterized (Linzell 1964; Turner and McIlwraith 1982). Cotton or gauze is then placed over the wound while the second horn is removed. Then an electric dehorner or firing iron can be used to cauterize smaller bleeders. Blood clots should be carefully removed from the sinuses and an antibiotic or disinfectant powder or spray applied.

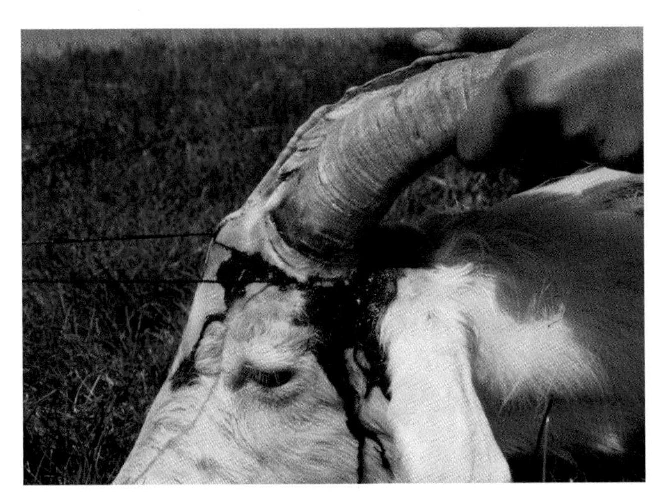

Figure 18.5. Use of a wire saw to removed the horns of an adult doe. (Courtesy Dr. M.C. Smith.)

An owner who watches the dehorning of an adult goat for the first time is impressed by the quantity of blood shed and the size of the holes left in skin and skull by the surgery. This is an excellent time to mention how much less stressful disbudding is than dehorning. If the owner does not observe and great efforts are made to clean up the goat and bandage its head, the owner may be left with the false impression that dehorning is normally postponed until goats mature.

Cosmetic dehorning of adult goats reduces the risks of sinusitis and myiasis, especially in warm climates (Mobini 1991). The technique is most applicable to animals with a small horn base. The skin is incised 1 cm from the base of the horn. Skin is then undermined and pulled away from the horn to permit slightly deeper placement of the obstetrical wire and facilitate subsequent skin closure. After the horn has been removed, hemorrhage is controlled and the surgical site is flushed to remove bone dust and blood clots. An antibiotic powder is dusted into the frontal sinus. Skin closure is achieved with horizontal mattress tension sutures placed well back and simple interrupted sutures at the wound edges, using nonabsorbable suture material. General anesthesia, postoperative penicillin for five to seven days, and bandaging for ten to fourteen days until the sutures are removed are all advised. It may not be possible to close the incisions in goats that had very large horns. Another description of cosmetic dehorning under tranquilization and local anesthesia (Hague and Hooper 1997) suggests leaving a rim of only 1 to 2 mm of skin attached to the horn and extending the skin incision 5 to 10 mm at the craniomedial and caudolateral aspects to facilitate undermining of the skin. After removing the horn with a wire saw, the frontal bone is contoured to a smooth shape using rongeurs to allow skin closure with minimal tension and a Ford interlocking pattern.

Elastrator bands are not recommended for dehorning goats. It is difficult to keep the band in position on skin; if it slips upward, the tip of the horn falls off but growth continues at the base. Six to eight weeks are required for a mature doe's horns to fall off; pain may be intense during much of this time. Also, the risk of tetanus is increased in unvaccinated animals.

Some owners request removal of only the horn tips, to avoid the pain and prolonged healing time associated with complete dehorning. Other reasons for partial horn removal are to prevent misdirected horns or scurs from penetrating the skin, or to make meat goats eligible for showing. A radiograph identifies the extent of the horn sinus and bony cornual process. Vascularized corium extends slightly farther into the horn than the bone, and the horn should be transected distal to the corium. If there is no radiograph to guide the surgery, make an initial transection at a location where the horn feels cool to the touch, meaning that large blood vessels are not present. If an even shorter horn is desired, small sections are sawed off, working in from the tip, until a satisfactory length is obtained or a few drops of blood are observed. Xylazine tranquilization simplifies the procedure.

Postoperative Care

Antibiotic therapy is normally not necessary but should be instituted if the goat develops anorexia or fever. Routine use of a broad-spectrum antibiotic such as long-acting oxytetracycline has been suggested to prevent bacterial invasion of the brain through damaged bone after disbudding by heat cautery (Thompson et al. 2005). An analgesic such as flunixin meglumine or ibuprofen (see Chapter 17) is appropriate, especially if surgical dehorning rather than heat cautery was performed.

Bandaging

Whether the older goat's head should be bandaged depends on many factors. If the animal is to be transported home in a compact car, a bandage is certainly in order. One is likewise needed if bleeding cannot be controlled by pulling arteries and applying cautery. If the goat will be fed from an overhead hay rack, the bandage will keep hay out of the sinuses. On the debit side, any bandage that extends under the jaws is apt to make eating and rumination painful. Sinusitis may develop unnoticed under the bandage, and a dry scab cannot form until the wounds are left exposed to the air. Many dehorning wounds heal well without any bandage. In Greece, beeswax is used to cover the opening to the sinus when an adult goat is dehorned (G. Christodoulopoulos, personal communication).

If the decision is made to bandage, many options are available. One possibility is to hold the wound dressing in place with a length of orthopedic stockinette (Bowen 1977); eye holes are cut after the two ends of the stockinette are taped around the goat's head and neck. Also easy to apply is a 2- or 3-inch wide elastic bandage (Elastikon, Johnson and Johnson, New Brunswick, N.J.) over a nonadhesive dressing; the first turn of tape around the head extends onto the skin rostral to the dehorning wounds and the second turn comes up behind one ear, then extends forward to the forehead between the eyes. Notches are cut in the tape to uncover the eyes and permit free movement of the eyelids. After one or two days, the "chin strap" (portion of the bandage below the level of the eye and ear) should be removed to lessen the tug on the wounds during chewing. The remainder of the bandage can be removed after one week (Figure 18.6). Continued use of a fly repellant is appropriate in warm seasons. Final

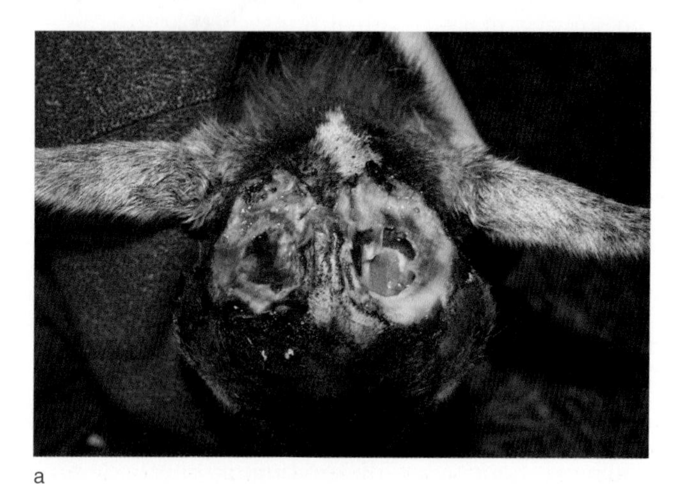

a

Figure 18.6a. Dehorning wound at time of bandage removal six days after surgery. (Courtesy Dr. M.C. Smith.)

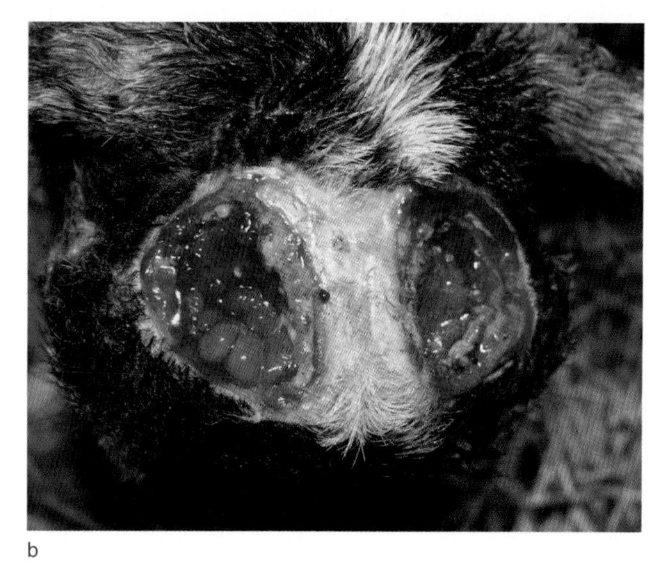

b

Figure 18.6b. Same goat nineteen days after surgery. The head has been left uncovered. Note smaller wounds and healthy wound edges. (Courtesy Dr. M.C. Smith.)

healing of the wound typically occurs in six to eight weeks, though even more time is required for large bucks. Sometimes when mature bucks are dehorned, the large holes that are created never close (Williams 1990).

Tetanus Prophylaxis

The practitioner should never dehorn a goat whose tetanus vaccination status is unknown without administering tetanus antitoxin: 250 to 300 IU to a kid and 500 IU to an adult. Death from tetanus can occur before antibodies are produced in response to an initial vaccination. Tetanus toxoid and antitoxin can be given simultaneously, as long as different syringes and different injection sites are used.

If the goat is known to have been vaccinated with toxoid (not antitoxin—many owners don't understand the distinction) then a booster dose should suffice. It is good policy to administer (and record in writing) a dose of tetanus toxoid or tetanus-enterotoxemia vaccine at the time an appointment is made for future dehorning of an adult. This permits giving the second dose in the series at the time of surgery. When the vaccination is a booster, maximum protection from a rise in titer is achieved for surgery.

Young kids normally receive adequate protection if the dam received a tetanus booster late in pregnancy and large amounts of colostrum were consumed. In disease eradication schemes that replace caprine with bovine colostrum, this protection is lacking unless a point is made of repeatedly vaccinating the donor cows. (If this is done, both tetanus and enterotoxemia vaccine should be given to the cows.) When the owner performs both vaccination of does and disbudding of kids, full dependence is generally placed on colostral protection. The practitioner who offers the service of disbudding kids might well prefer to administer tetanus antitoxin routinely rather than have to worry about the consequences of occasional failure of passive transfer.

Problems Associated with Dehorning

Tetanus is not the only disaster than can result from dehorning. Except in the very young kid, the procedure is accompanied by much stress to the goat. Selecting the time for optional dehorning of adults requires careful balancing of the relative dangers of dehorning at different times. Times to be avoided if possible include lactation (because of a likely drop in milk production) and late pregnancy (risk of pregnancy toxemia) (Bowen 1977). Winter is preferable to summer, assuming the local winters are cold enough to inhibit flies (Wright et al. 1983). In general, however, it is better to dehorn a two-month-old goat in the summer than to wait six months for winter because wound size and stress on the goat increase as the animal grows.

Heat Meningitis

Prolonged application of a hot iron to a young kid's horn buds can damage the underlying bone, meninges, or brain (Linzell 1964; Wright et al. 1984; Sanford 1989; Thompson et al. 2005). The frontal bone is thin and the frontal sinus is not yet developed at the time ideal for disbudding. Coagulative necrosis of meningeal vessels can result in thrombosis and infarction of the underlying cerebrum (Thompson et al. 2005). Problems are most apt to occur when a dehorner is not hot enough to rapidly sear the skin (Williams 1985). The longer the iron must be applied, the more heat will penetrate to deeper layers. Allowing the head to cool before finishing the disbudding is advisable if the dehorner is not very hot. Goat kids that appear unresponsive or are unable to nurse at one or two days after disbudding may have reversible damage or may be able to relearn with undamaged portions of the brain. Owners should be instructed to keep these kids warm and tube feed them if necessary. Antibiotics (in case the bone is necrotic) and anti-inflammatory agents should also be administered.

Brain Abscesses

Heat cautery or paste dehorning may destroy bone overlying the brain, thereby permitting entrance of bacteria (Figure 18.7). Too low a saw cut on a mature goat can also penetrate to the brain. The animal that develops neurologic signs referable to the cerebral hemispheres several weeks after dehorning may have a brain abscess, as discussed in Chapter 5. The prognosis is grave.

Sinusitis

Even when great care is taken to prepare the skin for surgery, infection of an opened sinus may occur. This infection may ascend from the nasal passages or result from foreign matter falling into the wounds. Nasal discharge, head shaking or rubbing, or an abnormal odor suggest sinusitis in the bandaged goat or in one whose sinus has already scabbed over (Turner and McIlwraith 1982). Pus in the sinus is more quickly noticed when the wounds are left unbandaged. Bandage, scabs, and any fragments of necrotic bone should be removed. The sinus should be rinsed with a mild disinfectant solution to remove all pus. Topical antibiotics (spray or mastitis infusion products) and regular cleaning usually control the infection. Depressed or febrile animals should also receive systemic antibiotics, such as penicillin.

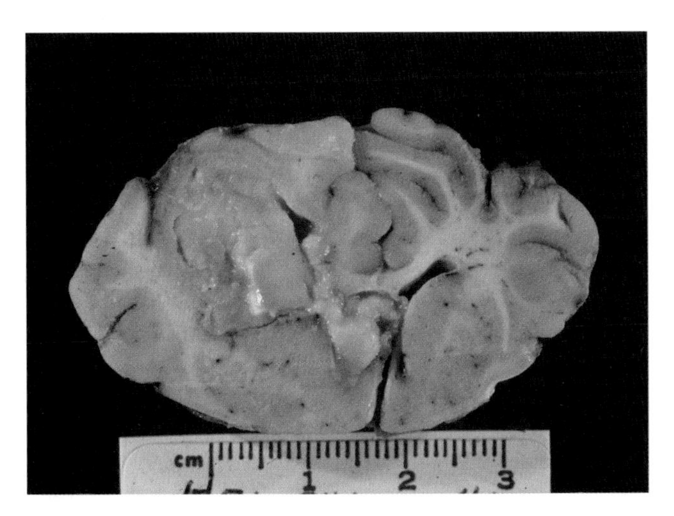

Figure 18.7. Brain abscess subsequent to bone damage by use of disbudding paste. (Courtesy Dr. M.C. Smith.)

Loss of Social Status

It is difficult to quantify the social stress experienced by the newly dehorned goat, but owners report radical upheavals and alterations in rank order in the herd as a consequence. This is especially true if a dominant individual is dehorned because it has been attacking and injuring others in the herd. When this goat has lost the means of enforcing its dominance over others, it may find itself in turn the victim of aggression. In some instances the herd behavior resembles revenge. The emotional effects on the dehorned goat may cause it to stop eating and "give up." In other circumstances, the dehorned goat is able to bite its way back to the top of the social order.

Ketosis

Decreased feed consumption, whether related to pain, infection, or loss of social status, is very dangerous to the doe in late pregnancy or early lactation. If ketosis develops, the resultant further decrease in food intake may be fatal. Does should be monitored closely in the first few days after surgery and given analgesics (aspirin 100 mg/kg orally twice daily, phenylbutazone 10 mg/kg orally once daily, flunixin meglumine 50 mg intramuscularly or orally as needed, all extra-label) if they appear to be severely depressed or in pain. Penning separate from (but within sight of) other goats and hand-feeding may encourage feed consumption. Ketosis is discussed in detail in Chapter 19.

Listeriosis

It is the author's experience that occasional goats develop clinical signs of listeriosis (i.e., depression, facial nerve paralysis, ataxia, torticollis, etc.) a few days after surgery. Presumably a latent infection has been activated by stress. Early treatment with penicillin or oxytetracycline, before signs are unequivocal, is indicated.

Scurs

The regrowth of small, deformed horns or large but rather blunt horns is a common phenomenon if corium

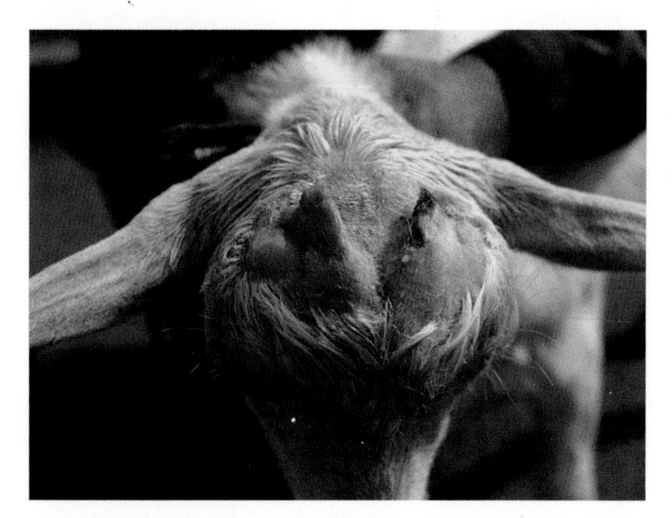

Figure 18.8. Scurs from incomplete disbudding of a buck kid. (Courtesy Dr. M.C. Smith.)

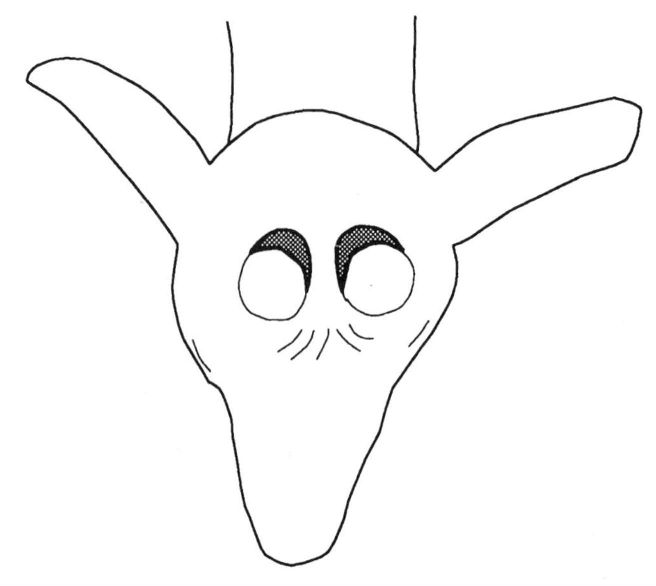

Figure 18.9. Location of skin to be cauterized or extirpated for descenting.

is incompletely removed (Figure 18.8). Practitioners or owners lacking experience with the disbudding procedure should expect their initial efforts to be accompanied occasionally by these aesthetically displeasing scurs. This is especially true when dealing with bucks and intersex goats. For this reason, buck kids should generally be disbudded at an earlier age than doelings, and a wider ring of skin should be removed from around the horn base of adult bucks.

The author always warns the owner at the time of surgery that scurs may occur. The first signs of regrowth are usually visible by the time the initial wound has healed. If the scur is in the form of a thin strip, like a piece of ribbon candy, the owner is instructed to keep it trimmed with hoof trimmers. Otherwise, the scur may grow around in a circle and press against the skull or the eye, requiring trimming with a (wire) saw as far back toward the head as the scur feels cool. If the scur has a broad base and is accompanied by outgrowth of bone, a second operation is performed; this, too, may be followed by scur formation. Poorly attached scurs are commonly dislodged during fighting and the skin may bleed profusely, but medical attention is rarely required. These scurs also regrow.

DESCENTING

Much of the odor of intact male goats emanates from multilobular sebaceous glands located caudomedially to the horns or the bosses of a polled goat (Figure 18.9). These scent glands are testosterone responsive, and one chemical produced has been identified as 6-trans nonenal (Smith et al. 1984). The odor of the buck is most rank during the fall breeding season (Jenkinson et al. 1967; Van Lancker et al. 2005). The scent glands and other sebaceous glands in the skin on the neck and shoulders are more active at this time of year, because of increased testosterone secretion. The sexually active buck also urinates on his head and forelegs, but the buck odor is absent from urine. Toggenburg bucks have a stronger buck odor than pygmy goats (Van Lancker et al. 2005). Does and castrated males only rarely produce noticeable buck odor. The odor is very marked in intersexes, which are genetically female but produce testosterone.

The skin over the scent glands can be kept clipped and scrubbed to remove as much secretion as possible. If owners or neighbors have sensitive noses, the scent glands can be destroyed, although the buck is not rendered odor-free by surgery (Bowen 1981) and may be less efficient at detecting and stimulating signs of estrus.

Descenting is easiest to do at the time of disbudding. An additional crescent of skin is burned caudomedial to each horn. Some owners choose to do this to doe kids also, theorizing that the occasional doe develops a slight buck odor.

When an adult buck is dehorned, additional skin can be removed to extirpate the scent glands. During the breeding season, this hairless skin is elevated and shiny, with large pores. If dehorning is not desired or has already been done, the glands should be located and a crescent of skin surgically removed. Tranquilization and local infiltration with lidocaine provide analgesia. The edges of the wound may be cauterized to control hemorrhage. If much skin is removed, the wound edges can be sutured (Bailey 1984). Sometimes the scent glands extend to an increased distance from the horns and may be easier to locate if a triangular flap of skin (apex of the triangle on the midline 3 to 4 cm in front of the anterior aspect of the horns) is

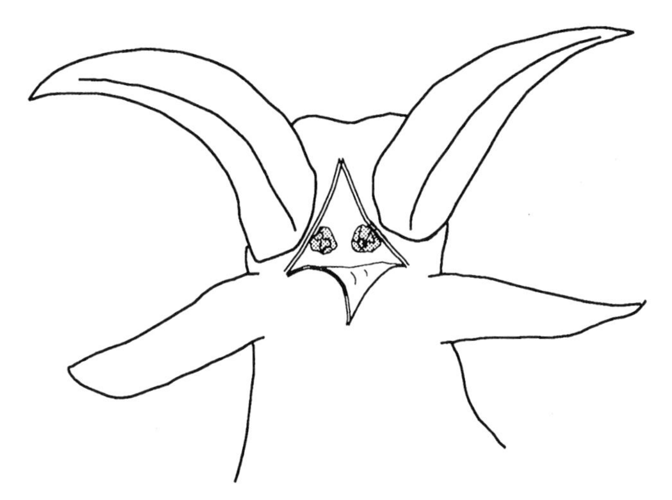

Figure 18.10. Surgical reflection of skin to locate scent glands of mature buck. (Redrawn from Johnson and Steward 1984.)

reflected caudally (Figure 18.10). The glands are then located underneath the flap and extirpated and the skin flap is sutured back into place (Johnson and Steward 1984).

REFERENCES

Anonymous: Freezing process may revolutionize disbudding, tattooing and other operations. Dairy Goat J., 55(10):14 and 77, 1977.

Anonymous: Caprine Supply 1988 Catalog. P.O. Box Y, 33001 West 83rd St., DeSoto, KS 66018.

Bailey, D.E.: The skin and subcutaneous tissue. Sheep and goats. In: The Practice of Large Animal Surgery Vol. 1. P. B. Jennings, Jr., ed. Philadelphia, W.B. Saunders Co., 1984.

Baker, J.S.: Dehorning goats. Bovine Pract., 2(1):33–39, 1981.

Baxendell, S.A.: Demonstration notes—disbudding. In: Refresher Course for Veterinarians, Proceedings No. 73, Goats, The University of Sydney, The Post-Graduate Committee in Veterinary Science, Sydney, N.S.W., Australia, Update 1984, pp. 561–562.

Bowen, J.S.: Dehorning the mature goat. J. Am. Vet. Med. Assoc., 171:1249–1250, 1977.

Bowen, J.S.: On descenting goats. Reply from a goat practitioner (letter). Vet. Med. Small Anim. Clin., 76:6, 1981.

Buttle, H., Mowlem, A. and Mews, A.: Disbudding and dehorning of goats. In Practice 8:63–65, 1986.

Elmore, R.G.: Food-animal regional anesthesia. Caprine blocks: cornual. Vet. Med. Small Anim. Clin., 76:555–556, 1981.

Hague, B.A. and Hooper, R.N.: Cosmetic dehorning in goats. Vet. Surg., 26:332–334, 1997.

Jenkinson, D.M., Blackburn, P.S. and Proudfoot, R.: Seasonal changes in the skin glands of the goat. Br. Vet. J., 123:541–549, 1967.

Johnson, E.H. and Steward, T.: Cosmetic descenting of adult goats. Agri-Practice, 5(9):16 and 20–21, 1984.

Koger, L.M. and McNiece, L.: Using the Hyfrecator for dehorning the kid. Proc. 3rd International Conf. on Goat Production Disease. Dairy Goat Journal Publ. Corp., Scottsdale, AZ, p. 530, 1982.

Linzell, J.L.: Dehorning goats. Vet. Rec. 76:853–854, 1964.

Lush, J.L.: Inheritance of horns, wattles, and color in grade Toggenburg goats. J. Hered., 17:73, 1926.

Mackenzie, D.: Goat Husbandry. 1st American Ed. Levittown, New York, Transatlantic Arts, Inc., 1975.

Mobini, S.: Cosmetic dehorning of adult goats. Small Rum. Res., 5:187–191, 1991.

Pieterse, M.C. and van Dieten, J.S.M.M.: [The dehorning of goats and kids.] Tijdschrift v. Diergeneeskunde, 120:36–38, 1995.

Reed, C.A. and Schaffer, W.M.: How to tell the sheep from the goats. Field Museum Nat. Hist. Bull., 43(3):2–7, 1972.

Ricordeau, G. and Bouillon, J.: Variation de l'âge d'apparition du cornage dans les races caprine alpine saanen, alpine chamoisée et poitevine. Ann. Génét. Sél. Anim., 1:397–401, 1969.

Sanford, S.E.: Meningoëncephalitis caused by thermal disbudding in goat kids. Can. Vet. J., 30:832, 1989.

Skarda, R.T.: Techniques of local analgesia in ruminants and swine. Vet. Clin. N. Am. Food Anim. Pract., 2:621–663, 1986.

Skarda, R.T.: Local and regional analgesia. In: Principles and Practice of Veterinary Anesthesia. C.E. Short, ed. Baltimore, Williams and Wilkins, 1987.

Smith, P.W., Parks, O.W. and Schwartz, D.P.: Characterization of male goat odors: 6-trans nonenal. J. Dairy Sci., 64:794–801, 1984.

Spaulding, C.E.: Procedure for dehorning the dairy goat. Vet. Med. Small Anim. Clin., 72:228 and 230, 1977.

Thompson, K.G., Bateman, R.S. and Morris, P.J.: Cerebral infarction and meningoencephalitis following hot-iron disbudding of goat kids. N.Z. Vet. J., 53:368–370, 2005.

Turner, A.S. and McIlwraith, C.W.: Techniques in Large Animal Surgery. Philadelphia, Lea and Febiger, 1982.

Van Lancker, S., Van den Broeck, W. and Simoens, P.: Morphology of caprine skin glands involved in buck odour production. Vet. J., 170:351–358, 2005.

Vitums, A.: Nerve and arterial blood supply to the horns of the goat with reference to the sites of anesthesia for dehorning. J. Am. Vet. Med. Assoc., 125:284–286, 1954.

Williams, B.M.: Disbudding kids. Vet. Rec. 116:480, 1985.

Williams, C.S.F.: Routine sheep and goat procedures. Vet. Clin. N. Am. Food Anim. Pract. 6:737–758, 1990.

Wright, H.J.: Disbudding technique not yet proved satisfactory. Vet. Med. Small Anim. Clin., 78:830, 1983.

Wright, H.J., Adams, D.S. and Trigo, F.J.: Meningoencephalitis after hot-iron disbudding of goat kids. Vet. Med. Small Anim. Clin., 78:599–601, 1983.

19

Nutrition and Metabolic Diseases

Goat keepers must assimilate much information regarding nutrition to raise healthy, productive animals. At least in the United States, some owners begin with absolutely no agricultural background. Their concept of nutrition has been molded by years of simply opening cans or bags of commercial pet food.

As a first step, one needs to learn the various nutritional requirements of the goat (i.e., energy, protein, fiber, vitamins, major minerals, trace minerals, and water) for whatever production is to be required of the goat. Types of production include maintenance, growth, finishing, gestation, milk production for raising kids, maximum milk production, and mohair or cashmere production. The educated owner can easily see analogies with regular dog food, puppy chow, and the limited diet necessary to stave off obesity in an older pet. But very rarely are goats fed a commercially prepared complete ration. After all, the importance of the goat in many parts of the world depends on its ability to subsist and produce on whatever grows there. It becomes necessary, then, to learn the nutritional value and relative cost of feeds available locally. This information can be gained from standard references, where concentrates are concerned, but forage quality is highly variable. The American goat keeper must either learn to accurately distinguish different types and maturities of forages or make use of feed analyses to determine the nutrient content of hays and silages.

Voluntary dry matter intake is another important consideration. What is the capacity of the goat to consume various feeds? Even more important, how much can the goat eat without deranging rumen function or the goat's own metabolism? Feeding any ruminant is first and foremost a question of properly feeding a rumen vat full of bacteria and protozoa. The energy, nitrogen, and all other requirements of bacteria must be met, and all nutrients must be provided in suitable proportions and at appropriate intervals to avoid malnutrition of the microbial population or its destruction via rumen acidosis. The ruminant needs a steady diet; unlike the situation with a monogastric animal (such as man) it is not enough to just be sure that a certain number of "servings" of hay or grain, energy or protein, have been consumed during one week or even one day. Even the physical form of the feed is important because grinding and pelleting of forages tend to decrease digestibility by decreasing the time the particles remain in the rumen.

As an additional complication, the digestibility of a given feedstuff varies with the energy and protein content of other components of the ration. Also, the energy content of a given feed or ration depends on the production function for which it is to be used. These and other problems give trained nutritionists much to argue about and go far beyond the scope of this book. The current chapter can only offer a brief overview of nutrition while trying to make the specific requirements of the goat understandable to the veterinarian or owner. As the level of production of the goat increases, the feeding must also be improved, and therefore other sources of information must be consulted to permit fine-tuning of a ration. Recently, the nutrient requirements of small ruminants, including goats, have been summarized (NRC 2007). An online ration balancer and calculator for the energy, protein, calcium, and phosphorus needs of the individual animal based on the equations used by the NRC is also available (Gipson et al. 2007) and makes the data more accessible to the potential user.

One final concern is the difference between the nutrient value of the feed offered and of the feed actually consumed (Brown and Weir 1987). Normal feeding behavior of a goat involves continual picking and choosing. When high production is required, the goat must be allowed enough extra feed that it can choose what it eats. It thereby achieves an increased level of feed intake and a richer ration, but at the expense of leaving perhaps 15% to 20% of the offered forage in the manger. Knowing the analysis values for a certain alfalfa hay is not the same as knowing the nutrient content of the leaves that were picked one by one off the stems (Morand-Fehr 1981a)! Furthermore, because of normal caprine behavior, the "choosiness" of a goat usually varies with its social status in the herd unless it is housed and fed individually. The dominant goat in the herd can stand for hours at the manger, eating what she will. Meanwhile, subordinate does and kids have to grab a mouthful and run, or even pick up discarded hay off the floor. Putting enough high quality forage into the manger to exceed the requirements of all the animals present does not ensure that one or more goats will not die of starvation.

ENERGY

All discussions of nutrition seem to begin with energy, probably because this is the best defined requirement of farm animals and is expensive. In addition, shortages of energy are translated immediately into a drop in production in dairy animals. Over a longer period of time, other effects such as retarded growth, delayed puberty, and decreased fertility become apparent.

Energy Systems

Energy is expressed in many different ways and units, which vary from system to system and country to country. This lack of uniform methodology slows the acquisition and application of knowledge relative to goat nutrition (Morand-Fehr 2005). American goat keepers should become familiar with total digestible nutrients (TDN). This system assumes that the energy value of a feed depends only on its content in terms of digestible elements. Thus, TDN (expressed as a weight or as a percentage of the feedstuff) is the sum of digestible crude protein, digestible carbohydrate, and 2.25 × digestible crude fat. A single predetermined yield in energy is assumed to apply to all types of feeds, whether forages or concentrates. With this system, energy requirements can be expressed in terms of grams of TDN, kcal of digestible energy (DE), or kcal of metabolizable energy (ME).

These units are interrelated as shown in Figure 19.1 and Table 19.1. In this example, 1 kg of TDN represents 4,409 kcal of DE, and 76 kcal DE yields 62 kcal ME (NRC 1981b). In fact, the numerical relationships vary from feed to feed. From this point, a lumper can use a global yield in net energy (NE), for instance that 62 kcal ME gives 35 kcal NE. Splitters, who are prevalent in dairy nutrition, admit that the energy losses associated with various types of production vary. Within the TDN system, one can distinguish net energy for maintenance (NE_m) with a yield of 0.72 × ME, NE for lactation (NE_l) with a yield of 0.60 × ME, and NE for growth or fattening (NE_g), with a yield of 0.45 × ME (Sauvant 1981). This compares rather poorly with the global estimate of 0.56 cited above and demonstrated in Table 19.1. However, as long as care is taken to express requirements and nutritional content in the same type of NE, the results should be the same. The system does overestimate the energy value of forages compared with concentrates.

The French system, like newer American systems for cattle, is based on NE_l and NE_g, and recognizes that different feeds have different yields in energy at each stage in the digestion/metabolism process (Vermorel 1978). For instance, long stem forages are associated with more energy losses in the form of heat of fermentation and methane gas (eructated from the rumen) than are concentrates. As in the TDN system, NE_m can be approximated by 0.72 × ME (although the actual range is 0.66 to 0.76). Similarly, NE_l is often assumed to be 0.60 × ME (actual range 0.54 to 0.68), which corresponds to the actual yield given a typical dairy ration in which 0.57 of the ingested energy appears as metabolizable energy. For all rations, the NE_l yield is proportional to the NE_m yield, such that net energy requirements for both maintenance and lactation can be expressed in terms of NE_l. Current French tables of nutrient composition and requirements use a new unit, the UFL, which is equivalent to 1,700 kcal of net energy for lactation (INRA 2007). The corresponding unit for net energy for growth is the UFV, equivalent to 1,820 kcal of net energy for growth.

The energy requirements for goats that will now be outlined follow French recommendations because much work has been devoted in that country specifically to the nutrition of the dairy goat. In addition, much of the original research has been summarized in one text (Morand-Fehr 1991), and updated tables are available (INRA 2007). Forage analysis reports currently available in the United States through the Dairy Herd Improvement Association and many computerized ration calculation programs also deal with NE_l. Readers who prefer the TDN system may refer to the National Research Council (NRC) publication Nutrient Requirements of Small Ruminants (2007). If goats differing greatly from European dairy breeds are to be fed, or if the climate is not temperate, then the estimates of other authors may be more appropriate (Rajpoot et al. 1981).

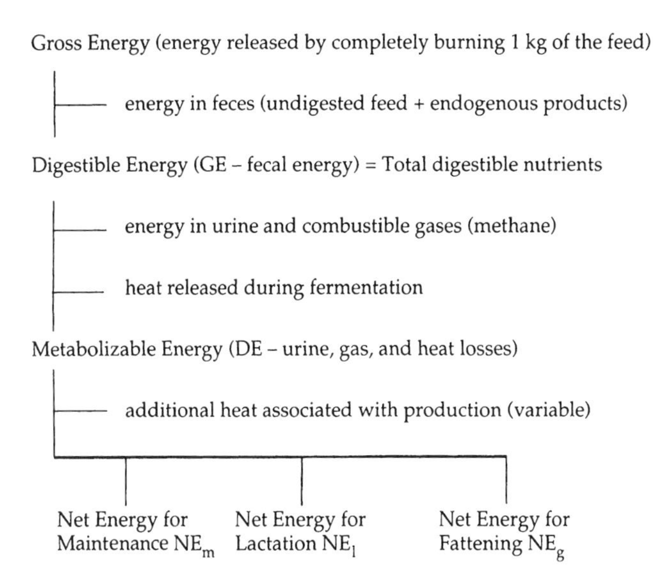

Figure 19.1. Energy categories.

Maintenance

The energy required for maintenance of a goat depends in a specific way on the bw of the animal. However, this is not a linear relationship and most people without access to calculators prefer consulting a table such as NRC (2007) or INRA (2007) to working through the arithmetic. Numerous studies for various breeds and ages of goats have each produced a different equation meant to represent the energy requirements. These equations may calculate either metabolizable energy or net energy and energy units may be in either kcal (total digestible energy system) or kilojoules (SI or International System) units. One such equation (Vermorel 1978) demonstrates that the daily NE_l needed in kcal for maintenance is proportional to the metabolic weight. The weight is expressed in kilograms (1 kg is equal to 2.204 pounds) and this is raised to the 0.75 power.

$$\text{Maintenance } (NE_l) = 65.3 \times W_{kg}^{0.75}$$

Table 19.1. Interrelationships of energy units in the total digestible nutrient system.

GE (kcal)	100					Gross energy
TDN (kg)		1	0.227	0.278	0.492	Total digestible nutrients
DE (kcal)	76	4409	1000	1226	2171	Digestible energy
ME (kcal)	62	3597	816	1000	1771	Metabolizable energy
NE (kcal)	35	2030	460	564	1000	Net energy

Table 19.2. Maintenance energy requirements for goats.

Weight (kg)	*Weight (lb)*	*Metabolic Wt (kg)*	*Daily NE_l (kcal)*	*Daily NE_l (MJoule)*
10	22	5.62	367	1.536
20	44	9.46	618	2.586
30	66	12.82	837	3.502
40	88	15.91	1039	4.347
50	110	18.80	1228	5.138
60	132	21.56	1408	5.891
70	154	24.20	1580	6.611
80	176	26.75	1747	7.309
90	198	29.22	1908	7.983
100	220	31.62	2065	8.640

Table 19.2 indicates the metabolic bodyweights and NE_l requirements for goats of various weights using this equation as an example. It can be used in conjunction with NRC requirement tables, with 1 Mcal equal to 1,000 kcal. For countries using SI units, note that 1 kilojoule = 0.239 kcal, and 1 kcal = 4.184 kilojoules.

Recently, many equations have been summarized and used as the basis for the energy recommendations in the 2007 NRC tables (Luo et al. 2004c; Nsahlai et al. 2004a; Sahlu et al. 2004). The factor by which the metabolic weight is multiplied depends on the age and breed of goat under consideration. This in turn makes the resultant tables more accurate when applied to a given class of goats.

Environment

The energy requirements for maintenance also vary with environmental conditions (such as temperature, humidity, and wind) and with exercise. The heat of fermentation normally lost during digestion helps to maintain body temperature of ruminants in a cold environment. In fact, a goat on a high roughage diet has the benefit of an internal hot water bottle, the rumen, to keep it warm. Supplemental grain feeding further increases the heat production from the rumen, even though the proportion of the digestible energy of concentrate feeds released as heat is less. Animals without active rumen function must shiver to maintain body temperature. For this reason a "goat coat" (i.e., a sweatshirt) or a blanket is often beneficial to an animal off feed because of illness or surgery.

The thermoneutral zone (TNZ) is the temperature range in which the animal is most productive with least stress and is approximately 32°F to 86°F (0°C to 30°C) in goats (Constantinou 1987). The upper critical temperature is the upper limit of the thermoneutral zone; above this temperature the animal experiences heat stress. High producing animals, with increased metabolic heat, are more susceptible to heat stress (NRC 1981a). The lower critical temperature is the lower limit of the thermoneutral zone. The lower critical temperature varies between animals and depends on hair coat, presence of insulating fat, and level of feeding. Shearing during cold weather increases the energy needs of hair goats and often leads to deaths.

Energy requirements need to be adjusted for very cold weather. When a goat is outside its thermoneutral zone, more energy is required for maintenance. For instance, for every degree centigrade below the thermoneutral zone, an additional 0.7 could be added to the 65.3 factor in the equation given above (figure used for beef cattle) (Simons and Hand 1986). The effect of wind velocity can be crudely estimated to be equivalent to a decrease of 0.6°C (1.08°F) for each mile per hour. Thus, for a temperature 10°C (18°F) less than the TNZ in the presence of a 20-mph wind, the equivalent temperature difference would be 10 + 0.6 (20°F) or 22°C, equivalent to a difference of 39.6°F. The maintenance requirement for a 50-kg goat would then be $(65.3 + 22\ (.7)) \times 50^{0.75}$ or (65.3 + 15.4) (18.8) = 1,517 kcal rather than the usual 1228 kcal. Wetness causes an additional decrease in "effective temperature" below that calculated by the wind chill factor. These corrections need to be verified for goats. Perhaps an increase of 1% in the maintenance energy for each degree C below the thermoneutral zone is a reasonable starting estimate.

Adjustment in the energy density of the diet may be required, because even though voluntary intake increases in cold weather, the energy requirement for maintenance usually increases more rapidly (Ames 1987).

Activity

An increase in NE_l of 20% to 25% more than the maintenance requirements for stabled animals has been suggested for goats engaged in light grazing. Animals traveling longer distances to find food and water need substantially more, but the exact amount is hard to quantify. An additional 40% more than simple maintenance is suggested for distances of four miles a day (6.5 km), and 60% for six miles (Morand-Fehr and Sauvant 1978). The increase suggested by NRC (1981b) for long distances and great changes in altitude is 75%. Thus, a goat weighing 60 kg is estimated to need 1,408 kcal a day if it stays in the barn, 1,690 if it grazes nearby, and approximately 2,250 if it travels six miles. Activity level and energy expenditure among goats in a single herd are actually quite variable.

Lactation

The proportion of ME that is used for lactation is independent of the level of production. However, it is necessary to adjust the NE_l requirements as the fat, protein, and lactose content of the milk changes. Using a reference milk containing 3.5% fat, 3.1% protein, and 4.3% lactose, the energy requirement per kg of milk produced is 676 kcal NE_l (INRA 2007). If the fat content of the milk differs markedly from 3.5%, the NRC (1981b) recommendation to change the ME needed by 16.28 kcal for each 0.5% fat would translate to adjusting the NE_l by 12 kcal.

Growth and Weight Gain

Yearling goats are still growing during lactation, and need extra nutrients to support this growth. In addition, high producing goats lose weight (up to 7 kg [INRA 2007]) during the first months of lactation because they mobilize body reserves to produce milk. They will eventually need to regain this weight. Approximately 6 kcal NE_l is needed for each gram of live weight gain. The average mature Alpine goat replacing her reserves needs 270 kcal/day extra for this purpose (Morand-Fehr and Sauvant 1978). This represents a weight gain of 45 g/day. By way of comparison, NRC (2007) uses values of 5.52 kcal ME/g daily gain of meat and dairy kids and 6.81 kcal ME/g of weight gain for mature animals.

Gestation

There is no extra energy requirement until the last two months of pregnancy. French workers use the bw at breeding time to calculate maintenance energy for a doe and then add 830 kcal NE_l /day for the last two months. In the experimental data used to derive this, the average weight of the kids at birth was 7.6 kg; 1 kg of kid thus required 109 kcal/day extra energy. In general, if the supplemental energy for pregnancy is dropped to less than 500 kcal the goats will be prone to pregnancy toxemia, while above 1,100 additional kcal of NE_l there will be digestive accidents, difficult births, and poor milk production in the subsequent lactation (Sauvant 1981). These situations are discussed in detail later in this chapter. The current French recommendation is to multiply the maintenance energy requirement by 1.15 to 1.30 for the last two months of gestation (INRA 2007). The current NRC tables (2007) distinguish between dairy and nondairy does carrying singles, twins, or three or more kids when determining the energy (and protein) requirements.

PROTEIN

Proteins are needed throughout life for growth and repair of the body and for synthesis of products such as enzymes, hormones, mucin, milk, and hair. As is true of monogastric animals, the ruminants' protein requirements consist mainly of amino acids that are absorbed from the small intestine. However, these amino acids come from two sources. The first is dietary protein that escapes degradation in the rumen but is digested to amino acids in the intestine. The second source is microbial protein. Almost all soluble protein, any nonprotein nitrogen, and approximately one-third of the insoluble protein in the diet are broken down in the rumen to release ammonia. This represents 40% to 70% of the nitrogen in green forages and 45% to 65% of the nitrogen in mixed rations. If energy supplies are adequate, this ammonia is then built into protein by rumen microbes. The microbes pass out of the rumen and are killed by the acidity of the abomasum. The dead microbes become available for digestion into amino acids in the intestine.

Because the rumen microbial population synthesizes all of the amino acids essential to a goat, sheep, or cow from dietary protein and nonprotein nitrogen and sulfur, the amino acid composition of the feedstuffs is relatively unimportant. However, for maximum milk production it is advantageous to supply some additional amino acids in the form of rumen undegradable protein or rumen protected amino acids. For dairy cattle, methionine and lysine are considered to be the most limiting amino acids relative to high milk production. Fishmeal as a bypass protein is a good source of methionine but heat treated soybean meal is not. Zinc-methionine and zinc-lysine chelates have been used to supplement these amino acids in dairy cattle (Kung and Rode 1996). There is very limited evidence that supplementation with protected methionine or lysine improves milk production in goats that are not deficient in zinc (Salama et al. 2003; Madsen et al. 2005; Kholif et al. 2006; Poljicak-Milas and Marenjak 2007). The possible benefits of additional cysteine and methionine for fiber growth are discussed below, under Special Consideration for Feeding Angora and Cashmere Goats.

Protein Systems and Requirements

Protein requirements for the goat were originally expressed in terms of total crude protein, which is simply determined by multiplying the nitrogen content of the feed by 6.25. This figure is used because most proteins contain 16% nitrogen. Nonprotein nitrogen

(NPN) substances in the feed thus enter into the calculation as if they were true protein, but this is not a serious flaw because the rumen microbes can transform NPN into protein. The previous NRC for goats (1981b) computed protein requirements from a simple calorie-to-protein ratio. Thus, the tables in this publication required 32 g of total protein for each Mcal of digestible energy. Efforts to express requirements in terms of digestible protein (apparently digested protein, determined by subtracting fecal nitrogen from dietary nitrogen) are not believed to be more accurate because metabolic fecal nitrogen (i.e., digestive enzymes, sloughed epithelial cells, etc.) comprises a variable proportion of the total fecal nitrogen. Also, ammonia released in the rumen in excess of what the microbial population can use for synthesis is absorbed into the bloodstream. This ammonia is converted by the liver to urea, some of which is recycled into the rumen by diffusion or via saliva so that it may be used between meals when the rumen ammonia levels fall, but some is lost in the urine.

When high production is desired it is necessary to refine the protein requirements beyond crude protein and digestible protein. Ruminants need both rumen degradable and rumen bypass protein (Waldo and Glenn 1984; Eastridge 1990). Newer systems for goats specify protein requirements in terms of metabolizable protein (MP). MP is defined as the true protein, derived from a combination of dietary and microbial protein, that is digested postruminally and from which the constituent amino acids are absorbed from the intestine (NRC 2007). The recent NRC (2007) determines metabolizable protein (MP) requirements from equations summarized by Sahlu et al. (2004) and others (Luo et al. 2004a; Nsahlai et al. 2004b) and available online (Gipson and Goetsch). The protein requirement for goats of various classes is expressed in grams MP/day but also converted to a crude protein requirement that depends on the proportion of the dietary protein that is rumen undegradable (UIP, undegradable intake protein). The formula used for the conversion of metabolic protein to crude protein is

$$CP = MP/((64 + (0.16 \times \%\ UIP))/100)$$

Beyond the protein required for maintenance (expressed on a metabolic weight basis), goats need additional protein for growth (0.29 g MP/g average daily gain for dairy and indigenous goats, 0.40 g MP/g daily gain for meat goats). Each g of milk protein requires 1.45 g MP, while each g of clean mohair fiber requires 1.65 g MP. Further protein is required for growth of the mammary gland, uterus, and fetuses during pregnancy.

The 2007 NRC composition tables specify CP, MP, and often UIP for each feedstuff. For forages, actual values determined by laboratory testing often give a better approximation of protein content than do book values. Overheating that occurs when hay is stored too wet or silage is stored too dry results in complexing of sugars with amino acids that reduces the digestibility of nitrogen. This nitrogen ends up in the acid detergent fiber fraction during forage analysis (Eastridge 1990). Some laboratories determine available protein (or adjusted crude protein) on forages to reflect this loss in feed value.

The amount of microbial protein formed with each feed actually depends on whether energy or nitrogen is the limiting factor for microbial reproduction and growth. Thus, with most concentrates, there is more than enough energy in the feed to fix ammonia released from rumen digestion into microbial protein; the nitrogen supply is what limits bacterial growth. With many forages not all of the ammonia liberated can be fixed because of an energy shortage, and the unused nitrogen is lost to the body, mainly through the urine.

Recent French composition tables give two metabolizable protein figures for each feedstuff (Morand-Fehr and Sauvant 1978; INRA 2007). One indicates the sum of digestible protein escaping the rumen and of the microbial protein that could be formed if all of the nitrogen released in the rumen could be converted into protein (PDIN in French usage, i.e., if energy were not limiting). The other (PDIE) is the sum of alimentary protein digested in the intestine and of the microbial protein that could be formed if all of the energy available for the rumen organisms could be used for their growth (i.e., if nitrogen were not limiting). When a single feed is fed, it is the smaller of the two values that represents the metabolizable protein. However, when feeds are combined, the ruminant (and the nutritionist) can add up all the PDIE values to give a global PDIE for the ration and can likewise obtain a global PDIN. If PDIE exceeds PDIN, it may be possible to add NPN to make use of the excess available energy, assuming that this can be done in such a way that the ammonia supplied and the energy released from digestion of carbohydrates are present simultaneously in the rumen. If PDIN exceeds PDIE, the diet could be better balanced by adding more energy or removing some nitrogen, depending on which of these options gives better economic results. Protecting some of the dietary protein from degradation in the rumen (as by heat or formaldehyde treatment) so that it can be digested in the intestine is one way of avoiding nitrogen losses associated with excess PDIN.

Milk Urea Nitrogen

Dairy cattle nutritionists pay close attention to milk urea nitrogen (MUN), the portion of the measured milk protein that is derived from blood urea nitrogen rather than casein or whey proteins. Ammonia produced during digestion that is not converted into microbial protein is absorbed from the rumen and converted to urea in the liver. This urea is recycled via saliva into the rumen but diffuses into milk. High MUN values are seen when too much crude protein or rumen degradable protein is fed relative to fermentable carbohydrate (Roseler et al. 1993) or when rumen acidosis slows microbial protein production. Low MUN values suggest that there is not enough ammonia produced in the rumen for optimum microbial growth, as might occur with inadequate rumen degradable protein intake. High MUN has also been associated with reduced conception rates in cows, though some say that this adverse effect actually reflects the presence of phytoestrogens in the soybean products that are typically the source of excessive dietary protein in the dairy cow studies (Piotrowska et al. 2006). Normal MUN values for cows are approximately 8 to 14 mg/dl. A brief report of MUN evaluation in dairy sheep on varying diets produced a range of average MUN values from 26 to 56 mg/dl (Cannas et al. 1995).

Little research has been done relative to interpretation of MUN in goats. Brun-Bellut et al. (1991) proposed a normal range of 28 to 32 mg/dl. A study comparing Alpine goats fed alfalfa hay or pasture and varying levels of concentrates found a range of MUN values of 18 to 22 mg/dl (Min et al. 2005). When varying amounts of tallow were added to the diet in another study, the MUN varied from 24 to 26 mg/dl (Brown-Crowder et al. 2001). In a long-term study that compared a forage based diet with one formulated with sunflower seeds, cassava, coconut meal, and cottonseed, the MUN was lower for the forage diet (approximately 15 mg/dl) than for the nonforage diet (approximately 30 mg/dl), even though milk yield was similar (Bava et al. 2001). It seems apparent that MUN values in goats are generally higher than those reported for dairy cattle. A French study that evaluated 2083 milk samples from 260 goat herds found an average MUN of 47 mg/dl, with 90% of the values falling between 35 and 55 mg/dl (Jourdain 2005). The author concluded that the average MUN values were too similar across feeding systems and the individual values too variable among goats on the same diet for the test to be useful for guiding ration adjustment. Some laboratories routinely test goat milk for this component without calibrating the equipment for goat milk, which further complicates interpretation of results.

How nutrition might influence true milk protein content in dairy goats has been reviewed by Chamberlain (1997).

Urea Toxicity

As is commonly done with dairy cattle, urea can be fed to goats as a nonprotein nitrogen source because rumen organisms can convert it to microbial protein if adequate energy sources are available (Harmeyer and Martens 1980). Much of the urea that reaches the plasma (absorbed from the gastrointestinal tract or produced in the liver) is recycled to the rumen via saliva.

Pathogenesis and Epidemiology

Toxicity is expected to occur if 30 to 50 g urea/100 kg bw is consumed in a single meal by an unadapted or hungry ruminant. This is because the urea is degraded to ammonia and excessive nonionized ammonia in the rumen diffuses out into the bloodstream. Toxic levels are reached when the liver's ability to convert ammonia back into urea is overwhelmed. The citrate cycle is inhibited by the ammonia (Lloyd 1986).

Improperly mixed feed and urea fertilizers are potential sources for toxicity. Nonprotein nitrogen is particularly dangerous when animals are fed high fiber diets lacking readily digestible carbohydrate. In one instance, a goat and other livestock at a fair died after drinking water contaminated by transport in a tanker that usually hauled a liquid fertilizer composed of urea and ammonium nitrate (Campagnolo et al. 2002).

Clinical Signs

Toxicity in small ruminants (Fujimoto and Tajima 1953; Obasju et al. 1980; McLennan et al. 1987; Ortolani et al. 2000) typically occurs within one hour after ingestion, and death after a few hours. Signs include muscle and skin tremors, salivation, frequent urination and defecation, incoordination, dyspnea, loud bleating, bloat, tetany or convulsions, and death. Laboratory findings include elevations in blood packed cell volume, potassium, phosphorus, and urea nitrogen. Sometimes, but not always, the rumen fluid pH exceeds 7.5 (Lloyd 1986), and ammonia concentration in rumen fluid exceeds 500 ppm (Ortolani et al. 2000, Campagnolo et al. 2002).

Treatment

The best antidote available is 0.5 to 1 liter of vinegar (typically 5% acetic acid), which may be given by stomach tube to decrease rumen pH (Osweiler et al. 1985). A potentially equivalent vinegar dosage is 10 ml/kg. At a lower pH, the ionized ammonium ion diffuses less readily through the rumen wall into the circulation, and free ammonia already in the blood may actually return to the rumen. If the goat is already in tetany, emergency surgery to empty the rumen has been suggested as the one method that might possibly save the animal's life (Bartley et al. 1976). Intravenous lactated Ringer's solution (for its acidifying effect) and B vitamins have also been proposed, among other treatments, as beneficial in treating animals with chronic consumption of excess urea (Hazarika et al. 2002).

Prevention

In the absence of PDIN/PDIE values for dietary components used by French nutritionists, other guidelines may be used to predict a safe level of urea use. For instance, in American literature there is often a statement that urea should not exceed 1.5% of a finished (total) ration (Adams 1986). It has also been recommended that urea supply no more than one-third of the total crude protein (CP) in forage or roughage diets and that it be no more than one-half of the CP in the concentrate part of the ration (NRC 1981b; Fernandez et al. 1997). At least three weeks are required for the rumen microflora to adapt to such a high level of urea feeding, and therefore, gradually increasing the concentration of urea in the feed is advisable. Not all goats are willing to eat grain containing so much urea (Skjevdal 1981).

FIBER

Insoluble dietary fiber is indigestible or slowly digesting organic material of feeds that occupies space in the digestive tract (Mertens 2003). Fiber is mostly cell wall material consisting of cellulose, hemicellulose, and lignin. Different roughages contain different amounts of these constituents. During analysis procedures, roughages are subjected to several treatments that distinguish these constituents (Figure 19.2). Thus, acid detergent fiber (ADF) is a measure of cellulose plus lignin, while neutral detergent fiber (NDF) represents the total cell wall content. Because pectin in the cell wall is highly soluble and lost from the NDF fraction, fiber is underestimated in pectin-rich feeds such as alfalfa or citrus pulp. The difference between ADF and NDF is essentially the hemicellulose content of the roughage. Laboratories usually calculate the energy value of a feed from the ADF and a formula appropriate for the class of feedstuff.

The goat, like other ruminants, is able to digest fiber such as cellulose and hemicellulose into volatile fatty acids by means of fermentation in the rumen. There is conflicting evidence whether goats are more efficient at digesting fiber than are other species of ruminants. In some instances, the apparent superiority of the goat to survive on poor roughages is because of its ability to choose the most digestible parts of the plant. Lignin in the cell wall bonds to cellulose and imparts structural strength to the plant as it matures, but markedly reduces its susceptibility to microbial digestion in the

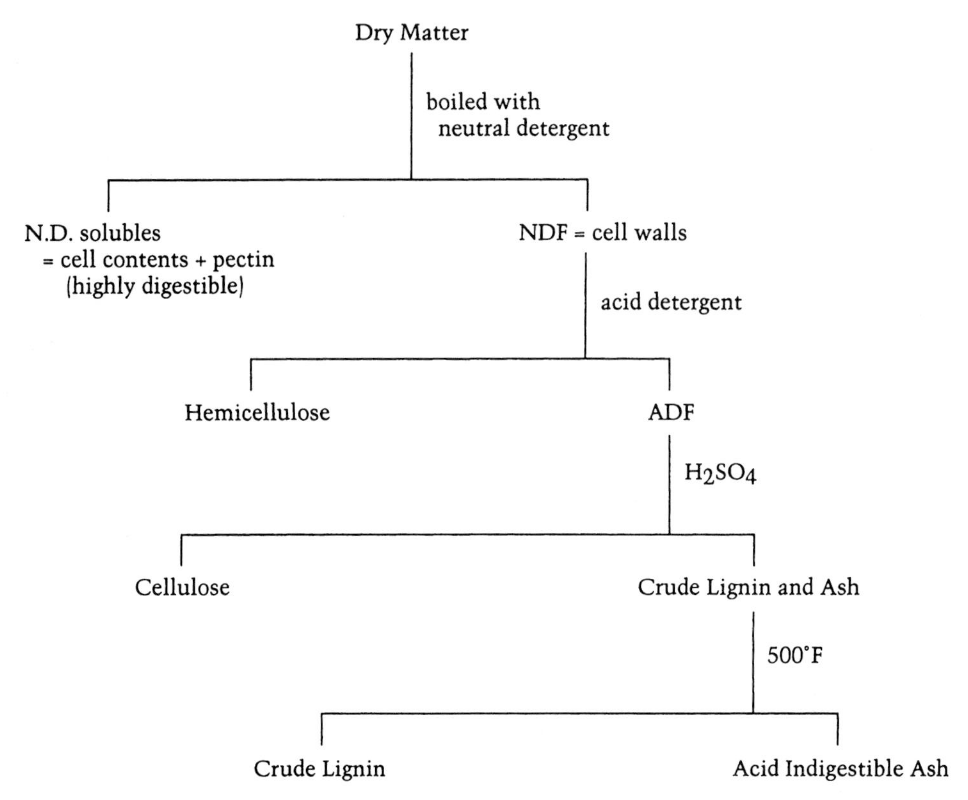

Figure 19.2. Laboratory scheme for fiber analysis. ND = neutral detergent, NDF = neutral detergent fiber, ADF = acid detergent fiber.

rumen (NRC 2007). Mature grasses with increased lignin content have lowered digestibility.

Goats undoubtedly have a requirement for fiber to maintain healthy rumen function and butterfat production (Santini et al. 1991, Lu et al. 2005). Little research data is available to document exactly how much NDF or ADF should be included in a goat's rations. Meanwhile, recommendations for dairy cows (more than 25% NDF and more than 19% ADF) may be used as a starting point. One recent paper suggests 18% to 20% ADF or 41% NDF for high producing lactating dairy goats, and 23% ADF for growing kids (Lu et al. 2005). Particle size is also important, because it determines the time required for mastication and the amount of saliva produced to buffer rumen contents.

VITAMINS

The fat-soluble vitamins are important in goat nutrition, as they are in the feeding of other domestic animals and humans. Water-soluble vitamins other than thiamine and niacin are generally ignored when formulating caprine rations.

Vitamin A

Beta-carotene is the standard dietary precursor of vitamin A, although some other carotenoids also have biological activity. Previously (NRC 1981b), 1 mg of beta-carotene was judged to be equivalent to approximately 400 IU vitamin A. Currently recommended conversions are 671 IU of vitamin A/mg of beta-carotene and 436 IU/mg of other common carotenoids such as cryptoxanthine in yellow corn (NRC 2007). As little as 10% of dietary beta-carotene escapes degradation in the rumen. Absorption, metabolism, and storage of the remainder require a healthy digestive epithelium and liver (Ferrando and Barlet 1978).

Vitamin A can also be expressed as retinol equivalents (RE), where 1 IU = 0.3 μg of retinol. The biopotency of 1 RE for goats is expressed as the vitamin A activity of 1 μg of all-*trans* retinol, 5 μg of all-*trans* beta-carotene, or 7.6 μg of other carotenoids with vitamin A activity (NRC 2007). The vitamin A requirement tables in this reference book use the RE unit. The RE can be converted back to IU of vitamin A by multiplying by 3.33, thus 1 RE = approximately 3.33 IU of vitamin A.

Signs of Deficiency

Poor appetite, weight loss, unthrifty appearance with a poor hair coat, night blindness, and a thick nasal discharge have resulted from experimental vitamin A deficiency in goats (Schmidt 1941). Especially in young animals, a deficiency predisposes to diarrheal and respiratory disease and to parasitism. To further compound the problem, kids with coccidiosis have an increased vitamin A requirement because of impaired absorption. Adult goats may have a decreased fertility rate (related to inadequate steroid hormone synthesis) in addition to an increased susceptibility to disease. Vitamin A deficiency may promote desquamation of urinary epithelium and nidus formation with subsequent urolithiasis (Schmidt 1941).

Dietary Recommendations and Supplementation

The NRC applies sheep requirements to goats. According to its 2007 recommendations, the daily maintenance requirement is 31.4 RE/kg body weight or 104.7 IU/kg. The 50-kg goat at maintenance should receive 1,570 RE or approximately 5,235 IU of vitamin A/day while the 90-kg goat needs approximately 9,423 IU. To this is to be added 45.5 RE/kg (152 IU/kg)/day for late pregnancy and 100 RE/kg (333 IU/kg) for growing goats. The NRC 2007 additional requirement for lactation is now 53.5 RE/kg and disregards the level of milk production. A simplified recommendation from the French is 5,000 IU vitamin A/kg dry matter of feed across the board (Morand-Fehr 1981b). Browse and green leafy hays are good sources of vitamin A, while old or weathered hay is a poor source. After six months of storage, all beta-carotene in hay has been destroyed (Ferrando and Barlet 1978). Vitamin A palmitate is commonly added to mineral mixes and commercial concentrates. Because vitamin A is fat-soluble and stored in the liver and other body fat, the adult goat can tolerate several months of low carotene intake without developing clinical signs of deficiency. Vitamin A toxicity does not occur when natural diets are fed but could occur with mixing errors. A maximum of 6,000 μg of retinol/kg bodyweight/day is recommended (NRC 2007).

Colostrum is a very rich source of vitamin A, and before its consumption kids have minimal stores. When kids receive colostrum from does that are primiparous (decreased concentration of vitamin A), or only limited amounts of colostrum, an oral vitamin A palmitate supplement is desirable. Injectable vitamin A is less valuable because of rapid peroxidation at the injection site.

Vitamin D

There are two principal forms of vitamin D. The first is vitamin D_2 (ergocalciferol) that is obtained from irradiation of the plant sterol ergosterol. Vitamin D_2 is thus abundant in sun-cured hay. The second form, vitamin D_3 (cholecalciferol), is found in liver oil from marine fishes, but it is also synthesized in the mammalian epidermis under the influence of ultraviolet light. One mg of either D_2 or D_3 is ascribed an antirachitic activity of 40,000 IU.

The metabolism of vitamin D_3 involves several steps. First, it is carried from the skin or digestive tract to the liver, where it is transformed to 25-hydroxycholecalciferol. Next, it passes to the kidney where a second hydroxylation creates 1,25-dihydroxycholecalciferol. This metabolite acts as a steroid hormone in increasing phosphorus absorption and inducing synthesis of calcium binding hormone in the intestine. Synthesis of 1,25-dihydroxycholecalciferol is stimulated by any decrease in blood calcium or phosphorus levels and by parathyroid hormone.

Signs of Deficiency

The effect of 1,25-dihydroxycholecalciferol on bone metabolism is important but complex. It stimulates both the fixation and release of calcium and phosphorus from the skeleton. Young, growing animals raised in dark conditions, whose dams were similarly housed and deprived of a vitamin D supplement, develop rickets. Signs include bowed limbs, enlarged joints, stiffness, and a rachitic rosary on the ribs. Growth rate and body condition are poor. Adults deficient in vitamin D develop osteomalacia or osteoporosis, especially if dietary Ca and P are not properly balanced. Blood calcium and phosphorus levels may be decreased, but this is not a consistent finding (Ferrando and Barlet 1978). See Chapter 4 for further discussion of metabolic bone diseases.

Dietary Recommendations and Supplementation

The exact vitamin D requirements for goats have not been determined. A level of 5.6 IU/kg bw/day has been recommended for both sheep and goats (NRC 2007). The NRC recommends an additional 54 IU/day for every 50 g daily weight gain and 213 IU/day for late pregnancy, and allows 760 IU/kg of milk produced. Colostrum is rich in vitamin D_3, and goat milk contains approximately 20 IU/liter. If adults are on pasture or fed much sun-cured hay, their needs should be easily met. Stabled animals fed much concentrate, especially if high milk producers, need a supplement.

Vitamin D Toxicity

Excess vitamin D activity from certain toxic plants (Mello 2003) such as yellow oat grass (*Trisetum flavescens*, Braun et al. 2000) in Europe and day-blooming jasmine (*Cestrum diurnum*) in the southeastern United States causes calcinosis of tendons and other soft tissues. The same effect can be had by large overdoses of oral or injectable vitamin D supplements (Singh and Prasad 1989).

Vitamin E

Vitamin E (1 mg dl-alpha tocopheryl acetate = 1 IU) is present in colostrum, milk, and many natural feeds, especially green forage. Ruminants do not synthesize vitamin E, but require it in their diet (Van Metre and Calan 2001). Its main action is as an antioxidant; it stabilizes polyunsaturated fatty acids, vitamin A, and various hormones and enzymes. Vitamin E and selenium are closely interrelated; a deficiency of one can be at least partially offset by increasing the intake of the other.

Signs of Deficiency

Vitamin E deficiency alone can cause nutritional muscular dystrophy (white muscle disease). This is most likely to occur with feeding of silage or old hay, because the vitamin is lost in storage. Kids may have muscle disease at birth and be too weak to suckle (Kolb and Kaskous 2003). Sudden death related to Zenker's necrosis of heart muscle or diaphragm may occur, even in kids with normal selenium status (Byrne 1992). Inhalation pneumonia can also result from muscle weakness of the larynx and pharynx. Affected kids are sometimes noted to cough or have milk run out the nose after drinking. Kids may also develop muscle stiffness after exercise. The diagnosis of nutritional muscular dystrophy is discussed in Chapter 4. Fastest growing animals are at the greatest risk.

Adults may show poor uterine involution and retained placenta. Undesirable milk flavors related to oxidation of milk fat might be expected to occur with vitamin E/selenium deficiency. Ventral edema of Angora goats (see Chapter 3) has also been associated with vitamin E deficiency.

Vitamin E is also very important for optimizing immune responses. Beneficial effects have been demonstrated in ruminants on phagocytosis by polymorphonuclear cells and on cell mediated immunity (NRC 2007). Obviously, increased incidence or severity of infectious diseases is a very nonspecific sign of vitamin E deficiency, but is part of the reason for recent increases in the dietary recommendation.

Plasma vitamin E concentrations of less than 1.5 μmol/l (65 μg/dl) in preparturient does and less than 1 μmol/l (43 μg/dl) in suckling kids have been associated with increased risk of myopathy (Jones et al. 1988). A normal range in goat serum of 60 to 150 μg/dl has been proposed by the Colorado Veterinary Diagnostic Laboratory (Van Metre and Callan 2001). Note that the blood sample needs to be handled very carefully (no hemolysis, rapid refrigeration and removal of the plasma or serum from the erythrocytes) if accurate results are to be obtained. Liver vitamin E concentration can also be determined and may better reflect the nutritional status of the animal (Liesegang et al. 2008). A normal caprine liver concentration of greater than 250 μg/100 g wet weight has been proposed (Van Metre and Callan 2001).

Dietary Recommendations and Supplementation

In the absence of selenium deficiency, the daily requirement of vitamin E for preventing nutritional muscular dystrophy in preruminant lambs and calves, and presumably, kids was previously given as 0.1 to 0.3 IU/kg bw (Ferrando and Barlet 1978). This was to be doubled when feeding milk replacers. Later, it was advised to add 25 to 50 mg of vitamin E/kg of concentrate for adults and 50 to 100 mg/kg of concentrate for kids (Ferrando and Barlet 1978). Note that vitamin E is relatively nontoxic and 75 IU/kg bw daily is presumed safe (NRC 2007). The current recommendation of 10 mg/kg bw daily (NRC 2007) takes into account the diverse functions of the vitamin beyond prevention of mypoathy.

Vitamin E is oxidized by iron (or copper) in the feed, and thus diets with high iron content may have less vitamin E available. Rapidly growing green plants have a high content of polyunsaturated fatty acids (PUFAs) and animals on lush pasture also have a higher need for antioxidants such as vitamin E because of increased incorporation of PUFAs into cell membranes and thus increased susceptibility to lipid peroxidation (Van Metre and Calan 2001). Oil seeds also contain high concentrations of PUFAs.

The vitamin E content of colostrum depends on the nutrition of the dam during pregnancy. At the end of the winter, when most goats in temperate climates kid, the hay cut the previous year is very low in vitamin E. Supplementation of the pregnant doe is important for optimizing kid health.

Some injectable preparations such as vitamin A and D include vitamin E as an antioxidant to stabilize the other fat-soluble vitamins; the quantity of vitamin E is inadequate for therapeutic purposes. Similarly, some vitamin E/selenium preparations contain relatively little vitamin E. Injectable preparations of vitamin E alone are available, with labeled recommendations of 600 to 900 IU to lambs at birth or weaning and 1,200 to 1,500 IU to ewes prepartum or at lambing.

B Vitamins

B vitamins are normally synthesized in adequate amounts by rumen microbes and thus supplementation of the adult goat's diet is not required. Colostrum is a good source of B vitamins. Older kids that do not yet have a fully developed rumen may need a dietary source of B complex vitamins, and supplementation of milk replacers is advisable. B vitamins also should be added to the diet or administered by injection to sick animals and those with poor rumen function or marked change in diet (NRC 1981b). Dietary supplementation with niacin is sometimes recommended for prevention of pregnancy toxemia (see below). There is currently no evidence that additional biotin promotes hoof health in goats (NRC 2007). Supplementation of periparturient does with rumen-protected choline may increase milk production, although the effect likely reflects dietary methionine availability (D'Ambrosio et al. 2007).

There are two instances in which B vitamin deficiency assumes primary clinical importance. The first is when a cobalt deficiency prevents synthesis of adequate vitamin B_{12}; this is discussed under cobalt requirements. The second problem is polioencephalomalacia, which can be caused by a thiamin (vitamin B_1) deficiency and results in severe neurologic signs. In this disease, rumen microbes fail to synthesize adequate thiamin or a toxic fern provides a thiaminase (Pritchard and Eggleston 1978) or, more commonly, an abnormal population of rumen microbes produces a thiaminase (Thomas et al. 1987). An excessive proportion of concentrates to roughage in the ration predisposes to polioencephalomalacia, as described under indigestion and rumen acidosis. In addition to the changes in rumen microbes that occur with grain feeding, decreased rumen pH values optimize the action of bacterial thiaminase (Brent 1976). Polioencephalomalacia is considered in detail in Chapter 5.

MAJOR MINERALS

The major minerals to be discussed are calcium, phosphorus, magnesium, potassium, sulfur, sodium, and chloride. The literature on mineral nutrition of dairy goats has been reviewed by Haenlein (1980) and Kessler (1991).

Calcium

Approximately 99% of the calcium in the body is found in the skeleton in combination with phosphorus (Ca:P ratio of 2.2:1). The remainder of the calcium is very important for diverse body functions, including muscle contraction, neuromuscular excitation, and blood coagulation. Absorption of calcium in the proximal small intestine involves calcium binding protein. Absorption is regulated by 1,25-dihydroxycholecalciferol, which is synthesized in the kidney from vitamin D. Parathyroid hormone increases osteolysis, while calcitonin (from the thyroid gland) decreases osteolysis. These hormones are in turn regulated by the blood calcium concentration. The normal serum calcium concentration for goats is approximately 9 to 11.6 mg/dl (4.5 to 5.8 mEq/L).

Signs of Deficiency or Excess

Young, growing kids are subject to retarded growth and rickets if calcium intake or vitamin D is inadequate, as discussed in Chapter 4. If doelings are bred when too young or too small, especially if they are carrying the weight of multiple fetuses, it is common to have bowing of the limbs and lameness develop because of high calcium requirements and inadequate calcium intake.

Veterinarians must be aware of related and clinically similar problems in the same type of animal (Anderson and Adams 1983) and in young, rapidly growing kids (Baxendell 1984). In this instance, the animals develop metabolic bone disease (epiphysitis) because of excessive calcium intake, often in the form of oyster shell or similar supplement to a legume hay.

A severe imbalance of calcium and phosphorus (relatively too much phosphorus from a mostly grain diet) can cause osteodystrophia fibrosa in goats, discussed in Chapter 4. The lower jaws are enlarged but soft and rubbery, with medial angulation of the crowns of the cheek teeth (Andrews et al. 1983). Rarefaction of all bone and long bone fractures may also occur. Clinically, this problem often occurs when the owner increases the grain in the diet with the thought of speeding the young goat's growth.

The occurrence of milk fever (periparturient hypocalcemia) in goats is discussed below. Lactation diets low in calcium lead to decreased milk production.

Dietary Requirements and Supplementation

Intestinal absorption of calcium is quite efficient for preruminants but probably less than 40% in adults when forage is the calcium source; realistically, the figure is approximately 30% (Kessler 1991). The most recent NRC (2007) uses an absorption coefficient of 0.45. Absorption rates are increased from inorganic sources such as calcium monophosphate and calcium chloride. When calcium intake is decreased, absorption efficacy increases (though usually not above 45%). Absorption decreases rapidly if intake is high. Legumes and cruciferous plants are typically rich in calcium, as are bone meal and fish meal. Dicalcium phosphate, ground limestone, and oyster shells are alternate sources. Little is known regarding calcium absorption in goats, and thus values established for sheep are used. It is best to include a wide margin of safety in stating mineral requirements in general, and this is particularly true of calcium, which is relatively inexpensive.

The calcium contained in milk is readily absorbed by the kid, but forages and concentrates are less available sources. After weaning, the calcium requirement of kids depends markedly on expected growth rate. For instance, according to the NRC (2007), a 20-kg dairy doeling needs 1.4 g calcium/day at maintenance but 5.1 g/day if gaining 150 g body weight/day. As a doeling matures and its growth rate drops, so does the daily calcium requirement. The absorbability of calcium (and phosphorus) varies with the feedstuff, and recent French composition tables report both total and absorbable values, rather than assuming one generic absorbability coefficient. According to the French (INRA 2007), doelings need 2.3 g absorbable calcium/day during the first three months of life. They need approximately 1.8 g absorbable calcium/day during the sixth month, for maintenance and growth. A mineral supplement must never be recommended for the growing goat without first ascertaining if the current dietary intake is deficient or excessive. A good quality mixed legume/grass hay and modest quantities of grain usually provide balanced calcium and phosphorus intake.

Adult goats at maintenance need approximately 3.5 to 6 g of calcium in the diet/day for goats weighing 50 to 100 kg (Morand-Fehr and Sauvant 1978). This requirement can be expressed on a metabolic weight basis as 0.19 g calcium per $kg^{0.75}$ (Kessler 1981). Skeletal growth, mineralization of the fetuses, and milk production all increase the goat's need for calcium. The NRC (1981) allows only 2 grams per day extra for late pregnancy, while French recommendations have varied from an extra 6 grams total dietary calcium per day (Morand-Fehr and Sauvant 1978) to 1 to 1.1 g additional absorbable calcium (INRA 2007). Current NRC (2007) recommendations take into account the litter size. If dietary sources are inadequate during pregnancy, the goat can draw on its skeletal reserves at this time, as long as an increased intake during lactation permits repletion of the reserves.

Goat milk contains approximately 1.4 g of calcium/kg (NRC 1981b), and the NRC (1981) suggests feeding 2 to 3 g/liter, depending on the fat content of the milk. This assumes a more efficient absorption of calcium than might be expected from forage sources, and thus the French use a value of approximately 4 g/liter to calculate requirements. Others have made a similar recommendation of 4.3 g per kg milk (Kessler 1981). (See Table 19.3.)

Phosphorus

Phosphorus is required for both soft tissue and bone growth. It plays an important part in nucleic acid synthesis, energy metabolism, and acid-base balance. The normal serum phosphorus concentration is approximately 4.2 to 9.8 mg/dl for adult goats and 8.3 to 10.3 mg/dl for juveniles (Sherman and Robinson 1983).

Signs of Deficiency

Clinical signs of a deficiency include slowed growth, pica (appetite for abnormal substances), an

Table 19.3. Summary of major mineral requirements for dairy goats (Kessler 1981).

	Daily Requirement (g)			
	Ca	*P*	*Mg*	*Na*
Maintenance per $kg^{0.75}$	0.19	0.14	0.045	0.045
Lactation per kg milk	4.3	1.7	0.7	0.5
Late pregnancy supplement	6	1.5	0.5	0.5

Ca: calcium; P: potassium; Mg: magnesium; Na: sodium.

unthrifty appearance, and decreased serum phosphorus levels. As with calcium, a temporary phosphorus deficiency in the adult can be met from body reserves, but milk production decreases with a prolonged deficiency.

Dietary Recommendations and Supplementation

Phosphorus is absorbed mainly from the small intestine but also from the stomachs. Phosphorus absorption is much more efficient than and is independent of calcium absorption. The true absorption coefficient of phosphorus for goats seems to be higher than for sheep. The NRC (2007) uses a value of 65%, Meschy (2000) uses 70%, and other texts propose that 64% to 75% of dietary phosphorus is typically absorbed. Some natural phosphates are relatively insoluble and poorly absorbed. Goats recycle phosphorus efficiently through saliva (NRC 2007).

The maintenance requirement is 2.5 to 5 g dietary phosphorus/day for goats weighing 50 to 100 kg (Morand-Fehr and Sauvant 1978). On a metabolic weight basis, this has been expressed as 0.14 g phosphorus per $kg^{0.75}$ (Kessler 1981). For late pregnancy, an additional 1.5 grams per day is in order. Goat milk contains 0.84 to 2.1 g P/liter, which can be supplied by adding to the diet 1.4 to 2.1 g P/liter milk produced. A suitable average is 1.7 g P/kg milk. The growing doeling needs a total of 1.4 g absorbable P/day during the first month of life and 2.4 to 2.5 grams absorbable P/day from months three to six (INRA 2007) or 1.4 g total P/day above maintenance to support a weight gain of 150 grams per day (NRC 1981b, 2007).

Animals fed a large quantity of concentrates, which typically contain 3 to 5 g P/kg, usually have adequate phosphorus intake, and in this instance a relative calcium deficiency may occur. In general, the Ca:P ratio in the diet should not be less than 1.2:1 (2:1 for males). Grazing goats rarely develop a phosphorus deficiency because of their tendency to browse varied and phosphorus-rich plants.

Magnesium

Magnesium has received far less study than have calcium and phosphorus, although the metabolism of these minerals is interrelated. Approximately 62% of body magnesium is deposited in bone, 37% in cells, and 1% in extracellular fluid (Stelletta et al. 2008). Magnesium is required for many enzyme systems (including those necessary for energy metabolism and for synthesis of RNA and DNA) and for normal neuromuscular function (Hoffsis et al. 1989).

Signs of Deficiency

The normal serum magnesium concentration for goats is 2.8 to 3.6 mg/dl (see Chapter 4). Hypomagnesemic tetany typically occurs if the serum level drops below 1.1 mg/dl (Stelletta et al. 2008). An average serum concentration of 0.79 mg/dl was reported in five goats with uncharacterized clinical signs of hypomagenesemia in India (Vihan and Rai 1984). Serum calcium may be low because magnesium is required for the release and action of parathyroid hormone (Hoffsis et al. 1989).

A magnesium deficiency may lead to anorexia or hyperexcitability. Hypomagnesemia is sometimes referred to as grass tetany. Although review articles such as Martens and Schweigel (2000) report clinical signs in dairy animals that include decreased production, teeth grinding, salivation, tetany, seizures, recumbency, and death, actual case reports in goats are lacking. Experimental magnesium deficiency has caused poor growth and reduced feed efficiency in West African dwarf goats (Aina 1997). Goats can compensate somewhat for a dietary magnesium deficiency by decreasing output of both milk and urine.

Dietary Recommendations and Supplementation

The percent magnesium absorption probably varies considerably with the diet and is not regulated by a hormonal feedback system (Martens and Schweigel 2000). NRC (2007) has proposed using an absorption coefficient of 0.20. Much is thought to be absorbed from the forestomachs (Poncelet 1983; Martens and Schweigel 2000), and transit time that is too rapid or a potassium excess may hinder magnesium absorption. A wide margin of safety is desirable. The possible contribution of a magnesium excess to urolithiasis in males, however, must not be ignored. Grasses growing rapidly in cool, wet weather or after heavy fertilization are often low in magnesium and high in potassium. Forages containing less than 0.2% Mg on a dry matter intake (DM) basis have been associated with hypomagnesemic syndromes in ruminants (Hoffsis et al. 1989). Whole goat milk also occasionally supplies inadequate magnesium, and kids might develop tetany if not supplemented (Hines et al. 1986).

There is little goat specific data available from which to calculate dietary requirements. AFRC (1998) and the French suggest using the levels indicated for sheep. For an animal that weighs 60 kg, then, total daily intake of magnesium is 1 g for maintenance (approximately 0.045 $g/kg^{0.75}$), plus 1.5 g for late gestation. The approximate magnesium supplement needed per kg of milk is 0.7 g (Kessler 1981). When additional magnesium is needed in the diet, it is often supplied at MgO, although $MgCO_3$, $MgSO_4$, and $MgCl_2$ are other, although less palatable or more laxative possibilities. On spring pastures, provision of NaCl in loose or block form helps to counter high dietary potassium and maintain absorption of magnesium from the rumen. A magnesium source can also be mixed with the salt.

Potassium

Potassium is the major intracellular cation in the tissues of the goat. Although large amounts of potassium are required for health, this mineral is normally present in abundance in forage-based diets and is well absorbed.

Signs of Deficiency

Possible signs of potassium deficiency include reduced feed intake, poor growth, and reduced milk production. Severe deficiencies may cause emaciation and muscle weakness. Dietary potassium is also important in the maintenance of plasma sodium concentration.

Dietary Recommendations and Supplementation

Potassium levels of 0.5% of the diet for growing kids and 0.8% for lactating goats have been recommended, based on requirements for other ruminant species. Lush forages with high potassium content can contribute to the development of hypocalcemia and hypomagnesemic tetany by antagonizing magnesium absorption from the rumen (Underwood and Suttle 1999).

Salt, Sodium Chloride

Ordinary diets are more apt to be deficient in sodium than in chloride.

Signs of Deficiency

Goats that lack sodium may lick dirt. They also may show reduced growth and feed intake and reduced milk production with increased butterfat concentration (Schellner 1972). Goat milk from European breeds contains approximately 0.4 g/kg sodium.

Dietary Recommendations and Supplementation

Dietary sodium recommendations of 0.045 $g/kg^{0.75}$ and 0.5 g/kg milk have been specified (Kessler 1981). The goat normally will eat salt to supply its sodium requirement, then stop. Sodium chloride can be provided free choice or mixed with the feed at 0.5% of the complete ration dry matter. A higher inclusion rate in feed is often used to promote water intake and diuresis to prevent urolithiasis. Either blocks or loose salt can be used. Consumption is typically increased with a loose salt but the goat that needs more salt is willing to chew on a block to get it. A mild excess only leads to increased water consumption and urination. However, high consumption of salt results in high salt content in the manure, which in turn can inhibit plant growth when the manure is used as a soil amendment. Excessive consumption of salt prepartum may contribute to udder edema, as it does in cattle.

When salt is used as a vehicle for trace minerals or medicaments and is fed free choice, it is important that the goat have no other source of sodium (plain salt or bicarbonate of soda) to satisfy its cravings. Goat keepers who offer a smorgasbord of supplements are ascribing greater nutritional wisdom to the goat than it actually possesses.

Sulfur

Sulfur is important in body proteins because it occurs in sulfur-containing amino acids such as methionine and cystine. The sulfur content in hair is especially high. Dietary supplementation of cashmere goats with dl-methionine increased hair yield much more than it increased cashmere yield (Ash and Norton 1987).

Signs of Deficiency

Salivation, lacrimation, and alopecia are reported with marked sulfur deficiency (NRC 1981b, 2007). A less severe deficiency may cause poor growth rate.

Dietary Recommendations and Supplementation

An S:N ratio of 1:10 is commonly recommended (NRC 1981b). This is necessary to meet the growth requirements of rumen microorganisms and thereby assure increased production by the goat. The presence of increased levels of tannins in certain range plants may interfere with sulfur availability (Gartner and Hurwood 1976). Likewise, if feeds are grown on certain deficient soils or if a high proportion of NPN is fed (Bhandari et al. 1973), supplementation of the ration with sodium sulfate or ammonium sulfate may be required. A sulfur concentration of 0.15% of ration dry matter with classic rations and 0.20% with rations high in NPN is appropriate. More recently, the estimated sulfur requirements have been increased to 0.22% for maintenance, gestation, and growth of goats and 0.26% for lactating goats, with a S:N ratio of 1:10.4 (NRC 2007).

Large excesses of sulfates interfere with trace mineral (copper and selenium) absorption and have been implicated in the development of polioencephalomalacia (Rousseaux et al. 1991; Gould 1998). Extrapolating from recommendations for cattle and sheep, the maximum tolerable dietary sulfur level in high concentrate diets is 0.30% and 0.50% if the diet contains at least 40% forage. Drinking water should contain less than 600 mg sulfate/L for high concentrate diets, whereas 2,500 mg sulfate/L is acceptable with higher forage intake (NRC 2005).

TRACE MINERALS

Trace minerals are needed in smaller quantities than are major minerals, but are still indispensable for the health of the goat. Requirements have been reviewed by Lamand (1981) (see Table 19.4). Other authors make slightly different suggestions. In particular, the AFRC

Table 19.4. Summary of trace mineral requirements of goats (Lamand 1981; Kessler 1991; Meschy 2000).

Element	*Deficiency limit*	*Diet requirements, standard diet*	*Diet with interference from other minerals*
Cobalt	0.07	0.1	0.1
Copper	7	10	14
Iron	15	30	30
Iodine	0.15	0.6	1
Manganese	45	40–60	120
Molybdenum	0.1	0.1	0.1
Nickel	0.1	1	1
Selenium	0.1	0.1	0.1
Zinc	45	45–50	75

Measured in mg/kg dry matter (parts per million).

Technical Committee (1998) proposes similar levels for most of the trace minerals but a lower requirement of only 0.05 mg/kg diet for selenium.

Cobalt

Cobalt is a component of vitamin B_{12}, and in the absence of cobalt rumen microorganisms cannot synthesize this essential vitamin. Vitamin B_{12} is required as a coenzyme for methyl malonyl-CoA mutase, needed for the transformation of propionate to succinyl CoA, which then can enter the citric acid (Krebs) cycle. Methionine synthase is also vitamin B_{12} dependent (Underwood and Suttle 1999).

Signs of Deficiency

Signs of cobalt deficiency include inappetence, poor production, weight loss, weakness, and anemia. Diarrhea is noted and is related to disequilibrium of the digestive flora, which also need cobalt, and to increased susceptibility to strongyles. White liver disease (i.e., hepatic lipodystrophy associated with low vitamin B_{12} levels in sheep; see Chapter 11) has been reported in young goats in New Zealand and responded to vitamin B_{12} injections and pasture topdressing with cobalt (Black et al. 1988). The condition has also been produced experimentally in young goats (Johnson et al. 2004).

Dietary Recommendations and Supplementation

For sheep, 0.1 mg/kg DM (ppm) of cobalt in the diet is probably adequate and 1 mg/kg ensures maximum vitamin B_{12} levels. Goats presumably have similar requirements, although several authors have found goats to be less sensitive to cobalt deficiency than sheep (Clark et al. 1987). A dietary level of 0.11 mg/kg DM has been specifically recommended for goats (NRC 2007). Some studies suggest that this level is marginal, as demonstrated by improved growth of young goats when supplemented with injectable vitamin B_{12} (Kadim et al. 2006). In regions where the soil is deficient in cobalt, commercial trace mineralized salt mixtures may not supply enough cobalt to meet the goat's needs (Mackenzie 1975). Cobalt chloride or cobalt sulfate can be added to the salt at a rate of 12 g/100 kg salt (NRC 1981b). Slow release rumen bullets or boluses may be an alternative to dietary supplementation or top-dressing of deficient pastures with cobalt salts (Underwood and Suttle 1999; Radostits et al. 2007).

Copper and Molybdenum

These two minerals are closely interrelated. High molybdenum (above 3 mg/kg) in the feed results in a relative copper deficiency, probably through formation of copper-molybdenum complexes in the tissues.

Signs of Deficiency

Inappetence, poor growth, weight loss, and decreased milk production are nonspecific signs of copper deficiency (Anke et al. 1972) related to decreased cytochrome oxidase activity. Anemia occurs because ceruloplasmin is required to mobilize stored iron for synthesis of hemoglobin and myoglobin. Decoloration of the hair occurs because a copper-containing enzyme is necessary for melanin production. Swayback and enzootic ataxia in kids (see Chapter 5) are related to defective myelination. Cardiac insufficiency is probably due to a combination of problems, including inadequate cytochrome oxidase activity and anemia. Osteoporosis and spontaneous bone fractures are also related to effects on copper-dependent enzymes. Abortions and stillbirths also occur. In addition, copper is required for proper function of the immune system.

Dietary Recommendations and Supplementation

Deficiency symptoms occur when dietary copper is less than 7 mg/kg and molybdenum is normal. A suitable level for ration formulation is 10 to 20 mg/kg DM (Lamand 1978; AFRC 1998), and it is generally recommended to keep the Cu:Mo ratio above 2:1 and below 10:1 (Buck 1986). Excessive calcium and sulfur both interfere with copper absorption (Senf 1974), as does excessive dietary iron (Schonewille et al. 1995). With feeding of corn silage or sulfur, dietary copper should be at least 14 mg/kg. Note that copper oxide is only one-third as digestible as copper sulfate. When the basal diet is deficient in copper or contains markedly excessive amounts of molybdenum, copper oxide wires (Copasure, Butler, Columbus, Ohio) administered orally in a gelatin capsule provide long-term (six-month) supplementation because they lodge in the abomasum and release copper slowly (Lazzaro

2007). An injectable supplement containing chelated copper is available in the United States labeled for goats (Multimin USA Inc., Porterville, California).

Copper Toxicity

Adult goats are not as susceptible to copper toxicity as sheep (Søli and Nafstad 1978), in part because of lower uptake by the liver (Meschy 2000). Liver copper stores are approximately ten times lower in normal goats than in sheep and cattle. In a toxicity study, hepatic copper concentrations were six to nine times higher in three-month-old lambs than kids (Zervas et al. 1990). A deficiency of molybdenum (less than 0.1 mg/kg (Kessler 1991), then, does not generally induce copper toxicity but rather interferes with normal growth and fertility (Anke et al. 1978). Also, goats can safely consume a trace mineralized salt preparation formulated for cattle or a horse grain mix, whereas this is dangerous for sheep. Young kids, however, are sensitive to increased copper levels in the feed (Morand-Fehr 1981c). One example of copper toxicity was reported in young Angora goat kids receiving milk replacer formulated for calves (10 mg/kg copper on a DM basis) in New Zealand. The kids died of a copper-associated hemolytic crisis (Humphries et al. 1987). It is likely that the preruminant kid absorbs copper more efficiently than does the adult goat. Fatal hepatic necrosis without hemolysis has also occurred in adult goats fed an improperly formulated mineral mix (Cornish et al. 2007), as discussed in Chapter 11.

Fluorine

Although fluorine is now viewed as an essential mineral (Kessler 1991), deficiency apparently does not occur under natural conditions. Excessive fluoride compounds from feed, water, and soil cause a chronic toxicosis in goats. Fluorosis is discussed in Chapter 4.

Iodine

In the absence of adequate iodine, the thyroid gland synthesizes an uniodinated inactive prehormone rather than thyroxine. In response to lower thyroxine levels the pituitary gland secretes thyroid stimulating hormone (TSH). As a result, the thyroid gland hypertrophies and produces the clinical condition goiter.

Goats may produce kids with goiter on the same property where sheep and their lambs remain healthy. This is because the goats' browsing habits result in less soil ingestion compared with the grazing sheep.

Signs of Deficiency

In addition to the goiter, signs of deficiency include birth of weak or dead kids and a poor hair coat. Kids may appear "dumb" or unwilling to suckle. Growth rate of kids is reduced, as is the fertility of does. These problems are discussed in Chapters 3 and 13.

Dietary Recommendations and Supplementation

The requirements of ruminants can usually be met by feeding 0.8 mg/kg iodine to lactating females and 0.5 mg/kg to the remainder of the herd (Lamand 1978; NRC 2007). Cruciferous plants increase the iodine requirement to 2 mg/kg in the ration dry matter for lactation and 1.3 mg/kg for other animals. Iodized salt is a simple way to prevent deficiency, but it should not be force fed. A maximum tolerable dietary iodine level of 50 mg/kg has been established for cattle and sheep, with the proviso that the iodine concentration in the milk of animals on such a diet may be undesirable for humans (NRC 2005). Owners should likewise be discouraged from feeding large quantities of kelp and other concentrated iodine supplements.

Iron

Hemoglobin and myoglobin contain iron, as do some enzyme systems such as cytochrome oxidase and catalase. Grazing animals rarely develop iron deficiency except in association with continual blood loss. Bloodsucking strongyles (*Haemonchus*) and bloodsucking lice (especially in Angoras) can create such a situation. An increased proportion of *Allium* (onion-type) plants in the diet can also cause iron deficiency because *n*-propyl disulfide in these plants induces hemolytic anemia.

Signs of Deficiency

An iron deficiency causes a microcytic or normocytic hypochromic anemia (reduced mean corpuscular hemoglobin concentration in anemic animals). Appetite is often reduced. A copper or cobalt deficiency may cause similar signs. Anemia is discussed in Chapter 7.

Dietary Recommendations and Supplementation

The current recommendation for dietary iron for goats is 35 mg/kg dry matter (ppm) in the ration of pregnant and lactating goats and 95 mg/kg diet for growing goats. An additional 5 mg/kg has been proposed for Angoras to support mohair production (NRC 2007). If supplementation is necessary it is useful to know that the iron in ferrous sulfate and ferric citrate is more available than that in ferric oxide. The maximum tolerable dietary level of iron is 500 mg/kg (NRC 2005).

Young kids on an all milk diet routinely become deficient and can be treated with injectable iron dextran if diet modification is not possible. A dose of 150 mg iron dextran/kid at two- to three-week intervals has been recommended (Bretzlaff et al. 1991). Such supplementation is not needed if the kids have access to solid feed (Wanner and Boss 1978). Anaphylaxis occasionally occurs after repeated injections of iron dextran and can be fatal (Ladiges and Garlinghouse 1981).

Manganese

Signs of manganese deficiency in goats include reluctance to walk, deformed forelimbs (caused by defective cartilage formation), excessively straight hocks, and reduced fertility (including silent estrus) or abortion in does (Anke et al. 1977a). Buck kids appear to show a greater depression in growth rate than doe kids when fed an extremely manganese-deficient diet (1.9 mg/kg) (Hennig et al. 1972). The recommended dietary level for goats by various authors has ranged from 20 to 120 mg/kg (NRC 2007), but 60 mg/kg allows for interference with absorption, as by excess calcium.

Nickel

Nickel is required by goats, but a deficiency is unlikely to occur under normal management conditions. Signs of experimental deficiency include skin disease typical of zinc deficiency, death of kids, and decreased first service conception rate in adults (Anke et al. 1977a, 1977b). An increase in feed intake and hence in growth rate was seen in kids when a basal corn based diet containing 0.3 mg/kg nickel was supplemented with chelated nickel (Adeloye and Yousouf 2001).

Selenium

Selenium deficiency occurs when the soil in a locality is deficient (less than 0.5 mg Se/kg of soil) and locally harvested feeds are fed (less than 0.1 mg Se/kg of feed) (Meschy 2000; Radostits et al. 2007). Selenium deficiency has occurred in animals and humans (Levander 1988) in many parts of the world, including the United States, China, Finland, New Zealand, and Australia.

Signs of Deficiency

Many selenium deficiency signs are identical to those of vitamin E deficiency, as mentioned earlier. Nutritional muscular dystrophy, which can be caused by either vitamin E or selenium deficiency, is discussed in detail in Chapter 4. Experimental selenium deficiency (less than 38 µg/kg DM) has produced lowered reproductive efficiency (apparent lowered conception rate) and decreased production of milk, milk fat, and milk protein in the following lactation (Anke et al. 1989). Selenoproteins act as antioxidants and are also involved in the conversion of T_4 to T_3 (Underwood and Suttle 1999; Surai 2006).

Increased supplementation with vitamin E masks a mild selenium deficiency. Potential selenium deficiency problems can be identified in clinically normal animals by evaluating their glutathione peroxidase status, because selenium is required for GSH-Px formation (Radostits et al. 2007). The activity of this enzyme in erythrocytes declines under conditions of selenium deficiency. Normals have not been well established for goats, but are discussed in Chapter 4. Analysis for glutathione peroxidase is typically performed on blood collected in EDTA and kept refrigerated until processed by the laboratory. Serum can be tested instead of erythrocytes, and serum GSH-Px activity changes more rapidly in response to alterations in selenium status (Wichtel et al. 1996).

Some diagnostic laboratories determine whole blood selenium instead; deficiency can be suspected if the goat has less than 5 µg selenium/dl blood (less than 0.05 mg/kg). Serum selenium concentrations less than 0.05 mg/kg have also been deemed to indicate deficiency (Puls 1994). Liver selenium content of animals that die or are slaughtered can be used to monitor the selenium status of the herd. Concentrations of 0.25 to 1.20 mg/kg wet weight are adequate, while concentrations of 0.01 to 0.10 mg/kg wet weight are deficient (Puls 1994). Maternal liver stores of selenium are decreased in advanced pregnancy as transfer to the fetus occurs (El Ghany-Hefnawy et al. 2007). When conversion of units is necessary for interpretation of laboratory reports, it helps to know that 1 µg selenium/dl is equivalent to 0.127 µmol/l.

Dietary Recommendations and Supplementation

Selenium should be present in the diet at a minimum of 0.1 mg/kg of feed. Some but not all commercial ruminant feeds are supplemented with selenium, but the level of supplementation in the United States is controlled by law. Sodium selenite and sodium selenate are permitted. Feed mills cannot add more than 0.3 mg/kg selenium to a complete ration for cattle or sheep or 90 mg/kg to a sheep salt-mineral mix, nor should the maximum daily intake of added selenium for sheep exceed 0.7 mg/head/day (Federal Register 1987; FDA 2004). A feed mill also cannot "fill a prescription" for an increased level of selenium supplementation.

Organic forms of selenium are more bioavailable than inorganic compounds for cattle, sheep, and goats, and transfer better into blood, colostrum, and milk (Aspila 1991; Surai 2006). Supplementation of goat diets with selenium yeast is specifically permitted in the United States, with up to 0.3 mg/kg added selenium in this form allowed in complete feeds (FDA 2005). In the European Union, the maximum allowed selenium inclusion rate in the ruminant diet is 0.568 mg/kg, and feeding selenium yeast at ten times this level did not result in toxicity (Juniper et al. 2008). However, dairy goats receiving 0.5 mg/kg dietary selenium had markedly elevated glutathione peroxidase concentrations, suggesting that this level of supplementation is excessive (Dercksen et al. 2007).

When the soil, and hence the roughages and grains grown on it, are deficient in selenium, several methods have been used to improve selenium content of feeds for goats. One is to use sodium selenate in fertilizer mixes applied to the fields. In Finland, this practice has increased the selenium content of feeds from 0.02 mg/kg DM to 0.2 mg/kg DM (Aspila 1991). Another technique is to use a foliar application of sodium selenite to growing plants approximately one week before harvest (Aspila 1991).

In selenium deficient regions, selenium by injection has been used as an alternative to oral supplementation (Kessler et al. 1986). It is common to incorporate a prescription vitamin E/selenium preparation into a herd health program at the times of year just prior to when deficiency symptoms are most likely to develop. These include shortly before breeding and four and/or six weeks before parturition for does, twice a year for bucks, and at birth and one month of age for kids. The dose administered is typically one to two times the labeled sheep dosage, with kids of normal size receiving the "minimum" dose at birth instead of two weeks of age. Because injectable selenium preparations available in the United States are not labeled for goats and are labeled as not for use in pregnant sheep, practitioners should be cautious about prescribing them for pregnant goats without informed owner consent. Excretion of injectable selenium supplements is rapid and this route of administration does not provide the even and dependable supply ensured by daily dietary selenium.

Selenium Toxicity

There is a relatively narrow margin of safety with selenium; the maximum tolerable level in the feed of ruminants is currently estimated to be 5 mg/kg (NRC 2005). Certain soils are termed "seleniferous" because of an increased selenium content, and certain indicator plants require and accumulate increased concentrations of the mineral. Some of these plants found in the United States are *Stanleya*, *Haplopappus*, and some species of *Astragalus*. They are very useful for indicating that the soil is dangerous, but they are not the only plants that accumulate toxic levels. Most crop plants, grasses, and weeds can accumulate as much as 50 mg/kg selenium when grown on seleniferous soils (James and Shupe 1986). The map in Figure 19.3 gives an approximation of where selenium deficiency or toxic-

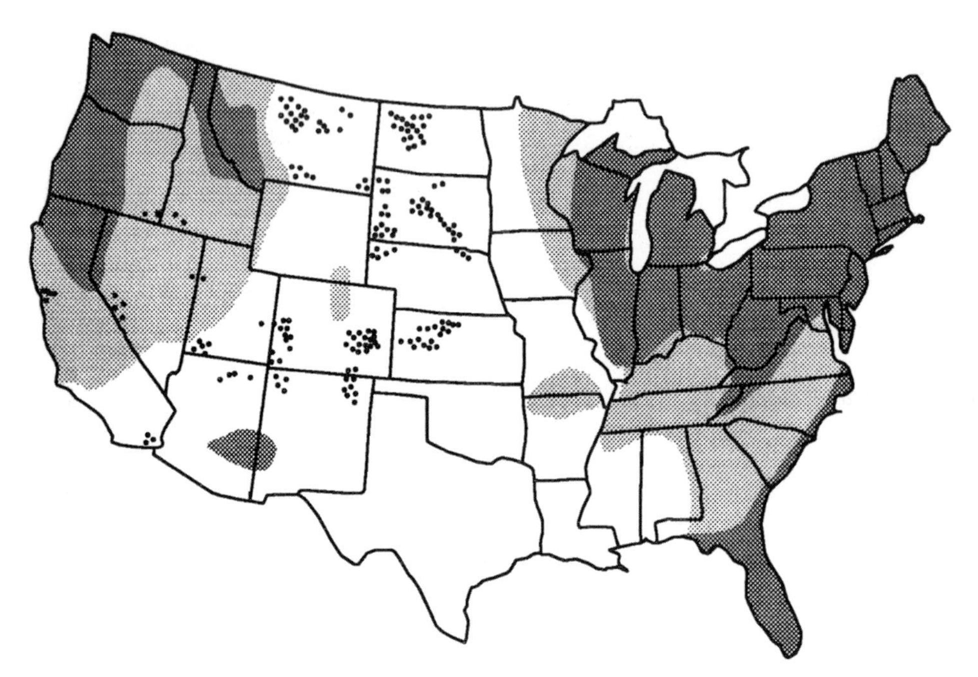

Selenium availability:

■ Low--80% of all forage and grain contains less than .05 ppm

▒ Variable--approximately 50% contains more than .1 ppm

□ Adequate--80% contains more than .1 ppm selenium

• Local areas where accumulator plants contain over 50 ppm

Figure 19.3. Regions of the United States with deficient or toxic levels of soil selenium. Redrawn from: Ammerman and Miller (1975).

ity might be expected to occur in the United States (Ammerman and Miller 1975). Local extension services can usually supply more detailed soil maps to guide the decision for or against selenium supplementation, when locally grown feeds are fed.

Acute selenium toxicosis (depression and dyspnea) has been produced experimentally in sheep with injections of 0.4 mg Se/kg bw, and the LD_{50} in this study was 0.7 mg Se/kg. Necropsy lesions included pulmonary edema and myocardial necrosis (Blodgett and Bevill 1987). Practitioners must guard against accidentally substituting an injectable selenium product marketed for adult cattle for the lower concentration calf and sheep product when small kids are treated. Selenium is less toxic when given orally. Daily oral doses of sodium selenite at 1 mg/kg body weight/day were nontoxic to growing Nubian goats, whereas a single dose of 40 mg/kg or two daily doses of 20 mg/kg were rapidly fatal (Ahmed et al. 1990).

Adverse reactions (deaths and abortions) in several flocks of pregnant sheep have led to the relabeling of injectable selenium in the United States as not for use in pregnant sheep. These products are not approved for goats, and thus the practitioner who prescribes injectable selenium for pregnant goats may be at increased risk of legal action should any adverse reactions or unrelated abortions occur.

Zinc

Zinc is required for formation of certain metalloenzymes, including alcohol dehydrogenase, alkaline phosphatase, carbonic anhydrase, and superoxide dismutase (Underwood and Suttle 1999).

Signs of Deficiency

The major metabolic abnormalities associated with a deficiency are caused by a blockage of protein synthesis, DNA synthesis, and cell division. Zinc deficiency in goats is reported to cause parakeratosis (see Chapter 2), joint stiffness, excessive salivation, swelling of the feet and deformities of the hooves, small testes, and low libido. Reduced feed intake and weight loss also occur. Appetite is said to return within a few hours after zinc supplementation.

Dietary recommendations and supplementation

Minimum dietary zinc requirements seem to be 10 mg/kg ration. Addition of excess calcium to the diet (but not the calcium in legumes) interferes with zinc absorption, as does excess sulfur. Male goats may require more zinc than female goats. Rapid intestinal transit time decreases absorption (young grass, ground feed). A reasonable feeding level to allow for variable absorption in different rations is 45 to 50 mg/kg. Organic forms such as chelated zinc methionine are not superior to inorganic salts as dietary sources of zinc (NRC 2007).

A proposed maximum tolerable level in the feed is 300 to 500 mg/kg (NRC 2005). Note that a 20% solution of zinc sulfate, as used in footbaths for sheep, can cause acute abomasal necrosis if drunk, apparently because the solution causes closure of the esophageal-reticular groove and the zinc passes directly into the abomasum (Dargatz et al. 1986). In sheep, a single dose of 200 mg zinc/kg bw may be fatal.

WATER

The normal body water content of a goat exceeds 60% of its live weight. With certain desert-adapted breeds water may reach 76% of body weight (Shkolnik et al. 1980). These goats can graze far from a water hole because they can store a three- to four-day supply of water in the rumen. Extracellular water includes blood, lymph, and water in the digestive tract. Intracellular water is rather constant, while extracellular water decreases with conditions that cause dehydration.

Water requirements are met by drinking but also from water in ingested feed and metabolic water released as energy stores are oxidized. Water is lost from the body in feces, urine, and milk. Evaporation of water from the lungs and skin is very important for temperature control in hot climates. Water intake increases markedly with elevated ambient temperature, while dry matter intake decreases under these conditions. Very cold water or eating snow as a water source increases energy requirements. The temperature of the rumen fluid may not return to normal until more than two hours after a cold drink. Water consumption increases with salt intake.

Goats in confinement generally drink three to five times daily. Lactating goats typically ingest 3.5 to 4 kg of water for each kg of dry matter consumed at environmental temperatures below 59°F (15°C) (Jarrige et al. 1978). Water ingested per kg DM consumed increases by 30%, 50%, and 100% at temperatures of 68°F, 77°F, and 86°F (20°C, 25°C, and 30°C), respectively (Jarrige 1988). A lower value (2 to 2.8 kg/kg DM) is observed for nonlactating goats in early gestation. Nonlactating animals on lush pasture can survive without additional water. In fact, in some tropical regions, goats may not learn to drink water unless owners make a conscious effort to introduce the animal to water at weaning time. These goats will be at a disadvantage if later moved to a drier region.

Kids raised in confinement systems should have water available to drink from a pan or bucket from a week of age, to assist with rumen development. Milk drunk bypasses the rumen because of closure of the esophageal groove, so plain water must be provided to mix with grain and hay in the rumen for best digestion. Supplying water from a nipple bottle can lead to hemolysis because too much is consumed by the kid at one time (Middleton et al. 1997).

Water requirements are difficult to specify, because they depend on breed, environmental factors, and diet. See NRC (2007) for a review. Maintenance levels of 107 g/kg metabolic weight have been suggested for European goats in temperate climates (Giger-Reverdin and Gihad 1991). These same animals have an additional requirement of 1.43 kg of water/kg of milk produced (Giger et al. 1981). Limited water supplies limit milk production. In general, goats should be provided with clean water ad lib (Figure 19.4). Goats are reluctant to drink from foul tasting water sources. This helps to protect them from water-borne infections and undesirable mineral intake, but may limit milk production and dry matter intake. Unpalatable or frozen water supplies also increase the risk of urolithiasis in male goats because water excretion through the urine is limited and minerals in the urine may not stay in solution.

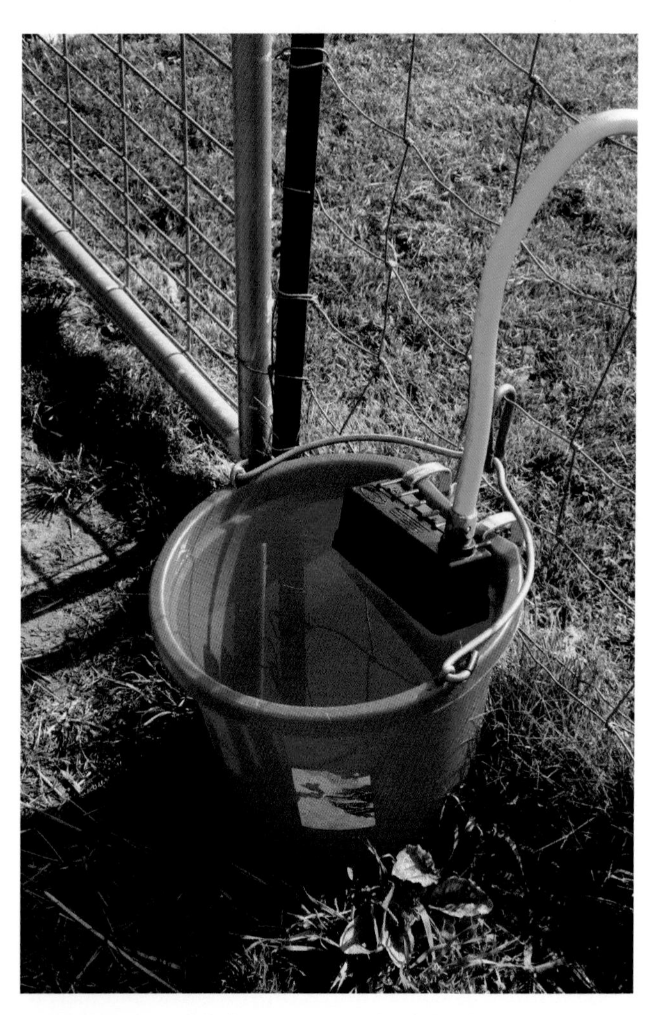

Figure 19.4. A fill float mounted in the bucket ensures that water is available ad lib. (Courtesy Dr. M.C. Smith.)

DRY MATTER INTAKE

The nutrient values of feeds and the requirements of animals are usually converted to a dry matter basis to simplify ration calculation. Dry matter is also important in its own right.

Forages

The quantity of feed that an animal is actually capable of ingesting in a day often limits the nutritive value of a ration, even if it is offered free choice. This is especially true of forages. The rumen is normally filled with a mass of feed in the process of being digested. The volume in the body cavity that the rumen can occupy and the distension of the abdominal wall possibly are limiting factors in feed consumption. Individual particles can only leave the reticulorumen and pass to the omasum and abomasum when they have been reduced to a certain small size by mastication and microbial digestion. The quicker the feed can be broken down, the sooner it exits, and the larger the volume of feed that can be consumed at the next meal. Thus, the capacity of ingestion is limited by the digestibility and especially the fiber content of the feed in question. The cellulolytic activity of the microbial population is also important, and this depends in a major way on the energy in the diet available to support growth of the microbes. With some forages such as mature grass hay or straw, it is the nitrogen available in the rumen that limits microbial growth and thus the total dry matter intake (TDMI). In other instances, trace minerals become limiting. The quantity of water in a feed is usually unimportant unless green chops are harvested at an immature stage (less than 18% DM).

Concentrates

Concentrates are generally ingested and digested more rapidly than forages, such that the substitution on a DM basis of grams of grain per grams of forage is not 1 : 1. In moderate amounts, concentrates improve the digestibility of poor forages by supplying energy needed for growth of the microbial population. If consumed rapidly in large quantities, concentrates decrease the rumen pH level to a point at which activity of cellulolytic bacteria is compromised and digestion of the forage is slowed (see Indigestion and Rumen Acidosis, below). Dividing the concentrate portion of the ration into several smaller meals is thus desirable because acidosis is prevented. The consumption of hay can only be increased in a limited fashion (less than 10%) by offering multiple meals, but it is important that the forage be available for many hours each day to encourage consumption (Jarrige et al. 1978). A total mixed ration is ideal, but few goat farms can afford the equipment required to combine hay or silage and grain intimately and even then the goat may sort out preferred components of the ration.

Intake Limits

Some feeds are eaten in smaller than expected quantities because the goat finds them unappetizing. This is often true of heavily fermented silages or moldy feeds. Many goats refuse to eat hay that has fallen to the ground and been walked on. When the ration is adequately ingestible and digestible for the ruminant to meet its nutritional needs, the level of production often becomes the factor limiting ingestion. High-producing animals voluntarily consume a larger quantity of DM. For this reason, tables ordinarily increase the TDMI for each kg of milk produced or gram of bw gained.

Voluntary dry matter intake is often expressed based on bw or metabolic weight, depending on whether animals are of similar or very different sizes. This is not a very accurate approach because it ignores the variations in digestibility and substitution. It does, however, permit discussion of gross trends in DM intake. During growth of a goat kid, the TDMI increases as the bw increases. This is because both maintenance requirements and volume of the rumen increase. The TDMI relative to bw decreases during growth. This is especially true at the end of the finishing period, when internal body fat limits rumen volume. It remains nearly constant when expressed in terms of metabolic bw. Similarly, in late pregnancy, the increased volume of the uterus results in a relative decrease in TDMI, although high estrogen levels are also involved. After kidding, TDMI increases as the volume available for the rumen is increased by the involution of the uterus and the rumen epithelium develops to improve absorption of the end-products of digestion. However, the requirements for high milk production increase even more rapidly than does TDMI, and thus the goat must either mobilize body reserves or give less milk.

The maximum dry matter intake for goats approaches 5 to 6 kg/100 kg bw, and animals with such elevated intake are naturally the best producers in the herd (Morand-Fehr 1981a). In goats fed alfalfa hay and grain during lactation, the average dry matter intake varies from 2.8 to 4.2 kg DM/100 kg according to the stage of lactation. During lactation, daily dry matter intake as hay may reach 3% to 3.5% of live weight. Intake is decreased during gestation. Typically the total DM intake is 2.2 to 2.8 kg/100 kg bw during the last eight weeks of pregnancy. Intake of hay varies from 1.7 to 2.3 kg/100 kg bw during this time.

These figures were obtained from Alpine dairy goats. For the same type of goat, a regression equation has been constructed based on 11,600 daily rations consisting of alfalfa hay and grain (Morand-Fehr and Sauvant 1978).

$$\text{Total DM} = 423.2 \times \text{Milk} + 27.8 \times W_{kg}^{0.75} + 13.2 \times \text{Gain} + 6.75 \times \text{Forage}$$

where

DM = dry matter intake in g/day
Milk = kg/d of 3.5% milk
Gain = weight gain in g/day
Forage = percent of roughage in the ration

Such an equation only applies to the particular forage for which it was constructed. Similar trends have been demonstrated in West African Dwarf goats, in which voluntary intake of pelleted alfalfa during peak lactation was almost double that of nonlactating goats of a similar age. Goats suckling twins had greater TDMI levels than goats suckling singles (Adenuga et al. 1991). Recently, many studies have been summarized to produce predictions of the voluntary dry matter intake of lactating, Angora, growing, and mature goats, independent of the forage consumed (Luo et al. 2004d).

Encumbrance

French nutritionists have proposed a unit of encumbrance or fill unit system as a better way of determining TDMI of various rations (Demarquilly et al. 1978; Jarrige 1988; INRA 2007). In this system each category of animal has a single value for capacity of ingestion, while each forage has several ingestability values, determined by the category of ruminant. At first, "standard" sheep (wethers at the end of their growth period) were used to determine ingestibility values. The quantity of a forage eaten by the sheep was then divided into the amount of a reference forage consumed (young pasture grass of a certain energy density) to obtain the encumbrance value, EV. Ingestibility values were later determined for lactating dairy cattle (units of encumbrance for lactation, UEL, or milk fill units, MFU) and also fattening cattle. Encumbrance has been applied to dairy goats (Morand Fehr and Sauvant 1988; INRA 2007). The "standard" goat weighs 60 kg and produces 4 kg of milk with 3.5% butterfat. It consumes 2.65 MFU per day. Capacity is adjusted by 0.23 MFU for each kg of 3.5% fat corrected milk. Voluntary dry matter intake increases in a nonlinear fashion after parturition until its maximum at approximately eight weeks of lactation. For dairy goats, the DMI is approximately 72%, 85%, 92%, 95%, and 98% of the maximum value during weeks one, two, three, four, and five, respectively, of lactation (Sauvant et al. 1991b; INRA 2007).

Tables have been constructed for goats of varying bodyweights, weeks in lactation, and levels of milk production. Selected values have been compiled from the INRA 2007 tables to create Table 19.5. These numbers presume a refusal level of 15% and digestible forage.

Encumbrance values are not routinely included in American feed tables. They are most useful when

Table 19.5. Daily dry matter intake (in kg) and capacity for ingestion (MFU).

Live weight of goat	*50 kg*		*60 kg*		*70 kg*	
	DM	*MFU*	*DM*	*MF*	*DM*	*MFU*
Last month gestation	1.16	1.14	1.32	1.30	1.49	1.46
After peak lactation (milk production)						
1 l	1.57	1.38	1.74	1.54	1.90	1.70
2 l	1.90	1.62	2.06	1.78	2.22	1.94
3 l	2.22	1.86	2.38	2.02	2.54	2.18
4 l	2.54	2.10	2.70	2.26	2.86	2.42
5 l	2.86	2.34	3.02	2.50	3.18	2.66
6 l	3.18	2.58	3.34	2.74	3.50	2.90

DM = dry matter intake, MFU = capacity for ingestion in milk fill units.

forages of variable quality are fed. These principles can be demonstrated by several examples. A 60-kg goat at maintenance can consume 1.30 MFU. An early cut grass hay might have an EV of 1.06 MFU/kg DM if it was cut in good weather. Hay from the same field cut late and rained on might have an EV of 1.25 for dairy cattle and goats (but 1.98 for sheep). For the first hay, the goat can eat 1.30/1.06 = 1.51 kg DM. For the weathered hay, she would eat only 1.30/1.25 = 1.04 kg DM. The French tables for TDMI (as given in Table 19.5) are constructed for a ration based on alfalfa hay or corn silage supplemented with concentrates (Morand-Fehr and Sauvant 1988). The NRC tables, on the other hand, indicate not the capacity for TDMI, but the amount of DM to be consumed when a ration has a certain energy density, to meet the energy requirements of the goat at maintenance. The ability of the goat to do this is not considered.

Substitution

When feeding concentrates in addition to the forage, it is helpful to know by how many grams the ingestion of forage DM decreases for each 100 g of concentrate DM consumed. This depends on the forage and the percent of the final ration that will be grain. The substitution rate is appreciably less than 1 when small amounts of concentrates are combined with energy-poor forage. In fact, when feeding weathered grass hay with an EV of 1.9 and an energy density of 0.76 Mcal NE_1/kg DM (0.35 Mcal/pound), the substitution rate varies from 0.02 to 0.21, depending on whether 10% or 70% of the diet is grain. Thus, the TDMI increases substantially. The substitution of one feed for another on a dry matter basis also seems to depend on stage of lactation. For instance, if 100 g more grain is fed to a goat in gestation, she will eat 62 g less alfalfa hay. In early lactation, for 100 g more grain the goat will eat 78 g less hay. After the first two months of lactation there is almost an equivalent substitution of grain for good hay on a dry matter basis.

Conclusions Concerning Dry Matter

Out of all this confusion comes one clear message. Anyone constructing on paper or computer a ration for goats must subsequently verify that the animals in question will actually consume it. This means weighing forage fed, refusals, and the grain consumed. If the animals are not eating as much forage as they need, the amount of grain must be decreased or the forage quality improved. Of course, the situation with pastured goats is trickier. Here, the goat raiser needs both experience and experimentation to feed the herd properly.

GENERAL RATION BALANCING CONSIDERATIONS FOR GOATS

In large herds, it is generally impractical to feed each goat individually. The milking process is slowed and the risk of indigestion is increased if all of the concentrate ration is fed in the parlor. Inevitably, some goats fed in a group are overfed and others are underfed. A measure of control can be maintained by grouping goats according to age and production (Skjevdal 1981). Using locking stanchions or short chains that clip onto collars and manger dividers permits each goat to consume its allotted share of concentrates without gross interference by more dominant does. The goats are then released because they normally consume more hay if they can move freely from hay to water or salt block and back to hay (Morand-Fehr 1981a).

Another problem associated with large herds that have gone beyond the hobby stage is that grain is sometimes cheaper (on a kcals of energy basis) than high quality forage, and grain is certainly easier to store and feed than hay. Thus, owners may choose to overfeed concentrates without considering the adverse effects on health related to this practice.

Zero-Grazing

Zero-grazing is an important step toward intensification of goat raising. The grazing goat eats slowly, carefully choosing young stems and leaves. It wastes a lot of forage, and does not achieve maximum dry matter intake unless supplemented in the barn. Some of these problems can be avoided by careful grazing management, including high density stocking, frequent rotation, and adequate rest periods for the pastures. Even under such a system, goats do not graze as closely as sheep (Jagusch et al. 1981). A much greater production of milk per acre often can be obtained by cutting the forage and bringing it to the goats. This forage can then be analyzed and it becomes possible to identify deficiencies and excesses in the total ration. At the same time, there is no need to maintain fences, the energy requirements for maintenance of the goats are reduced, and there should be less trouble with predators and internal parasites other than coccidiosis. However, an exercise lot at least twice the area of the stable is still desirable (Toussaint 1974).

Even in total confinement, goats often waste more than 40% of forage in the manger. The goal should be to limit the leftovers to no more than 20% of the feed offered. This means not distributing a plethora of forage and constructing mangers that impede the goat's tendency to remove its head and drop part of every mouthful on the ground. Slanted manger bars are preferable to keyhole feeders. On the other hand, goats do not achieve maximum intake if they are not allowed to exhibit their normal choosiness in eating; a bare manger indicates submaximal consumption. If hay is of poor quality, a greater excess should be distributed to encourage intake. Ideally, another livestock species (such as a pony or sheep) should be available on the farm to make use of the daily manger hay-sweepings. Goats spend more time eating each day than do sheep. They ruminate approximately eight hours a day, six of which occur at night.

Traditionally, dairy goats have been offered a basal ration of forage (such as hay) free choice, with concentrates fed individually, according to production. Hay should be fed before concentrates, to decrease the risk of low rumen pH resulting from rapid digestion of nonstructural carbohydrates in the grain. A total mixed ration can be fed to avoid excessive wasting of the forage and indigestion associated with "slug" feeding of concentrates and to improve consumption of less palatable feeds (Rapetti and Bava 2008). Chopped hay, grain, minerals, and vitamins are mixed with ensiled products (haylage, beet pulp) to obtain a final dust-free mixture. The formulation of the mixture is readjusted frequently during lactation to ensure that each goat consumes adequate fiber (optimum 1 kg hay) even when production and intake have dropped in late lactation (Hervieu 1990).

Forage Quality

Grasses and legumes typically give the highest yield in net energy and protein if they are harvested at the early budding stage (Fick and Mueller 1989). In more advanced stages of maturity, the proportion that is stem increases, as does indigestible fiber such as lignin, while the amount that can be consumed daily decreases. Mineral content also decreases in mature forages. Because of the increase in digestible energy and protein, a smaller quantity of concentrate with a lower protein level can be fed when forage is cut early.

Owners purchasing hay should use both subjective and objective evaluations. Hay should be bright green (not yellow or brown), leafy, sweet-smelling, and free of mold or weeds. If possible, the cutting number, cutting date or weeks of regrowth, and year should be ascertained. First cutting hay can be very early to very late cut, depending on local weather and farming practices. Moldy, weedy, badly weathered, or severely overripe hay should be rejected. Large round hay bales that have been stored uncovered in rainy climates are suspect, because the outer moldy part is a large proportion (often 25% to 30%) of the bale and rain water will have leached soluble nutrients out of the hay in the center of the bale. If the hay appears palatable but its nutritional value is questionable, crude protein, available protein, ADF, and NDF should be determined by a forage testing laboratory. This is especially important with grass hays in which stage of maturity is more difficult to judge than with alfalfa hays.

Owners of small herds probably do not buy at auctions, where hay has been analyzed and graded to reflect nutritional value. Some are fortunate and find a local, well-managed farm where representative twenty core hay samples have been taken and analyzed from each batch of hay (Putnam 2002). Alternatively, a cooperative extension office might lend the equipment and the hay seller might be willing to share the cost of the hay testing or pay for the testing with the understanding that the price of the hay will be determined by its quality. Sellers unwilling to cooperate often have poor hay.

Stored forages have decreased vitamin content. Thus, supplementation with vitamins A, D, and E is usually imperative when hays or silages are fed many months after harvest.

Silage

Because of weather constraints, it is often easier to make young herbage into ensilage than into good quality hay. For best results, including highest intakes, a preservative such as formic acid (0.2% to 0.5% added to the direct cut crop) is used (Nedkvitne and Robstad 1981). When silage is fed, it is still important to offer an excess of feed, allowing at least 10% to 15% refusals, to obtain maximum dry matter intake. Bunks should be cleaned daily to prevent spoilage. Though good milk production can be obtained when goats are fed silage in place of hay, the danger of listeriosis associated with silage feeding must be kept in mind. The herbage must be free of dirt that might carry *Listeria* organisms, and the silage must be properly made so that it maintains an acid pH (less than 5) unfavorable for additional multiplication of the bacteria. In small herds, ensiling is often impractical unless plastic bags are used. A few animals do not eat enough to prevent spoilage at the leading edge of a pile or conventional silo.

Corn silage (stalks, leaves, and ears chopped together) is commonly fed to livestock in the United States. When kernels are well developed at the time of harvest and moisture content of the plant is appropriate, there is adequate carbohydrate to permit good fermentation and attainment of a low pH. Contamination with soil (during harvest or packing) and surface spoilage can still permit dangerous growth of *Listeria*. Manger sweepings of corn silage from cattle farms should not be fed to goats. Additionally, goats pick the corn kernels out of the silage by choice and eat proportionately less roughage or else eat the roughage portion of their diet after the grain has been consumed.

Palatability

Goats show great individual differences in what they prefer to eat. Texture and taste are both important. Thus, goats generally dislike dusty feeds. Molasses makes a grain mixture more appetizing (Morand-Fehr 1981a). However, feeds with more than 5% to 6% molasses should be avoided (Adams 1986) because of possible adverse effects on rumen function. Coarse textured grains (i.e., rolled, cracked, crimped, flaked) and pellets are more acceptable than finely ground meals.

Past dietary experience is also important in determining what an individual goat will eat. This is important in range situations, when more palatable forages may be scare or potentially toxic secondary metabolites are present in many plant species. Goats appear to adjust their intake of available plant species to maximize nutritive value while avoiding toxicity (Papachristou et al. 2005). Young goats may learn which species to consume in part by observing more experienced members of the herd, and feed preferences developed in the second to fourth months may persist for life (Biquand and Biquand-Guyot 1992; Provenza et al. 2003). For this reason, converting a herd to a new feed resource base (different plant species, new region of the country, hay to silage, silage to cubes, etc.) may require a full year or even a full generation before previous productivity is restored.

Body Condition Scoring

In the adult goat, proper body weight is a function of breed, frame size, and stage of gestation or lactation. Accurate scales on which to weigh goats are often not available. The frame size of an individual adult is constant, but deposition of fat and muscle (body condition) varies with nutritional and physiologic status. Body condition is a measure of the animal's lipid and protein reserves. These reserves are used in late gestation, early lactation, and times of environmental adversity.

Although sophisticated methods to determine body composition based on slaughter or biopsy techniques have been developed for goats (Morand-Fehr et al. 1992), a practical method must rely on palpation and visual assessment of the animals. A lumbar score has been applied to meat goats in Australia, using scores of 1 (very lean), 2 (lean), 3 (medium), or 4 (fat) (Mitchell 1986; McGregor and Butler 2008). A similar scheme using one-fourth or one-half-point increments from 1 to 4 has been developed for indigenous goats of the Small East African type (Honhold et al. 1989). In score 1 goats, there is almost no muscle covering the intervertebral articulations; a score of 4 corresponds to muscle completely covering the vertical and horizontal processes of the lumbar vertebrae. In these animals, a change of 1 in the condition score represents an average of a 12% change in body weight.

Lumbar systems originally designed for sheep and cattle are not directly applicable to dairy goats because most of the dairy goat's body fat is stored in the omentum and perirenal tissues (Chilliard et al. 1981). Even obese animals have little subcutaneous fat. A system has been developed specifically for dairy goats but is appropriate for all breeds. This body condition score is an average of lumbar and sternal scores, each of which is divided into 0.25-point divisions. Integer scores from 0 to 5 used in this method are described in Table 19.6 (Morand-Fehr et al. 1989; Santucci et al. 1991; Hervieu and Morand-Fehr 1999).

The goat is evaluated while relaxed and standing evenly on all four feet. The sternal score correlates better with the proportion of adipose tissue in the goat, while the lumbar score (determined over the second to fifth lumbar vertebrae) better reflects body protein (Morand-Fehr et al. 1992). Each 0.25 change in the final score corresponds to approximately 1.5% lipid content of the body (Morand-Fehr et al. 1992). Owners are advised to select and score fifteen lactating goats one to two months before breeding will begin. Three of these animals should be high producers, nine average producers, and three low producers. The same fifteen goats are scored again at the end of lactation and

Table 19.6. Body condition scoring scheme for dairy goats.

Lumbar score	
0	The animal is extremely emaciated. The intervertebral articulations are easily felt and the skin seems to be in direct contact with the bones.
1	Muscle extends at most two-thirds of the distance out along the transverse spinal processes. Intervertebral articulations are still palpable but barely visible.
2	Dorsal and transverse spinous processes are prominent, and the skin forms a concave line between them.
3	Spinous processes are still easily felt. The space in the vertebral angle is filled with muscle and the skin determines a straight line between dorsal and transverse processes.
4	Dorsal and transverse spinous processes are difficult to detect and the skin forms a convex line between them.
5	There is a prominent groove down the back line and the fat and muscles mound up on each side of this groove.
Sternal score	
0	Costo-sternal articulations are very prominent. The bony surface of the sternum is easily felt. The skin callous over the sternum lacks mobility.
1	Costo-sternal articulations are more rounded but still easily felt. The depression over the sternum is not filled in but the callous is movable.
2	Costo-sternal articulations are difficult to feel. Internal fat pads develop under the muscle layers on each side of the sternum, and subcutaneous fat partially fills the central depression.
3	The central depression is completely filled with a thin and mobile mass of subcutaneous fat. Distinct depressions are palpable on each side between the mass of fat and muscle and the bones. The costo-chondral articulations are palpable.
4	Sternum and ribs are no longer palpable but a depression is still palpable on each side of a thick mass of subcutaneous fat.
5	Subcutaneous fat is no longer mobile. No depressions are palpable laterally or caudally.

immediately after parturition. A sick or injured goat is replaced with an animal of equivalent milk production. The lumbar score for Alpines and Saanens in France averages 2.5 to 2.75 at dry off, 2 to 2.25 at parturition, and 2.25 to 2.5 before the breeding season. The average sternal scores for the same time periods are 3 to 3.25, 2.5 to 2.75, and 2.75 to 3. The combined score should not drop by more than 0.5 points during the dry period (Herview and Morand-Fehr 1999). A group of ten doelings can be followed in a similar fashion to monitor the nutrition and well-being of that age group.

A very similar scoring system for meat goats also takes into consideration the degree of fat deposition over the rib cage. This body condition scoring system has been illustrated with videos and photographs of individual goats with each whole integer score (Langston University 2000).

Body condition scoring is useful for monitoring the adequacy of the feeding program under intensive and extensive conditions. Critical times for scoring goats might include dry-off, the last two weeks of gestation, six weeks into lactation, at turn-out onto pasture, at the beginning of the dry season, and at the beginning of the breeding season (Morand-Fehr et al. 1989). Dairy goats need body reserves at parturition to support maximum milk production in the subsequent lactation. Angoras kidding in good body condition also produce more milk, thereby limiting kid losses because of starvation. Under French intensive dairy goat conditions, the body condition score should be more than 2.25 and less than 3.5 at dry-off, and more than 2.75 and at or less than 3.5 at parturition. The score should not be less than 2 at peak lactation (forty-five days) nor should it have decreased more than 1.25 points from parturition (Morand-Fehr et al. 1992).

Target scores need to be established for extensively managed goats to obtain satisfactory production and reproduction (Santucci et al. 1991). For instance, recently shorn Angora goats with a low body condition score have a greater risk of dying during inclement weather (McGregor and Butler 2008). Body condition also should be considered when implementing a selective deworming program (see Chapter 10).

Apparent Starvation in the Face of Plenty

When an individual in the herd appears to be malnourished despite free access (including protection from competition) to a palatable and nutritious ration, other reasons for reduced consumption or utilization of nutrients must be investigated. These include dental disease, lameness, blindness, and chronic infectious and parasitic diseases. The clinical approach to such an animal is described in Chapter 15.

FEEDING PREGNANT GOATS

During gestation goats accumulate protein, fat, minerals, and vitamins beyond what is incorporated into fetuses and placenta. The magnitude of this net bodyweight gain varies from less than 1 kg to 8 kg and is strongly influenced by the level of nutrition. Protein, but not energy, is accumulated more efficiently during gestation than when the goat is not pregnant.

Seventy percent of the weight of the kid is acquired between the one hundredth day of gestation and parturition. The weight of kids at birth as a percent of the doe's weight at breeding is twice the corresponding ratio of calf to cow. Undernourishment during late pregnancy results in the birth of smaller kids that will in turn show increased mortality and slower growth rates (Bajhau and Kennedy 1990). Subsequent milk production will also be compromised (Sahlu et al. 1995). Particularly important is the potential adverse effect of an energy deficient diet on colostrum in the udder at delivery, as demonstrated in ewes (Banchero et al. 2006). The kids may die of hypothermia or starvation before adequate colostrum is produced.

If the doe is carrying multiple kids, especially three or more, then it will have to mobilize its fat reserves just before parturition to meet its own energy needs. This is because appetite often drops off at this time and the volume of the gravid uterus and of internal fat stores limits the volume of feed that can be consumed. When propionate supplies are inadequate, the acetate coming from mobilization of fat will be transformed into ketone bodies. Pregnancy toxemia may result, as discussed below.

A high quality, palatable hay should be fed during pregnancy. This permits limiting the grain to 200 g/day late in gestation. Goats that eat a lot of hay during gestation maintain that ability to ingest increased levels of roughage during lactation. Also, high concentrate consumption in pregnancy has been associated with slow parturition and poor cervical dilation and with poor persistence of lactation (Fehr et al. 1974). Recent reports suggest that protein should be fed to dairy goats at approximately 11.5% of ration dry matter during late gestation for fetal well-being (Sahlu et al. 1992) and for subsequent milk production (Sahlu et al. 1995), and supplying 14% crude protein did not improve performance. A supplement rich in rumen bypass protein is desirable at this time (Morand-Fehr and Sauvant 1988).

A recent experiment with a small number of late pregnant goats showed that they were capable of increasing dry matter intake and protein in the diet at this stage. In the last weeks before parturition, if allowed to choose from several hays and concentrates offered free choice, the goats increased their forage and protein intake by increasing consumption of alfalfa hay and chickpeas while decreasing grass hay and barley consumption. In the same study, goats fed only alfalfa hay and flaked barley increased their dry matter intake by the substitution effect of increasing consumption of the concentrate and protein consumption by eating only the more digestible portions of the hay (Fedele et al. 2002).

Abortion

Abortion as the result of inadequate nutrition has received the most attention in the Angora breed. Small, poorly grown animals or old does are most prone to abort. During inclement weather or after shearing, ad lib supplementation with whole grain treated with an alkali and ionophore prevents the spate of abortions that normally follows such stressful conditions, without causing rumen acidosis (Wentzel 1987). Lime, ionophore, and as much as 1.2% urea are mixed with molasses and water, then poured over whole grain and mixed in well. The final product contains 2% (by weight) slaked lime (calcium hydroxide, not calcium carbonate or field lime) and 20 mg/kg ionophore such as rumensin, salinomycin, or lasalocid. According to one recipe (Van der Westhuysen et al. 1988), 12.5 kg calcium hydroxide, 8 kg urea, 16 liters molasses, and the appropriate amount of ionophore are mixed with 20 liters of water, then poured over 560 kg of grain.

Native breeds are often observed to be less apt to abort than imported animals, especially dairy breeds, with higher nutritional demands (Mellado et al. 2006). It is difficult to separate the adverse effects on the placenta and fetus of nutritional deficiencies in high producing goats from lack of resistance to enzootic abortion diseases. However, within a herd in which feed or manger space is limited, the smaller, younger pregnant does whose nutritional needs cannot be met in the face of competition with mature, socially dominant adults are prone to abortion. Feeding these animals as a separate group alleviates the nutritional and social stresses.

Mineral and vitamin deficiencies and toxic plants that have been associated with abortion are reviewed in Chapter 13.

Pregnancy Toxemia

Goats are at risk of developing the metabolic condition termed "ketosis" at two stages: at the end of gestation (pregnancy toxemia) and during early lactation (i.e., lactational ketosis, as discussed later).

Etiology

Pregnancy toxemia is usually limited to the last six weeks of gestation, although one Indian study detected ketonuria in 3% of 120 inappetent lethargic does in the third month of pregnancy. By comparison, 24% of 160 does with a similar presentation in the fifth month of pregnancy were positive for acetoacetate in the urine (Lalitha et al. 2001). Its immediate causes can be crudely divided into undernutrition and overnutrition. In starvation ketosis, the animal has not been permitted access to enough nutrients, especially energy, to meet the demands of itself and its (usually) multiple fetuses. Low quality roughage is a particular risk because not enough can be consumed to meet requirements when the volume of the rumen is reduced by the presence in the abdomen of a large uterus (Bostedt and Hamadeh 1990). Secondary ketosis is similar, except that some other disease temporarily interferes with feed consumption by an otherwise properly fed doe. In overnutrition ("estate") ketosis, the goat has been overfed until its massive internal fat stores plus the full uterus occupy so much of the body cavity that dry matter intake is severely curtailed at a time when increased energy consumption is required. Leptin, a hormone produced by adipose cells, may also contribute to a reduction in feed intake by decreasing the obese animal's appetite (Kolb and Kaskous 2004).

Excessive grain feeding itself can lead to pregnancy toxemia because the goat that eats inadequate roughage is apt to go off feed at this critical time. When goats are heavily fed on corn silage in late gestation they become obese. Their level of ingestion then decreases dramatically before parturition. Rumen acidosis from energy-rich silage may contribute to the development of pregnancy toxemia.

Figure 19.5 shows various determining factors for ketosis (Sauvant et al. 1984). Etiologic factors involved in the development of pregnancy toxemia have been reviewed (Sauvant et al. 1991a).

Pathogenesis

The central metabolic events are fat mobilization and the availability of glucose (Caple and McLean 1986; Herdt and Emery 1992). Pregnancy toxemia is typically more common than lactational ketosis, and occurs predominantly in "improved" breeds with high prolificacy. It is not a disease expected to occur in native breeds carrying a single kid under extensive management conditions. With proper management and nutrition, even the doe carrying quadruplets can remain clinically healthy, although concentrations of ketone bodies in the blood can be expected to be higher in those goats carrying large litters. In a study of 514 native goats managed under a semi-intensive pasture and concentrate system in India, no clinical ketosis was observed but about 10% of the animals had subclinical ketosis based on laboratory findings of hypoglycemia (<30 mg/dl serum glucose) and hyperketonemia (>4.5 mg/dl ketones) (Gupta et al. 2007).

The developing fetuses depend upon glucose (maternal hepatic gluconeogenesis) for their energy needs. Ketone bodies and free fatty acids do not cross the placenta in any substantial quantities (Reid 1968). Insulin levels in the late pregnant doe are decreased; this spares glucose for fetal needs while at the same time stimulating lipolysis and gluconeogenesis. Placental lactogen levels are greatly increased when multiple fetuses are present (Sardjana et al. 1988). Placental lactogen has growth hormone as well as prolactin activity and is probably crucial to meeting the metabolic needs of the fetuses at the expense (if necessary) of the dam. Thus, the late pregnant doe is often subclinically ketotic.

Clinical Signs

The early signs of pregnancy toxemia are vague. They probably originate from decreased glucose utilization by the doe's brain. The goat may be slow to get up or may lie off in a corner. It eats less and its eyes are dull. There is often a noticeable subcutaneous edema of the lower limbs. Teeth grinding and generalized weakness progress to more apparent neurologic abnormalities (blindness, loss of menace response, star gazing, nystagmus, ataxia, tremors), then to coma. The fecal output is reduced to a few small, dry, mucus coated pellets.

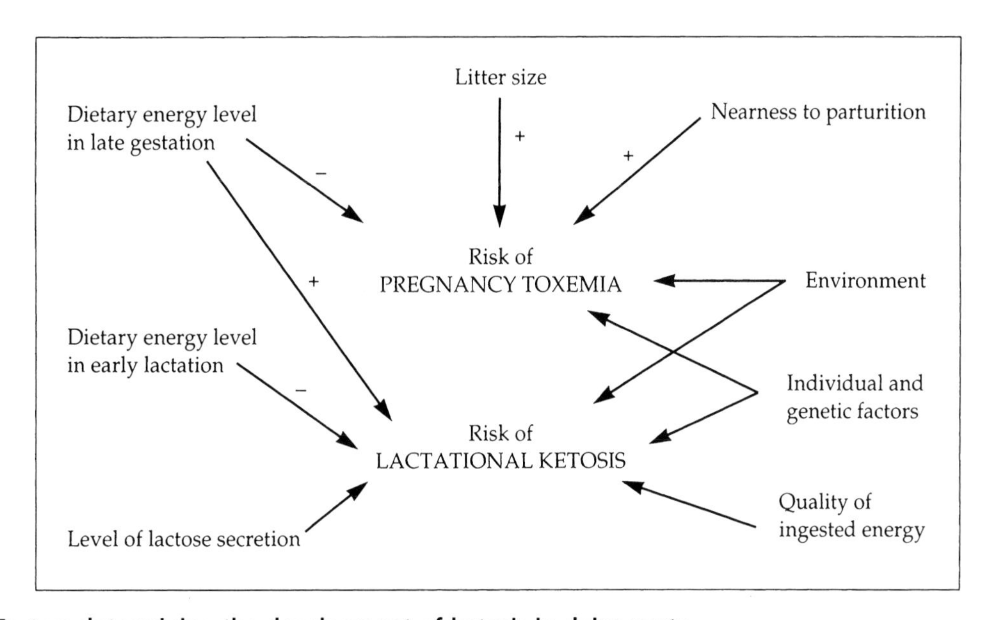

Figure 19.5. Factors determining the development of ketosis in dairy goats.

As metabolic acidosis develops the animal may breathe more rapidly. Thus, advanced primary ketosis may be difficult to distinguish from a primary pneumonia which has caused the goat to go off feed and develop a secondary ketosis. A careful physical examination is also necessary to identify other problems such as parasites, lameness, and bad teeth that might have contributed to the animal's present state.

In the terminal stages of pregnancy toxemia, the doe becomes recumbent. Death of the fetuses at this stage releases toxins and hastens the demise of the doe. Pulse and respiratory rates increase as endotoxic shock develops. The course of the untreated disease varies from twelve hours to one week.

Goats with pregnancy toxemia that do not die tend to have dystocias and higher kid mortality. They do not come to milk well. Similar problems are noted in obese goats, even when clinical pregnancy toxemia does not occur; in addition, these animals are at high risk of developing lactational ketosis.

Laboratory Tests

There are three major ketone bodies produced in the course of this metabolic disease: beta-hydroxybutyrate (BHB), acetoacetate, and acetone. In the past, these were sometimes measured together in a poorly defined way and reported as total ketones. Currently, BHB, which is the most stable ketone in blood and accounts for approximately 85% of the total ketones in sheep with pregnancy toxemia (Bostedt and Hamadeh 1990), receives the most attention in the laboratory.

Some people can detect an odor of ketones on the breath of ketotic animals. Others must depend on simple diagnostic reagents or laboratory tests. In the early stages of pregnancy toxemia, ketone bodies are easily detectable in the urine. The commonly used test strips and pills containing nitroprusside (Rothera reagent) turn purple in the presence of acetoacetate but react minimally with acetone and BHB. If the doe has only a trace ketonuria (physiologic when late pregnant with multiple fetuses), some other cause for its illness should be sought, but supportive treatment to prevent worsening of the ketosis should be given. Late stages are usually accompanied by renal failure; marked proteinuria, epithelial casts, and ketonuria are present (Kaufman and Bergman 1978). The veterinarian should have a collection cup close at hand whenever examining a late-pregnant goat. A doe often urinates when it first stands up on the approach of a stranger, as part of preparing for flight. If urination has not yet occurred by the end of the examination, then occluding the nostrils while an assistant holds the cup under the goat's vulva may be tried. However, even healthy goats rarely urinate in response to this stimulus, and the toxemic animal is typically dehydrated. The attempt must be abandoned before the goat is asphyxiated.

When urine is not available, plasma or serum can be checked with the ketone pills, powders, or strips. Recently, with the advent of hand-held meters for testing human blood for beta-hydroxybutyrate and glucose, precise BHB testing on farm has become possible. The test strips are inexpensive and the results determined rapidly. Unfortunately, specific BHB reference values have not been established for goats (Stelletta et al. 2008), but values established for sheep (Clarkson 2000) can be used by default. Thus, BHB values less than 1 mmol/l can be considered normal, values of 1.5 to 3 mmol/l can be considered indicative of severe undernutrition, and animals with pregnancy toxemia often show a BHB concentration greater than 3 mmol/l. For conversion to other units, note that BHB in mmol/l × 10.3 = BHB in mg/dl. If the animal is recently dead, aqueous humor or cerebrospinal fluid can be tested instead of blood (Scott et al. 1995), but the accuracy of the hand-held meters using these fluids has not been established.

Other laboratory tests are not commonly performed on field cases of pregnancy toxemia. Cortisol-induced changes in the hemogram (neutrophilia, lymphopenia, eosinopenia) and evidence of dehydration (elevated hematocrit and total protein) can be expected. Blood glucose levels are variable; severe hypoglycemia or terminal marked hyperglycemia are both possible (normal range 50 to 75 mg/dl; see Chapter 11).

Necropsy Findings

The doe that dies of pregnancy toxemia usually has multiple fetuses in the uterus, unless these were removed just before death. The fetuses may be fresh or decomposed. The doe's liver is enlarged and yellow because of infiltration with fat (Tontis and Zwahlen 1987). The doe's adrenal glands are enlarged. The carcass appears dehydrated. If urine remains in the bladder, it shows a strong ketone reaction.

Treatment

The treatment and prognosis depend on the stage of the disease. In the earliest clinical form, the goat readily eats offered grain. Its diet should be improved to include better quality roughage and increased concentrates. Propylene glycol is given orally by dosing syringe, at the rate of 60 ml two or three times daily as a glucose precursor. Although some authors suggest as much as 175 to 250 ml of propylene glycol twice a day (Bretzlaff et al. 1991), this dosage seems excessive and likely to overwhelm the ability of the rumen flora of an already sick goat to digest it. Overdoses of propylene glycol can be fatal, creating plasma hyperosmolality that impairs neurologic function. A commercial product that contains niacin as well as propylene glycol has been recommended, or the goat can be injected with enough mixed B vitamins to supply 1 gram of niacin/day (Bowen 1998). Calcium borogluconate (60 ml of a 23% to 25% solution) is given subcutaneously to counteract any concurrent hypocalcemia; approximately 20% of sheep with pregnancy toxemia are also hypocalcemic (Kolb and Kaskous 2004). Some authors recommend the use of insulin, up to 40 units of protamine zinc insulin twice daily subcutaneously (Matthews 1999), but an approved veterinary product is not available in the United States.

If the animal is unwilling to eat or to rise, the prognosis is guarded. Intravenous glucose (25 to 50 grams, preferably as a 5% to 10% solution), mixed B vitamins, and force feeding are added to the regimen. One author has suggested giving 5 to 7 g glucose as a 50% solution six to eight times a day via an indwelling jugular catheter (Marteniuk and Herdt 1988). If the goat is breathing rapidly, acidosis is likely and intravenous therapy should be extended to 3 to 4 liters of fluid including 15 grams or more of sodium bicarbonate. Antibiotic therapy is begun for primary or secondary pneumonia.

If the goat is known to be within one week of its due date, hormonal induction of parturition (see Chapter 13) with 10 mg of prostaglandin F2 alpha will end the energy drain to the fetuses. If the due date is uncertain and the owner desires to save doe and kids, 20 to 25 mg dexamethasone may be preferred for its gluconeogenic effects and beneficial stimulus to appetite. Late gestation fetuses are born in approximately two days after corticosteroid administration, while more immature fetuses are not always aborted but may instead be carried to term successfully if the doe responds to medical management. If possible, transabdominal ultrasound examination of the uterus for evidence of fetal movement or heartbeat should be performed to verify that the fetuses are still alive. Dexamethasone induction requires a live fetus, and slaughter or euthanasia may be more appropriate in commercial situations if the kids are already dead.

If the valuable goat is down and very depressed or has failed to improve by the day after initiation of treatment, then a cesarean section should be performed immediately. Severely toxemic animals do not kid rapidly or dependably after receiving hormones, but dexamethasone on the first visit may prepare the lungs of marginally immature kids and thereby increase their chances of surviving a cesarean operation that can be delayed for twenty-four hours. Even with surgery and extensive fluid therapy, the prognosis is poor for survival of the recumbent goat in the late stages of pregnancy toxemia. The kids from these does also frequently are delivered dead or die within a few hours of surgery.

Prevention

If goats are already obese when the last trimester is reached, it is too late to propose a weight-reducing diet. Instead, animals must be fed high quality roughage and as much as 500 g of concentrate daily. Any conditions that disturb the comfort of the goat, such as lack of exercise, poor ventilation, or drafts, should be corrected. This means that the stall should be dry, well-bedded, and uncrowded. The goats should be let loose for at least two to three hours per day. Timid does and slow eaters should be housed separate from dominant, aggressive animals that might drive them away from the feeder. If fetal numbers have been determined by real-time ultrasonography (see Chapter 13), the goats can be grouped and fed according to litter size. Goats carrying three or more fetuses should receive the best quality roughage available in addition to adequate concentrate.

When one doe develops pregnancy toxemia, the diet of the rest of the herd must be evaluated and corrected as necessary. Concentrates should be introduced gradually and under strict control, to avoid indigestion. It is unrealistic to expect a large herd of commercial goats to be totally free of pregnancy toxemia. Routine monitoring of all late-pregnant does for urinary ketones is also unrealistic. Healthy does carrying large litters can be expected to excrete small quantities of ketones yet do not need treatment. Drenching with prophylactic propylene glycol (60 ml orally twice a day) is in itself a stress to a goat and should be reserved for those showing abnormal behavior or diminished appetite.

Some authors have recommended supplementing ruminant diets with niacin to help protect against the development of a ketotic state. Niacin (nicotinic acid) is antilipolytic and causes blood glucose and insulin to increase (Herdt and Emery 1992). There are anecdotal reports that 500 mg niacin/pound of grain fed works well for preventing pregnancy toxemia in goats (Bowen 1998). Published research documenting a beneficial effect of feeding niacin appears to be lacking in goats, but the practice does not appear to carry any risks.

Parturient Paresis (Milk Fever), Hypocalcemia

Although various authors, especially in lay publications, talk about the occurrence of milk fever in goats, this condition is apparently rare (Linzell 1965; Kessler 1981).

Pathogenesis

Parturient paresis is a failure of calcium homeostasis, which depends in turn on intestinal absorption and skeletal reserves. Intestinal absorption requires calcium binding protein. The synthesis of this transport protein is controlled by vitamin D_3 availability (Sauvant et al. 1991a).

There is a sudden increase in calcium and phosphorus requirements at the onset of lactation, and the capacity for intestinal absorption of calcium increases more slowly than the requirement. Normal parturition in goats is accompanied by mild hypocalcemia. For instance, six healthy Alpine goats had an average plasma calcium concentration of 6.6 mg/dl three days after parturition, as compared with 8.4 mg/dl six days before and six days after kidding (Barlet et al. 1971). In another intensive study of healthy goats (six Saanens and one Alpine), plasma calcium concentrations as low as 6.7 mg/dl were encountered (Linzell 1965). When the hypocalcemia is extreme, milk fever can be expected to occur.

High producing dairy goats occasionally develop a severe hypocalcemic syndrome clinically similar to milk fever, except that the goat is one to three or more weeks after parturition (Barlet et al. 1971; Øverby and Ødegaard 1980; Ødegaard and Øverby 1993). The tendency of goats undergoing a high degree of lipid mobilization to have a significant increase in calcium and phosphorus content of their milk may be involved (Sauvant et al. 1991a).

Of forty Norwegian goats with hypocalcemia, seven were prepartum (two more than a week before kidding), ten were affected during kidding or the first day after kidding, eight more were within three weeks after kidding, and fifteen were more than three weeks into lactation. Older goats were affected; thirty-four of forty were starting their fourth or later lactation (Ødegaard and Øverby 1993).

Clinical Signs

Signs include a decrease in appetite, mild bloat or constipation, unsteady gait, and weakened uterine contractions, then an inability to rise and a decreased body temperature (Guss 1977; Øverby and Ødegaard 1980; Ødegaard and Øverby 1993). Affected goats are often somnolent and lie in sternal recumbency with the head turned back along the side of the body. Occasional goats lie in lateral recumbency, showing muscle spasms and screaming. There may be mucus at the nostrils or signs suggestive of pulmonary edema.

In forty Norwegian goats diagnosed as clinically hypocalcemic, the average plasma calcium concentration was 3.75 mg/dl (range 2.9 to 5.1), compared with an average of 9.91 mg/dl in thirty-six normal goats (Øverby and Ødegaard 1980). In an Indian study of nine mature goats of various breeds, in which the clinical signs of hypocalcemia were not described but diagnosis was based at least in part of response the therapy, the average calcium concentration was 6.66 mg/dl (Vihan and Rai 1984).

Treatment

The recommended therapy for either periparturient or lactational hypocalcemia is slow intravenous infusion of 50 to 100 ml of 23% calcium borogluconate. Rapid response to calcium therapy confirms the diagnosis if laboratory testing is not available. Additional calcium is sometimes administered subcutaneously or oral milk fever preparations are given. Calcium chloride gels should be avoided because of the risk of severe mucosal damage. Owners sometimes feed flavored calcium carbonate antacid pills to their does as a further calcium supplement, although this form of calcium is poorly absorbed until it is dissociated by acid in the abomasum (Thilsing-Hansen et al. 2002).

Most authors agree that the best response is achieved with early treatment. On the other hand, periparturient goats with clinical signs of excitability, posterior paresis, and constipation may not respond to calcium infusions (Kessler 1981). Perhaps some of the goats diagnosed as having milk fever are in fact victims of rumen acidosis caused by inadequate roughage consumption in late pregnancy.

Prevention

In dairy cattle, the avoidance during late pregnancy of feeds rich in calcium, such as alfalfa hay, was long considered central to preventing milk fever. More recent work in both cattle (Oetzel et al. 1988; Thilsing-Hansen et al. 2002) and goats (Fredeen et al. 1988) has shown that adjusting the cationic/anionic balance ((Na + K)/(Cl + S)) by acidifying the late pregnancy diet with added anionic salts also prevents the condition. Dietary magnesium must be adequate for calcium mobilization from bone to occur.

Alfalfa has a cation excess which may be associated with decreased calcium absorption from the diet prepartum. In regions where alfalfa is plentiful or indeed the only hay readily available, the prevalence of milk fever in goats does not seem to be increased. This may be because goats tend to come into milk production more gradually than do dairy cows. A very low calcium diet is not needed in goats and in fact might lead to hypocalcemia, as it does in ewes.

Because the etiology of lactational hypocalcemia is poorly understood, prevention centers on avoiding anything that upsets feed intake or gastrointestinal function (Ødegaard and Øverby 1993).

FEEDING LACTATING GOATS

In the past, the best producing goats in a herd were usually the ones that consumed the most forage. This may be because of intensive selection pressure in herds in which little or no grain was fed. As feeding practices change, goats may adapt to using grain in preference to forage. However, it remains true that goats have an aptitude to consume much forage, a characteristic that makes them well adapted to many extensive agricultural situations.

The forage-to-concentrate ratio should always be kept in mind (Kawas et al. 1991). With an alfalfa hay/grain ration, a forage:concentrate (F:C) ratio of 2:1 gives excellent results. With mediocre hay, F:C ratios of 1:1 to 1:2 are more appropriate. For best production of milk and butterfat, hay consumption should be maximized while still maintaining a positive energy balance. This requires good forage that is not overmature and lignified. As the proportion of concentrates in the ration increases (especially above two-thirds), butterfat percentage drops. It is not economically sound to force hay consumption if the hay is of poor quality. Green chops and dehydrated forages are better than most hays.

In early lactation, when goats are mobilizing body fat as an energy source, it is important to feed adequate protein to support milk production. A crude protein concentration of 17% to 18% of DM has been recommended for high producing goats at this stage (Skjevdal 1981). During midlactation, total crude protein in the ration should be 13% to 16% of DM.

Lactation Curves

In recent years, numerous researchers have taken production data acquired in the course of milk recording schemes and attempted to fit mathematical functions to the data to describe dairy goat lactation curves (Gipson and Grossman 1990; Macciotta et al. 2008). Factors affecting the lactation curve include breed, parity, season of kidding, and level of production (Gipson and Grossman 1990). First parity does have decreased peak yields, peak later, and are more persistent than later parity does. Higher producing does are less persistent than low producers; milk production declines more steeply after peak yield. Does freshening with two kids produce more milk than does with singles, whether suckled or not (Macciotta et al. 2008). The mathematical equations permit prediction of the total milk yield for the entire lactation from a few tests in early lactation and are thus useful for selection and culling decisions.

Figure 19.6 depicts lactation curves (total milk) for goats of different parities freshening at different times of the year. These curves were derived from the original data of Gipson and Grossman (1989).

Lactation curves describing total milk, fat, and protein have been used by dairy cattle consultants as indicators of nutritional status of individual animals or herds. The validity of such an approach for goat herds needs additional evaluation (Gipson 1992). Comparison of lactation curves generated during research trials is useful for demonstrating the beneficial effects of providing appropriate dietary energy and protein (Sahlu et al. 1995) or other nutrients. Looking at the curves from a commercial herd and then trying to predict the adequacy of the diet is more problematic.

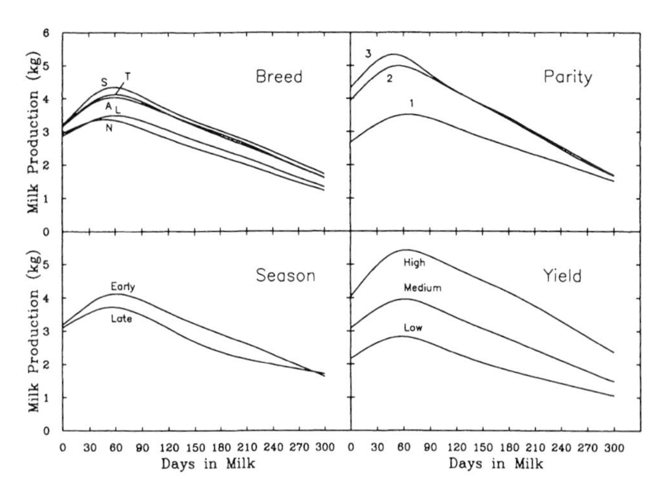

Figure 19.6. Lactation curves for dairy goats. Redrawn from: Gipson (1992).

Ketosis

Cows and goats have comparable milk production when the quantity of fat-corrected milk per kg metabolic body weight is considered. Goats and cows also have similar body reserves which are mobilized to support milk production (Sauvant et al. 1991a). Goats selected for high production but improperly fed may develop lactational ketosis.

Pathogenesis

Glucose is required by the mammary gland for synthesis of lactose. After parturition, the quantity of milk produced and thus the nutrient requirements of the goat increase more rapidly than does the level of intake. Plasma glucose is significantly influenced by digestibility of the diet, whereas the level of lipomobilization is more independent of the quality of the diet, increasing instead exponentially with production potential.

Older goats are generally larger and heavier and have an increased potential dry matter intake than yearlings. However, this increased intake is inadequate to compensate for their higher requirements which reflect higher milk production. The increased mammary uptake of glucose in high producers is not adequately offset by increased hepatic gluconeogenesis and increased absorption of glucogenic precursors. Thus, high producers tend to be hypoglycemic (Sauvant et al. 1984).

Clinical Signs and Treatment

In view of the typical signs of lactational ketosis in cattle, decreased appetite (especially for concentrates) and decreased milk production are to be expected in goats with ketosis. Ketonuria is present and some people can detect the odor of ketones on the animal's breath. Treatment consists of corticosteroids (2 to 6 mg dexamethasone [Braun 1989] or more) for their gluconeogenic and appetite-stimulating effects and oral propylene glycol (60 ml two to three times daily). Intravenous dextrose may also be given, as discussed under pregnancy toxemia. Provision of tempting browse or force feeding with a slurry of pelleted complete horse feed is used if needed to increase feed consumption.

A more severe syndrome sometimes occurs in which the best producing goat in the herd suddenly collapses. A severe hypocalcemia frequently accompanies ketonuria. Dramatic recovery often results from "shotgun" therapy with intravenous fluids, dextrose, calcium, and B vitamins. The exact pathogenesis remains obscure. An indigestion or acidosis from excessive grain consumption when hay is of poor quality may be involved.

Prevention

It is important to limit the early lactation energy deficit as much as possible, to avoid clinical ketosis. This can be done by stimulating appetite and feeding a balanced ration that includes grain early in lactation. The quantity of grain is increased by 0.1 kg every three days until requirements are met. Peak energy intake can be achieved several weeks earlier than peak dry matter intake if concentrates are fed judiciously. This is because the capacity to ingest concentrates rises more rapidly than does the capacity to ingest forages. Normally the goat achieves a positive energy balance during the second month of lactation.

Indigestion and Rumen Acidosis

When a high proportion of concentrates is fed in the ration, indigestion can lead to a marked day to day variation in feed consumption. The goat has subacute ruminal acidosis, a metabolic disease which is considered to be economically important in dairy cattle but is poorly described in goats (Stelletta et al. 2008). With even higher concentrate intake, life-threatening rumen acidosis may occur. Nutritionally induced rumen bloat, which is also potentially life-threatening, is discussed in Chapter 10.

Pathogenesis

In general, roughages have an increased fiber content compared to concentrates and stimulate long periods of rumination. This in turn results in buffering of the rumen fluid by bicarbonate in saliva. The rumen pH remains in a range (6.0 to 6.8) favorable for cellulolytic bacteria. The major end product of roughage digestion is acetate. Grains lack long fiber. Because of a decreased rumination rate, less saliva reaches the rumen and the pH of the rumen contents drops when grain is consumed. This is desirable within limits, because the bacteria for degrading starches and sugars multiply best at a pH of 5.5 to 6.0. Also, the volatile fatty acids propionate and butyrate are produced in large quantities by digestion of concentrates and are absorbed faster at lower pH levels.

If too much grain is eaten at one time (improper diet or forced entry into the feed room), lactic acid producing streptococci overgrow in the rumen and the pH decreases even more to a point where lactobacilli can proliferate. The ensuing lactic acid production lowers the rumen pH below the physiologic limit of 5.5 and kills the normal flora and fauna. Bacteria produce both dextro- and levo-rotatory isomeric forms of lactic acid, but the mammalian liver is only able to efficiently degrade the L form. This allows the D form to build up in the blood, causing a systemic acidosis. Increased production of histamine and other toxins is associated with the occurrence of laminitis in some animals. Deranged synthesis of B vitamins or production of thiamine antimetabolites can lead to polioencephalomalacia (see Chapter 5). It should be noted that liver abscesses in goats are usually caused by *Corynebacterium pseudotuberculosis*, rather than other bacteria passing through a rumen epithelium damaged by toxic indigestion, as in cattle.

Clinical Findings and Clinical Pathology

Mild overeating of grain results in an off feed condition. Rumen motility decreases but does not stop. The goat may grind its teeth. Milk production decreases and diarrhea may develop. Because the goat stops eating for one or two days, the rumen pH levels increase to a near-neutral range and recovery follows.

Severe overloading is accompanied by a systemic and often fatal acidosis. Rumen motility ceases and the contents are initially firm; mild bloat may be present. Constipation followed by diarrhea, muscle tremors, teeth grinding, groaning or blatting, increased heart and respiratory rates, and even a low fever may be noted. As the disease progresses, splashy (abnormally liquid) rumen contents, abdominal distension, and dehydration (evidenced by sunken eyes, decreased skin turgor, and increased packed cell volume) develop. This is because the rumen contents become hyperosmotic and pull water from the systemic circulation into the rumen. The urine is acidic and blood pH and bicarbonate values may be markedly decreased. Blood lactate levels greater than 40 mg/dl can occur in severe cases, with levels in normal goats of 8 to 10 mg/dl. Significant decreases in blood calcium sometimes occur. Some cases are fatal within twenty-four hours, while less severe cases may develop over twenty-four to seventy-two hours.

Diagnosis and Necropsy Findings

Rumen acidosis should be suspected when a goat is depressed and off feed and has had chronic or acute

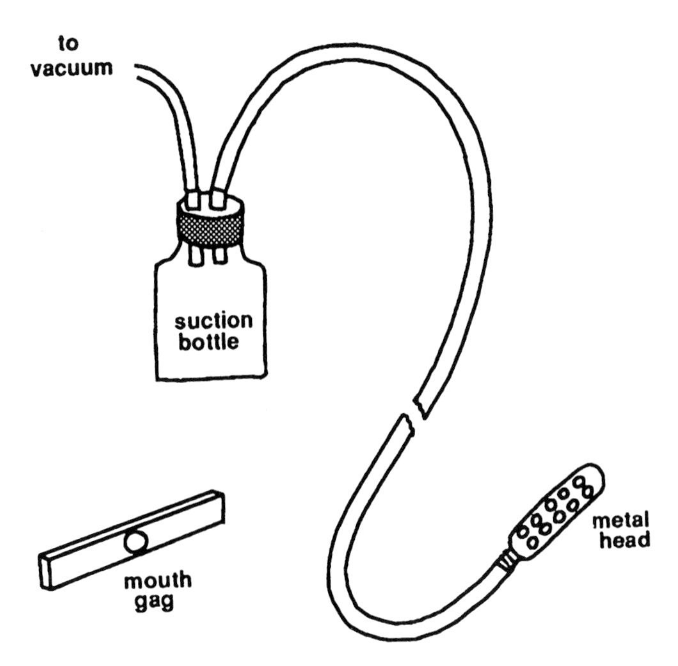

Figure 19.7. Homemade sound for obtaining rumen fluid from an adult goat.

access to large quantities of readily fermentable carbohydrates (i.e., grain, bread, sugar beets, apples) (Braun et al. 1992). If diarrhea is present, fecal pH may be reduced; in one experimental study feeding wheat flour, fecal pH dropped from above 7.0 to below 5.0 at twenty-four hours (Aslan et al. 1995).

A sample of rumen fluid obtained with the aid of a stomach tube (up to 1 cm diameter) or a specially designed device (a metal sound with many perforations; see Figure 19.7) or even a needle aspirate can be helpful both for establishing a diagnosis and for determining if a rumenotomy is justified. Ruminocentesis carries risks of peritonitis or localized abscesses, but these risks can be lessened by shearing and disinfection of the chosen site over the ventral rumen, restraining the goat to prevent sudden movement during the procedure, and avoiding needle insertion during a contraction of the ventral sac of the rumen (Stelletta et al. 2008).

A milky gray fluid with a sour smell and a pH level less than 5.0 is conclusive evidence of rumen acidosis. Slightly increased pH levels may result from contamination of the rumen fluid sample with saliva during collection. A pH level in the normal range (5.5 to 7.0) does not rule out rumen acidosis because absorption of acid, passage of ingesta to the abomasum, and flow of saliva cause increase of the pH level if the goat survives long enough. A Gram-stained smear of rumen fluid demonstrates an overwhelming preponderance of Gram-positive organisms when rumen acidosis has occurred. Rumen protozoa are dead or absent (Nour et al. 1998). In dairy goats in early lactation, the advanced stages of rumen acidosis may mimic toxic mastitis or milk fever. Animals recumbent with milk fever are not dehydrated or diarrheic and respond to parenteral administration of calcium salts. Enterotoxemia occurs under similar circumstances of accidental or excessive exposure to carbohydrates and may have a similar clinical appearance. Enterotoxemia generally has a more rapid clinical course and the degree of systemic acidosis and dehydration is not as severe.

At necropsy, the same changes in rumen fluid are apparent. Additionally, there may be evidence of large quantities of grain in the rumen or of rumenitis and localized peritonitis. Abomasal ulcers, sometimes perforating, have been produced experimentally by grain overload (Aslan et al. 1995). Dehydration is evidenced by sunken eyes.

Treatment

When the indigestion is judged to be mild, offering hay is sufficient treatment, and mixed B vitamins may be given "on general principles" and to protect against development of polioencephalomalacia.

Early in the course of the indigestion, oral antacids (Baumgartner and Loibl 1986) should stop progression of the disease. Various suggested adult dosages include 10 to 20 g magnesium oxide, 50 g magnesium hydroxide, or 20 g sodium bicarbonate. In an experimental model that produced ruminal acidosis by feeding 80 g of wheat flour per kg bw, oral sodium bicarbonate at 1 g/kg twenty-four hours later was an effective treatment, whereas oral baking yeast at 1 g/kg was not helpful (Aslan et al. 1995). Oral tetracycline (single dose of 0.5 to 1 g) also helps to inhibit additional bacterial proliferation. Concentrate is withheld and palatable forage is offered free choice.

A rumenotomy to remove the rumen contents and rinse the mucosa may be life-saving in acute, severe cases. If the rumen fluid pH is near neutral, and especially if the rumen contents have a splashy consistency, rumenotomy is no longer of great benefit. Instead, as much fluid as possible is drained off with a stomach tube. Then warm water, antacids, and (if available) rumen fluid from a healthy animal are administered through the tube.

If available, determination of acid-base status is helpful in guiding therapy; the severely affected goat has a metabolic acidosis. The base deficit is multiplied by 0.3 × bw in kg to determine the milliequivalents of bicarbonate (HCO_3^-) needed. Each gram of sodium bicarbonate supplies 12 mEq of bicarbonate. Even when clinical laboratory support is lacking, dehydrated goats should be treated intravenously with 3 to 5 liters or more of physiologic saline with added bicarbonate. A goat weighing 50 kg with moderate acidosis (base deficit of 12) needs approximately 15 g of sodium bicarbonate.

Thiamine (300 to 500 mg several times a day), other B vitamins, and calcium gluconate administered subcutaneously are commonly given. Glucose solutions are not necessary, and lactated Ringer's solution is contraindicated. Repeated oral administration of a liter of rumen fluid from a healthy cow, sheep, or goat (obtained fresh from a slaughterhouse or from a fistulated cow or with the aid of a rumen fluid sampling device) is very beneficial in restoring normal rumen flora and fauna (Braun et al. 1992).

Prevention

If the goat has two to (preferably) four weeks to adapt to gradually increasing quantities of grain, then many cases of indigestion can be avoided. Adaptation occurs in two ways. First, the rumen microorganisms that digest readily fermentable carbohydrates to volatile fatty acids increase in number. At the same time, certain bacteria (such as streptococci) produce lactic acid from starches and sugars, but still other species of bacteria with the ability to metabolize lactate to propionate have time to proliferate (Ogimoto and Giesecke 1974). Second, increased concentrations of propionic and butyric acid stimulate the development of rumen papillae so that there is an increased surface area for absorption of fatty acids. Rapid removal of volatile fatty acids from the rumen helps to keep the pH within physiologic bounds.

Another management technique that is very helpful with high concentrate feeding is to distribute the grain over three or more meals a day of 0.3 kg (2/3 pound) (Broqua 1990) per meal or slightly more. This results in a less drastic pH level decrease after each meal than if all the grain is fed at once. Grains that are digested very rapidly (e.g., wheat and high moisture corn) can be replaced by slower digesting grains (e.g., sorghum, dry corn). Whole grain is digested more slowly than finely ground grain that has more surface area for bacterial attack. Roughage should be fed before grain, first thing in the morning. Regular supplementation with buffers (bicarbonate of soda or calcium carbonate at 1.5% to 2% of concentrate) and magnesium (0.2% to 0.3%) (Broqua 1990) also reduces the risk of acidosis. Producers sometimes offer bicarbonate of soda free choice to goats on high grain diets. Corn silage should also be distributed three or more times a day; otherwise, the goat may initially select out a large quantity of corn grain from the silage, risking acidosis.

When individual feeding of grain is not possible, as when supplementing animals on range because of drought conditions, the use of alkali-treated grain with an ionophore has permitted feeding of relatively large quantities of grain to unadapted goats, as described above for prevention of abortion. Dried beet pulp, citrus pulp, and soybean hulls are other energy sources that carry less risk of acidosis than do standard grain products, because they are high in fermentable cell walls and support healthy rumen fermentation (DiTrana and Sepe 2008).

Enterotoxemia

Clostridium perfringens type D is a normal inhabitant of the goat's intestinal tract. Sudden changes in diet (consumption of unaccustomed quantities of grain or of lush pasture when first turned out in the spring) can result in incomplete digestion in the rumen. The ingesta that passes to the small intestine then favors overgrowth of the clostridia and production of epsilon toxin. This toxin is activated by trypsin and absorbed. The syndrome produced is called enterotoxemia or overeating disease and is described more fully in Chapter 10. Sudden death is common.

Because many of the same factors predispose to both enterotoxemia and to rumen acidosis, the two conditions can occur in the same outbreak and can be confused clinically. Necropsy findings (pH level less than 5.5 in rumen fluid for acute acidosis; fluid and fibrin in the pericardial sac, glucosuria, epsilon toxin in ingesta for enterotoxemia) can usually distinguish between the two diseases. Presence of epsilon toxin without other signs is not proof of enterotoxemia.

Milk Fat Depression

When a poor quality roughage is supplemented with concentrate, intakes of both dry matter and energy increase and milk production is increased. However, the amount of butterfat produced increases less than does the amount of milk, and thus butterfat percentage tends to drop (Morand-Fehr and Sauvant 1980). High concentrate, low roughage diets are associated, as discussed earlier, with decreases in rumen fluid pH and in the ratio of acetate to propionate produced in the rumen (Lu et al. 2005). These changes in turn are associated with decreased butterfat production, because acetate rather than propionate or butyrate is the main precursor of milk fat (Davis et al. 1964) and propionate stimulates insulin secretion, which inhibits release of fatty acids from adipose tissue (Emmanuel and Kennelly 1984). In many places where high-producing dairy goats are raised, good quality roughages to support production are unavailable or else very expensive. In select instances, it may be necessary to add a buffer, such as sodium bicarbonate at 4%, to the concentrate portion of the ration to maintain butterfat production (Hadjipanayiotou 1982). Other causes of milk fat depression are discussed in Chapter 14.

FEEDING NEWBORN KIDS

Depending on the intensification of the operation and the need to implement various disease control procedures, kids are either raised on the doe, switched to artificial rearing at the end of the colostrum period, or fed by hand from birth. If the doe is well fed and has a healthy, well-suspended udder, the "natural" approach of leaving kids with the doe gives good results. Milk is clean, warm, and waiting whenever the kid is hungry. Introduction to solid foods occurs as the kid samples what its dam eats.

Colostrum

Proper colostrum feeding is critical to health and survival of goat kids (Mellor and Murray 1986; Kolb and Kaskous 2003). If the doe dies or is too sick or malnourished at parturition to produce colostrum (Banchero et al. 2006), or if kids are removed from the dam at birth, then the owner must understand the principles of colostrum feeding. The first is to give enough, and enough is probably 50 ml/kg four times during the first day after birth. For owners who are not comfortable with the metric system, 1 ounce/pound three times is a comparable total amount. These rules of thumb are equivalent to feeding approximately 20% of body weight. The second principle is to give the first feeding of colostrum soon, preferably within the first hour after birth, and certainly within six hours. The antibodies in colostrum need to be consumed before the kid sucks on dirty, pathogen-loaded parts of its mother or stall. Death from hypoglycemia or hypothermia is also likely in cold weather if feeding is delayed. The colostrum should be of good quality, nonmastitic, and not contaminated with environmental or milk-borne pathogens. Only first milking colostrum from healthy animals should be frozen for later feeding, and the colostrum from older animals that have been on the premises for several years is typically higher in antibody content against endemic pathogens than is colostrum from first fresheners. Revaccination of the doe against tetanus and enterotoxemia two to four weeks before the due date is commonly used to improve the protective value of the colostrum against these conditions. Failure of passive transfer is discussed in Chapter 7.

Owners should be taught to tube feed kids that are not suckling well. This avoids both delays in colostrum consumption and the risks of inhalation pneumonia associated with pouring liquids into a weak kid's mouth. An 18 French feeding tube or urethral catheter long enough to reach the last rib can be safely passed without a gag in a newborn kid. It can be palpated between trachea and cervical vertebrae as proof of proper positioning. Gravity flow through the barrel of a 60-ml syringe or slow, careful injection is used to administer colostrum or milk as needed. Tube feeding does not encourage a kid to imprint on people, so it does not interfere with nursing of the dam. The tube must be cleaned and sanitized between kids.

Heat treating of colostrum is an important part of control programs for several diseases, such as caprine arthritis encephalitis and mycoplasmosis. In some instances, first-milking cow colostrum is substituted for goat colostrum. Consideration should be given to pasteurizing cow colostrum to prevent diseases such as paratuberculosis, salmonellosis, and cryptosporidiosis. In addition, substituting cow colostrum may leave young kids susceptible to enterotoxemia, tetanus, caseous lymphadenitis, and contagious echthyma.

Low quality "colostrum substitutes" described in many lay publications should be avoided because they fail to provide antibodies to the kid (Scroggs 1989). In one study, feeding a total of 480 ml of heat treated goat colostrum was associated with an increase of mean serum immunoglobulin levels more than twenty-four hours after birth of 1,549 ± 425 mg/dl, whereas a powdered bovine whey concentrate gave an increase of 90 ± 80 mg/dl and a dried colostrum and whey bolus increased immunoglobulins by 290 ± 557 mg/dl (Sherman et al. 1990). Commercial products based on bovine plasma offer more promise, because adequate immunoglobulin is absorbed in lambs (Quigley et al. 2002).

Hypothermia and Hypoglycemia

The normal healthy neonate has a body temperature above 102°F or 39°C. Hypothermia occurs if the neonate, especially a small, wet one, is exposed to cold, wet, or windy conditions. A secondary hypothermia develops if the kid does not obtain enough colostrum and milk to replenish its body reserves in less inclement weather. If the hypothermic kid is less than five hours old, it should be dried and rewarmed (forced warm air, heating pad on low, or very cautious use of a heat lamp to avoid overheating the kid or burning the barn), then given colostrum at 50 ml/kg. Body temperature should be monitored closely during rewarming, because overheating is rapidly fatal.

If the kid is beyond five hours of age, the brown fat stores around kidney and heart, used for nonshivering thermogenesis, have probably been depleted. The older kid that can hold its head up is fed by stomach tube and rewarmed, but if it is too weak to hold up its head, hypoglycemia is likely and fatal convulsions may occur during rewarming. To prevent this, the kid is given an intraperitoneal injection of glucose (dextrose) before being rewarmed (Eales et al. 1984; Matthews 1999). Commercial 50% dextrose is diluted with sterile or boiled water to make a 20% solution (two parts 50% dextrose mixed with three parts water). This solution is warmed to normal body temperature before use. The kid is held suspended by its front legs and a spot one inch lateral to and 1 inch caudal to the umbilicus is treated with a disinfectant such as iodine. A 1-inch (25 mm) 20-g needle is inserted through the body wall at the marked location and directed at a 45-degree angle to the skin and toward the kid's rump.

After the glucose solution has been injected somewhere into the abdomen where it can be rapidly absorbed, an antibiotic injection is given and the kid can be safely rewarmed, then tube fed when it is stronger. Providing a coat made from a sock with toe removed or a sweatshirt sleeve with holes cut for the front legs helps to maintain body temperature over the next few days.

First Weeks

The normal birth weight of kids, and how it is affected by breed, sex, and litter size, have been summarized by Morand-Fehr (1981c).

There are many schemes for raising young kids (Morand-Fehr 1981c). Breed, climate, and nutritional resources for both goat and owner must be considered. With larger dairy breeds, one schedule involves feeding 1 liter of milk/day by one week of age and 1.5 to 2 liters by three weeks of age, with no further increase. Other authors recommend substantially less milk per day (0.75 to 1 kg) (Adams 1986) but fail to allow for less than perfect environmental conditions, poor quality roughage, or inadequate concentrate consumption. An intake of 250 g fluid milk (13% solids) per kg live weight has been reported to give daily gains of 150 g (Jagusch et al. 1981). Intake of milk replacer dry matter needs to be 10% to 25% more than that of dry matter from goat milk, probably because of decreased digestibility (Morand-Fehr 1981c).

Milk replacer may be fed warm (95°F to 104°F, 35°C to 40°C) or cold (43°F to 50°F, 6°C to 10°C). Cold milk offers the advantages that the kid consume smaller and more frequent meals and there is limited opportunity for pathogens to grow in cold milk, but if the environment is cold, kids do better on warm milk. After the colostrum feeding period, milk may be fed one to three times per day or ad lib. Acceptable milk replacers are 20% to 28% protein and 16% to 24% fat (Morand-Fehr 1981c). One study showed improved consumption and rate of gain (but not feed efficiency) when dairy kids were offered ad lib milk replacer containing 23% protein and 26% fat, as compared with a milk replacer with a lower protein: energy ratio of 20% protein and 30% fat (Yeom et al. 2002). Soybean should be avoided as a source of protein, unless roasted or otherwise processed to improve digestibility and reduce immunoreactive properties (Ouédraogo et al. 1998).

Pygmy goat kids being reared artificially require less milk per day than larger breeds, but 15% of bodyweight is still appropriate. During the first two weeks after birth, a 3-ounce bottle of milk is fed four times per day. The feeding frequency is maintained but the quantity fed per meal is increased to 4 ounces at two to six weeks of age and 5 ounces from six weeks until weaning at eight to twelve weeks of age (Kinne 2008). Fresh green grass or mixed grass/legume hay and water are supplied free choice from the first week. Because male and castrated pygmy goats are at particular risk of urolithiasis, even as nursing kids, grain feeding of the male kid is usually avoided. These kids need early cut, high protein hay to meet their protein requirements. Some sources suggest feeding up to one cup of grain per day to growing pygmy goats (National Pygmy Goat Association 2006), but this practice is extremely risky.

Floppy Kid Syndrome

A poorly understood metabolic acidosis in young kids was first recognized in North America in the late 1980s and the first detailed clinical report was published in Canada (Tremblay et al. 1991). Owners in the United States and Canada soon named this the floppy kid syndrome. The names for the condition in French (chevreau mou), Portuguese (cabrito mole), and Spanish (borrachera de los cabritos) are equally descriptive of the poor muscle tone or softness and ataxia or apparent drunkenness that these kids display.

Etiology and Epidemiology

Kids of dairy, meat, and fiber breeds in confinement (but not on pasture) have been affected. Kids have been dam reared or fed goat milk, pasteurized goat milk, or milk replacer. There is usually no history of diarrhea or previous oral electrolyte therapy. The syndrome is a metabolic acidosis without dehydration. Morbidity approaches 100% on some farms in some years and mortality is very high if appropriate treatment is not given. A similarity with human infant botulism was noted early on, but researchers were unable to find botulinum toxin in affected kids and the observed response to just correction of acid-base status discounts botulism as a likely etiology. No association has been found with specific viral or bacterial pathogens of the neonatal kid (Bleul et al. 2006).

One proposed pathogenesis for the condition involves the over-consumption of milk (Riet-Correa et al. 2004), because kids are fed better or they nurse does that produce more milk than in previous seasons. The large amounts of milk in the digestive tract allow overgrowth of bacteria that then produce D-lactate and unidentified toxins. The observed increase in morbidity near the end of the kidding season supports an infectious etiology and buildup of pathogens in the environment. Often, the disease disappears from the farm the next year, adding to the mystery surrounding its etiology and complicating on-farm research efforts. Similar syndromes have been reported in calves (Kasari and Naylor 1986) and a llama cria (Shepherd et al. 1993).

Clinical Signs

Kids are born healthy, usually have received colostrum, and are not affected until three to fourteen days of age or occasionally up to one month (Bleul et al. 2006). Reported clinical signs include depression, reluctance to suckle, ataxia, weakness or muscle flaccidity, trembling or shaking, and abdominal distension (Tremblay et al. 1991; Riet-Correa et al. 2004; Bleul et al. 2006). A sudden buckling of the limbs is responsible for the syndrome name of floppy kid. Diarrhea is conspicuously absent, and the kids are not dehydrated. As signs progress, extremities become cold and the body temperature drops. The kid may become comatose and die after twenty-four to thirty-six hours if not treated. There are anecdotal reports of spontaneous recoveries and relapses in a small percentage of affected kids.

Diagnosis

Diagnosis depends on finding a metabolic acidosis without dehydration. If venous blood gases can be analyzed, previously untreated kids will be found to have a blood pH below 7.2 (sometimes as low as 6.8) and a base excess of less than −5.0. Ketones and L-lactate are not elevated, but D-lactate is substantially elevated (Bleul et al. 2006). The D-lactate averaged 7.43 mmol/L in affected kids but only 0.26 mmol/L in control kids in this study. The D-lactate only partially explained the anionic gap observed in these kids, suggesting the involvement of some other organic acid absorbed from the gastrointestinal tract. Serum potassium is low or normal, averaging 4.2 mmol/L in forty-nine affected kids and 5.1 mmol/L in thirty-five control kids (Bleul et al. 2006). Chloride may be slightly elevated. Packed cell volume is below 38%.

For a diagnosis of floppy kid syndrome, the kid should show no antemortem or post mortem evidence of hypoglycemia, septicemia, meningitis, white muscle disease, severe pneumonia, enterotoxemia, or dehydration with acidosis secondary to neonatal diarrhea. Owners tend to over-diagnose the condition, because the weakness that is the most prominent clinical sign can be present with many other diseases (Cebra and Cebra 2002). Rapid response to bicarbonate therapy is often considered diagnostic of floppy kid syndrome.

Necropsy is important to rule out other conditions, but findings are usually minimal. The abomasum may be distended with clotted milk and small hemorrhages may be present in the mucosa (Riet-Correa et al. 2004).

Treatment

The most important and often only required treatment is correction of the acidosis. This can be accomplished by intravenous administration of 1.3% sodium bicarbonate, 125 to 200 ml over one to three hours. If laboratory testing has been performed, the initial treatment is based on the following formula:

Body Weight in kg $\times$ 0.5 $\times$ (– Base Excess) = mEq Sodium Bicarbonate

Other authors have recommended that a factor of 0.6 or even higher be substituted in this formula in place of 0.5, at least for calves with changes in posture and demeanor due to severe D-hyperlactataemia (Lorenz and Vogt 2006).

Owners treat kids successfully with oral bicarbonate of soda, using 2.5 to 3 grams (a little more than one-half teaspoon) mixed with cold water. If the condition is not complicated by another problem, kids respond dramatically to one treatment, although a second oral treatment is sometimes needed twelve hours later and the occasional kid requires repeated treatments for up to four days (Bleul et al. 2006). Other oral alkalinizing agents such as Pepto-Bismol® have also been used successfully, but the dose used has not been reported.

Another apparently important part of treatment is to restrict milk intake for twenty-four hours, offering oral electrolytes instead. Additionally, a broad-spectrum antibiotic to treat or prevent septicemia in compromised kids has been advocated (Tremblay et al. 1991; Riet-Correa et al. 2004).

Prevention

It is difficult to propose a means of preventing a disease whose etiology is not understood. However, moderating the amount of milk consumed if this is judged to be excessive seems to be a reasonable starting point. When kids are reared artificially, keeping the milk or milk replacer cold with frozen jugs of water discourages slug feeding. Maintaining good hygiene to limit the buildup of potential pathogens in the kid rearing area is of course desirable on any farm. During an outbreak, owners should be advised to watch closely for well fed kids that sleep more than usual or are slow to suckle, so that they can be treated early.

FEEDING GROWING KIDS

A distinction is generally made between diets for meat kids and for doe kids being raised as replacements. In many parts of The United States the market for chevon (cabrito, goat meat) is very seasonal, being linked to religious holidays such as Easter. Although 10 kg is often the preferred weight at slaughter, both lighter and heavier kids are sold at the same time. After the holiday, it may be impossible to recover feed costs, let alone labor, involved in raising kids.

When kids are raised for meat, it is possible to produce an acceptable carcass on a diet of milk alone. In one study in which buck kids were grown for twenty weeks (to a final weight of approximately 20 kg), carcass characteristics were acceptable but cholesterol and saturated fatty acid levels were higher in meat from milk-fed kids when compared with conventionally reared, weaned kids (Potchoiba et al. 1990).

Castration is of limited benefit when bucks are slaughtered at a few months of age. Intact males have an increased daily rate of gain, while castrates lay down more fat and the fat contains relatively lower percentages of branched and odd-chain fatty acids and increased stearic acid (Bas et al. 1981). Older bucklings and mature males have a strong "buck odor" and meat taint that many people find highly objectionable. Thus, male meat goats that are to be raised until sexual maturity are often castrated even though there will be a resultant decrease in rate of gain. When weaned kids and yearlings are raised for meat, concentrate feeding has little effect on palatability of the meat because the fat is deposited in the kidney and pelvic regions rather than in the muscle (Smith et al. 1978).

Before Weaning

Fine-stemmed, pliable hays are ideal for encouraging roughage consumption before weaning. Chopping the hay increases consumption. Concentrates should be offered as pellets or rolled grains, rather than as ground meals (Morand-Fehr 1981c). Free choice water is necessary to optimize consumption and digestion of hay and concentrates, because milk bypasses the rumen, whereas water enters the rumen.

The time to wean is often determined by existence of other markets for the milk to be fed. Weight, rather than age, is the best indicator of how well a goat kid will withstand the shock of weaning. There is almost no growth retardation in Alpine kids weaned at 10 kg, whereas weaning at lighter weights leads to reduced growth rates for one week or longer. For other breeds, weaning when kids have achieved a weight equal to two and a half times birth weight has been recommended (Morand-Fehr 1981c). If economics do not demand early weaning, dairy breed kids grow quite well while at the same time learning to eat solid food if provided with 1.5 liters of milk/day until three or four months of age. Delaying weaning of replacement doelings also aids in reaching breeding weight at a younger age (Palma and Galina 1995). The growth rate of kids is influenced by the initial birth weight and by breed and feeding programs (Bajhau and Kennedy 1990).

After Weaning

Older kids, after weaning, can be grown easily on a concentrate or corn silage based ration, as long as proper consideration is given to preventing urolithiasis (see below and Chapter 12). Male Alpine kids, for instance, can have a daily gain of 180 to 190 g. This gives a dressed carcass of 10 kg or more by one hundred days of age. If no roughage is provided and castration is not practiced, the subcutaneous fat may be undesirably soft. This phenomenon is less important than with lambs because of the limited quantity of subcutaneous fat on a goat carcass. Female kids (Alpine breed) weaned by five to six weeks onto hay and grain have an average daily gain of 170 g for the first twelve weeks, but then growth slows (Morand-Fehr 1981c).

Most goats raised for meat live in regions where subsistence farming is practiced and nutritional conditions are poor. When feed intake is low or dietary energy and protein concentrations are inadequate, the growth rate is decreased and the feed conversion rate is high. Most goat breeds other than the Boer also have not been selected for increased growth rates (Nandé and Hofmeyr 1981). Nutritional strategies which may improve meat production include increased use of crop residues including sweet potato vines, use of urea-molasses licks, and increased cultivation and feeding of forage plants such as *Leucaena*, *Manihot* (cassava), and *Sesbania* (Devendra 1987). Constraints on *Leucaena* feeding are discussed in Chapter 10.

Doelings raised as replacements should not be overfed on concentrates or other energy sources. There is limited evidence that high energy intake in prepubertal goats results in decreased secretory tissue and increased fat deposition in the developing udder (Bowden et al. 1995). It is important, however, that they be well grown at the time of breeding. The French recommend attaining 55% to 60% of adult weight by seven months for natural breeding at that age. A figure of 70% is preferred if synchronization and artificial insemination are to be used. To achieve both good growth and a low percentage of concentrates in the ration, it is once again necessary to feed a good quality roughage. With poor hays, energy and protein intake do not support adequate growth.

Available nutrient requirement tables usually express requirements in calories of energy and grams of protein. Using this information to formulate an appropriate diet is laborious and depends strongly on the desired rate of gain and the dry matter intake achieved. The following examples of rations for replacement kids are calculated from the NRC 2007 tables of requirements and DM intake, using the online calculator (Gipson and Goetsch). A 15-kg kid approximately three months old and gaining 150 g/d needs 1.80 Mcal/d of metabolizable energy (ME) or 0.50 kg of TDN. Its metabolizable protein (MP) requirement of 67 g/d can be met with a diet that contains 2.87 kcal/kg ME and 16.7% crude protein (CP), assuming a DMI of 3.79% of bodyweight and a forage plus concentrate diet with 40% undegradable intake protein (UIP). A 30-kg dairy kid in its seventh month gaining 100 g/day needs 2.19 Mcal/day of ME or 0.61 kg of TDN. Its MP requirement of 68 g can be met with a diet that contains 2.39 kcal/kg ME and 10.7% crude protein, assuming a DMI of 3.03% of bodyweight and a similar diet with 40% UIP. Naturally, these levels must be increased to allow for activity or cold weather. Calcium and phosphorus recommendations for growing kids at varying growth rates have been summarized by Morand-Fehr (1981c) and the NRC (2007).

FEEDING BUCKS AND PET GOATS

Adult male goats and wethers should in general be fed a ration similar to what is appropriate for nonpregnant, nonlactating does. The energy requirements for maintenance are probably somewhat more for males than for females of equivalent metabolic body size. The French recommend an increase of 10% for males. An additional increase of 15% in energy and in protein and minerals is desirable beginning four to six weeks before the breeding season (Morand-Fehr and Sauvant 1978; Rankins et al. 2002). This normally needs to be supplied as grain (approximately 0.5 kg or 1 pound) because the buck may be so overexcited by the presence of his does that he does not take time to eat enough hay. Even with a supplement it is common for bucks to stop growing or lose weight during the breeding season (Louca et al. 1977; Gall 1981; Walkden-Brown et al. 1994). Feeding a poor quality ration (poor hay) to bucks is associated with a decreased scrotal circumference and poorer semen motility (Arbeiter 1963; Walkden-Brown et al. 1994).

Good quality grass forage and minimal grain, when supplemented with a trace mineralized salt and abundant fresh water, should generally meet most nutritional needs of goats at maintenance. Access to legumes should be limited to avoid calcium and protein excesses and nutritional bone disease (Adams 1986). Because forage quality is highly variable, owners should be encouraged to record the weight or girth tape measurement of their pets once a month. Restricted feeding or energy/protein supplementation can then be prescribed before the animal becomes either obese or emaciated.

Urolithiasis

Young male kids, breeding bucks, and wethers kept as pets or for fiber production are susceptible to urinary calculi. Commonly, when high concentrate feeding is practiced, a relative phosphorus excess predisposes to the precipitation of struvite (calcium, magnesium, and ammonium phosphates) crystals in the bladder. Urolithiasis is discussed in detail in Chapter 12.

Dietary recommendations to prevent the condition can be briefly summarized as follows. Dietary calcium : phosphorus should be at least 2 : 1; some authors recommend 3 or 4 : 1 (Van der Westhuysen et al. 1988). Excessive phosphorus is undesirable, even if additional calcium is incorporated in the diet to adjust the ratio. Ideally, the total ration fed to a buck should not contain more than 2.5 g P/kg dry matter, though this level is exceeded by many roughages. Likewise, the magnesium in the diet should not exceed the requirement for proper growth or maintenance. If attention is only given to the calcium : phosphorus ratio, the total quantity of minerals to be excreted in urine often exceeds what can be kept in solution. In general, mature males should not receive dairy concentrates or large quantities of alfalfa or subterranean clover, because these feeds contain excessive calcium and protein. Good quality grass hay is ideal for bucks.

French recommendations specify that the quantity of grain fed to a buck should not exceed 500 grams/day (Morand-Fehr and Sauvant 1988). Feeding more roughage and avoiding pelleted feeds may also help to maintain a fiber mat in the rumen and increase fecal (as opposed to urinary) output of phosphorus (NRC 2007). Ammonium chloride may be added at 0.5% to 1% of the ration or 2% of the concentrate to acidify urine and thus discourage precipitation of struvite. Clean water should be available at all times. Salt can be added to the ration at 4% to 5% to increase water intake and diuresis.

Posthitis

If excessive dietary protein is fed to a male goat, especially a castrated animal, the quantity of urea in the urine is increased. Urea-splitting corynebacteria within the prepuce can then release free ammonia, which scalds the external skin and preputial mucosa and produces "pizzle rot," described in Chapters 12 and 13.

Arthritis

Diets containing excessive calcium have been associated with calcification of periarticular tissues, ankylosis, and a stiff gait (Guss 1977), although experimental reproduction of the syndrome in goats is lacking. The pathogenesis is considered to be hypercalcitoninism induced in nonlactating animals (such as heifers and breeding bulls [Rostkowski et al. 1981]) by dietary calcium levels appropriate for lactating animals. Published descriptions of the syndrome in goats mostly predate discovery of the caprine arthritis encephalitis virus; it is also possible that excess calcium speeds dystrophic calcification of periarticular tissues damaged by the CAE virus, as discussed in Chapter 4. To avoid both metabolic bone disease and exacerbation of CAE in bucks and nonlactating pet goats, dietary calcium should be limited to 4 to 6 grams daily for mature animals weighing 70 kg (NRC 1981b).

SPECIAL CONSIDERATIONS IN FEEDING ANGORA AND CASHMERE GOATS

When Angoras are selected for high mohair production, their resulting higher nutrient requirements leave them only marginally capable of meeting their needs under normal foraging conditions in the dry climates to which they are best adapted (Huston 1981). Supplemental protein and energy are typically needed for early growth, at breeding, during mid- and late gestation, and after parturition. Supplemental feeding and shelter are also important for prevention of "freeze loss" after shearing, as discussed in Chapter 2.

Mohair Production

To allow for growth of the fleece (1.8 to 6 kg/year, Di Trana and Sepe 2008), Angora goats should be fed additional nutrients above those specified for maintenance, activity, gestation, and lactation of other breeds. The NRC (1981b) recommended a daily energy supplement of 30 kcal of ME (which could be approximated by $0.72 \times 30 = 21.6$ kcal NE_l) per kg of annual fleece. The protein supplement for the same kg of fleece (calculated from a protein-to-energy ratio) is 4.3 g TP or 3 g DP. More recently, regression equations have been developed to try to predict the requirements of Angora goats for energy and protein (Luo et al. 2004b) but do little to help an owner with diet formulation. However, ration calculators are available online to convert the formulas into a diet for the goats (Gipson and Goetsch).

Increased sulfur in the diet is also necessary (Adams 1986; Bretzlaff 1990; Qi et al. 1994). Feeding inorganic sulfur is beneficial as long as the rumen microbes are supplied with adequate nitrogen and energy to synthesize sulfur-containing amino acids, especially methionine and cystine, which are required for keratin production. Feeding of rumen bypass proteins high in sulfur-containing amino acids such as rapeseed and fish meal has also been proposed (de Simiane 1990). Supplementing yearling Angoras averaging 47.5 kg bodyweight with 2.5 g/day of a commercial rumen protected methionine product increased mohair production by 46% (Galbraith 2000). However, feeding of zinc methionine to supply a rumen bypass form of this important amino acid had minimal effects on mohair production (Puchala et al. 1999).

It has been estimated that mature females require 9%, 10%, and 11% crude protein when they are, respectively, nonpregnant, late pregnant, and lactating. Except during dry years and in winter, the range diet is adequate. At times of increased need and decreased availability, a supplement of 40% cottonseed meal and 60% sorghum grain (24% crude protein and 3.25 Mcal digestible energy/kg) has proven adequate (Huston 1981). To avoid indigestions and metabolic diseases, the proportion of grain in late gestation should be limited to 40% of DM (0.3 to 0.4 kg for a 35 kg doe). During lactation, the proportion of concentrates (DM basis) in the total ration should never exceed 60% (de Simiane 1990).

It is often noted that the diameter of the mohair fiber increases slightly with better nutrition. Thus, in one study of yearling males, the fiber diameter for a ration protein of 12% was 36 microns while for a ration protein of 18%, fiber diameter was 38 microns (Huston et al. 1971). In this same study, clean fleece weight increased from 6.5 to 9.9 pounds and pounds of feed per pound of mohair decreased from 84 to 61 with the higher protein. A later study showed that yearlings produced 31% more mohair when fed 16% protein as compared with an 8% protein diet (Jia et al. 1995). In another study using mature wethers, increasing the dietary crude protein level from 10% to 19% (DM basis) resulted in an 83% increase in live weight gain and a 38% increase in mohair produced over a 112-day feeding period (Calhoun et al. 1983). Intentionally depriving the Angora goat of protein is thus false economy, and causes negative effects on health, reproduction, feed conversion, and mohair yield. A more recent study reported that increasing stocking rate of mature Angoras on pasture can decrease fiber diameter by 4 microns via a decrease in bodyweight. Regression analysis showed that fiber diameter decreased 0.4 microns for each kg fasted live weight lost (McGregor 1986). Nutrition has minimal if any effects on medullation of mohair (Lupton et al. 1991).

When does are in poor body condition, flushing (feeding increased energy) at the beginning of the breeding season can markedly increase the number of kids produced, and best quality mohair is obtained from young animals. When grazing is poor, feeding a markedly increased energy to Angora does before mating increases the kidding percentage by 20% to 25%. This can be achieved by feeding 500 g of "chocolate grain" (whole grain treated with alkali-ionophore; see discussion of feeding the pregnant doe to prevent abortion) per day per doe from two weeks before to two weeks after introduction of the buck (Van der Westhuysen et al. 1988). Wheat treated with 2% slaked lime has been used in a similar fashion in Australia (McGregor 1998). Other flushing recommendations include feeding 250 to 500 g of corn/day or moving to fresh pasture (Bretzlaff et al. 1991).

Another management practice that affects both the nutritional status and the reproductive efficiency of Angoras is the selection for open faces. Hair-blind animals on range cannot forage selectively or reproduce well (Shelton 1961; Van Tonder 1975). However, length of facial hair is positively correlated to length of the fleece overall, and trimming the hair on the head to expose the eyes ("wigging") three months after each body shearing is currently preferred to genetic selection for an open face.

Vitamin and mineral requirements for Angoras should be similar to those for other goats. Phosphorus is sometimes deficient in range forage, and mineral supplements offered should not have a calcium: phosphorus ratio more than 2:1 (Huston et al. 1971).

Angora Kid Growth

The growth rate required of Angora kids is less than what many producers desire for dairy kids. This is because the Angora typically is not bred until eighteen months of age, when it should weigh 25 kg. Adult females are expected to weigh 30 to 60 kg. It has been estimated that kids should weigh 15 kg by weaning and 20 kg by April 1 in the United States. A supplement is imperative to achieve even this moderate gain on winter range in Texas.

Cashmere Production

Cashmere fiber, a fine, downy fiber produced as an undercoat (see Chapter 2), is produced seasonally and in far smaller quantities per goat than is mohair. Annual production is often 300 g/head or less, and the requirements for amino acids are more easily met on a daily basis (Galbraith 2000). Increasing the dietary protein or providing sulfur containing amino acids above the requirements for maintenance and fleece production does not improve the quantity or quality of cashmere produced (Jia et al. 1995; Di Trana and Sepe 2008) and may cause an undesirable increase in fiber diameter. Likewise, feeding increased amounts of energy or decreasing the stocking rate do not increase cashmere production, although body weight and guard hair growth are increased (Russel 1992). McGregor (1998) has pointed out, however, that goats with a good genetic potential for fiber production produce more cashmere if they gain weight over summer and fall, with a total weight gain of 1 to 2 kg being desirable on an economic basis. Heavier animals produce more cashmere but as cashmere production increases, the fiber diameter increases. Wethers over 55 kg should be culled because of the lower price paid for coarse fiber (McGregor 1998). It is important to meet maintenance and growth requirements, which are similar to those of other breeds, for young goats during the anagen phase of fiber growth.

POISONOUS PLANTS

Goats, by their curiosity, browsing habits, and inhabitation of some environments where food is very scarce, are exposed to a myriad of plants containing toxic compounds. Often these are secondary metabolites that have evolved in perennial plants for protection against herbivores, especially insects. The NRC (2007) includes in its feed composition table 15–12 (Composition of pasture or range forage, browse, and other novel feedstuffs) a number of plants that are potentially toxic to goats. The goat's ability to assume a bipedal stance and its mobile upper lip contribute to its ability to use tree leaves for feed (Malecheck and Provenza 1981). This can be especially important in drought conditions when grass is no longer available. Grazing and browsing goats tend to move from plant to plant and species to species; thus, they are less apt to eat a fatal quantity of a given plant than is the more confined animal with sudden access to a single bush or tree. The hurried browsing of a hungry goat increases the risk of plant poisoning. Supplementing the diet of goats on range with additional energy and protein also decrease the risk of toxicity (Provenza et al. 2003).

For a plant to be called poisonous for goats, it needs to cause toxicity under natural settings, not just in laboratory experiments. The goat must eat enough of the plant to become ill when raised in the environment where the plant grows. Without proof from experimental feedings, a plant likewise cannot be firmly said to be toxic to goats. The absence of many species from the list of species toxic to goats in Table 19.7 represents, in part, a paucity of literature documenting plant poisonings in goats. Where information is largely limited to experimental studies, this is indicated by "exp" in the table. Other plants with reports of just spontaneous or experimental toxicity have been summarized by Dobereiner et al. (1987). When the plant (but not necessarily a report of toxicity) exists in the United States, this is indicated in the table. Most plants are not restricted to the countries mentioned.

Because the same toxic compounds are often present in multiple members of a genus or family of plants, practitioners in all countries should be suspicious of plants closely related to those in Table 19.7. However, even though this table omits some species names, not all members of a genus are equally or invariably toxic. A computer database on poisonous plants in the United States has been established and should help to keep information relative to goats up to date (Wagstaff et al. 1989).

When plants cause well recognized clinical signs they are discussed further and more references are supplied under the appropriate body system. Texts by other authors should also be consulted (Kingsbury 1964; Howard 1986; Dobereiner et al. 1987; Tokarnia et al. 2000; Burrows and Tyrl 2001; Frohne and Pfänder 2005; Kellerman et al. 2005). Cyanide and nitrate poisoning are discussed in Chapter 9 and plants causing oxalate poisoning in Chapter 12. When the identity of a suspect poisonous plant or its toxic principle is unknown, oral dosing of the sick goat with activated charcoal is appropriate.

Even the partial listing of poisonous species given here could confuse the veterinarian searching for an

Table 19.7. Plants poisonous to goats.

Plant	*Family*	*Comments*
Amanita phalloides	Agaricales	France; colic, liver necrosis (Cristea 1970).
Galenia africana	Aizoaceae	South Africa; ascites, liver, and cardiac disease.
Agave lecheguilla	Amaryllidaceae	U.S.A.; liver disease, icterus, photosensitization.
Nerium oleander	Apocynaceae	U.S.A.; weakness, muscle tremors, irregularities in heart beat; cardioactive glycosides.
Sarcostemma viminale	Apocynaceae	South Africa; hypersensitivity, tonic muscle spasms, opisthotonos.
Aristolochia bracteata	Aristolochiaceae	Sudan; enteritis (exp) (El Dirdiri et al. 1987).
Asclepias spp.	Asclepidaceae	U.S.A.; depression, weakness, seizures.
Acanthospermum hispidum	Asteraceae	Sudan; icterus, liver necrosis and portal fibroplasia, anemia (exp) (Ali and Adam 1978).
Baileya multiradiata	Asteraceae	U.S.A.; anorexia, emaciation, regurgitation, inhalation pneumonia (Dollahite 1960).
Chrysocoma ciliata = *Chrysocoma tenuifolia*	Asteraceae	South Africa; alopecia (kaalsiekte), hairballs, diarrhea of kids if dam eats plant.
Fluorensia cernua	Asteraceae	U.S.A.; abdominal pain, reluctance to move; unpalatable, fruits toxic (Mathews 1933).
Geigeria spp.	Asteraceae	South Africa; regurgitation, dilated esophagus, pneumonia, paralysis.
Gutierrezia microcephala	Asteraceae	U.S.A.; abortion, necrosis of liver and kidney (exp).
Hymenoxys spp.	Asteraceae	U.S.A.; gastrointestinal and neurologic signs.
Isocoma wrightii (*Aplopappus heterophyllus*)	Asteraceae	U.S.A.; trembling, recumbency, constipation, pale liver; tremetol excreted in milk (Bretzlaff 1990).
Sartwellia flaveriae	Asteraceae	U.S.A.; weight loss, ascites, liver cirrhosis (exp) (Mathews 1940).
Senecio (several species)	Asteraceae	U.S.A.; centrolobular liver degeneration, megalocytes, bile duct proliferation (Goeger et al. 1982). Goats are resistant enough to *S. jacobaea* to be used for biological control.
Vernonia mollissima	Asteraceae	Brazil; acute liver necrosis (exp) (Stolf et al. 1987).
Brassica spp.	Brassicaceae (Cruciferae)	U.S.A., Europe; Congenital goiter.
Descurainia sophia	Brassicaceae	U.S.A.; Congenital goiter (Knight and Stegelmeier 2007).
Lobelia spp.	Campanulaceae	U.S.A.; depression, coma, death; may survive if force fed.
Cadaba rotundifolia	Capparidaceae	Sudan; enteritis, liver and kidney necrosis (exp) (El Dirdiri et al. 1987).
Capparis tomentosa	Capparidaceae	Sudan; posterior paresis and ataxia, renal and hepatic necrosis (exp) (Ahmed and Adam 1980).
Drymaria spp.	Caryophyllaceae	U.S.A.; diarrhea, rapid death (McGinty 1987, Mathews 1933).
Celastrus scandens	Celastraceae	U.S.A.; central nervous system disturbance, gastroenteritis.
Ipomoea spp.	Convolvulaceae	Brazil, Sudan, South Africa; nervous signs including ataxia, nystagmus, and opisthotonos; anemia.
Coriaria myrtifolia	Coriariaceae	Mediterranean; convulsions, rapid death (Anonymous 1973).
Cotyledon orbiculata	Crassulaceae	South Africa; krimpsiekte; cardiotoxicity (bufadienolides) (Tustin et al. 1984).
Kalanchoe spp. (*Bryophyllum*)	Crassulaceae	Africa, Australia; bufadienolide cardiac glycosides, also neurotoxicity.
Tylecodon spp.	Crassulaceae	Africa; krimpsiekte (bufadienolides).
Cycas media	Cycadaceae	Australia; ataxia; neuronal swelling and demyelination (Hall 1964).
Dichapetalum spp.	Dichapetalaceae	Nigeria, South Africa; extreme depression, dyspnea, convulsions, sudden death. Monofluoracetate.
Kalmia and *Rhododendron* spp., *Pieris japonica*	Ericaceae	U.S.A.; grinding of teeth, colic, vomition (grayanotoxins) (Puschner et al. 2001; Plumlee et al. 1992).
Clethera arborea	Ericaceae	New Zealand; depression, ataxia, salivation, projectile vomition (Gibb and Taylor 1987).

Table 19.7. ***Continued***

Plant	*Family*	*Comments*
Codiaeum variegatum	Euphorbiaceae	Sri Lanka; severe colic and ruminal distention.
Manihot spp.	Euphorbiaceae	Brazil; cyanide poisoning.
Abrus precatorius	Fabaceae	U.S.A., Sudan; bloody diarrhea, abdominal pain, hepatic and renal necrosis (exp; Barri et al. 1990).
Acacia berlandieri	Fabaceae	U.S.A.; ataxia, posterior paralysis after exclusive diet for nine months (Sperry et al. 1964).
Acacia leucophloea	Fabaceae	India; dyspnea, ataxia, bellowing, convulsions; HCN.
Acacia nilotica	Fabaceae	South Africa; methemoglobinemia, abortion.
Astragalus emoryanus	Fabaceae	U.S.A.; muscular incoordination and weight loss; toxicity may vary with soil type.
Cassia spp.	Fabaceae	U.S.A.; muscle degeneration and red urine (exp) (Dollahite et al. 1964; El Sayed et al. 1983).
Crotolaria burkeana	Fabaceae	South Africa; unknown toxin produces laminitis without liver disease.
Gymnocladus dioica	Fabaceae	U.S.A.; severe colic (Howard 1986).
Leucaena leucocephala	Fabaceae	Australia and Africa; mimosine toxic if not degraded by rumen microbes (Semenye 1990). Hypothyroidism (Jones and Megarrity 1983).
Lupinus formosus	Fabaceae	U.S.A.; cleft palate and skeletal deformities (exp).
Oxytropis ochrocephala	Fabaceae	China; depression, ataxia, dysphagia, weight loss; swainsonine causes α-mannosidase inhibition (Cao et al. 1992a).
Prosopis julifora	Fabaceae	Brazil; head tremors, difficulty chewing, salivation, emaciation after long-term consumption of pods (exp) (Tabosa et al. 2004).
Senna spp.	Fabaceae	U.S.A.; myopathy (exp).
Sesbania vesicaria	Fabaceae	U.S.A.; diarrhea, grinding of teeth, necrosis of abomasum, liver, and kidney.
Sophora spp.	Fabaceae	U.S.A.; muscle tremors, coma; seed very toxic if ground.
Quercus spp.	Fagaceae	U.S.A.; rumen stasis, constipation, gastritis, nephritis.
Brachiaria decumbens	Gramineae	Malaysia, Nigeria, Brazil; liver disease, photosensitization, icterus.
Cynodon dactylon	Gramineae	U.S.A.; ataxia and tremors (exp).
Pennisetum clandestinum	Gramineae	Australia; ataxia, abdominal pain, rumenitis; oxalates (Peet et al. 1990).
Trisetum flavescens	Gramineae	Europe; enzootic calcinosis from high vitamin D activity (Braun et al. 2000).
Dipcadi glaucum	Hyacinthaceae	South Africa; nervous signs and diarrhea.
Ornithogalum toxicarum	Hyacinthaceae	South Africa; cardiac glycosides.
Hypericum spp.	Hypericaceae	U.S.A.; primary photosensitization.
Persea americana	Lauraceae	U.S.A., Australia; cardiotoxicity, noninfectious mastitis.
Nolina texana	Liliaceae	U.S.A.; liver and kidney damage, secondary photosensitization; flowers and fruit toxic.
Stypandra imbricata and *S. glauca*	Liliaceae	Australia; degeneration of retina, optic nerve, and optic tract; "blindgrass."
Veratrum californicum	Liliaceae	U.S.A.; cyclopia if consumed on thirteenth to fifteenth day of pregnancy; collapse.
Mascagnia rigida	Malphighiaceae	Brazil; sudden death after eating plant for a long time.
Sida carpinifolia	Malvaceae	Brazil; ataxia, hypermetria, muscle tremors, lysosomal storage disease (Driemeier et al. 2000).
Clidemia hirta	Melastomaceae	Indonesia; tannins; liver and kidney degeneration (exp) (Murdiati et al. 1992).
Camptotheca acuminata	Nyssaceae	China; alkaloid camptothecin causes hemorrhagic diarrhea, coma, death (Cao et al. 1992b).
Tephrosia apollinea	Papilionaceae	Sudan; posterior paresis, ataxia, diarrhea, renal and hepatic necrosis (exp) (Suliman et al. 1982).
Plumbago scandens	Plumbaginaceae	Brazil; bloat, foamy salivation, dark urine, epithelial necrosis (Medeiros et al. 2004).

Table 19.7. ***Continued***

Plant	*Family*	*Comments*
Fagopyrum spp.	Polygonaceae	U.S.A.; primary photosensitization.
Notholaena sinuata	Polypodiaceae	U.S.A.; trembling, ataxia, may die if forced to exercise; "jimmies" (Kingsbury 1964).
Portulaca oleracea	Portulacaceae	U.S.A.; diarrhea, muscle weakness partially due to oxalate content (Obied et al. 2003).
Karwinskia humboldtiana	Rhamnaceae	U.S.A.; degeneration of cardiac and skeletal muscle fibers, demyelination and Wallerian degeneration; "limberleg."
Prunus and *Malus* spp.	Rosaceae	U.S.A.; cyanogenic glycosides.
Fadogia spp.	Rubiaceae	South Africa; chronic fibrotic cardiomyopathy.
Pachystigma spp.	Rubiaceae	South Africa; cardiac insufficiency, sudden death.
Pavetta spp.	Rubiaceae	South Africa; cardiac insufficiency, sudden death.
Thamnosma texana	Rutaceae	U.S.A.; primary photosensitization.
Atropa belladonna	Solanaceae	Europe; excitement, dilated pupils, rumen atony (Ogilvie 1935).
Cestrum laevigatum	Solanaceae	South Africa, Brazil; apathy, ptyalism, mydriasis, gastrointestinal stasis, liver necrosis.
Solanum spp.	Solanaceae	U.S.A.; neurologic or enteric signs.
Solanum malacoxylon	Solanaceae	Brazil; enzootic calcinosis due to excess vitamin D (exp) (Górniak et al. 2007).
Vestia foetida	Solanaceae	New Zealand; ataxia, mydriasis, seizures, liver necrosis (McKeogh et al. 2005).
Taxus spp.	Taxaceae	U.S.A.; sudden death (Van Gelder et al. 1972, Casteel and Cook 1985).
Conium maculatum	Umbelliferae	U.S.A.; colic, diarrhea, convulsions (Copithorne 1937); teratogenic (exp) (Panter et al. 1992).
Ferula communis	Umbelliferae	Mediterranean; hemorrhagic syndrome (coumarins) (Girard 1934).
Lantana camara	Verbenaceae	U.S.A., South Africa.; liver disease (Pass 1986).
Kallstroemia spp.	Zygophyllaceae	U.S.A.; knuckling at fetlocks, paresis, convulsions (Mathews 1944).
Tribulus terrestris	Zygophyllaceae	U.S.A., South Africa; hepatogenic photosensitization (in combination with *Pithomyces chartarum*).

etiology for an undiagnosed illness. It is guaranteed to terrify the average goat owner. Dozens of species of plants that contain toxic principles are found on most pastures and ranges. The quantity consumed is a critical factor in determining if poisoning occurs, but both the quantity required for signs to occur and the amount eaten by an individual animal are usually imprecisely known. The stage of growth and the availability of alternative forage are other important factors. In general, most plant toxicities can be avoided by supplying supplemental hay and grain in times of drought, not overstocking pastures (Taylor and Ralphs 1992), not turning hungry animals out to forage, and preventing access of goats to ornamental plants (including trees and shrubs) and their clippings. Overgrazed pastures, snow coverage of more desirable forages, and unsanctioned entry into a garden or planted field are common situations in which poisoning occurs. Goats used for weed or brush control (Popay and Field 1996) or handfed potentially toxic plants in a cut and carry system are also at risk.

REFERENCES

Adams, R.S.: Dietary management in goats. In: Current Veterinary Therapy Food Animal Practice 2. J.L. Howard, ed. Philadelphia, W.B. Saunders Co., pp. 264–271, 1986.

Adeloye, A.A. and Yousouf, M.B.: Influence of nickel supplementation from nickel sulphate hexahydrate and nickel-sodium monofluorophosphate on the performance of the West African dwarf kids. Small Rumin. Res., 39:195–198, 2001.

Adenuga, M.K., et al.: Effect of pregnancy and lactation on live weight, feed intake and feeding behavior in West African Dwarf (WAD) goats. Small Rumin. Res., 4:245–255, 1991.

AFRC: The Nutrition of Goats. Agricultural and Food Research Council Technical Committee on Responses to Nutrients Report no. 10, New York NY, CAB International, 1998.

Ahmed, K.E., et al.: Experimental selenium poisoning in Nubian goats. Vet. Hum. Toxicol., 32:249–251, 1990.

Ahmed, O.M.M. and Adam, S.E.I.: The toxicity of *Capparis tomentosa* in goats. J. Comp. Pathol., 90:187–195, 1980.

Aina, A.B.J.: Effect of dietary magnesium supplementation on serum magnesium concentration and performance of female West African dwarf (Fouta djallon) goats. Indian J. Anim. Sci., 67:890–893, 1997.

Ali, B. and Adam, S.E.I.: Effects of *Acanthospermum hispidum* on goats. J. Comp. Pathol., 88:533–544, 1978.

Ames, D.R.: Effects of cold environments on cattle. Agri-Practice, 8:26–29, 1987.

Ammerman, C.B. and Miller, S.M.: Selenium in ruminant nutrition: a review. J. Dairy Sci., 58:1561–1577, 1975.

Anderson, K.L. and Adams, W.M.: Epiphysitis and recumbency in a yearling prepartum goat. J. Am. Vet. Med. Assoc., 183:226–228, 1983.

Andrews, A.H., et al.: Osteodystrophia fibrosa in young goats. Vet. Rec., 112:404–406, 1983.

Anke, M., Groppel, B. and Lüdke, H.: Kupfermangel bei Wiederkäuern in der DDR. Tierzucht., 26:56–58, 1972.

Anke, M., Grün, M., Partschefeld, M. and Groppel, B.: Molybdenum deficiency in ruminants. In: Trace Element Metabolism in Man and Animals, 3. M. Kirchgessner, ed. Weihenstephan, Arbeitskreis für Tierernährungsforschung, pp. 230–233, 1978.

Anke, M., et al.: Der Einfluss des Mangan-, Zink-, Kupfer-, Jod-, Selen-, Molybdän- und Nickelmangels auf die Fortpflanzungsleistung des Wiederkäuers. Wissenschaftliche Zeitschrift Karl-Marx-Universität Leipzig, Mathematisch-Naturwissenschaftlich Reihe, 26(3):283–292, 1977a.

Anke, M., et al.: Nickel—ein essentielles Spurenelement. 1. (Nickel, an essential trace element. 1. Effect of nickel intake on live weight gain, feed intake and body composition of growing miniature pigs and goats.) Arch. Tierernähr., 27:25–38, 1977b.

Anke, M., et al.: The effect of selenium deficiency on reproduction and milk performance of goats. Arch. Anim. Nutr. Berlin, 39:483–490, 1989.

Anonymous: Une plante dangereruse: le redoul. La Chèvre, 76:38–39, 1973.

Arbeiter, K.: Untersuchungen über den Einfluss verschiedener Heuqualitäten auf die biologische Samenbeschaffenheit von Ziegenböcken. Zuchthyg., 7:349–362, 1963.

Ash, A.J. and Norton, B.W.: Effect of dl-methionine supplementation on fleece growth by Australian cashmere goats. J. Agric. Sci., Camb., 109:197–199, 1987.

Aslan, V., et al.: Induced acute ruminal acidosis in goats treated with yeast (*Saccharomyces cerevisiae*) and bicarbonate. Acta Vet. Scand., 36:65–77, 1995.

Aspila, P.: Metabolism of selenite, selenomethionine and feed-incorporated selenium in lactating goats and dairy cows. J. Agric. Sci. Finland, 63:1–73, 1991.

Bajhau, H.S. and Kennedy, J.P.: Influence of pre- and post-partum nutrition on growth of goat kids. Small Rumin. Res., 3:227–236, 1990.

Banchero, G.E., et al.: Endocrine and metabolic factors involved in the effect of nutrition on the production of colostrum in female sheep. Reprod. Nutr. Dev., 46:447–460, 2006.

Barlet, J.-P., Michel, M.-C., Larvor, P. and Thériez, M.: Calcémie, phosphatémie, magnésémie et glycémie comparées de la mère et du nouveau-né chez les ruminants domestiques (vache, chèvre, brebis). Ann. Biol. Anim. Biochem. Biophys., 11:415–426, 1971.

Barri, M.E.S., et al.: Toxicity of *Abrus precatorius* in Nubian goats. Vet. Hum. Toxicol., 32:541–545, 1990.

Bartley, E.E., et al.: Ammonia toxicity in cattle. 1. Rumen and blood changes associated with toxicity and treatment methods. J. Anim. Sci., 43:835–841, 1976.

Bas, P., Hervieu, J., Morand-Fehr, P. and Sauvant, D.: Facteurs influençant la composition des graisses chez le chevreau de boucherie: Incidence sur la qualité des gras de carcasses. In: Nutrition and Systems of Goat Feeding. Volume 1. International Symposium, Tours, France, 1981. ITOVIC-INRA, pp. 90–100, 1981.

Baumgartner, W. and Loibl, A.: Erkrankungen bei Schaf und Ziege.-2. Pansenazidose; Pansenalkalose; Pansenfäulnis. Wien. Tierärztl. Mschr., 73:375–379, 1986.

Bava, L., et al.: Effects of a nonforage diet on milk production, energy, and nitrogen metabolism in dairy goats throughout lactation. J. Dairy Sci., 84:2450–2459, 2001.

Baxendell, S.A.: Caprine limb and joint conditions. In: Refresher Course for Veterinarians, Proceedings No. 73, Goats, The University of Sydney, The Post-Graduate Committee in Veterinary Science, Sydney, N.S.W., Australia, Update pp. 369–372, 1984.

Bhandari, D.S., Sawhney, P.C. and Bedi, S.P.S.: Influence of sulphur and urea on growth and nutrient digestibility in goat kids. Indian J. Anim. Sci., 43:936–939, 1973.

Biquand, S. and Biquand-Guyot, V.: The influence of peers, lineage and environment on food selection of the criollo goat (*Capra hircus*). Appl. Anim. Behav. Sci., 34:231–245, 1992.

Black, H., Hutton, J.B., Sutherland, R.J. and James, M.P.: White liver disease in goats. N. Z. Vet. J., 36:15–17, 1988.

Bleul, U., et al.: Floppy kid syndrome caused by D-lactic acidosis in goat kids. J. Vet. Intern. Med., 20:1003–1008, 2006.

Blodgett, D.J. and Bevill, R.F.: Acute selenium toxicosis in sheep. Vet. Hum. Toxicol., 29:233–236, 1987.

Bostedt, H. and Hamadeh, M.E.: [Importance of ketonuria associated with pregnancy in sheep and goats.] Tierärztl. Praxis 18:125–129, 1990.

Bowden, C.E., et al.: Negative effects of a high level of nutrient intake on mammary gland development of prepubertal goats. J. Dairy Sci., 78:1728–1733, 1995.

Bowen, J.: Feeding niacin may prevent disease. Dairy Goat J., 76 :117, 1998.

Braun, U., Rihs, T. and Schefer, U.: Ruminal lactic acidosis in sheep and goats. Vet. Rec., 130:343–349, 1992.

Braun, U., et al.: Enzootic calcinosis in goats caused by golden oat grass (*Trisetum flavescens*). Vet. Rec., 146:161–162, 2000.

Braun, W., Jr.: Ketosis or pregnancy toxemia? Dairy Goat J., 67:768–769, 1989.

Brent, B.E.: Relationship of acidosis to other feedlot ailments. J. Anim. Sci., 43:930–935, 1976.

Bretzlaff, K.: Special problems of hair goats. Vet. Clin. N. Am. Food Anim. Pract., 6(3):721–735, 1990.

Bretzlaff, K., Haenlein, G. and Huston, E.: The goat industry: feeding for optimal production. In: Large Animal Clinical Nutrition. J.M. Naylor and S.L. Ralston, eds. St. Louis, Mosby-Year Book, Inc., pp. 339–350, 1991.

Bretzlaff, K., Haenlein, G. and Huston, E.: Common nutritional problems. Feeding the sick goat. In: Large Animal

Clinical Nutrition. J.M. Naylor and S.L. Ralston, eds. St. Louis, Mosby-Year Book, Inc., pp. 351–355, 1991.

Broqua, C.: Ration d'hiver: quels aliments utiliser? La Chèvre, 190:25–29, 1990.

Brown, D.L. and Weir, W.C.: Increasing efficiency of goat production. Available resources and strategies. Problems, challenges, and required nutritional base. Proceedings, Fourth International Conference on Goats, Brasilia, Brazil, EMBRAPA, pp. 43–53, 1987.

Brown-Crowder, I.E., et al.: Effects of dietary tallow level on performance of Alpine does in early lactation. Small Rumin. Res., 39:233–241, 2001.

Brun-Bellut, J., Lindberg, J.E. and Hadjipanayiotou, M.: Protein nutrition and requirements of adult dairy goats. In: Goat Nutrition. P. Morand-Fehr, ed. Wageningen, Netherlands, Pudoc, EAAP Publ. No. 46, pp. 82–93, 1991.

Buck, W.B.: Copper-Molybdenum. In: Current Veterinary Therapy Food Animal Practice 2. J.L. Howard, ed. Philadelphia, W.B. Saunders, pp. 437–439, 1986.

Burrows, G.E. and Tyrl, R.J.: Toxic Plants of North America. Ames, IA, Iowa State Univ. Press, 2001.

Byrne, D.J.: Vitamin E deficiency in a flock of Angora goats. Goat Vet. Soc. J., 13:55–62, 1992.

Calhoun, M.C., Bassett, J.W., Baldwin, B.C., Jr. and Stobart, R.: Effect of monensin and protein on fiber production in Angora goats fed a high roughage diet. In: Sheep and Goat, Wool and Mohair. Tex. Agric. Exp. Stn. CPR-4171, 1983.

Campagnolo, E.R., Kasten, S. and Banerjee, M.: Accidental ammonia exposure to county fair show livestock due to contaminated drinking water. Vet. Hum. Toxicol., 44:282–285, 2002.

Cannas, A., Pes, A. and Pulima, G.: Effect of dietary energy and protein concentration on milk urea content in dairy ewes. J. Dairy Sci., 78, Suppl. 1:277, 1995.

Cao, G.R., et al.: The toxic principle of Chinese locoweeds (*Oxytropis* and *Astragalus*): Toxicity in goats. In: Poisonous Plants, Proceedings of the Third International Symposium. L.F. James, et al., eds. Ames, IA, Iowa State Univ. Press, pp. 117–121, 1992a.

Cao, G.R., et al.: Studies on *Camptotheca acuminata* leaves: main toxic principle, poisoning, and treatment in goats. In: Poisonous Plants, Proceedings of the Third International Symposium. L.F. James, et al., eds. Ames, IA, Iowa State Univ. Press, pp. 506–508, 1992b.

Caple, I.W. and McLean, J.G.: Pregnancy toxemia. In: Current Veterinary Therapy Food Animal Practice 2. J.L. Howard, ed. Philadelphia, W.B. Saunders Co., pp. 320–323, 1986.

Casteel, S.W. and Cook, W.O.: Japanese yew poisoning in ruminants. Mod. Vet. Pract., 66:875–877, 1985.

Cebra, C. and Cebra, M.: Diseases of the hematologic, immunologic, and lymphatic systems (multisystem diseases). In: Sheep and Goat Medicine. D.G. Pugh, ed. Philadelphia, W.B. Saunders, pp. 359–391, 2002.

Chamberlain, A.T.: Manipulation of milk protein content in dairy goats. Goat Vet. Soc. J., 17(1):8–18, 1997.

Chilliard, Y., et al.: Importance relative et activités métaboliques des différents tissus adipeux de la chèvre laitière. In: Nutrition and Systems of Goat Feeding. Volume 1. International Symposium, Tours, France, 1981. ITOVIC-INRA, pp. 80–89, 1981.

Clark, R.G., Mantleman, L. and Verkerk, G.A.: Failure to obtain a weight gain response to vitamin B12 treatment in young goats grazing pasture that was cobalt deficient for sheep. N. Z. Vet. J., 35:38–39, 1987.

Clarkson, M.J.: Pregnancy toxaemia. In: Diseases of Sheep, 3rd Ed. Martin and I.D. Aitken, eds. Oxford, Blackwell Science, pp. 315–317, 2000.

Constantinou, A.: Goat housing for different environments and production systems. Proceedings, Fourth International Conference on Goats, Brasilia, Brazil, EMBRAPA, Vol. 1, pp. 241–268, 1987.

Copithorne, B.: Suspected poisoning of goats by hemlock (*Conium maculatum*). Vet. Rec., 49:1018–1019, 1937.

Cornish, J., et al.: Copper toxicosis in a dairy goat herd. J. Am. Vet. Med. Assoc., 231:586–589, 2007.

Cristea, I.: Intoxication par les champignons du genre *Amanita* chez la chèvre. Rec. Méd. Vét., 146:507–512, 1970.

D'Ambrosio, F., et al.: Effects of rumen-protected choline supplementation in periparturient dairy goats. Vet. Res. Commun., 31(Suppl. 1):393–396, 2007.

Dargatz, D.A., Miller, L.M., Krieger, R.I. and Gay, C.C.: Toxicity associated with zinc sulfate footbaths for sheep. Agri-Practice, 7:30–33, 1986.

Davis, C.L., Brown, R.E. and Beitz, D.C.: Effect of feeding high-grain restricted-roughage rations with and without bicarbonates on the fat content of milk produced and proportions of volatile fatty acids in the rumen. J. Dairy Sci., 47:1217–1219, 1964.

de Simiane, M.: Stratégie d'alimentation adaptée à la production de fibres. La Chèvre, 176:34–38, 1990.

Demarquilly, C., Andrieu, J., Sauvant, D. and Dulphy, J.P.: Composition et valeur nutritive des aliments. In: Alimentation des Ruminants. R. Jarrige, ed. Versailles, France, INRA Publications, pp. 469–518, 1978.

Dercksen, D.P., et al.: [Selenium requirements of dairy goats.] Tijdschr. Diergeneeskd. 132:468–471, 2007.

Devendra, C.: Feed resources and their relevance in feeding systems in developing countries. Proceedings, Fourth International Conference on Goats, Brasilia, Brazil, EMBRAPA, Vol. II, pp. 1037–1062, 1987.

Di Trana, A. and Sepe, L.: Goat nutrition for fibre production. In: Dairy Goats Feeding and Nutrition. A. Cannas and G. Pulina, eds. Cambridge, MA, CAB International, pp. 238–262, 2008.

Dobereiner, J., Stolf, L. and Tokarnia, C.H.: Poisonous plants affecting goats. Proceedings, Fourth International Conference on Goats, Brasilia, Brazil, EMBRAPA, pp. 473–487, 1987.

Dollahite, J.W.: Desert baileya poisoning in sheep, goats and rabbits. Tex. Agric. Exp. Stn. Prog. Rep. 2149, 1960.

Dollahite, J.W., Henson, J.B. and Householder, G.T.: Coffee senna (*Cassia occidentalis*) poisoning in animals. Tex. Agric. Exp. Stn. Prog. Rep. 2318, 1964.

Driemeier, D., et al.: Lysosomal storage disease caused by *Sida carpinifolia* poisoning in goats. Vet. Pathol., 37:153–159, 2000.

Eales, F.A., et al.: Effectiveness in commercial practice of a new system for detecting and treating hypothermia in newborn lambs. Vet. Rec., 114:469–471, 1984.

Eastridge, M.L.: Interpreting feed analyses: protein fractions relevant to ruminant nutrition. Comp. Contin. Educ. Pract. Vet., 12:1800–1803, 1990.

El Dirdiri, N.I., Barakat, S.E.M. and Adam, S.E.I.: The combined toxicity of *Aristolochia bracteata* and *Cadaba rotundifolia* to goats. Vet. Hum. Toxicol., 29:133–137, 1987.

El Ghany-Hefnawy, A., et al.: The relationship between fetal and maternal selenium concentrations in sheep and goats. Small Rumin. Res., 73:174–180, 2007.

El Sayed, N.Y., Abdelbari, E.M., Mahmoud, O.M. and Adam, S.E.I.: The toxicity of *Cassia senna* to Nubian goats. Vet. Q., 5:80–85, 1983.

Emmanuel, B. and Kennelly, J.J.: Effect of propionic acid on kinetics of acetate and oleate and on plasma and milk fatty acid composition of goats. J. Dairy Sci., 67:1199–1208, 1984.

Federal Register: Food additives permitted in feed and drinking water of animals. 573,920 Selenium, 52(65):10888, 1987.

FDA (U.S. Food and Drug Administration): Title 21. Food and Drugs: Food additives permitted in feed and drinking water of animals. Sec. 573.920 Selenium. 2004. http://a257.g.akamaitech.net/7/257/2422/12feb20041500/edocket.access.gpo.gov/cfr_2004/aprqtr/21cfr573.920.htm. Accessed April 19, 2008.

FDA (U.S. Food and Drug Administration): FDA permits the use of selenium yeast in sheep and goat feed. March 8, 2005. http://www.fda.gov/cvm/CVM_Updates/SEsheep.htm. Accessed April 19, 2008.

Fedele, V., et al.: Effect of free-choice and traditional feeding systems on goat feeding behaviour and intake. Livestock Prod. Sci., 74:19–31, 2002.

Fehr, P.M., Hervieu, J. and Delage, J.: Effet du niveau alimentaire en fin de gestation et en début de lactation sur le déclenchement de la lactation. In: Journée d'Étude sur l'Alimentation de la Chèvre Laitière, 1974. Paris, ITOVIC-INRA, pp. 88–105, 1974.

Fernandez, J.M., et al.: Production and metabolic aspects of nonprotein nitrogen incorporation in lactation rations of dairy goats. Small Rumin. Res., 26:105–117, 1997.

Ferrando, R. and Barlet, J.-P.: Vitamines. In: Alimentation des Ruminants. R. Jarrige, ed. Versailles, France, INRA Publications, pp. 161–176, 1978.

Fick, G.W. and Mueller, S.C.: Alfalfa: quality, maturity, and mean stage of development. Cornell Univ. Information Bulletin 217, 1989.

Fredeen, A.H., DePeters, E.J. and Baldwin, R.L.: Characterization of acid-base disturbances and effects on calcium and phosphorus balances of dietary fixed ions in pregnant or lactating does. J. Anim. Sci., 66:159–173, 1988.

Frohne, D. and Pfänder, H.J.: Poisonous Plants, 2nd Ed. Portland OR, Timber Press, 2005. Translated from the German 5th edition of Giftplanzen, Ein Handbuch für Apotheker, Ärzte, Toxikologen und Biologen, 2004.

Fujimoto, Y. and Tajima, M.: Pathological studies on urea poisoning. Jpn. J. Vet. Sci., 15:125–134, 1953.

Galbraith, H.: Protein and sulphur amino acid nutrition of hair fibre-producing Angora and Cashmere goats. Livestock Prod. Sci., 64:81–93, 2000.

Gall, C.: Husbandry. In: Goat Production. C. Gall, ed. New York, Academic Press, pp. 411–432, 1981.

Gartner, R.J.W. and Hurwood, I.S.: The tannin and oxalic acid content of *Acacia aneura* (mulga) and their possible effects on sulphur and calcium availability. Aust. Vet. J., 52:194–195, 1976.

Gibb, M.C. and Taylor, A.: Lily of the valley poisoning in an Angora goat. N. Z. Vet. J., 35:59, 1987.

Giger, S., et al.: Facteurs de variation et modèles de prévision de l'ingestion d'eau par la chèvre en lactation en climat tempéré. In: Nutrition and Systems of Goat Feeding, Volume 1. International Symposium, Tours, France, 1981. ITOVIC-INRA, pp. 254–262, 1981.

Giger-Reverdin, S. and Gihad, E.A.: Water metabolism and intake in goats. In: Goat Nutrition. P. Morand-Fehr, ed. Wageningen, Netherlands, Pudoc, EAAP Publ. No. 46, pp. 37–45, 1991.

Gipson, T.A.: Using the lactation curve as a management tool for dairy goats. Proceedings, National Symposium on Dairy Goat Production and Marketing, Oklahoma City, OK, pp. 43–60, 1992.

Gipson, T.A. and Goetsch, A.L.: Nutrient requirements for goats. Langston University. http://www.luresext.edu/goats/research/nutreqgoats.html. Accessed May 4, 2008.

Gipson, T.A., Goetsch, A.L. and Hart, S.: Ration balancer and nutrition requirement calculator. Langston University. http://www2.luresext.edu/goats/research/nutritionmodule1.htm, accessed May 4, 2008.

Gipson, T.A. and Grossman, M.: Diphasic analysis of lactation curves in dairy goats. J. Dairy Sci., 72:1035–1044, 1989.

Gipson, T.A. and Grossman, M.: Lactation curves in dairy goats: a review. Small Rumin. Res., 3:383–396, 1990.

Girard, F.: Le férulisme dans la région de Meknès. Thesis, École Nationale Vétérinaire de Lyon, 1934.

Goeger, D.E., Cheeke, P.R., Schmitz, J.A. and Buhler, D.R.: Toxicity of tansy ragwort (*Senecio jacobaea*) to goats. Am. J. Vet. Res., 43:252–254, 1982.

Górniak, S.L., et al.: Effect of *Soalnum malacoxylon* in goats: a prenatal study. In: Poisonous Plant: Global Research and Solutions. K.E. Panter et al., eds. Cambridge, MA, CABI Publ., pp. 141–146, 2007.

Gould, D.H.: Polioencephalomalacia. J. Anim. Sci., 76:309–314, 1998.

Gupta, V.K., et al.: Prevalence of ketosis in goats maintained under organised farming system. Indian Vet. J., 84:1169–1172, 2007.

Guss, S.B.: Management and Diseases of Dairy Goats. Scottsdale, AZ, Dairy Goat Journal Publ. Co., 1977.

Hadjipanayiotou, M.: Effect of sodium bicarbonate and of roughage on milk yield and milk composition of goats and on rumen fermentation of sheep. J. Dairy Sci., 65:59–64, 1982.

Haenlein, G.F.W.: Mineral nutrition of goats. J. Dairy Sci., 63:1729–1748, 1980.

Hall, W.T.K.: Plant toxicoses of tropical Australia. Aust. Vet. J., 40:176–182, 1964.

Harmeyer, J. and Martens, H.: Aspects of urea metabolism in ruminants with reference to the goat. J. Dairy Sci., 63:1707–1728, 1980.

Hazarkia, T., et al.: Therapeutic studies on induced urea poisoning in goats. Indian Vet. J., 79:909–911, 2002.

Hennig, A., et al.: Manganmangel beim Wiederkäuer. 1. Der Einfluss des Manganmangels auf die Lebendmasseentwicklung. Arch. Tierernähr., 22:601–614, 1972.

Herdt, T.H. and Emery, R.S.: Therapy of diseases of ruminant intermediary metabolism. Vet. Clin. N. Am. Food Anim. Pract., 8:91–106, 1992.

Hervieu, J.: Mélanger les aliments: quels avantages? La Chèvre, 176:18–21, 1990.

Hervieu, J. and Morand-Fehr, P.: Comment noter l'état corporel des chèvres. Réussir. La Chèvre, 231:26–32, 1999.

Hines, T.G., Jacobson, N.L., Beitz, D.C. and Littledike, E.T.: Effects of dietary calcium, vitamin D3, and corn supplementation on growth performance and mineral metabolism in young goats fed whole milk diets. J. Dairy Sci., 69:2868–2876, 1986.

Hoffsis, G.F., Saint-Jean, G. and Rings, D.M.: Hypomagnesemia in ruminants. Comp. Contin. Educ. Pract. Vet., 11:519–523 and 526, 1989.

Honhold, N., Petit, H. and Halliwell, R.W.: Condition scoring scheme for Small East African goats in Zimbabwe. Trop. Anim. Health Prod., 21:121–127, 1989.

Howard, J.L. (ed.): Current Veterinary Therapy 2 Food Animal Practice. Philadelphia, W.B. Saunders Co., 1986.

Humphries, W.R., Morrice, P.C. and Mitchell, A.N.: Copper poisoning in Angora goats. Vet. Rec., 121:231, 1987.

Huston, J.E.: Feeding of goats under extensive range conditions in Texas, USA. In: Nutrition and Systems of Goat Feeding. Volume 1. International Symposium, Tours, France, 1981. ITOVIC-INRA, pp. 496–505, 1981.

Huston, J.E., Shelton, M. and Ellis, W.C.: Nutritional Requirements of the Angora Goat. Texas A&M University Bulletin B-1105, 1971.

INRA: Alimentation des bovins, ovins et caprins: Besoins des animaux—valeurs des aliments: Tables INRA 2007. Versailles, Quae, 2007.

Jagusch, K.T., Kidd, G.T. and Lynch, R.: Commencing a dairy enterprise based on the grazing of ryegrass-white clover pasture. In: Nutrition and Systems of Goat Feeding. Volume 1. International Symposium, Tours, France, 1981. ITOVIC-INRA, pp. 383–391, 1981.

James, L.F. and Shupe, J.L.: Selenium accumulators. In: Current Veterinary Therapy Food Animal Practice 2. J.L. Howard, ed. Philadelphia, W.B. Saunders, pp. 394–396, 1986.

Jarrige, R.: Ingestion et digestion des aliments. In: Alimentation des Bovins, Ovins et Caprins. R. Jarrige, ed. Paris, Institut National de la Recherche Agronomique, pp. 29–56, 1988.

Jarrige, R., Morand-Fehr, P. and Hoden, A.: Consommation d'aliments et d'eau. In: Alimentation des Ruminants. R. Jarrige, ed. Versailles, France, INRA Publications, pp. 177–206, 1978.

Jia, Z.H., et al.: Effects of dietary protein level on performance of Angora and cashmere-producing Spanish goats. Small Rum. Res., 16:113–119, 1995.

Johnson, E.H., et al.: Caprine hepatic lipidosis induced through the intake of low levels of dietary cobalt. Vet. J., 168:174–179, 2004.

Jones, D.G., Suttle, N.F., Stevenson, L.M. and Hay, L.: Observations on the diagnostic significance of plasma alpha-tocopherol (vitamin E) estimations in goats. In: Animal Clinical Biochemistry—the Future. D.J. Blackmore, et al., eds. Cambridge, Cambridge Univ. Press, pp. 340–345, 1988.

Jones, R.J. and Megarrity, R.G.: Comparative toxicity responses of goats fed on *Leucaena leucocephala* in Australia and Hawaii. Aust. J. Agric. Res., 34:781–790, 1983.

Jourdain, L.: Lait de chèvre: le taux d'urée est-il un indicateur fiable? La Chèvre 266:34–35, 2005.

Juniper, D.T., et al.: Tolerance of ruminant animals to high dose in-feed administration of a selenium-enriched yeast. J. Anim. Sci., 86:197–204, 2008.

Kadim, I.T., et al.: Comparative effects of low levels of dietary cobalt and parenteral injections of Vitamin B_{12} on body dimensions in different breeds of Omani goats. Small Rumin. Res., 66:244–252, 2006.

Kasari, T.R. and Naylor, J.M.: Further studies on the clinical features and clinicpathological findings of a syndrome of metabolic acidosis with minimal dehydration in neonatal calves. Can. J. Vet. Res., 50:502–508, 1986.

Kaufman, A. and Bergman, E.: Renal function studies in normal and toxemic pregnant sheep. Cornell Vet., 68:124–137, 1978.

Kawas, J.R., Lopes, J., Danelon, D. and Lu, C.D.: Influence of forage-to-concentrate ratios on intake, digestibility, chewing and milk production of dairy goats. Small Rumin. Res., 4:11–18, 1991.

Kellerman, T.S., et al.: Plant Poisonings and Mycotoxicoses of Livestock in Southern Africa, 2nd Ed. Cape Town, Oxford University Press, 2005.

Kessler, J.: Éléments minéraux majeurs chez la chèvre: données de base et apports recommandés. In: Nutrition and Systems of Goat Feeding, Volume 1. International Symposium, Tours, France, 1981. ITOVIC-INRA, pp. 196–209, 1981.

Kessler, J.: Mineral nutrition of goats. In: Goat Nutrition. P. Morand-Fehr, ed. Wageningen, Netherlands, Pudoc, EAAP Publ. No. 46, pp. 104–119, 1991.

Kessler, J., et al.: [Influence of a parenteral vitamin E/selenium application on the vitamin E/selenium-status of the goat and their kids.] J. Anim. Physiol. Anim. Nutr., 56:41–51, 1986.

Kholif, S.M., Foda, M.I. and Kholif, A.M.: Effect of ration supplementation with lysine and methionine in two different forms on goat's milk protein. Indian J. Dairy Sci., 59:281–286, 2006.

Kingsbury, J.M.: Poisonous Plants of the United States and Canada. Englewood Cliffs, Prentice Hall Inc., 1964.

Kinne, M.: Personal communication, 2008.

Kolb, E. and Kaskous, S.: [Constituents of the colostrum and the milk of goats and their significance for the health of kids (A review).] Tierärztl. Umschau, 58:140–146, 2003.

Kolb, E. and Kaskous, S.: [Patho-biochemical aspects of pregnancy ketosis in sheep and goats.] Tierärztl. Umschau, 59:374–380, 2004.

Kung, L. and Rode, L.M.: Amino acid metabolism in ruminants. Anim. Feed Sci. Technol., 59:167–172, 1996.

Ladiges, W.C. and Garlinghouse, Jr., L.E.: Iron dextran-induced anaphylaxis in a goat (*Capra hircus*). Lab. Anim. Sci., 31:421–422, 1981.

Lalitha, K., Rao, D.S.T. and Suryanarayana, C.: Epizootiological studies on pregnancy toxaemia in does. Indian Vet. Med. J., 25:391–392, 2001.

Lamand, M.: Oligoéléments. In: Alimentation des Ruminants. R. Jarrige, ed. Versailles, France, INRA Publications, pp. 143–159, 1978.

Lamand, M.: Métabolisme et besoins en oligo-éléments des chèvres. In: Nutrition and Systems of Goat Feeding, Volume 1. International Symposium, Tours, France, 1981. ITOVIC-INRA, pp. 210–225, 1981.

Langston University: Body Condition Scoring of Goats. http://www.luresext.edu/goats/research/bcshowto.html. Accessed April 20, 2008.

Lazzaro, J.: Basic information on copper deficiency in dairy goats in southern California. http://www.saanendoah.com/copper1.html. Accessed April 12, 2008.

Levander, O.A.: The global selenium agenda. In: Trace Elements in Man and Animals 6. L.S. Hurley et al., eds. New York, Plenum Press, 1988.

Liesegang, A., et al.: Effect of vitamin E supplementation of sheep and goats fed diets supplemented with polyunsaturated fatty acids and low in Se. J. Anim. Physiol. Anim. Nutr. (Berl) 92:292–302, 2008.

Linzell, J.L.: Milk fever in goats. Vet. Rec., 77:767–768, 1965.

Lloyd, W.E.: Urea and other nonprotein nitrogen sources. In: Current Veterinary Therapy Food Animal Practice 2. J.L. Howard, ed. Philadelphia, W.B. Saunders Co., pp. 354–356, 1986.

Lorenz, I. and Vogt, S.: Investigations on the association of D-latate blood concentrations with the outcome of therapy of acidosis, and with posture and demeanour in young calves with diarrhoea. J. Vet. Med. A, 53:490–494, 2006.

Louca, A., Economides, S. and Hancock, J.: Effects of castration on growth rate, feed conversion efficiency and carcass quality in Damascus goats. Anim. Prod., 24:387–391, 1977.

Lu, C.D., Kawas, J.R. and Mahgoub, O.G.: Fibre digestion and utilization in goats. Small Rumin. Res., 60:45–52, 2005.

Luo, J., et al.: Metabolizable protein requirements for maintenance and gain of growing goats. Small Rumin. Res., 53:309–326, 2004a.

Luo, J., et al.: Prediction of metabolizable energy and protein requirements for maintenance, gain and fiber growth of Angora goats. Small Rumin. Res., 53:339–356, 2004b.

Luo, J., et al.: Prediction of metabolizable energy requirements for maintenance and gain of preweaning, growing and mature goats. Small Rumin. Res., 53:231–252, 2004c.

Luo, J., et al.: Voluntary feed intake by lactating, Angora, growing and mature goats. Small Rumin. Res., 53:357–378, 2004d.

Lupton, C.J., Pfeiffer, F.A. and Blakeman, N.E.: Medullation in mohair. Small Rumin. Res., 5:357–365, 1991.

Macciotta, N.P.P., et al.: Mathematical modelling of goat lactation curves. In: Dairy Goats Feeding and Nutrition. A. Cannas and G. Pulina, eds. Cambridge, MA, CAB International, pp. 31–46, 2008.

Mackenzie, D.: Goat Husbandry. 1st U.S. Ed. Levittown, N. Y., Transatlantic Arts, Inc., 1975.

Madsen, T.G., Nielsen, L. and Nielsen, M.O.: Mammary nutrient uptake in response to dietary supplementation of rumen protected lysine and methionine in late and early lactating dairy goats. Small Rumin. Res., 56:151–164, 2005.

Malecheck, J.C. and Provenza, F.D.: Feeding behaviour and nutrition of goats on rangelands. In: Nutrition and Systems of Goat Feeding. Volume 1. International Symposium, Tours, France, 1981. ITOVIC-INRA, pp. 411–428, 1981.

Marteniuk, J.V. and Herdt, T.H.: Pregnancy toxemia and ketosis of ewes and does. Vet. Clin. N. Am. Food Anim. Pract., 4(2):307–315, 1988.

Martens, H. and Schweigel, M.: Pathophysiology of grass tetany and other hypomagnesemias—Implications for clinical management. Vet. Clin. N. Am. Food Anim. Pract., 16(2):339–368, 2000.

Mathews, F.P.: The toxicity of *Drymaria pachyphylla* for cattle, sheep, and goats. J. Am. Vet. Med. Assoc., 83:255–260, 1933.

Mathews, F.P.: The toxicity of *Sartwellia flaveriae* to goats. J. Agric. Res., 61:287–292, 1940.

Mathews, F.P.: The toxicity of *Kallstroemia hirsutissima* (carpet weed) for cattle, sheep, and goats. J. Am. Vet. Med. Assoc., 105:152–155, 1944.

Matthews, J.: Diseases of the Goat. 2nd Ed. Oxford, Blackwell Science, 1999.

McGinty, A.: Toxic Plant Handbook for Pecos County. Fort Stockton, Texas, Texas Extension Service, 1987.

McGregor, B.A.: Live weight and nutritional influences on fibre diameter of mohair. Proc. Aust. Soc. Anim. Prod., 16:420, 1986.

McGregor, B.A.: Nutrition, management and other environmental influences on the quality and production of mohair and cashmere with particular reference to Mediterranean and annual temperate climatic zones: a review. Small Rumin. Res., 28:199–215, 1998.

McGregor, B.A. and Butler, K.L.: Relationship of body condition score, live weight, stocking rate and grazing system to the mortality of Angora goats from hypothermia and their use in the assessment of welfare risks. Aust. Vet. J., 86:12–17, 2008.

McKeough, V.-L., Collett, M.G. and Parton, K.H.: Suspected *Vestia foetida* poisoning in young goats. N. Z. Vet. J., 53:352–355, 2005.

McLennan, M.W.: Treatment of induced urea toxicity in sheep. Aust. Vet. J., 64:26–28, 1987.

Mellado, M., et al.: Factors affecting the reproductive performance of goats under intensive conditions in a hot arid environment. Small Rumin. Res., 63:110–118, 2006.

Mello, J.R.B.: Calcinosis—calcinogenic plants. Toxicon, 41:1–12, 2003.

Mellor, D.J. and Murray, L.: Making the most of colostrum at lambing. Vet. Rec., 118:351–353, 1986.

Mertens, D.R.: Challenges in measuring insoluble dietary fiber. J. Anim Sci., 81:3233–3249, 2003.

Meschy, F.: Recent progress in the assessment of mineral requirements of goats. Livestock Prod. Sci., 64:9–14, 2000.

Middleton, J.R., et al.: Hemolysis associated with water administration using a nipple bottle for human infants in juvenile pygmy goats. J. Vet. Int. Med., 11:382–384, 1997.

Min, B.R., et al.: The effect of diets on milk production and composition, and on lactation curves in pastured dairy goats. J. Dairy Sci., 88:2604–2615, 2005.

Mitchell, T.: Condition Scoring Goats. 2nd Ed. Agfact 47.2.3 New South Wales, Department of Agriculture, 1986.

Morand-Fehr, P.: Caractéristiques du comportement alimentaire et de la digestion des caprins. In: Nutrition and Systems of Goat Feeding. Volume 1. International Sympo-

sium, Tours, France, May 12–15, 1981. ITOVIC-INRA, pp. 21–45, 1981a.
Morand-Fehr, P.: Nutrition and feeding of goats: application to temperate climatic conditions. In: Goat Production. C. Gall, ed. New York, Academic Press, pp. 192–232, 1981b.
Morand-Fehr, P.: Growth. In: Goat Production. C. Gall, ed. New York, Academic Press, pp. 253–283, 1981c.
Morand-Fehr, P. (ed.): Goat Nutrition. Wageningen, Netherlands, Pudoc. (EEAP Publication No. 46) 1991.
Morand-Fehr, P.: Recent developments in goat nutrition and application: A review. Small Rumin. Res., 60:25–43, 2005.
Morand-Fehr, P., Hervieu, J. and Santucci, P.: Notation de l'état corporel: à vos stylos! La Chèvre, 175:39–42, 1989.
Morand-Fehr, P. and Sauvant, D.: Caprins. In: Alimentation des Ruminants. R. Jarrige, ed. Versailles, France, INRA Publications, 1978.
Morand-Fehr, P. and Sauvant, D.: Composition and yield of goat milk as affected by nutritional manipulation. J. Dairy Sci., 63:1671–1680, 1980.
Morand-Fehr, P. and Sauvant, D.: Alimentation des caprins. In: Alimentation des Bovins, Ovins et Caprins. R. Jarrige, ed. Paris, Institut National de la Recherche Agronomique, 1988, pp. 281–304.
Morand-Fehr, P., et al.: Assessment of goat body condition and its use for feeding management. In: Fifth International Conference on Goats, New Delhi, Pre-Conference Proceedings Invited Papers, Vol. II, Part I, pp. 212–223, 1992.
Murdiati, T.B., McSweeney, C.S., Campbell, R.S.F. and Stoltz, D.R.: Prevention of hydrolysable tannin toxicity by calcium hyroxide supplementation in goats fed *Clidemia hirta*. In: Poisonous Plants, Proceedings of the Third International Symposium. L.F. James, et al., eds. Ames, IA, Iowa State Univ. Press, pp. 431–435, 1992.
Nandé, R.T. and Hofmeyr, H.S.: Meat production. In: Goat Production. C. Gall, ed. New York, Academic Press, pp. 285–307, 1981.
Narjisse, H.: Feeding behaviour of goats on rangelands. In: Goat Nutrition. P. Morand-Fehr, ed. Wageningen, Netherlands, Pudoc, pp. 13–24, 1991.
National Pygmy Goat Association: Pygmy Goat Basic Owner's Manual. Revised edition. National Pygmy Goat Association, Inc., http://www.npga-pygmy.conm. 2006.
Nedkvitne, J.J. and Robstad, A.M.: Grass silage in dairy goat feeding in Norway. In: Nutrition and Systems of Goat Feeding. Volume 1. International Symposium, Tours, France, 1981. ITOVIC-INRA, pp. 352–356, 1981.
Nour, M.S.M., Abusamra, M.T. and Hago, B.E.D.: Experimentally induced lactic acidosis in Nubian goats: clinical, biochemical and pathological investigations. Small Rumin. Res., 31:7–17, 1998.
NRC (National Research Council): Effect of Environment on Nutrient Requirements of Domestic Animals. Washington, D.C., National Academy Press, 1981a. http://darwin.nap.edu/books/0309031818/html/index.html.
NRC (National Research Council): Mineral Tolerance of Animals, 2nd Rev. Ed. Washington D.C., National Academies Press, 2005.
NRC (National Research Council): Nutrient Requirements of Goats: Angora, Dairy, and Meat Goats in Temperate and Tropical Countries. Nutrient Requirements of Animals Number 15. Washington, D.C., National Academy Press, 1981b. http://www.nap.edu/books/0309031850/html/.
NRC (National Research Council): Nutrient Requirements of Small Ruminants: Sheep, Goats, Cervids, and New World Camelids. Washington D.C., National Academies Press, 2007.
Nsahlai, I.V., et al.: Metabolizable energy requirements of lactating goats. Small Rumin. Res., 53:253–273, 2004a.
Nsahlai, I.V., et al.: Metabolizable protein requirements of lactating goats. Small Rumin. Res., 53:327–337, 2004b.
Obasaju, M.F., Kasali, O.B. and Otesile, E.B.: Accidental poisoning of ruminants with the fertilizer, urea in Ibadan, Nigeria. Bull. Anim. Health Prod. Afr., 28:233–234, 1980.
Obied, W.A., Mohamoud, E.N. and Mohamed, O.S.A.: *Portulaca oleracea* (purslane); nutritive composition and clinico-pathological effects on Nubian goats. Small Rumin. Res., 48:31–36, 2003.
Ødegaard, S.A. and Øverby, I.: Hypokalsemi hos geit. Norsk. Veterinaertid., 105:207–212, 1993.
Oetzel, G.R., Olson, J.D., Curtis, C.R. and Fettman, M.J.: Ammonium chloride and ammonium sulfate for prevention of parturient paresis in dairy cows. J. Dairy Sci., 71:3302–3309, 1988.
Ogilvie, D.D.: Atropine poisoning in the goat. Vet. Rec., 15:1415–1417, 1935.
Ogimoto, K. and Giesecke, D.: Untersuchungen zur Genese und Biochemie der Pansenacidose. 2. Mikroorganismen und Umsetzung von Milchsäure-Isomeren. Zentralbl. Veterinärmed., A 21:532–538, 1974.
Ortolani, E.L., Satsuki, C. and Rodrigues, J.A.: Ammonia toxicity from urea in a Brazilian dairy goat flock. Vet. Hum. Toxicol., 42:87–89, 2000.
Osweiler, G.D., Carson, T.L., Buck, W.B. and Van Gelder, G.A.: Clinical and Diagnostic Veterinary Toxicology. 3rd Ed. Dubuque, Iowa, Kendall/Hunt Publ. Co., 1985.
Ouédraogo, C.L., et al.: Roasted fullfat soybean as an ingredient of milk replacers for goat kids. Small Rumin. Res., 28:53–59, 1998.
Øverby, I. and Ødegaard, S.A.: Hypokalsemi hos geit. Norsk. Veterinaertid., 92:21–25, 1980.
Palma, J.M. and Galina, M.A.: Effect of early and late weaning on the growth of female kids. Small Rumin. Res., 18:33–38, 1995.
Panter, K.E., James, L.F., Keeler, R.F. and Bunch, T.D.: Radioultrasound observations of poisonous plant-induced fetotoxicity in livestock. In: Poisonous Plants, Proceedings of the Third International Symposium. L.F. James, et al., eds. Ames, IA, Iowa State Univ. Press, pp. 481–488, 1992.
Papachristou, T.G., Dziba, L.E. and Provenza, F.D.: Foraging ecology of goats and sheep on wooded rangelands. Small Rumin. Res., 59:141–156, 2005.
Pass, M.A.: Current ideas on the pathophysiology and treatment of lantana poisoning of ruminants. Aust. Vet. J., 63:169–171, 1986.
Peet, R.L., Dickson, J. and Hare, M.: Kikuyu poisoning in goats and sheep. Aust. Vet. J., 67:229–230, 1990.
Piotrowska, K.K., et al.: Phytoestrogens and their metabolites inhibit the sensitivity of the bovine corpus luteum to luteotropic factors. J. Reprod. Dev., 52:33–41, 2006.

Plumlee, K.H., VanAlstine, W.G. and Sullivan, J.M.: *Japanese pieris* toxicosis of goats. J. Vet. Diagn. Invest., 4:363–364, 1992.

Poljicak-Milas, N. and Marenjak, T.S.: Dietary supplement of the rumen protected methionine and milk yield in dairy goats. Arch. Tierzucht, 50:273–278, 2007.

Poncelet, L.: La physiologie du magnésium chez les ruminants domestiques. Ann. Méd. Vét., 127:179–192, 1983.

Popay, I. and Field, R.: Grazing animals as weed control agents. Weed Technol., 10:217–231, 1996.

Potchoiba, M.J., Lu, C.D., Pinkerton, F. and Sahlu, T.: Effects of all-milk diet on weight gain, organ development, carcass characteristics and tissue composition, including fatty acids and cholesterol contents, of growing male goats. Small Rumin. Res., 3:583–592, 1990.

Pritchard, D. and Eggleston, G.W.: Nardoo fern and polioencephalomalacia. Aust. Vet. J., 54:204–205, 1978.

Provenza, F.D., et al.: Linking herbivore experience, varied diets, and plant biochemical diversity. Small Rumin. Res., 49:257–274, 2003.

Puchala, R., Sahlu, T. and Davis, J.J.: Effects of zinc-methionine on performance of Angora goats. Small Rumin. Res., 33:1–8, 1999.

Puls, R.: Mineral Levels in Animal Health, 2nd Ed. Diagnostic Data. Clearbrook BC, Canada, Sherpa International, 1994.

Puschner, B., et al.: Grayanotoxin poisoning in three goats. J. Am. Vet. Med. Assoc., 218:573–575, 2001.

Putnam, D.H.: Recommended Principles for Proper Hay Sampling. 2002. http://alfalfa.ucdavis.edu/+producing/forage_quality/hay_sampling/HAYSAMPLINGSTEPS.htm Accessed April 20, 2008.

Qi, K., et al.: Effects of sulfur deficiency on performance of fiber-producing sheep and goats: a review. Small Rumin. Res., 14:115–126, 1994.

Quigley, J.D.III, Carson, A.F., Polo, J.S.O.: Immunoglobulin derived from bovine plasma as a replacement for colostrum in newborn lambs. Vet. Ther., 3: 262–269, 2002.

Radostits, O.M., et al.: Veterinary Medicine. A text book of the diseases of cattle, horses, sheep, pigs, and goats. 10th Ed. Edinburgh; New York, Saunders Elsevier, 2007.

Rajpoot, R.L., Sengar, O.P.S. and Singh, S.N.: Energy and protein in goat nutrition. In: Nutrition and Systems of Goat Feeding. Volume 1. International Symposium, Tours, France, 1981, ITOVIC-INRA, pp. 101–124, 1981.

Rankins, Jr., D.L., Ruffin, D.C. and Pugh, D.G.: Feeding and nutrition. In: Sheep and Goat Medicine. D.G. Pugh, ed. Philadelphia, W.B. Saunders, pp. 19–60, 2002.

Rapetti, L. and Bava, L.: Feeding management of dairy goats in intensive systems. In: Dairy Goats Feeding and Nutrition. A. Cannas and G. Pulina, eds. Cambridge, MA, CAB International, pp. 221–237, 2008.

Reid, R.L.: The physiopathology of undernourishment in pregnant sheep with particular reference to pregnancy toxemia. Adv. Vet. Sci., 12:163–238, 1968.

Riet-Correa, F., et al.: [Floppy kid syndrome.] Pesq. Vet. Bras., 24:111–113, 2004.

Roseler, D.K., et al.: Dietary protein degradability effects on plasma and milk urea nitrogen and milk nonprotein nitrogen in Holstein cows. J. Dairy Sci., 76:525–534, 1993.

Rostkowski, C.M., et al.: Hypercalcitoninism without hypercalcitoninemia. Cornell Vet., 71:188–213, 1981.

Rousseaux, C.G., et al.: Ovine polioencephalomalacia associated with dietary sulphur intake. J. Vet. Med., A 38:229–239, 1991.

Russel, A.J.F.: Fibre production from sheep and goats. In: Progress in Sheep and Goat Research. A.W. Speedy, ed. Oxon, U.K., CAB International, pp. 235–256, 1992.

Sahlu, T., et al.: Influence of dietary protein on performance of dairy goats during pregnancy. J. Dairy Sci., 75:220–227, 1992.

Sahlu, T., et al.: Influence of prepartum protein and energy concentrations for dairy goats during pregnancy and early lactation. J. Dairy Sc., 78:378–387, 1995.

Sahlu, T., et al.: Nutrient requirements of goats: developed equations, other considerations and future research to improve them. Small Rumin. Res., 53:191–219, 2004.

Salama, A.A.K., et al.: Effects of dietary supplements of zinc-methionine on milk production, udder health and zinc metabolism in dairy goats. J. Dairy Res., 70:9–17, 2003.

Santini, F.J., Lu, C.D., Potchoiba, M.J. and Coleman, S.W.: Effects of acid detergent fiber intake on early postpartum milk production and chewing activities in dairy goats fed alfalfa hay. Small Rumin. Res., 6:63–71, 1991.

Santucci, P.M., et al.: Body condition scoring of goats in extensive conditions. In: Goat Nutrition. P. Morand-Fehr, ed. Wageningen, Netherlands, Pudoc, pp. 240–255, 1991.

Sardjana, L.K.W., Tainturier, D. and Djiane, J.: Étude de l'hormone chorionique somatomammotrophique dans le plasma et le lactoserum au cours de la gestation et du post-partum chez la chèvre (application au diagnostic tardif de gestation). Rev. Méd. Vét., 139:1045–1052, 1988.

Sauvant, D.: Alimentation énergétique des caprins. In: Nutrition and Systems of Goat Feeding. Volume 1. International Symposium, Tours, France, 1981. ITOVIC-INRA, pp. 55–79, 1981.

Sauvant, D., Chilliard, Y. and Morand-Fehr, P.: Etiological aspects of nutritional and metabolic disorders of goats. In: Goat Nutrition. P. Morand-Fehr, ed. Wageningen, Netherlands, pp. 124–142, 1991a.

Sauvant, D., Morand-Fehr, P. and Bas, P.: Facteurs favorisant l'état de cétose chez la chèvre. In: Goat Diseases, International Colloquium, Niort, France, INRA Publ., pp. 369–378, 1984.

Sauvant, D., Morand-Fehr, P. and Giger-Reverdin, S.: Dry matter intake of adult goats. In: Goat Nutrition. P. Morand-Fehr, ed. Wageningen, Netherlands, pp. 25–45, 1991b.

Schellner, G.: Die Wirkung von Natriummangel und Natriumbeifütterung auf Wafchstum, Milch-und Milchfettleistung und Fruchtbarkeit bei Ziegen. (Effect of sodium deficiency and sodium supplements on growth, yields of milk and milk fat and fertility of goats.) Jahresb. Tierer. Fütt., 8:246–259, 1972.

Schmidt, H.: Vitamin A deficiencies in ruminants. Am. J. Vet. Res., 2:373–389, 1941.

Schonewille, J.T., Yu, S. and Beynen, A.C.: High iron intake depresses hepatic copper content in goats. Vet. Q., 17:14–17, 1995.

Scott, P.R., et al.: Aqueous humour and cerebrospinal fluid collected at necropsy as indicators of ante-mortem serum

3-OH-butyrate concentration in pregnant sheep. Br. Vet. J., 151:459–461, 1995.

Scroggs, P.: Diary of tragedy. Dairy Goat J., 67:793–795 and 799 and 817, 1989.

Semenye, P.P.: Toxicity response of goats fed on *Leucaena leucocephala* forage only. Small Rumin. Res., 3:617–620, 1990.

Senf, W.: Beitrag zur Kupfermangelerkrankung-Swayback-bei Afrikanischen Zwergziegen und anderen Zootieren. XVI Internationalen Symposiums über die Erkrankungen der Zootiere, pp. 239–243, 1974.

Shelton, M.: Factors affecting kid production of Angora does. Tex. Agric. Exp. Stn., MP-496, 1961.

Shepherd, G., Petrie, L. and Naylor, J.M.: Metabolic acidosis without dehydration in a llama cria. Can. Vet. J., 34:425–426, 1993.

Sherman, D.M., Arendt, T.D., Gay, J.M. and Maefsky, V.A.: Comparing the effects of four colostral preparations on serum Ig levels of newborn kids. Vet. Med., 85:908–913, 1990.

Sherman, D.M. and Robinson, R.A.: Clinical examination of sheep and goats. Vet. Clin. N. Am. Large Anim. Pract., 5(3):409–426, 1983.

Shkolnik, A., Maltz, E. and Choshniak, I.: The role of the ruminant's digestive tract as a water reservoir. In: Digestive Physiology and Metabolism in Ruminants. Y. Ruckebusch and P. Thivend, eds. Lancaster, England, MTP Press, 1980.

Simons, J.C. and Hand, M.S.: Field calculations for ration formulation in food animals. In: Current Veterinary Therapy Food Animal Practice 2. J.L. Howard, ed. Philadelphia, W.B. Saunders Co., pp. 203–218, 1986.

Singh, S.K. and Prasad, M.C.: Cardiopathy associated with hypervitaminosis D in goats. Indian Vet. Med. J., 13:152–155, 1989.

Skjevdal, T.: Effect on goat performances of given quantities of feedstuffs, and their planned distribution during the cycle of reproduction. In: Nutrition and Systems of Goat Feeding. Volume 1. International Symposium, Tours, France, 1981. ITOVIC-INRA, pp. 300–318, 1981.

Smith, G.C., Carpenter, Z.L. and Shelton, M.: Effect of age and quality level on the palatability of goat meat. J. Anim. Sci., 46:1229–1235, 1978.

Søli, N.E. and Nafstad, I.: Effects of daily oral administration of copper to goats. Acta Vet. Scand., 19:561–568, 1978.

Sperry, O.E., Dollahite, J.W., Hoffman, G.O. and Camp, B.J.: Texas Plants Poisonous to Livestock. Tex. Agric. Exp. Stn. Bull., B-1028, 1964.

Stelletta, C., Gianesella, M. and Morgante, M.: Metabolic and nutritional diseases. In: Dairy Goats Feeding and Nutrition. A. Cannas and G. Pulina, eds. Cambridge, MA, CAB International, pp. 263–288, 2008.

Stolf, L., Gava, A. and Tokarnia, C.H.: Intoxicaçáo experimental por *Vernonia mollissima* (Compositae) em caprinos. Pesq. Vet. Bras., 7(3):67–77, 1987.

Suliman, H.B., Wasfi, I.A. and Adam, S.E.I.: The toxic effects of *Tephrosia apollinea* on goats. J. Comp. Pathol., 92:309–315, 1982.

Surai, P.F.: Selenium in Nutrition and Health. Nottingham U.K., Nottingham Univ. Press, 2006.

Tabosa, I.M., et al.: Intoxication by *Prosopis juliflora* pods (mesquite beans) in cattle and goats in northeastern Brazil. In: Poisonous Plants and Related Toxins. T. Acamovic et al., eds. Cambridge MA, CABI Publ., pp. 341–346, 2004.

Taylor, Jr., C.A. and Ralphs, M.H.: Reducing livestock losses from poisonous plants through grazing management. J. Range Manag., 45:9–12, 1992.

Thilsing-Hansen, T., Jorgensen, R.J. and Ostergaard, S.: Milk fever control principles: a review. Acta Vet. Scand., 43:1–19, 2002.

Thomas, K.W., Turner, D.L. and Spicer, E.M.: Thiamine, thiaminase and transketolase levels in goats with and without polioencephalomalacia. Aust. Vet. J., 64:126–127, 1987.

Tokarnia, C.H., Döbereiner, J. and Peixoto, P.V.: Plantas Tóxicas do Brasil. Rio de Janeiro, Helianthus, 2000.

Tontis, A. and Zwahlen, R.: Zur Graviditätstoxikose der kleinen Ruminanten mit besonderer Berücksichtigung der Pathomorphologie. Tierärztl. Prax., 15:25–29, 1987.

Toussaint, G.: Le zéro-pâturage en élevage caprin. In: Journée d'Étude sur l'Alimentation de la Chèvre Laitière, Paris, 1974. ITOVIC-INRA, pp. 131–141, 1974.

Tremblay, R.M., et al.: Metabolic acidosis without dehydration in seven goat kids. Can. Vet. J., 32:308–310, 1991.

Tustin, R.C., Thornton, D.J. and Kleu, C.B.: An outbreak of *Cotyledon orbiculata* L. poisoning in a flock of Angora goat rams. J. S. Afr. Vet. Med. Assoc., 55:181–184, 1984.

Underwood, E.J. and Suttle, N.F.: The Mineral Nutrition of Livestock 3rd Ed. New York, NY, CABI Publ., 1999.

Van der Westhuysen, J.M., Wentzel, D. and Grobler, M.C.: Angora Goats and Mohair in South Africa. 3rd Ed. NMB Printers, Port Elizabeth, South Africa, 1988.

Van Gelder, G.A., Buck, W.B., Osweiler, G.D. and Stahr, H. M.: Research activities of a veterinary toxicology laboratory. Clin. Toxicol., 5:271–281, 1972.

Van Metre, D.C. and Callan, R.J.: Selenium and vitamin E. Vet. Clin. N. Am. Food Anim. Pract., 17(2):373–402, 2001.

Van Tonder, E.M.: Notes on some disease problems in Angora goats in South Africa. Vet. Med. Rev., 1/2:109–138, 1975.

Vermorel, M.: Energie. Utilisation énergétique des produits terminaux de la digestion. In: Alimentation des Ruminants. R. Jarrige, ed. Versailles, France, INRA Publications, 1978.

Vihan, V.S. and Rai, P.: Studies on biochemical and haematological changes in metabolic derangements of sheep and goat. Indian J. Vet. Med., 4(1):9–12, 1984.

Wagstaff, D.J., Raisbeck, M. and Wagstaff, A.T.: Poisonous plant information system (PPIS). Vet. Hum. Toxicol., 31:237–238, 1989. System available online as FDA Poisonous Plants Database, http://www.cfsan.fda.gov/~djw/plantox.html. Accessed March 23, 2008.

Waldo, D.R. and Glenn, B.P.: Comparison of new protein systems for lactating dairy cows. J. Dairy Sci., 67:1115–1133, 1984.

Walkden-Brown, S.W., et al.: Effect of nutrition on seasonal patterns of LH, FSH and testosterone concentration, testicular mass, sebaceous gland volume and odour in Australian cashmere goats. J. Reprod. Fert., 102:351–360, 1994.

Wanner, M. and Boss, P.H.: [Parenteral administration of iron dextran to newborn kids.] Schweiz. Arch. Tierheilkd., 120:369–375, 1978.

Wentzel, D.: Effects of nutrition on reproduction in the Angora goat. Proceedings, Fourth International Conference on Goats, Brasilia, Brazil, EMBRAPA, pp. 571–575, 1987.

Wichtel, J.J., Thompson, K.G. and Williamson, N.B.: Serum glutathione peroxidase activity reflects short-term increases in selenium intake in goats. N.Z. Vet. J., 44:148–150, 1996.

Yeom, K.H., et al.: Effect of protein: energy ratio in milk replacers on growth performance of goat kids. J. Anim. Physiol. Anim. Nutr. (Berl), 86:137–143, 2002.

Zervas, G., Nikolaou, E. and Mantzios, A.: Comparative study of chronic copper poisoning in lambs and young goats. Anim. Prod., 50:497–506, 1990.

20

Herd Health Management and Preventive Medicine

In any livestock production system, certain diseases and production constraints can be anticipated on the basis of accumulated experience. Herd health management and preventive medicine programs are designed to minimize the potential adverse effects of these predictable constraints and to protect against unexpected ones. These goals are accomplished by timely and cost-effective application of suitable veterinary, nutritional, and management interventions before disease or lost production occurs.

The disease conditions and production constraints expected in any given livestock production system are a function primarily of the species of livestock kept, their intended use, and the management system in which they are kept. However, a range of geographic, climatic, cultural, and economic factors modify herd health and preventive medicine programs at the local level.

For example, free-ranging East African goats maintained for meat, milk, and hides in mixed herds with cattle and sheep by Maasai pastoralists in the savannahs of Kenya present quite a different set of circumstances from Saanen dairy goats maintained exclusively for milk production in total barn confinement in west central France. Yet, appropriate herd health management and preventive medicine programs can be designed and implemented for each situation. Appropriate means that the technology and methods employed are available, understandable, and implementable, that they are acceptable to the producer and the consumer, that they address a specifically identified disease or production problem which could potentially occur in the herd, and finally, that they produce a favorable cost/benefit ratio in terms of improved health or increased productivity relative to the labor and materials expended.

Because of their remarkable adaptability and utility, goats are maintained over a more diverse range of habitats and production systems than any other domestic livestock species. As a result, herd health recommendations for goats vary considerably and all possible situations cannot be covered here in the text. In general, intensified management not only allows, but also demands, more interventions than extensive management. As a result, there is a larger body of documented veterinary experience relating to herd health management of goats maintained intensively. In addition, as a general rule, veterinary services are more often available or used where goats are raised intensively rather than extensively. This also contributes to a greater knowledge of appropriate herd health programs in intensive management situations. Finally, specialization for the production of distinct commodities for established industries, such as milk for commercial cheese production or mohair for textile mills, helps to define and clarify meaningful health and production targets within well-defined economic constraints. Not surprisingly, the largest body of information about goat herd health relates to intensively managed dairy goats and Angora goats maintained under semi-extensive conditions.

The coverage of herd health and preventive medicine programs in this text focuses mainly on dairy goats and fiber-producing goats. There are also more general comments on health and production issues related to goats kept for meat, goats kept for skins, transgenic goats, and goats raised under organic farming systems.

DAIRY GOAT HERD HEALTH MANAGEMENT AND PREVENTIVE MEDICINE

It is useful to think of the dairy goat herd as divided into separate management subgroups, each with its own set of herd health and preventive medicine requirements. For the purpose of this discussion, the following groups of goats are identified: newborn kids to weaning, weaned kids to breeding, bred doelings and dry does, milking does, and bucks. For each group, the common and expected diseases are presented, followed by suggested routine management procedures appropriate for the group. This analysis of subgroups within the herd is preceded by a brief discussion of issues relevant to the herd in general.

General Comments about Dairy Goat Herd Health

In general, commercial goat dairies should be managed as closed herds to minimize disease problems. Taking goats to shows and fairs should be discouraged. If showing is necessary for the financial well-being of the farm through the sale of breeding stock, then isolation and quarantine procedures should be followed for animals returning from outside. A separation period of three weeks from the herd is warranted. From the disease control point of view, artificial insemination is preferable to introduction of bucks or trucking of does to other farms for breeding.

Goats are very clever about undoing fasteners and gate closings, so gates and doors must be very secure to avoid unwanted escape and accidental access to feed and chemical storage areas which could result in engorgement toxemia, bloat, or poisoning. Goats are also notorious for chewing on the materials from which their enclosures are constructed. Therefore, old barns with lead based paints should be avoided as goat housing. When new housing is constructed, lumber treated with potentially toxic chemicals such as pentachlorophenol, used as wood preservatives, should be avoided.

Goats are also very hard on fences because of their propensity for climbing, and improper selection of fencing materials can be costly to owners. Fences with horizontal rungs or slats encourage climbing and destruction of fences. Chain link fences predispose goats to catching their limbs in the fence, with possible fractures resulting. If vertical slats or bars are used on gates or fencing, the spacing should be carefully evaluated to be sure that goats cannot become trapped and strangled, especially horned goats. For these reasons, electric fencing for goats is gaining in popularity.

Goats, like sheep, are susceptible to predation due to their small size and lack of potent defenses. Kids are particularly defenseless and may fall prey to raptors and ground-dwelling predators. Because the main defense of small ruminants is fleeing, the practice of tethering goats can be deadly where predators are common. Various defenses against predation are discussed in Chapter 4.

Goats, like other livestock, can experience suboptimal performance or overt disease from mineral deficiencies in feedstuffs related to soil composition in different parts of the world. The veterinarian and producer must be aware of the mineral deficiencies occurring locally. Deficiencies well documented to cause financial loss in goats are selenium, iodine, cobalt, and copper. Fertilization, top dressing of pastures, supplemental feeding, provision of trace mineral salt licks, or parenteral administration of needed substances can be used to address these problems, as discussed in Chapter 19. Another potential local problem for goats is consumption of noxious or toxic plants. Plants toxic to goats are listed in Chapter 19 and are discussed throughout this book related to the organ systems most affected. Plants that can cause sudden death, those that cause primary or secondary photosensitization, and those that cause off-flavors in milk are of particular concern.

Veterinarians interested in goats should encourage herd owners to have regularly scheduled herd health visits. When a knowledgeable veterinarian becomes familiar with the routine practices and seasonal activities of the goat herd, he or she is better able to spot incipient problems developing in the herd and initiate appropriate interventions before costly losses occur. As with dairy cattle, reproductive consultation is a good place to begin to show the herd owner how the veterinarian can help improve production efficiency through pregnancy checking, heat synchronization practices, and out-of-season breeding programs. Mastitis control is an important area where veterinary inputs can improve herd productivity. Nutritional management of metabolic diseases such as pregnancy toxemia is another area of potential input. The development and implementation of practical and realistic CAE control programs are important concerns of goat producers that should involve the counsel of veterinarians. Veterinarians can also carry out necropsy examinations on all goats that die in a herd. This is an effective means of tracking unexpected disease developments in the herd.

Management of Newborn Kids to Weaning

Disease Problems

At birth, the major obstacles to survival are hypoxia, hypothermia, hypoglycemia, and susceptibility to infectious disease. The latter is exacerbated by delayed or inadequate intake of colostrum rich in maternal immunoglobulins. Failure of passive transfer of maternal antibodies to newborn kids leads to increased morbidity and mortality throughout the postnatal period, particularly from septicemia in the first week of life, and later, from pneumonia as kids reach weaning age and diminishing concentrations of maternal antibodies have not been fully replaced by immunoglobulins actively produced by the kid. Failure to disinfect the navel after birth and maintaining kids in a dirty environment also lead to increased incidence of omphalophlebitis, septicemia, polyarthritis, and pneumonia. Diarrheal diseases are common in this period. Numerous etiologic agents can cause neonatal diarrhea over the first two weeks of life, as discussed in Chapter 10. After two weeks of age, coccidiosis is an increasing threat. A pneumoenteritis complex is sometimes seen in young kids, suggesting poor husbandry, heavy environmental pathogen loads, and inadequate colostral intake. Contagious ecthyma also may appear clinically in this age group if endemic on the premises or recently introduced.

Newborn kids should be inspected carefully for congenital defects such as cleft palate, rectovaginal fistula, atresia ani, hydrocephalus, umbilical hernia, and ventricular septal defect. The intersex condition is especially common in goats. Beta mannosidosis and mucopolysaccharidosis IIID are genetic diseases of Nubian kids. Kids identified with congenital defects should be culled immediately or designated for meat production.

Caprine arthritis encephalitis (CAE) virus infection is a major concern of dairy goat producers worldwide. Although clinical disease is rarely seen in kids younger than two months of age, newborn kids are the focus of CAE control programs because the virus is spread primarily from infected does to susceptible kids via colostrum and milk. Current kid-rearing techniques are defined in large part by practices aimed at reducing transmission of CAE to neonates, as discussed in Chapter 4.

Management Practices

Kidding should be a well-anticipated event, not an unexpected surprise. Being prepared for routine processing of kids at birth and being ready to respond to emergencies reduce neonatal losses. A clean, warm, dry, well-lit, well-bedded, well-ventilated kidding area should be designated and maintained. Appropriate supplies should be on hand such as towels for drying kids, feeding tubes for kids that do not suckle, and tincture of iodine for dipping navels. A colostrum management program relative to CAE control should be developed and in place before the onset of the kidding season. Evaluation of colostrum quality and colostrum requirements are discussed with failure of passive transfer in Chapter 7. Colostrum management programs are discussed in the section on CAE in Chapter 4.

The timed induction of parturition using prostaglandin has become popular as a technique for assuring attendance at birth and facilitating CAE control activities. Protocols are discussed in Chapter 13 along with recognition and management of dystocia, resuscitation, and proper care of the neonate at birth.

Proper identification and record keeping are signs of a well-managed farm. For identification of neonates, the rubber rings from canning bottles marked with an indelible marker are sometimes used as identifying collars. Subsequent ear tattooing of kids is recommended for permanent identification and should be performed after three months of age. If done too early, the tattoo dots comprising individual numbers or letters expand and separate as the ear grows and the markings become difficult to interpret. Green ink is recommended because the skin of some goat ears is black, making black ink tattoos unreadable. For the LaMancha breed with minimal external ear, tattooing is performed on the underside of the tail.

Kids can be housed in group pens but should not be overcrowded. Pen design should allow easy and thorough cleaning. The spread of diarrheal agents is exacerbated by poor sanitation and overstocking. Early culling or marketing of unwanted male kids reduces kid populations and the attendant risk of increased environmental contamination and the spread of infectious disease.

Disbudding of kids to prevent horn growth is commonly practiced to prevent horn related injuries between goats and to handlers later in life. In the United States, purebred diary goats cannot be shown if they have horns. Disbudding is usually done between three and fourteen days of age, depending on breed, size, and sex of kids as described in Chapter 18. When buck kids intended for future reproductive use are disbudded, damage to the pheromonic scent glands adjacent to the horn buds may reduce the buck's breeding efficiency later on. However, when buck kids are to be raised for meat or as pets, destruction of the scent glands is indicated.

Extra teats are common on doelings. These can be easily removed at the same time kids are disbudded, using curved scissors. If there is any doubt about which teats are the functional ones, extra teat removal should be delayed. Wattles can also be removed from goats at a young age with minimal trauma using curved scissors. Though wattles potentially can become snagged or traumatized, this happens uncommonly and the decision to remove them is usually a cosmetic one.

Castration, when indicated, is best carried out between four and fourteen days of age. The reason for castration must be clearly defined. For meat kids, the intended market and the age at marketing determine the need for castration. In some ethnic markets, uncastrated goats are preferred. When the market calls for kids slaughtered by eight weeks of age, castration may not be required. If goats are kept longer for finishing, then they need to be castrated where the market will not tolerate a buck odor to the meat. If castrated males are destined to become pets, delaying castration until six to eight weeks of age may reduce later problems with obstructive urolithiasis, a common problem in pet wethers discussed in Chapter 12.

Vaccination and the timing of vaccinations of neonates depend a good deal on the overall herd vaccination program. If does have been vaccinated during the dry period and kids receive adequate colostrum from vaccinated does, then kids can be considered to be protected by maternal immunity for those specific diseases through the first six weeks of life. Because the waning of maternal antibody varies with initial concentration, vaccination of these kids should begin at four or five weeks of age with booster inoculations given at intervals prescribed for each vaccine.

Kids are immunocompetent at birth. If kids are born to unvaccinated does, vaccinations should begin during the first week of life and the kids should be boostered according to vaccine directions. Prophylactic antisera may be used during the first week concurrently with bacterin-toxoids to protect kids while active antibody is forming. Tetanus antitoxin and *Clostridium perfringens* type C and type D antitoxins are the products most commonly used in kids in this manner.

The vaccinations required for kids will vary with geography and management system. Nevertheless, a universal recommendation is the vaccination of kids for enterotoxemia due to *Clostridium perfringens* type C and type D as well as for tetanus. This is the minimum vaccination program for kids. Vaccination for contagious ecthyma is fairly common. The first time it is done, all goats on the premises should be vaccinated. In subsequent years, only kids need to be vaccinated because immunity persists in the adults. Maternal antibody may interfere with vaccination in kids vaccinated too early. Contagious ecthyma vaccination is discussed in detail in Chapter 2.

Other vaccines, such as paratuberculosis, foot and mouth, peste des petits ruminants or bluetongue vaccine may be mandated or recommended as part of national disease control programs. Still other vaccines, such as anthrax, blackleg, leptospirosis, or rabies vaccines, may be used on the basis of knowledge that the disease occurs commonly in a specific region. Specific details about vaccine availability and use in goats for various diseases are covered in each disease discussion throughout the text.

Indiscriminate use of vaccines should be avoided, especially the use of live vaccines not specifically designed for goats. For example, live intranasal infectious bovine rhinotracheitis (IBR) vaccine is sometimes given to goat kids in the United States to control respiratory disease problems without any confirmation of the role of IBR in the respiratory disease complex of goats.

Where soils are selenium-deficient, nutritional muscular dystrophy in young kids is a real concern, and parenteral administration of a combined vitamin E and sodium selenite injection to kids at birth or supplementation of the ration with selenium as discussed in Chapter 19 is indicated.

Feeding programs for kids are discussed in Chapter 19. Weaning may occur as early as six weeks or as late as twelve weeks of age, depending on the feeding system used and other management considerations. Regardless of the milk feeding regimen, it is important that kids be exposed to hay and grains early in life to promote proper rumen development. Abrupt cessation of milk feeding without adequate adaptation to solid feeds can predispose to indigestion, bloat, and possibly polioencephalomalacia.

Management of Kids from Weaning to Breeding

Disease Problems

Coccidiosis and pneumonia are the dominant problems in this age group, particularly under conditions of confinement housing. Regarding coccidiosis, the transition to a diet of solid feed encourages more ingestion of coccidial oocysts while feeding. With regard to pneumonia, the progressive decline of maternal antibodies and the stresses of weaning appear to predispose kids to respiratory infections after eight weeks of age. When kids are turned out to pasture during their first summer, they are very susceptible to gastrointestinal parasitism and lung worms due largely to the absence of a developed local immunity in the alimentary and respiratory tracts. The severity of clinical parasitism depends on the concentration of infective larvae on pasture, the stocking rate, weather conditions, and other factors as discussed in Chapter 10.

Other disease problems also may occur in this group. There is a recurrent risk of enterotoxemia when concentrates are fed. The neurologic form of CAE virus infection, a progressive paresis, is most often seen in kids between eight and sixteen weeks of age.

Management Practices

For housed kids, it is essential to maintain housing and feeding systems that minimize the incidence of pneumonia and coccidiosis, as discussed, respectively, in Chapters 9 and 10. Regarding coccidiosis, clinical disease can occur even on the most conscientiously managed farms. Therefore, in addition to good sanitary practices, it may be necessary to use a coccidiostat in the feed or water.

Currently, there are few, if any vaccines that can be confidently recommended for controlling respiratory disease in young goats. The role of viruses usually implicated in bovine respiratory disease is unclear, and the available *Pasteurella* and *Mannheimia* bacterins are of unproven efficacy. There are no goat-specific respiratory virus vaccines available. Reliable vaccines against mycoplasmal pneumonias are increasingly available in affected countries. In countries where vaccination for caprine brucellosis is carried out, kids are usually vaccinated between three and eight months of age.

Regarding pasture parasites, young goats should be turned out to pastures that have not been in use for at least one year, and should be kept on separate pastures from adults if possible. A broad-spectrum anthelmintic should be administered before turnout, and parasite loads monitored throughout the pasture season by microscopic examination of composite fecal samples collected at pasture or in the case of *Haemonchus contortus*, by application of the FAMACHA© system to identify clinically affected individuals as discussed in Chapter 10. Tactical anthelmintic treatments can be given accordingly as needed.

When spring kids are weaned properly, fed optimally, and kept healthy, they can reach proper breeding size by the autumn of their birth year and subsequently kid on their first birthday. In North America, the target is 70 pounds by seven months of age for heavy breeds (e.g., Alpines, Saanens, and Nubians) and 60 pounds by seven months of age for light breeds (e.g., LaMancha and Toggenburg). Male and female kids should be segregated by three months of age to avoid unwanted breedings among sexually precocious individuals. External genitalia of all kids should be examined before breeding to identify any intersexes present.

In temperate regions, goats are seasonal breeders induced to begin estrous cycles by decreasing day length. There is much interest in manipulating the hormonal signals for estrus to permit goats to cycle year-round. Year-round breeding is particularly important to large scale commercial milk producers who must provide a consistent volume of product on a year-round basis. The two main techniques for bringing does and doelings into heat during the normally anestrous period of the year are the use of progesterone supplements and the manipulation of day length through confinement and exposure to artificial light. These, and other useful techniques are discussed in Chapter 13 and elsewhere (Haibel 1990; Bretzlaff and Romano 2001). Breeding techniques and confirmation of pregnancy in doelings and does are also discussed in Chapter 13.

Management of Bred Doelings and Dry Does

Disease Problems

The major concerns in this group are pregnancy toxemia and abortion. Pseudopregnancies are also common in goats and may be recognized during this period by ultrasound evaluation or by the spontaneous release of uterine fluids with no attendant fetus or placenta. The lay term for this phenomenon is, appropriately enough, cloudburst. Goats that are obese when they enter the dry period are at increased risk for pregnancy toxemia, vaginal prolapses during late gestation, and dystocia at parturition.

Management Practices

Does in lactation are usually given a dry period coincident with the last two to three months of gestation. Bred doelings that have not yet milked are also nonlactating in advanced pregnancy. The key objective for these animals is proper nutritional management to avoid obesity in early gestation (late lactation) and to provide adequate nutrients to support the rapid growth of fetuses in the last trimester of pregnancy. This is particularly important regarding pregnancy toxemia. The disease can be avoided by curtailing grain in late lactation (early gestation) when milk production no longer justifies it. These goats can be carried through midgestation on a high quality legume hay and little or no grain. Grain feeding should be resumed at the beginning of the last trimester and gradually increased until term. In herds already experiencing a pregnancy toxemia problem, periodic checking of urine samples from does and doelings for ketones with commercially available powders or dipsticks helps to detect incipient cases.

There are many potential infectious and noninfectious causes of late abortion in goats, as discussed in Chapter 13. To protect pregnant does from infectious abortion, no new animals should be introduced into the herd when pregnant animals are present. This includes breeding bucks. Any animal that aborts should be isolated immediately and the area where the abortion occurred quarantined and disinfected. Attempts should be made to make a definitive diagnosis of the cause of abortion. All fetal tissues and placentas not submitted for diagnosis should be buried or incinerated. In herds with a history of chlamydial abortion or past vaccination, each year's new crop of doelings should be vaccinated before breeding.

The dry period is the appropriate time to vaccinate pregnant does to increase the concentration of specific antibodies in the colostrum and thereby enhance passive immunity in the kids. Vaccines, such as enterotoxemia, should be given to dry does three to five weeks before kidding.

Pregnant does with nematode gastrointestinal parasites may experience a periparturient egg rise with increased shedding of eggs around the time of kidding. This is a survival strategy of the parasite to enhance the likelihood of infecting a new generation of hosts. Therefore, pregnant does should be given a broad-spectrum anthelmintic two to three weeks before kidding. Though no anthelmintic at proper dose has been definitively shown to cause abortion or teratogenic effects in goats, levamisole and albendazole have been suspected to do so, thus inhibiting their use in pregnant does.

Management of Milking Does

Disease Problems

Not unexpectedly, mastitis is the major disease challenge in lactating does. A variety of pathogens has been identified in milking goats as discussed in Chapter 14. *Mycoplasma* mastitis can be epidemic in some herds with devastating results. Mastitis due to *Staphylococcus aureus* can also be costly and difficult to control if aggressive culling of affected goats is not practiced.

Caseous lymphadenitis can occur in goats of all ages but is particularly problematic in milking does. Abscessed lymph nodes most commonly occur on the head and neck. Restraining milking does in head catches for milking increases the risk of abscess rupture and transmission of the disease.

The mammary form of CAE virus infection often occurs at the onset of lactation. It is manifested by a distinct hypogalactia or agalactia associated with a firm udder. This is perhaps the most threatening form of CAE in that it strikes at the core of the animal's productivity. Herds with this problem must look carefully at implementation of CAE control programs as discussed in Chapter 4.

The arthritic form of CAE virus infection also shows up more frequently in does once they have entered the milk line. Epidemiologic studies in France suggest that clinical manifestations of swollen carpi are more likely to develop in infected goats that are subjected to conditions which increase trauma to the joints (Monicat 1989). Such conditions might include having to jump on to and off of milking stands, repeated banging of the carpi caused by improper stall or feeder design, hard floor surfaces, or being forced to rest for extended periods on the carpi because of stall confinement or tying up. Overgrown, inadequately trimmed hooves are another distinct predisposing factor.

Some weight loss is normal in early lactation, particularly in high-producing animals. The stresses of kidding and subsequent lactation, however, may trigger clinical manifestations of weight loss in carrier animals subclinically infected with *Mycobacterium avium* subsp. *paratuberculosis*. Animals that continue to lose weight during lactation should be tested for paratuberculosis, as discussed in Chapter 10.

When milking does are pastured, gastrointestinal parasitism must be anticipated as a potential problem. Though goats develop an age- and exposure-related resistance to parasites, it is not absolute. Even if adult milkers do not develop overt clinical parasitism, the subclinical effects of parasites on milk production may be significant (Farizy and Taranchon 1970; Hoste and Chartier 1998). Milk fever, or hypocalcemia, is uncommon in dairy goats relative to dairy cattle, but can be a recurring problem in certain herds. Management and feeding recommendations made for control of hypocalcemia in dairy cattle have not been proven applicable to goats, as discussed in Chapter 19. Abomasal displacement is another common problem in intensively raised dairy cattle that is virtually unknown in goats.

Management Practices

The major goal in managing lactating does is to maximize their milk output in a cost-efficient manner. To accomplish this, both general health and udder health must be maintained. The feeding program must optimize production and be tailored to suit the needs of individual goats, depending on their stage and level of lactation. In addition, a breeding and culling program that selects for superior milk production must be implemented. In support of these goals, health and production records, though they need not be elaborate, must be conscientiously maintained.

Preventive medicine procedures for milking does include vaccinations, foot care, and, when conditions dictate, deworming. Goats should be vaccinated at least twice a year for enterotoxemia, and, in problem herds, three times. Since one vaccination is given to dry does to enhance colostral antibody, these animals should receive one or two additional vaccinations during lactation. Vaccine products aimed at preventing abortion, such as chlamydial vaccines, are given before breeding.

Proper foot care in the form of regular hoof trimming is extremely important. It reduces the likelihood of foot rot, teat injuries, abnormal gait, and general sore-footedness leading to decreased feed intake. The technique for foot trimming is described in Chapter 4. The frequency of trimming depends to a large extent on the amount of exercise goats get. Natural wearing or trimming occurs through ambulation, especially on rough or rocky surfaces.

Pastured milkers should be checked periodically for nematode parasites by fecal examination. Milking does can be dewormed tactically as required but there are two concerns. One is that certain anthelmintics have antifungal and antibacterial properties that can damage cheese cultures and disrupt cheese making. The second is that regulatory agencies often set a milk discard requirement following any sort of drug administration, leading to economic loss to the milk producer. Anthelmintics used should be those approved for lactating animals and appropriate milk discard times must be observed.

Good udder health depends on selecting for does with good udder conformation and attachment, providing clean, well-bedded living quarters for milking does, properly functioning milking equipment, and an established protocol of udder hygiene during milking. Intramammary infusions of antibiotics at the beginning of the dry period can be used in herds with an active mastitis problem. Clipping the hair on the udder and hindquarters decreases sediment in the milk.

Milk quality is an important issue in goat dairies. Too often in the past, milk odors and taints have dampened consumer acceptance of goat milk as a wholesome, desirable product. Buck contact with milking does should be kept to a minimum and bucks should not be maintained near milking parlors or milk storage areas because buck odor permeates the milk. Milking does should not be allowed to forage indiscriminately in unimproved pastures or woodlands because many plants may lead to off flavors or odors in milk. Proper handling of milk after extraction from the doe is extremely important. Excessive agitation and delays in pasteurization promote lipolysis of the fat in goat milk, adding to the so-called "goaty" flavor of the milk. "Off" flavors in milk are discussed further in Chapter 14.

High somatic cell counts in goat milk are a serious concern. For a variety of reasons, not all of which are elucidated, goats tend to have higher somatic cell counts than cattle, even when udder infections are not present. This causes regulatory conflicts when somatic cell count standards set for cow milk quality are applied to goat milk. This, and other issues related to milking procedures and milk quality, are discussed in detail in Chapter 14.

Feeding for optimal milk production is discussed in Chapter 19. No matter what is fed, there must be adequate trough or feeder space for each and every doe in the milking herd so that submissive does are not deprived of feed by dominant does. In addition, dominant does may be so busy bullying other goats that they may not eat adequately themselves and may need to be culled. Another point related to feeding is that the feeding of silage is associated, though not consistently, with the development of listeriosis in goats.

Management of Bucks

The reader will note that bucks are the last subgroup to be considered in this discussion. This reflects the typical position of the bucks in the herd when it comes to the implementation of herd health practices. The buck, by virtue of his offensive odor, is too often neglected in herd health program. This omission should be conscientiously avoided because healthy bucks play a key role in reproductive efficiency and overall improvement of herd productivity.

Disease Problems

Disease conditions unique to bucks are limited. Obstructive urolithiasis is probably the most important. Though more common in castrated males, urinary calculi can also cause obstructive disease in intact males and may result in their loss as breeding animals. The condition is discussed in Chapter 12. Bucks become quite aggressive in the breeding season and can injure each other while fighting. They can also injure people, and workers should always exercise caution around breeding bucks. A common problem associated with fighting is the breaking off of a horn scur, with profuse bleeding from the poll. These poorly attached scurs occur when male kids are improperly disbudded and residual germinal horn bud tissue produces a regrowth of malformed horn. The profuse bleeding, though rarely serious, is a frequent cause of alarm. Proper disbudding prevents this problem, as discussed in Chapter 18.

In the breeding season, bucks acquire the habit of urinating on themselves, particularly on the face and the back of the forelimbs. This can cause severe urine scald and secondary bacterial dermatitis. Petroleum jelly applied to the back of the forelimbs inhibits the development of serious problems.

Management Practices

To obtain maximum performance from bucks, they should be "tuned up" before the onset of the breeding season. There is a definite tendency for bucks to become thin as the breeding season progresses. This appears to be physiologic rather than pathologic. Nevertheless, it underscores the need for bucks to be in excellent body condition before breeding begins. This requires regular deworming and proper feeding, as discussed in Chapter 19.

Of equal importance is proper foot care. Mounting does for breeding puts considerable strain on the back legs, and poorly trimmed feet can produce sufficient pain to inhibit the buck from performing properly, particularly if the buck is used heavily. Proper foot care is too often overlooked because herdsmen do not want to handle smelly bucks. Similarly, bucks should not be left out of herd-wide vaccinations simply because they are a nuisance to handle.

A complete reproductive examination should be performed on breeding bucks prior to use. This should include a general physical examination, genital examination, semen evaluation, and assessment of libido, as discussed in Chapter 13. This should not be done too long before the onset of the breeding season because semen quality may be diminished during the season of deep anestrus.

If bucks are housed in groups year-round, they get used to each other and even at the onset of the breeding season are unlikely to do serious damage to each other by fighting. However, introducing a brand new buck, especially a younger or smaller one, to the group during the breeding season could prove fatal to the newcomer.

Clipping the beards and hair of bucks, especially on the forequarters, may reduce the generally offensive odor of the buck that results from urine retention on the hair. This should be done before the onset of breeding activity. The presence of a buck near the does is quite helpful in detecting estrus. Fence line contact is adequate and the buck need not commingle with the does to elicit estrous behavior.

The above discussion is organized according to the needs of the various subgroups of animals within the dairy goat herd. Another approach to organizing herd health management activities is by the calendar. A typical seasonal calendar of herd health activities for dairy goats in North America is given in Table 20.1.

HAIR GOAT HERD HEALTH MANAGEMENT AND PREVENTIVE MEDICINE

The Angora goat is the source of the valued textile fiber mohair. Three main areas of mohair production in the world are the Anatolian plain of Turkey, where the Angora goat originated, the bushveld of the Karoo district of South Africa, and the Edwards Plateau region of Texas in the United States. All three regions are arid, with average annual rainfall generally less than 600 mm. They are also areas with elevations around 500 m above sea level. These attributes, among others, are highly favorable to the profitable exploitation of Angora goats for mohair under extensive or range management conditions. More recently, serious development and expansion of the mohair industries have successfully occurred in Australia and New Zealand. There have also been attempts to introduce Angora goats into colder, wetter climates such as are found in the upper midwestern United States. Success of these enterprises depends on a more intensive form of management.

Mohair production is a rather specialized agricultural enterprise, and an overall discussion of the indus-

Table 20.1. Seasonal herd health management and preventive medicine calendar for dairy goats in North America (Guss 1977).

Season	*Preventive activities*
Fall	Clean barn thoroughly before onset of bad weather.
	Clean and disinfect kidding pens and leave vacant.
	Administer anthelmintics to all goats coming off pasture.
	Use larvicidal anthelmintics.
	Check goats for lice; delouse entire herd if lice found.
	Check and trim feet as needed.
	Perform reproductive examination of bucks, including semen evaluation.
	Administer selenium prior to breeding if deficiencies expected.
Winter	Check goat housing for evidence of poor ventilation such as wet ceilings, wet bedding, or smell of ammonia.
	Correct ventilation deficiencies; identify and seal drafts.
	Check waterers for cleanliness and correct any leaks.
	Restock necessary kidding and kid rearing supplies.
	Deworm and vaccinate dry does three to five weeks prior to kidding.
	Clip hair on udder and hindquarters of pregnant does.
	Check and trim feet as needed.
Spring	Check and repair fences and gates around pastures and buildings.
	Remove sources of injury from lots and pastures.
	Administer anthelmintics at time of turnout to pasture.
	Check and trim feet as needed.
Summer	Ensure adequate shade and water for goats in hot weather.
	Monitor herd for parasites using composite fecal samples from pasture.
	Examine bucks for general condition and genital abnormalities; deworm and provide extra feed as needed.
	Check and trim feet as needed; include the bucks.

try is beyond the scope of this text. A good review of goat fiber production has been published (Shelton 1981). Health and reproductive problems related to fiber-producing goats in North America have been reviewed (Bretzlaff 1990). A history of the mohair industry in South Africa is available (van der Westhuysen et al. 1988), as is an overview of the health problems commonly seen in South African Angora goats (van Tonder 1975). A guide for mohair production under intensive management in cold climates is available (Drummond 1985), as is an excellent book on the developing goat fiber industry in New Zealand (Yerex 1986) and a good review of husbandry practices in the Australian Angora industry (Evans 1980).

One aspect of fiber production in goats rather unique to Australia and New Zealand is the capture and use of feral goats for crossing with Angoras to rapidly expand fiber production capacity in the face of limited access to purebred breeding stock. Feral goats, which tend to dwell in the mountainous regions of these countries, have a significant amount of hair that qualifies as cashmere on the basis of fiber diameter. The fiber from crossbred goats is known as cashgora.

The Cashmere goat, also known as the Kashmir or Pashmina goat, is the source of the textile fiber cashmere. As the name implies, the goat originated in the mountainous region of central Asia. The finest cashmere commercially available still comes from traditional sources in Mongolia and China. Coarser grades of cashmere have also been available in commercial quantities from Afghanistan, Iran, and the former Soviet Union. The remoteness of these regions from milling centers in Europe and North America, coupled with political instabilities in the region, have created increased demand for cashmere from other sources. As a result, nascent cashmere industries have developed primarily in Australia and New Zealand, but also in Europe and North America. Embryo transfer technology has played a significant role in the spread of cashmere production outside of traditional regions.

General Comments about Herd Health Management in Fiber-Producing Goats

Angora goats have a strong flocking instinct and a hierarchical social structure. The flock readily follows lead goats that can be trained to come by banging a grain bucket. Angoras do not respond well to herding dogs, especially if the dogs work in too close, in which case the flock may become disrupted and scatter. If goats and sheep are commingled and disturbed, sheep move downhill and goats uphill. Angoras do not readily jump fences, but assuredly find holes to go through or depressions to slide under. Fencing must therefore be kept in good repair. Electric fencing can be used to advantage with Angora goats. When working goats in pens or yards, care must be taken not to overcrowd or frighten them. Goats pack up in corners and are trampled or smothered.

At range, wethers should be kept separately from does and doelings because the wethers are more active and mobile. Females may follow and spend too much time traveling and not enough eating.

Fiber and Fleece Characteristics

The attractiveness of mohair and cashmere as textile fibers lies primarily in the fineness of the hair. These hairs represent the "down" or insulating undercoat of the goat produced by secondary hair follicles. The characteristics of the fibers are discussed in detail in Chapter 2. The quality of the fleece and its economic value are affected by a number of faults, including a high presence of "kemp" or guard hairs arising from the primary follicles; the presence of non-white fibers; contamination with plastic twine fibers, inks, marks, or dyes related to husbandry practices such as breeding harnesses; and the presence of vegetable matter such as seed heads and burrs. This latter must be controlled by timing shearing to precede the development of seeds and burrs on pasture or range. Carbonization, a process used to remove vegetable matter from a sheep fleece after shearing, damages the more delicate mohair fleece.

Shearing

Mohair grows at a rate of about 2.5 cm/month. The length of one year's growth, about 30 cm, presents manufacturing problems, and Angora goats are usually shorn two, sometimes three, times a year. Kids, yearlings, and adults should be grouped and sheared separately, and fleeces sorted separately. The younger the goat, the finer the fiber diameter. Sheep shears can be used but should be run at a slower speed (1,500 rpm). A 20-tooth goat comb head should be used. Various shearing techniques are used successfully in goats, including laying the animal down with the feet tied, standing the animal in a head catch, or tipping the animal up on its rump. Goats do not tolerate tipping as well as sheep, presumably because of their bony, unpadded rumps. To make the goat comfortable, its head should be allowed to fall back behind and between the handler's knees, with the goat's weight supported on the small of its back rather than its rump. With all methods, care must be taken not to cut the goat's loose skin or to traumatize teats or the penis during shearing.

Cashmere goats shed their down in the spring of the year. Traditionally, the down has been harvested by combing out the shed fibers from the hair coat. Cashmere goats can be sheared, however, and the guard hairs separated from the down at processing. Cashmere goats are sheared once a year in the spring.

The timing of shearing is an important issue in fiber production and animal health. Stress associated with shearing and the increased susceptibility to cold stress after shearing can lead to abortions or death losses in does, as discussed in Chapter 2. This is one reason that wethers are considered desirable for mohair production. Windbreakers have been designed for shorn goats and may be applied to valuable breeding stock, but their use in large commercial flocks is not practical.

Nutrition

The nutritional demands of fiber production are very high, especially with regard to protein. Yet, compared with sheep, the body size of fiber-producing goats is smaller, and their feed intake capacity is less. In does, gestation may increase nutritional demands beyond maintenance and hair production to the point that abortions readily occur.

Similarly, borderline nutritional status at breeding time may diminish prolificacy, leading to reduced kid crops. This is of particular importance in Angora goats because young animals produce better quality fiber. Both male and female kids are kept for production and the mean age of herds is kept young. Small kid crops make this difficult to accomplish.

Finally, future fiber yields appear to depend on adequate nutrition to the fetus in late gestation and to the newborn kid. The concentration of secondary hair follicles from which mohair arises is conditioned by fetal nutrition, while overall kid survival and growth depend on adequate milk supply from the dam.

To address these various management and production issues related to nutrition, does should receive supplemental feeding for four weeks before mating, four weeks before kidding, and four weeks after kidding.

Hair cover on the face is a common fault in Angora goats. Under extensive management conditions, impaired vision associated with facial hair can limit feed intake with adverse consequences. Ideally, breeding programs should select against facial hair, but a positive correlation between facial hair and total fleece weight limits this approach.

Reproductive Problems

Fiber-producing goats are seasonal breeders, with estrus beginning in the late summer/early autumn with decreasing day length. Poor reproductive performance, as manifested by low ovulation rates and reduced fecundity, is correlated with small body size in Angora does. As mentioned above, supplemental feeding, or flushing, of does may improve ovulation rates and prolificacy.

In addition to the broad range of infectious and noninfectious causes of abortion affecting other types of goats, Angora does are particularly susceptible to stress-induced abortion caused by cold temperatures, marginal or inadequate nutrition, and poor condition associated with parasitism. Good management is aimed at providing adequate shelter, nutrition, and parasite control. The frequency of abortion in Angora does increases as mohair production increases relative to body size.

A costly, inherited abortion syndrome of Angora goats associated with adrenal insufficiency occurs in South African Angoras. It is discussed in Chapter 13.

Cryptorchidism is common in Angora males. Such individuals should not be used for breeding. Overworking bucks should be avoided. Depending on nutritional status, health status, topography, and distance, the buck-to-doe ratio should be between 1:25 and 1:75.

Mothering

Angora does kidding at pasture or range have a distinctly different mothering pattern than sheep. Producers familiar with sheep and new to goats may not recognize this. The doe "plants" her newly born kid, leaving it camped by itself or with other kids while the doe goes off to graze. It returns to feed the kid in the afternoon. Though planting behavior is natural for goats, it increases the susceptibility of kids to predation. When predation is a problem, does should kid in areas where woods or rock formations allow some camouflage or protection for the kids.

Because dams spend a good deal of time away from their kids, early, strong bonding between dam and kid is very important to ensure proper recognition and nurturing of kids. To accomplish this, the pair need a critical five minutes of undisturbed contact after birth. Therefore, it is essential that the kidding process not be disturbed by human intervention. Foraging does return to protect their kids if the kids issue a distress call. To take advantage of this behavior, does should kid on somewhat restricted and familiar foraging grounds so they can readily find and return to their kids. Gradually, kids begin to follow does on their foraging forays and the goats can be moved to larger pastures.

Newborn kids, especially those of low bodyweight, can freeze to death easily. Providing shelter may be necessary when inclement or cold weather occurs in conjunction with kidding.

Dehorning, Castration, and Marking

Horns are a mixed blessing on fiber-producing goats. Under extensive management, they may help goats defend themselves against predators, but the more common result of horns is increased fighting among horned goats. Horns also increase the risk of goats becoming trapped in fences, especially mesh fences. Under intensive management, horns increase the requirement for bunk space and promote accidents and injuries. Angora kids can be disbudded by electrocautery at two to three weeks of age. Horns on mature goats can be cut back with a hacksaw, as described in Chapter 18. Intact horns are favored in show goats and breeding stock.

Open castration, elastrator bands, or clamping can be used. The time of castration is variable. In Texas, castration of buck kids is often delayed until one year of age to ensure good sturdy horn growth for defense against predators. In Australia, goats are routinely castrated at four to six weeks of age. On humane grounds, elastrator bands should not be used in kids over three weeks of age.

For improved record keeping and management, goats need to be identified. Ear tattoos are useful for permanent identification and are indicated for breeding stock. However, tattoos do not allow easy recognition of individual goats from afar. Ear tags are preferred for this purpose, but certain considerations apply. Any tag placed on the edge of the ear will readily tear out, especially metal tags. Penetrating, round button, flexible plastic ear tags are preferred, placed through the center of the ear. Tagging is best delayed until four to six weeks of age. Ear notching and horn branding are alternative methods of identification.

Parasitism

Fiber-producing goats are particularly sensitive to the adverse effects of gastrointestinal parasitism. The increased nutritional demand of hair production coupled with the limited feed intake allowed by their diminutive body size demands efficient use of nutrients for preserving health and productivity. The hypoproteinemia and blood loss associated with gastrointestinal parasitism can tip the nutritional balance against the doe, causing decreased fertility, abortion, increased susceptibility to disease, or outright death. Pasture management and strategic and tactical treatments with anthelmintic are integral parts of Angora goat management. Parasite control practices are discussed in Chapter 10.

Even though fiber-producing goats are usually managed extensively, there are times such as weaning, shearing, bad weather, and supplemental feeding when flocks are congregated in confined areas. This increases the risk of clinical coccidiosis in kids and weanlings. Conscientious attention to sanitation and hygiene, and the use of coccidiostats, are required to manage this problem, as discussed in Chapter 10.

Lice and keds are more than a nuisance on fiber-producing goats. They can cause itching, rubbing, and subsequent damage to the hair coat, as well as anemia. In cashmere goats, louse egg cases clinging to hair can alter the dyeing characteristics of the fiber. Routine louse control should be practiced as discussed in Chapter 2. Some pour-ons may stain the fleece. If sprays or dips are used, it is important that goats not be chilled when wet.

Other Disease Problems

Soremouth is common in fiber-producing goats. Affected kids may have difficulty nursing and does may contract mastitis. In extensive management systems in which bottle or tube feeding is impractical, kid losses can result. Vaccination is indicated. Foot rot and foot scald occur but less frequently than in sheep. Preventive measures are discussed in Chapter 4. Fly strike also occurs in goats, but less commonly than in sheep.

Wethers are extremely susceptible to the formation of urinary calculi and development of obstructive urolithiasis. The calculi are most often composed of phosphate salts and the main approach to control is to ensure a proper ratio of calcium to phosphorus in the overall ration, as discussed in Chapter 12.

Caseous lymphadenitis can be a serious problem in fiber-producing goats. As in sheep, the main route of transmission is through shearing, when cuts and abrasions in the skin are inoculated with bacteria from open abscesses on other sheared goats. The shearing equipment acts as a mechanical vector. Shearers must be knowledgeable about the disease and disinfect instruments between goats when necessary. Young, uninfected goats should be shorn first.

Pneumonia is a common occurrence in weanling goats and is exacerbated by changing, adverse weather or by housing, if ventilation is poor. Access to shelter in wet weather helps to reduce the incidence of pneumonia. Early recognition and mass medication are critical in controlling losses.

Hair goat breeds are susceptible to CAE virus infection. However, the prevalence of the disease is dramatically lower than in dairy goats. More must be learned about the epidemiology of CAE virus infection in hair goat breeds. At present, it is probably inadvisable to commingle hair goats with dairy goats. Milk or colostrum from dairy goats should not be used to raise orphaned hair goat kids unless the source herd is certified CAE free or the milk and colostrum have been properly heat treated to kill the virus.

As with dairy goats, the minimum vaccination program should include *Clostridium perfringens* types C and D combined with tetanus prophylaxis. In low-lying pasture areas, multivalent clostridial vaccines including protection against blackleg may be indicated. In selenium deficient areas, does should be drenched or injected with sodium selenite just before mating and again two to three weeks before kidding.

A herd health calendar for hair goat production is given in Table 20.2.

Table 20.2. Herd health management and preventive medicine calendar for fiber-producing goats in North America.

Season	*Preventive activities*
July and August	Check all goats for lice.
	Deworm spring kids.
	Vaccinate all goats for enterotoxemia.
	Begin supplemental feeding (flushing) of does to be bred.
	Ensure adequate number and quality of breeding bucks.
	Turn teaser bucks in with does if synchronized breeding is desired.
	Begin fall shearing.
September and October	Begin breeding; use marking harness and keep records.
	Check goats for parasites; deworm and delouse as needed.
	Check and trim feet.
November and December	Remove bucks from bred does.
	Perform pregnancy checks.
	Select rested pastures for kidding.
	Ensure adequate shelter facilities on kidding pastures.
	Begin preparations for indoor kidding, if an option.
January and February	Begin spring shearing; shear pregnant does three to six weeks prior to kidding; delouse goats after shearing.
	Boost feed levels to does due to kid four weeks prior to kidding date.
	Deworm and vaccinate does two to three weeks before kidding.
	Turn does out to kidding pastures to familiarize them with the pastures.
	Castrate buck kids from previous year.
	When kidding begins, keep accurate records of kidding activities.
March and April	Vaccinate kids at four weeks of age for enterotoxemia, tetanus, and soremouth.
	Place ear tags in goats at four to six weeks of age.
	Continue supplemental feeding of does for four weeks after kidding.
	When kids are following does, deworm goats and turn out from kidding pastures to larger grazing areas.
May and June	Wean kids and move does to a new pasture.
	Plan to cull does for poor health or poor reproductive performance.

MEAT GOAT HERD HEALTH MANAGEMENT AND PREVENTIVE MEDICINE

The use of goats for meat presents a paradox. On a worldwide basis, production of meat is the single most common usage of goats. However, goat meat production is the least developed aspect of goat husbandry in terms of an organized industry. This reflects the fact that the majority of goats intended for meat are found in the developing countries of the tropics and subtropics. These goats are maintained primarily by herders and smallholders and the goat meat they produce is used mainly for local consumption with relatively little marketing of meat outside the family or village. There is a limited but informative body of literature on the current status of goat meat production around the world and future needs for improvement (Dhanda et al. 2003; Alexandre and Mandonnet 2005).

Compared to the dairy breeds, comparatively little work has been done to breed goats specifically for meat production. Globally, the majority of goats used for meat are indigenous breeds in which little formal selection has been practiced. Historically, in North America, goats offered for slaughter were most commonly cull goats from dairy herds or fiber-producing flocks. In Australia and New Zealand, feral goats are harvested for meat.

There are two notable exceptions regarding selective breeding for meat production. In South Africa, a meat type goat, the Boer goat, has been developed (Mahan 2000). This animal has rates of feed conversion and weight gain and carcass characteristics approaching those of sheep. Advances with the Boer goat underscore the potential for improvement of meat production in other breeds. Indigenous breeds of African goats have been reported to have daily weight gains in the neighborhood of 90 g/day, while average Boer goat gains range from 170 to 200 g/day, with highly selected Boer goats on improved diets gaining as much as 290 g/day. A second meat type goat, the Kiko goat, has been developed in New Zealand by crossing feral does with Nubian, Toggenburg, and Saanen bucks (Batten 1987). Other breeds recognized with the potential for improving goat production are the Fijian breed from Fiji, the Katjang breed of Indonesia, the Ma'tou of China, the Sirohi of India, and the Sudan Desert breed of Sudan (Devendra 1999).

The high prolificacy of goats compared to cattle and even sheep makes them attractive ruminants for exploitation in meat production systems. Three kiddings every two years is a very reasonable goal. Selective breeding for meat production allows producers to take advantage of this potential in goats. Future advances and improvements in meat goat husbandry and production will depend a great deal on accurate market research to determine the desired characteristics of goat meat in varied markets. Production practices will be dictated to a large extent by such issues as the preferred age and weight of carcasses, preferences of taste and tenderness, preferences for live goats over slaughtered goats, preference for castrated over intact males, religious constraints on slaughter procedures, and potential of export markets compared to local markets.

The basic principles for herd health management of meat goats are similar to those for dairy goats. In general, emphasis must be placed on kid rearing techniques to reduce neonatal mortality. Excessive death losses in kids negate the advantage of prolificacy inherent in goats. In goats surviving the neonatal period, diseases which inhibit the rapid, efficient growth of young kids should be carefully controlled. The conditions most likely to disrupt normal growth are pneumonia, coccidiosis, and gastrointestinal helminthiasis. If finishing programs evolve and young goats are pushed on concentrate feeds, the risk of bloat, lactic acidosis, and enterotoxemia increases. Goats should always be vaccinated for the latter disease.

Conditions that could cause markdowns or condemnations at slaughter also need to be controlled. These include caseous lymphadenitis leading to lymph node and visceral abscesses, cestode infestations such as *Taenia ovis* or *T. multiceps* which produce cysts in muscle and viscera, and liver flukes which damage livers. Finally, when therapeutic efficacy is not compromised, drugs and vaccines should be given subcutaneously rather than intramuscularly to minimize damage to muscle tissue.

Since the 1990s, there has been a dramatic and robust increase in meat goat production in the United States, especially in the south. Texas, Tennessee, Oklahoma, Georgia, Mississippi, and Kentucky have been particularly active in this area. While Spanish, Angora, and dairy breed goats are being used for meat production, there has also been significant growth in the popularity and number of Boer and, to a lesser extent, Kiko goats. Both of these breeds were initially imported but are now bred in the United States. In addition, so-called fainting goats, i.e., goats with myotonia congenita, are heavily muscled in the hindquarters and have become desirable as a meat goat breed, particularly in Tennessee. Myotonia congenita is discussed in Chapter 4.

Because of the persistent warm climate and the heavy reliance on pasture grazing in meat goat production systems in the southern states, gastrointestinal parasitism, particularly haemonchosis, has emerged as a significant constraint on health and production and threatens the vitality of the meat goat industry. This issue is discussed further in the nematode gastroenteritis section of Chapter 10. Opportunities for veterinary participation in herd health management for meat goat production are increasing in the United States.

Langston University in Oklahoma has developed a Web-based training and certification program for meat goat producers which reflects the rapid advance of meat goat production in the United States since the first edition of this book was published in 1994. It is available on the Internet at http://www.luresext.edu/goats/training/QAtoc.html. The program provides a very informative overview of all aspects of meat goat production and marketing. It contains a useful and detailed module on meat goat herd health (Dawson et al. 2000) and another which provides an overview of the important diseases of meat goats (Olcott and Dawson 2000). A basic herd health calendar for meat goats in the United States is presented in Table 20.3. Additional links to useful information on goat meat production and marketing are available through the Website of the Agricultural Marketing and Resource Center at http://www.agmrc.org/agmrc/commodity/livestock/goats/meat+goats.htm.

MAINTAINING QUALITY GOAT SKINS

Goat skins are a valuable commodity in their own right as sources of high quality leather. The goat skin can represent as much as 15% of the total slaughter value of the goat. To maintain the highest value for skins, certain management and disease control efforts should be observed. Good nutrition throughout life improves the strength of the skin. Infectious skin diseases, such as goat pox, and external parasites, such as lice, keds, ticks, warbles, and mange, must be controlled in the live animal to avoid excessive damage to skins and subsequent downgrading. Any tattoos, fire branding, or injections should be performed on the periphery of the animal, avoiding the flanks and back. Animals should be handled gently during transport to market to avoid subcutaneous hemorrhages that can damage skins.

Table 20.3. Herd health management and preventive medicine calendar for meat goats in North America (from Brown and Forrest 2004).

January	Evaluate pasture and forage conditions.
	Monitor body conditions of does; supplement if necessary.
	Prepare for kidding.
February	Sort pregnant from open does.
	Begin feeding pregnant does.
	Evaluate does and bucks; sell unsound or inferior animals.
	Treat for internal and external parasites.
March	Begin kidding; check teats for milk flow; identify kids.
	Separate singles from twins; if possible, pen individual does with their kids; feed does to maintain milk production.
April	Finish kidding.
	Continue to supplement lactating does.
May	Consider weaning small, stunted kids.
	Discontinue supplement feeding to does.
	Monitor internal parasites through fecal samples.
June	Begin looking for replacement bucks with good conformation, structural correctness, muscling, and a high weight per day of age.
July	Continue selecting replacement bucks.
August	Treat for internal and external parasites.
	Vaccinate kids.
	Select replacement does and bucks.
	Wean kids; supplement replacement does and bucks with a high-protein (21%), high-energy feed.
	Evaluate does and bucks; sell unsound and inferior animals.
	Criteria for culling: Barren female: missed two seasons in a row. Bad teats or udders: too big or too small (mastitis). Bad mouths: smooth or broken mouth or over- or undershot jaw. Structural defects: bad feet and legs or back. Bad testicles: too small or infected (epididymitis). Unthriftiness: due to old age or disease.
September	Begin flushing does and bucks; flush with fresh green pasture or 1/2 pound feed/head/day for two to three weeks before and after buck turnout.
	Treat for lice if necessary.
October	Turn out bucks with does; breeding ratio 1 buck/20 to 25 does, depending on pasture size and breeding conditions.
	Continue to flush does for two to three weeks after buck turnout.
November	Evaluate pasture and forage conditions.
	Determine does' body conditions and plan winter supplemental feeding program.
	Monitor internal parasites through fecal samples. If heavy, treat after first hard freeze.
December	Remove bucks and feed to regain body condition.
	Evaluate pasture and forage conditions.
	Watch body conditions of does; supplement if necessary.
	Check for lice and use a pour-on lice treatment if needed.

HERD HEALTH MANAGEMENT FOR ORGANICALLY RAISED GOATS

Based on perceived health and environmental benefits as well as personal lifestyle choices, consumer demand for organically raised food has been steadily increasing over the last two decades in developed countries. In response, a growing segment of farmers, including livestock producers, have been switching to organic production systems to meet that growing demand. Veterinarians serving clients who raise livestock organically must be aware of the opportunities and constraints, as well as the rules and regulations, involved in maintaining animal health in an organic production system. It is suggested that veterinarians with clients raising goats organically read the section in Chapter 1 entitled "Special Considerations for Organic Goat Production" as well as this section.

The aim of organic farming is to establish and maintain soil-plant, plant-animal and animal-soil interdependence to create a closed and sustainable agro-ecological system based on local resources. To achieve this, organic farming uses what are considered environmentally friendly methods of crop and livestock production that exclude synthetic fertilizers, growth hormones, growth enhancing antibiotics, synthetic pesticides, and gene manipulation (Nardone et al. 2004). The focus of organic production systems is not on maximizing production, but rather on optimizing production in the context of the resources and management options available. As such, breeding programs for dairy goats, for example, might focus more on selection for disease or parasite resistance rather than increased milk production, while decisions on cropping and forage production might be driven by the decision not to include grains or concentrates produced off-farm in the animals' diet.

Livestock veterinarians used to working with clients in conventional farming systems may chafe at the constraints encountered in providing veterinary services to organic livestock producers, because many of the medicines routinely used in conventional livestock practice are not allowed in organically produced livestock. Most notable among these are the antibiotics. However, with an open mind, animal health care delivery for organic livestock production can offer opportunities for creativity and innovation in developing holistic herd health programs that place more emphasis on preventive medicine and progressive management designed to minimize the occurrence of disease and the need for antibiotics and other conventional therapies.

With regard to what is available for use in the treatment of organically raised livestock, the general rule is that all natural materials are allowed in organic agriculture, unless specifically prohibited, while all synthetic materials are prohibited unless specifically allowed (Karreman 2006). Synthetic materials allowed for use in organic livestock production under the regulations governing the National Organic Program in the United States are listed in the box titled "Synthetic Substances Allowed for Use in Organic Livestock Production." However, there is a petition process by which petitioners can approach the National Organic Standards Board (NOSB) to add additional approved materials, and this procedure has been used successfully. Some of the materials listed in Box 20.1 were added based on a petition initiated in 2001 (Karreman 2006).

Synthetic Substances Allowed for Use in Organic Livestock Production

From Section 205.603 of the United States Code of Federal Regulations at 7 CFR 205, National Organic Program. Items allowed as of December 12, 2007.

In accordance with restrictions specified in this section, the following synthetic substances may be used in organic livestock production:

(a) As disinfectants, sanitizer, and medical treatments as applicable:

(1) Alcohols
  (i) Ethanol: disinfectant and sanitizer only, prohibited as a feed additive
  (ii) Isopropanol: disinfectant only
(2) Aspirin: approved for health care use to reduce inflammation
(3) Atropine*
(4) Biologicals: Vaccines
(5) Butorphanol*
(6) Chlorhexidine: for surgical procedures conducted by a veterinarian
(7) Chlorine materials: disinfecting and sanitizing facilities and equipment; residual chlorine levels in the water shall not exceed the maximum residual disinfectant limit under the Safe Drinking Water Act
  (i) Calcium hypochlorite
  (ii) Chlorine dioxide
  (iii) Sodium hypochlorite
(8) Electrolytes: without antibiotic
(9) Flunixin
(10) Furosemide
(11) Glucose
(12) Glycerin: allowed as a livestock teat dip; must be produced through the hydrolysis of fats or oils
(13) Hydrogen peroxide
(14) Iodine
(15) Magnesium hydroxide*
(16) Magnesium sulfate
(17) Oxytocin: use in postparturition therapeutic applications
(18) Parasiticides—Ivermectin: prohibited in slaughter stock, allowed in emergency treatment for dairy and breeder stock when organic system plan-approved preventive management does not prevent infestation. Milk or milk products from a treated animal cannot be labeled as provided for in subpart D of this part for ninety days following treatment. In breeder stock, treatment cannot occur during the last third of gestation if the progeny will be sold as organic and must not be used during the lactation period of breeding stock.
(19) Peroxyacetic/peracetic acid: for sanitizing facility and processing equipment
(20) Phosphoric acid: allowed as an equipment cleaner, provided that no direct contact with organically managed livestock or land occurs

(21) Poloxalene: to be used only for emergency treatment of bloat
(22) Tolazoline*
(23) Xylazine*

(b) As topical treatment, external parasiticide, or local anesthetic as applicable:
(1) Copper sulfate
(2) Iodine
(3) Lidocaine: as a local anesthetic; use requires a withdrawal period of ninety days after administering to livestock intended for slaughter and seven days after administering to dairy animals
(4) Lime, hydrated: as an external pest control, not permitted to cauterize physical alterations or deodorize animal wastes
(5) Mineral oil: for topical use and as a lubricant
(6) Procaine: as a local anesthetic; use requires a withdrawal period of ninety days after administering to livestock intended for slaughter and seven days after administering to dairy animals
(7) Sucrose octanoate esters: in accordance with approved labeling

(c) As feed supplements: None

(d) As feed additives:
(1) Trace minerals, used for enrichment or fortification when FDA approved
(2) Vitamins, used for enrichment or fortification when FDA approved

*Federal law restricts this drug to use by or on the lawful written or oral order of a licensed veterinarian, in full compliance with the AMDUCA and 21 CFR part 530 of the Food and Drug Administration regulations. Additional restrictions may apply including extensions of meat and milk withdrawal times when the drug is used. For updates and specific restrictions, check Section 205.603 of the 7 CFR 205 directly at the Website of the National Organic Program at www.ams.usda.gov/nop/NOP/standards/FullRegTextOnly.html

Successful provision of animal health care in organic livestock production requires a strong partnership between the veterinarian and the producer. A "fire engine" approach to respond to disease problems after they occur is not effective, particularly with the constraints that exist on the drugs available for treatment. Instead, the producer and veterinarian should be proactive and develop an animal health plan for the operation. This should begin with a thorough review of existing facilities and management practices to identify situations conducive to the development of disease. Many conditions which require antibiotics for treatment, such as colisepticemia in kids, pneumonia and coccidiosis in weanlings, and mastitis in does, can be prevented or minimized with proper sanitation, housing design, ventilation, and management practices that promote good hygiene and minimize stress on the animals. In addition, veterinarians should recognize that the use of vaccines is not restricted in organic livestock production and vaccination represents a useful tool for preventing disease. Ration evaluation and nutritional counseling are also important because proper nutrition favors improved disease resistance.

The veterinarian should remain actively involved once the animal health plan is developed. Many farmers that enter organic production do so by making the transition from conventional production and have come to depend on conventional health interventions. The transition from conventional to certified organic farming may take three to four years, during which time unexpected health problems may arise due to the loss of familiar interventions and unfamiliarity with the new. The veterinarian should be ready to work through these difficult periods with the farmer and help with the transition.

Perhaps the biggest health challenge for organic goat production in the United States is control of gastrointestinal parasites, because the use of anthelmintics is currently limited to ivermectin and only under particular circumstances. The risk of parasitism in organic livestock production may be increased compared to conventional systems because organic production systems may depend heavily on use of pastures as a source of feed, and indirectly as a source of parasites. Interestingly, the accelerating development of anthelmintic resistance in recent years has spurred considerable interest and research in alternative parasite management strategies that depend less on anthelmintic use and more on alternative therapies and pasture management strategies.

Serendipitously, these approaches fit nicely with the objectives of organic livestock production systems, particularly goat production systems. Parasite control approaches compatible with organic livestock production include: grazing management strategies that minimize exposure to infective larvae at pasture, improved animal nutrition to promote parasite resistance, feeding or grazing of forages with high tannin content, selection and breeding programs for parasite resistance, biological control of parasitic nematodes using nematophagous fungi, and the development and use of vaccines against parasites. These options are discussed further in the section on nematode gastroenteritis in Chapter 10. In addition, there is renewed interest in a wide variety of traditional herbal and other phytotherapeutic remedies from around the world that have been reported to or are believed to control parasites. There is no doubt that some of these remedies are effective, and controlled studies are needed to identify those that are most efficacious.

A major component of organic animal health care is the use of alternative and complementary therapies including homeopathy, phytotherapy, acupuncture, immune augmentation, and vitamin and mineral supplementation. Herbs are used as treatments but may also be sown in pastures to provide both nutrients and prophylaxis against disease, most notably parasites. While modern day veterinarians may bemoan the lack of access to antibiotics in controlling disease for organically raised animals, it is useful to recall that before the advent of antibiotics in the 1940s, our professional predecessors had to depend heavily on botanicals and other natural therapies to effect cures in livestock. Veterinary textbooks published in the 1930s are good sources of information on therapies that were considered useful or reliable before the advent of antibiotics (Karreman 2006).

There is a steadily increasing amount of useful information available to veterinarians interested in organic livestock production. Symposia have been held on veterinary issues in organic farming with published proceedings (Thamsborg et al. 2001; Hovi and Vaarst 2002). In addition, national governments and producer groups have produced guidelines, some of which are available via the Internet (Australian Government 2007).

HERD HEALTH MANAGEMENT FOR TRANSGENIC GOATS

Because many transgenic herds are maintained for the purpose of producing recombinant biopharmaceutical proteins in the milk of goats for subsequent separation and preparation of commercial products, these transgenic herds can be viewed in essence as dairy goat herds and the principles of dairy herd health management discussed at the beginning of this chapter generally apply. However, because of regulatory concerns related to the purity of milk-derived pharmaceutical products, particularly with regard to the possible risk of zoonotic disease transmission, there are additional special considerations for the herd health management of transgenic herds, whether they produce recombinant proteins in milk or other body fluids or tissues. These considerations relate mainly to the importance of establishing and maintaining a closed herd, excluding specific diseases that can affect product safety, the types of vaccines used in the herd, and the use of medications in the herd. Each of these issues is discussed in the following sections.

The Importance of Establishing and Maintaining a Closed Herd

From the perspective of controlling diseases in goats, and particularly in transgenic goats, developing and maintaining a closed herd must be given significant consideration. There is no doubt that the number one threat to spread of disease between goats comes from new introductions of animals into a herd. Additionally, the continued spread of disease within a herd most certainly comes from the infected or carrier animal(s) within a given herd.

Developing a closed herd is not a minor undertaking and must take into consideration a number of factors. First, one must consider the source of the nucleus herd to be derived. This can be either from the original existing herd at a given site/farm or the goats can be obtained from an outside source. This outside source can be a known entity with a defined Specific Pathogen Free (SPF) population of goats or these animals can be obtained through the open market, either within one's own country or imported from a known disease-free country. Second, one must consider cost because this significantly impacts the extent to which one will go to derive a closed SPF herd. Third, the specific diseases for which testing is required, the type of testing/assays that will be performed, and the period of time involved in assembling and testing the animals needs to be given appropriate consideration.

A significant amount of disease testing needs to be performed on the potential incoming or existing animals to ensure, as best possible, their disease-free status when developing/starting a closed herd. However, not all diagnostic tests have 100% sensitivity and specificity. It must be remembered that even the most intensive pre-screening program is only a "snapshot" of the animal's/herd's disease status and does not ensure that a given animal or herd is negative for certain diseases with long incubation times, such as Johne's disease or caprine arthritis encephalitis (CAE). The list of diseases and/or disease agents to be considered in developing an SPF goat herd should include the following, at a minimum:

- Tuberculosis
- Brucellosis
- Caprine arthritis encephalitis (CAE)
- *Mycobacterium avium*, subsp. *paratuberculosis* (paratuberculosis or Johne's disease)
- Contagious ecthyma (Orf)
- Caprine herspesvirus-1 (CapHV-1)
- *Coxiella burnetti* (Q fever)
- *Neospora caninum*
- *Corynebacterium pseudotuberculosis* (Caseous lymphadenitis)

Once the closed herd is established, the testing regimen must continue for a specified period of time going forward in order to identify latent or chronic infections such as CAE and Johne's disease, which may have been undetected by initial screening tests.

Finally, once the closed herd is established, clinical monitoring and veterinary evaluations must be aimed at optimizing overall herd health, decreasing general morbidity/mortality, and removing those disease entities that are associated with production environments. Monitoring, detecting, and removing sources or animals that are carriers or contributors to clinical entities such as contagious mastitis, foot rot, certain bacterial or viral pneumonias are early priorities in a closed herd.

Specific Disease Implications for Transgenic Herds and Product Safety

For transgenic herds of goats producing recombinant human therapeutic proteins, the list of diseases one may want or need to test for most certainly is more extensive than the minimum set defined above. The rationale for screening for these additional entities is to identify agents that pose zoonotic risks or those that may be produced or detected in the tissue or fluid being used as a source material for recombinant protein production. There are additional viral- and prion-associated diseases, for example, scrapie, that need to be addressed due to the nature of the value-added product these goats are generating in a number of possible fluids or tissues. The following is a brief list of some of the additional viruses or family of viruses that should be considered, depending on the geographic region or emerging opportunistic nature of these entities around the world:

- Enzootic nasal tumor virus
- Ovine pulmonary adenocarcinoma virus (Jaagsiekte)
- Pestivirus (border disease)
- West Nile virus
- Respiratory syncytial virus
- Powassan virus
- Bunyavirus (Cache Valley fever)

Although the full list of potential viral problems may seem never-ending, the best approach to manage these possible threats is to first consider all viral agents that are known to infect goats. Second, address those that are known to be in the geographic locale of the flock or herd. Third, address those of specific concern for the herd, and last those which could potentially be found in the biological material being derived from the goats (milk, blood, serum, etc.). It may not be the intent of a given program for the SPF herd to be 100% viral free, and this may truly be unattainable, regardless of the type of operation.

Also, there are viruses, such as rotavirus and coronavirus, that may be manageable within a closed herd because they are typically found in young goats and are not problematic in the adult population from which biological materials are collected or harvested. This type of decision, as to which viruses will or will not be acceptable within a given herd, must be made on a case by case basis according on the nature of the operation, the type of biological product being produced, and the guidance of regulatory agencies involved, e.g., USDA and FDA.

Vaccine Issues in Transgenic Goat Herds

While vaccines are an important component of any herd health program, their use in transgenic herds needs to be evaluated carefully. The use of modified live viral vaccines can pose potential regulatory challenges to product safety when biopharmaceutical proteins are being produced in biological fluids such as milk, blood, or serum. Because many vaccines are produced in some form of culture system (egg, mammalian, bacterial, etc.), the vaccine production environment itself poses potential routes of viral/bacterial contamination that must be considered. The use of bovine serum, porcine trypsin, or other animal derived materials potentially allows for adventitious agents to inadvertently be introduced into the final product and ultimately into the animals being administered the vaccine. Therefore, strategic use of vaccine during times when the animal is not producing a biological material for recombinant therapeutic protein production may need to be considered.

Alternatively, the use of killed vaccines (e.g. Rabies) or toxins/toxoids (e.g. *Clostridium perfringens* types C and D and Tetanus) offers a slightly higher safety margin from a regulatory perspective. However, use of these products may limit the protective nature of the vaccination so that the frequency of administration may need to be modified. Additionally, as with all pharmacological agents administered to transgenic animals in production, one must consider all the subcomponents (adjuvant, animal-derived materials) of any vaccine being administered. Particular attention should be given ultimately to final product safety relative to human use. Finally, any vaccines to be used within a closed transgenic herd must come from approved and reputable manufacturers and sources and should have appropriate documentation upon receipt.

Medication Issues in Transgenic Goat Herds

Any and all pharmacological or medicinal agents used in the course of either preventative or clinical herd health management must be carefully considered and even scrutinized before use in transgenic animal populations. A thorough understanding of all the components within these materials is critical to avoid administering something to a goat that could negatively impact any biological material being produced/collected from the animal. One must consider the potential for adventitious agents (viral or bacterial) inadvertently being administered. There have been a number of historical cases in which this has happened in goat herds or other animals, with significant detrimental effects to the animals or the loss of product due to concerns of contamination. Reported examples include *inter alia*: sterile saline for injection contaminated with nonsteroidal anti-inflammatory drug (Gavin 2008); *C. perfringens* and *C. tetani* bacterintoxiod contaminated with *Staphyloccus intermedius*, which caused abscesses and abortion in vaccinated goats (Ayres, 2008); fetal calf serum for use in vaccine production contaminated with bovine polyomavirus (Kappeler et al. 1996); contagious ecthyma vaccine contaminated with pestivirus, which caused clinical border disease in goats (Løken et al. 1991); and a combined canine distemper, adenovirus, parvovirus vaccine contaminated with bluetongue virus that caused abortion and death in vaccinated dogs (Akita et al. 1994). All of these products were contaminated at the point of manufacture and not during use.

For transgenic goats, the judicious use of antibiotics or any pharmacological agent that could potentially produce a withdrawal period (meat, milk, etc.) must be considered relative to the biological material and product being produced. Following the prescribed withdrawal time at a minimum is prudent, but one must also consider those cases and circumstances in which the standard withdrawal time may not be sufficient. Finally, one may want to consider whether additional testing is warranted to ensure that the medicinal agent has cleared, what level of assay detection will be used (depending on what biological material is being collected), the product being produced, and the final product safety and use.

REFERENCES

Akita, G.Y., et al.: Bluetongue disease in dogs associated with contaminated vaccine. Vet. Rec., 134(11):283, 1994.

Alexandre, G. and Mandonnet, N.: Goat meat production in harsh environments. Sm. Rumin. Res., 60(1/2):53–66, 2005.

Australian Government: Going Organic—Organic Livestock Production—A conversion package for organic livestock production in the rangelands of western New South Wales. Rural Industries Research and Development Corporation, Kingston, Australia, 96 pp, April, 2007.

Ayres, S.: Personal communication. Dr. Sandra Ayres, Asst. Prof., Dept. Biomedical Sciences, Tufts Cummings School of Veterinary Medicine, No. Grafton, MA, April, 2008.

Batten, G.: A New Meat Goat Breed. Proceedings, IV International Conference on Goats, Volume II, Brasilia, Brasil, International Goat Association, p. 1330, 1987.

Bretzlaff, K.: Special problems of hair goats. Vet. Clin. N. Am. Food Anim. Pract., *6*:721–735, 1990.

Bretzlaff, K.N. and Romano, J.E.: Advanced reproductive techniques in goats. (Update on small ruminant medicine.) Vet. Clin. N. Am. Food Anim. Pract., 17(2):421–434, 2001.

Brown, K.R. and Forrest, C.: Meat Goat Selection and Care. Publication 2177, Mississippi State University Extension Service, 2004. http://msucares.com/pubs/publications/p2177.htm

Dawson, L., Allen, J. and Olcott, B: Meat Goat Herd Health—Procedures and Prevention. In: Web-based Training and Certification Program for Meat Goat Producers, Langston University Agricultural Research and Extension Programs, Langston, OK, 2000. 45 pp. http://www.luresext.edu/goats/training/QAtoc.html.

Devendra, C.: Goats: challenges for increased productivity and improved livelihoods. Outlook Agric., 28(4):215–226, 1999.

Dhanda, J.S., et al.: Goat meat production: present status and future possibilities. Asian–Australian J. Anim. Sci., 16(12):1842–1852, 2003.

Drummond, S.B.: Angora Goats the Northern Way. Freeport, Michigan, Stony Lonesome Farm, 1985.

Evans, J.V.: The Angora-mohair industry in Australia. The Angora goat—husbandry. Univ. of Sydney, Post Grad. Commun. Vet. Sci., *52*:143–162, 1980.

Farizy, P. and Taranchon, P.: Intérêt d'un traitement anthelminthique au thiabendazole chez la chèvre en lactation. Rec. Med. Vet., 146:251–260, 1970.

Gavin, W.G.: Personal communication. Dr. William G. Gavin, Vice President of Farm Operations and Chief Veterinarian, GTC Biotherapeutics, Framingham, MA. April, 2008.

Guss, S.B.: Management and Diseases of Dairy Goats. Scottsdale, AZ, Dairy Goat Journal Publ. Corp., 1977.

Haibel, G.K.: Out-of-season breeding in goats. Vet. Clin. N. Am. Food Anim. Pract., 6:577–583, 1990.

Hoste, H. and Chartier, C.: Response to challenge infection with *Haemonchus contortus* and *Trichostrongylus colubriformis* in dairy goats. Consequences on milk production. Vet. Parasitol., 74(1):43–54, 1998.

Hovi M. and Vaarst M.: Positive health: preventive measures and alternative strategies. Proceedings of the Fifth NAHWOA Workshop Rødding, Denmark—November 11–13, 2001, Network for Animal Health and Welfare in Organic Agriculture, Reading, UK, January, 2002. http://www.veeru.reading.ac.uk/organic/proc/FinalProceedingsDenmark.pdf

Kappeler, A., Lutz-Wallace, C., Sapp, T. and Sidhu, M.: Detection of bovine polyomavirus contamination in fetal bovine sera and modified live viral vaccines using polymerase chain reaction. Biologicals, 24(2):131–135, 1996.

Karreman, H.J.: Organic livestock production: veterinary challenges and opportunities. In: 2006 Convention Notes, 143rd AVMA Annual Convention, Honolulu, Hawaii, American Veterinary Medical Association, Schaumburg, IL. July 15–19, 2006.

Løken T, Krogsrud J, Bierkås I. Outbreaks of border disease in goats induced by a pestivirus-contaminated orf vaccine, with virus transmission to sheep and cattle. J. Comp. Pathol., 104:197–209, 1991.

Mahan, S.W.: The improved Boer goat. Small Rumin. Res., 36:165–170, 2000.

Monicat, F.: Arthrites des Caprins. Lyon, Centre d'Écopathologie, Conseil Regional Rhone-Alpes, 1989.

Nardone, A., Zervas, G. and Ronchi, B.: Sustainability of small ruminant organic systems of production. Livestock Prod. Sci., 90:27–39, 2004.

Olcott, B. and Dawson, L.: Meat Goat Herd Health—Common Diseases. In: Web-based Training and Certification Program for Meat Goat Producers, Langston University

Agricultural Research and Extension Programs, Langston, OK, 2000, 44 pp. http://www.luresext.edu/goats/training/QAtoc.html.
Shelton, M.: Fiber Production. In: Goat Production. C. Gall, ed. London, Academic Press, 1981.
Thamsborg, S.M., Albihn, A., Pedersen, M.A. and Christensen, B.: Veterinary Challenges in Organic Farming. Proceedings of the 14th Internordic Symposium of the Nordic Committee for Veterinary Scientific Cooperation (NKVet). Hveragerdi, Iceland, 5–8 October 2000. Acta Vet. Scand., 95 (Suppl.), 92 pp. 2001.
van der Westhuysen, J.M., Wentzel, D. and Grobler, M.C.: Angora Goats and Mohair in South Africa. 3rd Ed. Port Elizabeth, South Africa, NMB Printers, 1988.
van Tonder, E.M.: Notes on some disease problems in Angora goats in South Africa. Vet. Med. Rev., 1/2:109–138, 1975.
Yerex, D.: The Farming of Goats. Carterton, N.Z., Ampersand Publishing Associates Ltd., 1986.

Appendix A

Formulary of Some Drugs Used in Goats and Suggested Dosages

The appendix of the first edition of this textbook (Smith and Sherman 1994) assembled pharmacokinetic information on a diverse assortment of drugs. Many additional drugs and studies have become available in recent years, making the annotated bibliography format used in the first edition cumbersome. In addition, the advent of the Internet, with ready access to veterinary databases, has made retrieval of information on pharmacokinetic studies much easier. In lieu of providing pharmacokinetic data on selected drugs, this appendix lists the drug dosages discussed in each chapter of the current edition in tabular form for easy reference. Some of the drugs included are not available in the United States. Other available drugs are prohibited in goats because the species is classified as a food animal (Payne et al. 1999).

Information on pharmacokinetic terminology is retained from the first edition, to aid the reader in interpreting the literature. Pharmacodynamics, the study of the biochemical and physiological effects of drugs and the mechanisms of their actions, is a separate topic and beyond the scope of this appendix. It should be noted that knowledge of the pharmacokinetics of a drug in goats is helpful for selecting a route of administration and a dosing interval and for estimating withdrawal times but does not directly address the question of efficacy of a given dose. Clinical experience, in addition to pharmacokinetic data, must be taken into consideration (Martinez 1998d).

PHARMACOKINETIC TERMINOLOGY

Understanding of the literature in the field of pharmacology requires familiarity with a number of special concepts and terms. These are defined in textbooks (Baggot 1977; Riviere 1999) and review articles (Riviere 1988a, 1988b; Martinez 1998a, 1998b, 1998c, 1998d, 1998e), to which the reader is referred for additional information.

Pharmacokinetics is the mathematical description of concentration changes of drugs within the body. The drugs are described as distributing into and out of compartments, which are mathematical but not physiological entities. The drug distributes instantaneously and homogeneously into the central compartment when given intravenously. The central compartment is often equivalent to blood plasma and extracellular fluid of highly perfused organs. The peripheral compartment, into and out of which drugs may transfer more slowly, represents less well perfused tissues such as muscle, skin, and fat. Rate constants describe drug transfer between compartments and out of the body.

The volume of distribution (V_d) describes the relationship between the amount of drug in the body and its plasma concentration.

$$V_d(\text{ml}) = \frac{\text{Total drug in the body (mg)}}{\text{Concentration of the drug in plasma (mg/ml)}}$$

If the body appears to behave as a single homogeneous distribution compartment, drug disposition is described by a one-compartment open model. This model assumes that changes in tissue drug concentrations are reflected quantitatively by changes in plasma concentration. However, the drug concentrations are not necessarily the same in all body tissues at one time.

The term "open," when applied to a model, means that drug leaves the system.

The disposition of many drugs can be defined by a two-compartment open model, as depicted by the central and peripheral compartments, with elimination occurring only from the central compartment. With some drugs, a three-compartment open model is needed, because the plasma drug concentration over time can be best described by a triexponential curve.

The apparent volume of the central and peripheral compartments for each drug depends on blood flow, the drug's ability to enter the tissues from the circulation, and the extent of tissue binding. Increasing body water volume increases V_d, while dehydration or increasing the fraction of bound drug in the blood decreases the V_d. Drug binding in tissues can cause the apparent volume of distribution to exceed the real volume. Neonates have higher percent total body water than adults (Martinez 1998b). The volume of distribution tends to decrease with age.

In a two-compartment model, drugs are assumed to enter the system only via the central compartment and to leave it, by biotransformation and elimination, only from the central compartment. The rate of drug removal from a compartment is considered to be proportional to the concentration of drug in that compartment. During the initial or distribution phase, distribution to the peripheral compartment occurs simultaneously with elimination from the body. During the distribution phase, there is a rapid decline in plasma concentration described by an alpha rate constant or distribution half-life. After distribution is complete, elimination predominates, and the change in drug concentration is described by a beta rate constant or elimination half-life. In some drugs with extensive tissue binding, elimination slows later on during a gamma phase that is controlled by the rate of release of drug from its binding sites.

Total body clearance is a parameter that estimates drug elimination from the body by all routes relative to the concentration of drug in serum.

$$Cl = \frac{\text{rate of elimination}}{\text{serum drug concentration}}$$

It is expressed in terms of volume per unit time and represents the volume of serum completely cleared of the drug by all elimination processes per unit time. Serum protein binding influences clearance, as bound drug is often unavailable for glomerular filtration.

The elimination half-life is the time required for the total amount of drug in the body to decrease by half. The half-life in the body is directly related to the volume of distribution and inversely related to the clearance of the drug from the body by metabolism and/or excretion.

$$T_{1/2} = \frac{0.693 \times V_d}{Cl}$$

Although 97% of the drug is eliminated from the body in five half-lives, the half-life derived during pharmacokinetic studies depends on both the clearance and the volume of distribution and thus is altered by disease states.

The systemic availability, often expressed as a percent, is a measure of the extent of absorption of a drug given by something other than the intravenous route. For instance, the plasma concentration-time curve is plotted after oral (PO) and after intravenous (IV) administration. The area under the curve (AUC), expressed in µg/ml/hour, is calculated for the two curves and the ratio (AUC)PO:(AUC)IV gives the extent of absorption. Bioavailability also depends on the rate of absorption, which affects the peak plasma concentration achieved and the time to that peak. Absorption continues after the peak, but even if the drug has a high systemic availability, slow absorption may cause subtherapeutic plasma levels.

FORMULARY

Appendix A Table 1.1 is a partial list of drugs discussed in the text. Consult the chapter for details on duration of therapy and alternative treatments, as well as for warnings about use in meat or dairy animals. Numerous additional chemicals used to treat external parasites are listed in Table 2.1. Additional coccidiostats are listed in Table 10.7, anthelmintics in Table 10.8, and flukicides in Table 11.3. Supplements to correct nutritional deficiencies are discussed in Chapter 19. Additional antimicrobial and coccidiostat drug dosages have been compiled (Menzies 2000; Navarre and Marley 2006), although some of the suggested dosages for goats are empirical. Pharmacokinetic data for numerous antibiotics administered to goats have also been summarized (Navarre and Marley 2006).

MEAT AND MILK WITHDRAWAL TIMES

Relatively few studies have been conducted to determine drug metabolism and excretion in goats. Label information specifically for goats also is rarely available, because few drugs are approved by the Food and Drug Administration Center for Veterinary Medicine for use in goats in the United States (Webb et al. 2004). In the United States, whenever a drug is administered in any way that differs from the label directions (to a different species, at a different dosage, by a different route) its use is said to be extralabel. Only a veterinarian can legally use a drug in an extralabel fashion, and then only in the presence of a carefully defined veterinarian-client-patient relationship (U.S. Department of Health and Human Services 2005). The

Appendix A Table 1.1. Drug dosages used in goats.

Drug	*Dose*	*Indication*	*Chapter*
Acepromazine	0.2 mg/kg IM	Tetanus	5
Acepromazine	0.05–0.10 mg/kg IV	Preanesthetic sedation	17
Acetic acid 5% (vinegar)	0.5–1 liter PO	Urea toxicity	19
Activated charcoal	0.75–2 g/kg PO	Ethylene glycol poisoning	12
Albendazole	20 mg/kg PO divided into 2 doses of 10 mg/kg at 12 h	Gastrointestinal strongyles	10
Albendazole	10–15 mg/kg PO	Tapeworms, liver flukes	10, 11
Ammonium chloride	200–300 mg/kg/day	Urinary acidification	12
Ammonium chloride	0.5–1% of diet DM	Urolithiasis prevention	12
Ammonium molybdate	100 mg PO SID for up to 3 weeks in conjunction with 1 g sodium sulfate PO SID	Copper toxicity	7
Amoxicillin	One commercial bovine mastitis tube every 12–24 h, 2 or 3 treatments	Mastitis	14
Ampicillin	5–10 mg/kg IM BID	Bacterial pneumonia	9
Ampicillin	15 mg/kg SC TID	Prevention of cystitis	12
Ampicillin sodium	10–50 mg/kg IV or IM QID	Meningo-encephalitis	5
Amprolium	25–50 mg/kg PO SID for 5 d	Coccidiosis	10
Aspirin	100 mg/kg PO BID	Joint pain (CAE) Meningitis adjunct	4 5
Atipamezole	0.08–0.1 mg/kg slowly IV	Reversal of medetomidine	17
Atropine sulfate	0.6–1 mg/kg SC or IM, repeat as needed	Organophosphate poisoning	5
Butorphanol	0.2 m/kg IM	Post-surgical analgesia	17
Calcium borogluconate 23%	50–100 ml SC	Oxalate poisoning	12
Calcium borogluconate 23%	60–100 ml SC or slowly IV	Milk fever (hypocalcemia)	13, 19
Ceftiofur	1.1–2.2 mg/kg/d IM	Bacterial pneumonia	9
Charcoal, activated	1 g/kg PO	Chlorinated hydrocarbon toxicity	5
Chloramphenicol	Do not use in USA	Forbidden in USA	
Cloprostenol	0.125–0.250 mg IM	Luteolysis, correction of hydrometra	13
Closantel	10–20 mg/kg PO (risk of blindness with overdose)	Liver flukes	11
Closantel	7.5 mg/kg	*Haemonchus*	10
Clorsulon	7 mg/kg PO	Liver flukes	11
Clostridium perfringens C and D antitoxin	5 ml SC	Prophylaxis of enterotoxemia	10
Clostridium perfringens C and D antitoxin	15–20 ml IV, repeat every 3–4 h	Treatment of enterotoxemia	10
Colostrum	20% of body weight PO over first 24 h	Passive transfer	19
Danofloxacin	Do not use in USA	Forbidden in USA	
Danofloxacin	6 mg/kg SC, repeated in 48 h	Mycoplasmosis	4
Decoquinate	0.5–1 mg/kg/d PO in feed, continuously	Coccidiosis prevention	10
Decoquinate	2.5 mg/kg/d PO	Cryptosporidiosis	10
Detomidine	0.01–0.02 mg/kg IM	Moderate sedation	17
Dexamethasone	0.1 mg/kg/d IV	Adjunct–listeriosis	5
Dexamethasone	1–2 mg/kg IM or IV	Cerebral edema from polio-encephalomalacia	5
Dexamethasone	20–25 mg SC or IM	Induction of parturition	13
Dextrose		See Glucose	
Diazepam	0.5–1.5 mg/kg IV	Convulsions, tetanus	5

Appendix A Table 1.1. ***Continued***

Drug	*Dose*	*Indication*	*Chapter*
Diazepam	0.1–0.5 mg/kg IV	Urolithiasis, to relax urethra	12
Diazepam	0.5 mg/kg IV	Preanesthetic sedation	17
Diethylcarbamazine	40–60 mg/kg/d PO 1–6 d	Setariasis	5
Diminazene aceturate	3.5 mg/kg IM	Trypanosomosis	7
Dioctyl sodium sulfosuccinate (DSS)	15–30 ml PO	Bloat	10
Doxopram HCl	1–1.5 mg/kg IV or sublingually	Resuscitation of neonate	13
Enrofloxacin	Do not use in USA	Forbidden in USA	
Epinephrine	0.03 mg/kg IV	Anaphylaxis	10
Epinephrine 1:1000	1 ml IM	Uterine relaxation for obstetrical manipulation	13
Eprinomectin	1 mg/kg topical	Sarcoptic mange	2
Eprinomectin	0.4 mg/kg PO	Gastrointestinal strongyles	10
Equine chorionic gonadotropin (PMSG)	400–750 IU IM 48 h before progestogen withdrawal	Induction of estrus out of season	13
Fenbendazole	10 mg/kg PO	*Dictyocaulus*	9
		Gastrointestinal strongyles	10
Fenbendazole	15 mg/kg	Tapeworms	10
Fenbendazole	15–30 mg/kg PO	*Muellerius*	9
Fenbendazole	50 mg/kg/d for 5 d PO	Cerebrospinal nematodiasis	5
Florfenicol	40 mg/kg SC every 1–2 d	Bacterial pneumonia	9
Flunixin meglumine	1 mg/kg/d IV, IM or PO	Laminitis	4
Flunixin meglumine	1.1 mg/kg IV BID	Anti-inflammatory	12, 17
Flunixin meglumine	1–2 mg/kg IV or IM BID	Meningo-encephalitis	5
Furosemide	1 mg/kg IV	Cerebral edema	5
Furosemide	50–100 mg IM or IV	Udder edema	14
Glucose	25–50 g IV as 5% or 10% solution	Pregnancy toxemia, ketosis	19
Glucose 20% solution	25–50 ml IP	Hypoglycemia in neonate	19
Griseofulvin	25 mg/kg/d PO for 3 weeks	Ringworm, rarely justified	2
Imidocarb diproprionate	1–2 mg/kg once	Babesiosis	7
Isometamidium chloride	0.5–1.0 mg/kg IM	Trypanosomosis prophylaxis	7
Ivermectin	0.5–20 mg/100 kg SC	Warbles	2
Ivermectin	0.2–0.4 mg/kg SC, repeat in 2 weeks	Sarcoptic mange	2
Ivermectin	0.2 mg/kg PO	Nose bots	9
Ivermectin	0.4 mg/kg PO	Gastrointestinal strongyles	10
Ivermectin, adjunct to fenbendazole	0.2 mg/kg/d SC for 5 d	Cerebrospinal nematodiasis	5
Ketamine	6 mg/kg IV or 11 mg/kg IM	General anesthesia	17
Ketoprofen	3 mg/kg IV or IM SID	Post-surgical analgesia	17
Lasalocid	20–30 g/ton of feed	Coccidiosis prevention	10
Levamisole	12 mg/kg PO	Gastrointestinal strongyles	10
Levamisole	7.5 mg/kg PO or SC	*Dictyocaulus*	9
Lidocaine	Up to 5 mg/kg IM or SC	Local analgesia	17
Lidocaine 2%	2–4 ml	Caudal epidural	17
Lincomycin/Spectinomycin	5 mg/kg/d Lincomycin + 10 mg/kg/d Spectinomycin IM for 3 d	Mycoplasmosis (Contagious agalactia)	4
Magnesium hydroxide	50 g PO (adult goat)	Rumen acidosis	19
Medetomidine	0.005 mg/kg IV or 0.015 mg/kg IM	Deep sedation	17
Melengestrol acetate (MGA)	0.125 mg/head BID PO for 10–14 d, followed by a prostaglandin IM	Estrus synchronization in season (not permitted in USA)	13

Appendix A Table 1.1. ***Continued***

Drug	*Dose*	*Indication*	*Chapter*
Methocarbamol	22 mg/kg IV	Muscle relaxant (tetanus)	5
Methylene blue 1%	4–15 mg/kg IV	Nitrate poisoning	9
Midazolam	0.4 mg/kg IV	Preanesthetic sedation	17
Monensin	15–20 g/ton of feed	Coccidiosis prevention	10
Morantel tartrate	10 mg/kg PO	Gastrointestinal strongyles	10
Morantel citrate	6 mg base/kg PO	Paramphistomes	10
Moxidectin	0.4 mg/kg PO	Gastrointestinal strongyles	10
Niacin	1 g/animal/d IM or PO	Pregnancy toxemia prevention and treatment	19
Niclosamide	50 mg/kg	Tapeworms	10
Oxytetracycline	10 mg/kg IV BID at least 3 d	Listeriosis	5
Oxytetracycline	15 mg/kg/d IM at least 5 d	Mycoplasmosis	4
Oxytetracycline	5 mg/kg/d IV for 5 d (combined with intramammary therapy)	Gangrenous mastitis	14
Oxytetracycline, long-acting	20 mg/kg SC or IM once	Dermatophilosis	2
		Foot rot or foot scald	4
		Heartwater	8
Oxytetracycline, long-acting	20 mg/kg SC or IM every 3 d	Chlamydiosis, other abortion diseases	13
Oxytocin	5 IU IM BID–TID	Retained placenta, milk letdown	13
Oxytocin	50 IU IM BID for 4 d	Correction of hydrometra	13
Paromomycin	100 mg/kg/d PO	Cryptosporidiosis	10
Penicillamine	50 mg/kg/d PO	Copper toxicity	7
Penicillin G, procaine	20,000 IU/kg/d IM for 7–14 d	Staphylococcal dermatitis	2
Penicillin G, procaine	20,000–40,000 IU/kg/d IM	Bacterial pneumonia	9
Penicillin G, procaine	22,000 IU/kg IM BID	Prevention of cystitis	10
Penicillin G, procaine	25,000 IU/kg IM BID	Tetanus	5
Penicillin G, sodium	40,000 IU/kg IV QID followed by Penicillin G procaine 20,000 IU/kg IM BID	Listeriosis	5
Penicillin G, sodium	20,000–40,000 IU/kg IV or IM QID	Meningo-encephalitis	5
Pentobarbital	30 mg/kg IV	General anesthesia	17
Phenylbutazone	10 mg/kg/d PO	Joint pain (CAE), laminitis	4
Poloxalene	100 mg/kg PO	Bloat	10
Praziquantel	5–15 mg/kg PO	Tapeworms	10, 11
Praziquantel	25–60 mg/kg PO	Schistosomosis	8
Prednisone, prednisolone	1 mg/kg IM BID	Pemphigus foliaceus	2
Propofol	4–6 mg/kg IV	Anesthesia induction	17
Propylene glycol	60 ml PO BID or TID	Pregnancy toxemia, ketosis	19
Prostaglandin F2 alpha (Dinoprost)	5–10 mg IM	Luteolysis, correction of hydrometra	13
Pyrantel tartrate	25 mg/kg PO	Gastrointestinal strongyles	10
Selenite, sodium	1 mg/18 kg SC once (follow label for sheep on selenium-vitamin E product)	White muscle disease	4
Sodium bicarbonate	20 g PO (adult goat)	Rumen acidosis	19
Sodium bicarbonate 1.3%	125–200 ml IV	Floppy kid disease	19
Sodium bicarbonate (powder)	2.5–3.0 g PO (0.5 tsp mixed with cold water)	Floppy kid disease	19
Sodium iodide	20 mg/kg IV or SC, weekly 5–7 weeks	Actinobacillosis,	2
		Actinomycosis	3

Appendix A Table 1.1. ***Continued***

Drug	*Dose*	*Indication*	*Chapter*
Sodium nitrite	22 mg/kg IV	Cyanide poisoning	9
Sodium thiosulfate	660 mg/kg IV	Cyanide poisoning	9
Spiramycin	50 mg/kg IM then 25 mg/kg/d	Mycoplasmosis	4
Streptomycin	20 mg/kg/d 5–7 d	Actinobacillosis, Actinomycosis	2 3
Streptomycin	30 mg/kg/d IM at least 5 d	Mycoplasmosis	4
Sulfadimethoxine	75 mg/kg PO for 5 days	Coccidiosis	10
Tetanus antitoxin	10,000–15,000 units IV BID	Tetanus treatment	5
Tetanus antitoxin	250–300 IU SC/kid, 500 IU SC/adult	Tetanus prophylaxis	18
Tetracycline	5 mg/kg IM or SC SID or BID	Bacterial pneumonia	9
Tetracycline	0.5–1 g PO (single dose)	Adjunct–rumen acidosis treatment	19
Thiamine	10 mg/kg IV, IM, or SC QID	Polioencephalomalacia	5
Thiamine	300–500 mg IM or SC BID	Adjunct–rumen acidosis	19
Thiamylal sodium	10 mg/kg IV	Induction of anesthesia	17
Thiopental sodium	15–20 mg/kg IV	Induction of anesthesia	17
Tiamulin	20 mg/kg/d IM at least 5 d; severely irritating, toxic myopathy	Mycoplasmosis (CCPP)	4
Tiamulin	10 mg/kg IM BID	Mycoplasma mastitis	14
Tiletamine-zolazepam (Telazol®)	5.5 mg/kg IV	General anesthesia	17
Tilmicosin	Do not use	May be fatal	
Tolazoline	1.5 mg/kg IV	Xylazine reversal	17
Triclabendazole	10 mg/kg PO	Liver flukes	10
Trimethoprim-sulfonamide	16–24 mg/kg IV BID	Meningo-encephalitis	5
Trimethoprim-sulfonamide	15 mg/kg IV BID (trimepthoprim inactivated in rumen)	Salmonellosis	10
Tylosin	10–20 mg/kg IM SID or BID	Bacterial pneumonia	9
Tylosin	20 mg/kg/d IM at least 5 d	Mycoplasmosis	4
Vancomycin	Do not use in USA	Forbidden in USA	
Vitamin B_{12}	0.01–0.3 mg IM weekly	White liver disease	11
Xylazine	0.03–0.04 mg/kg IV	Light sedation	17
Xylazine	0.05 mg/kg IV or 0.1 mg/kg IM	Heavy sedation; combine with local anesthesia	17
Xylazine plus Ketamine	0.22 mg/kg IM Xylazine followed in 10 min by 11 mg/kg IM Ketamine	General anesthesia	17
Yohimbine	0.125 mg/kg IV	Xylazine reversal	17
Zinc sulfate	1 g/d/adult goat PO	Zinc deficiency dermatopathy	2

IM = intramuscular
IV = intravenous
IP = intraperitoneal
SC = subcutaneous
PO = orally
DM = dry matter
d = day
h = hour
SID = once a day
BID = twice a day
TID = three times a day
QID = four times a day
IU = international units
tsp = teaspoon